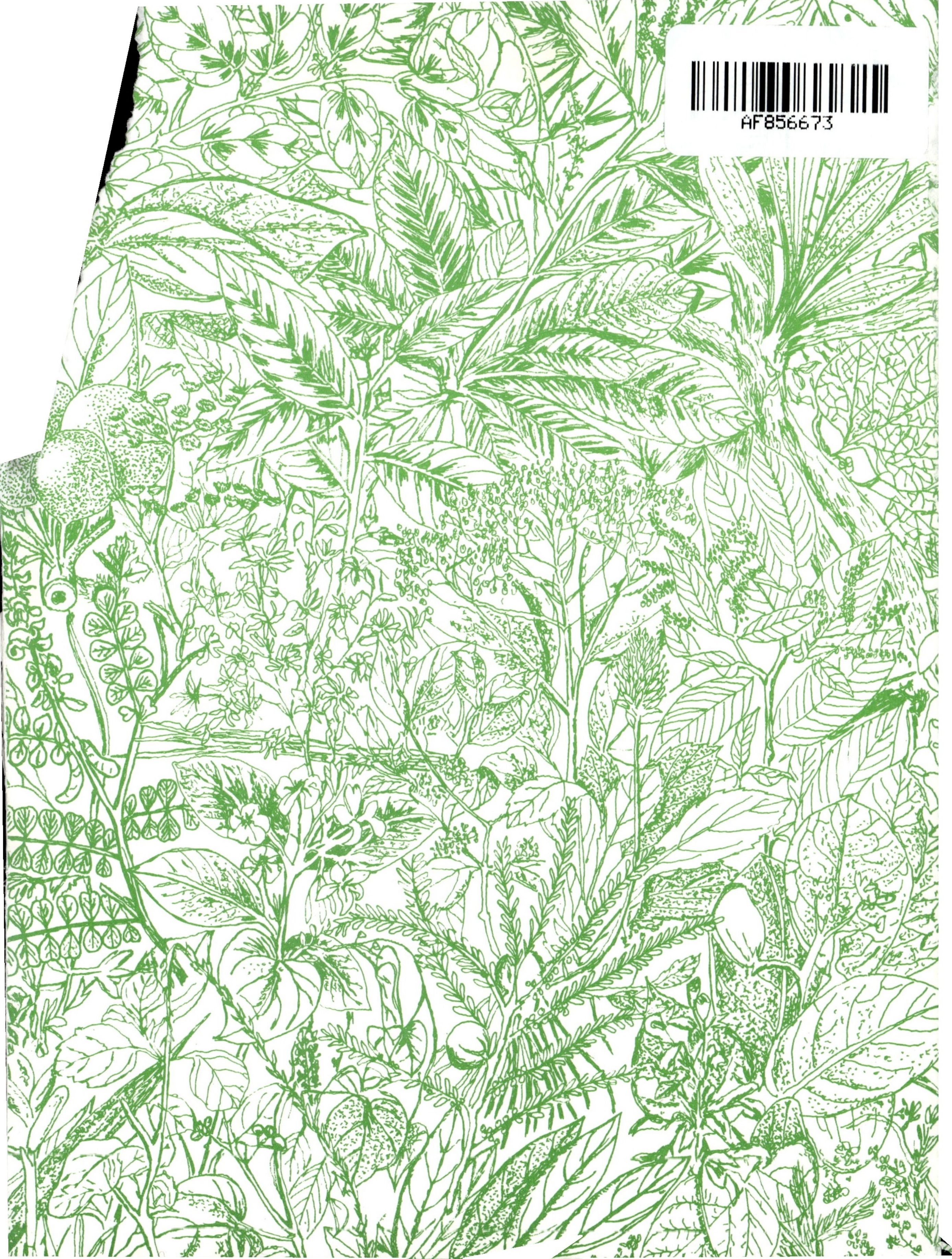

।। श्री धन्वन्तरये नमः ।।

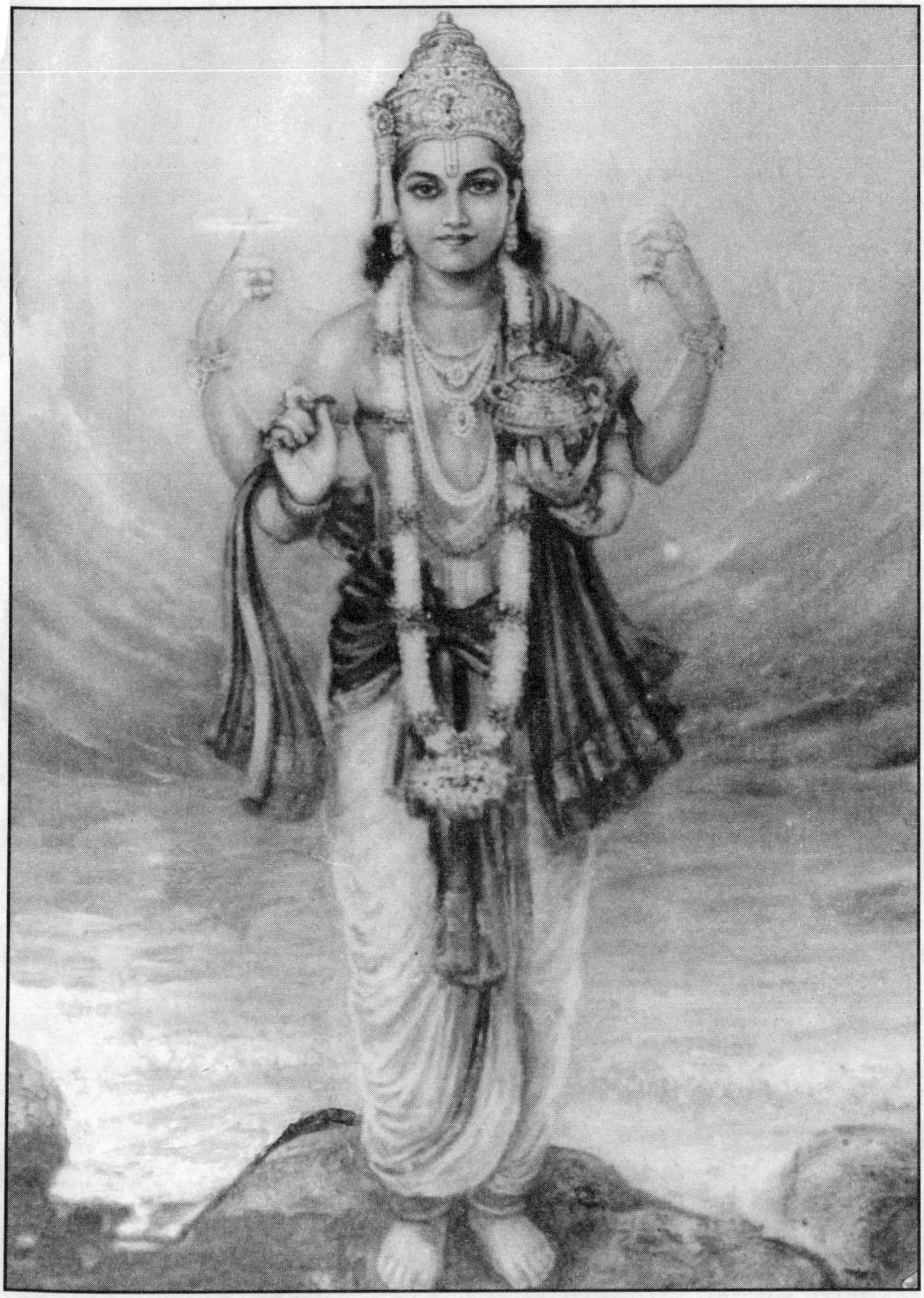

नमामि धन्वन्तरिमादिदेवं सुरासुरैर्वन्दित पादपद्मम् ।
लोके जरारुग्भयमृत्यु नाशं धातारमीशं विविधौषधीनाम् ।।

"धन्वन्तरी निघण्टु"

आ नो भद्राः क्रतवो यन्तु विश्वतः।

Let noble thoughts come to us from every side.

- Ṛgveda, I-89-i

BHAVAN'S BOOK UNIVERSITY

General Editor
S. RAMAKRISHNAN

AYURVEDIC PHARMACOLOGY AND THERAPEUTIC USES OF MEDICINAL PLANTS

(DRAVYAGUNAVIGNYAN)

VAIDYA V. M. GOGTE

BHAVAN'S BOOK UNIVERSITY

AYURVEDIC PHARMACOLOGY AND THERAPEUTIC USES OF MEDICINAL PLANTS (DRAVYAGUNAVIGNYAN)

VAIDYA VISHNU MAHADEV GOGTE

(1910 - 1987)

TRANSLATION :

THE ACADEMIC TEAM OF

BHARATIYA VIDYA BHAVAN'S

SWAMI PRAKASHANANDA AYURVEDA RESEARCH CENTRE (SPARC)

2000

BHARATIYA VIDYA BHAVAN

Kulapati Munshi Marg

Mumbai - 400 007

DRAVYAGUNAVIGNYAN
First Marathi Edition : 1982
Second Marathi Edition : 1997

First English Edition : Oct. 2000

ISBN 81-7276-192-9

Published By : Shri S. Ramakrishnan, Executive Secretary, Bharatiya Vidya Bhavan, Kulapati Munshi Marg, Mumbai - 400 007.
Permission for the Publication of the English translation granted by : Maharashtra Universities Book Production Board, Nagpur - 440 010, Maharashtra, India.

Typesetting : Deepa Rajput, Data Art Printers, 77/103, Padmaraj, Dahanukarwadi, Dattamandir X Road, Kandivli (W), Mumbai - 400 067.

PRINTED IN INDIA

By Surendra Shringi, Sharp-Em-Dense, 14, Ground floor, Municipal Ind. Estate, Vallabhbhai Road, Vile Parle (W), Mumbai - 400 056.

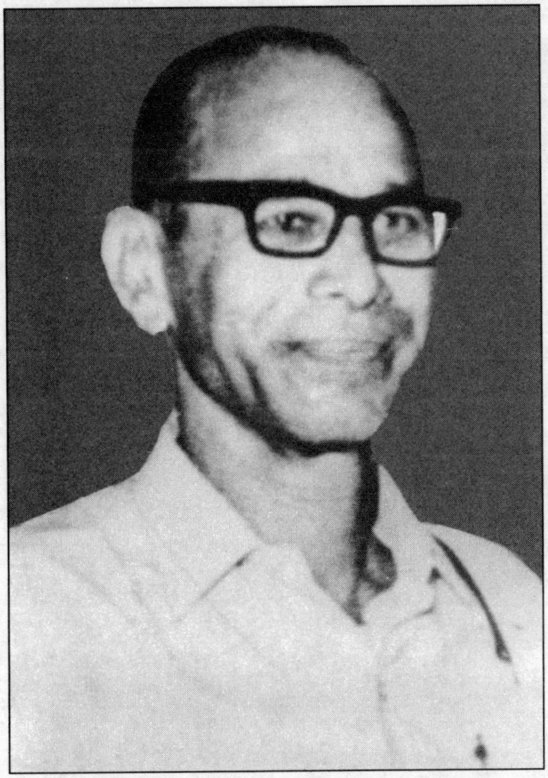

VAIDYA V. M. GOGTE
(1910-1987)

ACADEMIC TEAM : BHAVAN'S SPARC

TRANSLATION : **Dr. MANAS V. VYAS** B.A.M.S.
Dr. NEELAMBARI S. SAWANT B.A.M.S.
Dr. A. K. KOLWANKAR G.F.A.M., L.M.P., M.B.B.S.

SUPERVISION : **Dr. JAYA G. GOGATE** M.D., D.G.O.
Dr. RAMCHANDRA B. GOGTE G.F.A.M., A.V.V.
Dr. SATYAVATI M. SIRSAT M.Sc., Ph.D.
Dr. RAMA VAIDYA M.D., Ph.D.
Dr. S.I. NAGRAL G.F.A.M.
Dr. ASHWINIKUMAR RAUT M.D. (Ayu)
Dr. LALITA KOTHARI M.Sc., Ph.D.
Dr. RANJAN M. BHATT M.Sc., Ph.D.
Dr. PRALHAD PATKI M.D.

DIRECTION : **Dr. ASHOK D. B. VAIDYA** M.D., Ph.D.

PUBLISHER'S NOTE

In 1977, the Bhavan established the *Ancient Insights and Modern Discoveries* (AIMD) Project with the chief objective of drawing upon the spirit of and living up to the permanent values of **Bharatiya Vidya.** These values are treasured in the *Vedas*, the *Upanishads* and the *Puranas* as well as numerous books of great antiquity. The continuing striking parallels noticed between ancient insights, wisdom and modern discoveries during the course of our indepth research and study strengthened the belief that a systematic pursuit of correlative research would result in greater benefit to India as a whole and also to mankind the world over.

The Ancient Insights and Modern Discoveries Project has three wings: viz. (i) Science and Technology, (ii) Life and Health Science and (iii) Centre for the Synthesis of Science and Human Values.

In 1978, under the Life and Health Science Division, the Bhavan's AIMD Project set up the Bhavan's Swami Prakashananda Ayurveda Research Centre (SPARC) wherein work on medical service, research and education in Ayurveda is going on.

The SPARC has initiated and is executing action programmes for research, service and education in Ayurveda. A team of multidisciplinary experts from Ayurveda, Modern Life and Health Sciences, interact at SPARC for several priority oriented and well defined projects, short and long-term, which enhance the image of Ayurveda and also enrich modern biomedical sciences.

In the Life and Health Sciences Division, one of the research assignments was a comprehensive monograph on Ayurveda and modern medicine. Publication of research works on Ayurveda and Modern Medicine was started in 1986 with a view to making it useful to the practitioners of modern medicines with insights of Ayurveda and the Ayurveda physicians with modern achievements. Towards this end, the Bhavan had the privilege of so far publishing fifteen Research works namely:

1. ***Ayurveda and Modern Medicine*** by Dr. R.D.Lele (1986),
2. ***Selected Medicinal Plants of India,*** Chemexcil (1992),
3. ***Holistic Living*** by Prof. B.M.Hegde (1992),
4. ***Safe Motherhood*** by Dr. K.Bhaskar Rao (1995),
5. ***Hypertension—Assorted Topics*** by Prof. B.M.Hegde (1995),
6. ***Gita and Health*** by Vaidya Suresh Chaturvedi (1997),
7. ***Herbal Cosmetics in Ancient India with a Treatise in Plants Cosmetics*** by P.V.Bole & Kunda B.Patkar (1997),
8. ***Culture, Philosophy and Mental Health*** by Dr. A.Venkoba Rao (1997),
9. ***High Blood Pressure*** by Dr. Ashok B. Vaidya and Dr. Meenu Bhatt (1998),
10. ***Guggul Ani Guggulkalp Sarasangrah*** by Vaidya Vasudha Vijay Apte (1998),
11. ***Neem in Ayurveda*** by Vaidya Suresh Chaturvedi (1998),
12. ***Ayurveda for You*** by Vaidya Suresh Chaturvedi (1998),

13. ***Health is Wealth*** by K. Balan (1999),
14. ***Neem Aur Ayurveda*** (Hindi) by Vaidya Suresh Chaturvedi (2000) and
15. ***The Mind: Turbulent and Tranquil*** by Dr. A.Venkoba Rao (2000).

Vaidyaraj V. M. Gogte was entrusted by Maharashtra Universities Book Production Board, Nagpur, the task of preparing the textbook **"Dravyagunavignyan"** in Marathi for students of Ayurveda system of medicine. Over the years, almost all the students of Ayurveda have used and benefited from this excellent textbook.

The faculty at Bhavan's SPARC, thought appropriate that the English translation of this indepth textbook on herbal medicinal plants should be accessible to the growing and vast global readership and make available the knowledge embedded therein to seekers the world over.

We hope this book will be a worthy addition to our Ayurveda Sastra Series and will be warmly received by our esteemed readers in India and abroad.

Our hearty congratulations to the Gogte Parivar for their commendable contribution to this fine and informative work.

Vijayadashmi Day
October 7, 2000.

S. Ramakrishnan
Gen.Editor, Bhavan's Book University
Bharatiya Vidya Bhavan
Mumbai.

TRANSLATION : A CHALLENGE AND FULFILLMENT

Sanskrit, with its linguistic richness and phonetic excellence, is a language difficult to translate into English. The very method of the thought is different in these two languages. When a subject like Ayurveda, which is rooted in Sanskrit and which has Sanskrit derived words even in the regional versions, is to be translated, the translator is faced with a difficult task.

Ayurveda has a novel approach towards understanding the functioning of the body and genesis of diseases. To express these concepts aptly in English while retaining the depth and richness of the Sanskrit terms is next to impossible. For a beginner it would be convenient, to get a general idea, to say that 'pachan' means 'digestion'. But as one reads the texts and realises the broad sense in which this term is used, it becomes evident that equating 'pachan' and 'digestion' is like losing the depth of understanding and conceptualisation offered by the word 'pachan'.

Why then, did we undertake this exercise of translating the present work? The main purpose was to make available to a large number of readers the unique conceptual ideas of the author, Vaidya V. M. Gogte. English, in addition to being a global language, is also understood by a cross section of Indian population. We felt that an English version of "Dravyagunavignyan" would be helpful to those students who are not familiar with Marathi. Moreover, it can also help in creating awareness about Ayurveda in the global scenario.

Translating this book has been a learning experience for us. Sometimes, translation would appear effortless while at other times it would seem a herculean task. Nevertheless, it is a matter of joy and filfillment for us that we could complete this translation and thus pay tribute to the learned author, Vaidya V. M. Gogte.

The Academic Team, Bhavan's SPARC

FOREWORD
HEALTH–WISDOM OF INDIA

"It is quite possible that India is the real world, and that the white man lives in a madhouse of abstractions.....Life in India has not yet withdrawn into the capsule of the head. It is still the whole body that lives. No wonder the European feels dreamlike; the complete life of India is something of which he merely dreams. When you walk with naked feet, how can you ever forget the earth?"

- Carl Jung

Ayurveda is the art-science of health care, from India. It has been preserved, developed and now being globalised. The founder of Ayurveda - Lord Dhanwantari – manifested from the ocean, with Amritam (elixir of immortality) in one hand and Amrita (the plant – Tinospora cordifolia) in the other. From such an antiquity, India's quest for healthy life-style has centred around Nature and her rhythms. India's seminal contribution to the world of science is not only the discovery of zero and the decimal system, it has also been in the field of health-giving foods, medicinal plants, animal products and minerals. The world is waking up to the vast pharmacopoeia of Ayurveda.

The pharmacopoeia of Ayurveda was based on an understanding of the nature of the Dravyas (substances), which constitute human body-mind, the dynamic exchanges of these dravyas with the milieu and on how any disharmony be restored. The consensus on such a knowledge of several Rishis (seers), after meaningful debates, was capsuled in heuristic aphorisms-sutras of Ayurveda. A sutra is described by Charaka, as follows:

अल्पाक्षरमसंदिग्धं सारवद्विश्वतोमुखम् ।
अस्तोकमनवद्यं च सूत्रं सूत्रविदो विदुः ।।

"That is called a sutra, by the knowers of sutra, which has the least number of words; it is unambiguous, synoptical, all-embracing, devoid of redundant words and faultless". But it is difficult for those who do not know Sanskrit well to be able to read, grasp and utilize gainfully the capsuled health wisdom in Sutras. Hence the masters in Ayurveda, from time to time wrote commentaries, explanations and translations to make the process of learning Ayurveda easier. Vaidya V. M. Gogte belonged to this rich tradition of great teachers in Ayurveda. His book - in Marathi - of Dravyagunavignyan has been a popular text, in Maharashtra and for all those who know Marathi . But it was felt that an English translation would be of great value for service, education and research in global Ayurveda. Hence I first suggested to his daughter Dr. Jaya Gogate that the Bhavan's SPARC team and others should embark on this difficult but useful venture. We are happy that several years' efforts of the team have now provided this English translation – Ayurvedic Pharmacology.

The foundation of Ayurveda is constituted by several axioms of the basic philosophical systems (Darshanas) of India viz. Sankhya, Vaisheshik, Nyaya etc. Prof. Sathaye, in his book on Padartha-Vignyan, has cited how from Prakriti (nature), the Padarthas (substances) evolve:

प्रकृतेर्महान् ततोऽहंकार तस्माद् गुणश्च षोडशक: ।
तस्मादपि षोडशकात् पंचेभ्य: पंचभूतानि ।।

"Prakriti to Mahat then Ahankar (ego) and the sixteen gunas; from this sixteen are five-derived five bhootas (elements)" So Purusha (self) and Prakriti (nature), Kshetragnya (knower of the field) and Kshetra (field) constituted the primordial sources for the genesis and evolution of Mahabhootas and the resultant dravyas. In past it was a practical approach to incorporate the contemporary dominant philosophical system (Sankhya) as a foundation of a healing system. But what Jung calls "walks on the earth with naked feet" was also a bit lost in the abstractions of Sankhya and Panchikarana – five-fold genesis of materials.

While India was chafing under the foreign rulers, Ayurveda was ignored and derided too. The revolutions in physics, chemistry and biology almost went unnoticed by Dravyagunavignyan textbooks. The periodic table of elements, the structure and fission of the atom, the nature of the chemical bond, quantum chemistry, structure-activity relationship, pharmacokinetics and the central dogma of molecular biology etc. were and are still nonexistent in classical textbooks of Ayurvedic Pharmacology. But similarly, Rasa, Guna, Veerya and Vipak are absent in textbooks of Allopathic pharmacology. Are there any meeting grounds for a dialogue between these two separate ways of looking at the properties of useful remedies? There is an urgent need to list, debate and identify how reductionist and holistic modes of conceptualization and experimentation can judiciously be integrated for a better scientific understanding of drug action. For example, Rauwolfia serpentina served as a unique remedy from Ayurveda, which opened up new fields in basic and applied research in hypertension, depression and Parkinson's disease. Many such opportunities for research are described in the present textbook for the fundamental pharmacology and the remedies.

The present volume by Vaidya V. M. Gogate is a timely reminder to all pharmacologists and physicians that the men of renaissance lead us to intelligent correlation between ancient intuitive insights and modern discoveries of science.

The data on medicinal plants in the textbook have been a source of inspiration for the ongoing research at Bhavan's SPARC. It helped a lot in our compilation of the monograph on Selected Medicinal Plants of India. Gogteji, during his last years, was very happy the manner in which the multidisciplinary team at Bhavan's SPARC, conducted research on medicinal plants . He would have been pleased to learn how this work has progressed: (1) Mucuna pruriens for Parkinson's disease (2) Picrorrhiza kurroa for viral hepatitis (3) Curcuma longa as antimutagenic/cancer preventive (4) Saraca indica as antimenorrhagic (5) Panchvalkal as wound-healing agent and (6) Volatile oils of spices as antimicrobials.

All the scientists, physicians, vaidyas and students interested in "Green Medicine" will find a great friend, philosopher and guide in the form of this textbook for data-mining for new remedies and new uses. Many golden nuggets await the industrious, persistent and seeking minds. For us, over the years, this textbook in Marathi had served as an authentic reference. May many more who needed an English translation too derive benefits for research and therapeutics.

For this mammoth effort, the suggestions and guidance provided by Sri C. Subramaniam, the Bhavan's President, Sri S. Ramakrishnan, Executive Secretary and Director General and Sri Dhiru Mehta, Hon. Jt. Director of Bhavan have served as an inspiration to the Academic Team of Bhavan's SPARC, in the challenge of the work of translation.

We are also deeply appreciative of the brief opinions about the textbook, expressed by the eminent leaders of medicine, Ayurveda and phytopharmacology : Dr. P. K. Warrier, Dr. S. A. Dahanukar, Dr. S. S. Handa, Vd. D. S. Antarkar and Dr. B. M. Hegde.

Dr. Ashok D.B. Vaidya M.D., Ph.D., FAIM
Medical and Research Director
Bhavan's SPARC,
13th N.S. Road, Vitthal Nagar,
JVPD Scheme, Juhu,
Mumbai - 400 049.
Tel : 624 35 07/ 620 95 75

BRIEF REMARKS ON THE STRUCTURE OF THE MONOGRAPH

It has been generally agreed upon that education imparted to students in their mother tongue is more effective and useful. The number of students undergoing college education in Maharashtra is rapidly increasing. In the post - independence era there has been a considerable spread of education in the rural areas. The number of colleges has increased in all the ten universities of Maharashtra. Marathi is the medium of learning for most of the students in these universities. Some universities have even formally accepted Marathi as their medium of instruction. In short, with the advent of regional languages as the medium of instruction, the need of regional text books was urgently felt. Though the number of books in the regional languages has increased, books written by experienced and acclaimed authors on their respective subjects in regional languages are still scarce. Similarly, there are a few subjects which are elective and only for a small number of students. Hence publishers shy away from such subjects. One consequence is that the development of the subject itself is adversely affected.

The Ministry of Education at the centre has provided sizeable funds to all states with the noble aim of propagating the use of regional languages as medium of instruction for the development of necessary literature and terminology. The centre has outlined a strategy to publish textbooks in all the subjects in regional languages. However, details of the publication programme were to be formulated and inplemented by the respective state governments and universities.

Maharashtra accepted this programme and accordingly, on 19 March, 1969, an independent and autonomous Board called "The Maharashtra Universities Book Production Board" was constituted. The central committee of this Board comprised of the Deans of all the universities of Maharashtra as well as one representative each from the Central Education Department, University Grants Commission, Maharashtra State Education Department & Indian Institute of Technology.

The office of the Central Body was set up at Nagpur University. It was decided that the subjects would be distributed among the universities and these would take up the respective identified subjects. This is how the board started functioning.

For every subject, one specific committee was nominated from each university. One member was appointed in every subject committee who was either the Head of Department or a representative of the university. As a consequence, it was easier to identify and evaluate the needs of different universities with varying syllabi. This subject committee plays a crucial role in the choice and publication of these books. It provides an important forum for communication among the colleagues at the university, the professors in the associated colleges, expert authors and the Book Production Board. It was with the subject committee itself that the important work of the Book Production Board started.

The crucial functions of the subject committee include :

1) Modification of the existing syllabi in various universities.

2) Formulation of an outline of a common syllabus.

3) Selection of appropriate authors.

4) Proper guidelines for the authors as to the contents of the books and

5) Publishing the books in a stipulated time frame.

The subject committee also recommends various experts in the respective subjects for scrutiny of the text books as to their standard.

The Board has constituted an independent publication committee for printing and publication of text books.

Executive President,
Maharashtra Universities
Book Production Board.

PREFACE

Ayurveda, like the vedas, has existed and has been committed to memory in India since prehistoric times. Today, many institutions are engaged in teaching Ayurveda, either in its original form or integrated with modern medical subjects. People have been studying Ayurveda owing to their innate motivation as well as for the benefits derived thereby and this will continue in the future too. For hundreds of years, Ayurveda shouldered the responsibility of treatment of diseases and maintenance of health in India. It has admirably proved equal to this responsibility.

Notwithstanding the creditable performance, India, a multigeoclimatic sub-continent which was frequently invaded and fragmented, could never have a standard curriculum for the study of Ayurveda. Although the same textbooks were used, in a country like India, with different climate and conditions from Kashmir to Kerala and from Saurashtra to Assam, there was a marked diversity in Ayurvedic education and treatment methods. Different states had varying syllabi. As a consequence, Ayurveda was never able to achieve a consistent and organised image in the minds of the people. Barring a few exceptions, this led to a negation of Ayurveda. What was needed was organised unity of this science of health.

Eventhough based on firm philosophical foundations and its practical utility in day-to-day life, Ayurveda was neglected. Ayurveda had once treated and maintained health for 80% of the population. It was realised that to make Ayurveda again acceptable in the present day situation, it was extremely important to have a unified approach. With this aim, efforts were made throughout the country and a committee set up at the administrative level, which initiated work in this direction.

This committee, known as "Central Council of Indian Medicine", outlined a common syllabus so that all over India, a uniform education in Ayurveda would be imparted. Accordingly, acclaimed authors were asked to write books in their respective subjects. After evolving a common syllabus, the need for having text books in thirteen to fourteen Indian regional languages arose. "Dravyagunavignyan" is one of the important subjects included in the syllabus. It was the need of the hour to have a book on this subject, in Marathi, which would include the basic principles of Ayurveda, as found in the original texts, as well as experiences derived from generations of use of Ayurvedic medicines.

Vaidyaraj Bhalchandra Nanal, a member of the "Central Council of Indian Medicine", requested me to write a book on "Dravyagunavignyan" in Marathi, as he was acquainted with my work. I accepted the offer. It was in June 1973, that I started working on the book. After 26 months of continuous work, it was finally completed on 15th August, 1975. Before getting the book published, I thought it extremely important to have it approved by leading professors in the subject. The idea behind this was to overcome the shortcomings, resolving of perplexities and integration of new thoughts.

For this purpose, a workshop was organised which consisted of two senior professors each from every Ayruvedic college in Maharashtra. During this three day workshop, approximately thirty professors had lively discussions on the subject, provided valuable suggestions and finally approved the book. This contributed substantially towards the authenticity of the book.

This book contains sketches of almost 350 plants. References are provided from Ayurvedic texts. Out of the total number of pages, 284 pages have been devoted to principles of Dravyagunashastra. In the remaining part, medicinal plants, their Sanskrit and Marathi names, sketches and their kulas and families have been given. Latin names of the families have been provided along with their meaning as also the universally accepted binomial nomenclature.

Further, the Sanskrit synonyms, botanical description, chemical composition, properties, uses in various diseases, parts used, doses and formulations of the plants have also been described. Lastly, the dosha, dhatu and malagamitva of the herbs have been given.

Every page in the book carries a foot-note. These foot-notes, concerning every branch and section of Ayurveda, provide seminal material for thought and meditation. Many were drawn to this imaginative deployment of foot-notes. It has been my experience that these foot-notes convey the message far more effectively without the reader being burdened by volumious reading. This was the reason for providing foot-notes which elicit the basic principles of "Ayurveda - darshan".

Through this book, students, teachers, practicing vaidyas and even a casual reader will definitely grasp the fundamentals of the subject.

Presently, many books are available on "Dravyagunavigynan". Nevertheless, I am confident that this book, which is an extract of almost 50 years of my teachings on the subject, will fill the vaccum created by the lack of such a book. Moreover, information provided in the form of illustrations and pictures will be easily grasped by students.

Nobody can attain complete knowledge in any subject. The author is no exception to this rule. Evidently, the author is aware that there may be some errors, short-comings and printing mistakes in the book. If these drawbacks are generously brought to the notice of the author, it would enrich Ayurveda. This is a humble appeal to all the scholars on the subject, because

विद्वानेव विजानाति विद्वज्जनपरिश्रमम् ।
न हि वंध्या विजानाति तीव्रां प्रसववेदनाम् ।।

V. M. Gogte

Tryambak.

Dt. 3/11/1974.

GRATITUDE

My father, the late Mahadev Hari Gogte, was a vaidya. He worked as a Medical Officer in the Jawhar state and on retirement continued his private practice. It was my father who initiated me into the study of plants during this period.

Later, when I stayed at Dahanu for my higher secondary education for four years, the late Dr. Dadasaheb Phatak left a deep impact on my mind. In 1926, I joined the Ayurveda Mahavidyalaya of Ahmednagar. It was here that I achieved a thorough insight into the knowledge of various medicinal herbs and other dravyas under the guidance of my respected teachers late Ganeshshastri and late Gopalshastri Baivaru.

From 1930 to 1980, I was chiefly associated with teaching this subject. During this long span of 50 years, I was fortunate to have the whole-hearted cooperation of my colleagues and vaidyas who provided ample guidance. I visited many places in Nagar, Nasik, Pune, Thanĕ, Colaba (now known as Raigad), Ratnagiri and Kolhapur districts as well as some places in Kerala and collected information about medicinal plants from experts. Since I have been continuously guiding students on this subject in many colleges in Nagar and Nasik, my experience and knowledge of the subject increased.

The forest department, members of the Vana Mitra Mandal (Nasik) and many professors on the subject also enriched my knowledge.

Dr. Mrs. Shyamalatai Chitale (Nagpur), late Bapukaka Joshi (Devrukh), late Vaidya Ranade (Pune), late Vaidya Rambhau Rudrabhate (Phaltan), Late Vaidya Hiramanji Jangale (Waghadi), Vaidya Bapalalji (Surat), late Bhaushastri Jayil (Tryambakeshwar), Vaidyaraj Bhalchandra Nanal and others also enhanced my understanding of the subject.

The workshop on this book at Shree Kshetra, Tryambakeshwar, was attended by 35 vaidyas who scrutinized it and made important suggestions. The Maharashtra University Book Production Board, Nagpur, was indeed, instrumental in printing and publication of this book which was completed in 1975. Nevertheless, Mr. Anantrao Kulkarni, the Director of Continental Publications, his son Mr. Aniruddha as well as Mr. Jagtap, Mr. Tembhurnikar, Mr. Deshmane and Mr. Nathe of Janaseva Mudranalaya have taken considerable pains towards its publication. Mr. Dhaygude and Mr. Bhave took over the task of verifying the printed material. No words can aptly convey my gratitude to them. The block making was done by Shree Bhide Block Makers (Pune) and the sketches of some of the medicinal plants were drawn by Mr. Sunil Aherrao (Devlali).

The proof reading of hand-written copies was done by Vaidyaraj Sharadchandra Vasekar. The director of the Board, Mr. Vamanrao Chorghade and Mr. Vilas Andhare also extended their cooperation.

The honourable vaidyas present at the workshop were C.S. Kundle, C. C. Kundle, S. V. Dharmadhikari, C. V. Naik, S. P. Parker, J. V. Naik, V. K. Joshi, M. P. Nakade, A. M. Mohod, S. S. Gokhale, A. G. Dhondse, late Tryambak Gurujoshi, D. M. Joshi, M. R. Naik, P. M. Palshikar, Garge Upasni, A. P. Deshpande, S. G. Kulkarni, R. L. Shingare, G. B. Shukla (Tryambakeshwar), including the following from Ayurveda Seva Sangh (Nasik) namely M. D. Rajpathak, L. B. Kale, S. K. Karmarkar, Pandit, Shamrao Kulkarni, Pathak H. D., Rajpathak, R. S. Ware and others, experts and professors from Kolhapur Vanaspati Shibir, Vaidya Mrs. Yamutai Gogate, Vaidya T. M. Gogate, Vaidya D. M. Gogate, Dr. R. B. Gogate, Dr. Vikas Gogate, the teaching staff from Tilak Ayurveda Mahavidyalaya, Pune, Acharya Priyavrat Sharma, who made available his personal library for reference, Mr. Magar, all wellwishers who expressed their views on the introudction, Dr. Ashok D. B. Vaidya, who provided guidance about Latin nomenclature, Professor Sharangpani, Dr. D. G. Warhadpande of Pune University, Mr. Sathem, Mr. Marballi, Mr. Kale, Mr. Mitra, Mr. Gadgil and Mr. Dixit of the forest department as well as Dalit Mitra Mr. Gangaram Jame Awari who helped me considerably. Most importantly, it was my revered guru Vaidya P. V. Dhamankar, who was always there to encourage and guide me and help me in every possible way.

The credit of this book does not belong to me alone. Many people, including those whose names could not be mentioned here, have given their invaluable assistance in accomplishing this task.

I sincerely express my gratitude to all of them.

V. M. Gogte

CONTENTS

Foot-notes on every page are aphorisms which reflect Ayurveda-Darshan (Fundamental vision). They are meant to deeply impress messages on the mind of the readers.

PART I

BASIC PRINCIPLES OF DRAVYAGUNAVIGNYAN

CHAPTER ONE
INTRODUCTION TO DRAVYAGUNAVIGNYAN

Panchamahabhootas - ideological basis

The universe is as much a subject of curiosity as of research. It is a problem and a challenge to all intellectuals. Many philosophers have pondered over the universe as a mystery and have tried to understand it to the limits of their comprehension, though till now it deepens further with the striving. The world around is as perceived through our senses and mind. As a consequence, no one has any doubt over its existence, even though there are a few who do consider it to be false and ephemeral, an illusion! There is no intellectually convincing credible theory which can satisfactorily explain the origin of the universe. The only route is of paradoxical reality, viz. the seed first or the tree, the chicken first or the egg. This too is not easy to grasp. The mystery still remains unsolved and let it remain so! From the ancient scriptures, which claim to solve the mystery, to a recent visionary like H. G. Wells, who wrote "Riddle of the Universe", the problem poses a fresh challenge to Man. It is true that this universe is an inviting subject of learning but to attain complete comprehension of it is virtually impossible. As Charakacharya has said, "That which is directly perceptible is only a tip of the iceberg of reality." The non-perceptible and non-physical dimensions of the universe still remain to be explored.[1]

In spite of such a situation, after a careful deliberation of the diverse expert opinions regarding the origin of the universe, which has many visible-invisible, mobile-immobile, living - nonliving components, Ayurveda has adopted the then contemporarily relevant "Sankhya darshan" – an Indian school of philosophy.

Among the various stages of cosmogenesis described in the Sankhya darshan, Ayurveda has accepted the stages from avyakta to panchatanmatras ie. sukshmamahabhootas. Yet, Ayurveda believes in the principle of 'gunavat-dravya' – property-substance monad. Hence, after the stage of formation of panchamahabhootas which evolve from the panchatanmatras, Ayurveda has formulated its own basic principles. The stages from avyakta have practically no role to play in treatment of diseases or maintenance of health. These were then dropped and panchamahabhootas were accepted as the basis. Panchamahabhootas form the ideological foundation of Ayurveda. This is where dravyagunakarma (substance, property and action) started and developed. Since panchatanmatras do not have any guna-karma, it has laid emphasis on panchamahabhootas. From here starts the practical application of Ayurveda that the material things are constituted by panchamahabhootas.

In Ayurveda, the basic mode of classification and taxonomy utilizes groups of three. The initial classification of the body and drugs was done on the same triune basis. This marks the beginning of classification of groups. In fact, this idea of determining the properties of any substance as per its belonging to one of the three groups, became a prime basis of Ayurveda. This pervades the linguistic uniqueness involving dosha-dhatu-mala, swasthya and rogotpatti and dravyagunavignyan.

It is easy to study Ayurveda if one were to apply to it honest and straight forward intelligence with dedication.

Relationship between man and universe

Charakacharya categorises the foundation of philosophy and knowledge of the universe into six. These are commonality (samanya), specificity (vishesha), property (guna), substance (dravya), action (karma) and composition (samavaya).

The vast and endless universe falls within the orbit of these six categories.

The six existential phenomena (bhava padarth) according to Charaka are:-

1.	Commonality (Samanya)	Useful for obtaining broad fundamental knowledge.
2.	Specificity (Vishesha)	
3.	Property (Guna)	Useful for knowing the special properties of substance (dravya).
4.	Substance (Dravya)	This is prime matter on which the science of dravyagunashastra is based
5.	Action (Karma)	A substance is used for its actions; such effective actions are called karma.
6.	Composition (Samavaya)	Composition meaning how all the properties and actions of a matter are interrelated as to gunas etc.

[Charakacharya has not accepted non-existent entities (abhava).]

Whatever exists in the universe is included in these six categories. In vaidyak (ie. practice of Ayurveda) one deals with only existential phenomena (bhava padarth) and hence there is no need to consider non-existent entities (abhava padarth). It is an innate nature of matter, properties and elements to undergo entropy, alterations and decay.

Ayurveda has accepted a theory which states that every existential phenomenon after its genesis immediately leads to a similar homophenomenon (padarth) and then gets terminated soon. This theory is termed as the principle of ephemerality of existence or moment – fractional existence (Kshanbhangi Bhava Siddhant). As soon as a substance perishes, another similar bhava padarth arises. Therefore there is no need to allot a separate entity to abhava padarth (absence). The existence of abhava padarth is so closely embodied in that of bhava padarth, that Ayurveda has not accepted individual existence of abhava padarth. Consequently, in this world of mobile-immobile and living-nonliving components, there is nothing beyond these six padarthas. This is the fundamental difference between the basic padarthas as enumerated in Ayurveda and other schools of philosophy like Nyaya darshan. Charakacharya, in chapter 5 of Vimana sthana, has distinctly mentioned that the human body is constituted from these highly sublime components of the universe. The aphorism (sutra) reads -

Modern medicine has established its mastery in every branch of specialization. For Ayurveda, panchakarma is its unique contribution.

पुरूषोऽयं लोकसंमितः। यावन्तो हि लोके मूर्तिमन्तो भावविशेषास्तावन्तः
पुरूषे, यावन्तः पुरुषे तावन्तः लोके।

The sutra clearly states that what consitutes the universe also constitutes the human body This is satkaryavad.

असदकरणात् उपादानग्रहणात् सर्वसंभवाभावात् ।
शक्यस्य शक्यकरणात् कारणभावात् च सत्कार्यम् ॥ – Sankhyakarika

That which itself is non-existent can never create existent forms and that which is existent can never be made non-existent.

नासतो विद्यते भावो नाभावो विद्यते सतः। श्रीमद् भगवद्गीता अ.२/१६

Owing to these reasons, Ayurveda has not accepted "abhava padarth".

The following diagram shows how Ayurveda has derived its practical principles using Sankhya darshan as a foundation.

Avyakta (Prakruti)
|
Mahan
|
Ahankar (3 types)

Vaikarik | Taijas | Bhootadi

Through a combination of vaikarik and taijas ahankar, 5 buddhendriyas + 5 karmendriyas + 1 mana = 11 indriyas (senses) have been formed.

Through a combination of taijas and bhootadi ahankar, the panchatanmatras - akash, vayu, teja, aap and prithvi have been formed.
↓
From these were created the sense perceivable shabda, sparsha, roopa, rasa and gandha. Also from the panchatanmatras,
↓
akash, vayu, teja, aap and prithvi - the panchamahabhootas with their attributes were created.
↓
These panchamahabhootas, through various permutations and combina tions, gave rise to endless substances seen in this world.

The foundation of Ayurveda starts from this stage. →

Ayurveda and yoga are totally "communiant". Their goal is "equality" in all over.

Panchamahabhootas in the body are transformed into tridoshas by virtue of their union with the senses. Chaitanya is a pre-requisite for having senses and hence tridoshas are panchamahabhootas with chaitanya.

Endless dravyas are created from panchamahabhootas.

↓

For the study and knowledge of these dravyas, padarthvignyan shastra originated and later

↓

the doshas were defined

↓	↓	↓
akash + vayu	agni	aap + prithvi
↓	↓	↓
vata	pitta	kapha

Despite the doshas being constituted by all the panchamahabhootas, each dosha is dominated by a particular mahabhoota, as shown above. This dominant mahabhoota renders its attributes to that particular dosha.

Everything in this universe is preplanned

Man is a tiny replica of the vast universe. In the ocean of the universe, he is a drop of water or a particle of sand. But according to यत्पिण्डे तत् ब्रह्माण्डे theory, all that exists in the universe also exists in an individual. With such a vital relationship between the two, all the waves and vibrations occurring in the universe naturally have an impact on the individual. This impact, which occurs due to cause-effect relationship, is inevitable and sublime. The universe constantly undergoes changes and transitions owing to an innate tendency. As a consequence, these transitions occur in the individual as well, but in subtle form. Man has no control over these changes. He is totally dependent in this matter. Life, a complex entity comprising of the body, mind, senses, and soul, is always in a transitional phase undergoing minute changes which are universally controlled.

The world constantly undergoes transition

The body has to unite with the universe and it ceaselessly makes efforts to achieve this unity while alive and also after death. All changes in the universe have a corresponding impact on the human body which is easily identifiable because the five elements of the body are but a part of the panchamahabhootas of the universe. The body uses these panchamahabhootas as if obtained on loan. Once its time-frame is over, the panchamahabhootas are not destroyed but merge with those of the universe. Sant Kabir also meant to convey the same message when he said that the body is made up of soil and compared it with a frail piece of cloth. The universe is always eager to contribute its panchamahabhootas for the formation of the human body and therefore this cycle of change keeps on moving ceaselessly and will continue to do so. Similarly, the universe is also provided with a continuous flow of chaitanya (life-force).

All the good and bad characteristics of life are from the seeds of the very life process. Even death has its seeds in the same.

Will this problem be solved ?

The universe and the individual share such similarity that every part of the universe is represented in the individual in minute dimensions. That which is absent in the universe cannot have an existence in the individual. The body flourishes or perishes because of the universe. Life and death are also controlled by the universe. Since there exists such a close relationship between the universe and the individual, no knowledge of the individual can be obtained without a knowledge of the universe. Therefore, Man, equipped with the bliss of gnyana (truthful knowledge), started to study the universe for himself, for his knowledge and for his very survival.

Experiences started pouring in and got recorded. Some of these experiences which could be authenticated and established using praman (modes of authenticating knowledge) were formulated as principles. Using these principles as basis, a few scriptures were developed. These scriptures do not belong to any one person. Many people have put in endless efforts. This tradition is as eternal as it is old and long. These scriptures (shastras) give an organised form to various experiences. Padarthvignyan shastra (science related to knowledge of substances) was developed after inferences were drawn from reconsideration of these experiences. It became a science of the universe. From the study of this science, the problem of the universe was partially solved. Still, will this problem ever be completely resolved ?

The origin of tridosha siddhant

Since there exists a cause and effect relationship between man and universe, from the study of the universe (cause), better understanding of man and living creatures (effect) can be obtained. In this universe, resembling a continuously flowing river, various changes were studied. Even while undergoing these changes, how is the inherent resemblance maintained? How is the equilibrium maintained even after repeated changes? The answers to these important questions formed the fundamental principles of Ayurveda. In this universe, two forces – ushna (heat) and sheeta (cold) – are operational. (The human body has also originated from saumya shukra and ushna artava). These two forces operate continuously. Ushna and sheeta being antagonist forces, it was inferred that there has to be a third force which maintains an equilibrium between the two and keeps them controlled. The idea of tridosha siddhant arose from here (ushna force - pitta, sheeta force - kapha, the balancing force - vayu). The ushna and sheeta forces are complementary to each other and also act as antagonists but yogavahi (vayu) acts as controller for both of them. The same process takes place in the individual as man is a tiny replica of the universe. The balancing work is done by vayu and hence vayu is rightly called yogavahi.

The emergence of dravyagunavignyan

From this padarthvignyan shastra, man concentrated on the principles which maintained an equilibrium in the universe. These principles were studied in the light of padarthvignyan shastra for convenience and for maintaining a balance and this is how dravyagunavignyan emerged. Dravyagunavignyan not only agrees with the universal truths but it is based on principles of these truths. These principles have been derived through knowledge, through experience and through

The ultra-micro panchamahabhootas of the external universe give rise to the ultra-micro panchamahabhootas of the human body.

repeated elucidation of the findings.

Padarthvignyan and dravyagunavignyan are basically identical. The only difference is that of definitions. Dravyagunavignyan is based on the ideas of satva-raja-tama, panchamahabhootas and various experiences derived from the study of balance–imbalance of these basic components of the universe. Padarthvignyan shastra is based on panchamahabhootas. Dravyaguna shastra has also accepted this principle and so was evolved the basic principle of Ayurveda.

शीतांशुः क्लेदयत्युर्वी विवस्वान शोषयत्यपि।
तावुभावपि संश्रित्य वायुः पालयति प्रजाः ॥ सु. सू. ६/८.

Dravyaguna shastra has been formulated in context with swasthya (health) and the diseased (rugna). The basic ideas of the science have been developed keeping the patient in mind.

Health and dynamic equilibrium

At this point, one may raise a doubt that heat energy is the only form of energy and cold energy does not exist or is temporary. But in this world there can be no energy which is absolute. There is always another energy which antagonises it and neutralises it. Even the word heat is used in context with cold. No creature can survive in the presence of absolute heat energy. This is exactly what is meant by 'प्रवृत्तिरूभयस्य तु च. सू. १/४३. These antagonist forces constantly keep a check on each other and that is how equilibrium is maintained in the human body as well as in the universe.

Sheeta (cold), ushna (heat) and the third balancing force vayu (yogavahi) form the great processes into which the idea of panchmahabhootas was included to form a triad. Vayu does not have its own heat or cold and is basically non-aligned. This is the basis of tridosha-tridhatuvad. It is through these three basic elements that nature tries to rectify the dis-equilibrium caused by constant transitions.

The cold force (lunar force-sheeta shakti) is responsible for bestowal, the heat force (solar force – ushna shakti) is responsible for procurement and the third force maintains a balance between the two. These forces operate in the form of kapha, pitta and vata respectively. The formation of triads in Ayurveda like tridosha, triguna and tridhatu are inspired by these forces. This is the basis of study of the human body and its functioning.

Here, the outlook differs from that of padarthvignyan shastra. Ayurveda has developed a methodology to identify the panchamahabhoota content of various substances in the outer world and has used the same format everywhere. This format involves tridoshas. No branch of knowledge in Ayurveda is devoid of tridoshavignyan. From padarthvignyan shastra originated sharir - kriya vignyan and dravyagunavignyan. For the progress and use of these subjects, various definitions were formulated. The definition of tridosha was used on the practical basis of panchamahabhootas. This very principle of panchmahabhootas of padarthvignyan shastra is dealt with in sharir shastra and dravyagunavignyan. Without abandoning the basic principles of panchamahabhootas, sharir and dravyagunavignyan were created and definitions formulated to give a separate identity and demar-

The living body is a healing vehicle. Whatever we do or don't do are also the modalities of treatment.

cate the areas. The principles of both of these are based on the eternal principles of the universe.

The panchamahabhoota siddhant, doshadivignyan and dravyagunavignyan

The tridosha siddhant has originated and developed from the principles of panchamahabhootas. From these principles, the ideas of dosh-dhatu-mala were integrated after a study of the human body. Thus, the science of dosha-dhatu-mala developed. Basic principles of this science like the principle of samanya–vishesha were established and were based on dravyagunavignyan. Hence it is impossible to imagine dravyagunavignyan without the basis of panchamahabhoota and tridosha siddhant. It is necessary for a student to study padarthvignyan (study of the universe) and dosha-dhatu-mala vignyan (study of human body) before studying dravyagunavignyan. In dosha-dhatu-mala vignyan, the state of equilibrium (health) and the state of disequilibrium (disease) of the components of the body is studied. While undergoing the transition from panchamahabhootas to tridosha, the doshas achieve chaitanya (life force).

The triad in Ayurveda

Dravyagunavignyan is the science of medicine. Diseases, like health, have been considered in it. 'रोगमादौ परीक्षेत् ततोऽनन्तरमौषधम्' As said in this aphorism, "without a complete knowledge of diseases, it would not be possible to fully understand dravyagunavignyan." As the diseases are considered in context of health, it is impossible to know diseases without the knowledge of health. Since the ultimate goal of dravyagunavignyan is to maintain health, there exists such a live interrelation between these sciences that there cannot be a study of dravyagunavignyan in isolation. Therefore, while studying dravyagunavignyan, from time to time, panchamahabhoota siddhant, tridosha siddhant and the correlated samanya-vishesha siddhant are invariably mentioned. The science of dravyagunavignyan has been evolved from a holistic approach towards the working of the human body. Every component of the body is essential. The same idea forms the basis of dravyagunavignyan. The panchamahabhootas, in Ayurvedic terminology, have been modified into tridoshas. This triad is the subject of all considerations in Ayurveda.

Prior understanding of bhava padartha essential

It is seen that dravyagunavignyan is an extension of the principles of panchamahabhootas and their guna-karmas with respect to tridosha–siddhant. The aphorism हेतु लिग औषधिज्ञानम्' elicits complete Ayurveda. Here औषधिज्ञानम् means dravyagunavignyan. To understand dravyagunavignyan, the knowledge of hetu (cause of diseases) and ling (clinical features), is à prerequisite. For an understanding of these, it is necessary to know the six padarthas viz. samanya, vishesha, guna, dravya, karma and samavaya. On these six padarthas depends the practice of Ayurveda and dravyagunavignyan. A study of these six padarthas is the basis of the study of Ayurveda. After a complete and comprehensive knowledge of these six padarthas, there is not more in Ayurveda which remains to be known. Of these, the samanya-vishesha siddhant, which motivates the human intellect, is discussed first and other padarthas like dravya, guna etc. are dealt with later.

The practice of Rasayan and Vajikaran in Ayurveda are symbols of survival of one-self and origin as well as the continuity of the species.

The principle of samanya-vishesha

In the affairs of the universe, similar objects tend to bring about an increase in similar objects whereas dissimilar objects bring about a decrease. This principle of bestowal and procurement[2] is the basis of Ayurveda as well as of dravyagunavignyan. This phenomenon of increase and decrease is continuous in a living creature. To remain alive, a balance has to be struck between the two.

An imblance is indicative of disease. Although death is the result of gross imbalance, every individual has his own level of balance. There is no single standard by which a balance in all individuals can be evaluated. There cannot be such a standard. A balance is the cause of swasthya (health). Swasthya is an indication as well as a result of this balance. The importance of this balance can be comprehended by having a glimpse of the following definition of swasthya

समदोष: समाग्निश्च समधातुमलक्रिय: । प्रसन्नात्मेंद्रियमना: ।

The word समदोष: means that all the normal functions of the doshas are properly carried out. Also, the various sub-types of these doshas perform their normal functions, the gunas of these doshas are normal, and quantitatively, the dosha is in proportion. This is the meaning intended by the word समदोष: and the same applies to dhatus and malas. From the aphorism it is very clear that not only the well-being of the physical self is necessary for swasthya (positive health) but also the well-being of the atma (soul), indriya (senses) and mana (mind) as well as their non-attachment (स्थितप्रज्ञता) is equally important. The World Health Organisation has also included mana (mind) in the definition of swasthya.

In order to maintain this equilibrium, factors causing disequilibrium have to be avoided and those aiding equilibrium must be present. The practice of this duo is extremely necessary. Here, the idea of pathya-apathya (do's and dont's) should be clearly understood. For the maintenance of equilibrium, those substances which have increased have to be reduced and vice versa. To achieve this, one has to follow the samanya-vishesha siddhant and therefore it is observed that this principle is used everywhere in maintenance and generation of health. The samanya-vishesha siddhant does not belong to Ayurveda alone, but it is the law of nature.

Dravyagunavignyan–a truly natural science

Dravyagunavignyan is a science of treatment. It has not evolved spontaneously. Through centuries, the science has gradually developed with new experiences getting incorporated and old principles, which could not stand the test of authenticity, being discarded. This science has always been enriched by new and validated principles. Science involves an organised presentation of experiences. Many people know many remedies. Drinking water when thirsty, eating when hungry, use of heat when feeling cold and vice versa are all basically different forms of remedies. A man sleeps when tired.[3] This, again, is a remedy suggested by nature. From these elementary observations, through the experiences of tribal people (अविपाश्चैव गोपाश्च ये चान्ये वनवासिन: च.सू.अ. १/ १२०), by carefully noting various activities of animals when they are ill and through experiences registered from time immemorial, this great science of remedy (dravyagunavignyan) developed. [A pig, on having raktavriddhi (increase in quantity of blood), rubs his body against a rough surface like bamboo spikes or a stone

Just as negotiation, rewards, punishment and intelligence are used to get the work done, similarly sequentially, diet, strenthening medicines, potent remedies and toxic drugs are to be used in the management of diseases.

and loses some blood. On getting indigestion, cats and dogs eat grass and induce vomiting.] Dravyagunavignyan achieved the background of padarthvignyan and sharirvigynan and evolved into a meaningful science. In the vedas, which are the original source of all scriptures, it is observed that many substances are used for treating diseases and also as preventive medicine. Ever since, the tradition has continued and most of the conclusions drawn by them still hold true.

Changes according to times

Due to traditions getting shattered, and definitions not being understood in their correct perspective, sometimes facts appear to be irrelevant. Although, keeping pace with the change through ages, dravyagunashastra has started to obtain a new look. Keeping the basic principles intact, a change in the style of study and functioning in line with contemporary scientific advances is always welcome. For example, earlier, identification of various substances and plants was done only on the basis of their names and their synonyms. Dravyagunashastra was once called nighantu. Nighantu means a collection of synonyms. From these synonyms, information about various aspects of the plant or substance was obtained. Today, with the help of modern methods of classification, this information can be standardized. By doing this, there is no hindrance in giving many synonyms to plants. However, it is clear beyond doubt that contemporary methods of classification are necessary for definite identification of plants compared to the standardization achieved by giving different names to plants based on their morphology, attributes, properties, similarity with nature etc. Such a change was the need of the hour. Charakacharya has said that plants can be identified by their 1) name 2) morphology and 3) properties. Names of the plants can be helpful in identification by using nighantu. Modern methods help in understanding the morphology whereas a comprehensive study of these two will confirm the properties of plants thereby making dravyagunashastra a totally contemporary science. Earlier dravyagunashastra was called nighantu. It used to contain many names of plants. A plant was identified if all the names given in the nighantu exactly coincided with it. It was a huge collection. In fact, in a nighantu, efforts were made to describe a plant from all its aspects. The etymology of the plant names also gave considerable insight. From these, the properties and actions of the plant can be understood. But today, dravyagunashastra has at its disposal, the modern scientific methods of classification for identification of plants. Through this symbiosis, there will be no doubt in identifying a plant anywhere in the world and the sought-after plant would be available globally. It is true that this method will not follow the Ayurvedic style of classification ie. on the basis of properties and actions. But it would be useful in identification and standardisation. Even after such a classification, there is no problem in forming groups on the basis of properties and actions. These groups are useful in practical applications of Ayurveda. For the botanical classification of plants, modern classification techniques may be resorted to whereas the classification used by Charaka-Sushruta may be followed in properties and actions. In dravyagunashastra, classification according to properties and actions would be most useful. According to the Natural Order, vatsanabh (Aconitum ferox) and ativish (Aconitum heterophyllum) fall in the same family ie. Ranunculaceae but both vary considerably in their actions and properties. Vatsanabh acts as a poison whereas ativish is an antidote for poison.

Just as the skin is a good topographic indicator of the internal state of a person, the surface of the earth can give an indication of its subterranean structure.

Pratyakshadi praman for better understanding of shastra

Earlier, substances were classified on the basis of their medicinal properties. Contemporary classification provides a standardised methodology for identification. As a result, the same plant may be spotted anywhere "under the sun" without any doubt. This cleared all the confusion in identifying a plant and this change was urgently needed for giving dravyagunashastra, the status of a science. The acceptance of this change is indicative of close interaction, progressiveness and intellect; it is upgradation and not degradation. A science always has to be progressive. It will have to be accepted that the original source of all knowledge is aptavakya (an apta is a person who has gained authority over a subject and has risen above all worldly interests). Every branch of knowledge in life starts with an aptavakya. But, these too, have their own limitations. It is true that the origin of knowledge lies in aptavakya. But equally true is the fact that once the mastery is gained, further developments are achieved by pratyaksha, anuman and yukti praman. Ultimately, even the aptavakyas have to be tested by these pramans. Aptavakya alone can never become the basis of science. Perhaps, while considering the highly sublime or supernatural aspects of life, one has to resort to aptavakya. But for the development, progress and authenticity of dravyagunashastra, the use of other pramans is thoroughly justified. Hence, dravyagunashastra depends on various pramans and rightly so.

Concept of 'gamitva'

Like the human body, plants also have a definite structure. They too have dhatus and organs. They bear some resemblance to organs and structures in the human body. The parts of the plant body show more action on those parts in the human body which they resemble. This is called 'gamitva'. It can be illustrated by some examples. The seeds of certain plants act as 'vrushya'. The components used increase the corresponding components. But the substances showing similar 'gamitva' may have contradictory properties. The dravyas that are useful to the eyes and those that are harmful, both have 'gamitva' in the eyes, but their actions are totally opposite. Vrushya and avrushya dravyas act on the same site, both have the same gamitva but their actions differ. Dadhi (curd) produces abhishyanda in the liver and the path of pitta. Whereas pippali (Piper longum) which is also yakrutgami, reduces abhishyanda (abhishyanda is blockage of ducts due to excessive viscosity). Such gamitva has to be constantly considered in dravyagunakarma. The concept of gamitva is the soul of dravyagunashastra. Charakacharya has elucidated eight factors which are responsible for initiation of 'smruti'. Among these, like absolute similarity, absolute dissimilarity is also one of the factors. On watching an obese person, we are reminded of another obese person as also of a very thin person. Similarly, on watching a thin person, we may either remember a similarly thin person or a very obese person. Gamitva also works on a somewhat similar principle. It is not that gamitva is always directed towards similar aspects. It may be directed towards dissimilar aspects as well. Milk, which is similar in properties to 'ojas', consolidates ojas when consumed. Hence it is 'ojogami'. Similarly, poison, which is very contradictory in its properties to ojas, promptly disintegrates it and is fatal. In both these cases, the gamitva of the dravya plays a key role. The formulation of 'parpati' was introduced in Ayurveda so that the dravya becomes grahanigami. In fact, sharkara (sugar) is one of the causes of prameha. Yet, a combination of triphala and sugar is used in the treatment of prameha. The reason for this is

During the formulation of a churna we use two plants in combination. Can we use the same plants where one is grafted on other?

that sugar, through its gamitva towards the dosha-dushyas of prameha, provides an opportunity for triphala to act on them. One more example mentioned in the scriptures is as follows. Til (sesame) is known to produce kushtha. Eventhough, a combination of til and bhallatak (Semecarpus anacardium) is used as a remedy for kushtha. This implies that bhallatak, taking advantage of the gamitva of til, reaches those dosha-dhatu and malas which are responsible for generating kustha roga and cures the disease by improving their agni.

Selection of dravyas according to organogenesis

In order to understand the concept of gamitva, the chapters relating to the development of organs in a foetus given in the Sharir sthana of Sushruta samhita, would be helpful. It is important that whenever mention is made of any dhatu, at the same time the organs developing from that particular dhatu as well as its srotas must also be considered in depth. Similarly, while dealing with any organ, the dhatus from which it has developed must also be kept in perspective. In the Sushruta samhita this chapter relates to nidan and remedy ie. dosha-mala vignyan and dravyagunavignyan. This has been explained in detail later but a few examples have been cited below.

In any disease of the lungs, it is very important to consider rakta dhatu because in the gestation period, lungs are formed from the froth of rakta dhatu. Moreover, if the patient has epistaxis or haemetemesis connected with the lungs, then even more emphasis should be laid on rakta dhatu. Similarly, while dealing with diseases of the kidneys and other associated diseases, one has to first take into account rakta and meda dhatu since,

रक्तमेद: प्रसादात् वृक्कौ (सु.शा.अ. 4 / 31)

In the same way, liver and spleen have a close association with rakta dhatu. In the diseases of the raktajanya organs, raktasruti (blood letting) is one of the principal remedies. Also, those dravyas which are raktagami, prove useful. This is clear from the following aphorism given in the scriptures –

प्लीहामये पिप्पलि:

It is observed that pippali, which shows its gamitva on the spleen, improves the agni of rakta dhatu and acts as rasayana on it. (The author's experience of using vardhaman pippali rasayana has been very encouraging)

The constituent dhatus of various body organs

	The organs, substances, upadhatus etc. of the body	The constituent dhatu
1.	Intestine, rectum, bladder	From the prasad bhaga of rakta with kapha (with the help of pitta and vayu)
2.	Tongue	From the sara of kapha, rakta and mansa.

If we chew the root of Kuradu (Sunishannaka), then even sand can be crushed like the sugar crystals (Miracle of Forest) (Shri G.J. Aavari).

3.	Muscles	Mansa dhatu + vayu
4.	Sira - snayu	Sira = mridu pak, Snayu = khara pak, from the sneha of meda
5.	Kidney	Prasad of rakta and meda
6.	Testes	Mansa, rakta, kapha and meda
7.	Heart	Rakta and kapha prasad
8.	Pranvahadhamani	Rakta and kapha prasad
9.	Lungs	Froth of rakta
10.	Liver-spleen	Rakta
11.	Caecum	From the kitta bhaga of rakta
12.	Breast milk	Rasa
13.	Kandara, Sira	Rakta
14.	Skin	Mansa
15.	Sukshma snayu	Meda
16.	Teeth	Asthi
17.	Hair	Majja
18.	Oja	Shukra

While dealing with any of these organs, the corresponding dhatus must invariably be considered and vice versa.

Prime function of dhatus - malas and selection of dravyas

Similarly, while studying the dhatus, their malas and their prime functions and any change in them should always be considered. Even the upadhatus cannot be fully understood without a background of the dhatus. Accordingly, kapha and lasika as well as the function of prinana cannot be dealt with by overlooking the role played by rasa dhatu. An identical relationship exists between pitta, jeevaniya karma and rakta dhatu. Naturally, jeevaniya gana is raktagami. The chief function of rakta dhatu is ' jeevan'. There is a close relationship between rakta dhatu and jeevaniya gana. Mansa dhatu and mansagami dravyas should always be considered with all the srotas which have an external opening. If an excess of discharge occurs through nose and ears, then the pachana dravyas of mansa dhatu will be helpful. If a person becomes thin then his mansa and meda dhatu must be checked. The dravyas used in rajayakshma are mansagami and mansavardhak because it involves karshya (emaciation) because of mansakshaya. The pratishyaya in rajayakshma is also due to vitiation of mansa dhatu. Similarly, sweda (sweat) and meda dhatu are interrelated. If the skin becomes dry or sweats excessively, then it is important to think about meda dhatu. Deformities in the nail and hair point towards asthi dhatu as also the body posture. If the eyes or skin become dry, then it is mandatory to think of majja and majjagami dravyas. It may be remembered though, that the dhatu involved should not be thought of as isolated. It should be evaluated in a holistic perspective with regards to its precursor and its product dhatus. Hence rakta dhatu must be considered in context of its precursor rasa dhatu and its product mansa dhatu.

After chewing the root of Kokilaksha (Kolista), the teeth can also chew glass (seen in Adivasis).

Dhatus - their malas and chief actions

1.	Rasa - Kapha	Preenana
2.	Rakta - Pitta	Jeevana
3.	Mansa - The Malas in all srotas	Lepa
4.	Meda - Sweda	Sneha
5.	Asthi - Nails, hair	Dharan
6.	Majja - The sneha in eyes, skin, faeces	Poorana
7.	Shukra - Oja	Garbhotpadan

Dhatus		Organs/tissues developing from them
1.	Rasa	Stanya, artava, rakta
2.	Rakta	Antra, guda, basti, jivha, vrukka, vrushan, hridaya, pranvahadhamani, phuphus, yakrut, pleeha, unduk, kandara, sira and mansa
3.	Mansa	Jivha, peshi, vrushan, twak and meda
4.	Meda	Sira, snayu, vrushan, vrukka and asthi
5.	Asthi	Dant and majja
6.	Majja	Kesh and shukra
7.	Shukra	Oja (garbha)

Vayu - Antra, guda, basti, peshi
Pitta - Antra, guda, basti
Kapha - Antra, guda, basti, jivha, vrushan, hridaya

} While considering these organs it is necessary to consider the corresponding doshas.

Drugs targeting seven layers of skin

Moving a step further, it could be inferred that the dravyas used on sidhma and padmakantak act on the avabhasini layer ie. the first layer of the skin. These dravyas have their gamitva on the first layer. Similarly, those acting on tilkalak, nyachcha and vyang have their effect on the second layer, those used for charmadal–kustha on the third layer; kilas kustha is associated with the fourth layer whereas the remedies for kustha and visarpa are directed towards the fifth layer. The dravyas used in these disorders have more action on the fifth layer. Many dravyas mentioned in the texts on granthi, apachi, arbud, shleepad and galgand act on the sixth layer and those useful for bhagandar, vidradhi and arsh as well as procedures like shastra and ksharkarma have their action on the innermost ie. the seventh layer of the skin. It implies that the dravyas producing these diseases have their vitiating effect also on the corresponding layers.

In spite of giving multiple synonyms all the properties could not be exhausted. But the hints to other properties were not left out.

Such precise deliberation is possible in dravyagunavignyan. The word 'sharir' is not a mere indicator of the anatomical self but in this word is circumscribed a complete entity comprising of the outward appearance, the tendency, vitiation and elimination of the body. From the above definition it is clear why sharir is called as an entrance to the knowledge of treatment. Treatment in Ayurveda revolves around karmapurusha. How can one understand karmapurusha without the knowledge of sharir?

Akasheeya dravyas for srotas

The following illustrations given in the Sushruta samhita would be useful in determining the dhatu - upadhatu gamitva of various dravyas having the eminence of one or more mahabhootas. For example, when the intended site of action of any dravya is nakha, asthi, dant, mansa, charma, varcha, kesh, smashru, loma or kandara, then it would be more useful if eminent in prithvi mahabhoota. The reason for this is that these bodily substances have developed from dravyas prevalent in prithvi mahabhoota. The same principle applies to the aapya dravyas. The dravyas eminent in aap mahabhoota exhibit gamitva on rasa, rudhir, vasa, kapha, pitta, mutra and sweda. The taijas dravyas are useful for maintaining temperature, giving a shining appearance to the skin and improving vision.The dravyas that are eminent in vayu mahabhoota are useful for functions like throbbing of various structures, inspiration, expiration, blinking of the eyes, contraction, movement initiation and support. Various large and small srotas are made up of akash pradhan dravyas. Hence for a dravya to act on any of the large or small srotas, eminence of akash mahabhoota is a prerequisite. The body is made up of srotas and these srotas, in turn, are akashiya (akash is the chief constituent mahabhoota). Hence akash mahabhoota plays a major role in srotogamitva of a dravya. The pulsations of various body parts, the uninterruppted movement of vayu and the nonresistance to its movement are all essential indicators of the presence of life force (chaitanya). Since this nonresistance is possible by akash mahabhoota alone, it implies that akash is absolutely necessary for life and life force. To bring home this concept, an example of the nose is readily acceptable to the intellect. There are akashiya srotas which provide a passage to pranvayu. If these are compressed so as to obstruct them then what are the consequences? If a suitable amount of akash is not maintained in the pathways of faeces and urine then perhaps, even death would result due to udavarta. Life exists on account of the presence of nonresistent akash. When dyspnoea occurs due to the obstruction of the passage of air, the obstruction has to be cleared by a shodhan like vaman (shodhan is removal of vitiated doshas and vaman is medically induced vomiting) or by using dravyas like kapoor and hingu which clear the air passage.

Medicinal dravyas must target the respective malayanas

(Malayanas are sites in the body where malas are stored before excretion).

It is impossible to arrive at a decision about a remedy without due consideration to the roga samprapti (pathogenesis). The knowledge of samprapti forms a basis for further study of dravyagunavignyan. In any disease, the samprapti is first determined and then comes the choice of dravyas (रोगमादौ परीक्षेत् ततोऽनंतरमौषधम्). The general pathogenesis of all diseases is described in

The annual plants become ineffective within six months to a year, but the perennial plants should not be like this. Isn't it?

Ashtangsangraha as: (दोषा: दुष्टा: रसैर्धातून् दूषयन्त्युभये मलान् । मला: मलायनानि दूषयन्ति। यथास्वं तेषु (मलायनेषु) अतो गदा: । (वा.सू.).

The above quotation clearly states that every disease originates in some of the malayanas and the malayanas themselves are also vitiated. Obviously, the vitiation has to be taken care of by the remedies. The dravyas which are used as remedies will be effective only when they reach the srotas of those dosha, dhatu and malas which are involved in the samprapti and act on them as well as provide strength to the involved malayanas. The treatment involving sweda and swedayana (skin) in the samprapti of jvara, mala pitta in raktapitta, mutra and mutrayana in prameha, pureesh and pureeshayana in atisara etc. have been described in the scriptures. For example, abhyang (hot and cold) in jvara, treatment of liver in raktapitta, and basti in atisara and grahani have been indicated. These examples are provided to give a general idea. It is mandatory for the dravyas used in every disease to reach the malayanas involved and provide strength to it. A precise scrutiny of the interrelation of dravya and vyadhi (disease) is necessary.

The genesis of every disease is associated with some of the malayanas. The dravyas used as remedies should possess gamitva on these sites of origin of the disease. For example, in jvara, the causative dosha is pitta, the dooshya is rasa and both of them vitiate swedavahasrotas (the symptoms seen in jvara are those of sweda dushti)–treatment given is also sweda-vahasrotogami; the symptoms seen on resolution of jvara viz. स्वेदोलघुत्वं .... and दाह स्वेदो......... are also associated with swedavahasrotas. The remedies should also be directed towards swedavahasrotas. (लंघनं स्वेदनं.........वा.चि.अ. 1)

In this way, the malas are involved directly or indirectly in the pathogenesis of almost all the diseases related to the body. Even the malas and the malayanas associated with the dhatu which harbours the pathogenesis, have to be taken into account before arriving at a decision on the treatment. For a precise understanding of the choice of drug, it is necessary to consider the samprapti (pathogenesis) of the disease in great depth along with the proportionate involvement of the doshas. This is so because the main objective of treatment is to break the samprapti ie. the sequence of events leading to disease production and install the natural sequence which would result in health.

The ten antagonistic pairs of gunas

The concept of dravyas involves another thought which requires an understanding in the right context. Ten gunas, viz. guru (heavy), manda (slow acting), hima (cold), snigdha (oily), shlakshna (smooth), sandra (viscous), mridu (soft), sthira (steady), sukshma (fine) and vishada (non-sticky) have been mentioned. These, along with their antagonist twin-quality gunas, constitute the 20 gunas in Ayurveda. Thus there are 10 pairs of antagonist gunas, all of which exist simultaneously in the numerous cells of the living body (शरीरावयवास्तु परमाणुभेदेन अपरिसंख्येया: भवन्ति । अति बहुत्वात् अतिसूक्ष्मत्वात् अतीद्रियत्वात् च । चरक).

Even the smallest unit of the body ie. the cell, should be evaluated as to whether it is snigdha or ruksha. These gunas are interdependent and are scattered even in the minute parts of the body. It

Is it not possible that just as man thinks about plants, similarly plants, as living organisms, also are concerned about humans?

is necessary that various parts, dhatus and organs of the body maintain a normal proportion of the gunas. In Ayurveda, while stating an increase in the ruksha guna of a particular dravya, dosha, dhatu, mala or organ, it is understood that there is a corresponding decrease in the snigdha guna. While studying the gunas of various dravyas, a student must always remember that if a dravya is described as snigdha then it naturally implies that it would create snigdhata and thereby reduce rukshata. A student must meticulously try and achieve this attitude towards the study of dravyas. The gunas of all existent dravyas in the universe are inherent. The study of these inherent gunas is a part of the study of dravyagunakarma. The dravyas, possessing their respective gunas, constitute the dosha, dhatu and malas of the body. If a particular guna has been reduced then a dravya possessing that guna should be used. If an imbalance is caused due to an increase in any guna then a dravya that exhibits gamitva on the affected dosha-dhatu-mala but has opposite gunas should be used. Since all these concepts are based on existent gunas, there was no need to introduce the concept of abhava; but an even more important aspect should be examined. When any dravya is used, whether or not it would produce snigdhata or rukshata of some of the dhatus, parts or organs should also be determined in the light of its gamitva. This, precisely, is the study of dravyaguna.

'कायानां प्रकृतिर्ज्ञात्वात्वनुरूपा क्रियां चरेत् । सु. शा. अ. 4 / 98

In the Ayurvedic scriptures, the terms guna-dosha share a special relationship. Taking into consideration the cause and effect relationship between gurvadi gunas and vatadi doshas, the above statement holds true. It seems that the term 'dosha' must have come into existence only after a proper understanding of the gunas. Dravya itself does not have any action; all actions are the attributes of gunas. Such close relationship (and lively too) exists between guna and dosha. The identification, introduction, knowledge, existence and actions of all dravyas are known by their gunas but these gunas have no existence without dravya. Without the dravya, gunas have no separate entity and hence gunas have a subordinate status.

Maintenance of balance among ten pairs of gunas

1. Guru (heavy)	2. Laghu (light)
3. Mand (slow acting)	4. Teekshna (fast acting)
5. Hima (cold)	6. Ushna (hot)
7. Snigdha (oily)	8. Ruksha (non-oily, dry)
9. Shlakshna (smooth)	10. Khara (rough)
11. Sandra (viscous)	12. Drava (liquid)
13. Mridu (soft)	14. Kathin (hard)
15. Sthir (steady)	16. Chala (mobile)

At the beginning of Charaka-samhita, there is panchakarma and it ends also with panchakarma. Charaka Samhita is fully covered with panchakarma and that is the truth.

17. Sukshma (fine) 18. Sthula (gross)

19. Vishada (non-sticky) 20. Pichchil (sticky)

These ten pairs of antagonist gunas exist simultaneously in variable proportions in the body. There cannot be any substance which is 100% snigdha. If a substance is deemed to be snigdha then it only means that it has a predominance of snigdha guna. Nevertheless, ruksha guna would also be present. This is what is conveyed in the aphorism,

न हि एको वर्तते भावो । चरक

Nothing is absolute in this universe. This is what is meant by तस्मान्नैकरसं द्रव्यम्

A few rasas may be perceptible while others may be only slightly perceptible. In garlic, though imperceptible, five rasas are present which can be inferred upon through praman. This shows that all dravyas are constituted by mahabhootas.

नैक दोषास्ततो रोगा:

The above sutra means that these 20 gunas invariably represent some of the mahabhootas and all existent forms are made up of all the five mahabhootas. It implies that all the existent forms possess all the 20 gunas. Just as the universe contains these 20 gunas, in the same way, the human body, which has originated from this universe, possesses these gunas. The identification of these gunas is done by determining the prevalence of the related mahabhoota, rasa, guna and karma in the dravya. This remains the mode of determining the gunas of a dravya not only in Ayurveda but also throughout the universe, of which Ayurveda is an inseparable part.

Causes of diseases and dravyas effective on concerned dushya-srotas

The human body is an aggregation of different srotas. These srotas are instrumental in the origin, maintenance and destruction of the basic supporters of the body viz. dosha, dhatu and malas. It is a firm principle of Ayurveda that the srotas are responsible for origin, maintenance, increase or decrease of respective dosha-dhatu-malas. No disease can develop without a vitiation of the srotas. For any disease to progress, it is absolutely mandatory that a prior vitiation of the srotas of the dosha-dhatu-malas involved in the samprapti takes place. For example, let us consider jvara. In this roga, rasa (dhatu), pitta (dosha) and sweda (mala) have to be always vitiated. Without this there can be no jvara. This naturally means that the dravya which would be selected for treating jvara should be rasavahasrotogami, pittavahasrotogami as well as swedavahasrotogami. Only then will the dravya cure jvara completely. No matter what the causes or treatment of jvara are, they can produce or cure it only if they are pitta, rasa and sweda srotogami. The causes of prameha like a sedentary lifestyle and overeating of foods like curds and sugar can lead to prameha only if they can acheive a gamitva towards meda and similar components of the body (meda, mansa, kleda, drava, kapha, basti, ureters, mutrashaya etc.) Similarly, all attempts at curing prameha would be futile if the dravya used is unable to achieve gamitva towards the above mentioned dhatus (meda, mansa etc.)

It is not sufficient to have only the knowledge of plants. One should also know their applications and formulations of medicine. Similarly, one should also know the dose and proper time to employ the medicine.

Concurrent vitiation of doshas and weakness of their abodes

Furthermore, the dravyas which have been described as 'jvarahara' perform the function of rectifying the vitiation of rasa, pitta and swedavahasrotas and regulating their functions. This is why the treatment of disorders of swedavahasrotas is the same as that of jvara. The causes of various diseases, on account of their gamitva, produce a vitiation of the srotas of the associated dosha-dhatu-mala and thereby produce the disease. Similarly, the remedies of those diseases also have gamitva on the same srotas and become instrumental in the cure of the disease. This means that the dravyas responsible for the origin of disease as well as the remedies should possess gamitva towards the affected dosha, mala and organ. While dealing with the causative factors and the treatment of diseases, due consideration to the following criteria is unavoidable and inevitable:

a) यथा दुष्टेन दोषेण – Which dravyas vitiated the doshas and what is their dosha-dhatu-mala-gamitva

b) यथाचानुविसर्पता – Which dhatu-malas were the targets of the vitiated doshas

c) निर्वृत्तिरामयस्य – What was its consequence in terms of manifestation of the disease

The treatment of any disease would be right on target only if it can recreate the correct state of equilibrium which was disturbed by dosh-dushya sammoorchana. All other treatments are nothing but illusions. This is an example of Dehlideep Nyaya.

स एव कुपितोदोष: - समुत्थानविशेषत: - स्थानांतराणि च प्राप्य

In the above aphorism, the word समुत्थानविशेषत: applies to स एव कुपितोदोष: as well as स्थानांतराणि च प्राप्य. This means that when doshaprakopa occurs due to its causative factors, at the same time these factors affect other dhatus and avayavas and render them vulnerable. Thus the doshas find an abode in these sites. The causative factors induce doshaprakopa and vulnerability of the dhatus simultaneously. And therefore, the medicine used should be such that it nullifies the vitiation of doshas and also provides strength to the affected dhatus and organs. This is the idea behind

रोगमादौ परीक्षेत् ततोऽनन्तरमौषधम् ॥

Prameha and srotogamitva

To explain the above concept more vividly, the example of prameha would be helpful. Prameha involves vitiation of medovaha, mansavaha, kledavaha, kaphavaha srotas, basti (ie. the organs involved in the formation of mutra) as well as mutravahasrotas and mutra malayan. The causes of prameha are inactive and passive lifestyle, excess consumption of curds, meat of animals dwelling in watery regions, meat soup, milk, recently harvested foodgrains, refrigerated foods, unprocessed rain water and various preparations of jaggery. Because of these factors, the srotas of the dhatus

In Latin, plants are named after many scientists. Similarly, why could not there be names of plants after Ayurvedic scholars in nighantu? (One regret).

enumerated above, which perform the function of vahan (वहन) [ie. production, maintenance and destruction of dhatus] are unable to execute their normal functions and the disease which thereby ensues is called prameha. The treatment instituted for prameha, whether through diet or a change in lifestyle, has to have a normalizing and regulating effect on the srotas of meda, mansa, kapha and mutra and only then it would be successful. A combination of amalaki and haridra is capable of producing this effect. The rasayana, balya, pureeshshodhak and meda-mansa-balya karma of amalaki and the tikta rasa of haridra as well as the combined effect of the two results in the treatment of prameha. Besides, other treatments like walking a distance of 100 yojanas without carrying any money and bare foot and bare headed or productive exercise like digging a lake have been described. Also, administration of shilajit has been advised which is specifically used for prameha on account of its normalizing effect on the srotas of the dosha-dhatu-malas involved in prameha. All these treatments, when instituted, have a cumulative effect in the cure of prameha.

An intellectual seminal power

One more concept must be kept in mind while studying dravyaguna. All the dravyas should be considered in the context of the disease, the curing of which has been described as an attribute of the respective dravya. For example, 'loha' (iron) has been described as the chief dravya for panduroga (anaemia) in the Uttartantra of Ashtanghridaya (अ. 4 श्लोक. 48). While considering the sutra, one should try and correlate the effect of loha on all the dosha–dushyas as well as on all the stages of its samprapti. Pitta is the chief vitiating dosha while vayu is responsible for the movement of doshas. Hridaya is the main site of the disease process – धमनीर्दश संप्राप्य (spreading in all the ten directions) – the pitta flows through all the ten vessels and spreads throughout the body. Wherever the pitta goes, it vitiates the kapha, tvacha, rakta, mansa and finds a refuge between tvacha and mansa thereby producing various shades of colours on the skin. As a result, a laxity of all dhatus occurs along with ojakshaya, rakta and medakshaya. Taking into account the symptoms produced by ojakshaya (बिभेति - fearfulness, दुर्बल: - weakness), raktakshaya (अम्लशिशिर प्रीति - liking for sour and cold objects, सिराशैथिल्य - laxity of blood vessels) and medakshaya (स्वपन कट्या - pain in the flanks, प्लीहोवृध्दि - enlargement of the spleen), the list of the manifestations of panduroga becomes quite extensive. Symptoms like loss of refined dhatus, inefficiency of the senses etc. also develop. The purpose of the above explanation is to convey the message that the factors causing panduroga vitiate the srotas of all the dhatus involved in the samprapti. Only then panduroga develops and therefore it goes without saying that any dravya or combination of dravyas which is useful in panduroga must have a normalizing effect on all the srotas which are involved either in the samprapti or in the symptoms of panduroga. Such intense ideological possibilities lie in this sutra (aphorism).

Charakacharya, in Vimana sthana, has described various factors that vitiate the srotas carrying pran (vayu), ambu (kapha), anna (pitta), rasadidhatus, pureesh, mutra and sweda (च.वि.अ 5/10-22).

The word srotas includes all the minute, subtle, large, rounded or nonrounded structures of the body like sira, dhamani, rasayani, rasavahini, nadi, panthan, marg, sharir chhidra, sthana, ashaya, niket etc. When it is said that a particular dravya is specific for a particular disease then the obvious

While considering either the medicine or a constituent of the body, simultaneously their respective srotas must be visualised.

meaning derived from it is that the dravya increases the work-potential of all the srotas involved in the samprapti. These srotas, in turn, are instrumental in maintaining an equilibrium of the dhatus they carry.

Dravyagunavignyan–evolution through necessity

It is difficult to state when dravyagunakarma attained the status of a shastra (science). Man, who is constantly in search of happiness, has used infinite substances by virtue of his intellect and experiences to achieve happiness and eliminate sorrow. Man (effect), who possesses marked similarity with nature (cause), has tried to make his life happier by using many dravyas provided by nature. But human intellect and his intellectual efforts never allowed him to be satisfied. He accepted panchamahabhootas as the basis and started farming after observing that foodgrains are produced from their seeds. (That which can sprout and has the capacity to reproduce is called beeja whereas that which has lost the capacity of reproduction is called tandul. For example, apamarg beeja and apamarg tandul.) After the discovery of fire, man started eating grilled meat of hunted animals in order to make it more tasty and easily digestible. It is perfectly natural that the food which is artificially made tastier may be overeaten and subsequent necessity of measures to counteract the effect of overeating is also equally natural. As man continued with his artificial life, he must have increasingly felt the necessity of finding ways to deal with problems that arose from of his alienation from natural laws regarding food and lifestyle. It naturally follows that through these efforts, he might have obtained experience regarding remedies. Man sleeps, rests when tired, drinks water when thirsty and eats when hungry. These are the most primitive forms of remedies. Substances like food and water are eminent in rasas whereas medicines like sunthi, shatavari and chitraka are eminent in veerya. Remedies keep on being discovered through necessity. The number of remedies kept on increasing keeping pace with the ever increasing medical needs. Many medicines, not originally described in the scriptures, also started being used based on practical experience. Later on this information evolved into dravyagunashastra.

The importance of sanskar

संस्कारो हि गुणान्तराधानम् । च.वि. 1/22

For obtaining a special effect of any dravya at a particular site, it becomes necessary to perform a few sanskar on it (only if the dravya does not possess such innate property); then the dravya can yield the expected results. The concept of sanskar seems to have originated from panchavidh kashaya kalpana (वा.क.अ. 6). Various preparations of the same dravya like rasa (juice), kalka (pulp), shrut (decoction), sheeta (cold infusion) and phant (infusion) obviously have different applications. It would be incorrect to say that all of these have the same effect. Sanskar will definitely lead to an alteration in the gunas. Gunas, not earlier present in the dravyas, are imbibed in them after suitable sanskars. Dravya before sanskar and dravya after sanskar are two different entities even though they may be called by the same name for the sake of convenience. The science of cooking or dietetics as well as pharmacology are extensions of the concept of sanskar. A vaidya must be well-versed in the science of dietetics as also with pharmacology.

As garlic consists of five rasas and called rasona (minus one rasa), similarly haritaki and amalaki also consist five rasa.

If a dravya is subjected to a sanskar with another dravya having similar gunas then it will lead to an increase in the quality of the dravya. Better quality brings about better action. It is interesting to note that sanskar can also bring about a decrease in the undesirable attributes of a dravya. For example, if a dravya is a strong purgative (teevra virechak) and in a given situation, such strong purgative action is undesirable, then it may be treated with a pichchil dravya like shleshmatak (sanskar). The bhavana of shleshmatak on the dravya reduces the vibrations produced by it on the body and naturally, according to the sutra –

विरूध्द गुणसंयोगे भूयसाल्पं हि जीयते ॥ वा. स. 1

- the purgative dravya becomes mild and its purgative activity is reduced.[4]

Knowledge of dravyas only through gunas

In dravyagunashastra, dravyas are identified through their gunas. All the knowledge about dravyas is obtained from gunas. Other than this, there is no separate knowledge of dravyas. Through our senses we preceive the form, smell, touch, taste, weight, shape etc. of the dravyas. Such an entity which provides lodging to a compilation of gunas is termed as a particular dravya. Therefore dravyas do not have an independent identity (without gunas). A dravya is just an assumption. Dravya, as seen directly, is just an illusion; because without gunas, no matter can become a subject of our understanding. For example, it would be a mistake to state that we can directly perceive the panchatanmatra. In fact what we can perceive is the particular assembly of gunas and this is termed as a dravya. The dravya acts as a support for the gunas and therefore it has been given due importance in Ayurveda. But the very constitution of Ayurveda is such that it should be called gunavadi (a believer and follower of gunas). Is it possible to describe a dravya without the help of gunas? And if there is a change in the expected gunas of a dravya or if they are destroyed then would it be wrong to call it by its original name? Hence dravya is that particular substance which serves as a support for an aggregation of definite guna-karmas.

Any change in the composition of the dravya may cause an alteration in the gunas and therefore knowledge of gunas is given more importance in dravyagunashastra. Just as the identification of dravyas is done by gunas, the gunas are identified by karmas. In the chapter relating to gunas in Ashtangsangraha (वा. सू. अ. 1/18), the comments on the above aphorism points out the difference between gunas and explains how to identify gunas from their karmas. Generally, they are inactive. Only on special occasions do they get manifested. The human mind is trained to perceive knowledge and store images of past experience. Thus, an image of a previously experienced guna may also act as a guna. Therefore, by looking at a tamarind, one's mouth immediately starts salivating. A distinct point of difference between man and animals is that man can think or deliberate over perceived images. The thought process that follows after perception in human beings is absent in animals. In the absence of perceptible objects, there can be no perception. Like the state of health or of disease, dravya is also a subject of perception or knowledge. Who is eligible for acquiring this knowledge? An expert vaidya is the right choice for giving this knowledge. What will a lay man do with it?

The study of human and the plant organism cannot be independent of each other. It is not possible.

व्याधेस्तत्वपरिज्ञानम् वेदनायाश्च निग्रहः । एतत् वैद्यस्य वैद्यत्वम् ।

The same message is conveyed by Charaka in the above sutra. The vaidya is the right person eligible for acquiring knowledge and the body, medicines etc. are subjects of his knowledge. If there is nobody to acquire knowledge, there will be no subject of knowledge and if no subject of knowledge exists, the question does not arise of anybody acquiring it.

"Vibration" - most important concept

Ayurveda attributes the action of any dravya to its rasa, veerya, guna, vipak and prabhav. Any of the above may be responsible for generating the action of the dravya. But there is another substance which augments the rasa, veerya etc. and is necessary for generating the desired effect of the dravya; this substance is the "vibration" (praspand). The contact of a dravya with the body or the senses produces some vibrations and thereby the dravya has its action on the body. But sometimes even the sight or memory of a dravya may create its vibrations on the body. These vibrations may show different actions on the body depending upon their intensity, speed and site of action in the body. If the sight of a dravya can cause vibrations, then it is but natural that a direct contact of the dravya will definitely produce vibrations. Various effects produced on the body and mouth as a result of contact of madhur rasa with the tongue, are in fact, due to the vibrartions produced by the gunas of the dravya. The dravya still lies in the mouth, it has not been assimilated in the body, yet on contact with the tongue (which has predominance of aap mahabhoota) various vibrations are generated depending upon different potencies of the dravya. As an outcome, we perceive some of the qualities of the dravya. Amongst the various types of vibrations generated because of an interaction between the dravya and the body, the ones generated during the act of tasting are known as rasa. At the same time, other actions that occur on the body are due to its ordinary gunas or some other eminent gunas (ie. veerya). These vibrations arising after the digestion (pachan) of the dravya are of vipak. In foetal life, the earliest distinctly identifiable vibration is noticed at the start of the fourth month.

Vibrations in the body

Dravya, guna and karma have to be correlated with the concept of vibration. Whether a dravya is an ahar dravya (food item) eminent in rasa or a medicinal dravya eminent in veerya, the capacity to move throughout the body is possessed by vayu alone and the first and the most important attribute of vayu is vibration (throb, pulsation). प्रस्पंदनोद्वहन धारण पूरण विवेक लक्षणो वायुः । (चरक). A dravya has the capacity of producing various types of vibrations on the body. Such vibrations can be in the form of dravyagunakarma. Therefore according to satkaryavad, the dravya is able to generate such vibrations. Eventhough the body is receptive to the vibrations generated by varying stimuli like eating sugar or a chilli, these dravyas also originally possess such potency. Gunas like snigdha, sheeta, guru, pichchil etc., which are similar to kapha, or gunas like ruksha, ushna, laghu, vishada etc. which are contradictory to kapha or any other gunas, can have their respective effect on the body only with the help of vayu. Vayu alone has the ability to generate vibrations. This is what is meant by the "yogavahi" property of vayu and the apparently simple aphorism,

If one cannot identify a plant inspite of the detailed and industrious description involving many synonyms, isn't it a pity ?

पित्तं पंगु कफः पंगुः पंगवो मलधातवः । वायुना यत्र नीयन्ते ॥

also carries the same deep meaning, that is the concept of vibrations. All the states of the living beings due to health, diseases or the cure of diseases are due to these vibrations. The ability to move, which is an exclusive property of vayu, is nothing but vibrations वा - गति. This is why Charakacharya has called vayu as 'Bhagwan'. Yoga-vahi means a dravya, which in combination with another dravya, produces vibrations that carry the gunas of the combining dravya.

Vibrations – potency of dravyas

A dravya, which on consumption produces vibrations that bring about an increase in the dosha-dhatu-malas of the body, possesses the mahabhootas that are responsible for such an increase. When these dravyas are outside the body, they are considered on the basis of their panchamahabhoota content according to padarthvignyanshastra; but the same dravyas, on getting assimilated in the body, are known as dosha-dhatu-mala etc. The living body has an ability to convert these material dravyas into forms which are similar and acceptable to it. This ability is termed as 'agni'. In this way, padarthvignyanshastra and dosha-dhatu-mala vignyan are both combined in dravyagunashastra. Just as we call dosha-dhatu-mala as material substances, in the same way, the food items and medicines which produce these dosha-dhatu-malas are termed as vatakar, pittakar, kaphakar, rasakar, raktakar etc. as well as pureeshavardhak, mutral, swedal etc. Such close relation exists between the dravyas outside the body and vatadi doshas, rasadi dhatus and pureeshadi malas which are called as the basic supporters of the body. This relation has to be studied in dravyagunashastra. Like the dravyas, even the dhatus of the human body cannot generate vibrations when they become very old. This happens in old age when the 'ojas' cannot generate optimum vibrations and the face loses its glow.

Vrushyatva – a powerful vibration

As the body moves towards old age, normal vibrations start diminishing. As senility approaches, the vibrations responsible for the feminine appearance in women start diminishing and men start losing their vrushyatva gradually. Vrushyatva (potency) is also a powerful vibration. It is at its peak in youth and gradually diminishes under the influence of ageing and the man becomes 'harmless'. Numerous vibrations are generated in the living body at every moment. This is the real meaning of 'Kshanbhangi Bhava Siddhant'. The causes of diseases will produce abnormal vibrations and inhibit normal vibrations. In health, these normal vibrations are generated continuously. What else is done in treatment? In this body, which is always changing, we use various drayvas, which, by virtue of their gunas, produce new normal vibrations. Once these normal vibirations are generated, the disease is prevented. Abnormal vibrations aggravate the disease.

Hot and cold vibrations as therapy

These vibrations are the cause of various signs and symptoms manifesting themselves in the body and the mind. We have to generate vibrations while treating diseases. Every symptom is always related to some vibration. A thorough understanding of the symptoms invariably involves complete knowledge of associated vibrations. The action attributed to gunas while describing them are also established by their respective vibrations. In agnimandya, the vibrations of 'deepana' are absent whereas in 'bhasmak', these vibrations are generated in excess. The clue to the treatment of bhasmak by medicines and food items lies in these vibrations. Vibrations are special forces. The normal and abnormal actions of dosha-dhatu-malas are their vibrations. The gunas of all dravyas have a potency to generate vibrations. A few gunas possess higher potency to generate vibrations than others. These are called 'veerya'. A few possess even higher potencies. These are called 'prabhav'. The action may be accomplished by rasa, veerya, guna, vipak or prabhav but the real potency lies with these vibrations. As the human body becomes older, the capacity of its components to generate vibrations diminishes. [The description given by Kenneth Walker in his book 'Commentary on Age' becomes more clear by the concept of vibrations. His definition of old age is linked with vibrations.]

Independent existence of gunas

One more aspect of the vibrations that must be kept in mind is that these vibrations are positive forces and not negative. It is true that ten pairs of antagonist gunas have been mentioned. It is also true that these gunas have opposite actions but each one of these gunas enjoys a positive existence. 'Ruksha' guna does not imply an absence of 'snigdha' guna. On the contrary, ruksha is a padarth having an independent existence. This is 'satkaryavad'. Satkaryavad believes in positive existence and therefore Ayurveda has categorically ruled out 'abhava' padarth.

Its easy acceptability

Only a living body - one with a life force - can act as a medium of generating vibrations. This life force itself means vibrations. What type of vibrations need to be generated on the body that possesses life force and what dravyas must be used to do so is a subject of dravyagunashastra. During the summer season, due to the scorching heat, exhaustion, excessive sweating and other contributing factors, the sheeta guna in the body is proportionately reduced and ushna, ruksha gunas increase in the same amount. As a result, the naturally occurring soothing effect of sheeta guna decreases and thirst increases. In short, ushna vibrations are generated. In such a condition if a drink that is mildly sour and sufficiently cool is consumed then the ushna vibrations are replaced by sheeta vibrations and the body is rejuvenated. On the other hand, during the winter season, when parts of the body feel heavy and stiff, it is natural that one feels like taking strong drinks like alcoholic beverages. Once taken, the ushna vibrations produced replace the sheeta vibrations. Here also, the body is rejuvenated and the mind is pleased. According to the satkaryavad, in this body with life force, all the antagonist vibrations are continuously generated. It may be compared to a car which has been mounted on a jack. We have to decide whether to further elevate it or bring it down. Here, the example of antagonist vibrations generated by somal and mauktik may be cited. Whether a medicine is swedal, sara or hridayottejak, the concept of vibrations applies everywhere. In the experiment by Pavlov, what else is done other than generating vibrations?

Because of Rauwolfia serpentina, the industrialists became rich, but how did it benefit the science of Ayurveda?

Why Ayurveda has not accepted abhava?

The abhava padarth mentioned in the Vaisheshik darshan is totally dependent on bhava padarth for its identity. It has no individual status. It is always considered in reference to bhava padarth. Since it does not have any individual existence, Ayurveda has totally abstained from using abhava in its philosophy, and deals totally with bhava padarth only.

जायन्ते हेतुवैषम्यात् विषमाः देहधातवः । हेतुसाम्यात् समाः (जायन्ते) ।

In this aphorism the word जायन्ते points towards bhava padarth.

Abhava does not find place even in the aphorism सर्वदा सर्वभावानां...... Abhava is not mentioned in the Samanya–Vishesha Siddhant. The aphorisms प्रवृत्तिरूभयस्यतु and भूयसाऽल्पं हि जीयते also deal with bhava padarth only. No padarth is destroyed in this universe; it can only undergo a change in its appearance or be replaced by another padarth. A reduction in sheeta guna means that ushna guna is existent there. Thus bhava padarth is the basis of all Ayurvedic terminology. The principle of kshanbhangi bhava also emphasizes the phenomenon of replacement.

न ते तत्सदृशास्त्वन्ये पारंपर्यसमुत्थिताः । चरक शा १/४६.

The above aphorism by Charaka is also indicative of bhava padarth. Thus, to say that a particular vibration is absent in the body would be a mistake. In fact, one type of vibration is replaced by another antagonist vibration. In 'atisara' the 'sara' vibrations are expected to be replaced by 'grahi' vibrations. Our job is to bring about this change.

The plea of universe in man

The human body is a replica of the vast external universe. As in the universe so in this body composed of dosha – dhatu – malas. We have mentioned earlier that all that exists in the body also exists in the universe. The universe has given this body to atma (life force) for use on a 'loan'. The duration of every individual loan is different and nobody knows it. Once the duration is over, the body immediately moves towards unification with the universal panchamahabhootas.

पंचाभिभूतास्त्वथ पंचकृत्वः पंचेंद्रियपंचसु भावयन्ति । पंचेंद्रियं पंचसु भावयित्वा ।
पंचत्वमायान्ति विनाशकाले ॥ सु.शा. अ. 1/11

These panchamahabhootas may be known differently in padarthvignyanshastra; but once they assume the form of dosha – dhatu – malas, Ayurveda has its own individual outlook towards them. Yet their association with their universal parent components cannot be denied. Every body contains elements that represent the outside universe in it. The effects of diet and medicine generated within the body are indeed produced with the help of and in accordance with these representative elements of the universe. It is as if every element of the universe is advocating its use within the body. This plea takes care of the well being of the body. Those components which are present within the body may be instrumental in maintaining the equilibrium and well being of the body, but those are also controlled by the universal components. Therefore an alteration in the universal components

Manufacturing phyto-medicines is very costly due to the import of the plants. Why don't we cultivate these plants in India? Or why won't they grow here?

causes a corresponding change in the body components. When the body component (representative of the universal component) becomes ineffective, the universal component also fails to influence the body. The reason for any medicine not being effective is the absence of this representative force. The part of the body that loses its potency ie. its antagonist force is predominant, does not have any role to play in the functioning of the body. According to the sutra असद्करणात्......, no medicine is useful on these parts because no action can be obtained from padarth which has no existence. The disease becomes incurable. The universal components can influence the body only if their representatives in the body are operational and not otherwise. If a medicine does not yield the desired effect then it does not mean that it lacks guna – karmas. The guna-karmas are present but the targeted organs of the body have lost their ability to assimilate in them the potency provided by the medicine.

Treatment – not punishment but education

As our diet is 'rasapradhan' (predominant in rasa), it takes time for the effects of diet to be seen on the body. Medicines have quicker action on the body as they are veeryapradhan. Their vibrations are quicker in action. Our body is habituated to rasapradhan diet but not to veeryapradhan medicines; hence medicines act quickly; but even a medicine will not have adequate action once the body gets used to it. Single drugs are also less effective when administered for more than seven days. Maximum effect is obtained in the first few days of administration. Some medicines need to be given only once. Others have a limit of seven days. This limit must have been given keeping in mind the seven dhatus of the body. Rasayanas may be given for 15 days, a few for a month, others for six months while some have to be given for a year. More the grave nature or seriousness of the disease, greater is the time required to treat it. The diseases of antarmarg, bahirmarg and madhyamarg progressively take longer time to improve. The purpose behind administering medicines for a full year is to take care of the harmful effects of changing seasons and keep the body functions perfectly fit. Few medicines (in chronic diseases) are required for a life-time. Hence, the question arises whether this practice, if at all, can be called as treatment. Treatment is a process in which the capacity of maintaining equilibrium is generated within the body components. In a way, an administrator and treatment are similar. An administrator puts everything in order and creates a favourable environment and then the subordinates have to take up the work. The administrator cannot be always present. Same is the case with medicines. Through treatment, the body components have to be taught to remain in equilibrium.

The recipient has to be sound

Radio waves are transmitted in all directions but if the recipient instrument is not intact then no sound is heard. The universal components also have their effect on the body in a similar manner. The human body is a replica of the universe and all the known and unknown components have to be represented in this body. One cannot even imagine the minuteness of these representative components. We must try and assess the subtlety or minuteness of the dravyas so that they may have their effect on the representative components.

A life-saving weapon or science, if handled by a wrong person, can be deadly. Therefore medical sceince must be in the hands of worthy and trained persons.

Rasayanas for training

Treatment must be instituted for training and not for punishing these constituents. There is nothing wrong in saying that treatment is a training to the body constituents. Therefore, treatment must be given to the patients till the training of these components is completed. The diseases in which this training is quickly and easily completed are called 'sukhasadhya' diseases. Those diseases in which it is completed but with difficulty are 'kashtasadhya'. 'Yapya' diseases are those which show improvement only during the period in which this training is given and the diseases which do not show any improvement at all are called 'anupkramya' (asadhya). It is mandatory to consider this concept of 'training' while selecting a dravya for any disease.

Rasayana dravyas are specially meant for this training. Toxic dravyas have opposite action.

Concept of 'dhatubala' in pathogenesis

While treating any disease, the samprapti has to be taken into consideration.

आहारश्च विहारश्च यत् स्यात् दोषगुणै: सम: ।
धातुभिर्विगुणो यश्च स्त्रोतसां सप्रदूषक: ।। वा. शा. अ. 3/44

The above sutra indicates the causes of diseases. Avoiding the causes of disease is, of course, the first in treatment but the medicine which is instituted as treatment should not only reduce the vitiating power of the doshas but also increase the dhatubala (धातुबल).

This is so because dhatus have to perform the function of maintaining a balance between the doshas. If the dhatus are strong, the doshas would not be able to produce any deformity no matter what is the extent of vitiation of doshas. Hence, the dravya used for treatment of diseases must be such that it reduces the vitiating capacity of doshas and brings about an equivalent increase in dhatubala. A regimen of treatment that reduces dhatubala along with doshas cannot be considered ideal. A reduction in dhatubala necessarily means a condition favourable for the onset of disease. Treatment is done for achieving health and health depends on the strength (bala) of dhatus; hence the regimen of treatment must be so constituted that it increases the bala of all those dhatus which are involved in the samprapti. After treating every disease, the treatment regimen ends with a rasayana. In spite of all precautions, every medicine leaves its impact on the body and to compensate this effect, rasayana and rich nutritious food are necessary.

Decrease in vitiation of doshas and enhancement of dhatubala

While using various dravyas in diseases as well as in health, one more concept must be considered. The concept of strength of the doshas and dhatus in the affected part of the body is important. The real objective behind reducing the vitiating power of the doshas is to increase the dhatubala of the dhatus in which these doshas are situated by using various dravyas. Care must be taken to see that the dhatubala is not decreased. Due to any reason, if it is reduced, then remedies must be instituted to increase the same. Increased doshabala and decreased dhatubala inevitably give rise to

No two persons are totally identical; this is confirmed by the Ayurvedic concept as explained by " पुरुषं पुरुषं वीक्ष्य " - as per each individual.

disease. Therefore, the concept of dhatubala is important. According to the kshanbhangi bhava siddhant, all dravyas continuously undergo degeneration (be it dosha, dhatu or mala). This kshanbhangi bhava siddhant applies in disease as well as in health.

The vitiating dosha, while undergoing degeneration, gives rise to similar vitiated doshas and the cycle continues. न ते तत्सद्‌ शास्त्वन्ये (च.शा 1/46). Therefore, the choice of the dravya should be such that it breaks the vicious circle and consolidates the constituents which undergo degeneration according to the kshanbhangi bhava siddhant. A dravya is expected to generate such a chain of events.

How to fill in the gaps created by bhavas

Treatment consists of abstaining from the factors that induce vitiation of doshas (अपथ्यत्याग) and adopting a diet and other factors that induce equilibrium between the doshas (पथ्यसेवन). Since Ayurveda has accepted the principle of kshanbhangi bhava siddhant, the treated substance, immediately after its origin, undergoes degeneration and in its place a new substance is generated. At every moment, this natural (or supernatural) phenomenon of degeneration of all substances takes place incessantly. This phenomenon is not under one control but progresses on its own. It indicates that this universe is not stagnant but is always in a phase of transition. The existent substance which undergoes degeneration has the capacity to generate another substance which will take its place. This is the property which has to be taken advantage of while instituting remedial medicines and diet. It is our job to create a suitable condition which would allow origin of a substance which has the desired properties and actions.

व्याधेस्तत्वपरिज्ञानम् वेदनायाश्च निग्रह: । एतत् वैद्यस्य वैद्यत्वम् ।।

This sutra indicates the same phenomenon. न वैद्य: प्रभुरायुष:।

Treatment of diseases includes identification of these substances that originate incessantly and also methods to bring about desired change in them. It is to accomplish this goal that Ayurveda has included the concept of six padarthas viz. samanya, vishesha, guna, dravya, karma and samavaya. The concept of these six padarthas is sufficient for achieving a deep insight into identification and modification of the bhava padarth.

Concept of proportionate representation of gunas in a dravya

Although the twenty gunas explained in dravyagunashastra are primarily important, it is also necessary to take into account the proportionate presence of each of these gunas in the dravya. If two different dravyas are described as 'ushna' because of their 'ushna guna', it must be kept in mind that both these dravyas may be ushna in a varying proportion. Before using any dravya, a thorough estimation of its gunas is necessary because once a highly potent medicine (वीर्यवान औषधी) has been used, a low potency medicine may not have the desired effect. Therefore it is advisable to start with a low potency medicine and then proceed to high potency medicines if the low potency medicines are ineffective. If poisons are used frequently in medicines for their higher efficacy, then simple drugs

Considering the animal body as a laboratory, urine is its product which alleviates kapha, facilitates passage of vata and removes excess pitta. What a fine product it is!

are found to be ineffective. Hence proper estimation of the gunas is very important. Nevertheless, every regimen of treatment is terminated by tapering off the potency of medicines and the total charge is handed over to the strength of the body organs (bala). The treatment has to be ended by gradually decreasing the use of medicines and simultaneously increasing the use of diet. Hence while studying dravyagunashastra, the proportionate existence of various gunas in the dravya must also be considered. Sometimes dravyas having contradictory gunas have to be used alternately. This has to be done in diseases like kshayaj kasa. A single medicine given for a longer time may not be tolerated or the body may get used to it. While instituting a regimen of basti, anuvasan and asthapan basti are alternately given in yoga, kala and karmabasti and finally anuvasan basti is given for imparting strength (bala) to the body. Similarly, at the end of every regime of treatment 'balya' medicine and balya diet is necessary because teekshna dravya and visha dravya (poisonous dravyas) have a destructive effect on the constituents of the body.

Why are medicinal dravyas bitter ?

Every person, generally, hesitates to take bitter medicines. Medicines which are sweet, sour or salty are comparatively fewer. The sutras describe and emphasize the role of all the six rasas in maintenance of health. Noncompliance to the principles mentioned in these sutras may result in diseases (रसनिमित्तजा: रोगा:). Generally, people instinctively consume sweet-sour diets due to their pleasant taste. Bitter foods, due to their unpleasant tastes, generally do not find a place in our regular diet. (तिक्त: स्वयमरोचिष्णु: १ वा. सू.). Overindulgence in sweet–sour diets (मधुर रसात्मक आहार) and lesser consumption of bitter food leads to a particular group of diseases which can be controlled only by restricting sweet–sour diets and judicious use of bitter diets. A diet comprising of sweet–sour objects is prominant in rasa whereas bitter dravyas are prominant in veerya (veeryapradhan). There is no doubt that bitter and astringent dravyas have to be used in diseases caused by overnourishment (संतर्पणोत्थ). Without this, the overnourishment cannot be counteracted. But even in diseases caused by undernourishment, where sweet-sour dravyas are absolutely indicated, these must be given only after proper conditioning by bitter-astringent (तिक्त–कषाय) dravyas. Therfore, in dravyagunashastra, the bitter and astringent rasas of dravyas are given preference. Apart from this, tikta rasa (bitter) consolidates and provides strength to amashaya which is the main part of mahasrotas. Also, all medicines for rasa dhatu are bitter to taste. Only tikta rasa is amashayagami (acting on amashaya), balya (increasing the strength), laghu (easily digested) and rasadhatugami. Because of these qualities, tikta rasa is most effective in jvara.

Rasas of dravyas and concept of teja samyoga

Rasa is an important means of ascertaining the properties and actions of any medicinal herb. Once the rasa of a dravya is known, its veerya and vipak are automatically decided. However, there are exceptions to this rule. Dravyagunashastra not only involves a study of the doshas, properties, vipak, veerya etc. of the dravyas which invariably accompany the rasa, but it also primarily involves a knowledge of these exceptions. Thus the verdict given by Charakacharya that तस्मात् रसोपदेशेन न सर्वं द्रव्यम् आदिशेत । seems important. I may cite few examples. The fruit of temburni is kashaya but is laghu. A herb called 'hed' is pittasarak (enhances the secretion of pitta) but also stambhak (astringent). The

An Ayurvedic professional must introspect and cognize all the limitations. Only then he gets success.

fruits of hijjal are purgative and emetic but its leaves are grahi (prevent the loss of body fluids). The vipak of madayantika (Lawsonia inermis) is katu but it is sheeta veerya. Generally, shodhan dravyas are effective in worms, but a herb called 'sapsan' is effective on worms eventhough it is grahi; such exceptions are bound to occur. This is so, because eventhough the rasa is the main approach determining the properties of a dravya, the continuous transition occurring at every moment in every dravya results in an alteration in the properties of dravyas. The dravya may not necessarily always remain as an aggregation of the same mahabhootas in the same proportion which was originally responsible for its rasa. The comparative proportions of mahabhootas change continuously and the properties and actions of the dravya within the body may also change due to changes occurring in its mahabhoota composition. This change in the properties and eventually a change in the action is brought about by the action of 'agni'. The above principle is authentic. The properties of the dravya may change as and when it is acted upon by a dissimilar teja mahabhoota. If a similar teja majabhoota can cause a change in the dravya, then there can be no doubt that a dissimilar teja mahabhoota will also create a change. The contact of the dravya with teja mahabhoota which leads to this change is a result of the action of agni. The contact with agni or teja mahabhoota is similar if the properties of the dravya like its odour remain unchanged. If these properties show a change then it implies that the agni or teja mahabhoota was dissimilar. If a mango changes from green to yellow then the teja mahabhoota is dissimilar and if it remains green (even after ripening) then it indicates contact with similar teja mahabhoota. Every dravya that is consumed by the body continuously comes in contact with teja mahabhoota.

Signs and symptoms of diseases and actions of dravyas

The gunas mentioned in dravyagunakarmavignyan shastra are present in the constituents of the body as well. Since the same gunas are present in vatadi doshas, rasadi dhatus and pureeshadi malas and since these carry the same meaning in dosha-dhatu-mala vignyan and dravyagunavignyan, it is easier to make a comprehensive study of both. It is necessary to have uniform definitions in order to apply the samanya-vishesha principle. What are known as signs and symptoms in dosha-dhatu-mala vignyan are in fact the actions generated by the gunas of dosha-dhatu-malas at various sites. These actions are indicative of the useful and harmful properties of dravyas. The symptoms or the actions attributed to the doshas actually do not belong to the doshas but to the gunas present in the doshas. Similarly, the actions of the dravyas may be described as though these belong to the dravyas but these too are brought about by the gunas of the dravya and not otherwise. From the signs and symptoms, one can identify the properties of doshas just as we identify the properties of dravyas from their actions. After all, signs and symptoms are actions of diet and lifestyle and the actions of dravyas are the signs (manifestations) of that particular dravya. The actions are instrumental in identification of dravyas. This implies that the actions are signs of dravyas. In the treatment of diseases, we are meant to use the gunas which are capable of suitably altering the gunas that gave rise to the manifestations of doshas. The signs and symptoms of diseases are due to gunas. The actions of dravyas are also due to gunas.

Long time back near the Himalayas, Vaidyas gathered together at specific time, travelling distances of 2-3 thousand miles. What were their means to communicate?

Mahabhautik actions of dravyas

While dealing with dravyas, it is necessary to comprehend the prominence of various mahabhootas. The dravyas are said to be of a particular mahabhoota depending on which mahabhoota is present in maximum proportion according to the व्यपदेशस्तु भूयसा principle. This mahabhootatva (prominence of a mahabhoota) of dravya must be considered in treatment. When vivek (discrimination/isolation), saukshmya (subtleness) and laghav (lightness) are needed, akasheeya dravyas can be used. The dravyas which clear the blockage of srotas or dilate them are akasheeya. Raukshya (dryness), preran, dhatuvyaham (proper arrangement of the dhatu) are increased by vayaveeya dravyas. The taijas dravyas produce pachan (digestion) and aushnya (warmth). For generating shaitya (cold), mardav (softness), sneha (oiliness) and kleda (sliminess), aapya dravyas may be used. Parthiv dravyas can be used when gaurav (heaviness) and sthairya (firmness) are desired. One more thought that originates from this concept is that a child who has some disorder of mansa, rakta, majja, heart, umbilicus (nabhi), liver, spleen, intestines or anus and who is dependant on the mothers' breast milk, may be treated by giving medicines to the mother. This will prove more effective because the above mentioned parts are 'matruja' (resembling the mothers' body in their costitution). Sushruta, in his garbhayakshya, has mentioned mahabhootas which are responsible for producing various colours. For example, prominence of aap-dhatu results in white colour of the dravyas; whereas prithvi mahabhoota is needed in excess for producing black colour. A bluish-black colour is obtained by dravyas in which prithvi-akash mahabhootas are predominant and a greyish colour is obtained by dravyas predominant in aap-akash mahabhootas. Thus, excepting a few, in almost all cases it is possible to determine the predominance of mahabhootas and hence the qualities and gamitva of that dravya just by having a look at the colour. Earlier, there was a belief that the dravyas having the shape of heart are useful in heart disease and red coloured dravyas are useful in diseases of blood since blood is also red in colour. (Patient and Doctors – Kenneth Walker, 1957 page 17.)

Specific dravyas for doshas and diseases

In dravyagunashastra, the words 'doshanashak', 'dhatuvardhak' etc. are frequently used. These have to be understood in the correct perspective. No disease is produced without the vitiation of srotas. A diet and life style which is similar to doshas and at the same time having properties which are opposite to that of dhatus is the main cause of vitiation of srotas. This simply means that the dravyas which increase the 'doshabala' and simultaneously decrease the dhatubala will give rise to diseases. Similar diet and lifestyle will also produce diseases. If one observes carefully the sutras relating to the above concept, it would be clear that along with increase in doshabala, a decrease in dhatubala is absolutely necessary for the genesis of disease. If the dhatubala is intact, no disease can occur. If the support (dhatu) is unvitiated then what can the dependent vitiator (dosha) do? This is the difference between the general factors causing 'doshavardhan' and those causing 'rogotpatti' and hence the dravyas to be used in these conditions also differ. This is the point of differentiation between dosha-specific and disease-specific dravyas. The treatment of every disease must include dravyas which reduce the doshabala of vitiating doshas and at the same time increase the dhatubala of the dhatus involved in the samprapti. The treatment of all diseases must also conclude with a rasayana and it must be particularly effective on the dhatus involved in the samprapti. The rasayanas are helpful in 'रोगाणां अपुनर्भव (preventing the recurrence of diseases).

Suitable treatment for various symptoms

One more line of thought may be presented while pondering on the actions of dravyas. For example, if a dravya is described as kushthaghna (eliminating skin diseases) and keshavardhak (improving hair growth), it can be postulated that this dravya would be majjagami since keshavardhan is the function of majja dhatu. Therefore it naturally follows that this dravya would be more useful in majjagat kushtha. Similarly, if a dravya is described as medhya (improving the functions of the brain) and keshya, it should be understood that it will also be majjagami. A person having the 'sara' (optimally conditioned dhatu) of a dhatu will not easily contract diseases of that particular dhatu. When a particular dravya has been described as effective in one or more diseases and has also been called a 'rasayana', it is more logical to think that the dravya would be more useful in those diseases as a rasayana. For example, if it is mentioned that a particular herb is medhya and also rasayana then it should be understood that its rasayana property would be more pronounced on the brain. Generally, it has been observed that vrushya dravyas (improving the reproductive power) have madhur vipak. Of course, there are exceptions to this, but these are very few. Another important aspect of gamitva is that the dravyas possessing gamitva on distant dhatus are more potent than those possessing gamitva on proximal dhatus ie. a dravya which is shukragami is more potent than the one which is rasagami. This is so because these dravyas are able to retain their dhatugamitva even after the effects of the agni of all the preceding dhatus!

Dravyas undergo change at every moment due to action of body

Be it diet or medicine, as long as it does not come in contact with the body, it cannot have any effect on it. Nevertheless, when the dravya establishes contact with the live body (body with life force), it starts having its effects. The effect is generated even at the sight of the dravya. What more, even the noise of cups and saucers generates special vibrations in those who are addicted to tea. (Even the tingling sound of bangles produces immense sexual urge in some. Vibrations, of course, are instrumental in it.) The properties and actions of dravyas should be considered in the context of the changes that occur in the body after the dravya has come in contact with it. There is a big difference in the haritaki kept in a bottle, haritaki kept in the hand and haritaki kept in the mouth. When it comes in contact with the body, its action starts. Haritaki starts producing vibrations the moment it is kept in the mouth. The haritaki undergoes changes due to mixing with bodhak kapha (the kapha present in mouth which helps in the perception of taste). The rasa will also have properties corresponding to haritaki mixed with bodhak kapha. Further, the actions of haritaki will depend on the series of changes that it undergoes within the body. The haritaki that reaches the stomach would be different from the one that was present in the mouth. The form of haritaki keeps on changing as it reaches successive dhatus. The action of haritaki on rakta dhatu, mansa dhatu or for that matter any other dhatu would actually be the action of haritaki that has continuously undergone changes in the process of reaching that particular dhatu. Haritaki, as seen outside the body, is just instrumental in this action.

Man is a part of the universe. But for any part of the universe to get assimilated in man, the help of agni is very essential.

The use of single dravya

When we talk of a single dravya, the concept that is visualized is that of a dravya which is not in contact, combination or in mixture with any other dravya. 'Punarnava' as a single dravya means 'punarnava' alone which is not combined with anything else. This approach is correct from the point of view of practical considerations but the dravyas which we call 'single dravyas' are also an aggregation of constantly changing panchamahabhootas. Freshly grown punarnava and a fully grown punarnava can never be the same. There is a vast difference between a man in his childhood and the same man in his senility. The same rule applies here as well. Unripe 'kapittha' and ripe 'kapittha' are one and the same fruit but the properties differ greatly. Similar difference of properties is observed in 'bala moolak' (unripe radish) and 'pakva moolak' (mature radish) as well as in wet pippali and dry pippali (सा शुष्का विपरीता).

Extending the same logic, we can say that it would not be correct to randomly uproot a medicinal herb and store it in any season. During the rainy season, a medicinal herb may yield a larger quantity of juice but it would never be comparable to the properties of the juice obtained from the full grown herb with all its potency. The juice obtained from 'tridhari nivdunga' at the end of shishir ritu is far more enriched in its properties and actions than that obtained in any other ritu. The same statement, with minor alterations, can be applied to all plants.

Sanskar – basis of medication

Natural influences bring about a change in the properties and actions of dravyas. These changes have been successfully exploited. Similarly, desired changes may be produced in the dravya or herbs by sanskar (proper conditioning). This concept has given rise to panchavidh kashaya kalpana as also siddha sneha kalpana [panchvidh kashaya kalpana includes preparations like kalka (pulp), rasa (juice), shrut (decoction) sheeta (water in which the dravya has been kept overnight - cold infusion) and fant (boiling water in which the dravya is kept for some time - hot infusion)]. Siddha sneha kalpana is a preparation in which dravyas are boiled with ghee or oil. The ideas of samyoga, bhavana and anupan have arisen from this basic concept. [Samyoga is combination, bhavana–is a process in which a medicine is impregnated with the juice or decoction of another dravya so that its properties and actions also add to the medicine. The idea is to make the bhavana dravya reach the minutest particle of the medicine. Anupan is a dravya that has to be taken along with the main medicine as it catalyses the actions of the medicine]. It will not be an exaggeration if we say that this sanskar is the basis of all medication. Sanskar involves changing of properties of the medicinal dravya. A particular desired property, which was originally absent in the dravya, may be induced in that dravya and an undesired property may be deleted by instituting proper sanskar. Numerous preparations of medicines have been formulated on this basis.

Nevertheless, there remains a tremendous scope for using single drugs (herbs) which have been naturally imbued by various properties and actions. These herbs may be naturally single but even then these possess their own different guna, karma, veerya, vipak, prabhav, dushya gamitva and also efficacy on a particular disease. By virtue of these, the herbs can increase or decrease the

One cannot generalise the quantum of food required by all. It is relative to every man. Similarly the dose of medicine also must be decided to suit each patient.

properties of particular doshas situated in particular dhatus. There are herbs which have either restorative (rasayana) or depletive (apatarpan) actions on single doshas or dhatus.

Safe treatment necessary

Charaka, Sushruta, Vagbhatta and even more recent scholars have endorsed the use of single herbs or dravyas in their respective scriptures. वृष: सद्यो जयत्यस्त्रं - adulsa in a raktapitta; सर्वेषु श्वासकासेषु केवलं वा बिभीतकम् - bibheetaka in all respiratory disorders; मधुमेहित्वम् आपन्न: .... शिलाजतुतुलां अद्यात् - shilajatu in madhumeha; these and many other scattered examples indicating the use of single dravya may be cited. As if Vagbhatta, not satisfied with the number of uses he had indicated of these single dravyas or may be to summarize his vast book on chikitsa or perhaps to lay more emphasis on these single dravyas, has repeated the use of single dravyas in the last chapter of Uttartantra under the topic मुस्तापर्पटकं ज्वरे .... While doing so, he has even disregarded the criticism of being repetitive.

These medicines have been prescribed in such a way that once a preliminary diagonsis is made, then the appropriate dravya can be given to the patient without any possibility of harming the patient. These dravyas will only benefit the patient. Many of these herbs have a marked resemblence to the human body and each of these are specific for some disease. We may not have the time to study the complete science of vaidyak but Vagbhatta suggests that one may resort to the use of these simple herbs as the treatment without causing any harm to the patient.

Complete treatment

While treating diseases, sometimes a situation arises where there is little scope for improvement and yet, the treatment has to be continued. In such a situation care must be taken that the treatment does not create any adverse effect. For this, Vagbhatta has indicated many simple and harmless remedies in his Uttartantra. These include herbs, minerals and even animal products. Few are single dravyas while others are combinations. Nevertheless, it would be noticed that his combinations also do not have more than three dravyas. Many food items have also been indicated in the list of these medicines. These medicines have not only been used for oral administration but the same medicine can also be used for nasal administration, enema etc. This chapter contains remedies for diseases of people of all age groups and all types of diseases. The remedies have been selected in such a way that various formulations and combinations can be used. Even blood letting (asra-visruti) has been mentioned.

Various parts of the plants like gums, resins, juice, bark, roots, fruits, flowers, stem etc. have been described as medicine in this chapter. It contains procedures like basti (enema), virechan (purgation) and vaman (emesis) which are principally used for shodhan (removal of vitiated doshas from the body) and shaman dravyas (dravyas used for bringing about equality among the vitiated doshas) like oil, ghee and honey. Similarly, the list contains medicines which are kopan (induce vitiation of doshas), shaman and swasthahita (having a restorative effect). Along with the dravyas that show their effects immediately, it also contains dravyas which are rasayanas that take a longer time to have their effect on the body but create a long lasting effect. All the twenty gunas and six rasas mentioned in

The authorities, while writing the science of dravyagunashastra, simultaneously thought of dravya, guna, karma in the human body.

Ayurveda have been represented in these medicines. Various medicines useful in the morning, afternoon and evening and in the early, mid and late portions of the night have been mentioned. Also, various medicines useful in various seasons have been described. This chapter not only contains a list of medicines that act as a cure for diseases but also other medicines which prevent diseases by increasing the disease resistance capacity of the body and the mind. It also deals with various medicines that act on the mind along with those acting on the body.

Vagbhatta more inclined towards use of single dravya

The herbs which have been mentioned as the remedies of various diseases are in fact used as the basic drugs for their respective diseases and various formulations are made from these herbs. Approximately 55 diseases or conditions have been mentioned in this chapter. Among these, Vagbhatta has recommended the use of single herb or single remedy in 42 diseases or disease conditions. This is a clear indication that Vagbhatta was naturally inclined towards the use of single dravyas.

Perhaps, the main hypothesis of Vagbhatta must have been that the single herbs are capable of reaching the root cause lying in the srotas of the doshas and dhatus involved and rectifying the malfunction. Thus, a formulation prepared from the combination of various herbs may be used only on a selected few conditions.

अक्केचेन्मधु विन्देत किमर्थं पर्वतं व्रजेत् ?

In a complex situation of dosha dushya sammoorchhana, various combinations, conditionings and formulations are necessary. But if the dosha dushya sammoorchhana is simple then even the single dravya is capable of eliminating this sammoorchhana, reducing the doshabala, consolidating the organs of the body, regulating the functions of the srotas of the involved dosha-dushya and even has the ability to prevent reccurrence of the disease. Such confidence is generated by using these single herbs in practice.

Equation of remedies with diseases

The elaborate and concrete philosophy of Ayurveda involved in the use of these simple and harmless dravyas would be clear after considering the following examples. For any type of vomiting (emesis), ruksha lahi, laghu lahi and sheeta lahi (preparations useful in vomiting and diarrhoea) are indicated for reducing the inflammation of the stomach and for reducing the vitiated doshas. All these and others are simple dietary remedies! Shilajit in disorders of the bladder; here, the use of shilajit has been indicated only after careful deliberation. Prameha is one of the main diseases involving basti (bladder). Shilajit which is made up of various minerals, possesses gamitva on kapha dosha which is excessively fluid, on dhatus like meda, mansa etc., on mutra (which is a mala) and also on basti. By virtue of its gamitva, shilajit is capable of reaching these srotas and organs and thereby rectifying the abnormality. For this, it has to be taken as a rasayana. Vasa (adulsa) is used in raktapitta. Vasa reduces the vitiation of red coloured and fast acting pitta in the rakatavahi srotas of yakrut (liver) and lungs which develop from the froth generated by blood. Such is the efficacy of adulsa in raktapitta that it has become synonymous with raktapitta.

Ayurveda does not insist that the name of every disease must be known, but one must know Dosha-dushya-sammoorchhana.

A series of single dravyas

Because of its rasa, veerya, vipak and its amavaha srotogamitva, kutaja improves the functioning of amashaya and regulates the srotas that generate agni thereby acting as a remedy for atisara (diarrhoea) by reducing the toxicity of the faeces. On account of this property, it is universally observed that the statement made by Vagbhatta that "कुटजोऽतिसारे" holds true. In Konkan, the first and the final remedy for atisara and pravahika (some people misunderstand it as grahani) is a decoction of kutaja leaves. Iron, which has been accepted throughout the world as a remedy for anaemia, has been mentioned as a single drug by Vagbhatta. Spleen has been described as the chief and basic organ of raktavahasrotas. Vagbhatta has indicated a rasayana dravya like pippali in diseases of the spleen since pippali reaches the rakavaha srotas, optimizes the agni of rakta dhatu and reduces the excessive viscosity in the blood. By doing so, Vagbhatta has thrown open a whole new area for deliberation. Hundreds of preparations of laksha may be available for urahkshat but even if laksha alone is available there is no need to fear urahkshat. In medavrut vayu, guggulu which is also vatashamak is used since it digests meda. Bhallatak which is agnideepak (increases the agni), vibandhnashak (relieves constipation) and vatanulomak (enhances proper passage of vata) is used as a single drug for non-bleeding piles. Rasanjan which is extracted from daruharidra is used for obesity since it is medopachak, vidang for various parasites in the intestine and rectum, triphala for internal and external use in various eye diseases, guduchi which is a rasayana is used as a single drug in vatarakta which involves a vitiation of vatadosha within rakta dhatu as a result of obstruction of vata by rakta dhatu. Buttermilk is useful in grahani both as diet as well as medicine. Khadeer, which does not itself undergo putrefaction and at the same time also prevents putrefaction for kushtha, old ghee (10 years old) for mania, brahmi for epilespsy, buffalo's milk for insomnia, shreekhand for corryza, meat for debility, garlic for vata, gokshur for mutrakruchra,' roots of kantakari for cough, pushkarmoola for parshvashoola, amalaki for maintaining youth, honey for kapha, ghee for pitta and oil for vata. All these dravyas have been described as highly effective even when used as single drugs. This concluding chapter enumerates in a nutshell all the principles of Ayurveda. From this it would be clear that Vagbhatta was more inclined towards the use of single drugs.

Study of 25th chapter of Sutra sthana of Charaka samhita inevitable

It would be incorrect to say that the use of single drugs was a novel idea of Vagbhatta alone. Vagbhatta will never overrule Charakacharya either in ideology or in practice. Charaka, in the 25th chapter of Sutra sthan named यज्जः पुरूषीय अध्याय has emphasized the use of a single drug or diet by using the word प्रकृत्यैव. Charaka has given a long list which includes 152 single remedies from अन्नं वृत्तिकराणां श्रेष्ठम् to सर्वसन्यासः सुखानाम् । In this list also single food items, single medicinal dravyas and single procedures have been given more importance. Whether it is medicine or food, once we try to bring about a change in its gunas by way of sanskar (conditioning) or samyoga (combination), it is not easy to pin-point the exact change that takes place. Because मुनिरेव विजानाति द्रव्यसंयोगजम् फलम्।। Therefore, as long as a dravya is single, without any combination, ordinary human intellect can comprehend its properties and exploit them accordingly. Charaka – Vagbhatta have also recommended the use of single dravya as far as possible. We can evolve an effective treatment through this

A student of Charaka samhita should be true to the basic philosophy of Ayurveda. But he should also be ready to accept changes necessitated by scientific insights.

provided we make a sincere effort in this direction.

An addition to our experience

In Ayurveda, certain dravyas are administered in such a way that their dose is increased every day in a fixed amount until the whole body becomes influenced by its guna-karma. Pippali, nagbala, brahmi, yastimadhu, sunthi, bhallatak and garlic are a few dravyas which are used in this way.

Every medicinal plant has certain properties which are responsible for generating various actions. If it is required to increase the potency of this medicinal plant then certain fertilizers and atmospheric conditions can be provided to the plant which will enhance the required properties (gunas) and hence have better action.

A fine or coarse powder of herbs loses potency very quickly. If a powdered herb shows a reduction in its properties and actions after six months, then the herb is not to be blamed.

The reason why a particular herb is said to be specific for a particular disease is that it possesses a property of reversing or interrupting the dosha dushya sammorchhana ie. samprapti (sequence of events leading to the genesis of the disease).

The body is made up of vata, pitta, kapha, rasa, rakta, mansa, meda, asthi, majja, shukra and malas like pureesh, mutra and sweda. There are herbs, which by virtue of their special properties can mediate an increase or decrease in each of these. This concept is vital in dravyagunakarmashastra.

The classification of geographical terrain viz. jangal (dry, arid land), anup (wet, marshy land) and sadharan (intermediate between jangal and anup) has been done depending upon the growth of plants on these lands.

If, by using a particular part of a herb, some discomfort is produced, then it may be relieved by using some other part of the same herb. For example diarrhoea induced by consuming a mango fruit can be taken care of by the seed pulp of the same fruit.

Summary

This chapter mentions some seminal concepts on which further elaborations and deliberations have been made. Few observations have been given for further scrutiny and experimentation by experts. Let me humbly accept here that I do not staunchly and rigidly hold to my observations. All the statements that fail the test of pratyaksha (direct demonstrable evidence), anuman (logically arrived decision) and yukti (experimentation) and those that do not fall in line with the principles mentioned in the scriptures, may be changed. Shortcomings may be forgiven.

References –

1. प्रत्यक्षं हि अल्पं अनल्पम् अप्रत्यक्षम् - च. सू. अ. ११/७.

2. सर्वदा सर्वभावानां सामान्यं वृध्दिकारंणम् । -ह्रासहेतुर्विशेषश्च, प्रवृत्तिरुभयस्य तु । (च. सू.)

3. यदा तु मनसि क्लान्ते कर्मात्मान: क्लमान्वित: ।
विषयेभ्यो निर्वर्तन्ते तदा स्वपिति मानव: ॥
मेध्यानाडीमन:संयोगात् देहेंद्रियाणां सुखभोग: । सु. सू. अ. १।४.२५ (टीका).

4. अल्पस्यापि महार्थत्वं प्रभूतस्याल्पकर्मतां ।
कुर्यात् संश्लेष विश्लेष काल संस्कार युक्तिभि: । (वा. क. अ. २।६१)

CHAPTER TWO
THE CHARACTERISTICS OF DRAVYAGUNASHASTRA

Dravyagunashastra is that branch of knowledge that deals with the dravyas (drugs as well as diet) that help in the maintenance of health and alleviation of diseases in the purush (human body), which is a concomitance of panchamahabhootas and atma (the soul or the consciousness). It also deals with the properties, actions, dose, time of administration and various preparations of these dravyas.[1] Food items, like drugs, are also considered in these dravyas.

The word 'dravyaguna' may appear inapt at first sight, considering the variety of topics included in this subject. In practice, the actions of dravyas are inseparable from their properties (gunas). Since these properties are themselves responsible for generating the actions, everything like 'karma' is included in the word 'guna'.

Man has tried to make his life happier by using his intellect. For this, he made a big attempt to gain knowledge about the universe. He also tried to derive a logical conclusion about the genesis of the universe. Through this exercise he realised that he himself is a part of this universe which is made up of many visible and invisible components. Therefore all the major and minor events of the universe have an influence on the human being. Once this was realised, man first started studying the universe. For a study of the infinite phenomena existent in the universe, they have been classified on the basis of common properties. All existential phenomena were classified and a detailed and elaborate study of these was termed 'padarthvignyanshastra'. Nothing was left out from this study. All the phenomena of nature were included in it. Padarthvignyanshastra means a study of all visible and invisible creations.

This study is very elaborate, but since it provides the basic concepts required for further knowledge of dravyagunashastra and swasthavrittashastra, prior knowledge of padarthvignyanshastra is absolutely necessary. Dravyagunashastra has developed as a part of padarthvignyanshastra. Therefore the correct sequence of dealing with these two subjects is to first study padarthvignyanshastra and its principles. Once this is accomplished, then dravyagunashastra may be studied.

Dravyagunashastra is not only a useful factor for swasthya (maintenance of health) and chikitsa (treatment) but is also the chief factor involved. Thorough insight into the properties and actions of substances is necessary for treatment as well as maintenance of health. Various substances (and non-substances as well) are instrumental in vitiating health and creating disharmony in the equilibrium of body components. The use of dravyagunashastra is necessary for restoring this equilbrium.[2]

The body, the diet and the substances used as medicines have their panchamahabhoota constitution in common. If the equilibrium of these panchamahabhootas is achieved then health is maintained. If this equilibrium is disturbed then diseases are generated. Commonality between dravyas and dosha-dhatu-malas leads to an increase in dosha-dhatu-malas in the body whereas specificity

Not two particles of sand are exactly identical because when one particle occupies some space, the same cannot be occupied by the other.

leads to decrease in these. This process continues incessantly and their equilibrium or imbalance is produced. Imbalance means disease and to rectify this state, various substances (dravyas) which can restore equilibrium, have to be used.[3]

If drugs are to be used then a thorough knowledge of these is essential. Even though drugs are very useful, they can prove to be equally harmful. Therefore it is necessary for the physician to have complete knowledge of the drugs (useful and harmful effects). This has to be learnt and practised in dravyagunashastra.

Degradation due to environment, atmosphere and circumstances leads to an alteration in the normal properties of drugs and food items and results in an epidemic. Therefore a sound knowledge of appropriate and degraded drugs and food items is extremely important.[4]

The seven phenomena

For an easy knowledge of the universe, Nyayashastra has classified all the phenomena of the universe into substances, properties , actions, commonality, specificity, combination and absence. Everything present as well as absent in the universe is included in these seven phenomena. All phenomena which exhibited similarity were classified under one group and thus these seven types of phenomena were determined.

Charakacharya has strictly adhered to existential phenomena while classifying the universe. Therefore non-existential phenomena have no place in Ayurveda (this has been discussed earlier).

The seven phenomena in Ayurveda

Ayurveda, in its principles, has accepted seven phenomena viz. 1) Substance (dravya) 2) Property (guna) 3) Rasa 4) Veerya 5) Vipak 6) Prabhav and 7) Karma (actions). Every subject in Ayurveda is scrutinised in the light of these seven phenomena. These are the objects of deliberation in dravyagunashastra. These seven phenomena have been used to achieve the basic goal of Ayurveda which is to maintain health in the healthy and to reverse the disease process back to health in the sick. Therefore the definition of phenomena according to Ayurveda differs from that of other schools of philosophy. This definition of phenomena will fall within the area of dravya, guna, rasa, veerya, vipak, prabhav and karma. Their characteristics are explained in brief in the following paragraph. Details will be dealt with in subsequent chapters.

Dravya (substance)

A substance is defined as a phenomenon which acts as an abode for guna (property) and karma (action) in that guna and karma share an inseparable connection with it. In Ayurveda, the term 'dravya' applies to those phenomena which act as an abode for actions like emesis or pacification of doshas. For example, madanphala, vidang haritaki, chitraka, shatavari etc.[5]

Guna (Property)

समवायी तु निश्चेष्ट: कारणं गुण: च.स.अ. 1/51

An attribute, which is inseparable from the dravya and does not have any action of its own is

To excite a reflex or to purposefully control it - both are bad. But in the controlling of it, the energy of a man is continuously used therefore it is worse.

called guna (property). The word निश्चेष्ट: has been used in the characteristics of guna in order to differentiate it from karma (action), since karma is also inseparable from the dravya. The word 'karan' has been used while describing guna since other phenomena like commonality, specificity and combination are inseparable from the dravyas, yet they do not act as causative factor (karan) for any other phenomena (त्रयाणां अकार्यत्वं अकारणत्वंच सामान्य विशेष समवायानाते). Thus the attributes of dravyas like cold, heat, oily, dryness etc. are called as gunas (properties).[6]

Rasa (Taste) :

रस्यते आस्वाद्यते इति रस:

This is the etymology of the word 'rasa. When a substance is produced from panchamahabhootas, at that time different tastes develop in the substance depending on the proportion of panchamahabhootas. For example, sweet, sour, salty, bitter and astringent are all rasas (tastes).[7]

Vipak (Post-digestive rasa) :

Diet or drugs, both, as they get digested, undergo change. This does not mean that a food item which initially tastes sweet has an altogether different taste after digestion. Only, the sweetness of the substance would be transformed into a different type of sweetness that would be beneficial to the body. Eventhough the sweetness of the substance persists, after undergoing these conditionings, there occurs a change in the sweetness of the substance. It does not possess the same quality of sweetness as before. This occurs only after the digestion brought about by the jatharagni; this means that the initial dhatu ie. rasa dhatu becomes effective only after the action of jatharagni. Vipak is of three types viz. madhur (sweet), amla (sour) and katu (pungent). Some consider it to be of two types viz. guru (heavy) and laghu (light); but generally, vipak is considered to be madhur, amla and katu. (vipak is the taste of the substance generated after digestion). Vipak can only be predicted by logical inference, and by knowing the action on dosha-dhatu-mala.[8]

Veerya (Potency)

(वीर्यं तु क्रियते येन या क्रिया) (च.स.अ.२६/६५)

The effectiveness and potency of all gunas (properties) is known as veerya. A few acharyas believe that there are eight types of veerya viz. guru (heavy), laghu (light), snighdha (oily), ruksha (dry), hima (cold), ushna (hot), mridu (mild) and teekshna (fast acting). Yet, the accepted norm is to consider only two types of veerya ie. ushna veerya and sheeta veerya.

Eventhough, many scholars have enumerated eight types of veerya, they hardly make mention of these elsewhere in their texts. Thus, the concept of eight types of veerya lost its eminence in dravyagunashastra.[9]

Prabhav (Specific potency)

(रसादिसाम्ये यत्कर्म विशिष्टं तत् प्रभावजम्) (अ.हृ.सू.अ.१)

The innate and specific property of a dravya is known as prabhav. Prabhav cannot be described independently. This means that a specific action generated by prabhav may prove to be generated by

Plants in Ceylon (Sri lanka) are similar to the plants in India. But the Indian plants are not observed in Europe and Australia (Desha Vibhag).

it through circumstantial evidence but the exact mechanism by which prabhav brings about the action is hard to describe. A prabhav attributed to a particular dravya can be obtained only by using that particular dravya. Any other dravya with the same properties and actions will not be able to generate the same prabhav. In short, dravyas have their own exclusive prabhav.[10]

Karma (Action)

संयोगे च विभागे च कारणं द्रव्यमाश्रितम् ।
कर्तव्यस्य क्रिया कर्म नान्यद् अपेक्षते ॥

The changes brought about by the dravyas through their rasa, gunas etc. within the body are known as karma (action). For example, panchakarma, langhan, bruhan etc.[11]

All these have been described in detail in the following chapters.

Characteristics of dravya

यत्राक्षिता: कर्मगुणा: कारणं समवयि यत् तत् द्रव्यम्।।

A phenomenon which is an abode for gunas (properties) and karmas (actions) ie. gunas and karmas depend on it and which shares an inseparable concommitance with its causative substances and guna-karmas is called dravya (च.स.अ. १). This definition includes the entire spectrum of dravyas. It is complete and precise and is devoid of superimposition, under-purview and superannuation.[12]

According to this definition, prithvi, jala, teja, vayu, akash, kala, disha, atma and mana are classified as dravyas. These nine are called karan dravyas (causative substances) and the body, the diet and the medicinal substances that are produced from them and because of them are called karya dravyas (substances generated from karan dravya ie. effect). For example, items like wheat, rice etc., medicinal substances like sunthi, chitraka and amalaki are karya dravyas (produced from karan dravyas). From the above characteristics, it is clear that a wide range of substances fall within the category of dravyas. In Ayurveda, a study of only those substances is expected which have a cause and effect relationship with the panchamahabhootas. Kala, disha, atma and mana are also dravyas, yet they assume lesser significance in dravyagunashastra.

These substances have various tastes like sweet, sour, salty, pungent, bitter and astringent. They have various properties like heavy, light etc. as well as sheeta veerya and ushna veerya. Some of them also have prabhav. These substances have various actions like deepan (increasing the digestive capacity), pachan (increasing digestion) and bruhan (recuperative effect). These rasa (taste), guna (properties), veerya, vipak, prabhav, karma (actions) etc. have no independent existence without the support of dravya (substance). This is how, they have an inseparable interrelationship with each other. Only dravya has this capacity of providing abode or acting as a support for other phenomena. Other phenomena do not possess this capacity. Gunakarma etc can only become accessory causes but not the root cause like dravya.[13]

Nagarjuna has described dravya as a phenomenon which acts as a support for rasa, guna, vipak, veerya and karma.[14] One more definition of dravya is as follows :

रसोगुणास्तथा वीर्यं विपाक: शक्तिरेव च ।

What the adventurous man won't do - that cannot be said. Forests in the world are now occupying less than one-third part of the earth. (It is really a matter of major concern).

पञ्चानाय: समाहारस्तद् द्रव्यमिति कथ्यते ॥

Dravya is an aggregation of guna-karmas.[15]

Dravya in dravyagunashastra

Padarthvignyanshastra may have accepted the existence of nine dravyas viz. panchamahabhootas, kala, disha, atma and mana. As far as dravyagunashastra is concerned, Ayurveda includes only those substances which originate from panchamahabootas under the category of 'dravyas'. Kala and disha act as accessory causes for producing karya dravyas but they cannot be considered as the root cause. Atma and mana are not considered in the process of origin of karya dravyas; hence the dravyas used in dravyagunashastra are only those which have originated from the panchamahabhootas. Food and medicines are also constituted by Panchamahabhootas. Thus the word 'dravya' has a specific meaning in dravyagunashastra.

Panchamahabhoota constitution of dravyas

The karya dravyas of dravyagunashastra are constituted by panchamahabhootas. This has been explained in the earlier chapter. In this chapter, we will elaborate on the same point. The mystery of the origin of the universe has not yet been solved (and there are no signs that it will be solved); yet, the universe which is continuously in a state of transition, has evolved from some earlier state. When this process of transition started is difficult to predict even for astrophysicists. Various scientists have put forward various theories and hypotheses regarding the origin of the universe. Amongst these theories, Ayurveda has authenticated the one propagated by Sankhya philosophy.

According to this philosophy, Mahat-tatva evolves from Moola Prakruti. From this Mahat-tatva, Ahankar develops which is of three types 1) Vaikarik 2) Taijas and 3) Bhootadi. Through a combination of vaikarik and taijas ahankar, 11 indriyas (5 + 5 + 1) develop and through a combination of bhootadi and taijas ahankar, the panchatanmatra viz. akash, vayu, teja, jala and prithvi develop. Shabda, sparsh, roopa, rasa and gandha are the special properties of tanmatra. From these tanmatra, panchamahabhootas develop. Successive panchamahabhootas possess the properties of the previous mahabhootas. 8 prakruti = prakruti, mahat-tatva, ahankar + 5 tanmatra = 8.

Tanmatra

This is how, prakruti keeps on spreading its forms and ultimately leads to the formation of this universe. Further, panchamahabhootas originated from these most subtle panchatanmatras (Tat matra - meaning pure and non-dual tanmatra). Successive mahabhootas possess the properties of the earlier mahabhootas.[16] Various objects of the universe originate from these Panchamahabhootas. Therefore all substances of the universe are modifications of panchmahabhootas. (The difference between the building blocks of the universe as elicited by Sankhya and Ayurveda is discussed in the chapter titled Panchamahabhootas - an idealogical basis).

The difference as observed between various dravyas is actually due to the distinct variations in the constituents provided by the panchamahabhootas. Every substance will have a special property of each of the mahabhootas which is actually a perceptible property of a particular mahabhoota; few

It is estimated that in Maharashtra there are 150 families, 1200 genera and 3500 species of plants.

of them are actually evident while others are not so evident. Because of the variations in the proportion of panchamahabhootas, the dravyas are numerous. Their permutations and combinations are infinite and therefore the dravyas are also infinite. There are only seven basic sounds but from these basic sounds many ragas can be created. The numbers from 1 to 9 and zero can give rise to infinite numbers through various permutations and combinations. The value may change even if there is a change in the position of the numbers.

Various letters from A to Z can give rise to numerous words. Similarly, even though there are only five mahabhootas, they produce innumerable dravyas. Just as the numbers and letters give rise to infinite entities, the mahabhootas also, through various combinations give rise to infinite dravyas. Nevertheless, a dravya is considered to be of a particular mahabhoota if that mahabhoota is prominent in the constitution of that dravya.

The tanmatras cannot be perceived by our senses since they are not accompanied by perceptible guna karma. When the tanmatras evolve into mahabhootas, the gunas and karmas specific for the mahabhootas also develop in the mahabhootas thereby rendering them perceptible to the senses.

Ayurveda deals with panchamahabhootas; since the earlier evolutionary state i.e. the tanmatras fall outside the purview of perception by the senses, Ayurveda has felt it unnecessary to consider these tanmatras. The dravyas in Ayurveda are the ones which have originated from the panchamahabhootas; therefore when these tanmatras acquire perception through their association with guna-karma, the 'gunavad' of Ayurveda begins; because of this and also since Ayurveda believes in 'gunavat dravya', the concept of panchamahabhootas marks the beginning of the ideology of Ayurveda. In this way, the dravyas as referred to in Ayurveda, mean only panchamahabhootatmak dravyas. Those that produce dravyas are called panchamahabhootas. According to Ayurveda, dravya is a compilation of guna (property) and karma (action).[17]

Classification of dosha-dhatu-malas based on gunas

A dravya is known by its various properties like size, shape, weight, colour, touch, smell, sound, number, superiority, inferiority, combinations etc. Presence of a particular set of properties is indicative of a particular dravya. Thus, a dravya possessing particular properties is identified as that particular dravya. Of course, dravya is very important as it provides an abode for all the combinations of properties, but a dravya cannot be identified without its properties and hence the main characteristic of dravyas is that they imitate the gunas. This is why Ayurveda is 'gunavat dravya vadi'. Dosha-dhatu-malas are classified as dravyas because of their gunas (properties).

द्रव्यम् हि अनुमीयते ।

Dravyas cannot be perceived directly. They have to be inferred from their properties. Gunas are inferred from karmas and from these gunas dravyas are inferred. Dravyas come into existence before the gunas, yet they are identified by their gunas. A dravya has no existence devoid of gunas. Dravya is a compilation of gunas and karmas (samanvaya). Samanvaya means combination. This is why the characteristic of dravya is यत्राश्रिता: कर्मगुणा:। An introduction to dravya is possible only by prior knowledge of guna-karma.

In the subcontinent - entire India, there are 17000 species of plants (J.D. Hooker, 19th century).

The medicinal value of dravya

All the dravyas used for either medicinal purpose or as diet are considered to be panchabhautik. The body is also panchabhautik. The dosha-dhatu-mala of this body are also panchabhautik. If the natural balance of these dosha-dhatu-malas is disturbed, then the remedies also have to be panchabhautik.

According to the Samanya-vishesha siddhant, dravyas sharing commonality with each other tend to increase each other whereas those having specificity tend to deplete each other. Using this principle, various dravyas are used to increase their components which have been depleted and deplete those which have increased and achieve a balance. Thus, the main principle of treatment is 'क्षीणा: वर्द्धयितव्या: वृध्दा: ऱ्हासयितव्या: । समा: पालयितव्या: ।

The means by which this goal is achieved is known as 'medicine. A medicine has to be used considering its combination, dose, seasons, formulations etc.

It is perfectly logical that the body made up of panchamahabhootas can be treated by dravyas made up of panchamahabhootas. An increase or decrease in the panchabhautik vata, pitta, kapha, rasadi dhatus and pureeshadi malas can be brought about only by the panchamahabhootas which are the abode of all gunas. All the components of the body are made from the panchamahabhootas (through the presence of the soul (jeevatma) these components attain senses). Since all the dravyas are made up of panchamabhootas, there is no substance that cannot be used as medicine. Depending on the prominence of mahabhootas, dravyas may be parthiv, aapya, taijas, vayaveeya or akasheeya. Because of these gunas, they are used to create commonality or specificity with various body components. These dravyas must be used judiciously keeping the expected results in mind. For this, correct knowledge of the condition of the patient is necessary. This means that every dravya may be useful as a medicine.[18] There is no dravya which cannot be used as a medicine be it metals like gold, mica or biological wastes of animals like urine-faeces or soil, ashes etc. The group of medicinal dravyas in Ayurveda is so large that it is impossible for any dravya to be left out of it. The dosha-dhatu-malas which produce malfunctioning within the body are parts of the external universe (converted into body components) and are composed of panchamahabhootas accompanied by lifeforce. The human body which is formed from the external universe can be treated by components of the same universe and hence each and every constituent of the universe is a remedy. The remedy may be used internally or externally. Obviously, a person who can make judicious use of these dravyas has to be always there. Non-judicious use of medicines is totally unacceptable to Ayurveda. Ayurveda has condemned the non-judicious use of medicines at several places.[19]

Why is dravya of prime importance?

Among rasa, veerya, guna, vipak, prabhav, dravya etc., dravya is most important because it acts as an abode for all the rest. It is also a sustainer for all of these. Naturally, the dependent and sustained substance will be less prominent than the abode or the sustainer. Not only dravya but guna, rasa, veerya etc will have no sustainer if they are devoid of dravya. Therfore dravya is the most prominent and important of all. All the other phenomena are secondary. They do not have an independent existence. Apart from this, the scriptures have a few reasons consolidating the prominence

Generally, plants which are without stalk and a stem and have leaves with parallel venations and flowers having 3 or 6 petals are to be considered as monocotyledons.

of dravya. These are :

1. Vyavasthitatva : This means that, even though the guna-karma of a dravya may undergo a considerable change according to changes in conditions, there remains a type of continuity or stability within the dravya. Let us consider any fruit as an illustration. The appearance, taste, smell, and touch of an unripe fruit changes completely once it ripens. These qualities are replaced by others, yet the original dravya remains the same-and is known by the same name like mango, chikoo, pineapple etc. The taste, appearance etc underwent disorganisation because they changed in the course of time; but the dravya alone remained intact and organised. This organised nature itself is indicative of the eminence of 'dravya'.[20] A mango will be known as a mango, even if its colour changes to yellow from green.

2. Nityatva (Eternity) : Guna-karma are non-eternal. In comparison to these, dravya is eternal. Due to the effects of air, water and time, initially, the gunas like rasa, veerya etc. get depleted. For example, freshly prepared triphala churna does not have the same properties after six months, yet we call it triphala churna. It is true that even this churna will degrade after some time but compared to the guna-karmas it takes a longer time to perish. Here, eternity must be understood as undergoing degeneration after a comparatively long period.[21]

Since the eternity of the dravyas is subjective, dravyas do not enjoy eternity like atma, mana, disha, kala etc. In fact, gunas keep on changing as a result of conditioning due to time or due to some externally induced conditioning. The dravya, which undergoes subtle changes at every moment of time, cannot be addressed by a new name at every moment and hence dravyas are called nitya as compared to gunas. Lastly, since dravya is a karya dravya (effect), it has to perish but the eternity described even here is as compared to other phenomena.[22]

3. Swajati-avasthanat : Even if a dravya is acted upon by kala etc. it does not part with its parthiv, aapya, taijas, vayaveeya, and akasheeya nature. It is not so in the case of rasa, veerya etc. Once the rasa of a dravya changes then it completely loses its qualities of original rasa. Here, the illustration of curds can be given. Initially, curds is sweet to taste. After some time it becomes sour. This means that the sweetness of curds is replaced by sourness. Yet, the basic nature of curds does not change. All that is parthiv continues to remain parthiv. It cannot be converted into taijas or any other nature like aapya nature; this means that a dravya is the most eminent among all. This is called swajati-avasthan.[23]

4. Panchendriyagrahanat (perceptibility by the five senses) : Dravya can be perceived by all the five senses, e.g. the sound, touch, appearance, taste and smell. Thus the dravya forms an object of perception for the senses. Various sounds generated in the dravya like 'tat-tat' (taijas dravya), 'soo-soo' (vayaveeya) are forms of sound (shabda). Similar assessment can be made about roopa-rasa, gandh and sparsha. Rasa cannot be perceived by all the five senses. Rasa (taste) can be perceived by rasendriya, only forms by chakshurendriya, smell by ghranendriya and touch by tvagindriya only. Similarly guna, veerya and vipak are also perceived by single senses; not by all the five senses; and hence dravya is most important. Only dravya possesses the property of perceptibility by all the five senses simultaneously and not guna-karma etc. and hence dravya is the most important.[24]

Commonly, a plant with a stem, leaves having venation network and flowers having 4 or 5 petals, is considered as dicotyledon.

5. Ashrayatvat : Rasa, veerya, guna and vipak have no independent existence. They are sustained by the dravya. Since the dravya is independent and since rasa, guna etc. rely on the dravya, rasa-gunas are dependent. Since dravya is independent, it is the most important. Dravya is given so much of importance since it acts as an abode. The rasas-gunas are dependent and hence secondary. Rasa-veerya etc. are gunas; they are always secondary.[25]

6. Arambh-samarthyat : In treatment or even in our day-to-day practice, we use the decoction of roots, bark, leaves, and also pulp, powder etc. Here we do not say that we make the powder or decoction of a particular rasa, veerya or vipak. It is only the dravya which is selected initially and further considerations are made keeping in view the attributes of that dravya. The rasas-gunas etc. do not have the capacity of initiating such procedures. Only dravya possesses that capacity and therefore, only dravya is the most important. This is the sixth reason.[26]

7. Shastrapramanyat : This reason has also been described along with others. 'Shastra' means scriptural edicts. The gunas (properties) present in the drugs (medicines) are also present within the body. It is very evident that the properties present in the drugs have to be used to increase or decrease the corresponding properties within the body. Yet, the scriptures do not indicate the use of the properties directly but instead suggest the use of specific dravya. Because of this position of the dravya, it is the most important of all phenomena.[27]

8. Kramapekshitatvat : While discussing this reason also, the dependence of rasa-guna etc. on the various states of the dravyas has been emphasized. Unripe mango is sour; while a ripe mango is sweet; the rasa changed; dravya did not change; it is stable. Therefore, proper understanding of the dravya is essential for comprehending the existence of rasa-guna etc. Therfore, dravya is superior. The conditions like ripe and unripe fruit or the dry or wet conditions of pippali and ginger are important. The ripe-unripe, dry-wet states of the dravya are crucial. It is but natural that if the sustainer undergoes some deformity then the sustained will also undergo the same deformity. This is the reason why dravya is called superior. Dravya is addressed to initially and the rest are dealt with later. First comes the sustainer and only then the sustained.[28]

9. Ekdeshasadhyatva : Here the term 'desha' applies to parts of the dravya. For example, the latex of 'ark', the flowers of bakul, the fruits of haritaki and the roots of kantakari can be used independently. The roots, flowers, latex etc. are various parts of herbs. Rasas, gunas etc. do not have parts. It is impossible to use these singly. It is not so with dravya. We have the option of using any one of the 37 parts of the dravya. Thus, dravya is considered superior. Here 'Ek desha' refers to a particular part of a dravya.[29]

These nine reasons are enough to establish the superiority of dravyas over others. Yet, Nagarjuna has added three more reasons to these.

10. Tartamyoganuplabdhi : 'Tartamyog' is seen in the case of rasas. For example, there are states like sweet, sweeter, and sweetest. In gunas also there are states like heavy, heavier and heaviest. This is so, because the gunas present in the dravyas are variable. This is not applicable to karya dravyas. Since the karya dravyas are stable and fixed, there is no need to ascertain various dravyas of comparison between various states of the same dravya and thereby produce instability. We do not feel the

The human body is mainly made up fluid (Drava pradhan). Therefore solid food must also liquify in the mouth. "Eat what you drink and drink what you eat". The meaning of this is the same.

need of saying goldier or goldiest like heavier and heaviest since dravyas like gold are stable and non-changing. This also rates dravya as superior. Degrees of comparison are not applied to dravyas.[30]

11. Vikalp Samarthyat : Vikalp means various kalp (kalp = various preparations). For example - powder, decoction, juice, siddha ghrita, asava, arishta etc. Only dravyas can be used in these various forms. There is no such possibility in case of rasa, guna etc. This is also a chief reason for establishing the superiority of dravyas. A decoction of rasas and gunas is not possible.[31]

12. Pratighat Samarthyat : Dravya has a definite form. Two dravyas cannot simultaneously occupy the same space. This is called 'Pratighat Samarthya' of dravyas. This is not so in the case of gunas. Each guna does not need a separate space for its existence. The part of the dravya which sustains the rasa can also sustain 'gandha' (smell) at the same time. Every minute particle of a dravya occupies a separate space.[32] Among the twelve reasons mentioned above, the common factor is the role of the sustainer of the dravya. Rasa, guna, veerya, vipak are all dependent. Dependents are all inferior. The supporter or the sustainer is always superior. Therefore, dravya assumes more importance compared to others. It is appropriate to illustrate the superiority of dravyas in the chapter relating to dravyas. Keeping this in mind, the above discussion is apt. Sushruta has mentioned the following while concluding his chapter on dravyas.

1. There can be no vipak without veerya, veerya cannot exist without rasa and rasa has no existence devoid of dravya; hence dravya is superior amongst all. The gunas and veerya reside in the dravya (Sushruta) and not in the gunas.

2. Only the dravyas undergo vipak and not rasas. It is a common practice to say that madhur rasas undergo madhur vipak. But actually, it is the dravya with madhur rasa which undergoes madhur vipak. Therefore, dravya is superior.[33]

3. Apart from this, the padarth (phenomenon) called 'prabhav resides in the dravya only and is not influenced by the rasa, veerya, vipak etc. Specific dravya is necessary to obtain a particular prabhav. From this point of view also dravya alone is important and superior.

Because of this, Sushrutacharya has described the characteristics of dravya as under -

द्रव्यलक्षणंतु क्रियागुणवत् समवायिकारणम् ।

This means that dravya sustains karmas (actions) and gunas (properties) and is an essential prerequisite for the existence of guna, karma. Guna-karma accompanies a human being. Nagarjuna has described dravya as द्रव्यमाश्रयलक्षणं पञ्चानाम्.

Charakacharya has also mentioned the characteristics of dravya as

"यत्राश्रिता: कर्मगुणा: कारणं समवायी यत् ।

These quotations also illustrate the importance and superiority of dravya.

The meaning of the aphorism "किंचित् रसेन......

The body is made of panchamahabhootas. The dravyas are also made up of panchamahabhootas. These dravyas are used with the objective of obtaining some actions on the body. In our day to day

Body has to assimilate even water to make it congenial to our body with the help of agni (Digestive fire).

life, various natural actions are brought about in accordance with the universal law and satkaryavad and a constant state of equilibrium is thus maintained. The signs of health seen in a healthy person are indicative of this equilibrium. This state of equilibrium differs from person to person. No two persons or dravyas are exactly alike ("Man the Unknown" by Alexis Carrel). Their actions differ depending upon the dimensions of time and place.

रोगमादौ परीक्षेत (Diagnosis, the first step)

Throughout the twenty four hours various processes take place continuously within the body. This means that the guna-karma throughout the universe have theri effects on the body continuously, Due to some reasons,if the balance of these guna-karma is disturbed then the person loses his general state of health. The functions of the body may be intensified or depleted and accordingly one or a group of symptoms is produced. According to the satkaryavad, every manifested symptom has its active cause within this body which provides a stage for all the panchabhautik rasas, gunas, karmas, veeryas and prabhavas. When this active cause undergoes a change in natural 'satmya', its balance gets disturbed and symptoms of disease develop. Then priority must be given to find out which dravya-guna karma gave rise to such symptoms.

The capacity to generate symptoms lies within the body

The body has the causative factors of both atisara (diarrhoea) and baddhakoshtha (constipation). Both these factors act on the body. This is the meaning of "प्रवृत्तिरूभयस्य तु. This rule applies to each and every symptom, be it fever, headache, cough or anything else. The causative factor of fever is always present in the body. The natural tendency of pitta ie. its ushna dharma may increase as a result of depletion of its antagonist sheeta dharma and the body may experience warmth. Contrary to this, if various factors causing depletion of ushna dharma and increase in sheeta dharma occur, then the body will experience cold. In this manner, every symptom may be evaluated. This body has the potential of governing all the symptoms. The duty of the vaidya is to take into consideration this potential of the body and increase or decrease the associated actions and reinstate the state of equilibrium of the person.

एतत् वैद्यस्य वैद्यत्वम.

Pathology can be understood only after knowing physiology

A clear and vivid understanding of this concept is called for. The word diagnosis, which is a combination of two words, also bears the same meaning. (Dia - thorough, gnosis - (obtain) knowledge). The course of the treatment can be decided upon only after knowing which natural action has increased or decreased and due to what reasons. While doing this, it is necessary to assess the action potential of the body in the normal state and also any change in this potential. This is called 'Roga Nidan'. Once the problem is identified it becomes easier to find a solution; hence nidan has been given such importance. Once the 'prakruti' of the diseased person is ascertained, it becomes easier to evaluate the 'vikruti'. (The patient goes to the vaidya to get his prakruti exaimned whilst the vaidya looks for vikruti).

In the topic of Rasayana, the concept of Dosha has minor importance. The concept of Rasadi dhatus is dominant there.

The yogashastra of dravyagunashastra

Here, the considerations come under the review of dravyagunavignyan. A remedy has to be found which would restore the earlier state of equilibrium. The science of practical application of dravyagunavignyan begins from here and an aphorism like किंचित् रसेन कुरुते...... also has its beginning here. This is the basic principle in both, shodhan and shaman chikitsa.

Can these vibrations be created by rasas?

Once the main malfunctioning is identified, it is easier to decide on a future course of action. Then, a suitable dravya has to be selected and then starts the evaluation of the constitution and effectiveness of the dravya. If the desired action can be achieved by special vibrations generated by rasa, then the rasa should be used. If a dravya has been powdered two years earlier, then it may not be able to generate the special rasa vibrations. Such a dravya loses its utility as a remedy. A diet which is incapable of producing rasa vibrations is called stale diet. Similarly, the gross classification which divides dravyas into two groups viz. diet and drugs, also state that the dravyas which follow the "किंचित् रसेन कुरूते principle are predominantly ahar dravyas (diet). This is so because rasa is dominant in diet whereas veerya, vipak etc. are dominant in drugs.

Or will they be brought about by vipak?

If a particular action or the site of an action falls within the purview of vipak, then it becomes necessary to initially confirm whether the vipak potential of the dravya is intact or not. It can be taken for granted that if the capacity of a dravya to produce rasa vibrations is reduced as a result of alteration in its panchamahabhoota composition, then the dravya would be unable to create the expected vipak vibrations also. The diseases which develop in the organs undertaking 'sukshma pachan' can be treated suitably with vipak vibrations.

Individuality based on different combinations of gunas.

One more subject which must be paid attention to is the ten pairs of antagonist gunas which are always present within the body and are active in maintaining the equilibrium depending on the prakruti of the individual. Eventhough every person has some disequilibrium in his body, these gunas help in maintaining some balance relative to the constitution of the individual. This is what is meant by different prakruti (constitution). While trying to obtain the expected actions, these gunas must be considered and choice of the drug must be made accordingly.

Weak and strong gunas

Among these twenty gunas, eight gunas are stronger than the rest and are hence more effective. These are termed as veerya. Amongst these, again, the ushna and sheeta gunas are the strongest. As long as the dravyas within the body influence the body by their various gunas, the vibrations of gunas are produced and their respective actions are accomplished. Since these vibrations are of twenty types, the gunas are also twenty. These have twenty different actions in the living body. All these actions are brought about in order to maintain an eqilibrium. It is important that for these actions to become effective it is necessary to have the backing of the corresponding gunas.

The indices of proper digestion viz. smell-less eructation, enthusiasm, timely evacuation, lightness of the body and proper thirst and hunger are due to Pran, Udan, Apan, Vyan and Saman respectively.

Will the potency depend upon body acceptance?

The expected action may be obtained by the rasa vibrations, the guna vibrations (veerya) which superimpose on the vibrations of other gunas, vibrations generated by the rasa of a drug or diet after it has undergone digestion (vipak), or by the remaining 12 or 18 gunas. Whatever may be the cause of generating the action, vibrations play a major role in establishing the gunas. This means that for accomplishing this 'kinetic' action, it is necessary for the dravya to possess the 'potential' of generating all the four types of vibrations or atleast those which can bring about the necessary action. At the same time, the body must have the capability to extract these actions from the dravya (this capability is in agni). "किंचित् रसेन कुरूते – in this aphorism, other vibrations have also been enumerated, yet it is not observed that a particular action has been described as "द्रव्येण कुरूते. Why is it so ?

The limit of human manipulation

We have considered the four different types of potencies which can generate vibrations depending on the panchabhautik constitution of the dravya. This much deliberation is not enough as we have considered only a part of it. The dravya, in its complete and original form, has one more action which is above these four and cannot be explained. This is called 'prabhav'. The dravya works 'as a whole'. It is improper to say that the action was brought about by rasa, veerya, vipak, guna etc. If the action was generated by any one of these, then any other dravya having the same properties would have been used as a substitute. The word 'prabhav' indicates a special entity which is created even before the dravya is created by the universal force. The capacity of humans to generate ends at rasa, guna, veerya and vipak. But the vibrations generated by the universal force lie with the prabhav of the complete dravya. Some action is generated, but how? When a particular action cannot be attributed to rasa, guna etc., it is assumed that prabhav is the cause behind this action. There is a marked similarity between the ideas of 'Man as a whole' and 'dravya as a whole'.

Such is the aphorism and its meaning

For obtaining the vibrations of prabhav, the same dravya should be used and no substitution will work. Various aphorisms like "किंचित् रसेन कुरूते" have been mentioned in the scriptures which make us realise the limit of human ability to alter the properties of dravyas and also make us understand that there is much beyond this, which may remain concealed to the onlooker. The meaning of the sutra may be derived as shown above.

References -

1. द्रव्याणांगुणकर्माणि प्रयोगाः विविधास्तथा ।
सर्वशो यत्र वर्ण्यन्ते शास्त्रंद्रव्यगुणं हि तत् ।।

2. गुणा य उक्ता द्रव्येषु शरीरेष्वपि ते तथा ।
स्थानवृद्धिक्षयास्तस्माद् देहिनो द्रव्यहेतुकाः ।। (सु. सू. ४२),
द्रव्यरसगुणवीर्यविपाकनिमित्ते च क्षयवृद्धी दोषाणां साम्यञ्च ।" (सु. सू. ४६)

3. सुखहेतुर्मतस्त्वेकः समयोगः सुदुर्लभः ।" (च. शा. ९)
रोगस्तु दोषवैषम्यं दोषसाम्यमरोगता ।" (अ. हृ. सू. १)
येषामेव हि भावानां संपत् सज्जनयेन्नरम् ।

तेषोमेव विपद्व्याधीन् विविधान् समुदीरयेत् ।। (च.सू.२५)

4. ओषधय: स्वभावं परिहायापद्यन्ते विकृतिं,
तत उदध्वंसन्ते जनपदा: स्पर्शाभ्यवहार्यदोषात् । (च. वि. ३)

5. यत्राश्रिता: कर्मगुणआ: कारणं समवायि यत् । तद् द् व्यम्...." (च. सू. १)

6. समवाय तु निश्चेष्ट: कारणं गुण:" – (च. सू. १)

7. रस्यते आस्वाद्यते इति रस: ।

8. विशिष्ट: पाक: विपाक: । स च द्रव्याणां रसान्तरत्वेन परिणति: । (गंगाधर)
जाह्लरेणाग्निना योगाद्यदुदेति रसान्तरम् । रसानां परिणामान्ते स विपाक इत स्मृत: ।। (अ.हृ..सू.९)

9. वीर्य तु क्रियते येन या क्रिया" – (च. सू. २६)

10. रसादिसाम्ये यत्कर्म विशिष्टं तत् प्रभावजम्" – (वा. सू.९)

11. संयोगे च विभागे च कारणं द्रव्यमाश्रित् । कर्तव्यस्य क्रिया कर्म । कर्म नान्यदपेक्षते ।। (च. सू. १)

12. यत्राश्रिता: कर्मगुणा: कारणं समवायि यत् तद् द्रव्यम् (च. सू. अ. १)

13. क्रियागुणवत् समवायिकारणं । (सु. सू. अ. ४०)

14. द्रव्यमाश्रयलक्षमण् पञ्चानाम् । (र. वै.)
रसादीनां पञ्चानां भूतानां यदाश्रयभूतं तद् द्रव्यम् । (भा. प्र.)

15. गुणानां कर्मणाचेव समवायो द्रव्यमुच्यते ।

16. तेषामेकगुण: पूर्वो गुणवृद्धि: परे परे । पूर्व: पूर्वो गुणश्चैव क्रमशो गुणिषु स्मृत: ।। (च.शा.१ अ.)
आकाशादीनि भूतानि सर्वाण्येकगुणान्यथ । महाभूतेषु जन्येषु गुणवृद्धि: प्रजायते ।। एकद्वित्रि-
चतु:पञ्चगुणत्वं खादिषु स्मृतम् । गुणस्तत्रैक आत्मीय: शेष: संसर्गज: स्मृत: ।। अन्योन्यानुप्रविष्टानि
दृश्यभूतानि निर्दिशेत् । तस्मात् पञ्चगुणान्येव सर्वाणीति विनिश्चय: ।। (पं. भू.)
अन्योन्यानुप्रविष्टानि सर्वाण्येतानि निर्दिशेत् । स्वे स्वे द्रव्ये तु सर्वेषां व्यक्तं लक्षण मिष्यते ।। (सु.शा.१)
तत्र पृथिव्यप्तेजोवाय्वाकाशानां समुदायाद्द्रव्याभिनिर्वृत्ति:, उत्कर्षस्त्वभिव्यञ्जको भव-तिइदं पार्थिवम्,
इदमाप्यम्, इदंतैजसम्, इदंवायव्यम्, इदकामाशीयमिति । (सु. सू. ४१अ.)

17. सर्व द्रव्यं पाच्चभौतिकमस्मिन्नर्थे । (च. सू. अ. २६)
भवन्ति नित्य सत्तामनुभवन्तीति भतानि अथवा
भवन्त उपद्यन्ते येभ्य: द्रव्याणि इति भूतानि ।"

18. अनेनोपदेशेन नानौषधिभूतं जगति किंचिद् द्रव्यमुपलभ्यते तां तां युक्तिमर्थं च तं तमभिप्रेत्य ।
(च.सू.२६)
अनेन निदर्शनेन नानौषधीभूतं जगति किंचिद् द्रव्यमस्ति । (सु. सू. ४१)
रसादिभेदैरिति भेषजानां दिङ्मात्रमुक्तं न यतोऽस्ति किंचिद अनौषध द्रव्यमिह.... (अ. सं. सू. १२)
.... जगत्येवमनौषधम् । न किंचिद्विद्यते द्रव्यं वशान्नानार्थयोगयो: ।।" (वा. सू. ९)

19. च. सू. अ. १ श्लोक १२४ ते १३४, व च. सू. अ. ९।१४ ते १७.

20. व्यवस्थानात्" – (र. वै.१ सू. १०२) । व्यवस्थानादिति द्रव्यं व्यवस्थितं, गुणा: ह्यनवस्थिता: ।
उक्तं च – १दूर्वाङ्कुरनिभं भूत्वा फलं जम्वास्तत; पुन: । मेचकं भजते वर्णं पुनरञ्जनसंनिभम् ।"
इति । एवं तद्गताश्च स्पर्शरसगन्धाश्चानवस्थिता:५। जम्बूफलमिति द्रव्यम् सामान्यम् । (भा.)
केचिदाचार्या ब्रुवते – द्रव्यं प्रधानं, कस्मात्? व्यवस्थितत्वात्; इह खलु द्रव्यं व्यवस्थितं न रसादय:;

यथा – आमे फले ये रसादयस्ते पक्वे न सन्ति ।" (सु. सू. अ. ४०)

21. नित्यत्वाच्च, नित्यं हि द्रव्यमनित्या गुणाः; यथा कालादिप्रविभागात्तदेव संपन्नरसगन्धं व्यापन्नरसगन्धं वा भवति । (सु. सू. अ. ४०)

अनियतावस्थायिनो गुणा अनित्या उच्यन्ते, द्रव्यं च तदपेक्षया नियतावस्थायि नित्यमाख्यायते ।" (हारीत)

नित्यत्वं च द्रव्याणां कालपरिणामेनान्यताभावेऽपि तदेवेदमिति प्रत्यभिज्ञायमान-त्वादवगन्तव्यम् ।" (हारित)

22. यत्र यत्र कृतकत्वं तत्र तत्र अनित्यत्वम् । (तर्कसंग्रह)

23. स्वजात्यवस्थानाच्च; यथा हि–पार्थिवं द्रव्यमन्यथाभावं न गच्छत्येवं शेषाणि । म्हणजे पार्थिवांप्रमाणेच आप्यादिकांचे असते. (सु. सू. ४०)

24. पञ्चन्द्रियग्रहणाच्च, पञ्चभिरिन्द्रियैर्गृह्यते द्रवअयं न रसाद्याः ।" (सु. सू. ४०)
सर्वेन्द्रियोपलब्धेः" – (र. वै. १ सू. १०१) .... सवैः श्रोत्रादिभिरिन्द्रियैर्द्रव्यं गृह्यते, रसादयो ह्येकेन्द्रियग्राह्याः ।... एकमनेकेनद्रियग्राह्यत्वात् प्रधानं द्रव्यमिति । (भा.)

25. आश्रयत्वाच्च, द्रव्यमाश्रिता रसादयः" (सु. सू. अ. ४०)

अधिष्ठानादाश्रयात्" (र. वै. १ सू. १०३) – द्रव्यमाश्रयै आश्रयिणो रसादयः इति । आश्रयभूतः प्रधानः स्वामी दृष्ट इति ।" (भा.)

26. आरम्भसामर्थ्याच्च, द्रव्याश्रित आरम्भः, यथा 9विदारिगन्धादिमाहृत्य संक्षुद्य विपचेत् ।" इत्येवमादिषु न रसादिष्वारम्भः ।" (सु. सू. अ. ४०)

आरम्भसामर्थ्यात् । (र. वै. १ सू. १०४) – आरम्भश्चिकित्सायां क्रियारम्भः - मूलमाहरेत्यादि तस्मिन् द्रव्यस्यैव सामर्थ्यं न रसादीनामारम्भसामर्थ्यम् । अविकलेन्द्रियः पुरुषः प्रधानो दृ,टः पङ्गोरिति । (भा.)

27. शास्त्रप्रामाण्याच्च; शास्त्रे हि द्रव्यं प्रधानमुपदेशे हि योगानां, यथा 9मातुलुङगाग्निमन्थौ च" इत्यादौ न रसादय उपदिश्यन्ते ।" (सु. सू. अ. ४०)

शास्त्रोपदेशसामर्थ्यात्" (र. वै. अ. १ सू. १०७) – आगमादित्यर्थः । शास्त्र एवोपदिश्यते हि - य एव हि गुणा द्रव्ये शरीरेष्वपि ते स्मृताः । तान् द्रव्यैः तद्गुणैरेव प्रयोगेणाभिवर्धयेत् ।" इति सामान्य-प्रयोगवचने विशिष्टेन प्रयोगो निर्दिश्यते, इति । (भा.)

28. क्रमापेक्षितत्वाच्च रसादीनां, रसादयो हि द्रव्यक्रम ् पपेक्षन्ते – यथा तरुणे तरुणाः संपूर्णे संपूर्णा इति ।" (सु. सू. अ. ४०)

तदनुविधानाच्चेतरेषाम् (र. वै. अ. १ सू. १०९) इतरेषां रसादीनां द्रव्यस्यानुविधानात् । द्रव्यमनुवर्तन्ते हि रसादयः तारुण्ये तरुणाः संपत्तौ संपन्नाः, विपत्तौ विपन्ना भवन्तीति ये यमनुवर्त्तन्ते ते तस्मादप्रधाना दृष्टाः । तद्यथा, गुरोः शिष्या (अप्रधानाः) इति । (भा.)

9जन्म तु द्रव्यरसयोरन्योन्यपेक्षिकं स्मृतम् ।
अन्योन्यापेक्षिकं जन्म यथा स्याद् देहदेहिनोः ।। (सु. सू. अ. ४०)

29. एकदेशसाध्यत्वाच्च, द्रव्याणामेकदेशेनापि व्याधयः साध्यन्ते न रसादिभिः । कस्मात्? निरवयवत्वात्; यथा महावृक्षक्षीरेणेति; तस्माद् द्रव्यं प्रधानम् ।" (सु. सू. ४०) 9अवयवेन सिद्धेः" – (र. वै. अ. १ सू. १०८) अवयवेन एकदेशेन प्रदेशेन सिद्धेः;" प्रयोगेषु इति वाक्यशेषः यथा मूलत्वगादिना अवयवेन यः साधयति स प्रधानो दृष्टः । (भा.)

30. तरतमयोगानुपलब्धे :" – (र. वै. अ. १ सू. १००) तरतमयोगो रसादिषु दृष्ट:५।... मधुरतरो, मधुरतम:; शीततर:; शीततम:; छर्दनीयतरं, छर्दनीयतं, लघुतर:; लघुतम:; कर्मतरं, कर्मतमम् इति । द्रव्येषु नास्ति यष्टिमधुकतरो यष्टिमधुकतम इति । तस्मात् तरतमयोगाभावाद् रसादिभ्यो द्रव्यं प्रधानमिति (भा.)५।

31. विकल्पसामर्थ्यात्" – (र. वै. अ. १ पू. १०५) ९विविध: कल्पो विकल्प: कल्ककषायादिभेदेन, तस्मिन् विकल्पे सामर्थ्यात्, तत् सर्व द्रव्यस्यैव नान्यस्येति५।" (भा.) ।

32. प्रतीघातसामर्थ्यात् – (र. वै. अ. १ सू. १०६) प्रतीघात आवरणं, तस्मिन् सामर्थ् द्रव्यस्यैव भवति, मूर्त्तिमत्त्वात् ।... प्रतीघातसामर्थ्यात् स्वस्थानेऽन्यस्यानवकाशदानात् इति । रसादय: संपृक्तास्तिष्ठन्तीति । आवरणार्थोऽपि स एव घटते य: स्वस्मिन् स्थानेऽन्यस्यावकाशं निरुणद्धि स प्रधानो दृष्ट: चक्रवर्त्तीति । (भा.)

33. पाको नास्तिविना वीर्याद् वीर्य नास्ति विना रसात् ।
रसो नास्ति विना द्रव्याद् द्रव्यं श्रेष्ठमत: स्मृतम् ।। (सुश्रुत)

CHAPTER THREE
CLASSIFICATION OF DRAVYAS

In the universe, there are innumerable dravyas which are generated from panchamahabhootas. To be used, their identification and classification is necessary. In any science, the internal and external similarities of materials and their properties and actions form the basis of classification. Once classification is based on similarities, the understanding of dissimilarities automatically emerges which is also utilised in science.

Because of the absolute necessity of such a classification in Ayurveda, diverse classifications of dravyas based on different objectives have been done.

1. First classification is based on the cause and effect relationship.

Dravya

Causal dravyas (9)[1]	Effect dravyas (infinite)
↓	
The causal dravyas are natures' fundamental acts (panchamahabhootas, time, space, mind and soul 5+1+1+1+1 = 9)	Out of these entities, those infinite dravyas which arise from panchmahabhootas are called effect dravyas.

Karya dravyas (effect dravyas)

Parts of the body	Diet	Drugs

Though the causal dravyas are fixed and non-changeable, because of various combinations, and different properties, the karya dravyas are infinite.

Akash	Vayu	Teja	Jala	Prithvi
↓	↓	↓	↓	↓
Shabda	Shabda	Shabda	Shabda	Shabda
	Sparsha	Sparsha	Sparsha	Sparsha
		Roopa	Roopa	Roopa
			Rasa	Rasa
				Gandha

In the course of genesis of mahabhootas, first akash mahabhoota was created which had only shabda guna. The successive mahabhootas kept on adopting one extra guna. Thus, prithvi mahabhoota possesses all the five special properties. This is evident from the above table.

Praspanda of ushna, teekshna dravyas have to be of a high speed. This concept is wrong. Praspanda of snigdha, sheeta dravyas are not any less in the speed.

Classification of Karyadravyas

According to their constitution
1. Parthiv dravya
2. Aapya dravya
3. Taijas dravya
4. Vayaveeya dravya
5. Nabhas dravya

According to rasas
1. Madhur dravya
2. Amla dravya
3. Lavana dravya
4. Katu dravya
5. Tikta dravya
6. Kashaya dravya

According to veerya
1. Sheeta veerya
2. Ushna veerya

According to vipak
1. Madhur vipaki
2. Amla vipaki
3. Katu vipaki

According to their action
1. Doshaprashamanam
2. Swasthahitam
3. Dhatupradushanam

According to their prabhav
1. Drugs
2. Poison (Visha)
3. Diet

Depending on whether it is living or non-living
1. Antashchetanam
2. Bahirantashchetanam
3. Achetanam (without any senses or inorganic)

According to various modes of reproduction

Jangam	Audbhidam	Parthiva (minerals)
1. Jarayuj	1. Vanaspati	Gold, Silver, Copper,
2. Andaj	2. Vanaspatya	Lead, Mercury, Arsenic,
3. Swedaj	3. Virudh	Saindhav etc.
4. Udbhij	4. Oshadhi	

2. Dravyas are classified into two : living and non-living[2]

The difference between living and non-living dravyas is

living = with senses (organic)

non-living = without senses (inorganic)

A dravya which exihibits consciousness as a result of union with the soul, a dravya which allows manifestation to the soul is called chetan dravya. Humans, animals, birds, insects and other living entities which can move and other immobile life forms like trees, creepers etc. are included in chetan dravyas (possessing animation – life).[3]

If there is a definite sequence of using rasas in diet, then the same sequence must be applied to the plants as medicine as well.

Minerals like gold, which do not have life force and which do not manifest the soul in any form what-so-ever are called achetan dravyas.

Also, in our day to day life the dravyas like plants are used in their achetan form. But since these are basically alive, they are referred to as chetan.

The chetan dravyas are further classified into two groups.

1. Antashchetan

In these dravyas, the chaitanya is not clearly evident. Yet it is present. The audbhid dravyas (trees etc.) are included in this group. Their chaitanya is hidden inside.[4]

2. Bahirantashchetan

In these dravyas, the inner chaitanya present is evident outside. Such animals, whose chaitanya is evident in both ways are called bahirantashchetan.

The chaitanya of antashchetan plants has been experimentally proved by scientists. They can perceive various objects through their senses. For example –

Sight – If a plant grows in a dark place, then it tries to grow towards the source of light (heliotropism).[5]

Perception of forms –

वल्ली वेष्टयते वृक्षं सर्वतश्चैवगच्छति।
न ह्यदृष्टेश्च मार्गोऽस्ति तस्मात् पश्यन्ति पादपाः॥

Sound – Plants shed tears on hearing loud noises; leaves fall off from trees on hearing sounds of thunder. This happens because of their sense of hearing (वाय्वग्न्यशनि .... तस्मात् शृण्वन्ति पादपाः।).

Experiment carried out by Lord at Dresal University was as follows. Two plants were grown under similar conditions. One of them was subjected to a sound of 100 decibels (normally, the sound of a train is as high). That plant died. In another experiment, 12 siblings were allowed to grow for 11 days. Then they were subjected to high-pitched sound. The siblings started to 'shed tears' through their leaves and went dry.

Touch – The leaves of the "touch-me-not" plant (Mimosa pudica Linn) shrink as soon as they are touched. This is seen clearly. One more example of the sensitivity of touch is that of the "Ashoka" tree. If a young girl kicks the tree, flowers bloom. Similar examples can be cited regarding other senses also.

Plants also have sensation of touch.

उष्णतोम्लानपर्णानां त्वक्फल पुष्पमेव च ।
म्लायते चैव शीतेन स्पर्शस्तेन अत्र विद्यते ॥

All the above observations are supported by eminent scriptures. The writers of these scriptures have called plants as speechless creatures. Sir Jagdishchandra Bose has, through his experiments on plants, proved an inner consciousness in them.

The fundamental principle of Samanya-vishesha is not independent of the world. Nothing in the universe is outside it.

Sensation of smell -

पुण्यापुण्यैः तथा गंधैः धूपैश्च विविधैरपि ।

अरोगाः पुष्पिता सन्ति तस्मात् जिघ्रन्ति पादपाः ॥

More references on the sensation of smell -

पुण्यगंधाः कर्पूरचंदनादि रसगंधाः । अपुण्याः मत्स्यादिगंधाः ।

बीजं सुगंधरसेन अभ्यज्य अन्वितं सुगंधं अंकुरं जनयति ।

विविधैः धूपैः अरोगिणोभवन्ति (महाभारत विद्यासागर व्याख्या)

Perception of Taste -

पादैः सलिलपानंच व्याधीनामपि दर्शनम् ।
व्याधिप्रतिक्रियत्वाच्च विद्यते रसनं द्रुमे ॥
ग्रहणात् सुखदुःखस्य छिन्नस्यच विरोहणात् ।
जीवं पश्यामि वृक्षाणां अचैतन्यं न विद्यते ॥

(स्त्रीणां स्पर्शात् प्रियंगुः विकसति, बकुलः सीधुगंडूषसेकात पादाघातादशोकः – We cannot deny the possibility that these could be the imaginations of a poetic mind).

All the main factors in connection with absorption, transport and assimilation of food materials were known to the Hindus long before Stephen Hales demonstrated them in 1727 A.D. (Some aspects of Indian Civilisation in plant perspection - page 8 - Prof. Girija Prasanna Mujumdar).

अचोद्यमानानि यथा पुष्पाणि च फलानि च ।
स्वकालं नातिवर्तन्ते..............

(Mahabharat 12 - 174 - 12)

Where should a plant be planted?

फेनाघातो वल्लीफलानाम, परीवाहान्ताः पिप्पली मृद्रिका इक्षूणाम्, कूपपर्यन्ताः शाकमूलानाम्, हरणीपर्यन्ताः हरितकानाम्, पाल्यालवानाम् गन्धभैषज्य उशीर, ऱ्हीबेर पिंडालुकादिनाम् ।

(Mahabharat 2 - 24 - 22)

From this, it is proved that plant dravyas are antashchetan. The authors of the Ayurvedic scriptures believed the same and hence before uprooting the plants for medicinal purposes, they have instructed that the plants be informed about the act on the day before. Plants have birth, death, sleep, wakefulness, disease, activity, retirement, assets, drawbacks, infancy, youth, contraction, expansion, conception and all that occurs in other living organisms. They are also living organisms. They have emotions and experience joy and sorrow. (Nyaya darshan- The divya plants of Maharashtra - S.Y. Sawant, Ancient Sanskrit texts on trees and plants - Tilak Maharashtra Vidyapeeth, Pune, Research Group, 14th publication. Prof. V.M. Bedekers' article in the book titled Ancient Indian Science, 1st August 1974, is interesting and informative).

Teekshna-ushna gunas are not the only gunas to be tolerated in medical formulations. Sheeta-saumya gunas of pearl also must be tolerated.

Dravya

- Chetan (with sense organs)
  - Bahirantashchetan (jangam)
  - Antashchetan (audbhid, sthavar)
- Achetan (without sense organs) (minerals like gold and silver)

Among these, there is a limit to growth of jangam dravyas since they are movable; but there is no limit to the growth of audbhid dravyas as they do not have to move in search of nutrition (Commentary on Age; Kenneth Walker page 34).

Recently, Botany has made tremendous progress and emphasises that plants also have feelings. This science is known as "Epistemology". Many plants can express their emotions through their leaves and flowers - a polygraph can be made from the reactions to various emotions. Through these polygraphs it becomes evident that plants can express their likes and dislikes through their leaves. If a person destroys a plant in a room, then the remaining plants of the room can identify the person. If man can understand the language and emotions of animals then he can understand the emotions of plants also. (It is also presumed that perhaps, nature has endowed plants with even more senses than animals.)

There is one "Aushadhi ukta" in Rgveda (10-97). Atharvaveda also has aushadhi ukta. Bruhadaranyak Upanishad has a scientific description of trees and plants (3-9-38). Chandogya Upanishad also has description of plants. (The human body resembles a tree. The hair represent leaves of a tree. Just as a wound bleeds in man, latex is secreted from trees when cut. Flesh in human resembles the internal bark of the trees. Blood vessels in man are the thin layer on the inner side of the internal bark of trees. Bones in humans resemble the hard wood of trees. The marrow of trees is compared with the marrow in humans).

"Kautilya Arthashastra" includes scientific thought about plants. Other ancient texts like Seetadhyaksha and Mahabharat classify plants into vruksha, gulma, lata, valli, tvak and sara.

Indian culture considers trees as living and having inner consciousness. They definitely have likes and dislikes but since they are antashchetan, they are unable to express their joy or sorrow; they may even be expressing it but man is unable to perceive it.

3. Types of dravyas depending on their origin

Dravyas are constituted by panchamahabhootas. A dravya is said to be of a particular mahabhoota if it forms a major constituent of the dravya. Thus, there are five types of dravyas: 1) Parthiv 2) Aapya 3) Taijas 4) Vayaveeya and 5) Akasheeya. Due to the dominance of a single mahabhoota, naturally, specific actions and properties are seen in those dravyas. The table below will make the point clear.

Panchakarma, panchashodhan, shaman and brimhan produce the respective systemic vibrations in the body and bring about their actions.

Group of dravyas	Perceptible property	Rasa (taste)	Guna (property)	Karma (action)	Vipak
1. Parthiv	smell	sweet	heavy, hard, astringent immobile, juicy and bulky	heaviness slow acting,	guru
2. Aapya	taste	sweet, mildly astringent, sour and salty	cold, oily, slow acting and soft	oiliness, binding and softness	guru
3. Taijas	form	pungent, mildly sour and salty	hot, fast acting, subtle, light and dry	digestion and improving complexion	laghu
4. Vayaveeya	touch	astringent	light and	dryness sheeta	laghu
5. Akasheeya	sound	non-specific	soft and light	softness, lightness and porosity	laghu

4. Types of dravyas depending on their mode of origin

Dravyas are classified into three.[7]

1) Jangam 2) Audbhid 3) Parthiv (Bhaum)

1. **Jangam** - Dravyas obtained from jangam animals are called jangam dravyas. e.g. gorochan, kasturi etc.[8]

2. **Audbhid** - Dravyas that penetrate the earth and come out as plants. e.g. rice, chitraka etc.[9]

3. **Parthiv (Bhaum)** - Dravyas that do not fall in either of the two categories. e.g. minerals like mercury, sulphur, gold etc.[10]

उक्त प्रकारद्वयातिरिक्त: भौमम् । च. सू. 1/70, Commentary by Chakrapani).

Among these, jangam dravyas are further classified into four -[11]

1. **Jarayuj** - Jarayu is the amniotic membrane. Animals which are wrapped in an amniotic membrane during the intra-uterine life are called jarayuj. e.g. man, cow, horse etc.

2. **Andaj** - The animals which are born through eggs are called Andaj. e.g. birds like sparrow, reptiles like snakes etc.

(It has been observed that a female snake lays 15-20 eggs at a time and each one of these eggs can

Nature comprising of rivers, rivulets, streams, hills, hillocks, air, sunlight, cold and hot breeze truly makes a Botanical Garden.

give rise to 15-20 snakes).

3. Swedaj and **4. Udbhij** are both types which come into existence in special circumstances. Basically, these are andaj. Swedaj creatures are those which originate from vapours within the earth or from the sweat of animals. e.g. insects, lice, worms, ants etc.

4. Udbhij - These are also basically andaj. These creatures lie below the surface of the earth in hibernation period and then come on to the surface after a fixed time interval. e.g. indragopa insect and frog.

Just as jangam, audbhid dravyas are also classified into four groups-[12] 1) Vanaspati 2) Virudh 3) Vanaspatya and 4) Oshadhi.

1. Vanaspati - The trees which have very minute flowers and hence cannot be obviously seen are called vanaspati - apushpa, antahpushpa or guhyapushpa (banyan, peepal etc.) (अपुष्पा: फलिन:).

2. Virudh - Plants growing as creepers or growing in clumps or cluster are called virudh e.g. guduchi, patol, karvellak (प्रतानैर्वीरूध: स्मृता:) प्रतानशब्देन लता गुल्माश्च गृह्यन्ते । (च.स. 1/70 टीका).

3. Vanaspatya - The plants which bear visible flowers and then bear fruits also are called vanaspatya like mango.

4. Oshadhi - The plants which dry out once the fruits ripen are called oshadhi e.g. rice, wheat, barley etc. (फलपाकान्ता:).

(विनाऽपिफलं पाकेनैवान्तं येषां दूर्वादीनां तेऽपिगृह्यन्ते) (च.स. 1/72 टीका).

Two types of bhaum (parthiv) dravyas

1. Natural - These are found in the earth in their original form e.g. mercury, sulphur, gold, silver, hartal, mansheel, saindhav etc.

2. Artificial - Musk, vanshalochan, saindhav (saindhav available in the market is usually artificial because the mines which yielded saindhav are now situated in Pakistan and hence real saindhav is difficult to procure.) These are prepared from various parthiv dravyas by various procedures.

The karya dravyas which are used as diet or medicine are classified as follows -

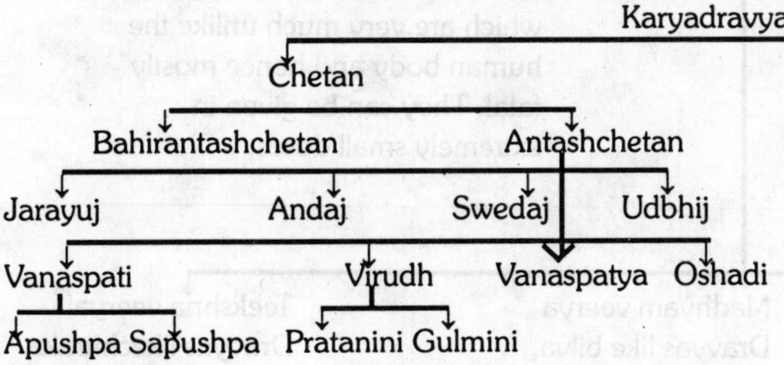

If we expect the plants to be rich in specific gunas, it is essential to grow the plants in the soil which is rich in respective particular gunas.

5. Types of dravyas depending on their use

Dravyas are classified into two types depending on their use:

1. Aushadh dravya (drugs) and 2) Ahar dravya (diet).[13] Charakacharya has put forth this classification while describing peya sanskar.

Among these, medicinal dravyas have dominant veerya. These dravyas cannot provide nutrition to rasadi dhatus. They can only pacify the vitiated doshas. Dravyas like chitraka, haritaki, bhallatak etc. fall in the category of medicinal dravyas.

Ahar dravyas (diet) - These have principally dominant rasas. The main action of these dravyas is to nurture rasadi dhatus and increase the strength and energy of the body. These also have sheeta-ushna veerya but they are mild as compared to those of medicinal dravyas. Dravyas like rice, wheat, jawar, bajri, barley etc. are ahar dravyas.[14]

Since the **medicinal dravyas** have dominant veerya, these are used in specific circumstances taking into consideration the roga-nidan (diagnosis). Drugs are used with the aim of creating a balance between the dhatus.

Ahar dravyas are used to maintain the equilibrium of the body and bring about necessary increase (vruddhi) or decrease (kshaya) in the dhatus. The aushadhi dravyas also have varying potencies.[15]

For example - dravyas like chitraka, maricha etc. are teekshna veerya dravyas (highly potent). Bilva, guduchi etc. have madhyam veerya (moderately potent) and dravyas like amalaki, rushabhak, jeevak etc. are mridu veerya (mildly potent). Amongst these, the mridu veerya dravyas closely resemble the ahar dravyas.

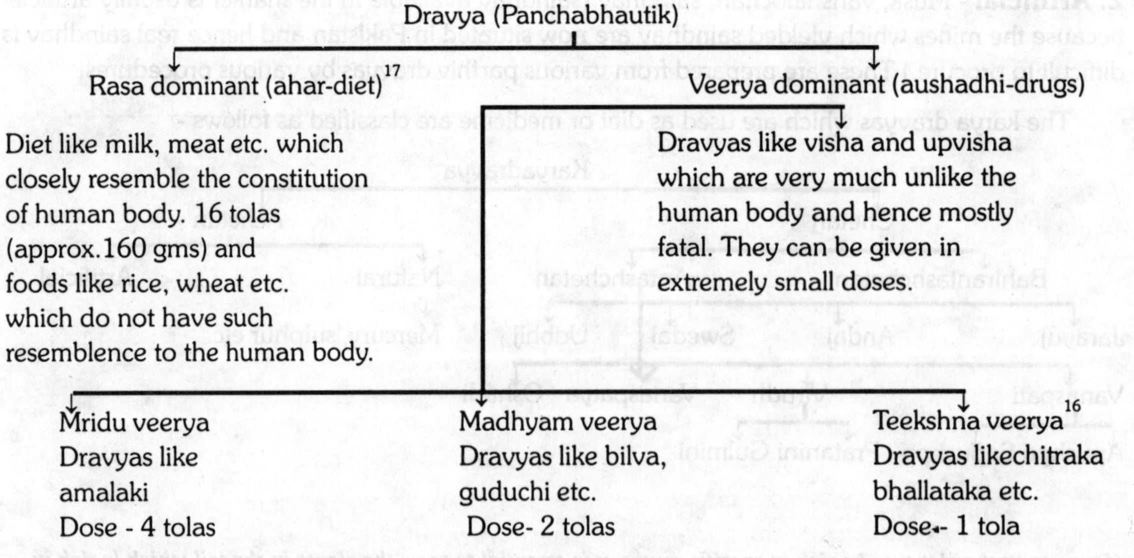

A human germ cell contains gold. Why only gold, it contains whatever in the universe.

Aushadhi dravyas are very distinct from ahar dravyas. They could have extremely contradictory effects on individuals and pose a threat to life. The choice of the drugs should be made after carefully evaluating the condition of the disease and the patient. On this is dependent the potency of the medicinal dravyas as well as the dose. If poisons are to be used then they should be given in extremely small doses. Poisons used properly may act as elixirs. योगादपि विषं तीक्ष्णं उत्तमं भेषजं भवेत् । च.स. 1/126.

All the dravyas starting from the ones which resemble the body and help by nurturing it, to extremely poisonous dravyas which are instantly fatal, are all made up of panchamahabhootas. At one end of the spectrum of dravyas is milk which nurtures ojas whereas at the other end is poison which destroys ojas. The other dravyas can be placed in between these two depending on their rasas and properties.

6. Six groups of dravyas depending on their rasas

There are infinite dravyas and each one has a different taste. Yet, all these various grades of tastes have been classified into six depending on their charateristics. Once rasa each is effective in each of the six ritus (seasons) of uttarayana and dakshinayana. Since ritus are six in number, the rasas are also six. The six rasas are madhur (sweet), amla (sour), lavana (salty), katu (pungent), tikta (bitter), and kashaya (astringent). Various groups (skandha) of dravyas have been formed which belong to these rasas.

Madhur varga (Group of sweet dravyas)

Ghee, jaggery, banana, milk, sugarcane, grapes, shaliparni, prushniparni, mudgaparni, mashaparni, jeevanti, jeevak, rushabhak, mohaphool, shatavari, kakdi, bala, atibala, nagbala, meda, mahameda, yashtimadhu, bhuikohla, shravani, mahashravani, ksheervidari, vansalochan, dudhi, shivanphala, ranshevanti, gokshur, gold etc.[18]

Amla varga (Group of sour dravyas)

Amalaki, chincha, mahalung, dalimb, buttermilk, curds, mango, kawath, karvand, amlavetas, silver etc.[19]

Lavana varga (Group of salty dravyas)

Saindhav, padelona, sanchala, bida lavana, samudra lavana, audbhid lavana, sambar lavana, kshar, lead etc.[20]

Katu varga (Group of pungent dravyas)

Hingu, maricha, sunthi, surana, onion, red onion, garlic, ginger, tulsi, rohish, marva, vidang, chitraka, chavaka, pippali, pippalimoola, bhallataka, pitta, mutra etc. (च.वि.अ. 8/142)[21]

Tikta varga (Group of bitter dravyas)

Haridra, parval, traymana, vala, black vala, chandan, kiratatikta, nimba, kutki, tagar, aguru, uda, sagargota, daruharidra, nagarmotha, morvel, vasa, pahadmoola, apamarga, guduchi, dhamasa, brihat panchamoola (bilva, shivan moola, tarkari, patla, tetu) kantakari, dorli, indravan, ativeesha,

Treatment should be such that the unwanted malas should be eliminated from dhatus. But during the process, if oja of dhatus is removed, nothing will be left.

vacha, kansya, loha etc. (सु.स. 42/11) (वा.सू. 10/28-29) (च.वि.अ. 8/143)[22]

Kashaya varga (Group of astringent dravyas)

Honey, bibheetaka, shireesha, kher, kadamba, kawath, moti, praval, anjan (surma), geru etc. (सु.स. 42/11) (वा.सू. 10/31-32) (च.वि.अ. 8/144)[23]

(Some minerals have also been included in these six groups. Sweet-gold; sour-silver; salty - lead; bitter - kansya (bronze) and iron; pungent - (no metal); astringent - gairik etc.

The rasas of these dravyas are not easily perceptible by the tongue, yet they are inferred upon by their actions. If milk is kept in a silver vessel then it perishes quickly; from this, we can infer that silver is sour to taste. The rasas of other metals also can be inferred upon from their actions.

7. Three types of dravyas depending on their vipak[24]

Even though there are six rasas, there are only three vipak 1) madhur vipak 2) amla vipak and 3) katu vipak

Madhur vipaki dravyas (Dravyas having madhur vipak)

The vipak of madhur (sweet) rasa is madhur and the sweetness of the madhur dravyas after madhur vipak is quite different. Yet, its basic nature of madhurya (sweetness) persists. Vipak can be known by anuman (inference). The action of vipak is generated in accordance with the rasa. The concept of vipak is more useful in understanding the subtle processes involved in digestion. The site of action of vipak is the terminal portion of the digestive system and the rasadi dhatus.

The vipak of sweet and salty dravyas is usually madhur (sweet). Similarly, pungent dravyas like sunthi, pippali etc., astringent dravyas like haritaki, sour dravyas like amalaki, dalimb etc. and bitter dravyas like patol also have madhur vipak. But there is a difference between the madhur vipak of madhur dravyas and the madhur vipak of non-madhur dravyas. Both do not have exactly identical actions.

Amla vipaki dravyas (Dravyas having sour vipak)

Dravyas included in the sour group as well as madhur dravyas like vrihi and astringent dravyas like kulattha also have sour vipak.

Katu vipaki dravyas (Dravyas having pungent vipak)

The dravyas belonging to the remaining three groups ie. groups of pungent, bitter and astringent dravyas predominantly have pungent vipak. Similarly, although oil is sweet to taste, it has a pungent vipak and salts like sauvarchal, though salty in taste, also have a pungent vipak.

8. Types of dravyas depending on their veerya

Dravyas are classified into two depending on their veerya viz. 1) sheeta (cold) and 2) ushna (hot).[25]

Charakacharya has accepted many types of veeryas. Some scholars believe that there are only eight types of veeryas (heavy, oily (unctuous) cold, soft, light, dry, hot and fast acting). Yet, since there are two major forces of hot and cold in this universe, veerya is also believed to be mainly of two types

Whether one wishes it or not, space and time continuously influence all matter and even you.

viz. sheeta veerya and ushna veerya.

Sheeta veerya dravyas[26]

Dravyas of the chandanadi varga - chandan, raktachandan, white vala, black vala, shatavari, shairal, rakta kamal, shweta kamal, neela kamal, kel, durva, murva, kakoli, ksheerkakoli, sariva, yashtimadhu, phalsa etc.

Ushna veerya dravyas[27]

Aguru, kushtha, haridra, kapoor, rasna, latakaranj, karanj, hindanbet, kadlavi, pippali, pippalimoola, chavaka, chitraka, sunthi and dravyas of sursadi, aragvadhadi, bruhatyadi, mushkadi and vachadi varga.

9. Three types of dravyas according to their action on doshas

1) shaman (dravyas that pacify doshas) 2) kopan (vitiating dravyas) and 3) swasthahita dravyas (dravyas that help in maintaining health).[28]

1) Shaman - The dravyas which equate the vitiated doshas without purifying the doshas or disturbing the equilibrium are known as shaman dravyas. The concept of shaman should be considered in the context of vitiation.

2) Kopan - The dravyas that vitiate the doshas in equilibrium are called kopan dravyas. This definition should be viewed in the context of health.

3) Swasthahita - The dravyas which have a tendency to increase or decrease vatadi doshas but do not produce vitiation of these doshas in a healthy person are known as swasthahita dravyas (complementary). These dravyas resemble the state of health of the body (the dravyas having contradictory properties are harmful). Swasthahita dravyas are considered in the context of health (swasthya).[29]

Charakacharya has classified all dravyas into three types :

1. Doshaprashaman (pacifying the doshas)
2. Dhatupradushan (vitiating the dhatus)
3. Swasthyakarak (maintaining and propagating health)[30]

(Here, the word dhatupradushan is very important).

What is the colour of water? What is the rasa of water? The answer to both these questions is the same. Water takes the colour and rasa of the substance with which it is mixed.

- Dravya
  - **Restoring health** — Shaman (dravyas having mild properties). (मंदः शमने शक्तिः)
    - Vata-shaman
    - Pitta-shaman
    - Kapha-shaman
  - **Detrimental to health** — Kopan (dravyas of fast acting properties).
    - Vatakopan
    - Pittakopan
    - Kaphakopan
  - **Propogating health** — The dravyas used as diet in condition of health as well as maintenance of health.

(Just as doshas, it is possible to have shaman, kopan and swasthahitatva of dhatus and malas).

The dravyas included in the swasthahita group are the ones which, eventhough belonging to a particular "rasa group", do not bring about an increase in the doshas that are generally increased by that rasa. For example, eventhough sugar is sweet to taste, it does not bring about an increase in kapha dosha. Other dravyas have to be consumed regularly in order to maintain health (वा.सू. 1/33 - 36). The dravyas which can be consumed regularly fall in the swasthahita group.

Vatashaman dravyas - Devadaru, tagar, kushtha, dashamoola, bala, atibala, dravyas of veertaradi and vedaryadi gana and dravyas having a strong odour.[31]

Vatashaman properties - The dravyas having antagonist properties to properties like unctuousness, cold, light, subtle, mobile, vishada (clear) and rough are vatashaman.[32]

Vatanashak rasas (tastes reducing vata) - Sweet, sour, salty. The guru pak (vipak of a dravya which has the property of heaviness in it) of a dravya reduces vata-pitta. Properties like ushna (hot) and snigdha (unctuous) reduce vata.[33]

Pittashaman dravyas - Chandan, durva, dhamasa, nimba, vasa, atmagupta, gundratruna, shatavari, shweta gunja, shalparni, prushniparni, kamal, fragrant dravyas and dravyas belonging to the nyagrodhadi and padmakadi gana are all pitta shamak dravyas (dravyas pacifying pitta).[34]

Pitta shamak properties - Dravyas having properties which are antagonist to properties like unctuous, hot, fast acting, liquifying, sour, fluid and pungent are all pittashamak dravyas.[35]

Dravyas possessing the property of heaviness in their vipak reduce vata and pitta. Properties like cold, soft and sticky act as pittashaman.

Pittashamak rasas - Rasas like sweet, bitter and astringent reduce pitta.[36]

Kaphashamak dravyas - Dravyas belonging to aragvadhadi, arkadi, mushkadi, asnadi, sursadi, mustadi and vatsakadi gana (वा.स.अ.15). Apart from this, dravyas having strong odour are kaphashamak.[37]

Kaphashamak properties - The dravyas which have properties antagonist to properties like

There are two types of purification, internal and external circum-ablution. The term circum (Pari) is important.

heavy, cold, soft, unctuous, firm and sticky are kaphashamak dravyas.[38]

Kaphashamak rasas - Pungent, bitter and astringent rasas are kaphashamak and dravyas having vipak which is light in property are also kaphashamak.[39]

Vatakopan dravyas - Pungent, astringent, bitter, ununctuous, light, sheetaveerya dravyas, dried vegetables, vallooraka, varak, uddalak, kodru, harenu, vatana and bhel are all vata prakopak dravyas. The body components which derive nutrition from these dravyas have increased properties of vata.[40]

Pittakopan dravyas - Pungent, sour, salty, teekshna, ushna, laghu, vidahi dravyas; kulathi, mohri, atsi, haritaki varga, meat of animals like goat, sheep, fish, curds, butter milk, milk products like koorchick, sauveeraka, various types of sura, sour fruits, tea, fried foods etc. are all pittaprakopak dravyas.[41] The body components that derive nutrition from these dravyas have increased properties of pitta (also, smoking and alcohol consumption are pittaprakopak).

Kaphakopan dravyas - Sweet, sour, salty, sheeta, snigdha, pichchila, abhishyandi dravyas, hayanak, yavak, naishadha, itkat, udid, mahamasha, wheat, sesamum, food items made from flour, meat of animals living in marshy land as well as of those living in water, substances made from sugarcane, fat, mrunal, kasheruka, shingada, sweet fruits of bilva, ice cream, fruit salad etc. are kaphaprakopak dravyas.[42] These dravyas increase the properties of kapha in the body components.

Swasthahita dravyas - Rice, wheat, barley, meat of animals living in arid areas, tender radish, chakvat, haritaki, amalaki, manuka, parval, sugar, ghee, rain water, honey, milk, saindhav etc. Generally, the dravyas which can be consumed regularly are swasthahita dravyas.

Dravyas which are conducive to health and at the same time help alleviate diseases are swasthahita dravyas e.g. लोहित शालय: (a variety of rice which is reddish in colour).

Charakacharya has mentioned the best swasthahita dravya of every group in Sutra sthana.[43]

10. Sanshodhan dravyas - The dravyas which remove the vitiated doshas - malas from the external apertures of the body like mouth, nose, anus, urethra, vagina etc. are called sanshodhan dravyas (उभयतो भागहर द्रव्य). For example, devadali causes emesis as well as purgation. (In Charaka samhita, सू. अ. 4/4 , six hundred such preparations have been given). These have been dealt with elaborately in the Kalpa sthana of Charaka samhita.

Sanshodhan dravyas are pungent, bitter and astringent to taste; they have teekshna and laghu gunas and have ushna veerya. These dravyas have predominance of prithvi, jala, vayu and teja mahabhootas.

Sanshodhan has been described as the prime and chief treatment in Ayurveda. Optimal removal of doshas from the body (सम्यक् शुध्दि) results in complete and total elimination of the disease (just as a tree dries up when the roots are cut). Thus the disease is not suppressed abruptly and since the causative mala-doshas are removed, there is no relapse of the disease.

Shodhana increases the strength of the dhatus as also the agni and slows down the ageing process. Ayurveda has therefore resorted to the five-fold purification procedures (panchakarma or

Kshanbhangi Bhava Siddhant encourages one to act. It says that if one does not give away things voluntarily then someday time will forcibly take these away.

panchashodhana). When there is an increase in the vitiated doshas, shaman alone will not yield the desired results. Prior shodhana karma is a must. Only then the relapse of the disease can be prevented.

दोषा: कदाचित् कुप्यन्ति जिता: लंघनपाचनै: । ये तु संशोधनै: शुध्दा: न तेषां पुनरूद्भव: ॥ (वा.स.)

Charaka has classified 500 dravyas on the basis of their actions and has thus created 50 ganas (groups) of dravyas which are useful in treatment. The terms used for various actions have been explained in the preceding chapter on karma.

The various groups are as follows :

Classification of dravyas on the basis of 50 different actions (Charaka)

1. Jeevaneeya
2. Bruhaneeya
3. Lekhaneeya
4. Bhedaneeya
5. Sandhaneeya
6. Deepaneeya
7. Balya
8. Varnya
9. Kanthya
10. Hridya
11. Truptighna
12. Arshaghna
13. Kushthaghna
14. Kandughna
15. Krumighna
16. Vishaghna
17. Stanyajanan
18. Stanyashodhan
19. Shukrajanan
20. Shukrashodhan
21. Snehopag
22. Swedopag
23. Vamanopag
24. Virechanopag
25. Asthapanopag
26. Anuvasanopag
27. Shirovirechanopag
28. Chardinigrahan
29. Trushnanigrahan
30. Hikkanigrahan
31. Pureeshasangrahaneeya
32. Pureeshavirajaneeya
33. Mootrasangrahaneeya
34. Mootravirajaneeya
35. Mootravirechaneeya
36. Kasahara
37. Shwashara
38. Shothahara
39. Jvarahara (These dravyas appear more Shonitprashaman)
40. Shramahara
41. Dahaprashaman
42. Sheetaprashaman
43. Udardaprashaman
44. Angamardaprashaman
45. Shoolaprashaman
46. Shonitprashaman
47. Vedanasthapan
48. Sangnyasthapan
49. Prajasthapan
50. Vayasthapan (वा.स. अ. 4/8).

Destruction (Entropy) of any dravya is a natural phenomenon. It is our arrogance to presume that we have destroyed it. But in treatment it is in our hands to suitably alter the locus of destruction.

11. Classification of medicinal plants on the basis of their habitat, family, morphology and life span

1. Audbhid dravyas are of four types depending on their habitat

a. **Sthalaj** (Terrestrial = land). The plants and trees that grow on land are known as sthalaj. e.g. haritaki, amalaki, bibheetaka, bhallataka, moha, vata, umbar, pippali etc.

b. **Jalaj** (Aquatic) (Aqua = water). The plants that grow in water are known as jalaj. e.g. kamal, spyrogyra etc.

c. **Vruksharuha** (Epiphytic, living on the surface of trees). The plants that grow on other trees but do not depend on that tree for their nutrition are called vruksharuha. e.g. rasana (Bengali) (Epi = above, phutan = plant).

d. **Vrukshadan** (Parasitic) - A plant which dwells on another tree and obtains its nutrition from its host is called vrukshadan [वृक्ष (tree) + अद् (to eat)] (An organism which obtains food or shelter from another host organism is called a parasite).

Morphological classification and its importance

This type of classification is very important for correct identification of plants for their medicinal use.

Since the main criterion of classification is similarity between dravyas belonging to the same family, this classification is called geneological.

Morphological classification

Depending on the shape and form, these udbhij plants are classified into four main groups.

a. **Vruksha** (tree) - plants which have a height ranging from 5 metres to 35 metres are called vruksha. These have a strong trunk while the branches grow upwards and, they too, are strong.

These are further divided into three sub-groups

Vruksha

Mahavruksha	Vruksha	Vrukshak
↓	↓	↓
Tall tree height more than approx 20 metres.e.g. deodar, pine etc.	Medium tree height ranging from approx. 13 metres to 18 metres. mango, jamun.	Small tree height ranging from5 to 10 metres . e.g. papaya, guava.

The simultaneous existence of two mutual impulses/ vibrations itself is the proof of life. If this phenomenon ceases to exist, there will be no life.

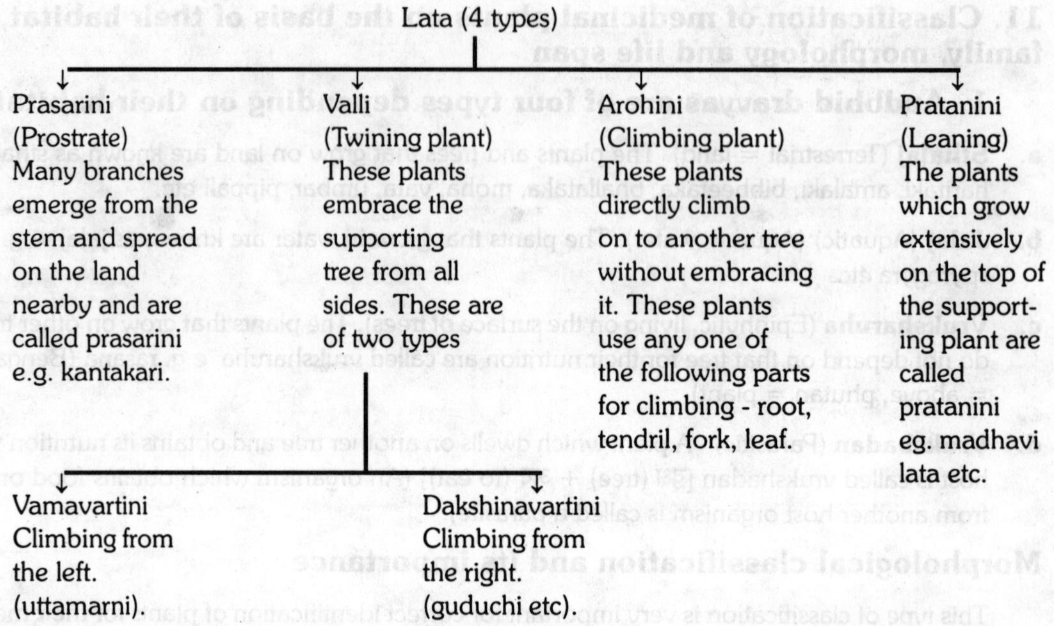

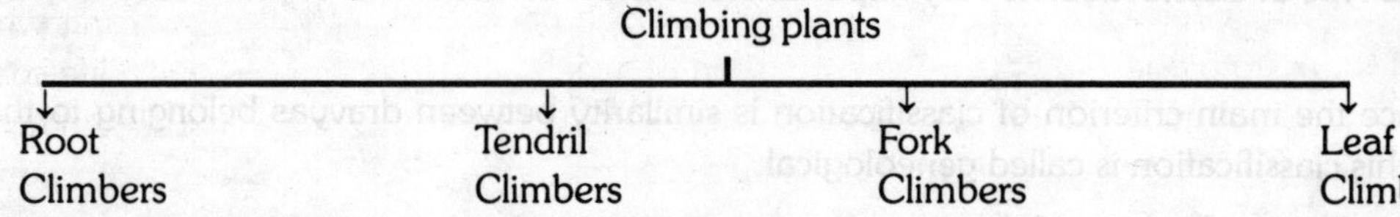

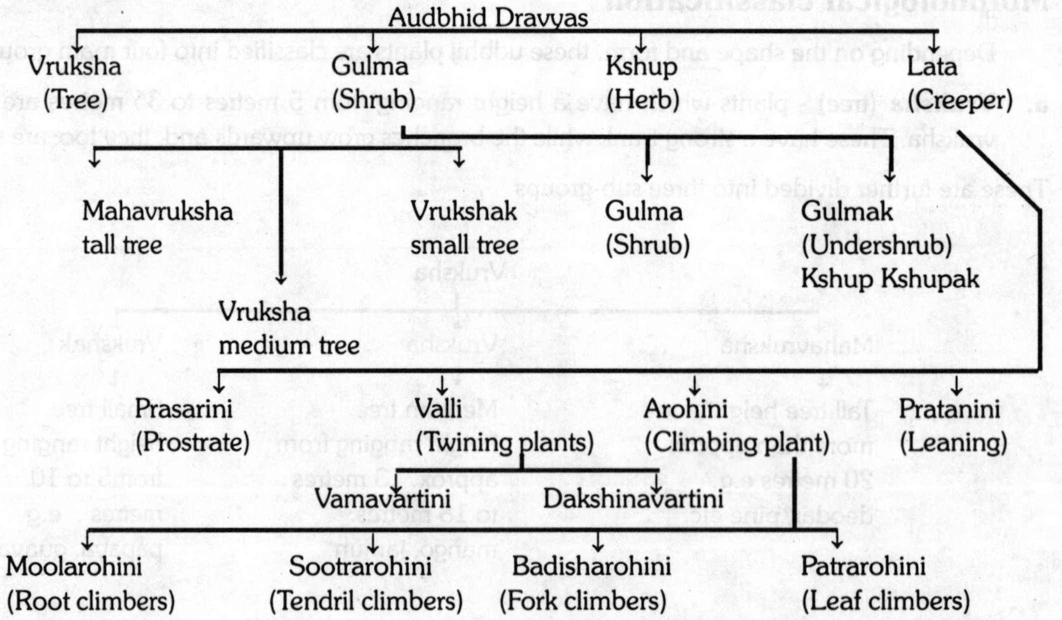

Vibrations of the opposite gunas are generated continuously throughout day and night i.e. ' प्रवृत्तिरुभस्य तु '

b. Gulma (Shrub) - The plants which have many small stems arising from a single root are known as gulma. eg. dhayti. Plants which are even smaller than these are called gulmak (undershrub). eg. bala, arka

c. Kshup (Herb) - These plants have a height ranging from 1 - 2 metres and have small roots. The branches are also very tender eg. prapunnad.

d. Lata (weak plants/creepers) - The plants which do not have a strong stem and hence cannot remain erect on their own but need the support of some other object to climb upon are called lata (weak plants).

4. The Udbhij dravyas are classified into three on the basis of their life span.

Udbhij

Ek Varshayu (Annuals)	Dwi Varshayu (Biennials)	Bahu Varshayu (Perennials)
The plants which have a life span of upto one season or maximum upto one year are called ek varshayu (annual).	The plants which have a life span of two years are called dwi varshayu (binennials) e.g. carrot, salgam	The plants which have a life span of more than two years are called bahu varshayu (perennial) e.g. vata, kadunimba, umbar, pipal etc.

Taking the 50 ganas given in Charaka samhita as the basis, the ganas given in Sushruta samhita have been compared. Following table shows the ganas given by Sushruta which resemble those of Charaka samhita.

Charaka Gana	Sushruta Gana
Jeevaniya	Kakolyadi
Bruhaneeya	Vidarikandadi
Lekhaneeya	Mustadi
Bhedaneeya	Shyamadi
Sandhaneeya	Ambasthadi, Priyangvadi
Deepaneeya	Pippalyadi
Balya	Laghupanchamoola
Varnya	Eladi
Kanthya	
Hridya	Parushakadi
Truptighna	Patoladi
Arshoghna	Mushkadi
Kusthaghna	Aragvadhadi, Salsaradi, Arkadi

Eventhough the concept of avrutta (covered), is not considered in sukhasadhya diseases, it should be considered in kashtasadhya diseases, but ....?

	Lakshadi
Kandughna	Eladi, Aragvadhadi
Krumighna	Sursadi, Lakshadi
Vishghna	Rodhradi, Aragvadhadi, Arkadi, Anjanadi
Stanyajanan	Kakolyadi
Stanyashodhan	Mustadi, Vachadi, Haridradi
Shukrajanan	Kakolyadi
Shukrashodhan	Vallipanchamoola, Kantak-
panchamoola.	Snehopag
Swedopag	
Vamanopag	
Virechanopag	Parushakadi
Asthapanopag	
Anuvasanopag	
Shirovirechanopag	
Chardinigrahan	Nyagrodhadi
Trushnanigrahan	Guduchyadi, Utpaladi, Sariwadi, Parushakadi
Hikkanigrahan	Bruhatyadi, Vidarikandadi
Pureeshagrahaneeya	Rodhradi, Priyangvadi, Ambashthadi
Pureeshavirajaneeya	Nyagrodhadi
Mootrasangrahaneeya	Nyagrodhadi, Salsaradi
Mootravirechaneeya	Trunpanchamoola, Veertarvadi
Mootravirajaneeya	Utpaladi
Kasahara	Vidarikandadi
Shwashara	Pippalyadi, Sursadi
Shothahara	Dashamoolagana
Jvarahara	Sarivadi, Patoladi, Amlakyadi
Shramhara	Parushakadi
Dahaprashaman	Sariwadi, Anjanadi, Utpaladi
Sheetaprashaman	Pippalyadi, Sursadi
Udardaprashaman	Salsaradi
Angamardaprashaman	Vidarikandadi
Shoolaprashaman	Pippalyadi
Shonitsthapana	Priyangvadi, Anjanadi
Vedanasthapan	Rodhradi
Sangnyasthapan	Priyangvadi
Prajasthapan	Vidarikandadi, Kakolyadi
Vayasthapan	Kakolyadi, Vidarikandadi

Ayurveda studies the human body from the time before birth till death and therefore it includes the study of morbid symptoms in sharir (anatomy).

Vaman	Urdhvabhaghara
Virechan	Adhobhaghara
Shodhan	Ubhayatobhaghara

The method of classification in other Ayurvedic texts

Charakacharya has classified plants on the basis of their actions like bruhaneeya, jeevaneeya etc. and has cited examples of 10 plants each in every group (varga). This is the simple method of classification (inductive method). Charakacharya had identified the inherent medicinal properties-actions of various dravyas and had formed groups accordingly for ready reference. Fifty groups were formed. Since each group (varga), has ten dravyas, 50 x 10 = 500 dravyas have been mentioned in this classification. Since a single dravya may have many different important actions, a single dravya falls in 2-3 groups. Thus the number of dravyas is less than 500. This type of classification is useful for the use of medicines according to their actions.

In Sushruta samhita, which has been written after Charaka samhita, this classification has been done in a special manner (deductive method). Rather than classifying dravyas according to their actions, Sushruta has laid more emphasis on the dravya itself. It can be presumed that the number of dravyas used by Sushruta might have been much larger than used by Charaka and hence for every action, the number of dravyas used might have exceeded ten. Therefore, Sushrutacharya resorted to a special method of classification and named the groups after specific dravyas (like pippalyadi, bruhatyadi etc.)

Moreover, since Charaka was a physician and Sushruta a surgeon, each of them classified the dravyas in a way which suited their branch of knowledge the most.

Ashtangsangraha and Ashtanghrudaya are both texts which are compilations based on Charaka and Sushruta samhitas. Both these texts have followed the classification methodology of Sushruta.

Eventhough Charakacharya has classified the dravyas on the basis of actions and Sushrutacharya on the basis of dravyas, yet there is remarkable similarity between the two methods of classification as is evident from the table given above.

It is not a rigid rule that all the dravyas of a group have to be used without disturbing the original composition of the group. In fact, one can even subtract an unwanted dravya and instead include a necessary drayva and use it along with other dravyas of the group. These groups should be used after taking into account the condition of dosha-dooshya. Various preparations of these dravyas (like juice, pulp, decoction, medicated ghee, pastes etc.) can be used internally and externally (oral or nasal administration, massages, oil-containing enemas, ointments etc.)

Apart from this, dravyas have also been classified on the basis of their rasas. This classification is helpful to those who use the rasas for treatment. In Sushruta samhita, classification has also been done on the basis of difference in vipak, veerya, vitiation and pacification of vata-pitta-kapha and swasthahita nature of dravyas.

Even in the era of Charaka, as in current times, various systems of medicines were popular among the masses.

Ashtanghrudaya

Vagbhatta, the compiler of Ashtanghrudaya, has classified liquid dravyas into five groups viz. 1) Jala varga (types of water depending on sources like river, lake, well etc.) 2) Ksheer varga (types of milk like cow's milk, goat's milk etc.) 3) Ikshu varga (various food items prepared from sugarcane juice) 4) Taila varga (various types of oils like groundnut oil, sesamum oil etc.) 5) Madya varga (various alcoholic beverages).[44] There is no mention of independent Mootra varga. Similarly, food items are classified into following groups:

1. Shookadhanya varga
2. Shimbidhanya varga
3. Krutanna varga
4. Mansa varga
5. Shaka varga
6. Phala varga
7. Aushadh varga[45]

Lavana, kshar, haritaki etc. are included in the aushadh varga

Dhanvantari nighantu (5th century)

In Dhanvantari nighantu, dravyas have been classified into seven vargas (groups). These are guduchyadi, shatapushpadi, chandanadi, karaveeradi, amradi, suvarnadi and mishrakadi.[46] It may be observed that this classification has been done on the basis of their actions like –

1. **Guduchyadi varga** - This includes dravyas which induce removal of doshas from the body (through purgation and emesis) as well as rasayan (rejuvenating) dravyas e.g. guduchi, madanphala, danti etc.[47]

2. **Shatapushpadi varga** - This group includes deepana (improving digestion), balya (increasing bodily strength) and mukhashodhana (having a cleansing effect in the mouth) dravyas e.g. shatapushpa, vacha etc.

3. **Chandanadi varga** - Fragrant dravyas like chandan, kumkum, usheer etc. are included in this group.

4. **Karveeradi varga** - This group includes many types of dravyas like karveer, tulsi, nakuli etc.

5. **Amradi varga** - This group includes phalavarga (various fruits), pushpavarga (various flowers) and plants having valkal e.g. amra, mallika, arjuna etc.

6. **Suvarnadi varga** - This group includes dhatuvarga (minerals), shookadhanya varga, shamidhanya varga, taila, ksheer, madya etc. It also includes mansa varga.

7. **Mishrakadi varga** - This varga includes triphala and other ganas (groups).

Madanpal nighantu (14th century)

This nighantu was written in 1375 AD. Following groups are seen in this nighantu.

Everyone wishes a long life, but if endowed with good health, it would be an added advantage.

1. abhayadi varga 2. shatyadi varga 3. karpooradi varga 4. suvarnadi varga 5. vatadi varga 6. phaladi varga 7. shaka varga 8. paneeyadi varga 9. ikshukadi varga 10. dhanyaguna varga 11. krutannadi varga 12. mansa varga 13. mishrak varga.

Raj nighantu (15th century)

Many groups have been included in this nighantu. But following groups have been formed of dravyas having medicinal value.

1. guduchyadi 2. shatahvadi 3. parpatadi 4. pippalyadi 5. moolakadi 6. shalmalyadi 7. prabhadradi 8. karveeradi 9. amradi 10. chandanadi 11. suvarnadi 12. paneeyadi 13. ksheeradi 14. shalyadi 15. mansadi 16. mishrakadi.

The classification of dravyas done in Dhanvantari nighantu and Raj nighantu does not seem to be very systematic. Though, at certain places, dravyas have been grouped together on the basis of similarity in their properties and actions, yet, in some groups, there does not appear to be any scientific basis for the classification. For example, taila, ghrita and mansa varga as well as other groups have been classified along with suvarnadi varga.

Keyadeva nighantu (16th century)

Dravyas have been classified into 9 groups in Keyadeva nighantu.[48] 1) aushadhi varga 2) dhatu varga 3) dhanya varga 4) drava varga 5) pakvanna varga 6) mansa varga 7) vihar varga 8) mishrak varga 9) nanartha varga.

Bhavaprakash nighantu (16th Century)

Dravyas have been classified into 21 groups in this nighantu

1) haritakyadi varga 2) karpooradi varga 3) guduchyadi varga 4) pushpa varga 5) phala varga 6) vatadi varga 7) dhatu varga 8) dhanya varga 9) shaka varga 10) vari varga 11) dugdha varga 12) dadhi varga 13) takra varga 14) navneet varga 15) ghrit varga 16) mootra varga 17) taila varga 18) madhu varga 19) ikshu varga 20) sandhan varga 21) mansa varga.

Bhavprakash has done systematic classification of food items. The classification in Bhavaprakash nighantu has been done on definite principles e.g. karpooradi varga includes only aromatic dravyas. Similarly only those trees which have a thick bark have been included in vatadi varga.

Other Nighantus

The successive nighantukars (authors of nighantu) have followed Bhavaprakash. These include Rajavallabh nighantu (1703), Nighantu sangraha (1758) Nighantu-ratnakar (1867), Shaligram nighantu etc.

Summary

From the above discussions it is clear that the ancient scriptures classified dravyas on the basis of

Infinite number of big and small pores in the human body fill up and empty throughout the twenty four hours of the day.

their actions and morphology whereas the nighantus laid more emphasis on "dravyatmak" classification. The authors of various nighantus relied on this type of classification for centuries.

References -

1. खादीन्यात्मा मनः कालो दिशश्च द्रव्यसंग्रहः ।" (च. सू. १)
2. तच्चतनावदचेतनञ्च ।" (च. सू. २६)
   सेन्द्रियं चेतनं द्रव्यं निरिन्द्रियमचेतनम् ।" (च. सू. १)
3. अत्र सेंद्रियत्वेन वृक्षादीनामपि चेतनत्वम् बोध्दव्यम् । (च. सू. अ. १) टीका.
4. गुच्छगुल्मं बहुविधं तथैव तृणजातयः । बीजकाण्डरुहाण्येव प्रताना वल्ल्य एव च ।।
   तमसाबहुरूपेण वेष्टिताः कमहेतुना ।। अन्तःसंज्ञा भवन्त्येते सुखदुःखसमन्विताः ।। (मनुस्मृति १४८।४९)
5. तेजोगमसंवलियता युक्ता चेतनाः वृक्षाः ।
   ग्रहणाच्च सुखादीनां छिन्नस्य च विरोहणम् ।
   जीवं पश्यामि वृक्षाणां अचैतन्यं न विद्यते ।। (महाभारत शांतिपर्व १८४)
   महाभारतमोक्षधर्मपर्व (१२-१७४) इत्येतैः पञ्चाभिः भूतैः युक्तं स्थावव जंगलम्५
6. तत्र स्थूलसान्द्रमन्दस्थिरगुरुकठिनगन्धबहुलमीषत्कषायं प्रायशो मधुरमिति पार्थिवं तत् स्थैय-बल-गौरव-संघोतोपचयकरं विशेषतश्चाधोगतिस्वभावमिति; शीतस्तिमितस्निग्धमन्दगुरुसरसान्द्रमृदुपिच्छिलं रसबहुल-मीषत्कषायाम्ललवणं मधुररसप्रायमाप्यम्; तत् स्नेहनल्हादनक्लेदनबन्धन-विष्यन्दनकरमिति; उष्णतीक्ष्णसूक्ष्म रूक्षखरतद्दहन-पचन-दारण-तापन-प्रकाशन-प्रभावर्णकरमिति; सूक्ष्मखरशिशिरलघुविशदं स्पर्शबहुलमीषत्तिक्तं विशेषतः खषायमिति वायवीयं, तद्वैशद्यलाघवग्लापनवि रूक्षणविचारकरमिति; श्लक्ष्णसूक्ष्ममृदुव्यवायिविशदविविक्तमव्यक्तरसं शब्दबहुलमाकाशीयं, तन्मार्दवसौषिर्यलाघवकरमिति ।" (सू. सु. अ. ४१) १तत्र द्रव्याणि गुरुखर... लाघवकराणि" (च. सू. २६)
7. तत्पुनस्त्रिविधं ज्ञेयं जांगमं भौममौद्भिदम्" । (च. सू. १)
8. जंगमप्रभवं जांगमम्, गोरसमध्वादि" । (यो.)
9. उद्भिद्य पृथिवीं जायते इति औद् भिदम् वृक्षादि" । (च. द.)
10. भूमेर्विकारः भौमम् सुवर्णादिकम् ।" (यो.)
11. जंगमाः खल्वपि जरायुजाण्डजस्वेदजोद् भिज्जाः ।" तत्र पशुमनुष्यव्यालादयो जरायुजाः खगसर्पसरीसृपप्रभृतयोऽण्डजाः कृमिकीटपिपीलिकाप्रभृतयः स्वेदजाः इन्द्रगोपमंडूकप्रभृतयः उद् भिज्जाः ।" (सु. सू. १)
12. ....औद् भिदं तु चतुर्विधम् । वनस्पतिस्तथा वीरुद्वानस्पत्यस्तथौषधिः ।।
    फलैर्वनस्पतिः पुष्पैर्वानस्पत्यः फलैरपि । औषध्यः फलपाकान्ताः प्रतानैर्वीरुधः स्मृताः ।। (च. सू. १)
13. यवागूसाधनद्रव्यं तावद् द्विविधं वीर्यप्रधानमौषधद्रव्यं, रसप्रधानमाहारद्रव्यच्च ।" (च. सू २ च. द.)
14. प्राणिनां पुनर्मूलमाहारो बलवर्णौजसां च स षट्सु रसेषु आयत्तः ।" (सु. सू. ४६)
15. तं तं युक्तिविशेषमर्थं चाभिसमीक्ष्य स्ववीर्यगुणयुक्तानि द्रव्याणि कार्मुकाणि भवन्ति । (सु. सू. ४१)
16. तत्नाप्यौषधद्रव्यं त्निविधं वीर्यभेदात् –तीक्ष्णवीर्यं यथा शुण्ठ्यादि, मध्यवीर्य बिल्वाग्निमन्थादि, मृदुवीर्यञ्चामलकादि ।" (सु. सू. २ च. द.)
17. तीक्ष्णानां कर्षः, मध्यानामर्धपलं, मृदूनां पलमित्युत्सर्गः ।... अन्त चतुःपलद्रव्याभिधानं रसप्रधानद्रव्याभिप्रायेणैव । (सु. सु. २ च. द.) (ह्या मात्रांचा फेरविचार व्हावा.)

18. तद्यथा जीवकर्षभकौ जीवन्तीवीरातामलकीकाकोलीक्षीर काकोल्यभीरुमुद्गपर्णी पृश्निपर्ण्यसनपर्णीमेदाम-हामे दाकर्कट शृङ्गाटिकाच्छिन्नरुहाछत्रातिछत्रा श्रावणी महाश्रावणीसहदेवाविश्वदे वाशुक्लाक्षीरशुक्लाब-लाविदारी क्षीरविदारीक्षुद्रसहामहासहर्ष्य गन्धाश्वगन्धापयस्यावृश्चीरपु नर्नवाबृहतीकण्ट कारिकैरण्डमोर-टश्वदंष्ट्रासंहर्षशिताव रीशतपुष्पामधूकपुष्पीयष्टिमधुमधूलिकामृद्वी काखर्जूरपरूषकात्म गुप्तापुष्करबीजक-शेरुकराजादनकतक काश्मर्यशीतपाक्योदनपाकीतालखर्जूरमस्तकेक्षुरिक्षु वालिकादर्भ कुशकाशशालिगुन्द्रे-त्कटकशरमूल राजक्षवकर्ष्यप्रोक्ताद्वारदारभारद्वाजीव नत्रपुष्पभीपत्नी हंसपादी काकनासाकुलिंगाक्षीक्षीरव-ल्ली कपोतवल्लीगोपवल्लीमधुवल्ल्यः सोमवल्ली चेति... मधुरस्कन्धः ।१ (च. वि. ८।१३९)

काकोल्यादिः क्षीरघृतवसामज्जशालिषष्टिकयवगो मधूममाषशृङ्गाटकशेरुकत्र पुषैर्वारुबूकार्कारूकालाबू-कालि न्दकतकगिलोड्याप्रियाल पुष्करबीजकाश्मर्यमधूकद्राक्षाखर्जूर राजादनताल नारिकेलेक्षुविकारबला-तिबलात्म गुप्ताविदारी पयस्यागोक्षुरकक्षीरमोरटमधूलिकाकूष्माण्ड प्रभृतीनि समासेन मधुरो वर्गः ।" (सु. सू. ४२।११)

19. आम्राम्रातकलकुचकरमर्द वृक्षाम्लाम्लवेतसकुवलबदर दाडिममातुलुंगकरीरमलकनन्दी तकशीतकतिन्तिडी-कदन्शशक्लैरावतककोषा म्रधन्वनानां फलानि, पत्राणि चाम्रातकाश्मन्तकचांगेरीणां चतुर्विधानां चाम्लिकानौ द्वयोः कोलयोश्चामशुष्कयोर्द्वयोश्च शुष्काम्लिकयोर्ग्राम्यारण्ययोः, आसवद्रव्याणि च सुरासौवीरतुषोदकमैरेयमेदकमदिरामधुसीधुशुक्तदधिदधिमंडो दश्विद्धान्याम्लादीनि च... इति अम्लस्कन्धः । (च. वि. ८।१४०)

दाडिमामलकमातुलुंगाम्रातकक पित्थकरमर्दबदरकोलप्राचीनामलक तिन्तिडीककोशाम्रक भव्यपारावतवेत्र-फललकुचाम्लवेतसदन्त शक्लदधितक्रसुराशुक्तसौवीर कतुषोदकधान्याम्लप्रभृतीनि समासेनाम्लो वर्गः ।" (सु. स. ४२)

20. सैन्धवसौवर्चलकालबिडपाक्यानूपकूप्यबालुकैलमौलकसामुद्ररोम कौद् भिदौषरपाटेयकपांशुजानीत्येवं प्रकाराणि चान्यानि... लवणस्कन्धः ।" (च. वि. ८।१४१)

सैन्धवसौवर्चलविडपाक्यरोमसामुद्रपक्तिमयवक्षारोषरप्रसूत सुवर्चिकाप्रभृतीनि समासेन लवणो वर्गः ।" (सु. सू. ४२)

21. पिप्पलीपिप्पलीमूलहस्तिपिप्पलीचव्यचित्रकशङ्गवेरमरिचाजमोदार्द्र कविडङ्गकुस्तुम्बुरुपीलुतेजोवत्ये लाकुष्ठभल्लातकास्थिहिङ्गुकि लिमूलकसर्षपलशुनकरञ्जशिग्रुक मधुशिग्रुकखरपुष्पाभूस्तृ णसुमुखसुरसकु-ठेरकार्जकगण्डीर कालमालकपर्णासक्षवक फणिज्जकक्षारमूत्रपित्तानाम्... इति कटुकस्कन्धः ।" (च. वि. ८।१४२) (किलिम् देवदार)

पिप्पल्यादिः सुरसादिः शिग्रु-मधुशिग्र-मूलक-लशुन-सुमुख-शीतशिव- कुष्ठ-देवदारु- हरेणुकावल्गुजफल-चण्डा-गुग्गुल-मुस्त-लाङ्गलकी -शुकनासा-पीलुप्रभृतीनि सालसारादिश्च प्रायशः कटुको वर्गः ।" (सु. सू. ४२)

22. चन्दननलदकृतमालनक्तमाल निम्बतुम्बुरुकुटज हरिद्रादरुहरिद्रामुस्तमूर्वाकिराततिक्तककटु रोहिणीत्राय-माणा कारवेल्लिकाकरीरकर वीरकेवुककठिल्लकवृ षमण्डूकपर्णीकर्कोटकवार्त्ताकर्कशकाकमाचीकाकोदु-म्बरिका सुषव्यतिविषा पटोकुलकपाठार गुडूचीवेत्राग्रवेतसविकङ्कतबकुलसोमवल्कसप्तपर्णसुमनार्कावल्गु-जव चातगरागुरुबालकोशीर... इति तिक्तस्कन्धः ।" (च. वि. ८।१४३)

आरग्वधादिर्गुडूच्यादिर्मण्डूकपर्णोवेत्रकरीरहरिद्राद्वयेन्द्रयव वरुण स्वादुकण्टक सप्तपर्णबृहतीद्वयशंखिनीद्रव-न्तीत्रिवृत्कृतवे धनकोंट ककारवेल्लकवार्ता ककरवीरसुमनः शङ्खपुष्प्यपामार्गत्रायमाणाशोकरोहिणीवैजय-न्तीसुवर्चलापुनर्नवावृ श्चिकालीज्योतिष्मतीप्रभृतीनि समासेन तिक्तो वर्गः ।" (सु. स. ४२)

23. प्रियङ्ग्वनंता म्रास्थ्यम्बष्ठकीकट्वङ्गलोध्रमोचरससमङ्गाधातकी पुष्पपद्मकेशरजम्ब्वाम्रप्लक्षवटकपी तनोदुम्ब-राश्वत्थभल्लातकाश्मन् तकशिरीषशिंशपासोमवल्कतिन्दुक प्रियालबदरखदिर सप्तपर्णाश्वकर्णस्यन्दनार्जु-

नासना रिमैदैलवालुकपरि पेलवकदम्बशल्लकीजिङ्गिनीकाश कशेरुकराजकशेरुककट्फलवंश पद्मकाशोकशालधवसर्ज भूर्जशणखरपुष्पाशमीकवर कतुर्गाजकर्णाश्वकर्णस्फूर्जक बिभीतककुम्भीपुष्करबीजबिसमृणालताल खर्जूरतरुण्य : इति कषायस्कन्ध: । (च. वि. ८/१४४)

न्यग्रोधादिरम्बष्ठादि : प्रियङ्ग्वादि : रोध्रादिस्त्रिफलाशल्लकी जम्बाम्रबकुलतिन्दुकफलानि कतकशाकफलपाषाणभेदकवनस्पतिफलानि सालसारादिश्च प्रायश : कुरुबककोविदारजीवन्तीचिल्ली पालङ्क्यासुनिषण्णकप्रभृतीनि वरकादयो मुद्गादयश्च समासेन कषायो वर्ग: ।" (सु. सू. ४२)

24. स्वादु : पटुश्च मधुरम् अम्लोऽऽम्लंपच्यते रस: ।
तिक्तोषणकषायाणां विपाक: प्रायश: कटु: (वा. सू. ९।२१.)

25. उष्ण शीतं द्विधैवान्ये वीर्यमाचक्षतेऽपिच ।। वा.स.

26. चन्दनभद्रश्रीकालानुसार्यकालीयकपद्मापद्मकोशीरसारिवामधुकप्र पौण्डरीकनागपुष्पोदीच्यवन्य पद्मोत्पलनलिनकुमुदसौगन्धिक पुण्डरीकशतपत्रबिसमृणालशालूकशै वालकशेरुकानन्ताकुशकाशेक्षुदर्भशरन लशालिमूलजम्बुवेत्रवेतसवानी रगुन्द्राककुभासनाश्वकर्णस्यन्दनवातपोथ शालतालधवतिनिशखदिरकदरकदम्ब काश्मर्यफलसर्जप्लक्षकपीतनोदुम्बरा श्वत्थन्यग्रोधधातकीदूर्वेत्कटकशृङ्गाटकमञ्जिष्ठा ज्योतिष्मतीपुष्कर बीज कौञ्चादनबदरकोविदारकदील संवर्तकारिष्ट शतपर्वाश्वेतकुम्भिकाशतावरीश्रीपर्णीश्रावणी महाश्रावणीरोहिणीशीतपाक्यो दनपाकीकालाबलापयस्याविदारीजीवकर्षभकक्षुद्रसहामेदामहामेदामधु र सर्ष्यप्रोक्तातृणशून्यमोचरसाटरूषक- बकुलकुटजपटोलनिम्बशाल्मली नारिकेलखर्जूरमृद्वीकाप्रियालप्रियंगु गुधन्वनात्मगुप्तामधूक ।" (च. चि. ३।२५८)

27. अगुरुकुष्ठतगरपत्रनलदशैलेयकध्यामकहरेणुकास्थौणेयकक्षेमकैला वरा ङ्गदलपुरतमालपत्रभूतीक रोहिषसरलशल्लकीदेवदार्वग्नि मन्थबिल्वश्योनाककाश्मर्यपाटलापुनर्नवावृश्चीरकण्टका रिकाबृहतीशाल पर्णीपृश्निपर्णीमाषपर्णीमुद्गपर्णीगोक्षुरकैरण्डशोभाञ्ज नकवरुणार्कचिरबिल्वतिल्व कशटीपुष्कर मूलगंडीरो रुबूकपत्तूराक्षीवाश्मन्तकशिग्रुमातु लुङ्गमूलकमूलकपर्णीतिलपर्णी माषपर्णीमुद्गपर्णीगोक्षुरकैरण्डशोभाञ्ज नकवरुणार्कचिर बिल्वतिल्व कशटीपुष्करमूलगंडीरोरुबूकपत्तू राक्षीवाश्मन्तकशिग्रुमातु लुङ्गमूलकमूलकपर्णीपीलुपर्णीतिलपर्णी मोरटमेषशङ्गीहिंस्राादन्त शैरावतक भल्लातकास्फोतकोण्डीरात्मजा काकाण्डैकेषीकाकार ञधान्यकाजमोद पृथ्वीकासुमुखसुरसकु रककालमालकपर्णासक्षव कफणिज्जकभूस्तृणशृङ्गवेर पिपल्लीसर्षपाश्वगन्धारास्नारुहारोहा वचाबलातिबला गुडूचीशतपुष्पाशीतवल्लीनाकुलीगन्धनाकुलीश्वेताज्योति ष्मती चित्रकाध्यण्डाम्लचाङ्गेरीतिलबदरकुलत्थ ।" (च. चि. ३।२६७)

28. शमनं कोपनं स्वस्थहितं द्रव्यमिति त्रिधा । (अ. सं., अ. हृ. सू. १।६७ च. सू. १)

29. किंचिद्दोषप्रशमनं किंचिद्धातुप्रदूषणम् । स्वस्थवृत्तौ मतं किंचित्त्रिविधं द्रव्यमुच्यते । (च. सू. १ - ६७)

30. यदाहारजातमग्निवेश ! समांश्चैव शरीरधातून् प्रकृतौ स्थापयति विषमांश्च समीकरोतीत्येतद्धितं विद्धि, । विपरीतमहितमिति ।" (च. सू. २५।३३)

31. तत्र भद्रदारुकुष्ठहरिद्रावरुणमेषशृङ्गीबलातिबलार्तगलकच्छु राशल्लकीकुबेराक्षीवीर तरुसहचराग्निमन्थवत्सादन्ये रण्डाश्मभेदकालकार्कशतावरीपुनर्नवावसुकवशिरकाञ्चन भाङ्गींकार्पासीवृश्चिकालीपत्तूरबदरयवकोलकुलत्थप्रभृतीनि विदारिगन्धादिश्च द्वे चाद्ये पञ्चमूल्यौ समासेन वातसंशमनो वर्ग: ।" (सु. सू. ३९)

32. रूक्ष: शीतो लघु: सूक्ष्मश्चलोऽथ विशद: खर: । विपरीतगुणैर्द्रव्यैर्मारुत: संप्रशाम्यति ।। (च. सू. १-५९)

33. तत्र मधुराम्ललवणा वातघ्ना: ।" (सु. सू. ४१)
गुरुपाको वातपित्तघ्न: ।" (सु. सू. ४१)

तत्र उष्णस्निग्धौ वातघ्नौ ।" (सु. सू. ४१)

34. चन्दनकुचन्दन-हीबेरोशीरमञ्जिष्ठाय पस्याविदारीशतावरी गुन्द्राशैवालकल्हारकुमुदोत्पल कदलीदूर्वामूर्वाप्रभृतीनि काकोल्यादि: सारिवादिरञ्जनादिरुत्पलादिर्न्यग्रोधादिस्तृण पञ्चमलमिति समासेन पित्तसंशयनो वर्ग: ।" (सु. सू. ३९)

35. सस्नेहमुष्णं तीक्ष्णं च द्रवमम्लं सरं कटु । विपरीतगुणै: पित्तं द्रव्यैराशु प्रशाम्यति ।" (च. सू. १.६०)

36. मधुरतिक्तकषाया: पित्तघ्ना: ।" (सु. सू. ४१)
गुरुपाको वातपित्तघ्न: ।" (सु. सू. ४१)
शीतमृदुपिच्छिला: पित्तघ्ना: ।" (सु. सू. ४१)

37. कालेयकागुरुतिलपर्णीकुष्ठ हरिद्राशीतशिवशत पुष्पासरलरास्नाप्रकीर्योदकीर्येङ्गुदीसुमन: काकादनीलाङ्गल-कीहस्तिकर्णमुञ्जातकला मज्जकप्रभृतीनि वल्लीकण्टकपञ्चमूल्यौपिप्पल्यादिर्बृहत्यादिर्मुष्ककादिर्वचादि: सुरसादिराग्वधादिरिति समासेन श्लेष्मसंशमनो वर्ग: ।" (सु. सू. ३९)

38. गुरुशीतमृदुस्निग्धमधुरस्थिरपिच्छिला: । श्लेष्मण: प्रशमं यान्ति विपरीतगुणैर्गुणा:।" (च. सू. १-६१)

39. कटुतिक्तकषाया: श्लेष्मघ्ना: ।" (सु. सू. ४१)
लघुपाक: श्लेष्मघ्न: ।" (सु. सू. ४१)

40. तत्रकटुतिक्तकषायरूक्षलघुशीतवीर्यशुष्कशाकवल्लरकउद्दाल ककोरदूष श्यामाकनीवार मुद्गमसूराढकीहरे-णुकलायनिष्पाव... वेगविघातादिभिर्विशेषै: वायु: प्रकोपमापद्यते । (सु. सू. अ. २१)

तत्रतिक्तकटुकषायरूक्ष लघुशीतविष्टंभिविरूढ कत्तृणधान्यकलायचणककरीतुम्बकालिंग चिर्भिटबिसशा-लूकजाम्बवतिन्दुक,.. शोकोत्कण्ठ्यादिभिरतिसे: वायु: प्रकोपमापद्यते । (अ. सं. नि. १)

41. कट्वम्ललवणतीक्ष्णोष्णलघुविदाहितिल तैलपिण्याककुल त्थसर्षपातसीहरीतकशाकगो धामत्स्यआविकमांसद धितक्रकूर्चिकामस्तुसौवीरकसुराविकाराम्लफलकट्वरप्रभृतिभि: पित्तं प्रकोपमापध्यते । (सु. सू. अ. २१)

कट्वम्ललवणक्षारोष्ण तीक्ष्णविदाहिशुक्तशाण्डिकी मध्यमूत्रमस्तुदधिधान्याम्लतैलकुलत्थ माषनिष्पावति-लान्नकट्वरकुळेरादिवर्गा म्रातकाम्लिकापीलुभल्लातका स्थिलाङ्गलिकामरिच... मैथुनोपगमनादिभि: पित्तं प्रकोपमापद्यते ।" (अ. सं. नि. १)

42. .... मधुराम्ललवणशीतस्निग्ध गुरुपिच्छिलाभिष्यन्दिहायनकयवकनैषधे त्कषमाषमहामाषगोधूमतिलपि-ष्टविकृतिदधिदुग्ध कृशरापायसेक्षुविकारा नूपौदकमांसवसाबिसमृणालकसेरुकशृङ्गाटकमधुरवल्लीफल... प्रभृतिभि: श्लेष्मा प्रकोपमापद्यते ।" (सु. सू. २१) १मधुराम्ललवणस्निग्धगुरु पिच्छिलाभिष्यन्दिन-वान्नपिष्टपृथुकस्थूल भक्ष्यशष्कुल्यामक्षीर किलाटमोरटकूर्चिकातक्रपिण्डकपीयूषेक्षुरसफाणितगुडानूपपिशि-तमो चखर्जूरभव्यनारिकेल... योगदिभि... श्लेष्मा प्रकोपमापद्यते ।" (अ. सं. नि. १)

43. लोहितशालय: शूकधान्यानां पथ्यतमत्वेन श्रेष्ठतमा भवन्ति, मुद्गा: शमीधान्यानाम्, आन्तरीक्षमदु-कानां, सैन्धवं लवणानाम्, जीवन्तीशाकं शाकानाम् ऐणेयं मृगमांसानां, लावपक्षिणां, गोधा बिलेश-यानां, रोहितो मत्स्यानां, गव्यं सर्पि: सर्पिषां, गोक्षीरं क्षीराणां, तिल तैल स्थावरजातानां स्नेहानाम्, वराहवसा आनूपमृगवासानां, चुलुकीवसा मत्स्यवसानां, पाकहंसवसा जलचरविहङ्गवासानां, कुक्कुट-वसा विष्किरशकुनिवसानाम्, अजमेद: शाखादमेदसां, शृङ्गवेरं कन्दानां, मृद्वीका फलानां, शर्करा इक्षुविकाराणआमिति प्रकृत्यैव हिततमानामाहारविकाराणां प्राधान्यतो द्रव्याणि व्याख्यातानि भवति ।" (च. सू. २५।३८)

तद्यथा – रक्तशालिषष्टिकङ्कुकमुकुन्दकपाण्डु कपीतकप्रमोदककालकासनपुष्प ककर्दमकशकुनाहृतसुगन्ध ककलमनीवारकोद्रवोद्दालकश्यामाकगोधूमवेणुयवादय: । एणहरिणकुरङ्गमृगमातृकाश्वदंष्ट्राकरालक्रकर कपोतलावतित्तिरिक पिञ्जलवर्त्तीकादीनां मांसानि मुद्गवनमुद्गमकुष्ठकलायमसूरमङ्गल्यचणकहरे ण्वाढकीसतीना: ।

चिल्लिवास्तुकसुनिषण्णक जीवन्तीतण्डुलीयकरण्डूकपर्ण्य: । गव्यं घृत सैन्धवदाडिमामलकमित्येष वर्ग: सर्वप्राणिनां सामान्यत: पथ्यतम् : ।" (सु. सू. २०)

44. तोयक्षीरेक्षुतैलानांवर्गैर्मद्यस्यक्रमात् । इतिद्रवैकदेशोऽयं उक्तो नित्योपयौगिक: ।। (वा. सू. ५)

45. शूकशिम्बीजपक्वान्नमांसशाकफलौषधे: । वर्गितैरन्नलेशोऽयमुक्तो नित्योपयोगिक: । (अ. हृ. सू. ६)

46. द्रवअयाण्युक्तानि गणशो मिश्रीकृत्य समासत: ।

47. गुडूचयादिरयं वर्ग: प्रथम: परिकीर्तित: । उर्ध्वाधोदोषहरण: सर्वामयविनाशन: ।।

48. इहौषधिधातुधान्यद्रवपक्वान्नमांसग: ।
सविहारो मिश्रकश्च नानार्थो नवम: स्मृत: ।। (के. नि.)

CHAPTER FOUR
THE GUNAS

Etymology of "Guna"

The Gunas are called so because :

1) They are dependent on the dravyas and have an inseparable relationship with the dravya 2) they are inactive 3) these are non-essential causes (असमवायि कारण) for the existence of the dravyas ie. the dravya may exist without the prior existence of gunas. Thus, these have a secondary or subordinate status and are called gunas (because of their गौणत्व). We use a dravya for its actions. Why then, do we need gunas ? The answer to this question is that gunas are necessary for the action itself. If a dravya does not have gunas (properties) it will not be able to carry out any karma (action). The gunas (properties) reside in the dravya (substance). From the point of view of generating karma (actions), the gunas (properties) cannot be underestimated. Karmas also reside in the dravya; and the dravya is essential for karma also. Since the gunas are inactive (ie. without karma) and since these are non-essential to the existence of drayvas, the gunas have a secondary or subordinate status as compared to dravyas and therefore they are called gunas.[1]

Characteristics of Gunas

"समवायी तु निश्चेष्ट. Here, the word निश्चेष्ट has been intentionally added to the characteristics of guna in order to differentiate it from karma. If only the word समवायी would have been used, it might have transgressed the characteristics of gunas since karmas also have an inseparable relationship to the dravyas and reside in the dravyas. To prevent this transgression and to clarify the characteristics of gunas from those of karmas, the word निश्चेष्ट is necessary कारणंगुण:[2] means that a phenomenon which has an inseparable closeness to the dravya, which does not provide an abode to the gunas, which is a non-essential cause and which is different from karma is called guna. समवायिकारणत्वं द्रव्यस्येवेति विज्ञेयम् । गुणकर्म मात्रवृत्तिज्ञेयमथाप्यसमवायिहेतुत्वम् ।।

Dravya sustains guna-karma, but guna cannot sustain guna-karma.[3] Karma also resides in the dravya; and it is a non-essential cause as well. Yet, it is the cause of aggregation and seggregation at the same time. Seggregation and aggregation are both gunas. This is the difference between guna-karma.[4] Guna is the cause of karma and karma is the cause of knowledge of gunas.

Various characteristics of the dravya are known as guna.

The author of the text Rasavaisheshik describes gunas as विश्वलक्षणगुणा : as these are responsible for the presence of various characteristics of padartha (substance).[5]

If a particular karma (action) is established, there must be a guna (property) within that particular dravya which has inspired this karma. The reverse is not true ie. if a guna is present in a dravya, the corresponding action has to be generated. Even though the dravyas are important as they provide support (abode) to the gunas, yet dravyas have no value in the absence of gunas.

The same substance may appear different depending on variations in its gunas. For example water is seen in the form (state) of water, steam and ice. The difference between these three states is felt because of difference in their gunas.[6]

Guna acts as a medium for understanding the peculiarities of the dravya.[7]

It is an acceptable principle that every guna has a definite action (karma). A single dravya may have many gunas (properties) and single specific guna may be present in many dravyas.

Classification of Gunas

Charakacharya has ennumerated 41 gunas. Chakradatta, a commentator of Charaka samhita, has subdivided these into three groups.[8]

1) Vaisheshik gunas 2) Samanya gunas 3) Atma gunas. Among these, samanya gunas are further divided into two groups.

गुणाः एकचत्वारिंशत् गुणाः

Atma gunas (आत्मगुणाः = आत्मनः गुणाः)

1.	Buddhi	-	intellect
2.	Ichchha	-	desire
3.	Dwesh	-	aversion (jealousy)
4.	Sukha	-	pleasure
5.	Dukkha	-	pain
6.	Prayatna	-	effort

Buddhi 1 + Prayatnant 5 = 6

Vaisheshik gunas (पञ्चमहाभूतानां विशेषगुणाः)

1.	Shabda	(sound)	-	[ear]	akash
2.	Sparsha	(touch)	-	[skin]	vayu
3.	Roopam	(shape/colour)	-	[eyes]	teja
4.	Rasa	(savour/taste)	-	[tongue]	jala
5.	Gandha	(odour)	-	[nose]	prithvi

Gunas

- Adhibhautik (35)
  - Samanya 30
    - Gurvadi gunas 20
    - Paradi gunas 10
  - Vishishta 5
    - Indriyartha 5 (shabda, sparsha, roopa, rasa, gandha)
- Adhyatmik (6)
  - Ichchha, dwesha, sukha, dukkha prayatna, buddhi

अर्थः गुर्वादयो बुधिः प्रयत्नान्ताः परादय :

5 + 20 + 1 + 5 + 10 = 41

Samanya gunas (सामान्य गुणा: पृथिव्यादिनां साधारणत्वात्)

1. Guru	antagonist	11. Laghu
2. Manda	"	12. Teekshna
3. Hima	"	13. Ushna
4. Snigdha	"	14. Ruksha
5. Shlakshna	"	15. Khara
6. Sandra	"	16. Drava
7. Mridu	"	17. Kathina
8. Sthira	"	18. Sara
9. Sookshma	"	19. Sthoola
10. Vishada	"	20. Pichchila

The gurvadi and paradi gunas are normally present in the mahabhootas[9] hence these are samanya gunas. And shabda, sparsha, roopa, rasa and gandha are the special gunas of these mahabhootas. Therefore these are called vishesha gunas or vaisheshik gunas[10] (special gunas) [vaisheshik = vishishtha]. Vaisheshik gunas are specifically helpful in identification and knowledge of dravyas.

Gurvadi 20, paradi 10 and vaisheshik 5 = 35 - these gunas are associated with the material world and hence these are called Adhibhautik gunas. The six atma gunas (buddhi 1 + prayatnanta 5 = 6), being associated with the soul (spirit), are called Adhyatmik gunas.

Adhyatmik gunas - 1) buddhi 2) ichchha 3) dwesha 4) sukha 5) dukkha and 6) prayatna are the six Adhyatmik gunas.[11]

Since the gunas like ahankar, chetana, medha, dhruti, smruti, mati, pratipatti etc are attributes of buddhi, these are included in buddhi itself.[12]

Chetana - consciousness, alertness (अहंकार बुध्दिविकारः) (च शारीर अ १/६३ टीका)

Medha - retentive faculty, retentiveness ग्रंथाकर्षणसामर्थ्यम् । धी धारणावति मेधा ।

Dhruti - firmness, steadiness मनः संतुष्टिः। नियमात्मिका बुध्दिः।

Smruti - memory, recollection पुर्वानुभूतस्य स्मरणम् (अर्थधारणाशक्तिः।)

Mati - understanding, sense, intellect अनागतार्थोद्देशः । त्रिकालविषयाबुध्दिरिति अन्ये)

Pratipatti - intelligence अर्थावबोधप्रागल्भ्यं अनुष्णनं वा ।

Bodily gunas

Gurvadi gunas are 20 in number. These gunas are closely related to the gross material body. These gunas are predominantly seen in the body constituents. Therefore these are also called shareer

There may be a vast difference in taking treatment by an Ayurvedic physician and that from Ayurvedic system of medicine.

gunas. These 20 gunas form 10 twin pairs of antagonist gunas.[13]

These antagonist gunas are present in all dravyas. Every dravya has all the twenty gunas in varying proportions. Even totally contradictory gunas may be present in a dravya. Yet, a drayva is said to be possessing a particular guna or to be made up of a specifie mahabhoota if that particular guna or mahabhoota is in abundance in that dravya. No dravya has absolute qualities.[14] (Even absolute alcohol is not absolute. That too, is so-called absolute. Every minute particle of a dravya always contains these antagonist gunas. These antagonist gunas are also present in each and every constituent of the body. All the existential phenomena present in the universe are also present within this body. This body as well as the dravyas outside this body are made up of panchamahabhootas and all the twenty gunas are present in these panchamahabhootas. This being so, these 20 gunas are present in every dravya and also in this panchabhautik body. This is what is meant by b प्रवृत्तिरुभयस्य तु । (च. सू. १)

Among these 20 gunas, guru, snigdha, hima, mrudu, laghu, ruksha, ushna and teekshna gunas are more potent and hence are known as veerya. (Nagarjuna has added vishada and pichchila gunas to this list and the number rises to ten.)

While classifying the gunas, Sushrutacharya has mentioned the pair of mridu-teekshna instead of manda-teekshna. This view is acceptable to Nagarjuna. Apart from this, there is a lot of difference between the list of gunas given by Charaka, Sushruta, Bhavaprakash and Vagbhatta.

Nevertheless, the view of those who state that there is no fixed number of gunas must also be given serious consideration. For example, sugandhi (fragrant), durgandhi (foul smelling), vyavayi, vikashi, ashukari, shuchi, vimal and visra gunas are very helpful in our day to day living.

Thus, the number of gunas is not fixed. As such, the number of gunas is not limited to twenty, but since these twenty gunas are most commonly used in our daily life, only these have been included in the chapter related to gunas. Neverthless, there is no opposition to the possible addition of more gunas to the list of gunas. (It is possible that due to the limitations of the human senses, all the gunas may not be perceptible and thus many gunas may be totally unknown to human beings. प्रत्यक्षं हि अल्पं अनल्पं अप्रत्यक्षम् - चरक).

Paradi gunas

These are 10 in number. The gunas like para, apara, yukti, sankhya, samyoga, vibhaga, pruthkatva, pariman, sanskar and abhyas are also material gunas and these are also used in our day to day living. Therefore, knowledge of these gunas is necessary (These gunas have been elaborately explained further on in this chapter).

Vishishta Gunas

These are material gunas. These are five in number viz. shabda, sparsha, roopa, rasa and gandha and are specific properties of akash, vayu, teja, jala and prithvi. The gurvadi gunas may be present in any dravya but a guna like shabda (sound) is an exclusive property of akash. There can be no shabda (sound) without akash. There can be no tangibility without vayu.

There is a specific sequence in mixing dravyas which are used for basti i.e. माक्षिकं...क्रमत् The significance of this sequence does not even cross our minds.

Teja mahabhoota is the cause of existence and discernibility of roopa guna. Rasa, which is a property of food and medicines, has no existence devoid of jala. Similarly, prithvi is the cause of gandha.The perception of these gunas also occurs only through those senses which have an abundance of the particular mahabhoota and not through other senses. Therefore, these are called Vishishta gunas. Among these, "rasa" is of prime importance in "dravyaguna" (ज्ञानेंद्रियाणि पंचानि न तु षष्ठ हि वर्तते)

Rasa is that property which has been utilised to the maximum in dravyagunashastra from 20 gurvadi gunas, 10 paradi gunas and 5 vishishta gunas. These varying gunas constantly act on the body. Some of the effects (actions) generated by these gunas are direct and demonstrable while others are known by inferential knowledge. Direct knowledge (कर्मभिस्त्वनुमीयन्ते नानाद्रव्याश्रयाः गुणाः) of gunas depends on the senses.

Now, let us consider the utility of gurvadi and paradi gunas in dravyagunashastra. All the gunas are important. We cannot conceptualise a dravya without these gunas. We have seen earlier that gunas can neither sustain the gunas nor actions; therefore, the actions which we feel are generated by the gunas, are in fact, generated by the dravya which imitates and acts in accordance with the gunas. In our daily life we state that a particular rasa is guru and so on. This is due to the close association between the two. The gunas are responsible for generating the actions, yet, gunas depend on the dravya. This is the reason for using adjectives like guru, laghu etc. for the dravya. In fact, the actions of the dravyas are not due to these adjectives but due to the dravya to which these adjectives apply. The gunas which appear to have an action on the body actually do so by increasing or decreasing the corresponding gunas of the body constituents. The increase or decrease thus induced is not possible without conjunction and disjunction (सयोग-विभाग) and this conjunction and disjunction is not of gunas but of dravya-components.

1. Guru - This means heavy by weight (but this is a coarse interpretation). The actual meaning of 'guru' is that it is heavy to digest. The estimation of the "guru" property should be done in context to the agnibala (digestive capacity). This guna creates heaviness in the body and reduces the digestive capacity (अग्निमंदता). Guru dravyas are digested slowly. Obviously, for digesting guru dravyas, the agni has to use considerable energy and thus the agni becomes weaker. This guru is principally found in prithvi mahabhoota.[15] It is also present in jala mahabhoota, but as a secondary guna. Teja, vayu and akash mahabhoota donot have this guna. This guna is responsible for the natural downward movement.[16] This guna reduces vata and increases kapha. Generally, guru guna is nutritive as it increases all the dhatus and it also produces heaviness in the malayanas and the srotasas (various channels) of the body.[17] Presence of this guna produces lassitude and laxity. Black gram and milk products are examples of guru dravyas. This guna is antagonist guna of laghu. Dravyas having madhur rasa are the heaviest. Generally, the dravyas of madhur varga are guru.

The dravyas which bring about bruhan of the body are guru.[18]

The components of guru dravyas are compactly arranged. The constituents of the body also become more compact on account of guru dravyas. Due to this compactness, pachak pitta cannot easily breakdown these dravyas. Therefore these are heavy to digest. The guru guna is more influential during the bestowal period (visarga kala) of the year and it gradually becomes more and more

Water is the best life-giving dravya for living creatures. But even a healthy man should drink it sip by sip.

influential as the period progresses.

2. Laghu - Laghu means light. Lighter by weight means laghu. Also, the guna, which, through its presence, brings about lightness of the body is called laghu.[19] This definition is relative to the action of agni. The word "laghu" is also used in context with "heavy".

Laghu dravyas relieve kapha and increase vata. This guna causes depletion of the dhatus of the body. It is also lekhana and facilitates healing of wounds (lekhan - reducing viscosity - Dalhan). Laghu dravyas clear the channels of the body of their wastes and bring lightness in the body. Laghu dravyas are easy to digest, increase the agni and relieve false sense of contentment (anti - saturative). Yet, over use of laghu guna is not desirable. Laghu dravyas induce a feeling of enthusiasm and alertness.[20] Laghu guna is the prime attribute of akash, yet vayu and teja mahabhoota also possess this guna. Laghu dravyas should be used in diseases generated by guru diet like aam, prameha, udar, jvara, grahani etc.

The property of lightness (laghu) can be created in food items by suitable conditioning; but rice flakes, moong and flesh of leva bird etc. are naturally laghu. This is so because the components of these dravyas are not compactly arranged.

Tikta rasa (bitter taste) is the lightest. This is the most approriate rasa in jvara roga (other rasas are contraindicated in jvara for different reasons). Laghu guna increases naturally during the procurement period of the year.

Akash is also of laghu guna. Presence of laghu guna does not imply absence of guru guna. Not only laghu guna but each and every guna also has an independent existence. The word सविपर्यय (meaning - along with its antagonist guna) has been deliberately used to emphasize the independent existence of each gunas.

3. Sheeta - Cold to touch. Naturally, it alleviates burning sensation (consequence of ushna [hot]). The guna which reduces the excessive heat in the body is known as sheeta guna. Sheeta guna reduces pitta (ushna guna) and increases vata-kapha (sheeta-guna). Generally, it increases all the dhatus of the body and acts as haemostatic. It increases the quantity of urine but induces constipation and acts as an anti-perspirant and as a mood-elevator. It reduces the symptoms produced by pitta like fainting, excessive thirst, burning sensation and pleases the mind.[21] Prithvi and vayu may appear cold bu-t this property does not belong to them. Sheeta guna is the exclusive property of jala mahabhoota. शीतस्पर्शवत्य: आप:।

Cold tangibility is the property of jala mahabhoota only, wherever it may be. Even the cold tangibility of iron is due to jala mahabhoota. Chandanadi varga, doorvadi varga etc. are examples of sheeta dravyas. This guna does not help in shodhana but is useful for shamana (pacification of doshas). The dravyas that induce stambhan action have sheeta guna.

Sheeta guna aids congestion. The constituents of the body also contract and thus the action of stambhan is produced. It propagates immobility. When, due to trauma, there is external or internal bleeding, sheeta guna is useful for haemostasis. Application of ice or cold water is found to be very useful for arresting external or internal bleeding due to trauma.[22]

An incompetent vaidya has been critisized badly and therefore a vaidya should be alert about his own abilities.

Hemant, shishir and varsha ritus are seasons having sheeta guna. Sheeta guna does not imply absence of ushna guna but sheeta guna has an independent existence.

4. Ushna - Hot touch is known as ushna. It is the antagonist of sheeta. Ushna guna has an innate tendency to increase burning sensation. It increases the heat of the dhatus of the body.[23]

Ushna guna increases pitta while sheeta guna increases kaphavata. Ushna guna reduces the fluidity of dhatus and causes their depletion. It is an adjunct to shodhana and bloodletting but is not advisable in raktapitta. Since ushna guna is inducive to shodhana, it facilitates excretion of faeces, urine and sweat. It produces fainting, giddiness, excessive thirst and burning sensation; it produces lassitude and is primarily seen in agni mahabhoota, prithvi, jala and vayu mahabhootas. Though it may feel hot to touch yet it is not the guna of these mahabhootas. It is as if these mahabhootas have taken the ushna guna on lease from teja mahabhoota. Ushna guna exclusively belongs to teja mahabhoota.[24]

Chitrakadi dravyas, maricha, pippali, sunthi, chillies are all ushna in property and action. The sun's rays, fire are examples of dravyas which are hot to touch. The guna which causes perspiration is ushna guna.[25]

Ushna guna is dominant during aadan kala (procurement period of the year) and sharad ritu. "Pachan" is the action of ushna guna.[26]

5. Snigdha - Due to this guna various parts of the body like skin become moist and unctuous. Snigdha guna is the exclusive property of jala mahabhoota.

Snigdha guna relieves vata and increases kapha which has a similar tendency. Snigdha guna strengthens all the dhatus. Sneha has an innate similarity with the constituents of the body and propagates the compactness between the components of various dhatus. This compactness relieves the laxity in dhatu components and thereby strengthens them. Snigdha guna brings about softness of srotas (various channels of the body) and thus there is better conveyance of dosha-dhatu-mala.

Regarding diet, it is said in the scriptures that स्निग्धं अश्नीयात् (food must have snigdha guna in it). The doshas get moistened on account of sneha and the removal of these doshas becomes easier. स्नेहात् क्लेदो विवर्धते snigdha dravyas have been used for snehana before instituting shodhana chikitsa. Snigdha guna is useful for shamana as well. Snehan is vajikar (aphrodisiac).[27]

Jala mahabhoota is the specific cause of snigdha guna. This guna is described as जलमात्रवृत्ति. Ghee, taila (oil), vasa (fats), majja (marrow) are representative dravyas of snigdha guna. Snigdha guna is the antagonist guna of ruksha. It has an independent existence too. Snigdha dravyas are guru.

Snigdha guna starts increasing gradually from the middle of visarga kala (bestowal period) and keeps on increasing till the end of hemant ritu. Further, ruksha guna starts increasing in shishir ritu.

6. Ruksha - This guna is the antagonist of snigdha. Presence of this guna brings about dryness. This guna has the capacity to absorb. That guna which brings about ununctuousness, hardness and dryness is called ruksha. Vayu mahabhoota possesses ruksha guna. Ruksha guna aggravates vata dosha. Ruksha guna has been mentioned first among all the other gunas of vata (तत्र रूक्षोलघु...) It

If a vaidya treats a patient successfully, there is no doubt about the fact that either money, friendship, religion, success or experience will be achieved.

reduces the snigdha guna of kapha dosha. The mild snigdha guna of pitta dosha also decreases by ruksha guna and as a consequence, teja mahabhoota, which is ruksha, increases.

Ruksha reduces laxity in the constituents of the body and strengthens them. Loose skin also improves. In fact this guna improves the skin in all such conditions which involve an increase in snigdha guna of the skin (as in madhumeha, prameha). In other conditions, ruksha guna causes depletion of strength. Due to this property, it reduces the water content in the body wastes and stagnates them. This guna is most useful for relieving kapha dosha.[28]

Vayu mahabhoota is the real abode of this guna. Food items like yava, vanshakareea, rajgeera, nagli etc. which are a part of our diet, and drugs like haritaki, chitrak etc. are examples of dravyas having ruksha guna.

Ruksha guna starts increasing from the beginning of the procurement period (adan kala) and subsequently the body also becomes ruksha. Shishir, vasant and greeshma ritus are more ruksha, in increasing order. (Vaisheshik darshan has equated ruksha guna with absence of snigdha guna; but Ayurveda has alloted independent existence to ruksha guna). Vata - vruddhi (aggravation of vata dosha) means the snigdha guna in each and every constituent of the body decreases and these constituents take up gunas like ruksha etc. which identify with vata dosha. Conversely, vata-kshaya (reduction of vata-dosha) means these constituents take-up gunas like snigdha, guru etc. (च. सू. अ. १२)

7. Manda - This guna is familiar to all. We use the word manda (dull) quite often as an adverb/ adjective for work, walking, fire, intellect and senility. This guna has the least amount of mobility; hence its action is also slow and mild. This guna is useless for shodhana but is good for shamana. It increases kapha, which has similar tendency. (स्निग्ध: शीतो गुरुर्मन्द:). Teekshna guna, which is the prime attribute of pitta dosha and an antagonist of manda guna, is pacified by manda guna. It increases all the dhatus of the body and since it slows down digestion, it acts as a nutritive.

Manda guna is acquired by the presence of prithvi and jala mahabhoota. All the manda dravyas like shatavari, doorva, anantamool are examples of shamana dravyas. These dravyas have properties anatagonist to teekshna guna.

While describing the properties of various dravyas in dravyagunashastra, manda guna has been used less often. Manda guna is in abundance in hemant ritu. It pacifies teekshna pitta which aggravates during sharad ritu (manda means that which acts mildly and gives stability to the body).[29]

8. Teekshna - In our day to day practice we use the word teekshna (sharp) for the edges of weapons and for describing the properties of old liquor, maricha etc. In dravyagunakarma also, teekshna guna has been mentioned in the gunas of mohari, maricha, chitraka etc. तीक्ष्ण : छेदने । The dravyas having teekshna guna have many actions and these are equally rapid as well. Generally, teekshna guna, induces shodhana.[30] Dravyas like danti (आताम्रश्यावतीक्ष्णोष्ण), tridhari nivdung, jayphal, mohri are teekshna, shodhana dravyas. Teekshna guna is an attribute of Agni mahabhoota. As this guna is similar to the gunas of pitta, it is natural that teekshna pitta will be increased by this guna. Kapha-vata are decreased by teekshna guna. Teekshna dravyas cause depletion of the dhatus and

A medical practitioner should know at what stage of the disease a medicine should be administered. However, it is more important for him to know in what conditions a particular medicine should not be given.

thereby emaciation of the body. Since the tendency of these dravyas is conducive to shodhana, these are used for removal of malas. This guna produces distress of the body constituents, burning sensation and putrefaction.[31] Among the panchamahabhootas, agni mahabhoota is the causal dravya of this guna. Generally, this guna co-exists with ushna guna. The dravyas having teekshna guna are lekhana (reducing viscosity). It alleviates kapha vata.[32]

Teekshna guna increases in sharad, vasant and greeshma ritus. Since pitta possesses teekshna guna, agni, which resides in pitta dosha is also teekshna. If kapha cannot control this teekshnagni, it may result in bhasmak roga (a disease characterised by abnormal hunger).[33]

9. Sthira - The guna which is immobile is called sthira guna. "Sara" guna is the antagonist of sthira. From this, one can have an idea about sthira. This guna has very little vibrations, tremors etc. It does not have unsteadiness. Sthira guna is essential for sustainability.

The body has both, mobile and immobile constituents. Among these, paternal constituents like hair, bones, nails, teeth etc which resemble bones, as well as other constituents like sira, snayu, dhamani and shukra are sthira constituents.[34]

All the dhatus are essentially sthira. If "shodhana" has been done properly, one of the parameters of knowing that shodhana has been done properly is "dhatu sthiratva". Yet, sthira guna should be seen in context with sara. The dhatus have an innate tendency towards vruddhi (increase) or kshaya (decrease). This continuous drift towards a state of either increase or decrease is not possible without saratva. Yet, dhatusara is predominantly believed to be of sthira guna. Their sthiratva is not absolute. Individuals in whom the dhatus are comparatively sthira do not undergo considerable change in their body weight which may remain unchanged for years. This is a sign of dhatu-shiratva as also of good health. "Buddhi" (intellect) should also be sthira.

From the point of view of doshas, it is kaphavardhak. (स्थिर: कफ:) This guna reduces pitta-vayu which are of sara and chala gunas. The chief action of this guna is to provide strength to the body by increasing the sthiratva of the malas and thereby stagnate vata and malas.[35]

This guna increases in hemant and shishir ritus. Among the mahabhootas, prithvi mahabhoota which possesses sthira guna, is the causal dravya of this guna. Dravyas like nutmeg, opium possess this guna.

10. Sara - This guna spreads because of its fluidity.[36] This guna has the capacity of "preran" (प्र + इरण). Sara guna is the antagonist of sthira guna. The dravyas having this guna provide impetus to vata, pitta, kapha and malas.[37] Sara guna causes mild attenuation of the dhatus. Similarly, it causes anuloman of the malas.[38]

In atisara (diarrhoea), the sara guna of the malas increases. The sara guna is produced by the drava guna of jala. Sara guna increases mobility.

Milk among food items and haritaki, bahva, kutki etc. among medicines are examples of sara dravyas. In atisara, the saratva in the malas and intestine increases.

In vasant ritu, the "sara" guna of kapha increases with an increase in its fluidity and this may

The surnames like Vaidya, Bhise (originated from Bhishak), Doctor, Hakim etc. are symbolic of the different systems of medicine to which their families belonged.

cause atisara.

11. Mridu - In our daily usage, it is termed as "soft". This guna is the antagonist of "hard". This is a tangible guna which is tender and soft to touch.[39]

The maternal organs of the body like mansa, rakta, meda, majja, hridaya, nabhi, yakrit , pleeha, antra (intestine), rectum etc. are soft (mridu) to touch.[40]

The guna which has the ability to produce laxity is called mridu. Presence of mridu guna generates tenderness, softness and laxity in the body.

Dravyas having this guna are kaphavardhak (increasing kapha) and pittashaman (pacifying pitta). One of the less prominent actions of this guna is vata shaman. Mridu guna is the antagonist guna of kathina (hard).[41] It softens the constituents of the body and alleviates burning sensation and putrefaction; it brings laxity in the malas as well.[42]

Just as jala mahabhoota is necessary for generating the softness of this guna, similarly akash mahabhoota is necessary for distinctiveness. Sweda (fomentation) is very useful for softening swelling etc. (स्वेदो मार्दवकराणां श्रेष्ठः । च. सू. अ. २५) Mridu guna is generated by akash and aap mahabhoota.[43] Mridu guna increases in sharad and hemant ritus.

12. Kathina - The word 'kathina" implies hardness. This guna, just like its antagonist mridu guna, is perceptible through touch. Presence of this guna brings hardness, firmness and steadiness in the constituents of the body.[44]

This guna is vatavardhak (increases vata). Sleeping on a kathina (hard) bed or sitting on a hard seat for a long period can bring on pain due to increase in vata. This guna is not so widely used in treatment. Yet the actions of this guna like stambha (stagnation) are quite evident. Signs of prithvi mahabhoota like strengthening the dhatus, reducing the water content of malas, making the faeces very hard, hardening the edges of wounds are induced by this guna.

Where else can this guna reside except in prithvi and vayu mahabhootas?[45]

The diet and medicines which alleviate the flaccidity or laxity of the body constituents possess this guna.

13. Vishada - Vishada means clean. If the hands are first washed by shikakai, soap, amalaki etc. and then by water, then the guna which is generated is "vishada" - pichchila guna is the antagonist of vishada. Pichchila is that particular guna which is present in nasal discharge, rakta, shukra, aam and pus. The antagonist of this Pichchila guna is vishada. "Kshalana" means washing; the dravyas which have this capacity are called vishada.[46] Kashaya rasa (astringent) has vishada guna.

The action of this guna is to increase vata by decreasing kapha. Internally, this guna causes depletion of the dhatus and externally it promotes early healing of wounds by cleaning the wounds.[47]

This guna alleviates the pichchila guna of aam, mala and makes them clean. All the four mahabhootas other than jala mahabhoota collectively generate this guna. Vishada guna is abundant in greeshma ritu and dravyas like kshar, honey, astringent dravyas, shikakai, ritha, amalaki and

In the 39th chapter of Uttar tantra of Vagbhatta samhita, it is mentioned that if one has to survive, one must change with time.

nyagrodhadi varga are examples of dravyas which have vishada guna.

14. Pichchila - Pichchila generally means that guna which we understand by the word mucilaginous. These dravyas have fibres. This guna is useful for coating (लेपन) of various body constituents.[48] It brings about heaviness in various body constituents. This guna with its adhesive properties, is kaphavardhak.

Dhatus are nourished and various tissues reunited by this guna. It is very useful in reunion of bones in fractures and promotes healing of wounds penetrating skin, muscles etc.

Presence of pichchila guna causes lubrication of the channels of the body and facilitates easy excretion of faeces. This guna is used for forming a coat over internal and external ulcers as well as intestinal ulcers. It is for this purpose that pichchabasti (a type of enema) is given in rectal fissures.[49]

Vishada is the antagonist of this guna. Just as all the four mahabhootas except jala are responsible for vishada guna, similarly jala mahabhoota is solely responsible for generating pichchila guna.[50]

Sanwar, isabgol, tender shoots of mohari, curd, dinka, recently harvested rice, mocharasa, lady's finger are all examples of dravyas with pichchila guna. This guna has a natural tendency to increase in hemant ritu.

15. Shlakshna - Shlakshna is that guna which we generally know as smooth. This guna is the opposite of rough. Both these gunas are perceived by the skin. The main action of this guna is ropana (healing). This is the power of shlakshna guna.[51]

This guna increases kapha. It is characterised by an ability to increase the dhatus, facilitate the excretion of malas and similarity in action with pichchila guna.[52]

Among the mahabhootas, teja mahabhoota is the causal mahabhoota of this guna.[53] Shankhajira, boric powder, sapeetha, face powder are examples of dravyas having shlakshna guna. The outer coat of sagargota, varatika, glass, carrom board, and bald head are all shlakshna (smooth) to touch.

16. Khara - Rough, irregular feeling to touch is called khara. This guna, which is perceived by the skin, is the antagonist of shlakshna. The feeling of this guna may be desirable while suffering from urticaria. Otherwise, the feeling of khara guna is not desirable. It brings about lekhana (depletion of dhatus).[54]

The action of this guna is to create vata vriddhi. This is so because vayu is also khara (rough) to touch. Wherever khara guna is present, the causal mahabhoota is always vayu.

Khara guna causes depletion of the constituents of the body. It absorbs the water content of the malas. The actions of this guna have some similarity with those of vishada guna. Vayu is the causal mahabhoota of this guna.[55]

Khara guna is present in the bones of the body. The leaves of sag, parijatak, kharvati and sandpaper, file etc are examples of khara sparsha (rough tangibility).

Students of treatises like Charaka and Sushruta samhita should appreciate their vast and subtle intelligence and minute observations.

The dravyas with this guna are widely used in rubbing the edges of a non-bleeding wound. This guna is also useful for rubbing the scabs of wounds. Khara guna is extensively seen in greeshma ritu.

17. Sookshma - The meaning of sookshma is extremely fine or minute. Due to their fineness, these dravyas can penetrate deep into the body. Thus this guna can reach the smallest of all the channels of the body and evacuate them of vitiated doshas (or carry with itself the desired actions to these channels).[56]

Vata is sookshma.[57] Sookshma guna increases vata, and causes depletion of the dhatus. It absorbs the water content of the malas. Dravyas having sookshma guna are easy to digest. The action of this guna is to clear the blocked channels (srotas). This guna is generated from agni, vayu and akash mahabhootas. Obviously, this guna is an antagonist of prithvi and jala mahabhoota. All poisons are sookshma. Alcoholic beverages, with properties similar to those of poisons, are also sookshma. But these must be old (दीर्घकालस्थित मद्य). Similarly, the meat of carnivorous animals also has sookshmagamitva. Dravyas like maricha are also sookshmagami. Coupled with teekshna guna, it becomes even more sookshmagami. After grinding pippali for 64 prahars (1 prahar = 3 hours) continuously, pippali becomes extremely sookshma. Thus, it becomes capable of removing the kapha which blocks the respiratory tract in respiratory tract diseases.

18. Sthoola - Dravyas which have an abundance of constituent components are called as sthoola dravyas. Sthoola guna can be appropriately described by the word "gross". Dravyas which are large in shape, which are not fine, which do not move easily and which cannot penetrate deep into the body, possess this guna.

These dravyas get digested very slowly and because of their grossness, these block the srotas. Dravyas which have the ability to form a layer or a coating possess this guna.[58]

Since this guna is similar to the gunas of kapha, it causes an increase in kapha. The action of sthoola guna is to increase the dhatus and make the body obese. Since, there is a quantitative increase in the malas also, it facilitates their excretion. Since the body becomes obese, various srotas (channels) which convey the dhatus, are obstructed. Prithvi mahabhoota is the sustainer and the causal mahabhoota of this guna.[59]

Examples-food items made of flour, butter, ghee, meat of animals dwelling in marshy land etc.

19. Sandra - This guna can be generally called as "viscous"[60] Sandra dravyas are sthoola as well as viscous.[61]

As this guna is similar to kapha, it is obvious that it causes kaphavriddhi. At the same time, the constituents of the body are increased. The malas are also increased and these become more viscous.

This guna is sustained by prithvi mahabhoota (which sustains the whole world). Milk, cream, butter and food items prepared from milk have this guna.

20. Drava - The fluidity of water, milk, sugarcane juice etc. is drava guna. The dravyas which are sookshma and get diffused very easily have drava guna.

Charaka has advised that one must imbibe knowledge not only from tribals but also from enemies.

This guna has the ability to moisten the constituents of the body and diffuse into these.[62]

These dravyas increase kapha, pitta and fluid dhatus of the body like rasa etc. The action of this guna is to increase the fluid malas like mutra, sweda etc. and facilitate their excretion.[63]

A normal human being generally drinks approximately 2.5 pints of water per day. The kidneys filter around 37 gallons of fluid per day. Jala mahabhoota is the only sustainer of this guna. Water, milk are examples of dravyas with this guna.

The human body, which appears solid to us, is actually made up of 60 to 70% of fluid. In our body, the circulation of dhatus is because of drava guna. Many litres of fluid is circulated through various organs of our body like heart, kidneys, liver, intestines etc per day. Pumping and supply of rasa dhatu from the heart to the various organs of the body is possible due to the drava guna of rasadhatu. Bones contain 20% fluid whereas plasma contains 95% fluid. Few dravyas have an innate property of drava (eg. water). But in some other dravyas it can be artificially created – ghee and metals like gold.[64]

Other physical properties

The twenty gurvadi gunas have now been dealt with in detail. Certain scriptures have mentioned a few other gunas. Due consideration must be given to these gunas as well. Sushrutacharya has illustrated five gunas viz. vyavayi, vikasi, sugandha, durgandha and ashukari in addition. Following is the description of these gunas –

1. **Vyavayi** - There are certain dravyas, like poisons, which on entering the body, bypass the natural course of digestion ie. these spread throughout the body without first getting digested. Their digestion begins after they spread throughout the body. Dravyas which possess this guna are called vyavayi. Vayu and akash mahabhootas are predominant in these dravyas. Generally, poisons, teekshna and potent drugs have this guna. Bhang, opium, strong liquor, narcotics[65] and few Siddha medicines are examples of dravyas having vyavayi guna.
2. **Vikasi** - Dravyas having vikasi guna, on reaching the body, cause depletion of oja. Vikasi dravyas are those dravyas which cause loosening of major joints between the constituents of various dhatus and bones, ligaments and also of numerous minor joints within the body. Thus, these dravyas bring about a considerable decrease in the strength of the body. Predominance of vayu is the cause of this guna. Vikasi dravyas act on the madhyam marg.

Dravyas like tobacco, supari etc. possess this guna. Because of these dravyas, the oja present in the dhatus gets separated from these dhatus. Even though Sushrutacharya has included the above two attributes in the category of gunas, he himself has mentioned these in the list of karmas (actions).[66]

3. **Sugandha** - Sugandha (fragrance) is that particular sense-object which is perceptible by the nose, subtle, pleasing, improves appetite and is mild. For example, the smell of chandan, vala, gulab etc. is sugandha. It acts as an adjunct to shaman (pacification of doshas). These dravyas are pittashamak and tranquilizers.[67]

To widen the horizon of knowledge and to get enlightened, Ayurveda should incorporate evolving science in a proper manner.

4. Durgandha - The guna (odour) which is the antagonist of sugandha and which causes anorexia and discomfort is called durgandha. It acts as an adjunct to vamana, a type of shodhana chikitsa. It reduces vata-kapha.[68]

(Sugandha and durgandha are both extremes of the same spectrum of odour. Hence there is no need to consider both these as independent gunas).

5. Ashukari - Ashu means quick. The ashukari guna of dravyas is responsible for producing prompt action of these dravyas. It is because of this ashu guna that a drop of oil spreads immediately on water. Bhavprakash has accepted ashu as a guna.

This being so, it is more logical to classify ashukari as a karma than as a guna.[69]

6. Shushka - Bhavaprakash has mentioned shushka guna as the antagonist of drava guna. Shushka is the opposite of drava (शुष्कस्तद्विपरीतक : I) This guna is generated due to predominance of prithvi, vayu and teja mahabhootas.[70]

These gurvadi gunas are material gunas. These gunas, originated from the panchamahabhootas are present in the human body, in the diet and in medicines (drugs) which are also made up of panchamahabhootas. According to the Samanya-Vishesha Siddhant (discussed earlier), dravyas having gunas similar to those of the dravyas within the body cause an increase in these dravyas. Whereas those with antagonist gunas cause depletion. The same principle applies to the genesis of disease, in the treatment of disease and even in maintenance of health. Few dravyas may have a higher degree of similarity with the body constituents. These dravyas will cause an increase in the body constituents more effectively. Those having lesser similarity will cause a comparatively minor increase in the body constituents. The same principle applies to the effect of dissimilar dravyas. It may not be always possible to find a dravya having absolute similarity with the constituents of the body. Yet, if due consideration is given to the permutation-combination of various gunas in the body, even a partially similar guna will have the desired result.[71] If these 20 gunas are broadly classified, it will be observed that 10 gunas act as adjunct to bruhan whereas the remaining 10 antagonist gunas act as adjunct to langhana. There are exceptions to this rule which have to be considered while studying dravyaguna.

While dealing with the gunas of the dravya, it has to be kept in mind that every dravya possesses all these gunas. It is quite likely that few gunas may be less while others may be more. Since the gunas are generated and constituted by the panchamahabhootas, all the gunas are always represented to varying extent in panchabhautik dravyas. Also, the term "snigdhatva" is a relative term. When we say that a particular dravya is snigdha, it means that the percentage of snigdhatva is more whereas the remaining percentage is of rukshatva. The percentage of guru guna is more in guru dravyas. If it is 70% then the percentage of laghu guna will be 30%. Laghu guna becomes ineffective because of the predominance of guru guna. But when we reduce the guru guna of these dravyas by heating or by any other procedure (or conditioning), we are in fact increasing the laghu guna in the same proportion. Both these actions occur simultaneously. It would not have been possible to increase the laghu guna had it been totally non-existent. The satkaryavad of Sankhya philosophy stands testimony to this. No dravya in this universe can be absolute (tanmatra). This principle is very important.

As time changes all the time, medical sciences also change with time.

The guna-karma of various dravyas have been described in relation to human life (प्राणि अदभिर्विनाग्लायमानप्राणानां एव प्राणित्वम्) Hence the purview of dravya-guna-karma gets limited. Minerals like gold, herbs and other animal products may possess many more properties in addition to those which are useful for treating disease and maintaining health in human life. These are not needed here.

Is the number of gunas fixed or variable? This question can be answered as follows – dravyas may have even more gunas, but how will one perceive these additional gunas? The perceptive abilities of an individual act as a limitation to the number of gunas. A blind person cannot perceive roopa, same is the case with other gunas. Eventhough the number of gunas is more, vaidyaka deals with only these twenty gunas. Hence the number of gunas, as far as vaidyaka is concerned, is twenty.

Paradi aadhibhautik gunas (10)

The word paradi guna implies the following 10 gunas viz. paratva, aparatva, yukti, sankhya, samyoga, vibhag, prithakatva, pariman, sanskar, and abhyas.[72]

In the day to day practice of dravyagunashastra, paradi gunas are used and accorded the same importance as the gurvadi gunas. A description of these gunas will answer the question as to why these gunas must be studied. (These gunas are described in detail later).

Vaisheshik darshan has considered paratva-aparatva in relation to kala (time) and desha (space). That which is nearer with respect to time and space is deemed "apar" (proximal) and that which is far is deemed "para" (remote). For example, a village situated at a distance of 10 miles from a particular place is apara when compared to another village situated at a distance of 20 miles from the same place. The village situated at 20 miles will be deemed para. Similarly, if the number 200 is considered apara with respect to 100, then number 300 will be para.

The paratva-aparatva in dravyagunashastra

Paratva (remoteness) - Chakradatta, in his commentary, has described paratva as superiority.[73] There may be many dravyas which are of similar type and have similar guna-karmas. It is necessary however to have a thorough insight to ascertain which one of these is most suited or superior and which is inferior with respect to the present state of health or disease. This concept is not widely utilised in vaidyaka and hence Chakradatta has said तच्च परत्वं प्रधानत्वम्. Thus according to this definition, all these dravyas which are proximal ie. beneficial, be it in the state of health or of disease, are para ie. superior. And all those dravyas which are less beneficial or are harmful are called apara. This point of view is more useful in Ayurveda and therefore easily acceptable. Detailed study of the paradi gunas in the correct perspective is extremely beneficial. Paratva-aparatva are very useful in treatment and preventive medicine while dealing with dooshya, desha (space), bala (strength), kala (time), agni, linga (signs and symptoms), prakriti (tendency), vaya (age), satva (mind), satmya (compatibility), ahar (diet), avastha (condition) and rasa, veerya, vipaka, guna etc of various dravyas.[74] For example the flowers and legumes of bahava plant produced during its flowering season are para whereas those produced in the off-season are apara.[75] All the gunas can be considered in this perspective and thus the concept of gunas can be logically developed.

One has to keep in mind that human body has been borrowed from the universe and has to be returned to the universe.

Aparatva - The idea of aparatva has been proposed along with paratva. This is so because both these gunas are mutually related. Aparatva = inferiority.[76] From the point of view of health, sugar which is made from sugarcane juice is superior whereas "kakvi" also made from sugarcane juice, is comparatively inferior. Cow's milk and ghee is para (superior) whereas sheep's milk and ghee is apara (inferior). This can be true for all groups (varga). The interpretation of paratva-aparatva, as emphasized by vaisheshik darshan, is not so useful in Ayurveda.

Yukti - The word "Yukti" is derived from the original Sanskrit root "Yuj". Yuj means coming together or bringing together. If an act is accomplished by bringing together many factors, it is said that, that particular act is accomplished by yukti.[77] Treatment (or even swathavritta) is also yukti. Institution of an appropriate regimen of treatment after due consideration of the dosha-dooshyas is called yukti.[78] Gunas like samyog (conjuction), sanskar (conditioning), parimaan (dimensions) etc are included in Bheshaja-kalpana. Yet, yukti has its own independent importance. The characteristic of yukti is that it originates as a result of combination of various factors. A regimen which is given indiscriminately, in improper doses, without proper timings, cannot be called yukti.[79] There is no dravya in this universe which cannot be used as medicine; but the treatment is successful only if the adminstrator makes judicious use of these dravyas and not otherwise.[80]

Even in dravyagunashastra, it is not enough just to know the name and identification of a particular dravya; knowledge of the judicious use (yukti or yojana) of dravyas is extremely important. "Yukti" is an intellectual faculty but it holds a specific meaning in dravyaguna and it is in this sense that yukti is considered as a guna.[81]

Actually, yukti can be included in samyoga, parimaan, sanskar etc. Yet, yukti has been mentioned independently since it has a special importance. In our daily activities, many times we say, "Do this work tactfully. The word 'tactfully' is also used in the sense of yukti.

Chanakya was well-known for his asset of yukti. When a certain work gets done without having to use yukti, we say the work was accomplished rather suddenly (अचानकपणे - the original word being अ-चाणक्यपणे).

A vaidya should know the names of medicinal dravyas as well as their identification. Besides, knowledge of beneficial (and harmful) effects of dravyas is also essential. A holistic approach towards all these details is called yukti.[82]

Sankhya

संख्यास्यात् गणितम् ।

One, two, three etc. are numbers for counting.[83] There are innumerable phenomena within the body. Yet, these have been classified in accordance to a definite number for convenience. For example-three doshas, seven dhatus, eight jvaras etc. For acquiring specific knowledge about diseases there is a type of samprapti (pathogenesis) called sankhya samprapti.[84] Sankhya means accurate measure. सम्यक् ख्यायते अनया इति संख्या ।[85]

Sankhya acts as a limiting factor for a multitude of entities like the weight of dravyas, their

If we think carefully, we will know that majority of the diseases seen today have resulted from pragnyaparadha.

volume, their gana and their actions. (sankhya = knowledge)

Yet, the numbers from one to parardha have to be used in vaidyak. परत्वं एकंदहंशतं चैव सहस्त्रमयुतं तथा । लक्षं च नियुतंचैव कोटिरबुदमेवच । वृंद: खर्वो निखर्वश्च शंकु:पदम्श्च सागर: । अंत्योमध्य: परार्धश्च दशवृदध्या यथाक्रमम् ॥

[Sankhya (number) has to be written from the right to the left. Writing numbers is called Kharoshti system. The system in which we write the numbers from the left to the right is the Brahmi system].

Samyoga (सं-योग)

युज् means coming together. Thus, when a minimum of two padarthas originally apart are brought together, it is called samyoga.[86] [The phenomena (padartha) which we know as sambandha (relationship) is only of two types viz. samanvaya and samyoga]. The guna known as samyoga is very useful in dravyagunashastra. Samyoga sambandha is temporary whereas samanvaya sambandha is permanent (indispensable). Therefore, while giving the characteristic of samyoga, it has been said that नित्य संबंध: समवाय: If a dravya is mixed with another dravya, it is called samyoga. This is frequently done in various medicinal practices. The gunas and karmas always have samanvaya sambandha with the dravyas even if they do not have a samyoga sambandha with each other.[87]

Samayoga is of three types based on combinations.[88]

a) **Dwandvakarmaj** -[89] When a minimum of two dravyas actively combine with each other, it is called dwandvakarmaj samyoga. For example, a combination of the actions of amalaki and haridra is useful in the treatment of prameha. This is dwandvakarmaj samyoga.

b) **Sarvakarmaj** -[90] When more than two dravyas combine together, it is called sarvakarmaj samyoga. For example - trikatu, panchakol etc.

c) **Ekakarmaj** -[91] In ekakarmaj samyoga one of the two combining dravyas is totally passive whereas the other dravya provides the necessary impetus. If some nasal drops are administered by a person to another unconscious paitent, it is called ekakarmaj samyoga.

Vaisheshik darshan has mentioned three types of samyoga 1) Anyatarkarmaj 2) Ubhayakarmaj and 3) Samyogaj.[92] Amongst these, the first two have been accepted by Ayurveda. Instead of sarvakarmaj samyoga, Vaisheshik darshan has mentioned samyogaj samyoga.[93]

(It is true that samyogaj samyoga is a type of samyoga described in the texts; but it has no direct application in our daily routine. Due to its relative non-utility, Ayurveda has not mentioned samyogaj samyoga).

Depending upon the actions generated after the combination, samyoga is classified into two important types. This classification is important in dravyagunashastra.

Dravya-samyoga

Bhautik (physical mixture) | Rasayanik (chemical compound)

Mukti - moksha is one of the aims of Ayurveda. To seek heaven, one has to die, but mukti can be enjoyed even while alive (Jeevan mukti).

Physical mixture (prakritisama samavaya) - When the combining dravyas retain their individual properties even after combination, then it is called bhautik samyoga. In this type of samyoga, new properties and actions are not produced. If water and salt are mixed, it is called samyoga. But what difference does it make? There will be no change in the gunas of either substances (white yarn fibres will only produce white cloth).[94]

Chemical compound (Vikritivishama samyoga) - Here, the combination of the original combining dravyas results in the production of new guna-karmas (properties-actions). For example - If an alkali and acid are mixed together, then the properties of both of these are lost and madhur rasa, originally absent, is generated. Calcium hydroxide on mixing with haridra (turmeric) gives red colour; or blue and yellow colours, when mixed together, yield green colour.[95]

Both these types of samyogas are widely used in dravyagunashastra. Samyoga has not been directly used in Ayurveda.

The characteristic of life has been given as 'शरीरेंद्रियसत्वात्म संयोग The term, samyog (conjunction) is used here in context to vibhaga (disjunction). The dravyas mentioned in the above sootra viz. shareer (body), indriya (senses), satva (mind) and atma (soul) have undergone vibhaga (disjunction) at some stage and only then can these be united again. When the mind is in conjunction with any of the senses, say eyes, it is in disjunction with all the other senses (ears etc). Here, the process of conjunction and disjunction is continuous. Wherever there is action, there is also conjunction and disjunction. Once the karma is accomplished, the object of karma is also automatically accomplished. Karma is the cause of conjuction and disjunction but production (genesis) of karma does not depend on any other factor.

Vibhaga (disjunction) - Vibhaga is that particular guna which ends the samyoga of drayvas. Vibhaga is the deaggregation of dravyas from their aggregate and is temporary.[96] This is so because samyoga, again, will bring an end to vibhaga. Just as samyoga is of three types, vibhaga is also of three types viz. 1) Dwandvakarmaj 2) Sarvakarmaj and 3) Ekakarmaj. Sarvakarmaj vibhaga is called vibhagaj vibhaga in Vaisheshik darshan. If a leaf falls off or detaches from a branch then it actually is detaching from the tree to which that particular branch belongs. This is an example of vibhagaj vibhaga.

There is a prevalent view that vibhaga is the absence of samyoga. Yet, we see that vibhaga can be directly demonstrated. If we assume that vibhaga is the absence of samyoga, then it implies that there is the existence of vibhaga between guna and karma as there is no samyoga between them. Both these reside in the same abode ie. the dravya and thus there is no vibhaga between guna and karma. Hence the assumption that vibhaga is the absence of samyoga, is wrong.

There is a difference between vibhaga and prithakatva. Presence of vibhaga means an end of samyoga; because vibhaga has been considered as a cause of "samyoganash'' (culmination of samyoga). But, prithakatva (distinctiveness) prevails during samyog as well as during vibhaga between dravyas. Prithakatva = distinctiveness

Prithakatva - The guna which enables us to differentiate one dravya from another is called as

Vaidyas living in the era of industrialization, unfortunately forget the importance of impregnating sutshekharrasa for 21 days in bhringaraj juice.

prithakatva.[97] Prithakatva guna is that particular set of circumstances which helps to make out the difference or distinctiveness between various dravyas. There are three causes which make this prithakatva evident.

1. Asamyoga (non-union) - Chakradatta has illustrated the following examples for asamyoga. Two different mountains like Meru and Himalaya, which by no means, will ever unite with each other, have prithkatva between them. Similarly, in no way can the eyes of the same person unite with each other.[98]

2. Vailakshanya (peculiarity) - The peculiarity of the dravyas belonging to different groups is also a type of prithakatva[99] (eg. the leaves of kanchan and apata).

3. Anekta (multiplicity) - The difference or distinctiveness between two individual grains in a heap of grains or the difference between two particles of sand on the seashore is because of the prithakatva guna.

According to Yogendranath Sen, asamyoga, vailakshnya and anekta have almost the same meaning as prithakatva; but this view does not seem to be acceptable to Chakrapani Datta, a commentator of Charaka samhita. Since there appears some amount of similarity between anyonyabhava and prithakatva, one is likely to get confused between the two. But in anyonyabhava, abhava (absence) is direct and demonstrable whereas in prithakatva a differing bhava padarth is demonstrable. This is the point of difference between prithakatva and anyonyabhava.

Abhava is conspicuous in anyonyabhava whereas bhava padartha is conspicuous in prithakatva. Therefore, anyonyabhava does not mean prithakatva and prithakatva does not mean anyonyabhava.

Anyonyabhava indicates that a particular dravya is not any other dravya. This is the difference between anyonyabhava and prithakatva.[100]

Pariman - The guna which enables us to carry out our usual chores like measurement and weighing of dravyas is called pariman (dimension). Pariman is of three types, a) measurement done by a tape like length, breadth, depth etc. b) measurement of volume in terms of litre etc. done by measuring vessels and c) measurement of the weight of various dravyas in terms of milligram, gram, kilogram etc.[101]

As one thinks of peaceful youth during childhood, one should also think of peaceful death since childhood.

Pariman (four types viz. small, large, long, short.)

- Dairghya (length)
  - Nitya (permanent or eternal)
    - Paramanu (smallest particle of a dravya)
  - Anitya[103] (temporary or non-eternal)
    - 1. Sankhyajanya (based on number) dwayanuk, trayanuk etc. (collection of two and three paramanu respectively)
    - 2. Parimanjanya-dravya which have been moulded into a definite shape - table, suitcase etc.
    - 3. Prachayjanya - cotton
- Gurutva (weight)[102]
  - Nitya dravya (permanent)
  - Anitya dravya (temporary)

Sanskar - The guna which enables the innate or inherent and dormant gunas (properties) of a particular dravya to manifest themselves is known as sanskar. For example, after performing various purification procedures on poisonous dravyas or dravyas like parad (mercury), many gunas, not evident earlier, are manifested. Same is the case with lahi or pohe prepared from rice. This is called sanskar. (Sanskar means instillation of new gunas.[104,105]

Sanskar

- Vega: Movements generated in material dravyas. (vibrations, impulse)
- Bhavana: This guna resides in the soul. It is the remembrance or recollection of a previously perceived object.
- Sthitisthapaka: If the condition of a dravya is altered then the guna by virtue of which the dravya regains its original condition is called Sthitisthapaka. eg. dog's tail and curly hair.

The sanskars mentioned in the Vaisheshik darshan do not have much resemblance to those mentioned in vaidyak. However, in vaidyak, sanskar has an extraordinary importance.

In sanskar, the sustainer (ie. the dravya) remains unchanged whereas the sustained (ie. the gunas) change. A change in gunas implies a change in karmas as well. This is the real purpose behind sanskar. If we say that the guna, karma and dravya, all change then one might ask - what remains?

It is said that the time is passing (lost) but in fact one is dying every moment and not the time.

There has to be some sort of perpetuity and it is the dravya which has it. It is true that after sanskar the dravya has to be identified from its altered guna-karmas but the continuity or perpetuity remains only in the dravya.[106]

Abhyas - Repetition, continuous practice is the meaning of the word "abhyas. This guna is widely used for treatment as well as maintenance of health. Any substance, taken continuously, is more effective. If a person is continuously exposed to the cause of a disease, then the possibility of the disease being produced is greatly increased. Same is the case with treatment. Even if the medicine is appropriate and is administered in an appropriate dose, at the appropriate time, to the right patient and by a right person along with correct "anupan, yet it needs to be taken for a few days, repeatedly and continuously. Only then will it have the desired result. Be it internal drugs or be it any other activity, if it is started abruptly without paying due attention to the tolerance of the mind and body, it will not have any beneficial effect; on the contrary, it will only prove harmful.[107]

In Ayurveda, continuous use of factors causing equilibrium of doshas has been indicated.[108] It should be kept in mind that abhyas has extraoridinary importance in both pathogenesis and treatment. The word अभ्यस्यमानै: is very important in the aphorism घातव: पुन: शरीरा:........ अभ्यस्यमानै: वृध्दि प्राप्नुवन्ति .... ऱ्हासंतु .... अपि अभ्यस्यमानै: .... in chapter 6 of sharir sthana of Charaka samhita.[109]

(Appendix)

Knowledge of the ten paradi gunas is extremely crucial from the point of view of both, dravyagunashastra and chikitsashastra. Revaluation and precise detailed description of these gunas will definitely help in overcoming many drawbacks in Ayurveda. Following description of these ten gunas will be found to be authentic as well as in accordance with modern times. New ideas can be evolved taking the basic principles as foundation.

1. **Paratva** - Superiority
2. **Aparatva** - Inferiority

The paratva or aparatva of any dravya can be ascertained on the basis of 1) desha (place) 2) kala (time) 3) vaya (age) 4) man (dimension) 5) pak (digestion) 6) veerya and 7) rasa.

In the context of dravyagunashastra, paratva-aparatva can be understood in the following way.

a) Desha - A condition or a place (habitat) which is ideal for the growth of a plant will be "para" condition or place (habitat) for that particular plant. For eg. chopchini (Smilex chinensis) has been found to grow naturally in China. Hence China is para or superior desha for chopchini. All other places (desha) will be apara, inferior for chopchini. In other words, the chopchini growing in China will possess superior gunas as compared to the ones growing in other places. (A detailed description of this can be found in various ecological studies. This guna called paratva will be useful in collection and preservation of dravyas. Similarly, it will also help in deciding the criteria for selection or rejection of dravyas - paratva - aparatva).

The proportion of various constituents within the same plant keeps on fluctuating depending on its place of origin and the climate.

b) Kala - Visarga kala (bestowal period) and adankala (procurement period). Visarga kala is para-superior for collection and preservation of dravyas whereas adan kala is apara-inferior. The word kala, with reference to plants, should be understood as the suitable time for collection and use (ie. para kala). The para kala of mangoes is greeshma ritu (summer season) whereas all the other seasons must be considered as apara kala. Ripe mangoes may be available in other seasons also but such fruits must be considered unsuitable - apara. This is so because these fruits are unseasonal.

c) Vaya (age) - While determining the paratva-aparatva of age, we must take into consideration the age of the dravyas. For example - only fully grown, mature dravyas should be used for the purpose of treatment. It will not be proper to use half-grown herbs since the rasa-veerya-vipaka will not have matured fully in these herbs. For example - it will not be appropriate to use partially matured pippali for pacifying kapha. Immature, wet pippali has madhur rasa and sheeta veerya and so will not be able to pacify kapha. Similarly, while selecting a particular part of a suitable dravya, care must be taken to choose only the fully grown parts (Sharangdhar). Ayurvedic scriptures have mentioned the time interval after which the stored dravyas become less potent. This aspect must also be studied in depth in relation to vaya (age).

d) Maan - Maan means (praman) measurement. While describing the human body, Sushrutacharya has used anguli praman (measurement of the parts of the body in fingers eg. length of the nose is four fingers). Thus, the patient whose body dimensions correspond exactly with those mentioned by Sushrutacharya, will need the exact dose of medicine as is prescribed in the Ayurvedic texts. A patient having smaller body dimensions will obviously require smaller doses of medicine. Two different patients of the same age may be in the same condition and may have the same disease, yet, the dose of the medicine will depend on the body dimensions of the individual patient. मात्राया: न व्यवस्थास्ति व्याधिं कोष्ठम् बलं वय: । आलोच्य देशकालौच योज्या तद्वच्च कल्पना।। (वा.क.अ.६)

The paratva-aparatva of pak - vipak, veerya and rasa should be understood in relation to the disease and the individual.

e) Pak - Dravyas like meat, which have madhur vipak and ushna veerya, as well as mansagami dravyas are para (most beneficial) for a patient suffering from "rajayakshma whereas other dravyas are apara.

f) Veerya - Dravyas having katu vipak and ushna veerya and which are conducive to removal of doshas from the body are para for a patient suffering from "udar roga whereas other dravyas are apara.

g) Rasa - For a patient of madhumeha (diabetes), tikta (bitter) rasa is para while all the other rasas, specifically madhur (sweet) rasa, are apara.

It seems that the study of paratva-aparatva from this angle is appropriate as it is useful in the treatment as well as collection and storage of dravyas.

3. Yukti - Yukti means institution of appropriate treatment. The regime of treatment started after

"All that is old is good and all that is new is bad" - this principle is wrong. This holds true for medical sciences too.

proper consideration of dosha, dooshya, vaya, bala, kala etc. is called yukti. It will not be wrong to compare yukti with 'prescription writing – it seems that this subject needs proper deliberation.

4. Sankhya - Sankhya is that particular entity which enables us to carry out our activities like counting and arithmetical calculations. Just as sankhya samprapti helps in differential diagnosis by ennumerating the types of diseases, knowledge of the number of dravyas makes it easier to determine the types of dravyas as also their utility.

For example - there are seven types of haritaki. Each one of these has its own specific properties which are useful in specific diseases. Knowledge of the sankhya (number) of haritaki will definitely aid in remembering their specific properties. Similarly, in case of a combination of various formulations, if the number of formulations used is known, then the proportionate increase in the properties of the combination can be easily predicted.

Example - The properties of trikatu churna, which is a combination of sunthi churna, maricha churna and pippali churna, are quite different from the individual properties of its ingredients and is useful in alleviating various groups of signs and symptoms.

5. Samyoga - Bringing together of two or more dravyas is called samyoga.

Types of Samyoga

Ekakarmaj | Dwandvakarmaj | Sarvakarmaj

The purpose of samyoga

Two dravyas are brought together or combined with the purpose of curing a disease. The correct method of implementing this samyoga and the characteristics of best samyoga have been described.

Ekakarmaj samyoga - This is a combination of two dissimilar dravyas. This combination of dissimilar dravyas should be done for treating specific diseases only when required. For example - if honey and ghee, which are dissimilar dravyas, are combined together in equal proportion then this combination is considered to be as harmful as poison. But this combination is used as an antidote for poisons in cases of poisoning. Ekakarmaj samyoga can be done keeping in mind the purpose of curing the disease.

Dwandvakarmaj samyoga - This is a combination of two similar dravyas having different guna-karmas. This samyoga is done with the aim of curing specific diseases. But it is not advisable to use this samyoga often.

For example - a combination of two dravyas having different guna-karmas like amalaki and haridra is beneficial in treatment of prameha. Eventhough amalaki and haridra have different veeryas, these have a common usage in the cure of prameha. Hence this samyoga can be done. This combination will not be useful in diseases other than prameha (madhyam samyoga).

Sarvakarmaj samyoga - Sarvakarmaj samyoga is a combination of similar dravyas having similar guna-karmas. This is a type of samyoga which is always beneficial and positive. Since various

Yoga, Ayurveda and Naturopathy have given prime importance to sharirshodhan (purification of body). All the three sciences are close to nature.

dravyas having similar guna-rasa-veerya are combined, this samyoga has certain, quick and positive actions. Among the various types of samyoga, this is the most useful samyoga. For example - triphala, trikatu etc.

(The concept of samyoga has some amount of similarity with the concept of compatibility of modern medicine)

6. Vibhaga - Vibhaga means taking apart two dravyas which were initially together. It is also of three types.

a) Ekakarmaj vibhaga - Separating two dissimilar dravyas (since samyoga of these dravyas hinders the cure of certain diseases).

For example - A combination of ghee and honey in equal proportions is not indicated for any patient if he/she is not suffering from poisoning. This means that this combination should not be used except in cases of poisoning. If it is used so, it may prove harmful. Such combination may only be used to induce emesis.

b) Dwandvakarmaj vibhaga - Separating two similar dravyas having different guna-karmas. When two similar dravyas having different guna - karmas are combined, these may not alleviate the disease and may even create other complications. Such dravyas must be kept apart. For example - madanphala and danti are both similar dravyas ie. both are shodhana dravyas. But their actions are different. It is not possible to alleviate diseases by a combination of these dravyas. And hence these must be kept apart (and should not be combined).

c) Sarvakarmaj vibhaga - If the combination of similar dravyas having similar guna-karmas is not beneficial then such combination should not be done as such a combination will not serve the purpose.

For example - Milk and water - as this combination is not viable, no purpose is likely to be served by it and hence it should not be done.

The concept of vibhaga has some degree of similarity with the concept of incomaptibility or antagonism of modern medicine.

a) Asamyogalakshan prithaktva (prithakatva characterised by non-union) - The prithakatva existing between two dravyas which can never unite due to difference in space, time, genesis and place. For example - The prithkatva between two separate mountains (Meru and Himalaya)

b) Vailakshamya Prithkatva (prithkatva characterised by pecularity) - The prithakatva existing between peculiar, dissimilar dravyas. For example - The prithkatva between a horse and a donkey which belong to two different species.

c) Anektaroopa prithakatva (prithakatva characterised by numerosity) - Prithakatva existing between similar dravyas eg. wheat, even though it is a single dravya each grain is different from the other. This prithakatva guna is important from the point of view of identification of dravyas as well as for knowing the properties of various formulations.

There is tremendous similarity in Yam-Niyam of Hathayoga and Sadvritta of Ayurveda.

For example - When two dravyas are brought forward for identification- the characteristics of asasmayogalakshan prithakatva, it should be determined whether the dravya is jangam, audbhid or parthiva. Once this is determined, the difference between the two dravyas is ascertained and it becomes easier to identify the dravyas.

For example - If one has to differentiate between kampillaka and brick powder, both the powders may be put in a vessel containing water and also tested by sprinkling the powders on fire. One which floats on water and burns with a crackling sound is kampillaka. The powder which sinks in water, does not burn, extinguishes the flame is brick powder. This is an example of asamyogalakshan prithakatva since kampillaka is a plant product (vanaspati dravya) whereas brick powder is a parthiva dravya.

Use of Vailakshanyaroopa prithaktva guna

This guna will be useful in identifying two audbhid dravyas belonging to different vargas.

For example - If a twig of tamarind with leaves, and another twig of gunja (also with leaves) are kept for identification, then knowledge of vailakshanyaroopa prithkatva will aid in differentiating the two.

7. Prithakatva - Here, the characteristics of these two are that these are audbhid and one is a twig of mahavruksha while the other belongs to veerudh varga.

Anektaroopa prithakatva - The difference between two similar dravyas. For example - Roses are of many colours. The difference between individual roses is an example of anektaroopa prithakatva.

Sahachara (koranti) is of four types depending upon the colour of the flowers. The difference is between these four types. Haritaki is of seven types. The difference between these seven types of haritaki is also anektaroopa prithaktva.

If the gunas are dealt with in this perspective, it is possible to use these gunas for confirming the identity of dravyas.

8. Pariman - Pariman is used for measuring. Pariman is used everywhere, in preparation of medicine, in determining doses of medicine etc.

9. Sanskar - A procedure which helps in bringing about a change in the gunas of dravyas are known as sanskar. Through the procedure of sanskar, the necessary gunas of the dravyas can be increased, the unnecessary gunas can be eliminated and thus only the beneficial effects of the dravyas may be obtained. For example- for eliminating the sedative guna of opium, it is given 21 bhavanas of ardraka juice.

10. Abhyas - Repeated, continuous use of a padartha is called abhyas. Abhyas guna appears to have some similarity with the concepts of habits and tolerance of modern science.

It is necessary for a vaidya to know the abhyas of a patient ie. the vaidya should know which medicinal dravyas the patient has been taking regularly; because once the patient gets used to a particular dravya due to regular intake then the normal dose of that dravya will not have the desired

Tridoshas are functional units but their strength is dependent on seven dhatus. Therefore, while treating, we should keep in mind the seven dhatus and the body parts which are formed by these.

effect on the patient. For example, a patient taking opium preparations regularly will progressively need higher and higher doses of the drug to have the desired effect; it is necessary for a vaidya to know this. A vaidya will not be able to do proper treatment unless he acquires knowledge of the abhyas of dravyas.

In this way, the ten paradi gunas have an important role to play in chikitsa and dravyagunashastra siddhanta.

The superiority of gunas

In the chapter on dravyas, the reasons for the superiority of the dravyas have been explained. In the chapter on gunas, it becomes imperative to list the reasons for the superiority of gunas ie. characteristics of gunas. Once the superiority of dravya has been established among dravya, guna, rasa, veerya, vipak, claiming superiority of each one of these padarthas in their separate chapters appears to be illogical. Hence Charaka-Sushruta have made no such separate mention. Yet, Nagarjuna has mentioned the superiority of gunas. Following are the reasons for this :-

Without contradicting the archaic view that compared to the dravyas, the gunas are inferior and secondary, it can be said that :-

1. **Rasabhibhava -** The rasas present in the dravyas are superseded by the gunas. For example, water is of madhur rasa and hence it should increase kapha. Yet, the same water, when hot, will be kaphavahasrotogami due to its hot tangibility, laghutva and property to liquify produced due to heating. This means that the madhur rasa has been superseded by ushna guna. Similarly, patola or brihat panchmoola should have been vatavardhak due to their tikta rasa; but these are actually vatahara because of their ushna guna. One who is strong supersedes the weak and thereby proves to be superior in comparison to the weak. Eventhough stars are present in the sky during daytime, these are not seen till the sun keeps shining.[110]

2. **Rasanugraha -** One more phenomenon is observed that if the gunas of the dravya are conducive to its rasas, only then the dravya is considered to be superior in the respective rasaskandha.

Ghee has madhur rasa, also gunas like sheeta, snigdha, mridu, pichchila etc. which are the gunas of those mahabhootas which are conducive to madhur rasa as well as to the causal mahabhootas of this rasa.

Ghee also has laghu vipaka and therefore ghee is considered to be superior to all the other dravyas in madhurvarga. The same can be said about other rasas also.

Amalaki - is sour, yet it is superior in its guna because it is mridu. sheeta, avidahi, kashaya-madhura and laghu-vipaki.

Saindhav - is salty but because of its gunas like natyushna, mridu, avidahi and snehanugami it is superior.

Pippali - is pungent to taste and is guru, does not increase vata-pitta and is also snigdha, vrushya. Hence pippali is superior.

Tikta parval - is tikta, yet, since it is vrushya, guru, pichchila and does not increase vata, it is superior.

Honey (Madhu) - is kashaya but vrushya, pacifies vata in (hiccups) and therefore it is superior.

In this way, the gunas which supersede the rasas prove to be superior to the rasas.[111]

3. Vipakakaranatva - During the digestion of the dravyas, the various stages of vipak through which the dravya passes are also dependent on the gunas of the dravya. There are two types of vipak viz. guruvipak and laghuvipaka. Of these - 1) guruvipak depends on sheeta, snigdha, guru and pichchila gunas 2) laghuvipak depends on gunas like ruksha, vishada, teekshna etc.

The vipak, which supersedes the rasas, depends on the gunas and therefore it follows logically that rasas also depends on the gunas. This is so because the cause is important while the effect is secondary. The dependent always proves to be secondary. For example, since the actions of dosha, dhatu and mala are dependent on vayu, it is superior amongst all.[112]

4. Sankhyabahulya - Those who are more in number prove to be superior (as in a democracy). Rasas are only six while the gunas are twenty in number. Therefore, when compared to rasas, gunas prove to be superior as they are more in number (sankhyabahulya).[113]

5. Prayogbahulya - The ancient scriptures have described the external use of gunas like sheeta, ushna, snigdha, ruksha, shlakshna, khara, vishada etc through various procedures like abyang, avagah, parisheka etc; but the use of rasas has been described only through the mouth. Because rasa is perceived by the tongue. Now, that which can be used in many ways will automatically and naturally attain superiority.[114]

6. Karmabahulya - Gunas, in association with the rasas, help in bringing about actions of these rasas. Thus various actions of these gunas can be observed. Because of this also, gunas are considered to be superior to rasas.[115]

7. Vishayabahulya - Dravyas, which are the sustainers of gunas, are superior. That which has many sustainers is superior. The senses like ear, eyes etc. which can perceive only one sense object from shabda (sound), sparsha (tangibility), roopa (form), rasa (savour) and gandha (odour) are inferior to mana (mind) which can perceive various sense objects like chintya (thought), vicharya (deliberation) etc. Thus, mana is superior amongst all senses. Same is the case here.[116]

8. Upadesha - means samhita grantha (scriptures). Even the scriptures mention gunas like guru, ushna, snigdha as vataghna. Thus, through aptopadesha (words of authoritative persons) also, gunas prove to be superior to rasas.[117]

9. Apadesha - means description. Even while describing an object, we mention gunas. For example, this particular gentleman is strict (teekshna), this song is melodius (mridu) etc.[118]

10. Anuman - The effect can be predicted from the cause (बीजात् फलमनागतम्). Dravyas are either sheeta or ushna. From this, we can predict whether the dravya will be pittaghna (alleviating pitta) or vataghna (alleviating vata). From the above mentioned exercise of anuman (prediction or

Diagnosis of a particular disease is not complete without examination of mala margas mentioned in that disease.

inference) it emerges that gunas are superior.

Therefore gunas are most important.

In all the ten reasons mentioned above, gunas have been considered superior in context to rasas and not dravyas. Yet, if the same dravya becomes old and gets spoilt then it loses the gunas and will not be able to generate its actions. From this point of view also, gunas have to be considered superior to dravyas.

Ayurveda believes that as are the gunas so is the dravya ie. the dravya imitates its gunas. All the considerations in Ayurveda revolve around the gunas. Rasa, veerya, vipak, prabhav are all gunas lying within the dravya. Knowledge of dravyas is derived from their gunas. As far as knowledge or perception is concerned, dravya has no independent existence. Dravyas can not be directly perceived whereas gunas can be perceived directly. From these (the gunas), the dravya is inferred upon. It is true that improper knowledge of gunas will eventually lead to improper knowledge of dravyas as well. Our understanding of dravya is in fact a reflection of the understanding of its gunas.

References -

1. द्रव्याश्रितत्वात् निश्चेष्टकारणत्वात्तथैव च । हेतुतोऽसमवायित्वाद् गौणत्वाद् गुण संज्ञका: ।।" (स्व.)
2. समवायी तु निश्चेष्ट: कारणं गुण: ।" (च. सू. अ. १)
3. द्रव्यं गुणकर्माश्रय: गुणस्तु गुणकर्म अनाश्रय: इति द्रव्यतो भेद: । (यो.)
   अथ द्रव्याश्रिता ज्ञेया निर्गुणा निष्क्रिया गुणा: ।" (कारिकावली)
4. द्रव्याश्रय्यगुणवान् संयोगविभागेष्वकारणमनपेक्ष इति गुणलक्षणम् ।" (वै. द. १, १ सू. १६)
   कर्म नान्यदपेक्षते ।" (च. सू. १)
5. विश्वलक्षणा: गुणा: ।" (र. वै. १ सू. १६८)
   गुणानामेवमेकलक्षणावरोधो नास्ति... तस्मादेवैतेषामतुल्यं विकीर्णलक्षणत्वमेव लक्षणम् इति...
   लक्षणलक्षितेष्वलक्षणलक्षितत्वाल्लक्षणप्रसिद्धिरिति ।" (भा.)
6. एकं हि गुणवैशिष्ट्यात् पृथक् त्वेनानुभूयते ।
   करकाचौंड्यबाष्पाणि स्वरूपाण्युदकस्यच ।।
7. अनुभूतद्रव्यवैशिट्ये नाम १गुण" इत्यभिधीयते ।। (आगस्त्यसंहिता).
8. अनेन त्रिविधा अपि वैशेषिका:, सामान्य:, आत्मगुणाश्चोद्दिष्टा: ।" (च.)
9. एते च सामान्यगुणा: पृथिव्यादीनां साधारणत्वात् ।" (च.)
10. एते च वैशेषिका:, यत: आकाशस्यैव शब्द: प्राधान्येन, वायोरेव स्पर्श: प्राधान्येन, एवमग्न्यादिषु रूपादय: ।" (च.)
    तस्य गुणा: शब्दादयो गुर्वादयश्च द्रवान्ता: ।" (च. सू. अ. २३)
    सन्निकर्षो भवेत् येन सहाभिज्ञायते गुण: । सुस्पष्टो वाप्यस्पष्टो वा गूढो दूरान्वितोऽपि च ।। (सन्निकर्ष – (इंद्रियार्था संनिकर्ष) - सुस्पष्ट, अस्पष्ट, गूढ व दूरान्वित असा असतो.) साहजिकच गुणज्ञान ४ प्रकारचे होते.
11. इच्छा द्वेष: सुखं दु:खं प्रयत्नश्चेतना धृति: बुद्धि: स्मृतिरहंकारो लिङ्गानि परमात्मन: ।। (च. शा. १)

प्रयत्नोऽन्ते येषां ते प्रयत्नान्ताः, एतेन चेच्छाद्वेषसुखदुःखप्रयत्नानां ग्रहणम् । (च.)

12. बुद्धिः ज्ञानम्, अनेन च स्मृतिः - चेतना- धृत्यहंकारादीनां बुद्धिविशेषाणां ग्रहणम्५। (च.)
इह चेतनादीनां बुद्धिग्रहणेनैव ग्रहणम् । (च.)

13. गुर्वादयस्तु-गुरुलघुशीतोष्णस्निग्धरूक्षमन्दतीक्ष्णस्थिरसरमृदुकठिनवि शदपिच्छिल शलक्ष्णखरस्थूलसूक्ष्मसान्द्रद्रवाः विंशतिः । (च.)
गुरुमन्दहिमस्निग्धश्लक्ष्णसान्द्रमृदुस्थिराः । गुणाः ससूक्ष्मविशदा विंशतिः सविपर्ययाः ।। (अ.सं.सू. १)
शीतोष्णस्निग्धरूक्षविशदपिच्छिलगुरुलघुमृदुतीक्ष्णा गुणाः कर्मण्याः । (र. वै. अ. ३ सू. १११).
दशाद्याः कर्मतः प्रोक्तास्तेषां कर्मविशेषणैः । दशैवान्यान् प्रवक्ष्यामि द्रवादींस्तान्निबोध मे ।। (सु.सू. अ. ४६)
तदिदानी पूर्वाचार्यप्रसिद्वेन क्रमेण द्वेधा विभज्य कर्मतः शीतादीन् गुणानुपदिदिक्षति ।
तेषां व्याचिख्यासितानां गुणानां मध्ये आद्याः पूर्वाचार्यैरादावुपदिष्टाः... । (हा.)
सुश्रुते तु गुणाः प्रोक्ता विंशतिस्तान् ब्रुवे शृणु । (भा.प्र.)
सत्यपि गुणो द्रव्ये योगाभावान्न ज्ञायते ।
किंचिन्न कुरुते कर्म संस्कारं न करोत्यपि ।।
सेंद्रिये नेंद्रिये चैव समाना हि व्यवस्थितिः ।।
(द्रव्यांची ओळख गुणांनी होते व गुणांची ओळख कर्माने होते.)
गुणानुसारी तत्कर्म समानं तेषु विद्यते ।।
विशिष्टश्च गुणो ह्येको विविधेष्वपि वर्तते ।

14. न हि एको वर्तते भावो (च. शा. १।५८).
केचिदत्र संख्याभंगभयाद् व्यवायिविकास्यशुकारिणामपाठमेव मन्यन्ते । (ड.)
य एतेऽतिरिक्ता गुणा दर्शिताः ते विंशतावेवान्तर्भूताः । (हे.)
गुर्वादय इति एते आविष्कृततमा एव यज्जःपुरुषीये उक्ताः, तेन गुणानामसंख्येयत्वादन्येऽपि ज्ञेयाः।
अत एव प्रमेहे श्लेष्मगुणेषु अच्छत्वादयो गुणाः पठ्यन्ते । (शि.)
एते विकासित्वादयो गुणा यद्यपि विंशतिगुणगणनायां न पठिताः, तथाप्यसंख्येयतया गुणानामेषामपि गुणत्वं सिद्धम्; ये तु तत्र पठितास्ते तावदाविष्कृततमाः ज्ञेयाः । (च.)
अधिकायामपि गुणविंशतावुक्तायां गुणा विंशतिरुक्ताः, न चात्र नियमो विंशतिरेवेति; व्यवायिविकास्याशुकारिणां तु स्वतंन्त्रे च परतन्त्रे च दर्शनात् पाठो न्याय्य एव । (ड.) परापरत्वे युक्तिश्च संख्या संयोग एव च । विभागश्च पृथक् त्वं च परिमाणमथापि च ।। संस्कारोऽभ्यास इत्येते गुणा ज्ञेया परादयः । सिद्ध्युपायाश्चिकित्साया लक्षणैस्तान् प्रचक्ष्महे ।। (च. सू. २६-३०)
गुणाः कर्मानुमेयाः वै ।
एते च सामान्यगुणा अपि नात्युपयुक्तत्वात्तथा बुद्धिप्राधान्याच्चान्ते प्रोक्ताः । (च.)
इति स्वलक्षणैरुक्ताः गुणाः सर्वे परादयः । चिकित्सा यैरविदितैर्न यथावत् प्रवर्त्तते ।। (च. सू. २६)
(ज्या गुणांशी सैनिकर्ष होईल तेवढ्याच गुणांचे ज्ञान होते.)
अर्थाः शब्दादयो ज्ञेया गोचरा विषया गुणाः । (च. शा. १)
कर्मभिस्त्वनुमीयन्ते नाना द्रव्याश्रया गुणाः । (सु. सू. ४६)
यावन्तो गुणविशेषाः कर्मसंख्याहि तावति ।

असंख्येया गुणाः द्रव्ये ततः कर्माण्यमितानिच ।
(जेवढे गुण तेवढी कर्मे – गुण असंख्य तर कर्मे ही असंख्यच.)
गुणाः गुणाश्रयाः नोक्ताः तस्माद्रसगुणान् भिषग् । विद्यात् द्रव्यगुणान् । (सु. सू.)

15. गौरवं पार्थिवमाप्यञ्च।" (र.वै.अ. ३ सू. ११६)

16. गुरुत्वं जलभूम्योः पतनकर्मकारणम् ।" (प्र. पा. भा.)

17. सादोपलेपबलकृद् गुरुस्तर्पणबृंहणः । (सु. सू. ४६।५१८)
गुरु वातहरं पुष्टिश्लेष्मकृच्चिरपाकि च । (भा.प्र.)

18. यस्य द्रवस्य बृंहणे कर्मणि शक्तिः स गुरुः ।" (हे.) वा. सू. १।१८
लघुर्गुरुस्तथा स्निग्धो रूक्षस्तीक्ष्ण इति क्रमात् ।
नभोभूवारिवातानां वह्नेरेते गुणाः स्मृताः ।। (भा.प्र.)

19. लङ्घने लघुः – (हे.) लाघवमन्यदीयम् – (र. वै. ३ सू. ११७)

20. लघुस्तद्विपरीतः स्याल्लेखनो रोपणस्तथा ।" (सु. सू. अ. ४६)
लघु पथ्यं परं प्रोक्तं कफघ्नं शीघ्रपाकि च ।" (भा. प्र.)

21. ल्हादनः स्तम्भनः शीतो मूर्च्छातृट्स्वेददाहजित् ।" (सु. सू. ४६)
शीतस्तु ल्हादनः स्तम्भी मूर्च्छातृट्स्वेददाहनुत् ।" (भा.प्र.)

22. स्तम्भने हिमः ।" (हे.)

23. स्वेदने उष्णः ।" (हे.)

24. तैजसमौष्ण्यं तैक्ष्ण्यं च ।" (र. वै. ३ सू. ११३)

25. उष्णस्तद्विपरीतः स्यात् पाचनश्च विशेषतः ।" (सु. सू. अ. ४६)
उष्णो भवति शीतस्य विपरीतश्च पाचनः ।" (भा.प्र.)

26. यस्य क्लेदने शक्तिः स स्निग्धः ।" (हे.)
स्नेहाऽपां विशेषगुणः ।" (प्र. पा. भा.)

27. स्नेहमार्दवकृत् स्निग्धो बलवर्णकरस्तथा ।" (सु.)
स्निग्धं वातहरं श्लेष्मकारि वृष्यं बलावहम् ।" (भा.)

28. यस्य शोषणे शक्तिः स रूक्षः ।" (हे.)
रूक्षस्तद्विपरीतः स्याद् विशेषात् स्तम्भनः खरः ।" (सु.)
रूक्षं समीरणकरं परं कफहरं मतम् ।" (भा. प्र.)

29. मन्दो यात्राकरः स्मृतः ।" (सु. सू. ४६)
यस्य शमने शक्तिः स मन्दः । १ (हे.)
मन्दः शमने शक्तिः ।
मन्दोगुणः यात्राकरः इति शरीर स्थायित्वाद्देहस्य यात्रावर्तनं करोति । (डल्हण)

30. यस्य शोधने शक्तिः स तीक्ष्णः । (हे.)

31. दाहपाककरस्तीक्ष्णः स्त्रावणः ।" (सु.)

32. तीक्ष्णं पित्तकरं प्रायोलेखनं कफवातहृत् ।" (भा.)

33. यस्य धारणे शक्तिः स स्थिरः" (हे.)

34. केशश्मश्रुलोमास्थिनखदन्तसिरास्नायुधमनीरेतः प्रभृतीनि स्थिराणि ।" (सु. शा. ३)

35. स्थिरो वातमलस्तम्भी ।" (भा.)
36. यस्य प्रेरणे शक्तिः स सरः ।" (हे.)
37. सरस्तेषां प्रवर्त्तकः ।" (भा.)
38. सरोऽनुलोमनः प्रोक्तः ।" (सु.)
सरो गुणः अनुलोमनः वातमलप्रवर्तनः।" (डल्हण)
39. यस्य श्लथने शक्तिः स मृदुः ।" (हे.)
40. मांसशोणितमेदोमज्जाहृन्नाभियकृत्प्लीहान्त्रगुदप्रभृतीनि मृदूनि ।" (सु. शा. ३)
41. मृदुरन्यथा ।" (सु.)
42. दारुणविपरीतः अदाहपाककरोस्त्रावणो मृदुः प्रोक्तः (सु. सू. ४६)
43. मार्दवमान्तरिक्षमाप्यं च ।" (र. वै. ३ सू. ११५)
44. यस्य दृढीकरणे शक्तिः स कनिः ।" (हे.)
45. कनित्वं पार्थिवम् ।" (र. वै. २ सू. ५८)
46. यस्य क्षालने शक्तिः स विशदः (हे.)
47. विशदो विपरीतोऽस्यात् क्लेदाचूषणरोपणः । (सु.)
क्लेदच्छेदकरः ख्यातो विशदो व्रणरोपणः ।" (भा.)
48. यस्य लेपने शक्तिः स पिच्छिलः । (हे.)
49. पिच्छिलो जीवनो बल्यः संधानः श्लेष्मलो गुरुः ।" (सु.)
पिच्छिलस्तन्तुलो बल्यः संधानः श्लेष्मलो गुरुः ।" (भा.)
50. पिच्छिलत्वमाप्यम् ।" (र. वै. ३ सू. ११२)
51. यस्य रोपणे शक्तिः स श्लक्ष्णः (हे.)
52. श्लक्ष्णः पिच्छिलवज्ज्ञेयः" (सु.)
श्लक्ष्णः स्नेहं विनाऽपि स्यात् कठिनोऽपि हि चिक्कणः ।" (भा.)
53. तैजसं श्लक्ष्णत्वं नाम ।" (र. वै. अ. २ सू. ५८)
54. यस्य लेखने शक्तिः स खरः । (हे.)
कर्कशो विशदो यथा ।" (सु. सू.)
55. कर्कशत्वं वायव्यम् ।" (र. व. अ. २ सू. ६०)
56. यस्य विवरणे शक्तिः स सूक्ष्मः ।" (हे.)
57. सूक्ष्मस्तु सौक्ष्म्यात् सूक्ष्मेषु स्रोतःस्वनुसरःस्मृतः ।" (सु. सू. अ. ४६।५२४)
देहस्य सूक्ष्मच्छिद्रेषु विशेद्यत् सूक्ष्ममुच्यते ।" (भा.)
58. यस्य संवरणे शक्तिः स स्थूलः । (हे.)
59. स्थूलः स्थौल्यकरो देहे स्रोतसामवरोधकृत ।" (भा.)
स्थूलः स्यात बंधनकारकः । (सु. सू. ४१)
60. यस्य प्रसादने शक्तिः स सान्द्रः । (हे.)
61. सान्द्रः स्थूलः स्याद् बन्धकारकः ।" (सू.)

62. द्रवत्वं स्यन्दने हेतुः निमित्तं संग्रहे तु तत् ।" (कारिकावली)
द्रवत्वं स्यन्दनकर्मकारणम् ।" (प्र. पा. भा.)
यस्य विलोडने शक्तिः स द्रवः । (हे.) 9द्रवः प्रक्लेदन ।" (सु.)

63. द्रवः क्लेदकरो व्यापी" (भा.) (स्यंदन, झीर्मर्दीूग्दह)

64. सांसिद्धिकं द्रवत्वं स्यात्, नैमित्तिकमथापरम्"
सांसिद्धिकं तु सलिले द्वितीयं क्षितितेजसोः ।।
नैमित्तिकं वन्हियोगात्तपनीयघृतादिषु ।" (कारिकावली)

65. व्यवायी चाखिलं देहं व्याप्य पाकाय कल्पते ।" (सु.)
पूर्व व्याप्याखिलं कायं ततः पाकं च गच्छति ।
व्यवायि तद्यता भंगा फेनञ्चाहिसमुद्भवम् ।।" (शा.)

66. विकासी विकसन्नेवं धातुबन्धान् विमोक्षयेत् ।" (सु.)
सन्धिबन्धाँश्च शिथिलान् करोति हि विकासि तत् ।"
विश्लिष्यौजश्च धातुभ्यो यथा क्रमुककोद्रवौ ।।" (शा.)

67. सुखानुबन्धी सूक्ष्मश्च सुगन्धो रोचनो मृदुः ।" (सु.)

68. दुर्गन्धो विपरीतोऽस्माद् हृल्लासारुचिकारकः ।।" (सु.)

69. आशुकारी तथाशुत्वाद्धावत्यम्भसि तैलवत् ।" (सु.)
आशुराशुकरो देहे धावत्यम्भसि तैलवत् । (भा.)

70. शुष्कस्तद् विपरीतकः । (भा.)

71. तत्रेमे शरीरधातुगुणाः संख्यासामर्थ्यकराःच तद्यथा-गुरुलघुशीतोष्णस्निग्धरूक्षमन्द तीक्ष्णस्थिरसरमृदुकठिनविशदपिच्छिलश्लक्ष्णखर सूक्ष्मस्थूलसान्द्रद्रवाः तेषु ये गुरवस्ते गुरुभिराहारविकारगुणैरभ्यस्यमानैराप्यायन्ते लघवश्च-हसन्ति; लघवस्तु लघुभिराप्यायन्ते गुरवश्च -हसन्ति; एवमेव सर्वधातुगुणानां सामान्ययोगाद् वृद्धिविपर्ययाद् -हासः ।"

तस्मान्मांसमाप्यायते मांसेन भूयस्तरमन्येभ्यः शरीरधातुभ्यः; तथा लोहितं लोहितेन, मेदो मेदसा, वसा वसया, अस्थि तरुणास्थ्ना, मज्जा मज्ज्ञा, शुक्रं शुक्रेण-गर्भ स्त्वामगर्भेण ।"

यत्र त्वेवं लक्षणेन सामान्येन सामान्यवतां आहारविकाराणामसान्निध्यं स्यात् सन्निहितानां वाऽप्ययुक्तत्वान्नोपयोगो घृणित्वादन्यस्माद्वा कारणात् स च धातुरभिवर्धयितव्यः स्यात्, तस्य ये समानगुणाः स्युराहारविकाराः असेव्याश्च, तत्र समानगुणभूयिष्ठानामन्यप्रकृतीनामप्याहारविकाराणामुपयोगः स्यात्; तद्यथआ-शुक्रक्षये क्षीरसर्पिषोरुपयोगो मधुरस्निग्धसमाख्यातानां चापरेषां द्रव्याणां, मूत्रक्षये पुनरिक्षुरसवारुणीमण्डद्रवमधुराम्ललवणोपक्लेदिनां, पुरीषक्षये कुल्माषमाषकुक्कुटाण्डाजमध्ययवशाकधान्याम्लानां, वातक्षये कटुतिक्तकषायरुक्षलघुशीतानां, पित्तक्षयेऽम्ललवणकटुक्षारोष्णतीक्ष्णानां, श्लेष्मक्षये स्निग्धगुरुमधुरसान्द्रपिच्छिलानां द्रव्याणाम्;... एवमन्येषामपि शरीरधातूनां सामान्यविपर्ययाभ्यां वृद्धि-हासौ यथाकालं कार्यो ।" (च. शा. अ. ६)

72. परापरत्वे युक्तिश्च संख्या संयोग एव च । विभागश्च पृथक्त्वं च परिमाणमथापि च ।।
संस्कारोऽभ्यास इत्येते गुणाः प्रोक्ताः परादयः ।" (च. सू. अ. २६)

73. तच्च परत्वं प्रधानत्वम् ।" (च. द.)

74. एकदिक्भ्यामेककालाभ्यां सन्निकृष्टविप्रकृष्टाभ्यां परमपरं च ।" (वै.द.)
किंवा परत्वापरत्वे वैशेषिकोक्ते ज्ञेये ।" (च. द.)

परत्वं सन्निकृष्टत्वम् उपयोगितामासन्नत्वम् ।" (यो.)
देशकालवयोमानपाकवीर्यरसादिषु । परापरत्वे ।" (च. सु. अ. २६)
तत्र देशो मरुः परः कालो विसर्गः परः, वयस्तरुणं परम्, मानं च शरीरस्य यथावक्ष्यमाणं शारीरे परम्, पाकवीर्यरसास्तु ये यस्य योगिनस्ते तं प्रति पराः ।" (च. द.)
आदिग्रहणात् प्रकृतिबलादीनां ग्रहणम् ।" (च. द.)

75. ऋतौ भवं आर्तवम् ।

76. तद्विपर्ययः अपरत्वम् ।" (यो.)
तत्र अनूपोऽपरः, आदानमपरः; अपरमितरत्, ततोऽन्यदपरम्, अयौगिकास्त्वपराः । (च. द.)

77. युक्तिश्च योजना यातु युज्यते ।" (च. सू. अ. २६।३१)

78. योजना दोषाद्यपेक्षया भेषजस्य समीचीनकल्पना ।" (च. द.)
या कल्पना यौगिकी भवति सा तु युक्तिरुच्यते ।

79. अयौगिकी तु कल्पनाऽपि सती युक्तिर्नोच्यते, पुत्रोऽप्यपुत्रवत् ।" (च. द.)

80. अमन्त्रमक्षरं नास्ति, नास्ति मूलमनौषधम् ।
अयोग्यः पुरुषो नास्तिः योजकस्तत्र दुर्लभः ।।

81. युक्तिश्चेयं संयोगपरिमाणसंस्काराद्यन्तर्गताऽप्यत्युक्तत्वात् पृथगुच्यते । (च. द.)
बुद्धिः पश्यति या भावान् बहुकारणयोगजान् ।
युक्तिस्त्रिकाला सा ज्ञेया त्रिवर्गः साध्यते यथा ।।" (च. सू. अ. ११।२५ व ३२)

82. न नामज्ञानमात्रेण रूपज्ञानेन वा पुनः । औषधीनां परां प्राप्तिं कश्चिद्वेदितुमर्हति । योगविन्नामरूपज्ञस्तासां तत्त्वविदुच्यते । (च. सू. १।१२१)
मात्राकालाश्रया युक्तिः सिद्धिर्युक्तौ प्रतिष्ठिता ।
तिष्ठत्युपरियुक्तिज्ञो द्रव्यज्ञानवतां सदा ।। (च. सू. अ. २।१६)
संख्या – १संख्यास्यात् गणितम्" गणना व्यवहारासी म्हणजेच एक, दोन, तीन इ.

83. संख्या स्याद् गणितम् ।" (च. सू. अ. २६।३१)
गणितं गणनाव्यवहार हेतुरेकद्वित्र्यादिसंख्या ।" (यो.)

84. संख्याविकल्पप्राधान्यबलकालविशेषतः । सा भिद्यते यथाऽत्रैव वक्षन्तेऽष्टौ ज्वरा इति । (नि.)

85. सम्यक् ख्यायतेऽनया इति संख्या ।" संख्या सम्यक्ज्ञानम् । (च. सू. १३।३ चक्रपाणी)

86. संयोगः पुनर्द्वयोर्बहूनां वा द्रव्याणां संहतीभावः ।" (च. वि. अ. १)
योगः सह संयोग उच्यते ।" द्रव्याणाम् – (च. सू. अ. २६)
अप्राप्तयोस्तु या प्राप्तिः सैव संयोग ईरितः ।"

87. समवायोऽपृथग्भावो भूम्यादीनां गुणैर्मतः । स नित्यः ट (च. सू. १)

88. द्रव्याणां द्वन्द्वसर्वैककर्मजोऽनित्य एव च ।" (च. सू. २६)
स च संयोगो द्रव्याणां द्वन्द्वसर्वैककर्मजः । द्वन्द्वस्य द्वयोः, सर्वेषां बहूनाम्, एकस्य च कर्मणः, जायते तेन त्रिविधः ।" (यो.)

89. तत्र द्वन्द्वकर्मजो यथा युध्यमानयोर्मेषयोः । (च. द.)

90. सर्वकर्मजो यथा – भाण्डे प्रक्षिप्यमाणानां माषाणां बहुलमाषक्रियायोगजः ।" (च. द.)
91. एककर्मजो या–वृक्षवायसयोः । (च. द.)
92. वैशेषिकास्त्वाहुः–9अन्यतरकर्मजः, उभयकर्मजः संयोगजश्च संयोगः ।" (वै. द. ७२।९२ इति)
93. संयोगजः संयोगो यथा–अङ्गुलीतरुसंयोगात् शरीरतरुसंयोगः ।" (यो.)
94. प्रकृत्या हेतुभूतया समः कारणानुरूपः समवायः कार्यकारणभावसम्बन्धः प्रकृतिसमसमवायः कारणानुरूपं कार्यमित्यर्थः, यथा शुक्लतन्तुसमवायारब्धस्य पटस्य शुक्लत्वम् ।
95. अम्लेन सह संयुक्तः स तीक्ष्णलवणो रसः ।
माधुर्य भजतेऽत्यर्थ तीक्ष्णभावं विमुञ्चति ।।" (सु. सू. ११)
विकृत्या हेतुभूतया विषमः कारणनानुरूपः समवायः विकृतिविषमसमवायः यथा हरिद्राचूर्णसंयोगे लौहित्यमिति ।" (मधुकोश)
96. विभागस्तु विभक्तिः स्याद्वियोगी भागशो ग्रहः ।" (च. सू. अ. २६)
प्राप्तिपूर्विका अप्राप्तिः विभागः ।" (यो.)
97. इदंद्रव्यं पटलक्षणं घटात् पृथक" इत्यादिका बुद्धिर्यतो भवति तत् पृथकत्वम् ।" (च. द.)
इदमस्मात् पृथक् अर्थान्तरमिति पृथक्प्रत्ययनिमित्त पृथक् त्वम् ।" (यो.)
98. यत् सर्वथाऽसंयुज्यमानयोरिवमेरुहिमाचलयोः पृथक् त्वम्, एतत् असंयोग इत्यनेनोक्तम् ।" (च. द.)
99. तथा संयुज्यमानानामपि पृथक् त्वं विजातीयानां महिषवराहादीनाम्, तदाह–वैलक्षण्यमित्यादि । विशिष्टलक्षणयुक्तत्वलक्षितं विजातीयानां पृथक् मित्यर्थः ।" (च. द.) एकजातीयेषु हि संयुक्तेषु न वैलक्षण्यं नाप्यसंयोगः, अथ चानेकता पृथक् त्वरूपा भवति । (च. द.)
पृथकत्वम्, असंयोगः वैलक्षण्यम्, अनेकता इत्यनर्थान्तरम् । इदमस्मात् पृथक्, इदमनेन न संयुक्तम्, इदमस्मात् विलक्षणं विशिष्टम्, इदमेतच्च नैकमितिप्रतीतीनां शब्द वैशिष्ट्येऽपि अर्थतोऽभिन्नत्वमेव ।" (यो.) । 9किंवा पृथक् त्वं गुणान्तरमिच्छन् लोकव्यवहारार्थमसंयोगवैलक्षण्यानेकतारूपमेव यथोदाहृतं पृथक् त्वं दर्शयति ।" (च. द.)
100. ननु अन्योन्याभाव एव पृथक् त्वम्... इति चेत्? न, पृथगादिशब्दानां पर्यायत्वेऽपि न अन्योन्याभावार्थत्वम्, तत्र पञ्चमीप्रयोगानुपपत्तेः। इदमस्मात् पृथक् इदम् इदं न भवति इति प्रतीत्याभिन्नविषयत्वाच्च । (यो.) अन्योन्याभावतो नास्य चरितार्थत्वमिष्यते । अस्मात् पृथगिदं नेति प्रतीतिर्हि विलक्षणा ।। (कारिकावली)
101. परिमाणं पुनर्मानम् । (च. सू. २६) । परिमितिव्यवहारकारणं परिमाणं मानं प्रस्थाढकादि । (यो.) । मानं प्रस्थाढकादि तुलामेयम् । (च. द.) । परिमाणं भवेन्मानव्यवहारस्य कारणम् ।" (कारिकावली)
102. अनित्ये तदनित्यं स्यान्नित्ये नित्यमुदाहृतम् ।
103. संख्यातः परिमाणाच्च प्रचयादपि जायते । अनित्यं, द्व्यणुकादौ तु संख्याजन्यमुदाहृतम् ।।
104. संस्कारोहि गुणान्तराधानम् । (चरक)
105. संस्कारस्त्रिविधः वेगो भावना स्थितिस्थापकश्च । (न्या. शा.)
106. पयोदधित्वं भजतेशीतमुष्णंक्रमेण ते । मूलतो एक-द्रव्यंहि गुणसंस्कार योगतः । धत्ते नानाविधं रूपं वैचित्र्यं गुणकर्मसु ।। संस्कारानुसरासृष्टिः तयानुमतो गुणः । गुणानुरूपवे कर्म वैभिन्य गुणकर्मणि ।
107. भावाभ्यसनमभ्यासः शीलनं सततक्रिया ।" (च. सू. २६।३४) । 9भावस्य षष्टिकादेर्व्यायामादेश्चाभ्यसनमभ्यासः ।" (च. द.) । 9भावानामभ्यसनं पुनः पुनरनुष्ठानं सातत्येन करणमभ्यासः

।“ (यो.)

108. त्यागाद् विषमहेतूनां समानां चोपसेवनात् । विषमानानुबध्नन्ति जायन्ते धातवः समाः ।।“ (च. सू. १६।३६)

109. समानगुणाभ्यासो हि धातूनां वृद्धिकारणमिति ।“ (च. सू. १२५)
नर्ते सन्तर्पणाभ्यासाच्चिरक्षीणस्तु पुष्यति ।“ (च. सू. २३।३१)
रसदोषसन्निपाते तु ये रसा यैर्दोषैः समानगुणाः समानगुणभूयिष्ठा वा भवन्ति ते तानभिवर्धयन्ति, विपरीतगुणा विपरीतगुणभूयिष्ठा वा शमयन्त्यभ्यस्यमानाः ।“ (च. वि. १), १धातवः पुनः शारीराः समानगुणैःसमानगुणभूयिष्ठैर्वाप्याहारविकारैरभ्यस्यमानैर्वृद्धिं प्राप्तनुवन्ति, -हासंतु विपरीतगुणैर्विपरीतगुणभूयिष्ठैरवाऽप्यभ्यस्यमानैः । (च. शा. ६९)

110. गुणाः प्रधाना इति केचित् ।“ १गुणाद् रसानामभिभवात् ।“ (र. वै. अ. १ सू. १२१)
१रसानभिभूय गुणाः स्वकार्यं निर्वर्त्तयन्ति । यथा उष्णोदकं श्लेष्माणं हरति माधुर्य मभिभूय, तथा पटोलश्च महत् पञ्चमूलं च तिक्तमौष्ण्याद् वातं जयति । यद् येनाभिभूयतेतत्तस्मादप्रधानं दृष्टम् । यथा भानोर्नक्षत्रम् इति ।“ (भा.)

111. गुणानुगृहीतानां रसानां प्राधान्यात् ।“ (सू. १२८) गुणैः शीतादिभिरनुगृहिता ये रसास्तेषां प्राधान्यदर्शनात् रसेभ्यो गुणाः प्रधानाः इति विदनः । कथं १शैत्यात् स्नेहान्मार्दवाच्च पैच्छिल्यादविभागतः । मधुराणां घृतं श्रेष्ठं विपाके लाघवेन च ।। अविदाहान्मृदुत्वाच्च कषायमधुरान्वयात् । अम्लेष्वामलकं श्रेष्ठं विपाके लाघवेन च ।। नात्युष्णत्वान्मृदुत्वाच्च स्नेहेनानुगमादपि । लवणानां स्मृतं श्रेष्ठमविदाहाच्च सैन्धवम् ।। मृदुत्वाच्च गुरुत्वाच्च वातपित्ताप्रकोपणात् । कटुकानां स्मृताः श्रेष्ठाः पिप्पल्यो गुणसंपदा ।। वृष्यत्वाच्च गुरुत्वाच्च मारुतस्याप्रकोपणात् । तिक्तानां तु स्मृतं श्रेष्ठ पैच्छिल्येन च कूलकम् ।। वृष्यत्वाद् बृंहणत्वाच्च हिक्कायां वातनिग्रहात् । कषायाणां स्मृतं श्रेष्ठ विविधैश्च गुणैर्मधु ।। (भा.)

112. वापाकरारणत्वात् ।“ (सू. १२३) । गुणाः विपाकयोः कारणं, शीतस्निग्धगुरुपिच्छिलाःगुरुविपाकस्य, लघुरूक्षविशदतीक्ष्णा लघुविपाकस्येति ।... रसानां कार्यनिर्वृत्तिः पाकायत्ता, स च पाको गुणायत्त इति । यदपेक्षयाऽन्यस्य वृत्तिस्तस्मात् तस्य प्राधान्यं दृष्टम् । यथा वायोर्दोषधातुमलानाम् । (भा.)

113. बाहुल्यात् ।“ (सू. १२४) रसेभ्यो बहवो गुणा दृष्टाः रसाः षट्, गुणाः विंशतिः इति, अल्पेभ्यो बहवो विशिष्टा इति लोकप्रसिद्धमेककर्मणि । (भा.)

114. बहुधोपयोगात् । (सू. १२५) किं च बहुधाऽभ्यङ्गपरिषेकावगाहरूपेण शीतादय उपयुज्यन्ते, रसास्तु मुखत एवेति गुणाः प्रधानाः, ये बहुधोपयोगं गच्छन्ति ते प्रधाना दृष्टा यथा कल्पवृक्षाः । (भा.)
(ज्यांचा विविध त-हेने पुष्कळ उपयोग होतो)

115. अनेककर्मत्वात् ।“ (सू. १२६) रसादिसाहितास्तेषां तेषां तत्तत्कर्मणि साहचर्यकरणादनेककर्माण इति । (भा.)

116. महाविषयत्वात् ।“ (सू. १२७)

117. उपदेशापदेशादनुमानात्“ (सू. १२९) १तेषां गुरूष्णास्निग्धा वातघ्नाः“ इत्यादि रुपदेशः ।

118. अपदेशः-तीक्ष्णोऽयं पुरुषः, मृदुरयं गीत इति ।“ (भा.)

CHAPTER FIVE
THE RASAS

Rasa

The etymology of "Rasa" - The word rasa is not only used in vaidyak, but is also used in diverse subjects including literature. The dictionary provides nine different meanings of rasa. With reference to Ayurveda, though, rasa has four meanings. Since the implications of these four are different, their etymology also differs.[1]

1) Rasa (dhatu) - रसति अहरह: गच्छति = रस:

Here, rasa refers to rasa dhatu which is the first among the seven dhatus of the body viz. rasa, rakta, mansa, meda, asthi, majja and shukra. It is called rasa as it circulates continuously throughout the body, 24 hours a day, and is always moving.[2]

2) Rasa (mercury) - रसति - भक्षयति सर्वान् लोहान् इति रस: ।

Since it has been claimed that parad (mercury) dissolves or amalgamates metals like gold, (ग्रासी), one meaning of the word rasa is taken as parad (mercury).[3]

3) Rasa (kalpana-preparation) - Various preparations of drugs have been used in Ayurveda while administering medicines. There are five basic preparations of medicines- rasa (juice), kalka (pulp), shruta (decoction), sheeta (cold infusion) and fant (hot infusion). Among these, that juice which is obtained by thoroughly crushing a fresh, green herb and then filtering it through a cloth or filter is called rasa. It spreads very quickly within the body. The etymology of rasa kalpana is as follows: रसति शरीरे आशु प्रसरति इति रस:।[4] The definition which is more relevant to dravyagunavignyan than the above three definitions is as follows:

4) Rasa (sense object) - रस्यते आस्वाद्यते रसनया रसनेंद्रियेण इति रस: ।

That particular sense object (artha, vishaya) which is perceived by the tongue is rasa. According to this derivation, the six tastes present in the dravyas viz. sweet, sour, salty, pungent, bitter and astringent fall in the category of rasas.[5]

The former three interpretations are used respectively in Ayurvedic physiology, rasashastra and pharmacology. The meaning accepted by dravyagunashastra is the one which is implied by the fourth. The impulses generated by the dravyas on the rasna-indriya (one of the five senses which perceives taste/savour) with the help of the tongue (acting as an instrument) are of six types and these are, in fact, the six rasas.

Characteristics of rasas - The sense object (artha or vishaya) of rasna-indriya is called rasa. That guna which can be perceived only by the rasna-indriya is called rasa. Though this tongue-perceptible sense object has many subtle grades and though every individual evaluates his experience of the rasas in a different way, yet, these can be broadly classified into six groups. Various grades of rasas have been classified into madhur, amla, lavana, katu, tikta and kashaya. Since all the above six have taste-perceptibility in common, these are called rasas. While perceiving these, the six groups which emerge (due to the impulses) give rise to a definite number of ras

The number of rasas with examples of each - Rasas are six ie. s
bitter and astringent. The examples are as follows-

1. Sweet - Sugar, banana, jack fruit, yastimadhu, mohaphoola, sugarcane,
   fruits or khirni etc.
2. Sour - Amla, tamarind, mahalung, buttermilk, curds, mango (unripe), un uka, ambada etc.
3. Salty - Saindhava (rock salt), black salt, sea salt, padelon etc.
4. Pungent - Sunthi, maricha, pippali, hinga (asafoetida). pitta (bile) etc.
5. Bitter - Neem, kirat-tikta, kutaki, kutaja, adulsa, guduchi, vekhanda etc.
6. Astringent - Haritaki, bibheetaka, kher, the bark of umbar, geru etc.[6]

Thus, the rasas have been classified into six groups based on types. Individual dravyas of each and every group differ from the dravyas of the same group in the grade of the rasas. Yet, owing to the similarity of their taste and action, these are placed in the same group inspite of their having varying intensities of rasas. There are many differences of opinion on the number of rasas. This is so because a rasa, which is a guna, is defined through subjective inference (experience) drawn after perceiving it by the rasna-indriya. Naturally, every individual classifies the rasas depending on his perception. Yet the ancient scholars have not accepted any unwarranted compromise and ultimately it was decided that rasas are only six as is evident from the detailed discussion given in Charaka samhita).[7] In fact, this was the conclusion arrived at after the discussion described in the chapter entitled AtreyaBhadrakapyeya adhyaya in the sutra sthana of Charaka samhita. In this chapter, the prima facie view or the first objection to an assertion is given first and then follows the answer to the objectionable argument. (This is the method and sequence in all discussions).

The perception of the rasas in a dravya is due to the constitution of rasna-indriya (tongue). As jala mahabhoota is predominant in the tongue, any dravya, after coming in contact with it undergoes a transformation and this transformed state of the dravya is then called its rasa. If sugar is given to two persons, one of whom is healthy and the other one is suffering from fever, then sugar, which is actually sweet, will taste bitter to the sick person. Therefore, even though the dravya is the cause of perception of rasas, the state of the rasna-indriya (tongue) of the consumer has also to be taken into account. In various stages of the vitiation of doshas, depending on the state of various parts of the body like mouth and tongue, one may feel the presence of sweet, sour, salty, pungent, bitter or astringent taste in the mouth irrespective of contact with any external dravya. Very often, one comes across such an experience. Therefore, these conditions have been included in the list of manifestations of the vitiation of doshas and their various stages.

The prima facie views (propositions) regarding the number of rasas-

1. Bhadrakapya rishi expressed the view that since rasa is the object of perception of rasna-indriya, jala mahabhoota and rasa are one and the same and therefore there is only one rasa.

Whichever work the body is supposed to do, the body should be trained to do the same.

ere are only two rasas - one that increases the bulk of the tissues (ie. bruhan) and the other that reduces the bulk of the tissues (langhan). This view was propagated by Shakunteya.

3. There are three rasas - chedaneeya (ie. langhan), upshamaneeya (ie. bruhan) and sadharan. This view was propagated by Poornaksha Moudgalya (He has made an addition of sadharan to the two rasas enumerated by Shakunteya).

4. Hiranyaksha Kaushik expressed the view that rasas are four viz. 1) savoury-beneficial 2) savoury-nonbeneficial 3) nonsavoury-beneficial and 4) nonsavoury-nonbeneficial.

5. According to Kumarshira Bharadwaj muni, there are only five rasas viz. bhaum, aapya, agneya, vayavya and akasheeya. These five are the rasas of the five panchamahabhootas respectively.

6. Rajarshi Vayorvid held the view that rasas are six viz. guru-laghu, sheeta-ushna and snigdha-ruksha. Thus, three gunas, along with their respective antagonist gunas, form six rasas in all.

7. Rasas are seven in number - madhur (sweet), amla (sour), lavana (salty), katu (pungent), tikta (bitter), kashaya (astringent) and kshara (corrosive). This was said by Vaideha Nimi Mahashaya.

8. Badisha Dhamargava made an addition of avyakta rasa (indistinct) and thus according to him rasas are eight in number viz - sweet, sour, salty, pungent, bitter, astringent, corrosive and indistinct.

9. Vaidya Kankayan of Balhik desha expressed the view that rasas are innumerable because just as the dravyas which sustain guna and karma are innumerable, similarly, rasas are also innumerable.[8]

These were the propositions made as prima-facie views - following are the answers to the objectionable propositions by which they are disposed off.

Answers to the objectionable propositions

The principle that rasas are only six in number was established by excluding all other possibilities (vyavrutti method). After listening to all these propositions and prima facie views, Atreya Punarvasu logically disproved these in the following manner -

1. It is improper to say that rasa and jala are one and the same. While jala is the sustainer, rasa is the sustained guna. The sustainer and the sustained can never be one. Therefore rasa is different from jala. Hence to say that these two are one was judged wrong. Rasa and jala are not identical.

2. Rasas are neither two nor three in number. The views of Shakunteya and Moudgalya are also wrong because chedaneeya (langhan) and upshamaneeya (bruhan) are karmas and not gunas. Sadharan, described by Moudgalya in addition to chedaneeya and upshamaneeya, is also a karma. Since rasa is a guna and since rasa and karma are totally different, the views of these two were not acceptable. Thus, rasas are neither two nor three in number.

3. Rasas are not four in number. Because the savoury-nonsavoury and beneficial-nonbeneficial types of rasas described by Hiranyaksha depend on individual likes - dislikes and the actions respectively. Therefore it was ruled improper to classify rasas into these types. This implies that

It should be understood that any positive or negative manifestation is influenced by functionality of srotas.

rasas are not four in number.

4. It is not correct to classify rasas as bhaum rasa, aapya rasa etc. saying that since panchamahabhootas are five, rasas are also five in number. This is so because the five mahabhootas are dravyas whereas rasa is a guna. Bhaum (parthiva), aapya etc. are actually types of dravyas and these can never be considered as rasas. Though rasas depend on and are sustained by the mahabhootas they are different padarthas (phenomena) from the mahabhootas.

Bhaum, aapya, agneya, vayavya and akasheeya are five types of dravyas and not rasas. In fact, rasa is sustained by the dravyas. The sustainer and sustained can never be the same, therefore dravyas are five in number whereas rasas are not. Dravyas constituted by the panchamahabhootas are influenced by prakriti (tendency), vikar (vitiation), vichar (combination with another dravya), desha (habitat) and kala (season). But rasa is totally different. Let us see how the concept of rasa differs. Mudga is innately laghu. It is madhur (sweet) and kashaya (astringent) to taste. Madhur and kashaya rasas are heaviest and heavier respectively ie. these are guru (heavy to digest), however, mudga is laghu (light to digest). Poha and lahya are two different items prepared from rice. Due to different ways of preparation (conditioning), lahya is laghu (lighter) as compared to poha. Both are sweet to taste but one (poha) is guru, whereas the other (lahya) is light. If this example is considered from the point of view of rasa alone, then as madhur rasa is guru, lahya should also be guru since it is sweet to taste. Similarly, honey and ghee, when mixed in equal proportions, are incompatible. This is due to the peculiarities of the dravyas and not rasas. Plants growing in the Himalayas possess superior gunas due to the effects which are exclusive to the Himalayan area. Tender and fully grown radish are both pungent but tender radish is doshaghna (alleviates the doshas) whereas a fully grown radish is tridoshakara (aggravates all the three doshas). This is the effect of kala (time) influencing the dravyas.

Thus, the five types of rasas as proposed by Kumarshira Bharadwaj are not rasas but are actually the effects of samyoga (conjunction), sanskar (conditioning), vichar (combination), desha (habitat) and kala (time) on the dravyas. Therefore the propositions made by him are not correct. This means that since rasas and dravyas are different, rasas are not five in number.

5. Rajarshi Vayorvid has listed six types of rasas like guru, laghu etc. These are among the twenty gunas sustained by dravya. These are not rasas. A rasa has to be necessarily perceptible through the tongue; but gunas like guru, laghu etc. are not perceptible through the sense organs and hence these are not rasas. From this it is correct to say that even though there are six rasas, the six gunas like guru, laghu etc. cannot be called as rasas.

6. Vaideha Nimi has described seven types of rasas. Among these, the first six – madhur, amla, lavana, katu, tikta and kashaya are in fact rasas. The inclusion of 'kshara' in the list of rasas as the seventh rasa is not correct; because kshara is a dravya prepared from many dravyas having many rasas and is chiefly katu (pungent) and lavana (salty) to taste. Apart from this, kshara is not exclusively perceptible through the tongue only, ie. other senses can also perceive kshara (a rasa is exclusively perceived through the tongue). In addition, kshara is prepared by a unique procedure called ksharavidhi. Therefore kshara is not a rasa.

Twenty gunas and their actions are constantly functional in a living being. These are not to be formed newly.

7. Badisha Dhamargava even accepted avyakta (indistinct) rasa as an independent rasa and thus put the number of rasas at eight. This is not acceptable, because vyakta (distinct/manifested) and avyakta (indistinct/unmanifested) are conditions of rasas, then how can one accept these conditions as rasas themselves? Rasa remains in the indistinct or unmanifested form in jala, in the state of anurasa and also in dravyas having anurasa. Therefore there can be no independent rasa as 'avyakta rasa'. Also, from the aphorism ''तत्र व्यक्तो रसः स्मृतः we can say that 'avyakta' cannot be an independent rasa.

8. By saying that rasas are innumerable, Vaidya Kankayan of Balhik desha has created confusion. This statement is totally unfair, because even though various dravyas which sustain madhuradi rasas, as well as gunas and karmas and similarly, their tastes, are innumerable, yet the number of rasas remains the same. The reason for this is that dravyas like milk, ghee, manuka which sustain madhur rasa have gunas like guru, snigdha, sthira, pichchila etc. All of these also have karmas like bruhan, tarpan etc. Also, it is beyond doubt that these have various gradations like less sweet, moderately sweet and extremely sweet. Yet, the characteristics (quality) of sweetness (madhuratva) remains common in all these dravyas. Therefore, the number of rasas does not change. It remains six only. To acquire knowledge of entities, it is essential to classify them into groups on the basis of their commonality.

One may say that due to the combination of various rasas there occurs a change in the taste, actions etc. and therefore rasas should be considered innumerable; but even this statement is not acceptable, because the guna-karmas of the rasas do not change even after combination of various rasas. After such combinations, the actions generated by the innate guna-karmas of the individual rasas are always evident in a mixed form and therefore it is not logical to say that rasas are innumerable. Just as vatadi doshas may combine through various permutations and combinations and yet the number of doshas remains three only, similarly, even though rasas have many grades, the number of rasas is only six. This is the reason behind not describing the actions of combined rasas.[9]

Conclusion

The conclusion of the above discussion is that rasas are only six in number. These six rasas are madhur, amla, lavana, katu, tikta and kashaya.[10]

One more proposition

It was proposed that since the dravyas falling in the madhur varga like sugar, jaggery etc. differ in their tastes, it is not appropriate to assume that rasas are only six. Rasas should be considered innumerable. Well, if 'taste' is considered as a criterion, then all the rasas will be of only one type considering that the 'taste perceptibility' is common to all; ie. the number of rasas will be only one. Therefore the proposition is that either accept that rasas are innumerable or that there is only one rasa.

Following is the dismissal of the above proposition (Ashtangsangraha)

The answer to this is that even though the tastes of these dravyas differ due to slight difference in their panchbhautik composition, yet there is not much difference in the effects generated by their madhur rasa. Even if the degree of sweetness varies in these dravyas, there is no difference in their kind, is there? One dravya may be the heaviest while another dravya may be lighter (laghutara) and a third may be the lightest (laghutama). Here, there is a difference in the degree of lightness and heaviness of dravyas but the basic quality or the natural disposition to lightness (laghutva) or heaviness (gurutva) has not changed, has it? Just as this quality remains unchanged, similarly, even though there is a difference in the tastes of rasas, yet, all of these fall in the same kind ie. madhuratva, kashyatva etc.

The sweetness of jaggery prepared in different factories is different or the taste of honey extracted from different flowers is different; this means that the slight difference in the degree is always there, but these grades are of one and the same rasa. Therefore each and every grade can not be considered as an independent rasa.

The characteristics of dravyas having the same rasas show similarity in their actions. For example, all the dravyas like manuka, jaggery and ghee will bring about actions like smearing the mouth and pleasing the mind. These gunas will be found only in other madhur dravyas. These gunas will not be found in sour dravyas like buttermilk, curds, amla, tamarind etc. and Therefore due to the commonality in the gunas, karmas and vargas, rasas are only six in number. If it is assumed that rasas are innumerable then comprehension of innumerable rasas is not possible and if it is assumed that there is only one rasa, then nothing can be elaborated further as nothing specific remains.

मधुरस्कन्धनिर्दिष्टघृततैलगुडादिषु ।
गुणास्वादादिभेदेन रसषट्कं न युज्यते ॥
अस्तु भेदादसंख्यत्वमैक्यं वाऽऽस्वादलक्षणात् ।
भूतोत्कर्षापकर्षेण भेदो योऽल्पेन कल्प्यते ॥
संकीर्णत्वात् फले चासौ तुल्यत्वान्न विवक्ष्यते ।
गुर्वादीनां विशेषऽपि स्वजातेरनतिक्रमात् ॥
संख्याभेदो यथा नास्ति रसानामपि स क्रमः ।
दृष्टं मुखोपलेपादि यत् सर्वेषु घृतादिषु ॥
न च तद्दाडिमाद्येषु षडेवातो रसाः स्मृताः ।
आनन्त्यैकत्वयोश्च स्थान्न विचित्रार्थतन्त्रणाम् ॥
(अ. सं. सू . १४)

The conclusion of the whole debate was that, as the authors of the scriptures have accepted the number of rasas as only six and as the number of savours is also six, there are only six rasas.
11

(The impulses generated after the contact of dravyas having various rasas with the rasna indriya- ie. the tongue, are only of six types. Due to this also, it is appropriate to consider that the number of rasas is only six).

(In Ayurveda, the word 'tikta' implies what we generally call as bitter in our day to day life. For example - quinine, karavellaka, seeds of methi etc. Similarly, the word 'katu' means pungent. For example, chillies, pippali etc. However, due to the similarity of pronounciation between 'tikta' and 'tikhat' as well as 'katu' and 'kadu', sometimes people misunderstand 'tikta' as pungent and 'katu' as

Analysing complex synthesized substances is not easy like resolving woven chord.

bitter. But this is not correct. While studying the scriptures, tikta should always be taken as bitter and katu as pungent.)

Nagarjuna has also ascertained the number of rasas at six. He has given two evidences in support. One is direct demonstrable evidence - we can perceive only six rasas and the second is the words of the rishis (apta). As the rishis (aptas) are devoid of raja-tama doshas, their words are always true and hence always acceptable. The words of the rishis are the basis of all evidence. Due to both these evidences it is established that there are only six rasas.

Concept of rasas according to modern science

According to modern physiology and modern psychology, rasa is of four types: 1) madhur (sweet) 2) amla (sour) 3) lavana (salt) and 4) tikta (bitter).

The remaining two rasas ie. katu (pungent) and kashaya (astringent) are perceptible through the tongue and also through the skin. These are not exclusively perceptible by the tongue and hence are of dual nature.

Eventhough modern science does not consider these two as independent rasas, yet, in pharmacology, astringent group of drugs and volatile, pungent group of drugs have been mentioned. Therefore there is no alteration in the number of rasas. (Every rasa has one pecularity of its own; every rasa is independent).

The panchabhautik basis of rasas

Just as the dravya is constituted by the panchamahabhootas, similarly, rasa which is a guna residing in the dravya, is also panchabhautik. From the point of view of rasas, jala is the most important among the panchmahabhootas. There cannot be rasa without jala. Yet, jala + prithvi is the essential (unavoidable/indispensable) cause of rasas (prithvi is the less dominant cause). Apart from this, the three mahabhootas viz. teja, vayu and akash have their subtle gradations. All these three mahabhootas are not the chief causes, only jala is. Prithvi, though essential, is a secondary cause compared to jala and the remaining three mahabhootas are merely instrumental causes. In this manner, all the five mahabhootas act as causes in the genesis of rasas. Since dravyas and rasas are both panchamahabhootatmak and since rasas are also panchamahabhootatmak, a dravya may have many rasas simultaneously. Nevertheless, the dominant or subordinate status of a rasa depends on its proportion. This is the main cause of genesis of subtlties like rasa and anurasa. Rasa is a guna, even though it is perceptible by the rasna-indriya, yet it is the exclusive property of jala mahabhoota. Therefore, there can be no genesis of rasa without jala. Dravyas predominant in rasas possess more characteristics of jala mahabhoota than any other mahabhoota. Jala mahabhoota is the essential, indispensable cause of rasa. Prithvi is the subordinate but basic cause while teja, vayu, akash are only instrumental causes.[12]

Rasa and anurasa

Rasa - That particular dominant guna which resides in the dravya and is perceived exclusively by the tongue is called 'rasa'. Following are the characteristics of this rasa 1) The rasa needs to be completely manifested, which means that it is necessary that it should be perceived directly and

Actions are of three types - kayik, vachik and manasik. The dravya which acts at all the three levels simultaneously is the best.

promptly. For example - sweetness of sugar, sourness of lime, saltiness of common salt, pungency of chillies, bitterness of kirattikta, astringence of alum. 2) The rasa which is manifested both in the wet and in the dried state of the dravya is the predominant rasa. (Reference: Dravyagunavignyan, Priyavrat Sharma - Guna khanda, 1955 edition, page 161). Ripe grapes are sweet to taste and the sweet taste remains even after drying the grapes (manuka). But, pippali is sweet when wet and tastes katu (pungent) on drying. Thus the ultimate rasa of pippali ie. the katu rasa, is the actual rasa of pippali. Its madhur rasa is not fixed. Therefore, it is not fit to be called rasa. (It may be called anurasa). 3) The guna which is perceived immediately after contact of the dravya with the tongue is called rasa.

For example - buttermilk, lime-juice, sugar, kutaki, salt.

Anurasa - Anurasa is the opposite of rasa. Rasa is predominant. This predominant rasa supersedes the other subordinate rasas and thus these rasas are not manifested first. This happens in accordance with the principle of 'भूयसा अल्पं हि जीयते.' Even if these subordinate rasas get manifested, the manifestation occurs either after the rasas in minute proportion or in the end.

The entity which we call as a dravya's rasa does not belong to the dravya alone but is the overall perception generated after the contact of the rasna-indriya (tongue) with a combination of jala mahabhoota, bodhaka kapha etc. Here, if jala, which is a padartha residing in the tongue, is not available to the dravya, then no taste will be perceived. Rasas cannot be perceived by a dry tongue. For the perception of rasas, the almighty (nature) has provided ample supply of jala mahabhoota to the tongue. The jala derived from this supply, on combining with the dravya to be perceived, gives rise to a transformed dravya and that is its rasa. It will not be the whole truth to say that this taste belongs to the transfomed state of the dravya. Nevertheless, it is true that the dravya is the stimulator of rasa.

Various tastes are felt in the mouth in various diseases. The reason is that the aapya dravya of the tongue assumes that particular taste. Continuous feeling of sweetness or any other taste in the mouth is an important criterion for the diagnosis of diseases. Here, the taste felt in the mouth does not belong to any external dravya but to the body constituents. Sometimes, in fever, one experiences a bitter taste of anything eaten. This is because the tikta rasa supersedes all the other rasas. This condition is indicative of an increase in pitta dosha in rasa dhatu. In this way, precise correlation can be established among rasas and in turn anurasas as well.

Characteristics of anurasa

Anu means after, anu-inferior, lower in value or importance. Following meaning of the word anu is given in the dictionary - आयामेऽपरभावेच (पश्चादर्थे) वीप्सायां संनिधौ तथा । इत्यंभूते लक्षणेच भागसादृश्ययोरपि । योग्यतायां तथा हीने तृतीयर्थे ह्यानुक्रमे । अर्थेष्वेतेषु बहुश: अनु शब्द प्रयुज्यते। When the prefix 'anu' is used before rasa, addition of the prefix imparts many meanings to the word 'anurasa'. Many of these meanings apply in the present context-

1) Anurasa is either unmanifested or is manifested in small proportion.

2) Anurasa does not remain in the dravya in its dry state. For example - the sweet anurasa of wet pippali does not remain the same in the dry state.

Medicines prepared with scientific methods have high safety profile, but the process of 'Amrutikaran' is a boon for human kind. It is the speciality of Ayurveda.

3) Anurasa is perceived after the prominent rasa ie. in the end. For example, haritaki, when put in the mouth, initially tastes extremely astringent but in the end it tastes sweet.

Comparison

Rasa	**Anurasa**
1. is manifested	1. either is unmanifested or is manifested in very small proportion.
2. remains intact even after the dravya is dried (as in grapes)	2. does not remain intact in the dry state of the dravya (for example, pippali tastes sweet when wet but on drying it is pungent. Thus 'madhur' is the anurasa of pippali. Same is the case with maricha.
3. is the first to get manifested	3. is manifested later or in the end.

Actually, as soon as the dravya comes in contact with the tongue, the rasa, which was dormant till the time of contact, starts generating impulses. These impulses create more impulses on the rasna-indriya. Simultaneously, due to the addition of bodhaka kapha and similar substances, the dravya keeps on changing at every moment even though it is called by the same name. The taste of the combination may remain the same or may change. But the changed taste will be perceived only after the rasa. This is anurasa. Since anurasa is one among the six rasas and is manifested due to various reasons like time-gap and change in dravya, there is no reason to consider anurasa as the seventh rasa.

व्यक्त: शुष्कस्य चादौ च रसोद्रव्यस्य लक्ष्यते (च.सू.२६)
तत्र यो व्यक्त: रस: । यस्तु रसेन अभिभूतत्वात् न व्यज्यते, व्यज्यते वा किंचित अन्ते स: अनुरस: ॥ (यो.)
तत्र द्रव्ये कश्चिदन्ते व्यक्त: । तेष्वाद्यो रसाख्य:, इतरे त्रयोऽनुरसाख्या: । (हि.)
विपर्ययेणानुरसो रसो नास्तीह सप्तम: । (च.सू.२६)
तत्र व्यक्तो रस: । अनुरसस्तु रसेनाभिभूतत्वादव्यक्तो व्यक्तो वा किंचिदन्ते । (अ.सं.सू १७)
तत्र व्यक्तो रस:स्मृत: । अव्यक्तोऽनुरस: किंचिदन्ते व्यक्तोऽपि चेष्यते ॥ (अ.ह.सू.९)

Characteristics of rasas

Although it is true that the bodies of all animals are made up of panchamahabhootas, yet these are of innumerable types due to different of permutations and combinations and varying proportions of the mahabhootas. Even two people belonging to the same race are not exactly identical (Man The Unknown-by Dr. Alexis Carrel). Similarly, the specific rasas within the dravyas are produced due to innumerable combinations and varying proportions of mahabhootas and therefore the genesis of these rasas also appears to be an infinite process.[13]

Jala mahabhoota is the most important cause in the genesis of rasas. This mahabhoota itself has indistinct rasa but while falling from the sky as rain drops (आकाशात् पतित), it comes in contact with

The terminology "Vichitrapratyayarabdha" is self explanatory. It dictates cause-effect relationship.

other mahabhootas to a varying extent. Also, when this jala mahabhoota actually falls on the ground and comes in contact with it, the gunas of all the mahabhootas get incorporated in jala mahabhoota; thus all the six rasas are generated in it. According to the science of Ayurveda, two mahabhootas are responsible for the genesis of each rasa depending on their higher or lower proportion.[14]

1.	Madhur rasa	-	generated due to preponderance of jala + prithvi mahabhootas
2.	Amla rasa	-	Prithvi + agni (Charaka,Vagbhatta, Ashtangsangraha, Asthangahridaya) jala + agni (Sushruta)
3.	Lavana rasa	-	Jala + agni (Charaka, Ashtanghridaya, Nagarjuna) prithvi + agni (Sushruta)
4.	Katu rasa	-	Vayu + agni
5.	Tikta rasa	-	Vayu + akash
6.	Kashaya rasa	-	Vayu + prithvi[15]

Question No. 1 - If combinations of mahabhootas are responsible for the genesis of rasas then since ten such combinations are possible through various permutations and combinations, why are rasas only six in number? Why are rasas not produced from the remaining four combinations, namely jala + vayu, jala + akash, prithvi + akash and teja + akash ? Why are six rasas generated only from six combinations?

The second question which arises in one's mind is, what is the reason behind this combination of mahabhootas resulting in the genesis of rasas?

The answer to the first question is that 'this is the innate tendency of the mahabhootas'. There is no definite rule to determine which two mahabhootas will combine to generate a rasa. The answer to it is that this is the inherent disposition of the mahabhootas. This is how it is. There is no other explanation than the 'innate tendency' of the mahabhootas which can explain why mahabhootas combine only in this manner and not in any other way. The commentators have also given the same explanation. Very few diseases are caused due to vitiation of two doshas (dwidoshaj diseases). (Not all diseases are dwidoshaj). Just as the reason for this is the inherent disposition, similarly, the same applies here. Therefore, even though there are 10 combinations of two mahabhootas each, yet dravyas have only six rasas. Just like prabhav, there is no answer to this inherent predisposition of the mahabhootas.

The answer to the second question is that the various conditions in the six ritus (seasons), which divide one year in six parts, give rise to different rasas. Therefore it is logical to say that since there are six ritus, the rasas are also six in number. (The following table throws some more light on this concept). Shishir, vasant, greeshma, varsha, sharad and hemant are the six ritus (seasons) and in these ritus, tikta, kashaya, katu, amla, lavana and madhur rasas are generated respectively. The first three rasas are generated during the Adan kala (procurment period) and the remaining three during the

Forests are the real treasures of nations. Indian forest has reduced from 33% to 18% not because of natural calamities but due to greedy indulgent human beings.

Visarga kala (bestowal period). Their actions are similar to the effects of their respective seasons. If a dravya, naturally having apatarpana guna, also possesses santarpana guna, then it is the innate tendency of the dravya that these two gunas do not contradict each other due to their inherent compatibility.

Cycle of seasons & genesis of rasas

Seasons		Preponderance of mahabhootas	Genesis of rasas	Veerya
1. Shishir	Uttarayana	Vayu + Akash	Tikta	Sheeta
2. Vasant	Adankala	Vayu + Prithvi	Kashaya	Veerya
3. Greeshma	(Procurment period)	Vayu + Agni	Katu	
4. Varsha	Dakshinayana Visargakala	Prithvi + Agni	Amla	Ushna veerya
5. Sharad	(bestowal	Jala + Agni	Lavana	
6. Hemant	period)	Prithvi + Jala	Madhur	Sheeta veerya

There are exceptions to this general rule. Sometimes in some seasons, another mahabhoota may be dominant and this may give rise to another rasa. Apart from this, like the year, ritus are also divided into six parts.[16] Similarly, due to the rising and setting of the sun, one day-night (24 hours) is again divided into six parts just as the ritus. As a result of this (प्रहर), there are exceptions to this rule. Lastly, the 'unforeseen' is also considered as a cause for these exceptions.

There appears to be a difference of opinion among the acharyas over the mahabhoota composition of amla and lavana rasas. According to Charaka, amla rasa results from prithvi + agni mahabhootas whereas Sushruta opines that it arises from jala + agni mahabhootas. Considering the effects of these rasas, there is not much anomaly in the above disagreement. Secondly, the mahabhoota composition of the rasas would have been ascertained only on the basis of effects generated by the respective rasas. Thus, even if there is a minor difference, it is not a matter of grave concern. Whether it is amla rasa or lavana rasa, both will increase kapha and pitta and reduce vata.[17] Amla rasa is more bruhan compared to lavana rasa whereas lavana rasa is more langan compared to amla rasa. Because of this, the difference might have been created between the two.

Now, one may raise a doubt that agni and jala are mutually antagonistic. Rasa is created from jala and if agni and jala are antagonistic, then how can rasa be created from agni and jala? Similarly, how are mutually antagonistic rasas generated in a single dravya and why are mutually antagonistic gunas not created from mahabhootas ? There is only one answer to these questions–this is their svabhav (innate tendenty) and it always supersedes everything else. If anything has to be changed through 'sanskar' it can not be done without taking into consideration its svabhav. It is the tendency of dravyas that while they are being created, some gunas get manifested while others remain unmanifested. For example - matha is sweet but not unctuous. Similarly, saindhav is predominant in

The etiopathogenesis of dosha kshayaj diseases are not distinctly evident as that of dosha vruddhij. Why is it so?

agni + jala mahabhootas but is not ushna. The answer to all this is unforeseen tendency.[18]

(In this universe of known-unknown components, eventhough there is a cause-effect relationship behind each and every event, yet it is not possible to fully explain each of them. When the cause-effect relationship of a particular event falls beyond the ambit and purview of human intellect, then the possible answer to it lies in the svabhav and prabhav – 'प्रत्यक्षं हि अल्पं अनल्पमप्रत्यक्षम्. The purpose behind this aphorism is also the same. Therefore, sometimes it becomes inevitable to find refuge with the 'aptavakyas' (the words of the learned).

How to ascertain the panchabhautik origin of rasas?

What is the evidence to prove that all these rasas are formed by mahabhootas? This can be understood through inferential knowledge.[19]

The panchabhautik origin of rasas might have been ascertained after observing the actions of the rasas and comparing them with the guna-karmas of the mahabhootas.(This is also a type of inferential knowledge). Use of rasas will lead to an increase in similar components of the body and decrease in dissimilar components.

(सर्वदा सर्वभावानां सामान्यं........) It is on this principle that the causal mahabhootas of a particular rasa are determined. For example- madhur rasa causes an increase in aapya kapha and decrease in agneya pitta.

Considering this, it was concluded that madhur rasa is produced from jala and prithvi. The same principle can be applied to other rasas as well. Amla rasa increases kapha and pitta therefore it is produced from prithvi + agni mahabhootas, lavana rasa increases drava kapha and ushna pitta therefore this rasa is produced from jala + agni mahabhootas and katu rasa increases vata-pitta therefore vayu + agni are the causal mahabhootas. The domain of anuman praman (inferential knowledge) begins where the domain of pratyaksha praman (direct and demonstrable evidence) ends. (प्रत्यक्षपूर्वं अनुमानम् । च.सू.11)[20]

A few commentators hold the view that this issue should be solely decided on the basis of aptavakyas. Through aptavakyas, one knows about the panchabhautik composition of rasas whereas through anuman praman these findings can be confirmed. Aptopadesha is of three types - pratyakshartha (one that emerges from direct demonstrable evidence), anumeyartha (one that emerges from inferential knowledge) and shraddheyartha (one that depends on faith). Of these three, the authenticity of the first two can be confirmed through pratyaksha and anuman. The third type of aptopadesha is solely a subject of faith.[21]

The existence of mahabhootas can be inferred through various actions and effects generated by the use of the respective rasas. If a particular rasa or a dravya induces emesis, then it can be concluded that made up of agni and vayu mahabhootas as agni mahabhoota tends to move upwards and vayu mahabhoota tends to create the force behind emesis. If the rasa or dravya induces purgation, then it should be understood that it is made up of prithvi and jala mahabhootas as both these mahabhootas tend to move downwards. This is so because jala mahabhoota has a tendency to move downwards and prithvi mahabhoota also moves downwards due to gravity. If a single rasa

It is my strong belief that these footnotes will certainly enlighten a serious thinker of Ayurveda.

brings about all these actions then it should be understood that all the four mahabhootas are the causal mahabhootas. Similarly, various actions of the rasas also provide a clue to the mahabhoota composition of the rasas and direct evidence can also be obtained which verify the observations.[22]

If a particular rasa or a dravya produces an upward movement of gastric contents, direct or indirectly, then it should be said that the dravya is conducive to emesis. The reverse applies to purgation.

Dravyas dominant in akash mahabhoota produce the action of sanshodhan. Similarly, dravyas dominant in vayu mahabhoota are shoshan, agneya dravyas are deepan and dravyas dominant in vayu and agni mahabhootas bring about lekhan karma. Dravyas dominant in prithvi and jala mahabhootas bring about the action of bruhan.[23]

Among the six rasas, madhur and kashaya rasas are stambhak whereas all the other rasas help in shodhan. This is a general rule with no exceptions to it.

How are rasas perceived?

According to the Indian Darshanshastra (philosophy), knowledge can be acquired through three pramans. 1) pratyaksha 2) anuman and 3) aptavakya. Rasas can be known through all these three modes of knowledge. Yet, direct demonstrable knowledge is more widely used. If the dravya comes in contact with the tongue, then and only then direct perception of the rasa is possible. This is called रासन प्रत्यक्ष. The taste which is perceived as soon as the dravya is placed on the tongue is called as rasa. The rasas of some dravyas have to be ascertained through anuman only. The sweetness of gold, the sour taste of silver, salty taste of lead and the bitter taste of iron have all been ascertained through inference after carefully observing the effects of these dravyas on the body. Similarly, avyakta rasa or anurasa have to be specifically understood through aptopadesha and this knowledge is endorsed through anuman praman. According to some, a general knowledge of rasas is obtained through pratyaksha; anuman provides specific knowledge whereas aptopadesha provides experiential knowledge.[24]

The knowledge produced due to contact with the tongue is called pratyaksha knowledge. Experiencing a rasa which has been experienced earlier is anuman and the first hand knowledge that honey is kashaya and water is sweet is obtained through aptavakya. This means that it is only through aptavakya that we learn to call a particular perception as astringent, bitter etc. It is a universally experienced fact that the source of all knowledge is aptavakya. The perception generated immediately after a dravya comes in contact with the tongue is pratyaksha. Later on, the knowledge that it has tastes like sweet etc. is anuman. And finally the knowledge that a particular rasa is useful in certain conditions is obtained through aptavakya.[25] (A dravya, after coming in contact with the tongue, produces varying impulses which generates a general perception of the rasas. Various peculiarities of the rasas should also be understood through these impulses).

Disturbance in physical and mental homeostasis is scientifically considered as one of the major causes of diesase.

Conversion of rasas (Rasantar)

(अन्यो रस: रसान्तरम्)

The rasa of any dravya is never permanent. It always keeps on changing in subtler proportions. This means that a change in the rasas of dravyas is possible. Following are the reasons for this -

1. **Time-** If a dravya is kept for a longer period, then a change in its rasas is possible. e.g. cooked rice, on keeping for a long time becomes sour.

2. **Vessel** - If a dravya is kept in a particular vessel for some time then a change in its rasa is possible. Coffee kept in a bronze vessel becomes bitter. Milk kept in a silver vessel becomes sour.[26]

3. **Combination-** Combination of some different dravyas produces a change in their rasas. For example- a combination of salt and tamarind produces sweet taste.[27]

4. **Pak (ripening)** - Ripening (pak) means conditioning with teja mahabhoota. Due to the effects of teja mahabhoota, a mango fruit, which is intially astringent, becomes sour later on. And finally, on ripening completely, it becomes sweet.[28]

5. **Sunlight** - (This is also a type of pak-combination with teja mahabhoota). The astringent taste of tamarind changes to sweet on exposure to sunlight.[29]

6. **Bhavana (impregnation)** - The original rasa of a dravya changes after giving it a bhavana with some other dravya. For example - Sesamum seeds are astringent, bitter and sweet to taste; but on giving it a bhavana with yashtimadhu, (ie. impregnating sesamum seeds in the juice of yashtimadhu), the astringent and bitter tastes are eliminated.[30]

7. **Desha** - Environmental factors are also responsible for bringing about a change in the rasas. An amla fruit is sweet at some places (Priyavarat Sharma, Dravyagunavignyan, 1968 edition, page 195).[31]

8. **Kalapak** - By allowing some time interval (ie. through kalapak) to pass, astringent bananas turn sweet.[31]

9. **Parinam** - Parinam means transformation. For example, milk gets converted into curds thereby losing its sweetness, which is transformed into the sour taste of curds. Similarly, some fruits, transformed on becoming extremely ripe, become sour to taste. Bananas can be cited as examples of this phenomenon.[32]

10. **Upsarga** - If a dravya decays then its rasa may change. For example, if a sugarcane rots then its sweet taste changes to either bitter or sour.[33]

11. **Vikriya** - Vikriya means some special procedures. If some special procedures are done on a dravya then its rasa also changes. It has been cited in the texts that if a coconut is heated and then hit on the ground firmly then it loses its sweetness and becomes bitter to taste. Similarly, if pieces of jackfruit are rubbed in hands for some time then they become sour. The fruits of umbar when rubbed in hands, partly lose their astringent taste and become sweet.

Mere touch of Gloriosa superba by a woman immediately after delivery helps to expel placenta due to induction of uterine contractions.

(The fruits of umbar are always rubbed in the hands before eating in some parts of India).[34]

Classification of rasas - saumya & agneya

The whole universe is classified into two on the basis of its properties. One type is agneya and the other is saumya. The rasas in whom teja mahabhoota is the causal mahabhoota, ie. amla, lavana and katu rasas, are agneya whereas other rasas like madhur, tikta and kashaya are called as saumya. Obviously, the saumya and agneya properties of these rasas have their own gradations.[35]

Agneya rasas (amla, lavana and katu) are ushna, increase pitta and cause fainting and burning sensation. Saumya rasas (madhur, tikta and kashaya) are sheeta, reduce pitta and alleviate fainting and burning sensation.

The Characteristics of rasas

The impulses generated immediately after a dravya comes in contact with the tongue help in perceiving the taste of that dravya. From this it is called as madhur, amla etc. These characteristics are highly subjective. In science, it is not enough to define the characteristics only in subjective terms. Some other demonstrable properties are also required to be cited. Considering this, other idetifying features have also been described. Among these, certain local features and some other reflexs have been described. While describing the characteristics of rasas, the local effects generated by them have been described in each case. The systemic effects, other than the local effects generated by rasas, have also been described. A rasa is classified after taking into consideration all the effects generated by it (local as well as systemic).

Just by looking at an amla dravya (the amla rasa of which has been experienced earlier) like tamarind, certain impulses are generated in the body. These impulses have their impact initially on the tongue and later on this impact is felt on the whole body. If a person playing a flute sees someone eating a tamarind in front of him, then his salivary secretion increases and it becomes difficult for him to play the flute. If the tongue of a patient becomes excessively dry due to profuse emesis then the Ayurvedic texts have prescribed an unusual remedy. They ask another person to eat sour fruits in front of this patient.[36] This is to reduce the dryness of the tongue by creating suitable impulses.

Once the rasas of a dravya start getting perceived, the impulses are generated and their actions are seen. The actions of the rasas are generated while the rasa is being tasted (while eating). The criteria for identifying the rasas are those which are produced while the rasa is being tasted. Apart from this, the rasas can be identfied by looking at some other characteristics. These are described below -

Madhur rasa - Snehan, tarpan, alhadak (pleasing), mardavkar, mukhlepakar (smears the mouth) and increases kapha and is liked by ants and flies.

If there is sweetness in the urine then ants are attracted towards to it. If the sweetness in the body increases then flies are attracted towards the body. There is much similarlity in the appearance of a crystal of sugar and a crystal of alum, but the effects produced on the tongue are quite different.[37]

Madhur rasa is best suited for bruhan.

Ideally, antibiotics must be such that they have maximum antimicrobial activity while causing minimum hazard to the body.

Amla rasa - When dravyas of this rasa are kept in the mouth and they come in contact with the tongue, the teeth get sour and salivation increases. Amla rasa is swedan. Amla rasa clears the mouths is an appetizer, produces contraction of the eyes and eyebrows, produces burning sensation in the mouth and throat, and produces pitta.[38]

Since it is bhedan, it acts as anuloman. It is useful in diseases like udavarta; it will be seen that amla rasa has been used widely in dryness of mouth.

Lavana rasa - It dissolves immediately on putting in the mouth, produces moistness and softness, is an appetizer and produces burning sensation in the mouth, throat and cheek. Lavana rasa is the most dominant rasa. If any of the rasa among sweet, sour, bitter, pungent or astringent becomes excessive, then adding lavana to it counteracts the excessive rasa. Lavana rasa is the best for generating appetite in food articles.[39]

Katu rasa - This rasa produces irritation of the tongue immediately after putting it in the mouth. It creates foaming sensation and induces secretions from the mouth, nose and eyes.[40] Dravyas like sunthi and pippali, which have katu rasa, are used in rakta pitta; but otherwise katu rasa is contradicated in raktapitta.

Tikta rasa - Once a bitter dravya is placed in the mouth, it causes loss of sensitivity of the tongue to all the other rasas. Though this rasa is ordinarily not pleasing due to its natural properties, yet it has the property of producing appetite for other rasas. Similarly, it cleanses the mouth and clears the throat, produces dryness of the mouth, and has a soothing activity.[41] Tikta rasa is the best in jvara (fever).

Kashaya rasa - It cleans the tongue and produces a feeling of numbness and heaviness in it. Similarly, it produces numbness in the throat also. It produces dryness of the mouth, heart-pain and reduces kapha. It also produces heaviness.[42] Kashaya rasa is best suited in diarrhoea and raktapitta. The discomfort caused by areca nut to some people is because of its kashaya rasa along with its other properties.

Why are rasas only six? There are causes like six seasons along with other causes. The habitat, which is broadly classified into three types is also a cause for the number of rasas being six.

Habitat

Anoop	**Sadharan**	**Jangal**
Anoop=cause of madhur rasa Anoopsadharan is the cause of lavana and amla rasa.	In sadharan desha 4 rasas are produced viz. amla, lavana, tikta and kashaya.	Jangal=cause of katu rasa Jangalsadharan is the cause of tikta and kashaya rasas.

Apart from this, habitat is further divided into four types; among these, one rasa each is produced in 2 types of habitat and the remaining two types of habitats give rise to the remaning 4 rasas. Thus these four types are 1) anoop-madhur 2) anoopsadharan-amla 3) anoopsadharan -lavana 4) jangal-

For a disturbed mind, meditation is more safe, appropriate and effective treatment than medication.

katu 5) jangalsadharan-tikta 6) jangalsadharan-kashaya (अष्टांगसंग्रह सूत्र अ. 18 - श्लोक 32/33)

The properties of rasas

Rasa is a property (guna) which resides in the dravya. All the gunas reside in the dravyas only. Gunas cannot support other gunas. Then how can rasas have their own gunas? But this is just a convention. These gunas are not the gunas of the rasas but they belong to the dravyas in which these rasas reside. Rasa and guna, both reside and depend on the dravya. The dravya is the abode for both. There is no supporter-supported relation between rasa and guna. But since the dravya is the abode of both, there is a co-existence between the two. Because of this co-existence, it has become a convention to say that the gunas belong to the rasas. If a person's mouth gets burnt by drinking hot milk, it is said that the person got burnt by milk. But actually, milk does not have the natural property of causing burns; it is the heat of the milk which causes the burns, yet we say that the person got burnt by milk.[43] The gunas of the rasas are actually the gunas of the dravya which supports the rasa. Now let us see the gunas of each of these dravyas.

Madhur rasa - Since it is believed that madhur rasa is generated from jala and prithvi mahabhootas, it possesses the snigdha guna of jala and guru guna of prithvi mahabhoota. Apart from this, mardav (softness) is generated in madhur rasa due to jala mahabhoota. It has been advised in the Ayurvedic texts that food should be prominent in madhur rasa.[44]

Amla rasa - This rasa which is generated from jala + agni mahabhootas has snigdha guna of jala and laghu guna of agni.[45]

Lavana rasa - Since this rasa is generated by the predominance of prithvi and agni mahabhootas, it has the guru guna of prithvi mahabhoota as well as snigdha guna in small proportion along with the ushna guna of agni mahabhoota. (The snigdha guna of lavana rasa is far less than the snigdha guna of madhur and amla rasas. Yet, lavana rasa is best suited for making the snehas more effective). Thus this rasa has guru, snigdha and ushna gunas. In addition, it also has teekshna guna due to the presence of agni mahabhoota.[46]

Katu rasa - This rasa has ruksha and laghu gunas due to vayu and ushna guna due to agni. Due to the presence of agni mahabhoota, teekshna guna is produced in katu rasa.[47]

Tikta rasa - This rasa is ruksha and sheeta because of vayu and laghu because of akash.[48]

Kashaya rasa - This rasa is ruksha and sheeta because of vayu and guru because of prithvi mahabhoota.[49]

It is of no use merely knowing names and gross morphology of medicinal plants. It is important to know where, how and how much to be used.

Characteristics of rasas

No.	Rasa	Mouth & tongue	Senses	Body	Chest, throat and palate	Other
1.	Madhur	Smears the mouth and tongue	pleases the senses	pleases the body		very dear to ants & other insects
2.	Amla	Stimulates and increases salivation	causes contraction of eyes and eyebrows	produces a thrill even by loo-king at it	produces burning sensation	
3.	Lavana	Causes overflow	produces appetite		produces burning sensation	
4.	Katu	produces irr-itation on the tip of the tongue and produces burning sensation in the mouth	induces secretions from the eyes, nose, mouth	produces burning sensation		
5	Tikta	Clears the mouth and tongue	produces numbess in the tongue		Cleanses the throat	
6.	Kashaya	produces numbness and heaviness in the tongue			Creates pain in the region of the chest and a sensation of chocking	

From the above as well as the following tables, one point is understood. No two rasas have exactly the same gunas. Each one of the six gunas viz. snigdha, ruksha, sheeta, ushna, guru and laghu is found in three rasas.

While describing diagnostic aspects, miserability is dealt with but not while describing treatment, since in Ayurveda , no treatment in recommended for miserable diseases.

The proportion of gunas in rasas

Charakacharya and Vagbhatta have differed in mentioning the proportion of gunas in various rasas. According to Charaka, the maximum, moderate and minimum proportion of these gunas is as follows-

Guna	Maximum	Moderate	Minimum
ruksha	kashaya	katu	tikta
snigdha	madhur	amla	lavana
ushna	lavana	amla	katu
sheeta	kashaya	madhur	tikta
guru	madhur	kashaya	lavana
laghu	tikta	katu	amla[50]

Knowledge of the proportion of these gunas is very important in choosing the correct dravya for treatment. For example, if there is aam, then rasas like madhur should not be given since they are guru while rasas like tikta should be used.

The difference between the opinions of Charaka and Vagbhatta is that Vagbhatta has said that madhur rasa has the maximum of sheeta guna wheras kashaya rasa has moderate amount of sheeta guna.

Some experts believe that lavana rasa is the most laghu of all rasas.

The rule stated above is the general rule but there are certain dravyas which are exceptions to it. Following are the examples of such exceptions.

Madhur rasa - has to be sheeta, but the meat of marine animals and animals dwelling in marshy land is ushna.

Amla rasa - must be ushna, but amalaki is sheeta.

Lavana rasa - must be ushna, but saindhav is not ushna.

Katu rasa - should be ruksha and laghu, but pippali and lashun are snigdha and guru

Tikta rasa - should be sheeta, but aguru and guduchi are ushna inspite of being tikta rasatmak.

Kashaya rasa - should be sheeta and stambhan but haritaki is ushna and purgative.

Tiktakashaya rasa - should be sheeta but brihatpanchamoola is ushna inspite of being tiktakashaya.

There is a definite reason behind giving these exceptions. Once the rasa of a dravya is known then by applying the general rule, the related properties of that dravya can be easily understood. This

Properties of contradictory gunas are based on relativity. If there was no term "sheeta", the term "ushna" would not have originated.

is the property of the rasas. If the dravya possesses some attribute which supersedes the rasas then the properties may be different. Study of such special cases is a must in dravyagunavignyan. Therefore Charakcharya has pointed out these exceptions.[51]

The actions of rasas

Various dravyas having different rasas, on coming in contact with the body, produce varying effects. Every rasa has some effect on the innumerable components of the body having micro dimensions, as well as on the mind.[52,53,54,55,56] The substances having their properties and actions similar to those of dosha-dhatu-malas bring about an increase in the doshas-dhatus and malas whereas those having dissimilar actions cause a decrease. This is the most general principle called the samanya-vishesha siddhant. When the actions of the dravyas are brought about, this principle is extremely important. It is this the fundamental principle of dravyagunashastra. Rasas which are made up of mahabhootas, produce an increase in the constituents of the body which are made up of the same mahabhootas. Our body is made up of various systems. When the dravyas enter these systems of the body, the effects generated by their rasas are described in the following chapter. It is necessary to consider the dosha-dhatu-mala gamitva of the rasas.

These actions are brought about in accordance with the samanya-vishesha siddhant. Similar dravya-guna-karma increase similar dravya-guna-karma and dosha-dhatu-mala whereas dissimilar dravya-guna-karma bring about a decrease. The actions described as the actions of the rasas are in fact the actions of the gunas belonging to the dravya having that particular rasa.

Just as the rasas have their actions on various parts of the body and also on the dosha-dhatus, similarly, they have their effects on the malas as well as on the mind. On this basis rasas can be broadly classified into two 1) Snigdha rasa (unctuous) – madhur, amla and lavana 2) Ruksha rasa (ununctuous) – katu, tikta and kashaya.

Group I - Vatanulomak - facilitates excretion of urine and stool.

Madhur rasa is the best-vatanulomak where as lavana rasa is the least vatanulomak.

Group II - Vatapratilomak - produces stagnation of urine and stools.

Kashaya is the most powerful in this activity, whereas tikta is the least powerful.

Various dravyas, on coming in contact with the tongue, spontaneously create either strong or mild impulses. Only those actions which are generated spontaneously are the actions of the rasas. There are certain dravyas which are exceptions to the general rule of doshavruddhi through their rasas. These dravyas might have a secondary position in their group. This is so because these are unable to exhibit the complete naturual actions of these rasas. Yet, it is worth noting that such dravyas are said to be beneficial to health. Guduchi is an exception to this rule.

Eventhough body and mind are the basis of diseases and symptoms, mind is more important.

Diseases, symptoms & their genesis by rasas

अग्निसाद - madhur, अलसक - madhur, excessive sleep - madhur, sweetness of mouth - madhur, अभिष्यंद - madhur, convulsions - lavana and kashaya, आध्मान - kashaya, इंद्रियावरोध - lavana, urticaria - madhur, उदर्द - madhur, ओजोनाश - lavana and katu, skin diseases - lavana, cough -madhur, कफविलयन-amla, कार्श्य-katu, kashaya, कोड - lavana, parasites - madhur, tremors - katu, itching - amla, ulcers-lavana, गडमाला - madhur, diseases of the throat - madhur, गड-अर्बुद - madhur, emesis - madhur, fever-madhur, तोद - katu, thirst - amla, lavana, katu and kashaya, skin tears - amla, धातुक्षय - tikta, sinusitis-madhur, back pain - katu, पारूष्य - tikta, panduroga (anaemia) - amla, diabetes - madhur, malaise-lavana, tikta and katu, vertigo - amla, मद - katu, मद - lavana, fainting - lavana, tikta and katu, hallucinations - katu, constipation - kashaya, dysuria - kashaya, रक्तपित्त - amla and lavana, dementia -madhur, poison - lavana, विष्ठंभ - kashaya, erysepelas (traumatic) - amla, erysepelas - lavana, वातरक्त - lavana, वातव्याधि - tikta and kashaya, distension of the abdomen - kashaya, elephantiasis-madhur, dyspnoea - madhur, oedema (in the debilitated) - amla, laxity - katu and amla, शुक्रशोष -katu and kashaya, सन्ताप -lavana and katu, संकोच - katu, स्तभन - kashaya, स्रोतोरोध - kashaya, obesity-madhur etc.

Vatashamak - Sweet, sour, salty.
Vataprakop-pungent, bitter, astringent.
Pittashamak - astringent, bitter, sweet.
Pittaprakopak-pungent, sour salty.
Kaphashamak - pungent, bitter, astringent.
Kaphaprakopak-sweet, sour, salty[57]

The following table shows the exceptions to the general rule of the natural actions of rasas.

Sweet - increases kapha - **exceptions**: honey, sugar, meat of animals living on dry, arid land, old rice, barley, wheat and moong.

Sour - increases pitta - **exceptions** : pomegranate and amalaki.

Salty - increases pitta, harmful to the eyes- **exception** : saindhav.

Pungent - increases vata, adversely affects semen production- **exceptions** : sunthi, pippali, and garlic.

Bitter - increases vata, adversely affects semen production - **exceptions** : guduchi and patolpatra

Astringent - cold stambhan - **exception** : haritaki[58]

Priorities in the use of rasas in diet and medicine

In medicine : Medicines are used in treating the vitiation of various doshas. The rasas which are used in treating kapha, pitta and vayu should also be used after ascertaining certain priorities.

Disease caused due to an increase in kapha dosha may be treated with katu (pungent), tikta (bitter) and kashaya (astringent) rasas since these rasas alleviate kapha. Just as there are number of factors contributing to the increase of kapha dosha, similarly there is a variation in the mahabhoota constitution of these rasas and therefore it becomes necessary to use these rasas in the same order of priority. Thus, these rasas are used in the order viz. katu, tikta and kashaya. The reason for using katu rasa first is that it reduces the heaviness and stickiness of kapha. After that, tikta rasa should be used. Because of this rasa, the sweetness in mouth, produced by kapha is reduced and excess kapha is dried up. After this, kashaya rasa is indicated. This rasa reduces the unctuousness of kapha (कषायापहृतस्नेह). Because of this, expectoration of kapha is reduced and then it stops.[59]

There are three rasas which are used in disorders involving increase in pitta dosha. These are used in the following order - tikta (bitter), madhur (sweet) and kashaya (astringent). The reason for using tikta rasa first is that it brings about pachan of aampitta and increases the agni. Next comes madhur rasa. The gunas of this rasa like coldness, heaviness, unctuousness and sweetness pacify the pakva pitta. And finally, the reason for using kashaya rasa is that it reduces the fluidity of pitta through its dryness and astringent properties.[60]

While treating vata dosha, the order of using the rasas is lavana, amla and madhur. The reason for using lavana rasa first is that since it is abhishyandi (प्रक्लेदी) it reduces the blockage of vata. Due to its ushna guna, the sheeta guna of vayu is reduced while the guru guna reduces the laghutva of vayu. Then comes the turn of amla rasa due to its teekshna, snigdha and ushna gunas. Among these, teekshna guna reduces the block of the srotas of vayu; this is so because dravyas of teekshna guna can penetrate deep and clear the passage of vayu. The snigdha and ushna gunas of amla rasa help in restoring the normal course of vayu. On using madhur rasa, its heaviness reduces the lightness of vayu, stickiness reduces the dryness whereas unctuousness also reduces the dryness. In this way, Kashyap samhita has indicated the use of rasas in preferential order to either eliminate or reduce the gunas of kapha, pitta and vata doshas.

For vata, snigdha-ushna gunas are used first, for pitta, ruksha-sheeta gunas and for kapha, ruksha and ushna gunas have been used first. The rasas used in the end in the case of all the three doshas are heavy and help in pacifying the doshas.[61]

The above explanation can be represented in tabular form as below :

Doshas	**First**	**Second**	**Third**
Vata	lavana	amla	madhur
Pitta	tikta	madhur	kashaya
Kapha	katu	tikta	kashaya

It may seem that kapha and aam are very closely related to each other but according to Kashyap, pitta (ie. agni) is more related to aam. The presence or absence of aam is more dependent on pitta (ie. agni).

Here, the generally accepted notions of vata, pitta and kapha have to be put aside. An increase or decrease in vata, pitta and kapha means that the gunas of these doshas have either increased or decreased in those body organs. Accordingly, certain symptoms are manifested. These conditions are

It is written in Eknathi Bhagwat that ingestion of patalgarudi relives the body of all kinds of pain. What is the meaning of this?

respectively called doshavruddhi and doshakshaya.

Vatavruddhi means that the concerned body organs become excessive in the gunas of vata like ruksha etc. The treatment of vatavruddhi also involves reduction of the gunas of vata in those parts of the body; this in turn involves use of the antagonist gunas and generating the basic dravyas in the affected parts of the body. The same principle applies to the vruddhi and kshaya of all the doshas.

The preferential use of rasas in diet

Rasas are extremely important in diet. In medicine, the veerya is predominant whereas in diet, rasa is predominant. The texts have instructed to always keep the habit of using all the six rasas. Similarly, consumption of a particular rasa in large quantities in particular seasons has also been advised. Diet should contain all the six rasas. Yet, it has been instructed that madhur rasa should be consumed first, amla and lavana rasas should be consumed in the middle of the meal and tikta, katu and kashaya rasas should be consumed at the end. Madhur dravyas do not indicate absolute sweet items like sugar, jaggery but other food items like wheat, rice, maize etc. are also considered as madhur dravyas. There is some ideological basis for this. When a person is hungry, the stomach is empty. Empty stomach causes an increase in vata dosha. To pacify this vata dosha, madhur rasa should be eaten first. Apart from this, kaphavruddhi is required to moisten the ingested food. This is accomplished by the madhur rasa. Since dravyas having madhur rasa are guru and hence difficult to digest, it is advisable to eat these dravyas first. After this, it is correct to use amla and lavana rasas. The reason for this is not only to pacify the remaining vata but also to aid digestion by improving the agni. Lastly, katu, tikta and kashaya rasas should be taken as these rasas increase the agni along with reducing the kapha which increases after ingestion of food.[62]

This rule applies in relation to health, but in pathological conditions this idea has to be modified accordingly. For example, in anorexia and similar kapha disorders, initially ginger and salt ie. katu and lavana rasa should be used. Of these, katu rasa pacifies the kapha while the lavana rasa moistens food and pacifies vata. Similarly, the order of using these rasas can be suitably altered taking into consideration the prakriti, individual preferences and the condition of the doshas.[63] At times, when rasas like lavana, amla and katu, which produce burning sensation, are used first, madhur rasa has to be used in the end in order to reduce the offending pitta.[64]

In tropical countries, there is a custom to eat some sweet preparation before starting the meal. This is useful in bringing about moistening of the annavaha srotas before ingestion of food. Contrary to this, in cold countries, there is a custom of taking soups of amla and katu rasas. There is a definite order even in arranging food items in the dish. Staple food like rice and chapati are kept in the centre of the dish. Then on the left side first sweet dishes are kept, then sour pickles and lemon. Lavana rasa is kept in the centre, right in front of the eyes and finally tikta and katu rasas are placed on the right side of the plate.

The predominance of rasas

It has been a convention to illustrate the peculiarities of each padarth in its chapter. Adhering to this convention, the peculiarities of dravyas were mentioned in the chapter on dravya. Similarly, it

It should be borne in mind that as machines require overhauling and decarboning, every human body has to undergo overhauling.

becomes necessary to enumerate the peculiarities of rasas in this chapter. Even if we accept the permise that dravya is the most important padarth, yet the dravya will not be able to have any action at all without rasa. Moreover, rasa is extremely important in identification of dravyas since it is perceptible. Apart from this, once the rasa of a dravya is known, from this knowledge generally, its mahabhootas, its associated gunas, its vipak, karma etc. can be easily inferred upon.

Nevertheless there are certain reasons which depict the peculiarities of rasa. These are -

1. Adhikar - The regimen of diet prescribed in swasthvritta and in treatment of diseases is constituted on the basis of the rasas. It is true that diet is the basis of life but that too is dependent on (six) rasas. Similarly, shodhan and shaman chikitsa are also based on the rasas.[65]

2. Updesha - The scriptures have described madhur, amla and lavana rasas as vatashaman and katu, tikta and kashaya as kaphashaman etc. This description is considered as a major reason for justifying the predominance of rasas.[66]

3. Anuman - Since the properties and actions of dravyas are inferred upon through their rasas, rasa is predominant. Therefore it should be understood that wherever rasa becomes weak, other properties and actions also become weak.[67]

4. Agam - In certain ancient scriptures, rasas have been used to indicate dravyas instead of using the names of dravyas. For example, instead of saying, "bring sugar" the scriptures declare, "bring sweet". There are descriptions which say that, "give some bitter taste." This convention might be used to emphasize that the action is brought about by the rasa rather than the dravya.[68]

5. Upsamhar - A few dravyas are classified in one group which is then known by the name of the rasa. For example, while describing vidarigandhadi dravyagana, it is said in the end that such dravyas having madhur rasa should be included in this group. This is called upsamhar. Here also rasas are mentioned.[69]

6. Vyapattinimittata - Vyapatti = vikruti (vitiation). If the rasa of a dravya gets vitiated, so does dravya and vipak. This means that rasa is the lifeline of a dravya. Therefore rasa is predominant.[70]

7. Apadesha - When two different objects are compared, rasas are used in such comparisons also. For example- 'sweet words' or "He spoke such bitter words!" or "He is sitting with a bitter face" etc.[71]

8. Anekvishayatva - A single rasa may have many abodes. For example, on mentioning sweet taste, one immediately thinks of sugarcane, sugar, milk, dates, ghee, banana, jackfruit etc. Since rasa has many abodes, rasa is predominant.[72]

9. Pravruttinimittata - It means – being the cause of human attraction. Why a person is drawn to food items is because these items have different rasas and therefore some persons develop a liking for sweet substances whereas others prefer sour substances. There are many people who enjoy eating 'sweet-n-sour' and 'salty' foods.

10. Ashukaritva - Dravyas generate their actions on the body through their rasa, veerya, guna,

All the small or big pores of the body can be used for sneha - sweda treatment.

vipak etc. Yet, the initial action is always brought about through the six rasas viz. sweet, sour, salty, pungent, bitter and astringent. These rasas have immediate action on the mouth. This has been ascertained as the criterion for identifying rasas. Therefore, since the dravyas can have their actions immediately through the rasas, rasa only is predominant.

11. Gunavyapadesha - Rasa is the means through which the guna, veerya, vipak etc. of the dravya can be known. Once the rasa is known, its veerya, its gunas, its vipak etc. can be easily known.

References -

1. मांसे, द्रवे, चेक्षुरसे, पारदे, मधुरादिषु ।,
बाले, रोगे, विषे, नारे, रसो नवसु वर्तते ।। (भा. प्र.)
2. तत्र ९रसगतौ" धातुः, अहरहर्गच्छतीत्यतो रसः (सु. सू. १४)
3. रसनात् सर्वधातूनां रसेंद्र इति कीर्तितः (र. र. स.)
4. रसः कल्कः शृतः शीतः फाण्टेश्चेति प्रकल्पना ।। (वा. क. अ. ६)
5. रस्यते आस्वाद्यते इति रसः (चक्रदत्त)
रसनार्थो रसः ।" (च. सू. अ. १)
रसनेन्द्रियग्राह्यो योऽर्थः स रसः ।" (शि.)
रसस्तु रसनाग्राह्यो मधुरादिरनेकधा ।" (का.)
6. रसास्तावत् षट्–मधुराम्ललवणकटुतिक्तकषायाः ।" (च. वि. १-४)
स्वादुरम्लोऽथलवणः कटुकस्तिक्त एव च । कषायश्चेति षट्कोऽयं रसानां संग्रहः स्मृतः ।।" (च. सू. १-६५)
रसाःस्वादुम्ललवणतिक्तोषणकषायकाः । षड्द्रव्यमाश्रितास्ते तु यथापूर्वं बलावहाः ।। (अ. सं. सू. १)
तत्र स्वादुर्मधुरो घृतगुडादिः, अम्लोऽम्लिकामातुलुङ्गादिः लवणः सैन्धवादिः, ऊषणः कटुको मरिचादिः तिक्तो भूनिम्बादिः, कषायो हरीतक्यादिः ।" (च. द.)
7. षडेव रसाः नोनाधिकाः । (इन्दुटीका)
8. एक एव रस इत्युवाच भद्रकाप्यः–यं पञ्चानामिन्द्रियाथनामन्यतमं जिव्हावैषयिकं भावमाचक्षते कुशलाः स पुनरुदकादनन्य इति । द्वौ रसाविति शाकुन्तेयो ब्राह्मणः– छेदनीयः उपशमनीयश्चेति । त्रयो रसा इति पूर्णाक्षो मौद्गल्यः–छेदनीयोपशमनीय साधारणा इति । चत्वारो रसा इति हिरण्याक्षः कौशिकः–स्वादुर्हितश्च, स्वादुरहितश्च अअस्वादुर्हितश्च, अस्वादुरहितश्चेति । पञ्च रसा इति कुमारशिरा भरद्वाजः–भौमौदकाग्नेयवायव्यान्तरिक्षाः । षड्रसा इति वार्योविदो राजर्षिः-गुरुलघुशीतोष्णस्निग्ध रूक्षाः । सप्त रसा इति निमिर्वैदेहः–मधुराम्ललवणकटुतिक्तकषायक्षाराः । अष्टौ रसा इति बडिशो धामार्गवः-मधुराम्ललवणकटुतिक्तकषायक्षाराव्यक्ताः । अपरिसंख्येया रसा इति कांकायनो बाल्हिकभिषक्-आश्रयगुणकर्मसंस्वादविशेषाणामपरि संख्येयत्वात् ।" (च. सू. २६-८)
9. तेषां षण्णां रसानां योनिरुदकं, छेदनोपशमने द्वे कर्मणी, तयोर्मिश्रीभावात् साधारणत्वं, स्वाद्वस्वादुता भक्तिद्वेषौ, हिताहितौ प्रभारौ, पञ्चमहाभूतविकारास्त्वाश्रयाः प्रकृतिविकृतिवाचार देशकालवशाः तेष्वाश्रयेषु द्रव्यसंज्ञकेषु गुणाः गुरुलघुशीतोष्णस्निग्धरूक्षाद्याः क्षरणात् क्षारः, नासौ रसः, द्रव्यं हि तदनेकरससमुत्पन्नम अनेकरसं कटुकलवणभूयिष्ठम् अनेकेन्द्रियार्थसमन्वितं करणाभिनिर्वृत्तम्, अव्यक्तीभावस्तु खलु रसानां प्रकृतौ भवत्यनुरसेऽनुरससमन्विते वा द्रव्ये; अपरिसंख्येयत्वं पुनस्तेषामाश्रयादीनां भावानां विशेषापरिसंख्येयत्वान्न युक्तम्, एकैकोऽपि ह्येषामाश्रयादीनां भावानां विशेषानाश्रयते

विशेषापरिसंख्येयत्वात्, न च तस्मादन्यत्वमुपपद्यते ; परस्परसंसृष्टभूयिष्ठत्वान्न चैषामभिनिर्वृत्तेः गुणप्रकृतीनामपरिसंख्येयत्वं भवति, तस्मान्नसंसृष्टानां रसानां कर्मोपदिशन्ति बुद्धिमन्तः ।" (च. सू. २६-९)

10. षडेव रसा इत्युवाच भगवानात्रेयः पुनर्वसुः-मधुराम्ललवणकटुतिक्तकषायाः ।" (च. सू. २६-९)

11. षट्सूत्रकारप्रामाण्यादास्वादाच्च ।" (र. वै. ३ सू. ५)

12. तस्य द्रव्यमापः क्षितिस्तथा । निर्वृत्तौ च विशेषेच प्रत्ययाः खादयस्त्रयः ।।" (च. सू. १) १द्रव्य-शब्दो ह्याधारकारणवाची...१अक्षिती" इति वक्तव्ये, १क्षितिस्तथा" इति वचनात् क्षितेराधार-कारणत्वममुख्यमिति दर्शयति । ... मधुरादिविशेषनिर्वृत्तौ निमित्तकारणं खवाय्वनलाः, न त्वाधारकार-णभूताः ।" (च. द. १-६४)

द्रवस्य पाञ्चभौतिकत्वाद् तदाश्रितरसोऽपि पाञ्चभौतिकः । ...रसोऽपां नैसर्गिकः, क्षितेस्तु अबनुप्रवेश-कृतः । तेन रसस्य योनिरापः, क्षितिश्चाधारः, तस्य निर्वृत्तौ निष्पत्तौ विशेषे मधुरादिभेदे च खादयः खं वायुरग्निश्च एते त्रयः प्रत्ययाः कारणानि । ... अनेन खादीनां त्रयाणां रसंप्रति कारणत्वमुपर्शितं भवति, अपां क्षितेश्च तदनिबोधमेव । एवं पञ्चानां महाभूतानां रसं प्रति कारणतया वर्त्तमानत्वाद्, रससेषुपाञ्चभौतिकत्व मुपपद्यते ।" (यो.) १तस्मान्नैकरसं द्रव्यं भूतसंघातसंभवात् ।" (अ. हृ. सू. ९) १सर्वं द्रव्यं पञ्चमहाभूतसमवायसंभवं, तस्मादनेकरसम् ।" (यो.)

13. एवमेषां रसानां षट्त्वमुपपन्नं न्यूनातिरेकाविशेषान्महाभूतानां, भूतानामिव स्थावर जङ्गमानां नानाव-र्णाकृतिविशेषाः ।" (च. सू. २६)

14. सौम्याः खल्वापोऽन्तरिक्षप्रभवाः प्रकृतिशीता लघ्व्यश्चाव्यक्तरसाश्च, तास्त्वन्तरिक्षाद्भ्रश्यमानाः भ्रष्टाश्च पञ्चमहाभूतगुणसमन्विता जङ्गमस्थावराणां भूतानां मूर्त्तोरभिप्रीणयन्ति, तासु मूर्त्तिषु षडभिमू-र्च्छन्ति रसाः ।" (च. सू. २६)

रसः खल्वाप्यः प्रागव्यक्तश्च । स षड्तुकत्वात् कालस्य महाभूतगुणैरूनातिरिक्तैः संसृष्टो विषमं विदग्धः षोढा पृथग्विपरिणमते मधुरादिभेदेन ।" (अ. सं. सू. १८) १आप्यो रसोऽव्यक्तोऽपि कालसहाय-भूमिवियदनिलानलसंसर्गेण परिपाकान्तरं गतः षोढा विभज्यते षट्प्रकारो भवति (इ.)

स खल्वाप्यो रसः शेषभूतसंसर्गाद् विदग्धः षोढा विभज्यते, तद्यथा-मधुरः, अम्लः, लवणः, कटुकः, तिक्तः, कषाय इति ।" (सु. सू. ४२)

15. तेषां षण्णां रसानां पृथ्वीसोमगुणातिरेकान्मधुरो रसः पृथिव्यग्निभूयिष्ठत्वादम्लः, सलिलाग्निभूयिष्ठत्वा-ल्लवणः, वाय्वग्निभूयिष्ठत्वात्कटुकः, वाय्वाकाशातिरिक्तत्वात्तिक्तः, पवनपृथिव्यतिरेकात् कषाय इति ।" (च. सू. २६)

क्ष्माऽम्भोऽग्निक्ष्माऽम्बुतेजः खवाय्वग्न्यनिलगोऽनिलैः ।
द्वयोल्बणैः क्रमाद्भूतैर्मधुरादिरसोद्भवः ।।" (अ. हृ. सू. १०।१)

16. षड्तुकत्वाच्च कालस्योपपन्नो महाभूतानां न्यूनातिरेकविशेषः ।" (च. सू. २६)
स षड्तुकत्वात् कालस्य महाभूतगुणैरूनातिरिक्तैः संसृष्टो विषमं विदग्धः विपरिणमते ।" (अ. सं. सू. १८)

कथं महाभूतानामूनाधिक्यम? उच्यते-कालस्य संवत्सराख्यस्य षड्तुकत्वाद्र सस्यापि षड्भेदत्वम् । तथा च शिशिरे वाय्वाकाशयोराधिक्याद्रसस्य तिक्तता, वसन्ते वायुपृथिव्योः कषायता ग्रीष्मेऽग्निवाय्वोः कटुता, वर्षास्वग्निपृथिव्योरम्लता, शरद्यग्न्युदकयोर्लवणता, हेमन्ते पृथिव्युदकयोर्मधुरतेति प्राधान्याद् व्यपदेशः, तेनाग्न्यर्तूद्भवानामपि रसानां यथोक्तमहाभूतद्वयाधिक्यमेव कारणं विज्ञेयम् ।" (इन्दुः) षड्तुकत्वाच्चेति चकारेणाहोरात्रकृतोऽपि भूतोत्कर्षो ज्ञेयस्तथाऽदृष्टकृतश्च, तेन हेमन्तादावपि रसान्तरो-त्पादः क्वचिद्वस्तुन्युपपन्नो भवति ।" (च. द.)

यद्यपि च ऋतुभेदेऽपि भूतोत्कर्षविशेष एव कारणं, यदुक्तं–तावेतावर्कवायू (सू. ६) इत्यादि, तथापि बीजांकुरकार्यकारणभाववत् संसारानादितयैव भूतविशेषर्त्वोः कार्यकारणभावो वाच्यः । (च. द.)

17. चरके तोयाग्निगुणबाहुल्याल्लवणः पठितः इह तु तोयाग्निगुणबाहुल्यादम्लः पठ्यते तदत्र प्रमेये विरोधो नास्त्येव, उभयथाऽपि वक्ष्यमाणरसगुणानामुपपत्तेःट (च. द.) ९एवं लवणेऽप्ययां कारणत्वं ज्ञेयम् । लवणस्तु सुश्रुते पृथिव्यग्न्यतिरेकात् पठितः, अस्मिंश्च विरोधे कार्यविरोधो नास्त्येव ।" (च. द.)

18. नात्र वस्तुस्वभावे युक्तयः क्रोशनीयाः, अपर्यनुयोग्यत्वाद्भावस्वभावानाम् ।" (च. द.) ९भूतानामयं स्वभावः, यत् केनचित् प्रकारेण सन्निविष्टाः कञ्चिद्गुणमारभन्ते न सर्वम् । यथा मकुष्ठकेऽद्भिर्मधुरो रसः क्रियते न स्नेहः, तथा सैन्धवे वन्हिनाऽपि नोऽणत्वमारभ्यते । अयं च भूतानां सन्निवेशोऽदष्टप्रभावकृत एव ।" (च. द.)

19. ते निर्धार्यन्तेऽनुमानात् ।" (र. वै. सू. ४४)

20. वर्धनात् समानजातीयस्य, असमानजातीयस्य क्षपणाच्च । (सू. ४५)
स च सन्निवेशः कार्यदर्शनेनोन्नेयः । तेन यत्र कार्यं दृश्यते तत्र कल्प्यते यथा-लवणे उषअणत्वादग्निर्विष्यन्दित्वाच्च जलमनुमीयते ।" (च. द.)
भूतेजोवारिजैर्द्रव्यैः शमं याति समीरणः । भूम्यम्बुवायुजैः पित्तं क्षिमप्रमाप्नोति निर्वृतिम् ।। खतेजोऽनिलजैः श्लेष्मा शममेति शरीरिणाम् । वियत्पवनजाताभ्यां वृद्धिमाप्नोति मारुतः ।। आग्नेयमेव यदद्रव्यं तेन पित्तमुदीर्यते । वसुधाजलजाताभ्यां बलासः परिवर्धते ।। (सु. सू. ४२)

21. आगमवेदनीयश्चायमर्थः नात्रास्मद्विधानां कल्पनाः प्रसरन्ति ।" (च. द.)
आगमेन पूर्वमुपलब्धानां प्रमाणान्तरेण दृढीकरणार्थमयमारम्भः, आप्तवचनस्य त्रैविध्यात्-श्रद्धेयार्थम्, अनुमेयार्थं, प्रत्यक्षार्थं चेति । श्रद्धेयार्थ-उत्तराः कुरवः, स्वर्गेऽप्सरस इति । अनुमेयार्थ प्रत्यक्षार्थ च यथा–चक्षुरित्यनुमीयते; प्रत्यक्षतश्च रूपमुपलभ्यते इति । इहाप्ययमागमोऽनुमानार्थ... नह्यायुर्वेदे प्रत्यक्षार्थानुमेयार्थाभ्यामागमाभ्यामन्यच्छ्रद्धेयार्थमस्ति, दृष्टिफलत्वादिति ।" (भा.)

22. तत्राग्निमारुतात्मकाः रसाः प्रायेणोर्ध्वभाजः, लाघवादुत्प्लवानाच्च वायोरूर्ध्वज्वलनाच्च वन्हेः, सलिलपृथिव्यात्मकास्तु प्रायेणाधोभाजः पृथिव्या गुरुत्वान्निम्नगत्वाच्चोदकस्य, व्यामिश्रात्मकाः पुनरुभयतोभाजैः ।" (च. सू. २६)
तत्र विरेचनद्रव्याणि पृथिव्याम्बुगुणभूयिष्ठानि पृथिव्यापो गुर्व्यस्ता गुरुत्वादधो गच्छन्ति तस्माद्विरेचनमधोगुणभूयिष्ठन्ति तस्माद्वमनमप्यूर्ध्वगुणभूयिष्ठयुक्तम् । उभयगुणभूयिष्ठमुभयतोभागम् ।" (सु. सू. ४२)

23. आकाशगुणभूयिष्ठं संशमनम्, संग्राहकमनिलगुणभूयिष्ठमनिलस्य शोषणात्मकत्वात् । दीपनमग्निगुणभूयिष्ठं, लेखनमनिलानलगुणभूयिष्ठं, बृंहणं पृथिव्यम्बुगुणभूयिष्ठम् ।" (सु. सू. ४२)

24. प्रत्यक्षतोऽनुमानादुपदेशतश्च रसानामुपलब्धिः ।" (र. वै. ३ सू. १०८)
रसो निपाते द्रव्याणाम् ।"

25. आस्वाद्य प्रत्यक्षत उपलभ्यते, अनुमानात् पूर्वोक्तं लिंगं दृष्ट्वा मधुरोऽयमित्युपलभ्यते । उपदेशात् आगमात् कषायं मधु, मधुरमुदकम् इत्यादि । अथवा आस्वादतो रसानां सामान्यत उपलब्धिर्भवति, अनुमानाल्लिंगपूर्वकाद् विशेषोपलब्धिर्भवति, उपदेशतः कर्मणि रसानां प्रवृत्तिरुपलभ्यते । अथवा सर्वमास्वादत एव रसो न गृह्यते, आगमतश्च क्वचित्, क्वचिदनुमानाच्चेति ।" (भा.)

26. अन्यथात्वगमनं स्थानात् । (र. वै. सू. २९)
स्थानम् अधिकरणं भाजनं तद्वेतोरपि रसान्तरं भवति ९ (भा.)

27. संयोगत:, क्षारोहि याति माधर्युं शीघ्रमम्लोपसंहित: । (वा. सू. अ. ३०)
28. अग्ने: पाकात् (सू. ३०)
29. आतपात् (सू. ३१)
30. भावनया (सू. ३२)
31. देशकालाभ्याम् (सू. ३२)
32. परिणामत: (सू. ३३)
33. उपसर्गत: (सू. ३४)
34. विक्रियात: (सू. ३५)
35. अग्नीषोमीयत्वाज्जगतो रसा द्विविधा:– सौम्याश्चाग्नेयाश्च । मधुरतिक्तकषाया: सौम्या: । कटु अम्ल लवणा: आग्नेया: ।
36. फलानि अम्लानि खादेयु: तस्य चान्ये अग्रतो नरा: । (वा. क. अ. ३।३०)
37. मार्दवं वर्तते यत्र तनोतिमृदुता सदा । माधुर्यं कुरुतेऽह्लाद: यत्रयत्रापि संश्रितम् । तत्तदस्य नियतं कर्म वर्तते यत्र यो गुण: ।।
स्नेहनप्रीणनाल्हादमार्दवैरुपलभ्यते । मुखस्थो मधुरश्चास्यं व्याप्नुवल्लिम्पतीव च ।।" (च. सू. २६)
तत्र य: परितोषमुत्पादयति, प्रल्हादयति, तर्पयति, जीवयति, मुखोपलेपं जनयति, श्लेष्माणं चाभिवर्धयति स मधुर: ।" (सु. सू. ४२)
तेषां स्वादुरास्वाद्यमानी मुखमुपलिम्पति, इन्द्रियाणि प्रसादयति, देहं प्रल्हादयति, षट्पदपिपीलिकादीनामभीष्टतम: ।" (अ. सं. सू. १८)
षट्पदपिपीलिकादीभिश्च शरीरमूत्राभिसरणम् ।" (च. वि. ४)
मक्षिकोपसर्पणेन शरीरमाधुर्यम् ।" (च. वि. ४) मधुर द्रव्याचे ल्हादन कार्य ते द्रव्य तोंडात असताना होते.
38. दन्तहर्षान्मुखास्त्रावात् स्वेदनान्मुखबोधनात् । विदाहाच्चास्य कण्ठस्य प्राश्यैवाम्लं रसं वदेत् ।।" (च. सू. २६)
यो दन्तहर्षमुत्पादयति, मुखास्त्रावं जनयति, श्रद्धां चोत्पादयति सोऽम्ल: ।" (सु. सू. ४२)
अम्लतु जिव्हामुद्वेजयति, उर:कण्ठं विदहति, मुखं स्त्रावयति, अक्षिभ्रुवं संकोचयति, दशनान् हर्षयति रोमाणि च ।" (अ. सं. सू. १८)
39. प्रलीयन् क्लेदविष्यन्दमार्दवं कुरुते मुखे य: शीघरं लवणो ज्ञेय: स विदाहान्मुखस्य च ।। १ (च. सू. २६) सर्वरसप्रत्यनीकभूत: (च. सू. अ. २६।४२।३)
यो भक्तरुचिमुत्पादयति, कण्ठकपोलं विदहति, अन्नं प्ररोचयति ।" (अ. सं. सू. १८)
40. संवेजयेद्यो रसनं निपाते तुदतीव च । विदहन्मुखनासाक्षिसंस्त्रावी स कटु: स्मृत: ।।" (च. सू. २६) ।
यो जिव्हाग्रं बाधते, उद्वेगं जनयति, शिरो गृहणीते, नासिकां च स्त्रावयति स कटुक: ।" (सु. सू. ४२) ।, कटुको भृशमुद्वेजयति जिव्हाग्रं चिमचिमायति कण्ठकपोलं स्त्रावयति मुखाक्षिनासिकं विदहति देहम् ।" (अ. सं. सू. १८)
41. प्रतिहन्ति निपाते यो रसनं स्वदते न च । स तिक्तो मुखवैशद्यशोषप्रल्हादकारक: ।। (च. सू. २६) ।
यो गले चोषमुत्पादयति, मुखवैशद्यं जनयति, भक्तरुचिं चापादयति हर्षं च, स तिक्त: ।" (सु. सू. ४२) । १तिक्तो विशदयति वदनं, विशोधयति कण्ठं, प्रतिहन्ति रसनाम् । (अ. सं. सू. १८)
तिक्तस्य हर्षणं, शैत्यमास्यस्य, गलद्वारशोषणं च ।" (र. वै. ३ सू. १८) । १तिक्तो रस: स्वयमरोचिष्णुरप्यरोचकघ्न: (च. सु. २६)
42. वैशद्यस्तम्भजाड्यैर्यो रसनं योजयेद्रस: । बध्नातीव च य: कण्ठं कषाय: स विकास्यपि ।। (च. सू. २६) । १यो वक्त्रं परिशोषयति, जिव्हां स्तम्भयति, कण्ठं बध्नाति, हृदयं कर्षति पीडयति च स

कषायः इति (सु. सू. ४२) कषायस्य मुखपरिशोषः। श्लेष्मसंवृत्तिः, गौरवं, स्तंभश्च। (र. वै. ३ सू. १८)

43. गुणा गुणाश्रया नोक्तास्तस्माद्रसगुणान् भिषक्। विद्याद् द्रव्यगुणान् कर्तुरभिप्रायाः पृथग्विधाः ।।" (च. सू. २६)। १गुर्वादयो गुणा द्रव्ये पृथिव्यादौ रसाश्रये। रसेषु व्यपदिश्यन्ते साहचर्योपचारतः ।।" (अ. हृ. सू. ९)। १गुर्वादयो गुणा द्रव्य एव न रसेषु। यस्तु मधुरो गुरुः, अम्लो लघुरित्यादिव्यपदेशः स साहचर्योपचारतः। एकस्मिन् आश्रये द्वयोरवस्थानं साहचर्यम्। ... द्रव्यं हि गुर्वादीनामिव रसानामप्याश्रयः। अत एकाश्रयत्वात् साहचर्यं तेन उपचारः अविद्यमानस्याप्याश्रयाश्रयिभावस्यारोपः।" (हे.)

44. तत्र मधुरो रसः... स्निग्धः शीतो गुरुश्च।" (च. सू. २६)। १तत्र मधुरो रसः.... स्निग्धः शीतो मृदुर्गुरुश्च।" (अ. सं. सू. १८) षड्सं मधुरप्रायम्। (वा. सू.)

45. अम्लो रसः... लघुः उष्णः स्निग्धश्च।" (च. सू. २६)।

46. लवणो रसः.... नात्यर्थगुरुः स्निग्धः उष्णश्च।" (च. सू. २६) १लवणः... नातिगुरुः तीक्ष्णोष्णश्च।" (अ. सं. सू. १८) स्नेहाश्च लवणोल्बणाः। (वा सू.)

47. कटुको रसः.... लघुः उष्णो रूक्षश्च।" (च. सू. २६)। १कटुको... लघुरूक्षतीक्ष्णोष्णश्च।" (अ. सं. सू. १८)

48. तिक्तो रसः.... रूक्षः शीतो लघुश्च।" (च. सू. २६)

49. कषायो रसः.... रूक्षः शीतोऽलघुश्च।" (च. सू. २६)

50. रौक्ष्यत्कषायो रूक्षाणामुत्तमो मध्यमः कटुः। तिक्तोऽवरस्तथोष्णानामुष्णत्वाल्लवणः परः ।। मध्योऽम्लः कटुकश्चान्त्यः स्निग्धानां मधुरः परः। मध्योम्लो लवणश्चान्त्यो रसः स्नेहान्निरुच्यते ।। मध्योत्कृष्टावराः शैत्यात् कषायस्वादुतिक्तकाः। स्वादुर्गुरुत्वादधिकः कषायाल्लवणोऽवरः ।। अम्लात्कटुस्ततस्तिक्तोलघुत्वादुत्तमोत्तमाः। केचिल्लघूनामवरमिच्छन्ति लवणं रसम् ।। गौरवे लाघवे चैव सोऽवरस्तूभयोरपि।" (च. सू. २६)।

तिक्तः कषायो मधुरस्तद्वदेव च शीतलाः।" (अ. हृ. सू. १०)
मधुरं किंचिदुष्णं स्यात् कषायं तिक्तमेव च। यथा महत्पंचमूलयथाऽब्जानूपमामिषम् ।।
लवणं सैन्धवं नोष्णमम्लमामलकं तथा। अर्कागुरुगुडूचीनां तिक्तानामुष्णमुच्यते ।।
पिप्पली च लशुनोऽपि स्नेहोष्ण्यगौरवैः।" (अ. सं. सू. १७)
....कषायःस्तम्भनः शीतः सोऽभयायामतोऽन्यथा।

51. ....तस्माद्रसोपदेशेन न सर्वं द्रव्यमादिशेत्। दृष्टं तुल्यरसेऽप्येवं द्रव्ये द्रव्ये गुणान्तरम् ।। (च. सू. २६)

तत्र मधुरो रसः शरीरसात्म्याद्रसरुधिरमांसमेदोऽस्थिमज्जौजःशुक्राभिवर्धनः आयुष्यः षडिन्द्रियप्रसादनः बलवर्णकरः पित्तविषमारुतघ्नः तृष्णादाहप्रशमनः, त्वच्यः केश्यः कण्ठ्यो बल्यः प्रीणनोजीवनः तर्पणः बृंहणः स्थैयकरः क्षीणक्षतसंधानकरः घ्राणमुखकंण्ठौष्ठजिव्हाप्रल्हादनः दाहमूर्च्छाप्रशमनः।" (च. सू. २६)। १शुक्रस्तन्यवर्धनः।" (सु. सू. ४२)

माधुर्यस्नेहगौरवशैत्यपैच्छिल्यगुणलक्षणः श्लेष्मा, तस्य समानयोनिर्मधुरो रसः, सोऽस्य माधुर्यान्माधुर्य वर्धयति, स्नेहात्, स्नेहं, गौरवाद् गौरवं, शैत्याच्छैत्यं, पैच्छिल्यात् पैच्छिल्यमिति।" (सु. सू. ४२)।

माधुर्यस्नेहगौरवपैच्छिल्यमार्दवशैत्यैः श्लेष्माणं वर्धयति मधुरः।" (र. वै. ३ सू. ६२)

52. अम्लो रसो भक्तं रोचयति, अग्निं दीपयति, देहं बृंहयति, ऊर्जयति, मनो बोधयति, इन्द्रियाणि दृढीकरोति, बलं वर्धयति, वातमनुलोमयति, हृदयं तर्पयति, आस्यमास्रावयति, भुक्तमपकर्षयति, क्लेदयति, जरयति, प्रीणयति।" (च. सू. २६)

पित्तं भृशविदाहित्वादुष्णत्वात्तीक्ष्णत्वाच्च विदाहयति कोपयति चाम्लः।" (र. वै. सू. ६८)

कोपयति क्लेदयति चैनमम्लः, औष्ण्यात् तैक्ष्ण्यात् गौरवात् स्नेहाच्च।" (र. वै. सू. ६५)

53. लवणो रसः पाचनः क्लेदनो दीपनः च्यावनः छेदनो भेदनः तीक्ष्णः सरो विकासी अधःस्रंसी, अवकाशकरी वातहरः स्तम्भबन्धसंघातविधमनः सर्वरसप्रत्यनीकभूतः आस्यमास्रावयति कफं विष्यन्दयति, मार्गान् विशोधयति, सर्वशरीरावयवान् मृदूकरोति, रोचयत्याहारम् आहारयोगी ।" (च. सू. २६) विष्यन्दयति चैनं लवणः । (र. वै. सू. ६६)

54. औष्ण्यतैक्ष्ण्यरौक्ष्यलाघववैशद्यगुणलक्षणं पित्तं, तस्य समानयोगिः कटुको रसः सोऽस्य औष्ण्यादौष्ण्यं वर्धयति, तैक्ष्ण्यात्तैक्ष्ण्यं, रौक्ष्याद्रौक्ष्यं, लाघवाल्लाघवं, वैशद्याद् वैशद्यमिति ।" (सु. सू. ४२)

कटुको रसो वक्त्रं शोधयति, अग्निं दीपयति, भुक्तं शोषयति, घ्राणं आस्रावयति, चक्षुर्विरेचयति, स्फुटीकरोतीन्द्रियाणि, अलसकश्वयथूपचयोदर्दाभिष्यन्द-स्नेह-स्वेदक्लेदमलानुपहन्ति, रोचयत्यशनं, कण्डूर्विनाशयति, व्रणानवसादयति, कृमीन् हिनस्ति, मांसंविलिखति, शोणितसंघातं भिनत्ति, बन्धांश्छिनत्ति, मार्गान् विवृणोति, श्लेष्माणं शमयति ।" (च. सू. २६)

तस्य पुनरन्ययोनिः कटुको रसः, स श्लेष्मणः प्रत्यनीकत्वात् कटुकत्वान्माधुर्यमभिभवति, रौक्ष्यात् स्नेहं लाघवात् गौरवं, औष्ण्याच्छैत्यं, वैशद्यात् पैच्छिल्यमिति ।" (सु. सू. ४२)

रौक्ष्मलाघवकाटुक्यैरेव वायुं कोपयति कटुकः ।" (र. वै. सू. ७२)

55. तिक्तो रसः स्वयमरोचिष्णुररोचकघ्नः, विषघ्नः, कृमिघ्नः, मूर्च्छादाहकण्डूकुष्ठतृष्णाप्रशमनः, त्वङ्मांसयोः स्थिरीकरणो, ज्वरघ्नो, दीपनः, पाचनः, स्तन्यशोधनः, लेखनः क्लेदमेदोवसामज्जलसीकापूयस्वेदमूत्रपुरीषपित्तश्लेष्मोपशोषणः ।" (च. सू. २६) १शैत्यरौक्ष्यवैशद्यलाघवमार्दवैरेनं कोपयति तिक्तः ।" (र. वै. सू. ७१)

56. कषायो रसः संशमनः संग्राही सन्धानकरः पीडनो रोपणः शोषणः स्तम्भनः श्लेष्मरक्तपित्तप्रशमनः शरीरक्लेदस्योपयोक्ता ।" (च. सू. २६) उपयोक्ता, आचूषकः । १तत्र शैत्यरौक्ष्यलाघववैशद्यवैष्टभ्यगुणलक्षणो वायुः तस्य समानयोनिः कषायो रसः, सोऽस्य शैत्याच्छैत्यं वर्धयति, रौक्ष्याद्रौक्ष्यं लाघवाल्लाघवं, वैशद्याद् वैशद्यं, वैष्टभ्याद्-वैष्टभ्यमिति ।" (सु. सू. ४२)

रसदोषसन्निपाते तु ये रसाः यैर्दोषैः समानगुणाः समानगुणभूयिष्ठा वा भवन्ति ते तानभिवर्धयन्ति, विपरीतगुणा विपरीतगुणभूयिष्ठा वा शमयन्त्यभ्यस्यमानाः ।" (च. वि. १)

त एते रसाः स्वयोनिवर्धना अन्ययोनिप्रशमनाश्च ।" (सु. सू. ४२) । १स्वयोनेरागमाद् विवृद्धिर्दोषधातुमलानाम्, क्षयः प्रतिपक्षस्यागमात् ।" (र. वै. ३ सू. ६३-६४)

57. स्वाद्वम्ललवणा वायुं कषायस्वादुतिक्तकाः ।
जयन्ति पित्तं, श्लेष्माणं कषायकटुतिक्तकाः ।।" (च. सू. १) ।
तत्राद्या मारुतं घ्नन्ति त्रयस्तिक्तादयः कफम् ।
कषायतिक्तमधुराः पित्तमन्ये तु कुर्वते ।।" (अ. सं. सू. १)
कट्वम्ललवणाः पित्तं स्वाद्वम्ललवणाः कफम् ।
कटुतिक्तकषायाश्च कोपयन्ति समीरणम् ।।" (च. सू. १)

तत्र दोषमेकैकंस्त्रयस्त्रयोरसा जनयन्ति त्रयस्त्रयश्चोपशमयन्ति । तद्यथा-कटुतिक्तकषायाः वातं जनयन्ति मधुराम्ललवणास्त्वेनं शमयन्ति-कट्वम्ललवणाः पित्तं जनयन्ति, मधुरतिक्तकषायास्त्वेनंशमयन्ति, मधुराम्ललवणाः श्लेष्माणं जनयन्ति कटुतिक्तकषायास्त्वेनं शमयन्ति ।" (च. वि. १६)

58. तत्र प्रायो मधुरं श्लेष्मलं, अन्यत्र पुराणशालियवगोधूममुद्गमधुशर्कराजांगलमांसात् । प्रायोऽम्लं पित्तलं अन्यत्र दाडिमामलकात् । प्रायो लवणं पित्तलमचक्षुष्यं अन्यत्र सैन्धवात् । प्रायस्तिक्तकटुकं वातलमवृष्यं च अन्यत्रामृतापटोलीनागरपिप्पलीलशुनात् । प्रायः कषायं शीतं स्तम्भनं च, अन्यत्र हरीतक्याः ।" (अ. सं. सू. १८)

59. कटुतिक्तकषायाँस्तु रसान् प्राज्ञो यथाक्रमम् । योगतः कफजे व्याधौ भैषज्यमवचारयेत् ।।
प्रयुक्तः कटुकः पूर्व पैच्छिल्यं गौरवं च यत् । श्लेष्मणस्तंनिहन्त्याशु तिक्तस्तमादनंतरम् ।।

ह्रसयत्यास्यमाधुर्यं कफं संशोषयत्यपि । संगृण्हाति कषायश्च स्नेहं चाप्यवकर्षति ।।

60. तिक्तस्वादुकषायाः स्युः क्रमशः पैत्तिके हिताः ।
आमान्वयत्वात् तु पित्तस्य पूर्व तिक्तोऽवचारितः ।।
पाचयत्याशु तं पक्वं ततस्तु मधुरो रसः ।
शैत्याद् गुरुत्वात् स्नेहाच्च माधुर्याच्च नियच्छति ।।
तद्द्रवत्वविघातार्थ कषायश्चावचारितः । रौक्ष्याद्विशोषिभावाच्च विशोषयति तैजसम् ।
वातिके क्रमशो योज्याः पट्वम्ललवणा रसाः वातिके लवणः पूर्वसयोगादवचारितः ।। प्रक्लेदिभावाज्जयति विबन्धं मातरिश्वनः । निहन्ति शैत्यमुष्णत्वाद् गुरुत्वाच्चापि लाघवम् ।।
तथैवाम्लो रसः पश्चात्तस्मिन्नेवावचारितः । जडीकृतानि स्त्रोतांसि तैक्ष्णदुद्घाट्य मारुतम् ।।
अनुलोमयति क्षिप्रं स्निग्धोष्णत्वाद् विमार्गगम् ।
अम्लादनन्तरं पश्चात् प्रयुक्तो मधुरो रसः ।।
वायोर्लघुत्वं वैशद्यं रूक्षत्वं च व्यपोहति । गुरुत्वात्पिच्छिलत्वाच्च स्निग्धत्वाच्च यथाबलम् । इत्युक्ताः सर्वदोषेषु रसानां प्रविचारणाः ।" (काश्यपसंहिता,)

61. पूर्व मधुरमश्नीयान्मध्येऽम्ललवणौ रसौ । पश्चाच्छेषान् रसान् वैद्यो भोजनेष्ववचारयेत् । "मधुरमधुरमादौ मध्यतोऽम्लैकभावः, कटुकटुकमथान्ते तिक्ततिक्तं तथैव । यदि सुखपरिणामं वाञ्छसि त्वं हि राजन्, त्यज खलजनसंगं भोजनं मा कदाचित् ।।" (क्षे. कृ.)

62. भोजनाग्रेसदा पथ्यं लवणार्द्रकभक्षणम् । अग्निसंदीपनं रुच्यं जिव्हाकंठविशोधनम् ।। (भा. प्र.)

63. लवणाम्लकटूष्णानि विदाहीन्यत्ति यानि तु । तद्दोषहर्तुमाहारं मधुरेण समापयेत् (भा. प्र.)

64. नेत्याहुरन्ये रसास्तु प्रधानं कस्मात्? आगमात्; आगमो हि शास्त्रमुच्यते, शास्त्रे हि रसा अधिकृताः- यथा-"रसायत्त आहार इति, तस्मिंस्तु प्राणाः" (सु. सू. १) इति; (सु. सू. ४०) । "रसानधिकारात्" (र. वै. १ सू. १११) केचिद् रसान् प्रधानान् ब्रुवतेऽधिकारात् । ते ह्यधिकृताश्चिकित्सायामिति । कथं-"षट्स्वेव युक्तं वमनं, षट्सु युक्तं विरेचनम् । षट्सु चास्थापनं युक्तं, षट्सु संशमनं हितम् ।।" इत्यादि यो यस्मिन्नधिकृतः स तस्मिन्नान्येभ्यः प्रधानो दृष्टः । यथा सेनायां सेनापतिः ।" (भा.)

65. उपदेशाच्च उपदिश्यन्ते हि रसाः, यथा "मधुराम्ललवणा वातं शमयन्ति" । (सु. सू. ४२) उपदेशात् ।" (र. वै. सू. ११४)

66. अनुमानाच्च रसेन ह्यनुमीयते द्रव्यं, यथा मधुरमिति ।" (सु. सू. ४०) अनुमानात्" (र. वै. सू. ११५)

67. ऋषिवचनाच्च, ऋषिवचनं वेदः, यथा किंचिदिज्यार्थं मधुरमाहरेदिति; तस्माद्रसाः प्रधानम् ।" (सु. सू. ४०) ।"आगमाच्च" (र. वै. सू. १२०)

68. तेनोपसंहारात् ।" (र. वै. सु. ११२) यथा विदारिगन्धादीन् द्रव्यगणान् उक्त्वा "यानि यान्येवंप्रकाराणि मधुरस्कन्धपरिसंख्येयानि भवन्ति ।" (भा.)

69. तद्व्यापत्तौ शेषव्यापत्तेः ।" (र. वै. सू. ११३) रसव्यापत्तिनिमित्तं शेषाणां द्रव्यादीनां व्यापत्तेः-यथा क्षीरस्य रसे दुष्टे क्षीरं न गृह्यते, तद्विपाकादयश्च विपन्ना इति । (भा.)

71. अपदेशात्" (र. वै. सू. ११५) अपदेशो नाम अन्येनान्योऽपदिश्यते उपमारूपेण... प्रधानेन... मधुर गान्धर्वं, मधुरा वाणी, कटुकः फणीति ।" (भा.)

72. नानाविषयत्वात् ।" (र. वै. सू. ११७) अनेकाधारत्वादिति मधुरस्य तावदिक्षुक्षीरशर्कराखण्डादयः एवमन्येषां च । बहु विषयं तत् प्रधानं दृष्टं, यथा मनः, अथवा चक्रवर्ती ।" (भा.)

CHAPTER SIX
VIPAK

Etymological interpretation of vipak

A specific rasa emerging at the end of the digestive stage is 'vipak'. This digestive end product which is not going to change is also called as 'nisthapak'. In vipak there is not only a conversion of rasa but also of dravya.[1]

The rasa that is formed at the end of the action of gastric juice is termed as vipak. Vipak means the end result. Ayurveda mentions two types of pak.[2]

1) Awasthapak - During the stages of digestion, the digestive juice is called awasthapak, which is subjected to change. It is non-specific and is also called as prapak.

2) Nishthapak - It is called nishthapak because it is not subjected to change like awasthapak.

Vipak is specific.

Any type of diet or drugs, when ingested orally, undergo constant and total change from the original state in form and appearance. On coming in contact with gastric juice the change takes place very rapidly. The stage of awasthapak begins when the action of rasa ends. The digestion begins as soon as the dravya is put into the mouth. A practical example is eating of salt and bread. If chewed for a longer period, they become sweet to taste.

The change in ingested diet or drug occurs at every stage in the digestive tract. After digestion, the separation of digested and residual undigested products begins. Digestive juice (chyme) and mala (stool and urine) are differentiated on further passage along the intestine. From the beginning the serially converted digestive juice (pak) is called awasthapak because it depends on the anatomical structure of the gastrointeslinal tract and the status of the organs of the tract. Awasthapak takes place in stages. The first stage begins in the stomach. Here, diet containing the six specific rasas (षड्रस) gets converted to madhur awasthapak (which is sweet). This gives rise to the formation of kapha. The second stage of digestion takes place from duodenum to jejunum, ilium and upto descending colon. During this stage, pitta is formed due to prominence of amla rasa. The third stage of digestion takes place from the descending colon to the anal region. In this stage due to the prominence of katu rasa, vayu is formed.

Diet of any rasa has to undergo these three stages. Proportion or quantity of the formed doshas definitely differ during the stages of awasthapak which depends relatively on different proportions of rasas (madhur etc.). This means that if diet contains excess madhur rasa dravya then during awasthapak more kapha is formed in the stomach. But Kapha will not be formed if dravyas are katu or bitter. Satiety and heavyness felt immediately after a meal is attributed to the formation of kapha at the time of awasthapak. Charakacharya has advised consumption of oily and ushna diet for the formation of liquid kapha.

Apertures of the body like anus can provide valuable information to an expert clinician. How can they avoid examining these?

The end result of rasa is a transformation to nishthapak. Vipak formed in such a mode of nisthapak or transformed rasa is circulated throughout the body with rasa dhatu. Due to this, all bodily dhatus are nourished and doshas are evolved.

Madhur vipak gives rise to kapha, amla vipak gives rise to pitta and katu vipak to vata.

In this way, nisthapak is a special kind of rasa (guna) and is produced after awasthapak. Rasa dhatu is formed during the stage of rasa mala vivek which is the end stage of awasthapak. This stage is marked as nishthapak.[3] But this digestive juice (पाक) does not remain in the lumen of the bowel (chyme). It is present in all the dhatus and channels leading to those dhatus. Therefore it cannot be factually observed. Awasthapak could be factual but not nishthapak. It is infered by its effect and action on dhatus and formation of the excreta (perception). Malas are formed in the lumen of the large bowel, extremities and midway in the channels.

Difference between the digestive stages is shown in the table below :-

Pak

Awasthapak	**Nishthapak**
1) Observed during different stages of digestion.	1) End result of digestion.
2) Basic doshas are formed by the awasthapak.	2) Malaroopa doshas are evolved.
3) Factually observed	3) By perception only.
4) Formation in the lumen of bowel. Therefore lasting action is limited to lumen.	4) Though formed in lumen, its effect is seen on dhatus and connecting channels. (Nistha - perfection, end, termination.)
5) Macrodigestion (in bowel)	5) Microdigestion (extremities and channels of digestion)

Vipak is responsible for the easy assimilastion of diet or drugs into dhatus. Food or drugs in awasthapak are digested, as ingested. In vipak, it is suitable for the digestion in dhatus. After vipak, the transformation of food is more towards body constituents. Digestion in awasthapak is in the lumen and on nonspecific base. While digestion after vipak is within the dhatu and is minute. To make the external food suitable to body constituents (धातुरूप), it is essential to transform it. It first becomes awasthapak and then nishthapak which takes it to various dhatus and channels.

Once the digestion begins in dhatus, kapha in excretory form is seen from rasa while pitta etc.

Achhapan sneha, anuvasan basti and kutipraveshik rasayana are very extensive and effective modes of therapy while vichar snehapan, matrabasti and vatatapik rasayana are minor modes.

are the excretory elements of the successive dhatus.

In the treatment of grahani, Charakacharya has quoted that, "Excreta of food is stool and urine while kapha is formed from rasa and pitta from blood (rakta)." Based on this, some vaidyas believe that awasthapak gives rise to increase in kapha-pitta in the form of dhatu within the lumen. Nishthapak gives excretory form of kapha - pitta as the end product.

3) Types of Vipak

Differences are found in literature about the types of vipak. Among them are four prominent types :-

1. **Shadvidha vipakvad** - Subdivided into two -
   a) Yatharasa vipakvad (synergic to rasa).
   b) Aniyat vipakvad (individual).
2. **Panchavidha vipakvad.**
3. **Trividha vipakvad.**
4. **Dwividha vipakvad.**

1. Shadvidha vipakvad - Some acharyas consider that there are six rasas and therefore vipak also should be six. This is further divided into a) Yatharas vipakvad and b) Aniyat vipakvad.

a) Yatharasa vipakvad - says that vipak of every rasa is according to type such as madhur vipak of madhur rasa, amla vipak of amla rasa and so on........ milk remains sweet even after heating or seeds of sali when sown give rise only to sali. This has exactly the same specificity. Rasa is an inherited property (or natural) and therefore cannot be 'given away' (त्याग).[4] Similarly, six vipaks are formed from six madhuradi rasas. This is Shadvidha vipakvad.

b) Aniyat vipakvad - Acharyas belonging to this school feel that any rasa will not form any vipak. A particular vipak will result depending on the prominence of a particular rasa during the active period of vipak. Therefore it is difficult to predict the vipak because of unpredictability of rasas predominant during vipak. However there will be only six types of rasas even if it is uncertain. In this way the number of vipak (ie. nishthapak) will be six according to anniyat vipakvad.[5]

2. Panchavidha vipakvad : According to Sushrutacharya, based on panchamahabhoota theory, vipak should also be of five types. Therefore they are called as parthiv, aapya, taijas, vayaveeya and akasheeya.[6]

Reasons for change in vipak : Vipak changes because of the following reasons. Guru vipaki dravyas turn to laghu vipaki and vice versa.

a) Dravya quantity - Guru vipaki dravyas when consumed in small or negligible quantities form laghu vipak and laghu vipaki dravyas eaten in excess get converted to guru vipaki.

b) Processing - Guru vipaki dravyas change to laghu vipaki and act as deepaniya. For example - red pumpkin (guruvipaki) after cooking becomes laghu vipaki. Laghu vipaki dravyas turn to guru vipaki e.g. papad if fried becomes guru vipaki and on roasting it becomes laghu vipaki.

c) Acceptibility or tolerance - (सात्म्य) Guru vipaki dravyas, if tolerable to a person, behave as laghu vipaki, For example - milk does not become guru vipaki to persons who can tolerate milk.

d) Power of agni - Person having powerful agni can digest guru vipaki dravyas like laghu vipaki. For example - roti stuffed with sweet dal and jaggery (पुरणपोळी) can be easily digested like laghu vipaki by a person of powerful agni.

e) Desha (land) - In cold countries guru vipaki dravyas behave like laghu vipaki. In tropical countries laghu vipaki behave (become) like guru vipaki.

f) Kala (time) - In rainy season, laghu dravyas become guru and in winter (हेमन्त), guru dravyas turn to laghu dravyas.

g) Combination (संयोगविशेष) - Guru dravyas become laghu when combined together e.g. milk + dry ginger (सुंठ)[7]

(3) Trividha vipakvad - Agnivesha, Vriddha Vagbhatta, Vagbhatta etc. have described vipak into three types viz. madhur, amla and katu. Among these madhur and lavana rasas have madhurvipak, amla rasa has amla vipak and katu, tikta and kashaya rasas have katu vipak.[8]

Parashar theory - This theory also classifies vipak into three but with different basis.

Katu rasa - Katu vipak.
Amla rasa - Amla vipak
and Madhur + Lavana + Tikta + Kashaya - Madhur Vipak

This is so because if the vipak of tikta and kashaya is considered to be katu then they cannot act as pittashamak. So, dravyas having tikta and kashaya rasa should be considered as having madhur vipak.[9]

Why are there only three types of vipak? As there are three main doshas, subset of these should also be three in vipak. In fact tridoshavad is the base of the three types of vipak. Tridoshas in the body are increased or decreased by diet and drugs. Life sustains on tridoshas which are related to dravya. Tridosha represent three vipaks. Madhur vipak increases kapha dosha, amla vipak increases pitta dosha and katu vipak increases vata dosha. Effect of vipak is similar to rasa and therefore brings about the desired effect of increasing or decreasing doshas.

(4) Dwividha vipakvad - Sushrutacharya and Nagarjuna, belonging to Dhanvantari tradition classify vipak into two types. (1) guru and (2) laghu. This classification is based on the prominent mahabhoota at the time of formation of vipak.

Just as a stationary living tree, if a human being starts growing, what would happen ? But in nature this does not happen.

Guru mahabhootas – Prithvi and Aap – Guruvipak.

Laghu mahabhootas – Agni, Vayu and Akash – Laghu vipak.

Even twenty gunas are further classified into two varieties.

Guru – snighdha, pichchila, manda, hima, sandra and sthira – Madhur vipak.

Laghu - Teekshna, ushna, vishada, drava and chala - Katu vipak.[10]

Dwividha vipakvad is based on panchamahabhoota just as trividha vipakvad depends on tridosha theory. Sushruta gives more importance to panchamahabhoota and though admits the panchavidha vipakvad, he does not contradict dwividha vipakvad. Dravyas can be classified by various means.[11]

Conclusion

By considering and evaluating the different views of classification, the following decisions are valid :

1. Shadvidha vipakvad -

a) Yatharasa vipakvad - Six vipaks because of six rasas. This is not accepted by many because vrihi rice of madhur rasa turns to amla vipak. Pippali of katu rasa turns to madhur vipak. Oil is sweet but katu vipaki and amalaki is sour but madhur vipaki. Patol of bitter rasa has a madhur vipak. Kulittha of kashaya rasa has amla vipak. Haritaki is kashaya but has madhur vipak. This proves that vipak does not follow rasa in property. Nagarjuna is also of the same opinion. He states that characteristics of rasa and vipak do not correspond and their site of actions are different. Rasa is factual and vipak is perceptible. If rasa and vipak are identical then there is no reason to call them as independent. Therefore rasa and vipak are not identical.[12]

(b) Aniyat vipakvad - This opinion is also not accepted by many because science does not believe in chaos, instability or indiscipline. If vipak exists as a substance and if it is acceptable to science then it should be based on some firm principles.

Science does not have any place for inconclusiveness and therefore it does not accept this aniyat vipakvad. It is unacceptable.

(c) Panchavidha vipakvad :- Basically panchavidha vipakvad is dwividha vipakvad and is based on panchamahabhoota which is also the basis of dwividha vipakvad.

d) Trividha vipakvad :- Charaka school accepts trividha vipakvad. Madhur, amla and katu vipak are the three basic vipak. However, there are exceptions to this theory. For example, pippali is pungent but madhur vipaki. Trividha vipak is based on the assumption of tridoshavad and therefore some acharyas have proposed a view that a combination of kapha and vata doshas gives rise to madhur vipak. Similarly, kapha and pitta give rise to amla vipak whereas vata and pitta produce katu

One has to be extremely careful during the first three months of pregnancy. Similarly, one has to be careful during the three stages of life i.e. childhood, young age and old age for enjoying death without stress.

vipak. But this is not true. Because dosha vardhan or kshaya (decrease) is a result of the effect of vipak. So vipak is responsible for the increased or decreased state of doshas and not vice versa.

Acharya Sushruta does not agree with this explanation of trividha vipakvad. Rasa of normal pitta is katu (pungent) but in vitiated state, its rasa is amla (sour) - which in pitta, is an abnormal property. Vipak is always ascertained after considering some actions based on the normal state of dosha. Kapha in vitiated state is salty and if vipak is ascertained on this vitiated state then one will have to accept lavana vipak as well. Sushruta also does not consider amla vipak (Aptavachan). We can predict that those rasas which are responsible for the increase of doshas also exist in doshas. When kapha vriddhi is caused by lavana (salt), it proves that lavana is already present in kapha dosha. Therefore it is wrong to consider three vipaks.[13]

Nagarjuna also does not accept the theory of trividha vipakvad. While discussing vipak, the following three reasons are essential to consider :-[14]

1. Some dravyas are digested earlier during the process of digestion. They are laghu or achirkalin (unstable) and the others are digested in the later stages of digestion (vipak); they are guru or chirkalin (stable). The third vipak does not exist.[15]

2. Even while considering gunas, only laghu and guru vipak are possible and none else.[15]

3. From the point of view of rasas also, vipak is only of two rasas. This is proved in tridoshavad as well as in panchamahabhootavad, because vata and pitta have katu rasa whereas and kapha has madhur rasa. Therefore katu vipak increases vata and pitta and madhur vipak increases kapha vata. Similarly madhur vipak alleviates vata and pitta while katu vipak alleviates kapha.[16]

4. Based on principles of mahabhootas, prithvi + aap = madhur vipak and agni + akash = katu vipak. Madhur vipak is guru and katu vipak is laghu.

Dwividha vipakvad

Acharyas of Sushruta tradition accept the above dual theory. Sushruta has described two vipaks based on agam pramanya (आगम प्रामाण्य) and panchamahabhootas. Nagarjuna considers the vipak as the end result of digestion. Digestion of laghu guna dravya and guru guna dravyas is again early and prolonged (delayed) respectively. Therefore vipak are also considered of two types.

This statement of Nagarjuna is debatable because early and delayed digestion depends on awasthapak and not on nishthapak, since nishthapak follows awasthapak. Principally the status of vipak is independent of early or delayed digestion. Nagarjuna has considered awasthapak as a part of nishthapak or vipak.

According to Charaka, the action of nishthapak is decided after the completion of awasthapak which is asserted by the increased or decreased effect on the doshas. Vipak is action-based (bound), therefore instead of measuring laghu and guru guna, it should be decided by shodhan and langhan

There is no evidence as strong as direct demonstrable evidence (pratyaksha).

effects or actions of gunas.

Similarity between trividha vipakvad and dwividha vipakvad

There is no basic difference between these two vipakvad. Trividha vipakvad is based on tridosha and rasa, while dwividha vipakvad on mahabhootas and gunas. Doshas are related to mahabhootas and classification of rasas depends on gunas. Therefore these two have a very close relationship.

Charaka and Sushruta both accept madhur or katu vipak with a slight difference. Madhur rasa is parthiv and aapya – similar to guru guna – therefore madhur means guru and katu vipak means laghu. Thus no difference exists between these two.

What is not clear is the question of amla vipak. Charaka accepts amla vipak while Sushruta not only denies it. but does not even mention amla vipak. Amla rasa is predominant in prithvi and agni mahabhoota and thus is both, laghu and guru. Vipak is also viewed from this aspect of laghu and guru. Also the different views on rasas of pitta are responsible for this conflict. According to Charaka, pitta is amla and katu while Sushruta describes it as katu.

This difference can be nullified by considering the actions based on gunas. The action of vitiation of pitta by amla is due to its ushna veerya.

Guna and karma of vipak (Charaka)

Vipak	Guna	Dosha	Dhatu	Mala
Madhur	Snigdha and guru	Increases kapha	Shukra vardhak	Laxative
Amla	Snigdha and laghu	Increases pitta	Shukra Nashak	Laxative
Katu	Ruksha and laghu	Increases vata	Shukra Nashak	Constipative

Sushruta :

Madhur (guru vipak)	Increases kapha, reduces vatapitta	Laxative
Katu (laghu Vipak)	Increases vatapitta reduces kapha	Consiipative

Guru dravyas in nishthapak nourish the dhatus slowly and after a delay as they are difficult to digest. Laghu dravyas are digested easily and nourish the dhatus rapidly. Vagbhattacharya describes the effect of vipak as similar to rasa. But rasa, when absorbed, shows different effects which are not seen with vipak on body and mind. This is an important point. Vipak will not produce those mental

Eventhough madhur is maximally opposite to tikta rasa, both do pittashaman.

and physical effects which are produced by perception of rasas.

According to Nagarjuna vipak does not always influence the doshas. Madhur, amla and katu vipak result in a definite aggravation (वर्धन) or amelioration (शमन) of doshas. Laghu and guru vipak do not show a definite effect of this kind. For example, water of laghu vipak results in increase of kapha while Alcohols, which have laghu vipak, decrease kapha.

Grades in vipak

Once we establish a definite relationship between rasa and vipak, it is obvious that vipak is similar to rasa in the sense that vipak will also have grades like rasa. Thus, vipak of a sweet dravya will be sweet, vipak of sweeter dravya will be is sweeter and that of sweetest will be the sweetest.

Comparatively, madhur vipak of madhur rasa is the best. Madhur vipak of amla rasa is second best, while madhur vipak of lavana rasa is inferior.

Similarly, katu vipak of katu rasa is the best, katu vipak of tikta rasa (bitter) is inferior and katu vipak of kashaya rasa is of medium quality. We can also predict that snigdha and ruksha gunas acting on vipak will affect the actions of vipak and will also change the quality of vipak.[17]

Perception of vipak

Vipak is formed after undergoing the transformation of digestion through madhur, amla and katu stages. Though we cannot assess or see it directly, its action is inferable. For example, kapha increases as effect on dosha or mansa meda increase as effect on dhatu. Similarlyy laxative activity may be seen as an effect on the malas. Thus, vipak can be inferred upon through these actions.[18]

Because of lack of perceptibility, vipak has become a subject of debate.

Rasa and Vipak

Rasa and vipak are two different entities. One cannot carry the action of the other. The following five differences prove the statement :-

1. **Difference in characteristics** - Both differ in their properties. Rasa is a subject of taste organ (tongue) and vipak is the transformed state of rasa.

2. **Difference in kala (time)** - Knowledge of rasa is experienced after its contact with taste organ while vipak is formed at the end of digestion. Rasa when tasted by a taste organ, lasts only upto awasthapak. The vipak follows thereafter.

3. **Difference in action** - Action of rasa is limited to some specific parts of the body whereas vipak acts on the whole body. That is why while describing rasa, local bodily actions are mentioned e.g. action of amla rasa on sight (eye) etc. But vipak acts on doshas, dhatus and malas.

4. **Differance in sites of action** - Action of rasa is dual, on body and mind. Vipak's action is

The discovery of sweet grass i.e. sugarcane was done by Vishwamitra. How many sugar industrialists know about it?

predominantly bodily action and secondarily on mind. After consuming a pleasant rasa, action is observed on the mind along with its action on the body. This is not so with vipak therefore actions of vipak are not considered to be the same as rasa. Their actions are only considered to have some similarity.[19]

5. **Difference in availability :-** The action of rasa is proved predominantly by special taste organ, while that of vipak is by inference.

Difference between rasa and vipak.

	Rasa	Vipak
1.	One can elicit taste	Can be elicited only by result.
2.	Quick action	Slow action (except visha dravyas).
3.	Local effect	Whole body.
4.	Action on body and mind	Primarily on body, secondarily on mind.
5.	Directly perceptible	Known by inference.
6.	Action on tongue	Effect from pakvashaya (colon) to anal canal - and then on dhatus at the time of micro-digestion.

Digestive chyme

Prapak	Vipak
1. Formed in the lumen of intestine and action is limited to bowel	1. Formed at the end of digestion in the lower colon and acts on (lumen). dhatus.
2. At the time of macrodigestion	2. At the time of microdigestion.

Vipak (Generally accepted view)

Rasa	Vipak
Madhur, lavana	Madhur
Amla	Amla
Kashaya, katu, tikta	Katu

In the universe and in man made by the universe, there is continuous duel between the gunas of opposing forces. Human life is one such contradiction.

Parashar's view

Rasa	Vipak
Madhur, lavana, tikta, kashaya	Madhur
Amla	Amla
Katu	Katu

Importance of vipak

Vipak is important among all the other qualities like rasa within dravya, because guna or dosha of dravya depends on proper or improper digestion. Gunas are evolved due to proper digestion of dravya by balanced digestive fire (समाग्नी) and doshas due to incorrect digestion.

According to some acharyas, the desired and undesired actions of the properly digested substances and improperly digested substances depends upon vipak. Thus properly digested chitraka produces agni-deepan (desired action) and constipation (undesired action) whereas undigested pippali generates excess of semen (desired action) and excess of kleda (undesired action).[20]

Vipak is important because both aggravation or amelioration of doshas is due to vipak.[21] Building up of dhatus by vipak also proves its importance.[22] All types of diets and medicines have their desired or undesired actions through vipak. Properly digested diet or medicine is beneficial while same, if wrongly digested, gives rise to dosha and disease.

For this reason vipak is important among all the qualities of dravya.[23]

Appendix - 1

Concept of vipak in Ayurveda

Vipak cannot be demonstrated directly. It is an inferential entity and such entities are always debatable.

In the universe, the tangible (evident or direct or obvious) is in minority as compared to what is not factually perceptible which is in a much greater proportion. Vipak falls in the latter category.

Assumed principles

According to geometrical definitions, we can not draw a line because it has length but no breadth. It is assumed, that it has some breadth. This is also true for a point. Geometry can progress further only if we accept these two tenets and not otherwise. Similarly, relationship between the universe and humankind should be assumed and can be known through inferential knowldedge only. Every constituent in the universe is represented within the atoms and molecules of the human body.

This is the basis of all thought. All the components of the universe are represented in the human body and their relationship is established through this advocacy.

To obtain knowledge about a speciality, fundamental or basic knowledge is essential.

Body changes at every moment

The human body exhibits constant transformation. The etymological meaning of sharir is one which is constantly degraded (शीर्यते इति). According to the theory of moment-fractional existence, the human body continuously experiences states of genesis, stasis and degradation. This is true for the universe as well as the human body formed of molecules of the universe. In living as well as in non-living systems every moment, each dravya assumes a fresh state from the previous one. From the invisible to the visible, the universe continuously demonstrates this transition. The word 'jagat' means moving.

Transformation through pak

A specific power brings about this constant change. Transformation is the action of pak which in turn is brought about by the effect of heat (उष्णशक्ती) . The effect of cold (शीतशक्ती) is the balancing power to ushna. Time, which has momentum, helps this duality of ushna-sheeta.

The constant transformation going on within the universe is only due to pak.

The body, constituted with different forms of panchamahabhootas, is formed by pak. Answers to the riddle of the universe lies in pak. Pak is responsible for the formation of the Himalayas from the seas and bringing about earthquakes. Human evolution from the universe is by pak. Everything from fertilization to death is by pak. Similarly the journey from disease to health and health to disease is attributed to pak. Rain water going back to the clouds and coming down as rain is a cycle of pak. Pak is responsible for maintaining the good or bad state of the formed dravya or substance. Pak is the reason behind transformation of the life of human beings. Pak sustains life by providing nourishment from diet. Old age and death are both natural forms of pak.

Kala and pak are both unavoidable. Pak is transformation with the help of ushna shakti. Pak and ushna shakti go together. Sheeta shakti is considered in relation to ushna shakti. Pak denotes the past, present and future condition of ushna shakti. Pak and ushna shakti cannot exist without each other. Even for generating heat some fuel has to undergo pak. Ushna shakti or the solar energy which is responsible for such pak, continuously affects the ever changing universe and the human body which is a replica of the universe.

Relationship of time and agni

In the living human system, ushna shakti brings about all the innumerable transformations which are taking place continuously at every moment. Agni is the cause of this. This agni which sustains life, is of thirteen types. This agni shakti is related to time. There is a lively bond between time and agni shakti. Agni is self digestive of all the molecules of the body. The presence of agni, in macro and micro constituents of the body, leads to continuous depletion and digestion of the whole body. Therefore, for survival, one has to compete or resist this agni and the only way is by ingestion of food.

In this world, nothing is stable and similarly, nothing is identical i.e. "गच्छति इति जगत्"

Imbibition of diet in the body

For the purpose of survival, only a balanced diet is not sufficient. The external constituents (macrocosm) should match the internal (microcosm) constituents. Diet has to be imbibed in the bodily constituents. This action is done by pachak pitta (जठराग्नी), bhautik agni and dhatu agni. This is the natural process going on in the body. It is the same as the process of pak. Though macro digestion takes place in the lumen of the intestine, the micro digestion continues in each and every atom and molecule of the body. Due to different stages, different times and different sites of digestion, dietary dravyas undergo physical and chemical changes. The part where the macro digestion takes place is called mahastrotas. Here, the dietary dravya is converted so as to faciliate its imbibition in the body by macro processing. This occurs at the stage of separation of digestive juice and excretory material.

Pak and prapak

Overall digestive juice is called pak (chyme) but the first part of digestion is termed as prapak (predigestive) stage. As this is subjected to different stages according to the time and site, it is also called awasthapak. This concept of prapak is very important regarding the dietary dravyas. Poisons, alcohols and dravyas having a specific potency, do not undergo a predigestive stage. Their actions start spontaneously.

Dietary and medicinal dravyas are both subjected to change during digestion. But both undergo mutually contrasting changes and hence this division into dietary dravyas and medicinal dravyas. Generally, dietary dravyas are rasa predominant and medicinal dravyas are veerya predominant.

Diet forms the main component of any treatment eventhough dietary dravyas are only the start of the treatment. It is clear that we cannot compare diet and medicine by the same norms. On the contrary, there is a marked difference between the two. Also, actions of medicinal dravyas are considered on the basis of time and site. Drugs act by either rasa, pak, guna, veerya or prabhav.

All these terms are time bound

रसोनिपाते means rasa is considered only at the time of contact with the toungue (निपात). Not before or after. Vipak is at the end of digestion which is also time related. Consideration of vipak is incorrect without specific digestion being completed. वीर्यं यावत् अधीवासात्।

Among all these properties, rasa is given importance. Just as by knowing the planet-star relationship of a person, one can predict 'nadi, yoni, guna, deity tree (आराध्यवृक्ष), type of donation to ameliorate disease, planet deity, stars, swagam etc. Similarly, by knowing the rasa of a dravya, prediction about effect, guna, veerya (ushna or sheeta) and vipak (madhur, amla and katu) becomes easy. If this would have been universally true then no intelligence would have been required. Study of nighantu would have been easy if it was general. But rasa behaves exceptionally (सापवाद) and nighantu contains a specific study of these. All actions do not follow the characters of rasas. Thought of vipak is born out of this concept.

Our intellectual capability doesn't match with that of the ancient philosophers. Then how can we challenge their decisions?

Vipak are only three

Though it is said that rasas are six in number due to six seasons, yet Ayurveda classifies the year into three main seasons. As this principle is universally accepted, all the topics in Ayurveda are based on the triad theory. Dosha-dhatu-mala based on panchmahabhootas of padarthvignyan are based on tridosha. Though the five mahabhootas form ten pairs of two mahabhootas each (through permutations and combinations), yet the number of rasas is kept at six. This is done keeping in view the triad theory whereby six rasas will bring about an increase or decrease in three doshas.

Though rasas are six, prapak and vipak can only be three as they are based on the tridhatu theory.

Sushrutacharya described only laghu and guru vipak considering the terminal effect. They do not fit well in the dosha theory as they are included in the twenty gunas. Parashar also turns down this classification of three types of vipak considering veerya as the single most important criterion for classification. For example - tikta, kashaya rasa - katu vipak but is sheeta veerya and therefore instead of increasing pitta, by its sheet veerya it ameliorates pitta.

It is proper to consider prapak and vipak in association with rasa as is done with guna, veerya, karma etc. Gaurav, laghav effect on dosha, dhatu and mala etc. are infered upon by taking rasa's property as the base because it is directly tasted by the tongue. While considering prabhav, it is worth considering veerya. Similarly, while considering the inferential vipak, it is correct to take into account the rasa which is perceived by the special senses. Vipak, when considered as a total transformation of rasa, no longer remains perceptible to the sense organ of taste. Therefore it is inferential and not directly perceptible.

Vipak is not factual but described by its action (कर्मानुमेय). Vipak is described in relation to diet and medicine, but with a difference that prapak stage exists in relation to diet and not to medicine. किंचित् रसेन कुरुते कर्म पाकेन – in this sutra, the word pak refers to all the entities like prapak, vipak, sthoolpak, sukshma pak, doshapak dhatupak, malapak, kalapak, vayupak, ayushyapak etc.

Grades of vipak

Knowledge of rasa is direct and that of vipak is by inference. But inference can follow only after direct knowledge. Hence inference of vipak follows the factual perception of rasa. Therefore, in vipak and rasa, the terminology is similar. Different tastes are experienced by tongue at different stages of digestion. What harm is there if we consider these taste - experiences as vipak? Taste of a medicine is experienced while it is in contact with the tongue, while vipak is known through inference at the time of separation of the metabolic juice and dhatu from the waste product at the end of the pak in the intestine. Both rasa and vipak exhibit grades in their intensities.

There is a big gap between the perception of rasa and the beginning of the vipak action.

When we say that macrodigestion takes place in the intestine then it implies that microdigestion

If these footnotes are read, one would come to know various facts of Ayurveda.

must be taking place some where else. It takes place in the external and middle channels (बाह्य मार्ग and मध्यम मार्ग) after the formation of vipak. Vipak is responsible for the expression of bodily elements (भाव). Oja formation is the last stage of microdigestion. Effect of vipak is seen by its actions on the srotas of the respective elements of the body.

As a rule, vipak of a dominant rasa will be similar to that dominant rasa. Rasa is superseded by vipak and vipak by veerya.

Madhur vipak of madhur rasa and lavana rasa show different effects. Pungent shunthi and pippali forming madhur vipak are used in rakta pitta while lavana (salt), though avidahi (अविदाही), is not used in rakta pitta. Dravyas which do not undergo prapak stage can be used for direct action on the dhatus.

A concept

If milk is boiled after adding a particular dravya and if it gets precipitated, then one can infer that the dravya is amla vipake. If it does not precipitate then the dravya is madhur or katu vipaki. It is essential to have such tests for deciding vipak. As soon as this dravya comes in contact with the tongue it gets converted into another form. This new substance emits various vibrations which bring about the action of rasa. This is the end of the existence of rasa. Action of rasa is limited to this stage only. Whatever action starts (or is observed) after this stage is attributed to other gunas contained in the substance. Similarly, veerya, guna, prabhav and vipak also generate vibrations affecting the sensitive body. The effect, whether beneficial or otherwise, can be ascertained from the result.

The dictionary meaning of vipak is ripening to maturity, fully developed etc. It implies that something has remained undigested after the prapak stage. The question viz. what next after vipak, does not arise. The function of prapak is generalised whereas that of vipak is specialised.

Life is judged by vibrations. Life ends if these vibrations stop. In this life, which is full of vibrations and rasa, veerya, vipak, guna and prabhav function at their own frequencies at different levels different sites. Vibrations are the base of all these. At the site of the tongue just as rasa works with its various frequencies, vipak also works at its own frequencies.

Similarity and differences between prapak and vipak

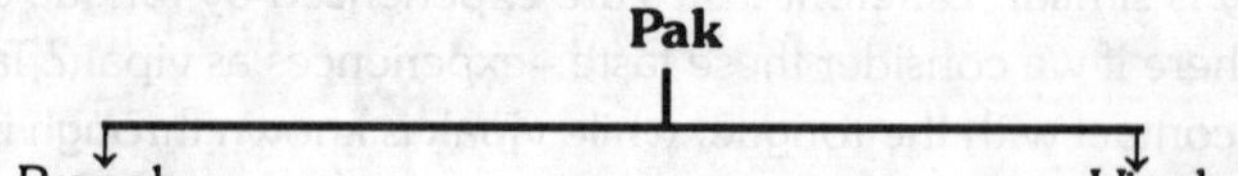

Prapak	Vipak
1) It is a relatively gross form of digestion (macrodigestion)	1) It is a relatively subtle form of digestion (microdigestion)
2) Designated as awasthapak.	2) Called nishthapak.

Generally, collection of plants for medicinal purpose is done during the month of Ashwin - Kartik of Hindu calender. On the other hand, plants used to induce vomiting and purgation are collected during Vaishakh and jyeshtha months.

3) The term prapak is used to denote a stage prior to vipak. It is unavoidable and is not always definite.	3) The term vipak is used in relation to the term prapak. It is specific and occurs after prapak. It is the final end result.
4) Every dravya undergoes madhur, amla and katu awasthapak, in that order.	4) Every dravya undergoes vipak depending on the final stage of transformation of that substance.
5) Prapak generates gross kapha, pitta, vata, excreta and chyle of food.	5) Vipak forms subtle rasadi dhatus and upadhatus and at the end, oja.
6) Its direct effects are observed locally on stomach, duodenum, small and large intestine.	6) Its effect is seen all over the body.
7) Prapak is named after rasas.	7) Vipak is also named after rasas.
8) Knowledge is obtained directly.	8) Knowledge is obtained by inference.
9) The basic philosophy of triads in Ayurveda applies to prapak as well.	9) Vipak also follows the philosophy of triads.
10) This converts food to a state acceptable to the body.	10) In vipak, molecular state of bodily dhatus are formed.
11) The rasas do not remain in the same state once they undergo vipak.	11) Rasas do not remain in the the same state because the dravya itself gets converted. The rasas may be of the same kind. The composition of the dravya, and hence its rasas, get altered in vipak.
12) This stage is useful for the separation of digestive and excretory part of the chyme.	12) Vipak is transformation into nutritive stable elements.
13) Jatharagni and bhootagni act predominantly in prapak.	13) Dhatvagni act predominantly in vipak.
14) Dietary dravyas containing	14) End result of the

Prior to rejuvenation therapy, formulations used for shodhan (purification) are prepared from dravyas having six rasas and seven colours.

rasas are transformed in prapak. elaborated further as signs	transformed rasa is altered further in vipak.
15) Awasthapak can be termed as a digestive process.	15) Vipak can be termed as a metabolic process.

This table describes the recognition of vipak by inference from its actions. It may be confirmed appropriately by observations in experimental work.

Appendix - 2

Vipak

The concept of vipak is explained in a modern view by Pandit C. Dwarkanath, the author of 'Digestion and Metabolism in Ayurveda.'

Transformation after ingestion of a diet containing six rasas taking place in the gastrointestinal tract is called awasthapak. Chakrapani terms this as prapak. In Ayurveda, it is described that rasa is perceived by bodhak kapha whose site is mentioned as the base of the tongue. Charaka and Sushruta have mentioned bodhak kapha but not of teja associated with bodhak kapha. Reference to bodhak kapha and associated teja is found in Ayurvedic sutras and commentary by Yoganandnath. Teja associated with bodhak kapha helps in breaking down madhur dravyas. Bodhak kapha is linked to salivary secretion of carbohydrate in a modern concept. Saliva is secreted by three salivary glands namely parotid, sublingual and submaxillary.[24] Saliva or bodhak kapha acts in two ways: (1) It helps swallowing by assisting bolus formation (2) by the action of ptyalin enzyme (teja in bodhak kapha), it breaks down the carbohydrate contents of the diet.

First stage of digestion in stomach - madhurbhav

The digestive action of saliva, started in the mouth, continues further into the stomach. In this process, insoluble starch is converted into soluble starch by the following steps:

Starch ® erythro dextrin ® stable dextrin. The end result of this dietary digestion in this first stage is madhur and therefore called as madhurbhav. Pran vayu helps the passage of the food from mouth to stomach according to Charaka and Sushruta.[25] The site of pran vayu is in the brain (head). In the modern concept, the centre of the act of swallowing is situated in the medulla oblongata.

Kledak kapha in madhurbhav

According to Charaka, after ingestion of a balanced diet, first madhur awasthapak is formed and frothy cough is evolved from it. According to the modern view, this kledak kapha can be compared to secretion of mucin. This is secreted by mucous cells through the pyloric and cardiac glands of the stomach. It is a thick, mucinous liquid. This secretion can be considered as kledak kapha. The action

It is seen that in Rasayan and Vajikaran tantra, doshas are not given much importance but dhatus are considered more important.

of this is softening the food, breaking down of the molecules and alteration to a liquid state. Charaka also mentions the evolution of frothy kapha. The word evolution is important because it is formed by cardiac and pyloric glands.

Amlabhav of awasthapak

Madhur rasa of the awasthapak ends by the amla rasa of stomach. Mucosal lining of the stomach forms this sour juice. This is the beginning of the sour state. There is no effect of this state on the madhur rasa formed in the first stage of digestion. In sour state, mainly protein and fat are acted upon. Insoluble proteins are converted into soluble proteins. The steps are as follows :-

Proteins → Proteases → Peptones

The amla state gives rise to amla dravya, which is called acidified chyme. Charaka and Vagbhatta mention this as vidagdha.[26]

Chakrapanidatta explains the meaning of vidagdha as a state which is mid way in digestion, or partly digested and partly undigested chyme. According to Charaka and Chakrapani, this acidified chyme is not fully digested therefore it is not ready for absorption in the body. After its full digestion, in the stage of Nishthapak, it gets ready to get transformed into various dhatus.

Digestion in the stomach and small intestine

After studying madhur and amla conditions of awasthapak (as described above) it is observed that various secretions responsible for digestion in the stomach and small intestine were first studied by Punarvasu Atreya. Not only was he precise about digestion of proteins and carbohydrates in the stomach but he has also mentioned the digestion in the small intestine. After considering the modern view of the stages of digestion, it proves without doubt that Charaka and Sushruta knew of the process 2000 years ago.

Charaka mentions that bile is secreted when the digested and undigested acidified chyme moves from the stomach to the duodenum. Chakrapani, in his criticism, says vidagdha means partly digested food and amla means a stage after it is acted upon by hydrochloric acid in the stomach. Such acidified chyme, when goes into the duodenum with the help of vayu (vata), results in the secretion of bile.

Observations of Punarvasu Atreya, made 2000 years ago, tally with the work of Pavlov, Starling and Baylis. This proves that acidified chyme, while passing from pylorus to duodenum, results (helps) in the secretion of bile and pancreatic juice into the duodenum. It helps the completion of digestion of food. The residual stool is minimal and hard in consistency.

Gastric juice

Digested material in the small intestine, treated by the various digestive enzymes is called chyme (जठरागनी पाक). Various terms are used for digestive enzymes viz. 1) pittagni 2) koshthagni 3) antragni

Some plants act through their appearance, taste, fragrance, sound and touch. Such actions are also called remedies.

4) kayagni and 5) audaryagni

Though food undergoes madhur and amla state, the total digestion takes place in the small intestine with the help of various digestive enzymes. The chyme then becomes suitable for absorption into the body. Charaka, Sushruta and Vagbhatta refer to this specific stage of chyme formation as vipak. Charaka and Vagbhatta consider three types of vipak viz. madhur, amla and katu whereas Sushruta considers only two types viz. madhur and katu.

Pungency of awasthapak (कटुभाव)

Katubhav is the third stage of awasthapak and this takes place in the large intestine. The large intestine is called as pakvashaya. When the chyme enters pakvashaya, it is converted into solid form due to absorption of its liquid part by the ushma (heat). This solid part is nothing but anna mala. Katu vayu is also formed in this stage. Chakrapani, in his comments on this stage of digestion, stresses the importance of the word 'shoshana' (absorption).

Liquid is absorbed in the large intestine while digested food, vitamins and minerals are absorbed in the small intestine. Generally the status of stool depends upon the amount of water absorbed in the large intestine. Similarly it also depends on the type of food consumed. In vegetarian diet the stool is abundant and soft while non-vegetarian people have smaller quantity of hard stool.

Saman and apan vayu

In the awasthapak described above, the actions of pran, saman and apan vayu are mentioned.[27] According to contemporary views and comparison to Ayurveda, the correlation is as follows :-

Saman vayu in Ayurveda means the nerves (plexus) distributed to the stomach and small intestine. These nerves are distributed into the submucosa and the muscular wall of the oesophagus and small intestine. Anatomically and physiologically, nerves of the spinal cord and brain are included.

Site of apan vayu is described as being in the large intestine and its function is evacuation of excreta, solid as well as liquid. The sympathetic and parasympathetic nerves and nerve plexuses are included in this process.

References -

1. पाक: पचनं द्रव्याणां स्वरूपरसयो: परावृत्ति: । सा च स्वरूपान्तरत्वेन रसान्तरत्वेन च परिणति:, तस्या विशेषो विपाक: ।" (ग.) । अवस्थापाकापेक्षया विशिष्ट: पाक: विपाक: ।" (शि.)

2. जाठरेणाग्निना योगाद्यदुदेति रसान्तरम् । रसानां परिणामान्ते स विपाक इति स्मृत: ।। (वा. सू. ९) । १रसानां परिणामान्ते जरणनिष्ठाकाले, यद् रसान्तरं रसविशेष: उदेति उत्पद्यते स विपाक:" । (अ. द.) १परिणामलक्षणो विपाक: ।" (र. वै. १ सू. १७०)

3. अन्नस्य भुक्तमात्रस्य षड्रसस्य प्रपाकत: । मधुराद्यात् कफोभावात् फेनभूत उदीर्यते ।।
परंतु पच्यमानस्य विदग्धस्याम्लभावत: । आशयाच्च्यवमानस्य पित्तमच्छमुदीर्यते ।
पक्वाशयं तु प्राप्तस्य शोष्यमाणस्य वह्निना । परिपिण्डितपक्वस्य वायु: स्यात् कटुभावत: ।। (च. चि. १५)

अवस्तापाकात् कफपित्तयोर्वृद्धिः तथा निष्ठापाकाच्च मलरूपतया उत्पादः ।" (च. द.) 9विपाकस्तु रसमलविवेकसमकालो भिन्नकाल एवावस्थापाकैः समम् इति न विरोधः ।ऌ (च. द.) । 9इमे मधुराम्लकटुरूपेण रसानां त्रयो विपाकाश्च सपरिणामाः रसाख्ये आद्यधातौ गुणा भवन्ति, न तु पाकारम्भचरमपर्यन्तं पच्यमाने षड्रसद्रव्ये प्रथममध्यमचरमावस्थासु मधुराम्लकटुरूपाः ।" (ग.) एवं कर्मभिश्चानुमित एकरूपावस्थो जाऌराग्निसंयोगाद् यो रसानां रसान्तरोद्भवः, स एव विपाकः, न तु यो जाऌराग्निसंयोगमात्राद्रसानामनेकावस्थः प्राङ्मधुरोऽनन्तरं स किट्टमन्नस्य विण्मूत्रं रसस्य तु कफोऽसृजः पित्तम् (च. चि. १५)

4. तत्राहुरन्ये–प्रतिरसं पाक इति । मधुरो मधुरस्याम्लोऽम्लस्यैवं सर्वेषामिति । दृष्टान्तं चोपदिशन्ति–यथा शालियवमुद्गादयः प्रकीर्णाः स्वभावमुत्तरकालेऽपि न परित्यजन्ति तद्वदिति ।" (सु. सू. ४०) प्रतिरसं पाक इति केचित् । अयमाशयः–यथा स्थालिस्थं तावत् क्षीरं पच्यमानं मधुरमेव स्यात्, यथा वा शालियवमुद्गादयः प्रकीर्णाः स्वभावं न परित्यजन्ति अर्थात् शालियवमुद्गादिबीजेभ्यः उप्तेभ्यः शालियवमुद्गाद्यंकुरा उत्पद्यन्ते, तद्वन्मधुरादयो जऌराग्नि पक्वाः स्वं स्वं रूपं मधुरादिकं न त्यजन्ति ।" (यो.) । इह केचिदाक्षते–प्रतिरसं पाकः मधुरो मधुरस्य, अम्लो अम्लस्य, लवणो लवणस्य, कटुकः कटुकस्य, तिक्तस्तिक्तस्य, कषायः कषायस्येति षडेव विपाकः । किमत्र प्रमाणमिति चेत्, उच्यते – यथा क्षीरमतिपच्यमानमपि मधुरमेव स्यात्, यथा वा शालियवाद्यः उप्ताः प्ररूढाश्च फलिताश्च शाल्यादिस्वरूपा एव भवन्ति, तथा मधुरादयोऽपि निष्ठापाकेऽपि मधुरादिस्वरूपा एव भवितुमर्हन्तीति । उक्तं च – उप्ताः षष्टिकमाषाद्याः बाह्यपक्वाश्च षड्रसाः । यान्ति नान्यत्वमित्येवं पाकः प्रतिरसं भवेत् । (शि.) । 9यथारसं विपाकमेके ब्रुवते ।" (र. वै. ४ सू. ३१)

5. केचित् पुनरबलवन्तो बलवतां वशमायान्ति, तस्मादनवस्थितः पाक इति । (सु. सू. ४०) 9अन्ये तु ब्रुवते–रसा द्विविधा बलवन्तोऽबलवन्तश्च; बलवत्त्वं च व्यक्तत्वेन मात्राबाहुल्येन वा, अबलत्वं पुनरेतद्विपर्ययेण; तत्राल्पतयाऽबलवन्तो रसा बलवतां वशमायान्तीति, तेन निष्ठापाके बलवता रसेन दुर्बलरसाभिभवान्न रसप्रतिनियमेन मधुरस्य मधुर एव पाकोऽम्लस्य चाम्ल एवेत्यादि; प्रतिनियमाभावाच्चानवस्थितः पाक इति । अनियतत्वपक्षेऽपि षट्कत्वमेव, कदाचित् कस्यचित् संभवात् इति । उक्तंच – 9बहवोऽभिभवन्त्यल्पान् बहिर्मिश्रीकृताः रसाः । तेनानिश्चितमेवैके पाकमाहुर्मनीषिणः ।।" (शि.)

6. पञ्चभूतात्मके देहे आहारःपाञ्चभौतिकः । विपक्वः पंचधआ सम्यक् स्वान् गुणानभिवर्धयत् ।। (सु. सू. ४६) इत्यनेन पञ्चधाऽपि विपाकस्तेनवोक्तः ।" (शि.) । पंचभूतात्मके देहे आहारः पाञ्चभौतिकः । विपक्वः पञ्चधा सम्यक् स्वान् गुणानभिवर्धयेत् ।। इत्यनेन पञ्चधा पाकोऽभिहितः ।" (च. द.)

7. द्रव्यप्रमाण-संस्कार-सात्म्याग्निबलाबल-देश -काल-संयोग-पाक विशेषैर्विपाकविषर्यासः । (र. वै. सू. अ. ४, ५५).

8. कटुतिक्तकषायाणां विपाकः प्रायंशः कटुः । अम्लोऽम्लं पच्यते स्वादुर्मधुरं लवणस्तथा ।।" (च. सू. २६)

9. पाकास्त्रयो रसानामम्लोऽम्लं पच्यते कटुः कटुकम् ।
चत्वारोऽन्ये मधुरं संकीर्णरसास्तु संकीर्णम् ।।
कटुतिक्तकषायाणां कटुको येषां विपाक इति पक्षः । तेषां पित्तविघाते तिक्तकषायौ कथं भवतः ।। (अ. सं. सू. १७)

10. वस्तुतस्तु दोषाणां त्रैविध्याद्विपाकस्यापि तदनुगुणतया त्रैविध्यमेवोचितम् ।" (यो.)

11. आगमस्त्वाह–द्विविध एव पाको मधुरः कटुकश्च, तयोर्मधुराख्यो गुरुः, कटुकाख्यो लघुरिति । तत्र पृथिव्यप्तेजोवाय्वाकाशानां द्वैविध्यं भवति तद्गुणसाधर्म्याद् गुरुता, लघुता च, पृथिव्यापश्चगुर्व्यः

शेषाणि लघूनि, तस्माद् द्विविध एव विपाक इति । भवन्ति चात्र–द्रव्येषु पच्यमानेषु येष्वम्बुपृथिवीगुणाः । निर्वर्त्तन्तेऽधिकास्तत्र पाकः कटुक उच्यते ।।" (सु. सू. ४०)

गुणा विपाकयोः कारणम्, शीतस्निग्धगुरुपिच्छिला गुरुविपाकस्य, लघुरूक्षविशदतीक्ष्णा लघुविपाकस्येति ।" (र. वै. भा. १ सू. १२३)

तस्योपयोगोऽभिहितश्चिकित्सां प्रति सर्वदा । भूतेभ्यो हि परं यस्मान्नास्ति चिन्ता चिकित्सिते ।।" (सु. शा. १)

भेत्ता हि भेद्यमन्यथा भिनत्ति, अन्यथा पुरस्ताद् भिन्नं भेदप्रकृत्यन्तरेण, भिन्दन् भेदसंख्याविशेषमापादयत्यनेकधा, न च पूर्वं भेदाग्रमुपहन्ति ।" (च. वि. ६)

पञ्चधापि विपाकस्तेनवोक्तः, तत्कथं न विरोध इति चेत्, नैवम्, उपाधिभेदेन, विरोधाभावात्, तत्र हि भूतभेदमवलम्ब्य पञ्चधात्वम् अत्र तु लाघवगौरवरूपं भूतगुणद्वैविध्यमाश्रित्य द्वैविधअयमुक्तमिति न विरोधः, यथा पञ्चभूतात्मकत्वेऽपि द्रव्याणां सौम्याग्नेयत्वाद्द्वैविध्यमिति ।" (शि.) । १यत्त्वत्र वक्तव्यम्" पंचभूतात्मके... परिवर्धयेत् ।" इत्यनेन पंचधा पाकोऽभिहितः, स द्रव्यस्वरूपचिन्तनीयो नैतत्पाकद्वयविरोधी; यथा पंचभूतात्मकत्वेऽपि द्रव्याणां सौम्याग्नेयत्वाद् द्वैविध्यं भवति । (च. द.)

12. यथारसं जगुः पाकान् षट् केचित्तदसांप्रतम् । यत् स्वादुर्व्रीहिरम्लत्वं न चाम्लमपि दाडिमम् ।। याति तैलं च कटुतां कटुकापि न पिप्पली । यथारसत्वे पाकानां न स्यादेवं विपर्ययः ।।" (अ. सं. सू. १७)

यथारसं वइपाकमेके ब्रुवते" (र. वै. ४ सू. ३१) । १न, भिन्नलक्षणत्वात्" (र. वै. ४ सू. ३२) १नायं पक्षः साधुः, कुतः? भिन्नलक्षणत्वात्; १आस्वादग्राह्यो रसः, परिणआमलक्षणो विपाक" इति । विपाकस्य मधुरता कथमास्वाद्यते? यद्यास्वाद्येत, रसलक्षणत्वात् रस एवेति विपाकाभावः । यदि नास्वाद्येत, कथं भवथा १मधुरं पच्यते" इत्युपलब्धमित्युक्तं भवति ।" (भा.)

किंच प्रतिरसं रससदृशः पाकस्तथा बलवत्पराधीनता च पाकस्य रसद्वारा प्रतिपाद्यमानकार्येणैव लभ्यते, तेनैतत् पक्षद्वयमपि न निष्ठापाके चिन्तनौयं, रसस्वरूपनिरूपणे नैवोकार्थत्वात् ।" (शि.)

13. केचित् त्रिविधमिच्छन्ति-मधुरम्, अम्लं, कटुकं चेति । तत्तु न सम्यक्, भूतगुणादागमाच्चाम्लो रिपाको नास्ति, पित्तं हि विदग्धमम्लतामुपैत्याग्नेयत्वात् । यद्येवं लवणोऽप्यन्यः पाको भविष्यति, श्लेष्मा हि विदग्धो लवणतामुपैतीति ।" (सु. सू. ४०)

कट्वम्ललवणं पित्तं स्वाद्वम्ललवणं कफः । कषायतिक्तकटुको वायुर्दृष्टोऽनुमानत्ः ।।" (क.)

14. कालतो गुणतो रसतश्चानुपपत्तिः त्रित्वस्य ।" (र. वै. १ सू. ५०)

कालतस्त्रित्व नोपपद्यते चिराचिरकालव्यतिरिक्तस्याभावात् ।" (भा.)

15. गुणतश्च त्रित्वं नोपपद्यते, गुरुभूतजनिता, लघुभूतजनिता इति गुणद्वैविध्यादिति । (भा.)

16. रसतश्च त्रित्वस्यानुपपत्तिः, कटुतिक्तकषायस्तु लघवः, गुरवः परे इति द्विविधःभेदावरोधात् इति ।" । (भा.)

आगमस्त्वाह–द्विविध एव पाको मधुरः कटुकश्च ।" (सु. सू. ४०)

द्वौ, द्वैविध्यदर्शनात् परिणामस्य । (र. वै. १ सू. ५०) । यथा खदिरसारादीनि चिरादग्निसंयोगे परिणामं गच्छन्ति, पललादीन्यचिरादिति । (भा.)

गुणकारणत्वाद् गुणद्वैविध्याच्च ।" (र. वै. १ सू. ५१)

परिणामोऽर्थान्तरभावः जीर्तिरित्यर्थः । एवं विदाहानामपि पाकावयक्त्वं युज्यते (भा.)

रसानां परिणामान्ते स विपाक इति स्मृतः ।" (च. सू. २६)
त्रिधा विपाको द्रव्यस्य स्वाद्वम्लकटुकात्मकः ।" (अ. सं. सू. १)
द्विविध एव पाको मधुरः कटुश्च ।" (सु. सू. ४०)
मधुरकटुकशब्दयोरर्थतत्त्वाभिधाने गुणभेद उक्तः... अत्राप्यस्ति सारूप्यमेकहेतुजन्यत्वं मधुरोऽपि पार्थिवाप्यः गुरुरपि गुणः पार्थिवाप्य इति ।" (भा.)
तयोर्मधुराख्या गुरुः कटुकाख्यो लघुरिति ।" (सु. सू. ४०) १मधुरो गुरुत्वात् लघुत्वाच्च कटुकः ।" (र. वै. १ सू. ५२)

अम्लपाकस्याभ्युपगमानभ्युपगमयोर्बीजं तु चरकनये पित्तं प्रकृत्याऽम्लं कटु च, सुश्रुते तु कटुरसं, यत् पुनरम्लतवं तदस्य विद्ग्धस्यैवेति सुश्रुतेन पित्तस्य प्राकृतस्याम्लत्वानङ्गीकारात्, सुतरामम्लपाकोऽपि नाङ्गीक्रियते, निष्प्रयोजनत्वात्, इह पुनरम्लपाकः सप्रयोजन एव ।" (यो.)
तेषां गुरुः स्यान्मधुरः कटुकाम्लावतोऽन्यथा ।" (च. सू. २६)
पृथिव्यम्बुगुणभूयिष्ठतया स्निग्धानां मधुराम्ललवणानां त्रणायां मधुरो विपाकः, वायुगुणातिरेकाद्रूक्षाणां कटुतिक्तकषायाणां त्रणायां कटुकः ।" (यो.)
अम्लकटुकतिक्ता अधममध्यमोत्तमा लघव उक्ताः ।... अम्लरसद्रव्यपाके अत्राग्नि गुणानामम्लरसव्यतिरिक्तानामाधिक्येनाभिनिर्वृत्तिर्भवति, अतोऽयं लघुपाक उक्तः । तत्राम्लो रसस्त्वम्ल एव पच्यते विशेषरूपेण तत्राम्लरसो न तोयगुणो न वाग्निगुणः, उभयगुणयोगे हि तोयस्याव्यक्तरसः परिणम्याम्लः पूर्वजातः पश्चाद्मलविशेषरूपेण पच्यते इत्यतोऽयंलघुपाकरूपः कटुपाको भूतगुणानाम्, अम्लरसस्य पुनरुभय एव पाक इत्यविरोधः ।" (गं.)
अम्लपट्वोः फलं विद्यात् स्वादुपाकः कटुः पुनः । कषायतिक्तयोरित्थं सुश्रुताचार्यसंमतः ।।" (शि.)
तथा चाम्लगता ह्यग्निगुणा विपाचकाग्निगुणैः सामान्यादभिवृद्धा, अल्पानां, स्थूलसारसान्द्रादीनां विरूद्धानां तत्रस्थानां भूमिगुणानामवजयाय भवतीत्यम्लो रसोग्नि गुणबाहुल्यात् कटु विपच्यते नैवाम्लम् ।" (हा.)

17. विपाकलक्षणस्याल्पमध्यभूयिष्ठतां प्रति । द्रव्याणां गुणवैशेष्यात्तत्रतत्रोपलक्षयेत् ।।" (च. सू. २६)
तेन मधुररसविपाको मधुरः श्रेष्ठो विण्मूत्रमोक्षे कफशुक्रवृद्धौ च, लवणरसविपाको मधुरस्त्वप्लसृष्टविण्मूत्रः कफशुक्रश्चाल्पः अम्लश्च मध्यमसृष्टविण्मूत्रः शुक्रनाशनश्च मध्यमः तिक्तकटुकषायाणां तिक्तरसविपाकः कटुरल्परूपेण शुक्रहा बद्धविण्मूत्रो वातलश्च, कटुरसविपाकः कटुर्मध्यमरूपेण, कषायरसविपाकः कटुरुत्तमरूपेणेति । एवं द्रव्याणां स्नेहरौक्ष्यादिगुणवैशेष्यादल्पमध्यश्रेष्ठतामुपलक्ष्य ब्रूयात् ।" (ग.)

18. विपाकः कर्मनिष्या ।" (च. सू. २६) । १कर्मणो निष्ठा निष्पत्ति... कर्मसमाप्तिः । रसोपयोगे सति योऽन्त्याहारपरिणामकृतः कर्मविशेषः कफशुक्राभिवृद्ध्यादिलक्षणः, तेन विपाको निश्चीयते । एतेन विपाको नित्यपरोक्षः, तत्कार्येणानुमीयते ।" (च. द.) । १विपाकः कर्मणः आहारपरिणामकृतस्य निष्ठा निष्पत्तिः दोषशुक्रवृद्धिक्षयलक्षणा, तया उपलभ्यते । (यो.) अयं च विपाकाधेयो रसो न रसनेंद्रियग्राह्यः, किन्तु तत्तत्कार्येणैवोन्नीयते–यथा कटुरसाया उष्णवीर्याया अपि शुण्ठ्या वृष्यत्वेन मधुरः पाकोऽनुमीयते, तथा लवणस्य सृष्टविण्मूत्रत्वेन मधुरः पाक उन्नीयते, तथा तिक्तकषाययोर्बद्धविण्मूत्रतया कटुपाक उन्नीयते । (शि.)

19. रसैरसौ तुल्यफलः ।" (अ. सं. सू. १७) । १अभ्यवहृतस्य मधुररसस्य जाठराग्निसंयोगाद् यद्रसान्तरं फलतया निष्पन्नं तद्रसैः सदृशफलम् । फलग्रहणेनैतत् प्रतिपादयति फलोपममेव वृष्यादिलक्षणं कार्यं सदृशं, न तु कुसुमोपमं देहाल्हादनादिलक्षणं कार्यमिति ।" (हे.)

20. नेत्याहुरन्ये, विपाकः प्रधानमिति । कस्मात्? सम्यङ्मिथ्याविपाकत्वात्; इह सर्वद्रव्याण्यभ्यवहृतानि

सम्यङ्मिथ्याविपक्वानि गुणं दोषं वा जनयन्ति ।" (सु. सू. ४०)

सम्यक् विपक्वानि गुणं, मिथ्याविपक्वानि दोषं जनयन्ति । सम्यक्पाकः समेनाग्निना, मिथ्यापाकस्तु हीनातिपाकरूपो यथाक्रमं मन्देन तीक्ष्णेन वाऽग्निना क्रियते । ... किंवा सम्यक् पाको द्रव्यानुगुणः पाकः यथा चित्रकः... मिथ्यापाको तद्द्रव्यगुणविसदृशः पाकः यथा पिप्पल्यः । तेन... यथोक्तं गुणं दोषं वा करोति ।" (च. द.) अत्र द्रव्यगुणानुरूपो निष्ठापाकः सम्यग्विपाक उच्यते, तद्विपरीतस्तु मिथ्याविपाकः । तयोराद्यः कटु कश्चित्रकः पाकेऽपि कटुक इत्यादौ, द्वितीयस्तु कटुका पिप्पली पाके मधुरा इत्येवमादौ बुभुत्सितव्यः । गुणं दोषं वा इति वा शब्दश्चार्थे, सम्यग्विपक्वानि मिथ्याविपक्वानि वा गुणं दोषं च जनयन्ति; मिथ्याविपक्वा पिप्पली याशुक्रवर्धनादिरूपं गुणं प्रक्लदजननादिरूपं दोषं च जनयति । यद्वा अग्निसाम्यान्न हीनं नापि चाधिकं निष्ठापाकः सम्यक् विपाकः तदन्यस्तु अग्निवैष-म्यान्मिथ्याविपाकः । तत्र सम्यग्विपाके यथोक्ता गुणाः मिथ्याविपाके चामादिदोषाः संभवन्तीत्यायुर्वेद-विदो भाषन्ते ।" (हा.)

21. तन्निमितत्वात् प्रशमन वर्धनयोः (र. वै. सू. १ सू. १४२)
22. धातूपदेहात् (र. वै. स. १ सू. १४३)
23. विपाकाक्षेपकत्वात् इतरेषां प्रायशोविपाकसाद्गुण्ये च गुणवतामप्यदोषात् । (र. वै. सू. १४४)
24. लालारूपो रसादिभेदान्विभजन् जिव्हा रसं गृहणाति ।
25. प्राणोऽत्र मूर्धगः ।
उरःकण्ठचरो बुद्धिहृदयेन्द्रियचित्तधृक् ।
ष्ठीवनक्षवयूद्गारनिःश्वासान्नप्रवेशकृत् । (अ. हृ. सू. अ. १२)
26. परं तु पच्यमानस्य विदग्धस्याम्लभावतः ।
आशयाच्च्यवमानस्य पित्तमच्छमुदीर्यते ।। (चरक चि. ५:१०)
27. समानोऽग्निसमीपस्थः कोष्ठे चरति सर्वतः ।
अन्नं गृहूणाति पचति विवेचयति मुञ्चति ।।
अपानोऽपानगः श्रोणिबस्तिमेड्रोरुगोचरः ।।
शुक्रार्तवशकृन्मूत्रगर्भनिष्क्रमणक्रियः ।। (अ. हृ. सू. अ.१९)

CHAPTER SEVEN
VEERYA

Etymological interpretation of the word 'veerya'

The word 'veerya' is derived from veer = vikrant. A dynamic property or potency of a substance which brings about the action is called veerya.[1] Actions of rasa and vipak are already described. The remaining actions are due to veerya.

Charactristics of veerya

The potency of a substance which brings about the action is called as veerya. Why is veerya effective? The answer to it is that it is present at the time of rasa as well as at vipak.

It is observed that drugs which effectively act on dosha, dhatu, mala at a particular time become ineffective after sometime. This is so because the potency of a substance or the veerya which is responsible for the effective action, is lost when old. For this reason all the samhitas advise use the fresh dravya instead of an old one.[2] Various preparations like churna, kashaya and tablet possess a potency for a limited period. After the expiry period, these substances become ineffective as they loose veerya (lack veerya). Roots of dashamoola (e.g. bel) have vataghna and shothaghna potencies which other parts of the same plant do not possess. Therefore only roots of Dashamoola are used for vataghna and shothaghna actions. Dhanyamla is sheeta to touch and teekshna-ushna by veerya. Liquid possesses a property of sheeta. But pitta, though liquid in form, is ushna. Different parts of the plant possess different properties. For example, the flowers of palash are sheeta veerya but seeds are ushna veerya.

Other synonyms for veerya are shakti, teja, prabhav and vikram, all of which convey the similar meaning ie. strength, power and influence. (Veerya = power to bring about the action).

A drug works through its veerya. If its veerya gets depleted due to the effect of adverse conditions it loses its dynamic potency because of which it becomes ineffective. Action only takes place if the drug possesses its veerya. In the absence of veerya, no action takes place.

Different opinions exist regarding the form of veerya. Some ancient acharyas mention veerya as substance (द्रव्य), others as guna and karma. Some vaidyas describe veerya as dynamic potency and therefore consider it as a part of guna. Modern scholars consider veerya as 'active principle' and hence a part of the substance. Therefore it is essential to know the exact form of veerya.[3]

Gunaveeryavad - Charakacharya is of the opinion that all the potencies present within the substance (or dravya) should be called veerya. Actions of rasa, vipak, veerya and prabhav of a dravya are due to its active principle or dynamic potency. Among the four cardinals, whichever is powerful and which brings about the action is considered to possess a dynamic potency. Sushrutacharya and Vagbhatta have mentioned such gunas containing potency as veerya. Guru, snigdha, hima, mridu, laghu, ruksha, ushna and teekshna are eight gunas which are called as veerya when they bring about the action by their potency. The remaining twelve are simply gunas.

Nearly thirty plants in their original forms are exported from Konkan area and the same are returned to India in the form of medicines.

Gunaveeryavad (2 types)

Veerya = Dynamic potency According to Charaka — Vriddha Vagbhatta-scientific concept of veerya

Veerya according to Sushruta - Vagbhatta — colloquial concept of veerya[4]

Karmaveeryavad - Nagarjuna differs from this concept of Gunaveeryavad.

According to Nagarjuna, it is wrong to call rasa or guna as veerya, because sometimes a totally different action is observed though a dravya possesses rasas and gunas having known actions. Therefore the potency of a dravya which brings about the action should be called as veerya. In spite of the presence of rasa and guna, no action takes place without veerya. On the contrary, the presence of veerya brings about the desired action even if rasa and guna are absent.

The power of mantra power can be attributed to this phenomenon. Therefore by logical conclusions it is inferred that veerya is action potential.[5]

It is absurd to call potentially enriched gunas as veerya because superiority and inferiority of any substance does not change the family or classification. Superlative madhur guna of a substance does not change the madhur class or family. Nagarjuna, admiring this principle, states that it is wrong to call active guna as veerya. And so guru, laghu etc. should not be considered as veerya but purgative and emetic action should be classified (attributed to) as veerya.

Dravyaveeryavad - Like guna and karmavad this is another school of thought which exists. Modern scientists and Shivdas Sen consider that the active principle (most essential part) of any panchamahabhoota is veerya. This brings about the action which is of two types. One which is justified by intelligence is called veerya and the other which can not be justified is called as prabhav.[6]

Considering all these views of various schools of thoughts we come to the conclusion that veerya is power. It is different from rasa and brings about the different actions while residing in the dravya. Though this belongs to the agreement in different schools of opinions

and even though it appeals to us as correct, more importance has to be given to intellectually convincing explanations.

According to Charakacharya, shakti (power) is called veerya but after all veerya is also a guna. Sushruta and Vagbhatta consider enhancement of guna as veerya. Veerya is responsible for bringing about many actions. Based on this principle, Nagarjuna called veerya as karmalakshan instead of gunalakshan, keeping in mind that veerya is associated with dravya. Modern scientists accept veerya as active principle of a dravya. Veerya is shakti and shakti is one of the most potent gunas. This guna

Usually trees grow leaves before they bear flowers (leaves, flowers and fruits grow in that order). But a plant, Vanapalandu is an exception to this rule.

associated with active principle of a dravya, is responsible in bringing about various actions.

Even though the action of a dravya is mainly brought about by its active principle, the dravya and its active principle cannot be separated. The shakti which brings about the action, is a guna. If we separate the active principle, the said dravya becomes ineffective due to lack of the active principle. We cannot remove only shakti (which is guna).

Therefore veerya is guna. It cannot be a dravya. It can be a part of the active principle of a dravya. Guru laghu etc. are gunas. Shakti also is a guna. Emetic and purgative are actions. Veerya is shakti and the active principle of a dravya is a base of this shakti. Therefore veerya is not dravya but a guna and emetic and purgative action are the expressions of this guna.

1. Effectivness - Eight gurvadi gunas are more effective and long lasting than all the other active principles of a dravya. Even the contact of jatharagni cannot change them easily.

2. Power - These eight gunas possess more shakti or action potential in comparison to rasas and the remaining 12 gunas.

3. Familiarity - In our daily activities as well as in clinicals practice, these gunas are refered to more commonly than others.

Number of Veeryas

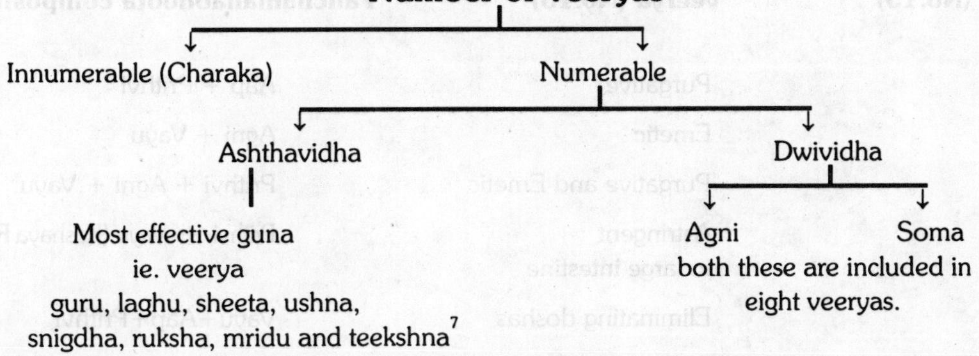

4. Frequency - Dravyas also contain these eight gunas more frequently than other 12 gunas.

5. Utility - These eight gunas are more useful and enduring while practising chikitsa.

6. Dominance :- Gurvadi eight gunas, being strong in action, supersede rasa, vipak and other 12 gunas. E.g. In a dravya having madhur rasa but ushna or teekshna gunas, the ushna, teekshna gunas supersede the action of madhur rasa. Sushruta, Dalhan and Chakrapani replaced laghu and guru by vishad and pichchil as veeryas. But this is deceptive because guru-pichchil and laghu-vishad are similar in action.

Some followers of gunaveeryavad consider only two veeryas viz. ushna and sheeta[8] because-

Agnihotra clears environment, but it is also very useful for the development of plants. This has been proven experimentally

1) Though the universe is panchamahabhautik, only agni and soma principles are predominant. Humankind and universe are designated as agnishomiya for the same reason.
2) In human reproduction, shukra is soma and artava is agneya, which gives rise to a human being.
3) Classification of kala as adan and visarga are based on agni and soma ie. ushna and sheeta shakti.
4) In tridoshas, pitta is agneya, kapha is soma whereas vata is ushna with pitta and sheeta with kapha (yogavahi). Therefore tridoshas are considered as agni-shomatmak.
5) Even twenty gunas are classified on an agnishomatmak basis.

Soma - Guru, snigdha, pichchil, hima etc. (10)

Agni - Laghu, ruksha, vishad, ushna etc. (10)

Therefore veerya is also either agni (ushna) or soma (sheeta) as no third type exists.

Nagarjuna considers veerya as action bound. This will lead to innumerable veeryas, similar to Charakacharya's veerya guna. But Acharya Nimi, who was a follower of Nagarjuna, has described 15 excellent actions (karmas) denoted as veerya based on panchabhautik composition.[9]

Karma (No.15)	Veerya (No.15)	Panchamahabhoota composition
(1)	Purgative	Aap + Prithvi
(2)	Emetic	Agni + Vayu
(3)	Purgative and Emetic	Prithvi + Agni + Vayu.
(4)	Astringent in large intestine	Prithvi + Vayu (Kashaya Rasa)
(5)	Eliminating doshas	Vayu+Aap+Prithvi
(6)	Deepan (Appetiser)	Prithvi+Agni
(7)	Jeevaneeya (Rakta)	Prithvi + Aap.
(8)	Pranaghna (Chest)	Vayu+Agni
(9)	Madan (Head)	Vayu + Agni
(10)	Soothing (all over)	Aap (soothing property is specific of aap.)
(11)	Shothakar (all over) (Inflammatory)	Prithvi + Aap (Mahabhootas producing obstruction)

One should pluck flowers by one's own hands for worshiping God. This helps to completely understand flowers 'स्वाहतानि पुष्पाणि'. The same holds true for gathering leaves.

(12)	Shothaghna (all over)	Akash + Vayu (Mahabhootas relieving obstruction)
(13).	Pachan (Digestive) (Pittashay Pakvashay)	Agni (Site of Pitta)
(14).	Daran (Mansa-skin)	Vayu + Agni (Katu rasa)
(15).	Ropan (Healing) (Mansa-gami)	Prithvi + Aap + Vayu.

N. B. Jeevaneeya action is a property of blood. Jeevan is a specific action of rakta dhatu. This action belongs to prithvi and aap mahabhootas. Therefore jeevaneeya action also belongs to rakta just as it belongs to prithvi and aap. Blood is also composed of prithvi and aap mahabhootas.

Even though these 15 types are described, veerya according to nighantus and Charakaharya should be classified into only two types (1) ushna and (2) sheeta. Those rasas which are generated by agni mahabhoota are ushna veerya while the others are called sheeta veerya.

Ashtavidha veerya - composition, action and effect on doshas.

No.	Veerya	Mahabhautik composition	Action	Effect on Doshas
1.	Sheeta	Prithvi + Aap	Pleasurable Stabilising Cleaning Life giving Coagulating Heavy	Pittashaman Vitiate Kapha Vata
2.	Ushna	Agni	Burning Digestion Fainting Loss of senses. Sweating Emesis Purgation Disintegration	Vata Kapha shaman Pitta Vardhan

Shlokas from 348 to 518 of Amarkosha are very useful as they describe the plant synonyms and various parts of the plants.

			Euphoric Thirst promoting Giddiness Laghu (Lightness) Anti-aphrodisiac	
3.	Snighdha	Aap	Snehan (Oleation) Nutrition Restorative Aphrodisiac Anti-ageing	Vatahara Kapha Vardhak
4.	Ruksha	Vayu	Constipative Painful Drying Heating	Vata Vardhan Kapha Shaman
5.	Guru	Prithvi + Aap	Applicative Promotive Mucous Aphrodisiac Supportive	Vatahara
6.	Laghu	Agni + Vayu	Scraping Absorption Drying Healing	Kaphahara
7.	Mridu	Aap+Akash	Blood and Mansa promoting Soft tangibility	Pitta Shaman
8.	Teeksna	Agni	Collective Aspiration Drying Oozing	Kaphaghna

Ayurveda describes plants which aid in all the eight types of surgical procedures (surgery and plants have inseparable relationship).

According to some, vishad replaces laghu and pichchil replaces guru veerya.

1.	Vishad	Agni Vayu	Absorbs fluid Drying Healing wounds Visible and Palpable	Kaphanashan
2.	Pichchil	Prithvi + Aap	Tissue generation in wound Promotive Coagulative aphrodisiac[10]	Kaphotpatti

How do we perceive veerya?

Veerya of a dravya is ascertained in three ways -

(1) Pratyaksha (2) Anuman (3) Pratyakasha + Anuman.

Among these knowledge obtained by keeping a dravya on the tongue (by taste) is pratyaksha e. g. teekshna guna of miri (black pepper). The same dravya on entering the gastrointestinal tract gives a feeling of ushna (heat). This is anuman as an act of inference. And the knowledge acquired by taste and inference is pratyaksha + anuman.

Examples - (1) Miri is ushna. On coming in contact with the tongue, it produces a burning sensation. This is called pratyaksha.

(2) Ushna veerya dravya - Animal meat generates heat which is felt or experienced for a longer period of its digestion - anuman.

(3) Taste of miri is pratyaksha, its heat felt in the body later on is through anuman.

So there is a combined effect. Pratyaksha is not only limited to taste but also is applicable to other special sensations. When a dravya is brought in contact with the special sense organs, it is identified by its action potential (veerya). For example, skin perceives sheeta, ushna or mridu gunas of a dravya on touch; this is also veerya. Similarly pichchil or vishad can be judged by sight or touch. Snigdha or ruksha veerya is recognised by sight (pratyaksha). Pratyaksha of teekshna veerya is by taste as perceived by the tongue.[11]

Relationship between rasa and veerya

Generally, dravyas having madhur, tikta and kashaya rasas are sheeta veerya and those having amla, lavana and katu rasas are ushna veerya. All those rasas[12] which are related to agni mahabhoota are ushna veerya and the rest are sheeta veerya. But there are exceptions. Even though rasa is useul in arriving at an inference about the veerya, vipak and guna, it is wrong to decide the veerya, vipak

A lovely rose bud decays within seven days but Akkalkara does not decay even in seven years. What is its secret?

and guna of any dravya based on its rasas.

Examples (Exceptions)

	Dravya	Rasa	Veerya
1.	Brihat Panchamoola	Kashaya Tikta	Ushna
2.	Meat (animal)	Madhur	Ushna
3.	Saindhav (Salt)	Lavana	Neutral
4.	Amla	Amla	Neutral
5.	Aloewood, guduchi, arka	Tikta	Ushna
6.	Haritaki	Kashaya	Ushna

Importance of Veerya

Dravya contains different entities like rasa, veerya, vipak, guna etc. Among all these, veerya is prominent because it brings about the action of a dravya. Also it supersedes the action of rasas by its presence.[13]

Some Examples -

	Dravya	Rasa	Veerya	Action
1.	Brihat Panchamoola	Kashaya tikta	Ushna	Vatashamak
2.	Horse gram (Dolichos biflorus)	Kashaya	Usshna	Vatashamak
3.	Onion	Katu	Sheeta	Vatavardhak
4.	Sugarcane juice	Madhur	Sheeta	Vatavardhak
5.	Piper	Katu	Mridu	Pittashamak
6.	Amla	Amla	Mridu	Pittashamak
7.	Saindhav	Lavana	Mridu	Pittashamak
8.	Garden night shade (Solanum nigrum)	Tikta	Ushna	Pittavardhak
9.	Fish	Madhur	Ushna	Pittavardhak
10.	Radish	Tikta	Snigdha	Kaphavardhak

Generally, plants which grow taller grow their roots deep in the ground. But the creepers keep spreading their roots.

11.	Kavath	Amla	Ruksha	Kaphanashak
12.	Honey	Madhur	Ruksha	Kaphanashak

Veerya is responsible for superseding the rasa and its presence suppresses the action of rasa.[14] For example, madhur, amla and lavana rasas are vatashamak but if they are accompanied by ruksha, laghu and sheeta veerya, then they will not act as a vatashamak.

Madhur, tikta and kashaya rasas are pittashamak but if they are accompanied by teekshna, ushna and laghu veerya then they are not pittashamak. Katu, tikta, kashya rasas are kapha shamak but if they are accompanied by snigdha, guru and sheeta veerya then they are not kaphashamak.[15] Here veerya is predominant.

Nagarjuna gives the following reasons for the predominance of veerya -

1. Only those drayas which are predominant in veerya are used in chikitsa (treatment) and not the others.
2. Action of a dravya is due to the presence of veerya.
3. Veerya supersedes rasa, vipak and guna. Therefore, even when the rasas, vipak and gunas of a dravya act in accordance with each other, veerya may being about a totally different action.
4. Veerya is mentioned as extremely importance even by aptavachan in literature.

   So veerya is prominent among rasa, vipak, veerya and guna.[16]

References -

1. येन कुर्वन्ति तद्वीर्यम् ।" (च. सू. २६, सु. सू. ४१)
   वीर्यं तु क्रियते येन या क्रिया । नावीर्यं कुरुते किंचित् सर्वा वीर्यकृता: क्रिया: ।" (च. सू. २६)
2. द्रव्याण्याभिनवान्येव प्रशस्तानि क्रियाविधौ ।" (प.)
3. अयं च वीर्यशब्द: पारिभाषिकवीर्यवचनो न भवति, किन्तु शक्तिमात्रवचन: तेन प्रभावरसादय: सर्व एव स्वकार्य कुर्वन्त: शक्तिपर्यायरूपवीर्यवाच्या इति ज्ञेया: (च. द.) १शक्तिमात्रं तु वीर्य स्यादिति केचिद् बुधा विदु: । तन्मते द्रव्यरसयो: पाकस्य च गुणस्य च ।। मृद्वादे: स्वक्रियोत्पादे शक्तिर्वीर्यमिति स्थिति: ।।"
4. गुर्वादयो गुणा द्रव्ये पृथिव्यादौ रसाश्रये । रसेषु व्यपदिश्यन्ते साहचर्योपचारत: ।।" (वा. सू. ९)
   मृदुतीक्ष्णगुरुलघुस्निग्धरूक्षोष्णशीतलम् । वीर्यमष्टविधं केचित् । (च. सू. २६)
   गुर्वाद्या वीर्यमुच्यन्ते शक्तिमन्तोऽन्यथा गुणा: । परसामर्थ्यहीनत्वाद् गुणा एवेतरे गुणा:।। (अ.सं.१७)
   गुर्वादीनां वीर्यसंज्ञा विशिष्टाम्नायविहिताऽपि लौकिकीति समुद्भाव्यते । (अ. सं. सू. १७)
5. कर्मलक्षणं वीर्यम् ।" (र. वै. सू. १ सू. १६९) रसगुणामात्रं वीर्यमित्येके (र. वै. सू. २ सू. ३०)
   न, तुल्यरसगुणेषु विशेषभावात् । (र. वै. सू. २ सू. ३१) ।
   रसगुणव्यतिरेकेण चोपलब्धे: कर्मणस्तस्य ।" (सू. ३५) ।

सत्सु तेषु तस्मिंस्तस्यैवाकरणात् कर्मणः सति सम्यक् प्रयोगे ।" (सू. ३६)
मधुरसं स्निग्धं शीतं च यष्टिमधुकं संदधाति, क्षीरं च तादृगेव स्रंसयतीति विशेषः५।
अस्य कर्मविशेस्य दर्शनादेतस्माद् रसगुणाख्यात् कारणमन्यद् विद्यते । अस्य विशेषस्य साधकं तद् वीर्यमिति जानीय इति । (भा.)

6. वीर्य शक्तिः, सा च पृथिव्यादीनां भूतानां यः सारभागस्तदतिशयरूपा बोध्या । सा च द्विविधा चिन्त्याचिन्त्यक्रियाहेतुत्वेन, तत्र चिन्त्यक्रियाहेतुर्या द्रव्यरसादीनां स्वस्वकर्मणि स्वभावसिद्धा शक्तिः, अचिन्त्यक्रियाहेतुश्च प्रभावापर्याया द्रव्याणां रसाद्यननुरूपकार्यकरणशक्तिः । उक्तं च १भूतप्रसादातिशयो द्रव्ये पाके रसे स्थितः । चिन्त्याचिन्त्यक्रियाहेतुवीर्यं धन्वन्तरेर्मतम् ।" (शि.)
परमार्थतः शक्तिरेव वीर्य, सा पुनर्बलवत् क्रियानिर्वर्तनक्षमा रसादिनाऽयोगान्निरूपाधिरिति तस्याः शीतोष्णदयो गुणा उपाधित्वेनांगीकृताः उक्त च -१गुणाः कर्मव्यवस्थार्य द्रव्याणां रसपाकयोः । शक्तेः कर्मसु शक्ता ये निरुपाधेरुपाधयः ।" (शि.)

7. तत्र य इमे गुणा वीर्यसंज्ञकाः शीतोष्णस्निग्धरूक्षमृदुतीक्ष्णपिच्छिलविशदाः ।" (सु. सू. ४१)

8. अन्ये तु गुर्वादीनामग्निषोमात्मकत्वादादानविसर्गविभागेन कालस्य चोष्णशीतात्मकत्वाद् द्विविधमेवामनन्ति । एवं चाहुः-नानात्मकमपि द्रव्यमग्निषोमौ महाबलौ । व्यक्ताव्यक्तं जगदिव नातिक्रामति जातुचित् ।। (अ. सं. सू. १ अ. हृ. सू. १) । १उष्णं शीतं द्विधैवान्ये वीर्यमाचक्षतेऽपि च । नानात्मकमपि द्रवअयमग्निषोमौ महाबलौ ।। व्यक्ताव्यक्तं जगदिव नातिक्रामति जातुचित् ।" (अ.हृ. सू. ९)

9. दश पञ्च च कर्माणि गुणानां पाञ्चभौतिकात् ।
द्रव्येष्वेवं विजानीयात् कर्माणि दशपञ्च च ।। (भा.)
अब्भूमिजमधोभागं तेजोवायुजमूर्ध्वगम् । वायुसोममहीजातं तथा संशमनं विदुः ।। पृथिव्यनिलबाहुल्याद्दीपनं परिचक्ष्महे । पृथिव्यपां गुणैर्युक्तं जीवनीयमिति स्थितिः५।।
वाय्वनिलस्वभावाच्च प्राणघ्नं मदनं मतम् । प्राणघ्नं तीव्रभावात्तु दोषधातुप्रकोपनम्५।।
मदनं चलधातुत्वाद् दोषकोपनमेव तु । अपां गुणबहुत्वात्तु शीतीकरणमिष्यते ।। (निमि)

10. तेषां मृदुशीतोष्णाः स्पर्शग्राह्याः, पिच्छिलविशदौ चक्षुःस्पर्शाभ्यां, स्निग्धरूक्षौ चक्षुषा, तीक्ष्णो मुखे दुःखोत्पादनेन ।" (सु. सू. ४१)

11. वीर्य यावदधीवासान्निपाताच्चोपलभ्यते ।" (च. सू. २६)
किञ्चिद् वीर्यमधीवा सादुपलभ्यते, यथा आनूपमांसादेरुष्णत्वं, किञ्चिच्च निपातादेव लभ्यते यथा मरिचादीनां तीक्ष्णत्वादि, किंचिच् निपाताधीवासाभ्यां यथा मरिचादीनामेव । एतेन रसः प्रत्यक्षेणैव, विपाकस्तु नित्यपरोक्षः तत्कार्येणानुमीयते; वीर्य तु किञ्चिदनुमाने न, यथा सैन्धवगतं शैल्यम्, आनूपमांसगतमौष्ण्यं वा, किञ्चिच्च वीर्य प्रत्यक्षेणैव, यथा–राजिकागतं तैक्ष्ण्यं घ्राणेन, पिच्छिलविशदस्निग्धरूक्षादयः चक्षुःस्पर्शनाभ्यां निश्चीयन्त इति वाक्यार्थः ।" (च. द.)

12. शीतं वीर्येण यद्द्रव्यं मधुरं रसपाकयोः । तयोरम्लं यदुष्णं च यद् द्रव्यं कटुकं तयोः ।। तेषां रसोपदेशेन निर्देश्यो गुणसंग्रहः । वीर्यतोऽविपरीतानां पाकतश्चोपदेक्ष्यते ।। यथा पयो यथा सर्पिर्यथा वा चव्यचित्रकौ । (च. सू. २६)

13. वीर्य प्रधानमिति । कस्मात? तद्वशेनौषधकर्मनिष्पत्तेः । इहौषधकर्माण्यूर्ध्वाधोभागोभयभाग संशोधनसंशमनसांग्राहिकाग्निदीप नपीडनलेखनबृंहणरसायनवाजी करणश्वयथुकविलयनदहन दारणमादनप्राणघ्नविषप्रशमनादीनि वीर्यप्राधान्याद् भवन्ति ।" (सु. सू. ४०)

14. एतानि खलु वीर्याणि स्वबलगुणोत्कर्षाद्रसमभिभूयात्मकर्म कुर्वन्ति–यथा तावन् महत्पञ्चमूलं कषायं तिक्तानुरसं वातं शमयति, उष्णवीर्यत्वात्; तथा कषायः कुलत्थः । कटुकः पलाण्डुः स्नेहभावात् च; मधुरश्चेक्षुरसो वातं वर्धयति, शीतवीर्यत्वात्; कटुका पिप्पली पित्तं शमयति, मृदुशीतवीर्यत्वात्; अम्लमामलकं लवणं सैन्धवं च । तिक्ता काकमाची पित्तं वर्धयति, उष्णवीर्यत्वात्, मधुरा मत्स्याश्च; । कटुकं मूलकं श्लेष्माणं वर्धयति स्निग्धवीर्यत्वात्, अम्लं कपित्थं श्लेष्माणं शमयति रूक्षवीर्यत्वात्, मधुरं क्षौद्रं च । तदेतन्निदर्शनमात्रमुक्तम् ।।

भवन्ति चात्र–

15. ये रसा वातशमना भवन्ति यदि तेषु वै । रौक्ष्यलाघवशैत्यानि न ते हन्युः समीरणम् ।।
ये रसाः पित्तशमना भवन्ति यदि तेषु वै । तैक्ष्ण्यौष्ण्यलघुताश्चैव न ते तत्कर्मकारिणः ।।
ये रसाः श्लेष्मशमनाः भवन्ति यदि तेषु वै । स्नेहगौरवशैत्यानि न ते तत्कर्मकारिणः ।। (सु. सू. ४०)

16. वीर्य प्रधानमित्येके, द्वीर्यप्राधान्याद् द्रव्याणाम् य। (र. वै. अ. १ सू. १३०)
तेन कर्मकरणात्"(र. वै. अ. १ सू. १३१) तुल्यरसगुणेषु विशेषात् । (सू. १३६) आगमाच्च ।"(सू. १४०) वीर्यतः कार्यसामर्थ्य द्रव्याणां भिषजो विदुः । (भा.)

CHAPTER EIGHT
PRABHAV

Etymology

"Due to its presence and combination, the substance (dravya) acquires a distinct activity that is called prabhav."

Characteristics of Prabhav

Substances may have similar rasa, veerya and guna but one substance may have a distinctive action. The cause of that is prabhav; that distinct pharmacodynamic property is called prabhav.[1]

For example -

	Rasa	Veerya	Vipak	Prabhav
Chitraka (Plumbago zeylanicum)	Katu	Ushna	Katu	-
Danti (Baliospermum montanum)	Katu	Ushna	Katu	Purgation (Virechan)

Both these plants have the same rasa, veerya and vipak. But chitraka is not a purgative, whereas danti is. If the purgation was due to rasa or veerya or vipak or their several permutations - combinations, then chitraka should also be a purgative. But what is present in danti is prabhav as seen in its distinct purgative action.[2]

Similarly the inorganic poisons are antidotes to poisons of biological origin and vice versa. Wearing semi precious stones, fever-medicines, precious stones, mantras etc. or wearing herbs [tying country mallow (sahadevi) to heal in quartran fever] - such actions have been described as being due to prabhav. One can give more examples; sesame seeds and Randia dumetorum (madanphala) both are sweet, astringent, pungent, unctuous etc. But madanphala is emetic whereas sesame seeds are not. Liquorice and grapes are sweet and cold, yet grapes are aperient but liquorice is not. Then the aperient effect of grapes is due to prabhav. It means that the effect of laxation is caused by prabhav.

Milk and ghee both are sweet and cold. But ghee is agni deepan (enhancing appetite and digestion) but milk is not. Hence ghee has a distinct property to increase agni. (घृतमग्निमेधे करोति च. सू. 1-44). Garlic is pungent in rasa and vipak, unctuous and heavy. Hence these properties should actually increase vata and kapha. Instead, it relieves vata and kapha. Similarly, Emblica officinalis and unpolished red rice are tridoshahara; yavak (a variety of rice) is tridoshakarak due to prabhav. Albizzia lebek (shirish) is a poison antidote, sleep enhances poison, vajikaran dravyas enhance semen quality,

A drug placed under the tongue gets absorbed directly and acts on the disease (sublingual absorption).

Convolvulus pluricans (shankhapushpi) improves intelligence (मेध्या विशेषेण शंखपुष्पी वा. उ. ३९), rasayanas work as longevity enhancing; all these actions are due to prabhav. What is novel in common actions? That is natural. But when distinctive effects occur then we have to believe that prabhav is responsible.[3]

Any effect has to have a cause. Even the word karya (effect) is not possible without karan (cause). These words are mutually related. Any effect makes one seek a cause. In spite of all efforts to determine the cause, when direct perceptible cause is absent, the effect is attributed to the unforeseen. Similarly, when dravyas, rasa, vipak and guna cannot explain an effect then the effect is attributed to prabhav.

The nature of prabhav

There are two energies in dravyas to which cause effect relationship can be ascribed. That conceivable energy is named as veerya. There is another inconceivable energy which coexists in a dravya. Its effect is seen but one cannot establish a causal relationship. That is called prabhav. Prabhav is that dravya's nature and supersedes all other properties. Only the cause is not known.[4] The effects due to properties other than prabhav can be obtained by representative dravyas with similar properties. But for prabhav–effects such representative dravyas do not serve the purpose. That dravya is indispensible for that action. Excluding all the effects of rasa - veerya - vipak, whatever action remains and can not be causally connected is considered to be due to prabhav. It is the inconceivable unique property of a dravya. No other dravya can be used instead.

In Sushruta samhita and other texts, prabhav is referred to as unthinkable, innate, undebatable, wellknown etc. For such inconceivable prabhav of a dravya, one has to refer to the authentic proof of a statement by an apta. Effect has to have a cause but it may not be evident. In such a situation 'unseen' (adrushta) has to be assumed. Similarly, where causality cannot be attributed to rasa-veerya-vipak etc., one has to believe in prabhav. Dravya's properties - adhobhagharatva, vrushyatva etc. are due to prabhav. When effects are seen but connecting a cause is not possible then the idea of prabhav emerges. Nagarjuna describes prabhav as intangible, non-cognizable etc.[5]

On the whole, Charaka, Vagbhatta etc. have alloted a separate entity to prabhav. Whereas Sushruta and Nagarjuna have considered veerya as of two types - thinkable and unthinkable. Amongst these, the unthinkable is prabhav.[6]

Prabhav can be the combined result of mahabhootas. These are not easily explained on the tridosha basis (that is why मुनिरेव विजानाति - only a muni knows the result of combination of dravyas). There are no two opinions that for every effect there has to be a cause. But that does not mean that the cause is always identifiable. Such statements apply to drug effects; limits do exist. Direct perception, association, correlation, experimental proof etc. are not always adequate as evidences for causality. In such cases, one has to take refuge with the aptavakyas. This certainly applies to prabhav.

Actions due to prabhav

Sushrutacharya has said that veerya has effects of sanshodhan, sanshaman, sangrahi, vajikaran

Arabian akkalkara, tobacco and marigold plants of Mexico, Australian eucalyptus, Japanese chopchini and Brazil's aayapan have all become a part of Ayurveda.

etc. Among these, deepan, brimhan etc. are explicable on cause-effect basis. So a specific property of the dravya is responsible for that effect. Hence, these are conceivable and thinkable actions and can be ascribed to veerya. But sanshodhan, visha-prashaman, madan etc. have not been ascribed to gunas clearly until now. These effects are due to inconceivable causes or prabhav. The effects of gems belong to this category as causality cannot be explained. And even the elements of the host on which the effects occur are still 'unknown'. So to explain fully how the cause brings about the effect is difficult.

The diverse actions can be categorized by modern classification as follows :-

1) **Pharmacological** - Danti (Baliospermum montanum), Dravanti (Ipomoea reniformis), Madanphala (Ramdia dumetorium Linn.)
2) **Antidotal actions** - Shirish (Albizzia lebeck)
3) **Antibacterial effects** - Guggulu (Commiphora mukul Linn), Ral (Shorea robusta), Mohari (Brassica nigra Linn), Vacha (Achorus calamus) etc.
4) **Psychodynamic effects** - on mania etc.
5) **Physical actions** - the effects are due to a physical property e.g. drawing of iron particles by a magnet.

Veerya is where the energy can be causally associated and where the effects are definite but a connection cannot be made, that is prabhav. Some people include prabhav as part of the effect. But prabhav is cause and cannot be grouped with effect. For a karma (effect), guna (property) is responsible, karma cannot be a cause of karma. Hence prabhav is not karma but a unique property of dravyas.

In the universe, the pratyaksha, perceivable sense objects are few and the imperceptible objects beyond the senses are numerous. To believe that everything should be proved by sensory evidence only, is an erroneous assumption. And if prior perceivable evidence is not there then even inference is not possible. If an effect is real then it must have a cause even though not demonstrable. Thus the concept of prabhav emerges. No individual can be beyond sensory perception. So for effects where causal connection is not possible but the effects are demonstrable, we have to be pragmatic. Empirical experience and shastriya reference should be contemplated upon for medicinal use. We can see the results clearly but the cause is not known. We should not be inactive. The poisonous effects described by apta have to be believed. It is not worth while to experiment on one's own self for proof.

Samanapratyayarabdha (Regular cause effect) and Vichitrapratyayarabdha (Anomalous cause effect)

Dravyas are evolved from a combination of specific ingredients. As mahabhoota combinations are infinite, dravyas are infinite too. These dravyas have two modes of physical phenomena or for-

Foreign food items like tea (China), custard apple (America), saffron (Asia Minor), dates (Middle east/Arabia), potato (Italy) etc. are eaten by Indians during sacred-fasts !

mations. One is of samanapratyayarabdha (regular cause effect) type and the other is of vichitrapratyayarabdha (anomalous cause effect) type. Pratyaya means cause. The effects and results generated by a dravya are dependent on the gunas of that dravya as causes. This means that the mahabhootas and their rasas etc. which constitute the dravyas are primal causes. When the effects of a dravya are congruent with the properties of its constituent mahabhootas then it will be called samanapratyayarabdha. But eventually this is a concept.

On the contrary, it is vichitrapratyayarabdha when a dravya having madhur rasa constituted by prithvi and jala mahabhootas does not have the effect of sweet rasa but different and of other mahabhootas. Dravyas which have effects as per their rasa are said to have samanapratyayarabdha. But when an effect is different from the rasa, vipak etc., that is vichitrapratyayarabdha. The distinction between vichitrapratyayarabdha and prabhav is that, for the latter cause effect connection cannot be made. Whereas for vichitrapratyayarabdha dravyas that is made possible by the very adjective. Samanapratyayarabdha and vichitrapratyayarabdha are relative terms as to the results. Those dravyas, as per rasa - veerya - vipak have comparable results then the term samana is used for them and for those not comparable, the term vichitra is used. But the connection is not applicable in all instances.

The concepts of samana and vichitra arise from rasa as this is perceptible. Rasa assists in attributing mahabhootas of a dravya. If the mahabhootas have harmonious and predictable effects then it is samanapratyayarabdha.

One can provide examples of both types as follows :-

	Dravya	**Guna**	**Karma**	**Prakara**
1.	Wheat	Sweet-heavy	Vatahara	Samanapra.
2.	Barley	" "	Vatakara	Vichitrapra.
3.	Milk		Sheeta veerya	Samanapra.
4.	Fish	" "	Ushna veerya	Vichitrapra.
5.	Wild Boar meat	" "	Madhur vipak	Samanapra
6.	Lion's meat	" "	Katu vipak	Vichitrapra.
7.	Ghee	Sheeta veerya	Deepan	Vichitrapra.
8.	Fat	Ushna Veerya	Agnisadan	"
9.	Moonga	Katu vipak	Pittashaman	"
10.	Udid	Madhur vipak	Pittavardhak	"

Ayurveda has survived through following eras; Charaka - Sushruta period (origin), Vagbhtta period (progress), Madhav-nidan period (spread), medieval period (regression) and contemporary period (reinstatement).

11.	Curds	Heavy	Deepan	Vichitrapra.
12.	Paravat	Heavy	Adeepan	"
13.	Dalimb	Amlarasa	Grahi	Vichitrapra.
14.	Amla	Amlarasa	Sara	Samanapra.
15.	Dhayatifula	Astringent	Sheetaveerya	Samanapra. Grahi.
16.	Harde	Astringent	Ushnaveerya	Vichitrapra. Rechan.

The connection to samana or vichitrapratyayarabdha can be attempted. The general directions are as follows :-

1) Wheat when ripening in the season of vasant is snigdha and kapha vardhak. Whereas barley carries the effects of greeshma, hence is ruksha and vata vardhak. So the difference may be due to the season when the cereals are ready for reaping (such correlations are possible).

2) Compared to wild boar, lion is very active and agile. Hence lion's meat is katu in vipak and wild boar's meat is madhur in vipak. The lion's body is vata pradhan, whereas boar is fatty and kapha pradhan.

3) Fish have to survive in water hence they have to counteract sheeta veerya with ushna. Milk has no such aspect and hence is sheeta.

Such an approach may open up a direction. Arsenic bisulphide (manshil) and arsenic trisulphide (hartal) are derivatives of somal (arsenic). But the formula of the compound has separate effects.

Dravyas are created first from distinct mahabhootas. But the dependent rasa etc. vary as per the fractional combinations of mahabhootas. Accordingly, dravya has diverse rasas etc. emerging from that combination mode.

During the use of dravyas - the mahabhoota which it manifests is expressed in rasa. Later the foundation dravya's mahabhoota manifests but if the rasa is not congruent then different effect can be seen. With such effects the dravya is called vichitrapratyayarabdha.

Those dravyas which have the constituent mahabhootas of one type and rasa etc. of different mahabhootas are vichitrapratyayarabdha. Whereas when the constituent mahabhootas and rasa etc. of the dravya are similar then these are samanapratyayarabdha.

The fundamental elements and their modes of combination and unique structures lead to infinite variety of dravyas. Innumerable dravyas result from synthesis and degradation. The concepts of samanapratyayarabdha and vichitrapratyayarabdha are not mentioned by Charaka or Sushruta. In

Brahmakamal (Epiphyllum crenetum - class of cactus) is a Mexican flower. These flowers blossom at night and wilt within an hour or two.

Ashtanghridaya, at the end, there is a passing reference to them.

The predominance of prabhav

Prabhav is the most important amongst padarthas like rasa, guna etc. belonging to the dravya. Prabhav can supersede all these padarthas but none of these can supersede prabhav. Rasa etc. reside in the dravya itself. Therefore, it is but natural that prabhav assumes the most important place among all. A single rasa may be found in two or more dravyas. Same is the case with guna, veerya etc. Hence, dravyas having similar rasa, guna, veerya may be used as substitutes. But for prabhav, there are no substitutes. It is imperative to have the original dravya for obtaining its prabhav.

Nagarjuna, in his description of prabhav, has mentioned the following reasons for the predominance of prabhav.

These reasons are :-

1. Prabhav is intangible.[7]

2. Prabhav is bactericidal; because some medicines destroy micro-organisms.[8]

3. The antitoxic activity of dravyas obtained by oral or topical administration is also a prabhav. Still, even the sight of those dravyas or even hearing about them brings relief. The reason for this is prabhav specifically.[9]

4. Prabhav has a special pharmacodynamic status. Though the rasa, guna etc. may have similar actions, yet it has an altogether different specific action.[10]

5. Adbhut karma - In instances where some therapeutic action has been generated by wearing certain gems or by chanting certain mantras, it is difficult to demonstrate the exact cause-effect relationship. Since such actions are generated by prabhav, this property is predominant.[11]

6. The scriptures also consider prabhav as the most dominant.[12]

   Because of these reasons, prabhav is predominant among rasa, guna etc.

Some of the arguments given above cannot be explained by simple reasoning. Such actions are generated by the action of the dravyas on the mind. This, again, is not physically demonstrable. That too, in the final analysis, has to be considered as the effect (prabhav) of the dravya on the mind.

A few dravyas have their action through their rasas. These dravyas can be substituted by other dravyas having the same rasa. In case sugar is not available, tea can be prepared by using jaggery also. Some act through their vipak. Here also, another dravya having the same vipak can be used as a substitute. While obtaining the actions of ushna and sheeta veerya, another dravya having the same veerya can be used as a substitute.

The same is true for the various gunas. Here also, a substitute may be used. But when a substitute does not have the desired action, then the original dravya is a must. Such an action of the dravya, which cannot be substituted, is brought about by the prabhav of the dravya. It should be said that dravya equals prabhav or prabhav can be produced by that specific dravya only.

How is the action of a dravya generated?

1. By generating impulses through rasas - immediately on putting in the mouth.
2. By generating impulses through veerya - immediately on putting in the mouth and till the dravya acts in the body.
3. By generating impulses through vipak - this is brought about after the digestion of that dravya.
4. By generating various impulses through other gunas.
5. By generating certain special impulses which can be exclusively generated only by that dravya.

(For prabhav, only that particular dravya is needed; no other substitute has the same prabhav).

PRABHAV
(Appendix)

It is said in the scriptures that the dravya acts through its rasa, vipak, veerya, guna or prabhav. The cause-effect relationship can be elicited in rasa etc., but the action in which the cause effect-relationship cannot be elicited is called "prabhav".

Precisely for this reason, prabhav has been called अचिन्त्य (inconceivable).[13] Prabhav has been described in detail in this chapter, yet a further description is given in this appendix with the aim of providing a better insight into the subject.

It is not only Ayurveda that has the concept of prabhav. It is wrong to assume that medicine is faced with such situations wherein it is impossible to demonstrate the cause- effect relationship; such situations arise in other fields of knowledge as well. This is so because the evident is limited while that which is not evident is very vast.[14]

Even in modern medicine there are instances where it is not possible to totally explain the pharmacological actions of certain drugs. The cause - effect relationship of the drug and its action has been indirectly established.

For example - ergot[15] is not included in the group of analgesic drugs. Yet, the pain in migraine is alleviated by it. Explanations such as the vaso-constricting property of ergot may be given to explain this phenomenon, but the fact remains that it has no direct analgesic action.

Second example - colchicine[16] is extremely useful in pain related to gout, but it is ineffective in other types of pain and arthralgia related to osteoarthritis. Its effectiveness only on gout can be thus related to its prabhav.

It is said that if Semecarpus anacardium is used as a fertilizer, white flower of dhattura becomes black. If salt is added as a fertilizer for growing garlic (which has five rasas), will it acquire sixth rasa?

The third example cited is of chlorthiazide.[17] It is used to increase the production of urine so that the extra fluid is drained off, reducing oedema. But in diabetes insipidus, the same medicine causes a reduction in the quantity of urine. This has to be considered as its prabhav.

One more example is that of sulphonamide.[18] The antibacterial activity of this drug has to be considered to be like prabhav in its nature.

Unani medicine has also accepted prabhav. They have included diet along with medicines in the list of substances having prabhav. They have also classified diet into gija[19]-e-faadjahari and gija-e-julkhasiyat which mean anti-toxic diet and a diet having a unique pharmacodynamic action respectively. Similarly, the medicines whose actions are brought about by their properties or their prabhav are called dava-e-julkhasiyat.

Modern medicine has admirably absorbed the discipline of phytochemistry. It is possible that we might find some explanation for prabhav through such analyses. Until and unless the cause-effect relationship can be demonstrated scientifically, the unexplained action should be considered as being produced by prabhav. Once the explanation is found, then there is no reason to call it as prabhav.

Thus prabhav is a relative term. Unless the tricks of a magician are understood, it remains magic. But once the mechanism underlying the trick is understood, it ceases to be magic. The same can be said about prabhav.

Ghee is sheeta veerya, yet is deepana (increases the agni-digestive power). If, in the future, the reason for this is discovered, then there will be no need to classify this action as prabhav. Similarly, ghee improves brain function.[20] This is also considered as prabhav until the cause-effect relationship is established. Same is the case with 'manidharana' and antipyretic activity of sahadevi. But, any action should not be attributed to prabhav outright; rather, the other causes like rasa etc. should be given due consideration and once these are ruled out, only then should one resort to calling it prabhav.

In ancient times, it was not possible to link the cause-effect relationship through disciplines like phytochemistry. Certain actions, in which the cause-effect relationship was not known despite its being present, were included under prabhav. This classification should not be considered unchangeable. Demonstrable causes must be sought first. Even if such demonstrable causes are not found, there has to be some cause to which that particular action can be attributed. Such a cause is called the undemonstrable cause, meaning "not found", invisible. Once found, its undemonstrability ceases to exist. Same is the case with prabhav.

It is true that haritaki and dhataki are both examples of dravyas having kashaya (astringent) rasa but haritaki acts as a laxative whereas dhataki causes constipation. It is the natural property of kashaya rasa to cause constipation; but chemical analysis of haritaki revealed the presence of anthroquinone which has laxative properties. Thus, laxative action of haritaki could be explained. It is possible to obtain similar explanations in case of danti and chitraka.

It is our shortcoming that we do not give much importance to plant and plant products. We have

Animals are either herbivorous or carnivorous. Same holds true for trees.

still not acquired optimum knowledge about chemical components and their actions on each other. Phytochemistry has now started discovering and understanding them. It is possible to illustrate the difference between two identical plants by analysing their molecules after enzymatic lysis. Various strong substances (acidic and non-acidic) having differing properties and actions have to be used to separate the molecules from their complex interrelated structures. This is similar to the number of minute instruments which a watchmaker has to use to place the spare-parts of a small watch in order.

Dravyas have to be tested in many ways viz. 1) their identification 2) their chemical composition 3) their in vivo action on the body and various organs of the body and 4) their use as medicines in diseases. Even if a single dravya like dinka (a gum) is taken from various species, all these will have different actions due to different chemical compositions, though all these will have the property of stickiness in common.

The chemical analysis of these dravyas may show the existence of 1) fatty acids 2) fixed oils, fats, waxes 3) phenols 4) tannins and related substances 5) proteins 6) alkaloids 7) carbohydrates 8) glycosides 9) gums, mucilages, pectins 10) volatile oils 11) resins, gum resins 12) colouring matters and 13) enzymes etc.

All these substances are further classified into smaller groups. These have their specific analytical tests which are highly complex. Various methods have to be used to differentiate minor changes in the structure and chemical composition. Two plants may have a single chemical component in common and yet the remaining chemicals may be slightly different. Even then, the required change in the analytical tests have to be made.

These advances in analytical tests will have an invaluable role to play in standardisation, determination of efficacy of active components and prevention of adulteration. For example, if fine wheat flour is mixed with butter, it can be easily identified by these tests and thus adulteration can be prevented. This has become all the more important in the case of plant products.

Not only this, but it is also without doubt that there will be considerable difference in the constituent phytochemicals. The efficacy of the same plant species which grow in the foothills of the Himalayas will change in Maharashtra. It has been observed that morphine growing in different countries has varying chemical constistuents.

This analytical knowledge can be used to determine whether or not a decoction should be made from the plant or ghee should be used in the preparation, whether it should be dried in the sun or in shade and whether it should be kept in the oven or in the refrigerator.

If there is really something like a 'miracle' then according to the Ayurvedic definition, it will have to be included in prabhav.

References -

1. रसवीर्य विपाकानां सामान्यं यत्र लक्ष्यते । विशेष: कर्मणां चैव प्रभावस्तस्य स स्मृत: ।।" (च. सू. २६)

रसादिसाम्ये यत् कर्म विशिष्टं तत् प्रभावजम् ।" (अ. सं. सू. १७, अ. हृ. सू. ९)
रसवीर्यविपाकादिगुणातिशयवानलम् । द्रव्यस्वभावो निर्दिष्टः यः प्रभावः स कीर्तितः ।। (अ. द.)
सर्वातिशायी द्रव्यस्वभावः प्रभावः ।" (अ. सं. सू. १७)

2. कटुकः कटुकः पाके वीर्योष्णश्चित्रको मतः । तद्वद्दन्ती प्रभावात्तु विरेचयति मानवम् ।।
विषं विषघ्नमुक्तं यत् प्रभावस्तत्र कारणम् । ऊर्ध्वानुलोमिकं यच्च तत् प्रभावप्रभावितम् ।।
मणीनां धारणीयानां कर्म यद्विविधात्मकम् । तत् प्रभावकृतं तेषां प्रभावोऽचिन्त्य उच्यते ।। (च. सू. २६)

3. दन्ती रसाद्यैस्तुल्यापि चित्रकस्य विरेचनी । मधुकस्य च मृद्वीका घृतं क्षीरस्य दीपनम् ।।
कटुपाकरसस्निग्धगुरुत्वैः कफवातजित् । लशुनो वातकफकृन्न तु तैरेव यद्गुणैः ।।
मिथो विरुद्धा वातादीन् लोहिताद्या जयन्ति यत् । कुर्वन्ति यवकाद्याश्च तत् प्रभावविजृम्भितम् ।।
शिरीषादि विषं हन्ति स्वप्नाद्यं तद्विवृद्धये । मणिमन्त्रौषधीनां च यत् कर्म विविधात्मकम् ।। शल्याहरणपुंजन्मर क्षायुर्धी वशादिकम् । दर्शनाद्यैरपि विषं यन्नियच्छति चागदः ।। विरेचयति यद् वृष्यमाशु शुक्रं करोति च । ऊर्ध्वाधोभागिकं यच्च द्रव्यं यच्छमनादि च ।। मात्रादि प्राप्य तत्तच्च यत् प्रपञ्चेन वर्णितम् । तच्च प्रभावजं सर्वमतोऽचिन्त्यः स उच्यते ।।" (अ. सं. सू. १७)

4. सर्वातिशायी द्रव्यस्वभावः प्रभावः" (अ. सं. सू. १७)
द्रव्यस्वभावो निर्दिष्टः यः प्रभावः स कीर्तितः" (अ. द.)
रसेन वीर्येण गुणैश्च कर्म द्रव्यं विपाकेन च यद्विदध्यात् ।
सद्योऽन्यथा तत् कुरुते प्रभावात् हेतोरतस्तत्र न गोचरीऽस्ति ।।" (अ. सं. सू. १७)

5. अमीमांस्यान्यचिन्त्यानि प्रसिद्धानि स्वभावतः । आगमेनोपयोज्यानि भेषजानि विचक्षणः । प्रत्यक्षलक्षणफलाः प्रसिद्धाश्च स्वभावतः । नौषधीर्हेतुभिर्विद्वान् परीक्षेत कदाचन ।। सहस्रेणापिहेतूनां नाम्बष्ठादिविरिचयेत् । तस्मात्तिष्ठेत्तुमतिमानागमे नतु हेतुषु ।। (सु. सू. ४०)

6. अत्र च वीर्यशब्देन द्रव्यस्य द्विविधापि चिन्त्याऽचिन्त्या च शक्तिरुच्यते । तत्राचिन्त्या शक्तिर्या तन्त्रान्तरे 9प्रभाव" इत्युच्यते सा ग्राह्या, तस्यैव च वीर्यस्य प्रभावस्य स्वतन्त्रे" तद्द्रव्यमात्मना किञ्चित्-" इत्यादिना निष्कृष्टद्रव्यप्रकारतयोक्तस्य एतदधोभागहरत्ववृष्यत्वादि प्रायः कार्य, न हीदमुष्णशीताभ्यां वीर्याभ्यामष्टाभिर्वोष्णादिभिर्वीर्यैरुपपद्यतेकार्यम् ।" (च. द.)

रसगुणभूतसमुदायाश्रयः एषामनवधारणीयः, तथारसभूतसमुदायानामन्येषावन्यथा वीर्यत्वात् ।" (र. वै. ४ सू. २४)

7. अचिन्त्यवात्" – (र. वै. अ. १ सू. १३२)
8. दैवप्रतीघातात्" – (र. वै. अ. १ सू. १३२)
9. विषप्रतीघातात् – (र. वै. अ. सू. १३४) दर्शनाच्छ्रवणात् – (र. वै. अ. सू. १३५)
10. तुल्यरसगुणेषु विशेषात्- (र. वै. अ. सू. १३६)
11. दर्शनाच्चाद्भुतादीनां कर्मणाम् – (र. वै. अ. सू. १३९)
12. आगमाच्च– (र. वै. अ. सू. १४०)
13. प्रभावोऽचिन्त्य उच्यते (च. सू. अ. २६)
प्रभवति सामर्थविशिष्टं भवति द्रव्यमनेन इति प्रभावः ।।
14. प्रत्यक्षंहि अल्पं अनल्पमप्रत्यक्षम् । (च. सू.)
15. Ergotamine is neither sedative nor analgesic and other forms of pain are not relieved by

the drug. (Goodman Gillman)

16. The machanism of dramatic relief afforded by Colehicine in acute attack of arthritis is not completely known. (Goodman Gillman p. 339)

17. "Chlorthiazide, usually diuretcs, gets anti-diuretics effect in diabetes insipidus." The mechanism of anti-diuretic, effect is yet not completely understood. (Goodman Gillman)

18. Many hyhothesis have been advanced to explain mechanism of antibacterial action of Sulphonamide,... The theory does not explain all the known facts concerning the action of Sulphonamide on bacteria.

19. गिजा=भोजन, खुराक

20. घृतं अग्निमेधे करोति । (च. सू. टीका अ. ९)

CHAPTER NINE

INTER-RELATIONSHIPS OF RASA, GUNA, VEERYA, VIPAK AND PRABHAV

Rasa, veerya, vipak, guna and prabhav are adhesives of dravya. Therefore these are dependant on the dravya. They not only bear equal but also maintain inter-relationship with each other. The scientific basis can be explained by the following four rules :-

First Rule : Dravyas having madhur rasa form madhur vipak and have sheeta veerya. Similarly, amla rasa forms an amla vipak and has ushna veerya. Lavana rasa forms madhur vipak but its veerya is ushna. Though tikta and kashaya rasas form katu vipak, their veerya is sheeta. This is the rule. Similarly, if the rasa of each dravya is known, one can derive its mahabhootas, vipak, veerya, guna etc. Generally, this is true but there can be exceptions too. Knowledge of rasa leads to the knowledge of many facts about the dravya and therefore rasa has its own importance.[1]

Second Rule : Generally, if the quality of rasadi padarthas (ie. rasa, veerya, vipak and guna) is equal or at par, then its rasas are superseded by its vipak while vipak is superseded by veerya. But all are superseded by prabhav (prabhav supersedes all the rest).[2] For example, katu rasa of piper is superseded by its madhur vipak and therefore it acts as a vrushya. Though brihat panchamoola (bilva, kashmari, tarkari, patala, tentu)have kashaya, tikta rasas and katu vipak, yet its ushna veerya supersedes rasas and vipak and therefore its action of amelioration of vata instead of its aggravation through rasas and vipak. Danti, by its prabhav, acts as purgative though it possesses katu rasa, katu vipak and ushna veerya similar to chitraka which is not a purgative. Two persons, though similar in appearance, differ in their personality traits.

Third Rule : The stronger always conquers the weaker. In case of a powerful rasa, it always dominates veerya and vipak. For example, rasa of flower of Calotropis procera (raktarka pushpa) is madhur and tikta, its vipak is katu and veerya ushna. Yet, it is very useful in haemorrhage due to the dominance of its rasa. Basically, tikta dravyas lack the property of vrushya. but dry ginger is a vitalizer by its powerful madhur vipak though its rasa is katu and veerya ushna. Experience and science tell us that dravyas having katu, tikta rasa and katu vipak aggravate vata, but asafoetida though of similar properties, acts in an opposite manner to ameliorate vata by its powerful property of ushna veerya. Though Emblica officinalis has amla (sour) rasa, madhur vipak and sheeta veerya, it acts as tridoshashamak by the presence of prabhav.[3]

Fourth Rule : The actions of dravyas are also brought about through their properties of rasa etc. In a person having satva prakriti, raja and tama gunas continue to act even in excess of satva guna. In a person having a constitution with excess pitta, it does not mean that vata kapha are totally inactive. They are also active. Some dravyas act by rasa, some by vipak, some by veerya and some by prabhav. Definitely the action of a dravya should be considered by the sum of the integrative action of rasa etc. Considering this view, none of the rasa etc. assume a secondary position. It is important in their field of action. According to their strength they acquire the chance of action in the body. For example, Tinospora cordifolia, by its property of tikta rasa, is kaphapittahara; by its ushna veerya it is vatahara, vitaliser because of madhur vipak and its prabhav leads to its use in gout.

Inter-relationship of rasa and vipak

Action of vipak is at its peak when conjugated with similar rasa. Madhur rasa intensifies the action of madhur vipak, amla rasa of amla vipak and katu rasa that of katu vipak.

Different sites of action

Action of rasa is on the tongue whereas the action of vipak is seen at the end stage of digestion. The stage of macrodigestion is the separating state between the sites of action of rasa and vipak. The action of rasa ends when the action of vipak begins. The action is enhanced when rasa etc. are complementary, but they may not nullify each other even though antagonistic.[4] A dravya is known by its gunas and gunas, in turn, are inferred upon by its actions and end results.

References -

1. शीतं वीर्येण यद् द्रव्यं मधुरं रसपाकयो: । तयोरम्लं यदुष्णं च यच्चोक्तं कटुकं तयो: ।
तेषां रसोपदेन निर्देश्यो गुणसंग्रह: । वीर्यतोऽविपरीतानां पाकतश्चोपदेक्ष्यते ।। (च. सू. २६)

2. रसं विपाकस्तौवीर्य प्रभावस्तान् व्यपोहति । वलसाम्ये रसादीनां इति नैसर्गिकं बलम् ।। (च. सू. २६)

3. किञ्चित् रसेन कुरुते कर्म वीर्येण चापरम् । द्रव्यं गुणेन पाकेन प्रभावेण च किञ्चिन ।।" (अ. सं. सू. १७)

पृथक् त्वदर्शिनामेष वादिनां वादसंग्रह: । चतुर्णामपि सामग्र्यामिच्छन् यत्र विपश्चित: ।। तद्द्रव्यमात्मना किंचित् किंचिद्वीर्येण सेवितम् । किंचिद्रसविपाकाभ्यां दोषं हन्ति करोति वा ।। (सु. सू. ४०)

द्रव्याणि हि द्रव्यप्रभावाद् गुणप्रभावाद् द्रव्यगुणप्रभावाच्च कार्मुकाणि भवन्ति ।" (च. सू. २६)

यद्यद्द्रव्ये रसादीनां बलवत्त्वेन वर्तते । अभिभूयेतस्तांस्तत्तत् कारणत्वं प्रपद्यते ।।

विरुद्धगुणसंयोगे भूयसाऽल्पं हि जीयते" (अ. सं. सू. १७)

4. विरुद्धा अपि चान्योन्यं रसाद्या: कार्यसाधने, नावश्यं स्युर्विघाताय गुणदोषामिथोयथा ।। (अ. सं. सू. १७)

A sure way to develop peptic or duodenal ulcer is to have hot exchange of words along with pungent food.

CHAPTER TEN
KARMA

Etymology of the word 'karma'

The word karma is derived from 'action'. The result is called the action or karma. Action is responsible for adhesion and separation of the particles of the dravya and is intimately associated with the dravya. Actions in the body are subject to change with the help of adhesion and separation properties just as in the universe.[1] In short, that entity of a drug which brings about changes in the body is called as karma (action). Action takes place only when the potential energy of a substance is changed. Karma (action) means a visible sign of an energy.

Characteristics of karma

Karma is described as action - a constant action taking place in health or the diseased state of a living body. In treatment, emesis and purgative actions are used. These procedures can be cited as good examples for beneficial actions. In Ayurveda, the word karma has also been used to describe the unforeseen (adrushta karma). But in dravyaguna, this meaning is not applicable and therefore it should not be considered. The procedures which are used for treatment are designated as karmas (actions).

The terms expulsion, impulsion, contraction, relaxation, motion etc. are used for action in Vaisheshik darshan. But in dravyaguna, the word action means emesis, purgation etc. Charaka, Sushruta and Vagbhatta use the word karma for various modes of treatment like emesis, purgation, enema, retention enema, nasya, deepan, pachan etc. included in pancha karma. In swasthavritta the word karma is used in the same context.[2]

How does a drug act?

One should observe the way in which various dravyas having different properties bring about their actions in the body because ultimately, these properties are known through their actions.[3] The dravyas which are composed of five elements (panchamahabhootas) are similar to the composition of tridosha, universe and purusha. The five elements (panchamahabhootas), which compose the body, dravyas and tridoshas, are responsible to bring about various actions. The energy of panchamahabhootas is expressed in the form of actions.[4]

The dravyas contain potential energy, which, on applying the stimulus, gets converted into kinetic energy and results in action. Impetus brings about the action.

Action of a dravya is always brought about in accordance with its gunas. There can be no action contrary to the gunas. The actions of dravyas depend on the number and permutations-combinations of their gunas.

Since the gunas can be predicted from their actions, it establishes the rule that the number of

If one gets conscious of any part of one's body, then it means that something is wrong with that part. A person with an ego is also a diseased person.

gunas are equivalent to the number of actions. Number of actions cannot be determined if the number of gunas is not known. Relative grades of these gunas and their permutations-combinations make the number of gunas infinite. So the number of actions also becomes infinite. Gunas cannot be described objectively. However it is said that mridu guna is the one which creates softness, while the one which cleans is called vishada guna. From these, it is clear that one can assertain gunas through their actions.

When the action takes place it is not possible that the guna responsible for bringing about this action does not exist within the substance.

If two drugs show similar actions then their gunas are similar. The action will depend on the relative strength of these gunas.

A guna which is superseded by another powerful guna cannot be effective. The dravya possessing gunas is always capable of bringing about the action. This is latent energy (potential energy). When it gets impetus it is converted to kinetic energy and results in action.

A usually cool person, when provoked, gets angry and suddenly reacts violently out of pattern. Similarly, the potential energy, which is in a quiescent form, when stimulated, gets active and brings about the action. Reflex action can be included in this category.

The actions mentioned in relation to the dravya are resultant of the energy existing within the dravya. Therefore the dravya is a support to this energy. No doubt that the action is secondary to the dravya but it is self-potent and independent in existence.

Dravya

Guna	**Karma**
(Static Energy)	(Kinetic Energy)
Gunas are manifested in the form of karmas. Therefore the characteristic of a particular guna is described as that particular entity which brings about that particular action.	Without guna, there is no karma and therefore karma has no independent existence. Gunas can act only with the support of the dravyas. Absence of dravya implies absence of guna and karma. That is why eventhough karmas are generated by gunas, yet gunas are considered attributes of the dravya.

When body constituents like dosha-dhatu-mala are not in balance the body suffers from a state called disease. The balanced form of the basic constitution is called the healthy state. According to Charaka the main aim of Ayurveda is to restore the balance desired between the dosha-dhatu-

A person with healthy srotasas experiences good health.

malas by the actions brought about by treatment. For this, various dravyas are used because the gunas of the body and that of the dravyas are the same. The use of dravyas can bring about an increase or decrease in the body constituents.

The composition of body and dravyas being the same, dravyas can also cause diseases. Similarly, the use of dravyas can cure them too.[5] Both the dravya and the body are formed by the macro cosmos.

Dravya and agni

Ayurveda has described thirteen 'agni' in the living human body - jatharagni (pachakagni, kayagni are the synonyms of jatharagni), seven agnis of seven dhatus and five agnis of five mahabhootas. Dravyas when consumed in the form of food or medicine are first acted upon by jatharagni. Then it is subjected further to panchamahabhootagni and saptadhatuagni. Due to the digestion by these thirteen agnis, the digested food nourishes the different dhatus in terms of panchmahabhootas. Chemical composition of the finally digested food or medicine gets conjugated with the respective chemical composition of the body constituents and brings about the desired result. The digestion of the dravya is brought about by the cumulative effect of bhautik agni of the dravya and the body. All the thirteen agnis continue to work in the body to bring about their actions.

The rasa of a dravya acts at local, general as well as at the level of the mind . All dravyas undergo the three consecutive stages of digestion namely madhur, amla and katu awasthapak. Kapha, pitta and vata are generated during these three stages of digestion respectively. Every dravya has its own definite nishthapak eventhough it undergoes various awasthapak. After the stage of nishthapak, when the digested juice comes in contact with dosha-dhatu-mala, these are either increased or decreased by the effect of the digested juice. Similar changes take place in the tridoshas by vipak because the creation of dravya and dosha is from panchamahabhootas.

The action of a dravya depends on the relative composition and strength of these five mahabhootas. Ayurveda mentions that some actions of dravyas take place by gunas, some by vipak, some by veerya, and some by prabhav.[6] Beyond these there is no other way of bringing about the action of a dravya. Generally the site of action of rasa is limited to the tongue and tastebuds. Action of rasa is followed by action of prapak and then of vipak. Though veerya is more effective and powerful than rasa and vipak, it is the prabhav that acquires the highest position in drug action. The action may take place through any one amongst rasa, guna, veerya, vipak and prabhav, but the action seen is because of its effect on the various elements of the innumerable cellular components of the body. This effect of molecular changes is seen on the body according to principle of peelupak. Through the various gunas of a dravya, its action is brought about in the body. The gunas of a dravya are ascertained from its actions on the body. Vibrations generated by the gunas are responsible for the action.

Types of action

Action of dravyas is mainly of two types: 1) localised and 2) generalised. Unpredicted effect is seen due to prabhav. Rasa, guna, veerya and vipak can bring either localised or generalised effect, while the dravyas applied externally show localised effect. Reverse effect is also observed.[7]

Though the dravyas cause different types of actions in the body, they are not of the same intensity. Some are strong while others are weak. Some actions are generated directly while others are generated through a chain of events. Katu rasa causes immediate burning sensation of the tongue but eventually results in lacrimation and running nose. Emesis and purgation can also cause effects on the other organs. The act of purification initiates purifying process which continues for some time. Associated procedures are important for this reason.

Even then, further research is required to decide the exact action of various dravyas or their parts, according to the priciple of panchamahabhootas. However, knowing the name, guna, karma, and its effect on the diseases, and with knowledge about the dravya, it is possible to predict the effect of such a dravya on dosha, dhatu, mala or organs concerned in a systematic manner. If the guna of a dravya is specially mentioned in the text as effective symptomatically or cures diseases due to its special action then it is wise to say that the said action takes place by its gamitva.

These actions can be classified as follows based on the consideration of the different systems, organs, diseases, doshas, dhatus and malas of the body.

(I) Actions on nerves / nervous system - (8)

1) Brain tonic
2) Intoxicant
3) Consciousness restoring
4) Sedative
5) Causing insomnia
6) Analgesic
7) Convulsant
8) Anticonvulsant.

II) Actions on the senses - (20)

1) Strengthening the eyes
2) Dilatation of the iris
3) Contraction of the iris
4) Useful to the ears
5) Shirovirechaka
6) Sweat promoting
7) Sweat adjuvant
8) Reducing sweating
9) Promoting hair growth
10) Controlling hair growth
11) Promoting hair growth and nourishment
12) Producing burning sesnsation
13) Unctuous
14) Adjuvant to unctuous
15) Dryness
16) Improves complexion
17) Anti-pruritic
18) Anti-dermatosis
19) Anti-urticaria
20) External anti-parasitic.

(III) Actions on respiratory system (Pranavaha srotas) - (9)

(1) Stimulating respiratory centre
(2) Depressant of respiratory centre
(3) Stimulating respiration
(4) Expectorants
(5) Suppressing cough
(6) Antiasthmatic
(7) Antihiccough
(8) Demulcent
(9) Antitussive.

(IV) Actions on alimentary system - (31)

(A) Oral cavity

(1) Promoting salivary secretion
(2) Decreasing salivary secretion
(3) Antidyspeptic
(4) Mouth freshener.
(5) Improving taste
(6) Beneficial to teeth

(B) Stomach

(1) Reducing the feeling of fullness of stomach
(2) Stomachic
(3) Appetizers
(4) Digestive
(5) Appetite depressants
(6) Producing burning sensation
(7) Anti - irritant
(8) Carminatives
(9) Constipative
(10) Emetic
(11) Adjuvant to emesis
(12) Antiemetic
(13) Absorbant

(C) Intestine

(1) Enhancing stool formation
(2) Purgatives
(3) Adjuvants in purgatives
(4) Constipative
(5) Maintaning the colour of stools
(6) Clearing the intestines
(7) Adjuvants in clearing the intestines
(8) Restoration of intestinal mucosa
(9) Adjuvants in restoration of intestinal mucosa
(10) Removing doshas from the intestine
(11) Antihelminthics
(12) Helminthicidal (vermicidal)

(V) Actions on lymphatics - (3)

(1) Oedema suppressant
(2) Oedema enhancing.
(3) Useful in enlargement of cervical lymphnodes.

(VI) Actions on circulatory system - (7)

(1) Cardiotonic
(2) Cardiostimulant.
(3) Cardiac depressant
(4) Hypertensive

Behind every tradition there is a scientific reason. Outward appearance of the traditions may change, but the core will not change.

(5) Hypotensive
(6) Blood coagulant
(7) Anticoagulant.

(VII) Actions on liver - (5)

(1) Cholagogue
(2) Biliary lithotripsic
(3) Glyconeogenesis
(4) Glycogenolytic
(5) Antihemorrhoidal

(VIII) Actions on spleen - (1)

(1) Curing splenomegaly

(IX) Actions on female genital tract - (9)

(1) Promotion of fertility
(2) Antifertility
(3) Oxytocic
(4) Uterine relaxants
(5) Emmenogogue
(6) Haemostatic
(7) Galactogogue
(8) Galactofuge
(9) Purifying breast milk

(X) Actions on male genital organs - (3)

(1) Aphrodisiac
(2) Reducing sexual urge
(3) Improving semen quality

(XI) Actions on urinary System - (5)

(1) Diuretic
(2) Restoring normal colour of urine
(3) Lithotriptic
(4) Antidiuretic
(5) Purifying urine

(XII) Antipyretic - (9)

(1) Febrifuge
(2) 'Ama' digestive
(3) Periodical fever preventive
(4) Refrigerant
(5) Anti-rigors
(6) Anti-inflammatory
(7) Antibiotic
(8) Deodorant
(9) Wound - cleansing

(XIII) Actions on general body tissues - (7)

(1) Tissue building
(2) Tonic
(3) Increasing oja
(4) Destruction of oja
(5) Rejuvenating body tissues
(6) Toxic
(7)Anti-toxic.

There is always a line of ants gathering food, because the first ant secretes pheromone and others follow. Is this pheromone a fragrant substance or is it a liquid?

(XIV) Target-specific actions (gamitva) - (21)

(1) Pramotion of rasa
(2) Control of rasa
(3) That which promotes blood clotting
(4) Haemolytic.
(5) Vitiating blood
(6) Purifying blood
(7) Increasing body tissues
(8) Decreasing body tissues
(9) Relieving fatigue
(10) Relieving body ache
(11) Wound healing
(12) Cleansing the skin
(13) Wound cleansing
(14) Increasing meda
(15) Reducing meda
(16) Increasing asthi
(17) Reducing asthi
(18) Increasing majja
(19) Reducing majja
(20) Increasing shukra
(21) Reducing shukra.

(XV) Actions on srotas of doshas - (6)

(1) Vitiating vata
(2) Pacifying vata
(3) Vitiating pitta
(4) Pacifying pitta
(5) Vitiating kapha
(6) Pacifying kapha

Description of some of the commonly used actions

(1) Deepan

In dyspepsia the appetite is reduced and less food is consumed. In such conditions the drugs which increase the appetite and remove the dyspepstic symptoms are called deepan. Deepan drugs do not help digestion but stimulate appetite. Deepan drugs possess the properties of teja mahabhoota and are pungent, sour, salty, ushna veerya, teekshna, ushna and laghu. Some acharyas consider these as predominant in vayu and prithvi mahabhoota (Bha.) but in fact agni and vayu should be predominant because vayu is associated with agni (fire). Saman vayu is a stimulant of appetite, therefore vayu stimulates agni. Action of deepan takes places in stomach. According to modern concept the vagus stimulates and controls the secretions of stomach. Stimulation of vagus increases the digestive secretions. Even the appearance and smell of food is enough for stimulation. Stimulation of vagus by sour, salty and pungent rasas induces the secretion of psychic and appetite juices in the stomach. Deepan drugs act from mouth to the pyloric end of the stomach. For example, tasty and pungent, bitter foods stimulate the salivary juice, pilocarpine-like drugs stimulate vagus and induce gastric secretion. Mansa rasa (mutton soup) helps to increase appetite as well as digestion not only in the intestinal lumen but also further in dhatus where agni exists.[8]

A mixture of 77% of alcohol and 23% of water is used to keep thermometer in hospitals, as it is the strongest antimicrobial agent.

(2) Pachan (Digestion)

There is a basic difference between appetite and digestion. Deepan drugs may stimulate appetite but do not help digestion. Similarly, digestive drugs may not stimulate appetite. Digestive drugs are predominant in agni and less in vayu. Digestive juices stimulated by these drugs bring about this action. Some drugs are both digestive as well as appetite stimulants like chitraka (Plumbago zeylanicum). Appetiser and digestive are two different entities, yet, Charakacharya has described appetiser group (deepaneeya gana) and not the digestive group for the simple reason that appetite and digestion are the two sides of the same coin and stages of the same action. Appetite and digestion are the two actions of gastric juice similar to the light and heating actions of the fire. For deepan, vayu associated with agni is required whereas for pachan (digestion) teja mahabhoota associated with agni is required. Malfunctioning within the digestive tract will subsequently result in the indigestion of the dosha-dhatu-malas and vice-versa. Thus in Ayurveda, whenever the word pachan is used, one should think of both, digestive tract as well as dosha-dhatu-malas.[9]

(3) Sanshodhan (Purification)

A drug that drives the vitiated doshas by ascending or descending pathways from the body is called as a purifying drug. For example, 'devdangari'. These drugs basically bear the properties of katu, tikta rasas, teekshna, laghu gunas, ushna veerya, prithvi, aap, teja and vayu mahabhootas. For purification, Ayurveda predominantly describes five procedures (panchakarma) and other purifying methods (fumigation, mouth wash, bath etc.) because a body subjected to continuously generated impurities through metabolism must be maintained in a clean condition.[10]

(4) Sanshaman

Without expelling the aggravated doshas of the body (without interfering with the balanced doshas) the drugs, which maintain a balance among the doshas by changing their gunas internally are called sanshaman. Tinospora cordifolia is an example of sanshaman dravya.. Different drugs exist for amelioration of every dosha. Sanshaman drugs are predominant in akash mahabhoota. According to Nagarjuna vayu, aap and prithvi mahabhootas predominate in sanshaman dravyas. Shaman is logical when done on a purified body but shaman carried out on an impure body should be considered as exceptional.[11]

(5) Anuloman (Carminative)

Doshas from the body, especially vayu, need expulsion by the nearest path with the help of drugs known as anuloman. Such drugs have the property of ushna veerya and oleation. For example, dravyas having pungent odour, camphor, alcohol, peppermint, asafoetida, dikemali and Allium sativam (garlic) are anulomann dravyas. The action of anuloman is generalised and not limited to the colon.[12]

Hydrogen peroxide, along with destroying microbes, harms other constituents of the body. Hence its use is discouraged.

(6) Sransan (Laxatives)

These are the drugs which cause purgation by smooth action and which are not very drastic purgatives. For example, trivrut, kalabol (of Aloe vera) and pulp of Cassia fistula are sransan dravyas. Since these drugs are not very irritant or very mild, they help to evacuate the bowel. These drugs cause excretion of excess of kapha and pitta doshas from the large intestine. Laxatives (and not very strong purgatives) are advocated in febrile conditions.[13]

(7) Bhedan (Strong purgative)

These drugs are drastic purgatives by their irritant action. They cause burning and griping pain and liquify the stools for excretion by rectal pathway, e.g. jayapal, kaduvrindavan, tridhari nivdung, kutaki, shyamatrivrut etc. These drugs are harmful to body tissues and therefore should be used cautiously.[14]

(8) Rechan (Purgative)

The drugs which enhance the excretion of solid or liquid stool through anal canal are called rechan. These drugs may be of any rasa and are ushna veerya, teekshna, sukshma, vyavayi and vikashi. They are predominant in prithvi and aap mahabhoota both of which are guru and acting in the direction of gravitational force. Since guru guna moves in the direction of gravity, it leads to excretion by anal pathway. The action is attributed to prabhav because all drugs having the above properties are not purgatives. These drugs not only excrete stools but also carry out the purification of vata, pitta and kapha doshas. In toxic and excessive dose, dhatus in ascending order are excreted by anal path, ie. rasa, rakta, mansa and meda.[15]

Different modes of action of purgative drugs

1) The drugs by their non-absorptive property increase the bulk of the stool (predominantly prithvi mahabhoota).

2) By interfering with the absorption of the water content in the bowel.

3) By irritating the mucosa of the small and large intestines.

4) By increasing the peristalsis of the intestine.

The time and duration of action of these purgative drugs differ because they act on different parts of the intestine to start the purgative action. Rubbing the oil of croton seeds on the skin can cause purgation. It also causes purgation even by holding the fruit in the hand or standing under the shadow of the tree. The drug which causes excretion of stool followed by pitta, kapha and vayu in that order is considered to be superior. Also it should not cause any complication but should stimulate the appetite. It creates body strength and makes the mind energetic and fresh. Clarity of thought, sharpness of special organs, stability of body tissues, improvement of appetite and enhanced longevity are the signs of good purgation.

Carbolic acid as an antiseptic for wounds was first used on 12/8/1965 by Dr. Joseph Lister.

(9) Chhedan

Chhedan literally means cutting. Those drugs, which, by their properties, actions and prabhav extract and excrete the doshas - kapha, pitta etc. - are called chhedaniya (dissociation from the body). Example - yavakshar, asafoetida and Piper nigrum (black pepper) are chhedan dravyas. These drugs are amla, lavana, katu and teekshna. The chhedan action is brought about in two ways (1) by secretion and (2) by expulsion. This is to increase the secretion and then expelling it out of the body. Watery constituent increases the secretion whereas vayu and agni bhootas by their property of teekshna expel it. Amla, lavana and katu rasas help this action of chhedan. The basic concept of surgical amputation underlies this process of chhedan which removes vitiated kapha from the organs.[16]

(10) Lekhan

Ruksha (rough) and chhedaniya drugs bring about this action. These drugs are effective on meda (fatty tissue). Khara and vișhada guna are very helpful for this action.

Examples - Shilajit, Commiphora mukul (guggula), cow's urine, triphala, iron, honey, ajawain etc.[17]

(11) Grahi

These drugs having ushna veerya, katu rasa and katu vipak help to increase appetite, digestion, and absorption of fluid resulting in solidification of stool. Heat reduces the increased vayu from the colon. These are further classified as ushna grahi and aam grahi. Grahi dravyas are useful in dysentry.[18]

(12) Stambhan

These drugs are ruksha, kashaya (astringent) and sheeta (cold) and therefore help to increase vata and absorb fluid in the colon. Astringent rasa results in the contraction of the contents and vayu absorbs fluids. Since these drugs do not digest aam, they are termed as pakvagrahi. Since they are sheeta (cold), they are called sheetagrahi. These drugs are useful in diarrhoea of digestive disturbances or colonic origin. Charaka's constipative drugs belong to this group. Dosha-dhatu-mala situated in any site accompanied with aam should not be subjected to stambhan.

Difference Between

	Grahi	**Stambhan**
Rasa	Katu (pungent)	Kashaya (astringent)
Veerya	Ushna	Sheeta
Action on Doshas	Vata shamak (amelioration)	Vata vardhak (aggravation)
Action	Deepan, pachan	Decrease appetite.[19]

Indigestion occurs on overeating even by one extra morsel.

(13) Madakari (Narcotics)

The drugs which cause abnormality in the central nervous system are called madakari dravyas (narcotic drugs). Alcohol, morphine and cannabis are predominantly made up of agni and vayu mahabhootas. They contain all the rasas and are teekshna, laghu, ushna, sukshma, amla, vyavayi, vikashi, ashu, ruksha and vishad. These gunas are exactly the opposite of oja. Therefore they cause irritation and destruction of oja. They have similar effect on the mind, making it euphoric. In the beginning, the action of these dravyas is predominantly agneya, followed by vayaveeya action ending in coma and death.

The effects of narcotic drugs show variation in different persons having different prakritis. Tamas and pitta prakriti individuals show immediate response.

Rajas and vata prakriti people exhibit intermediate response to these drugs.

Rajas and kapha prakriti individuals show very slow response.

Rajas-tamas diet mentioned in the dietary chapter of Bhagvad Geeta is narcotic in nature.[20]

(14) Pramathi

These drugs, on entering into the body, induce a feeling of churning sensation all over, cause irritation and separate wastes from the capillaries. Pramathi dravyas are katu (pungent) and teekshna (irritant). Example - piper, vacha (Achorus calamus). Mind, when affected by raja-tama, acts like pramathi. (Bhagvad Geeta)[21]

(15) Abhishyandi

Properties of drugs causing obstruction in the srotas (capillaries) are called abhishyandi. These dravyas are pichchil, guru and snigdha (unctuous). They increase kapha which causes obstruction to the flow of lymph. Obstruction results in the formation of kleda.

Curd is the best abhishyandi material. Viscous state is similar to the state of cooked rice where the water does not get separated from the rice and forms a paste. Jaggary, salt and tamarind showing wetness in rainy season belong to the class of abhishyandi.[22]

(16) Vyavayi

The drugs which get absorbed immediately before digestion and then undergo digestion during the circulation in the body are called vyavayi. They are predominantly made up of vayu and akash mahabhootas. Vayu produces motion and akash keeps the capillaries (srotas) open.

Example - Morphine, Cannabis sativa (Indian hemp) and poisons. These drugs being micromolecular and dispersible do not have to undergo the natural stages of digestion, absorption, spread and excretion.[23]

Asepsis, anaesthesia and artery-forceps are the three A's in surgery. Due to these A's, surgery has become easy and advanced.

(17) Vikashi

These drugs spread very rapidly into the body and destroy oja. All tissues and joint movements get sluggish. These drugs are predominant in vayu mahabhoota and are called vikashi.

Example - Areca nut and intoxication brought about by tobacco is due to its vikashi action.[24]

References -

1. वर्ततेहि गुणाः केचित्सुखदाः दुःखदाः तथा ।
सुखदुःखविरक्ताश्च तेषां कर्महि तद्यथा ।।
गुणानुवर्तिनं कर्म चाविरोधेन वर्तते ।
संयोगे च विभागे च कारणं द्रव्यमाश्रितम् । कर्तव्यस्य क्रिया कर्म कर्म नान्यदपेक्षते ।।" (च. सू. १)
एकद्रव्यमगुणं संयोगविभागेष्वनपेक्षकारणमिति कर्मलक्षणम् ।" (वै. द.)
क्रियालक्षणं कर्म ।" (र. वै. अ. १ सू. १७१) । १यत् कुर्वन्ति तत् कर्म ।" (च. सू. २६)
कर्तव्यस्य क्रिया कर्म ।" (च. सू. १) । प्रयत्नादि कर्म चेष्टितमुच्यते ।" (च. सू. १)
प्रवृत्तिस्तु खलु चेष्टा कार्यार्था सैव क्रिया, कर्म, यत्नः, कार्यसमारम्भश्च ।" (च. वि. ८)
उत्क्षेपणं ततोऽपक्षेपणमाकुञ्चनं तथा । प्रसारणं च गमनं कर्माण्येतानि पञ्च च ।।
भ्रमणं रेचनं स्यन्दनोर्ध्वज्वलनमेव च । तिर्यगगमनमप्यत्र गमनादेव लभ्यते ।।" (कारिका)
2. संयोगश्च विभागश्च वेगश्चैते तु कर्मजाः ।" (कारिकावली)
कर्म पञ्चविधमुक्तं वमनादि ।" (च. सू. २६) । १एतच्च प्राधान्यादुच्यते तेन बृंहणाद्यपि बोद्धव्यम् ।" (च. द.)
इहौषधकर्माणि ऊर्ध्वाधोभागोभयभागसंशोधनसंशमन सांग्राहिकाग्निदीपनपीडनलेख नबृंहणरसायनवाजीकरणश्वयथुकर-विलयन-दहन- मादन-प्राणघ्न-विषप्रशमनादीनि वीर्यप्राधान्याद् भवन्ति ।" (सु. सू. ४०)
3. यावन्तो गुणविशेषाः कर्मसंख्याहि तावति ।
असंख्येयाः गुणाः द्रव्ये ततः कर्माण्यमितानिच ।
गुणाः कर्मानुमेयाः वै ।
गुणानुरूपं वै कर्म ।
गुणानुज्ञापितं कर्म । कर्मभिस्त्वनुमीयन्ते नानाद्रव्याश्रयाः गुणाः ।।
4. शक्तिस्तु कर्मसामर्थ्य चेष्टितं कर्म भण्यते ।
शक्त्युत्कर्षघटितं यत् तत्तु कर्माभिसंज्ञितम् ।। (आगस्त्यसंहिता)
व्यक्तस्वरूपा या शक्तिः सा वै कर्माभिसंज्ञिता ।
5. बहुधाऽभ्यंगपरिषेकावगाहरूपेण शीतादय उपयुज्यते ।" (र. वै. भा.) ।
१रसदोषसन्निपाते तु ये रसा यैर्दोषैः समानगुणाः समानगुणभूयिष्ठा वा भवन्ति ते तान्अभिवर्धयन्ति । विपरीतगुणा विपरीतगुणभूयिष्ठावाशमयन्त्यभ्यस्यमानाः । (च. वि. १)
6. तद्द्रव्यमात्मना किंचित् किंचिद्वीर्येण सेवितम् ।
किंचिद्रसविपाकाभ्यां दोषं हन्ति करोति वा ।।
7. तत्रान्तःपरिमार्जनं यदन्तःशरीरमनुप्रविश्यौषधमाहारजातव्याधीन् प्रमार्ष्टि । यत् पुनः बहिःस्पर्शमाश्रि-

त्याभ्यंगस्वेदप्रदेहपरिषेकोन्मर्दनाद्यैरामयान् प्रमार्ष्टि तद्बहि:परिमार्जनम् ।।

8. दीपनाय वह्नेरुद्दीपनाय हितम् । (ग.)
दीपनं अन्तरग्नेः संधुक्षणं, तस्मै हितं दीपनीयम् । (यो.)
यदग्निकृत् पचेन्नामं दीपनं तद्यथा घृतम् । दीपनं ह्यग्निकृत्वामं कदाचित् पाचयेन्न वा ।। (अ. हृ. ७)
पचेन्नामं वह्निकृच्च दीपनं तद्यशा मिशि ।" (शा.) (बडिशेप)
दीपनमग्निभूयिष्ठं तत्समानत्वात् । (सु. सू. ४१)
पित्तलान् रसान् गुणांश्च दीपनीयम्, तदाग्नेयम् ।" (र. वै. ४)
कटुकाम्ललवणान् रसान्, तीक्ष्णोष्णलघून् गुणांश्चाश्रितमिति, तदग्निनैव निर्वर्त्यम् । (भा.) पाचन

9. पचन्तमग्निं प्रतिपक्षक्षपणेन बलदानेन च यत् पाचयति तत् पाचनम् ।" (च. द.)
पचतोऽग्नेः पक्तुं शक्तिमधिकां यदुत्पादयति तद् द्रव्यं क्रिया वा पाचनमुच्यते ।" (अ. द.)
पचत्यामं न वह्निं च कुर्यात्तद्धि पाचनम् । नागकेसरवत् विद्यात् ।" (शा.)
तच्च वाय्वग्निभूयिष्ठम्"-(च.द.) १अग्नेस्तु गुणबाहुल्यात् पाचन परिचक्ष्महे ।" (भा.)
चित्रो दीपनपाचनः ।" – (शा.)

10. संशोधन स्थानाद्बहिर्नदूर्ध्वमधश्च मलसंचयम् ।
देहसंशोधनं तत् स्याद् देवदालीफलं यथा ।।" (शा.)

9 वातलान् रसान् पित्तलांश्च गुणानुभयतोभागम् । तत् पार्थिवाप्यतैजसवायव्यम् ।।"
(र. वै. ४/६-७) १उभयगुणभूयिष्ठमुभयतो भागम् ।" (सु. सू. ४१)

9 वमनं रेचनं नस्यं निरूहश्चानुवासनम् ।
एतानि पञ्च कर्माणि कथितानि मुनीश्वरैः ।।" (शा.) शमन

11. न शोधयति यद् दोषान् समान्नोदीरयत्यपि । समीकरोति विषमान् शमनम् ।।" (अ. हृ.)
न शोधयति न द्वेष्टि समान् दोषांस्तथोद्धतान् ।
समीकरोति विषमान् शमनं तद्यथाऽमृता ।। (शा.)
आकाशगुणभूयिष्ठं संशमनम्" (सु. सू. ४१)
वायुसोममहीजातं तथा संशमनं विदुः । (र. वै.)
अनुलोमन

12. कृत्वा पाकं मलानां यद् भित्त्वा बन्धमधो नयेत् ।
तच्चानुलोमन ज्ञेयं यथा प्रोक्ता हरीतकी ।।" (शा.)
अनुलोमनो वातप्रवर्तनः (सु. सू. ४६ टीका)
सरोऽनुलोमनः प्रोक्तः (सु. सू.) स्रंसन

13. पक्तव्य यदपक्त्वैव श्लिष्टं कोष्ठे मलादिकम् ।
नयत्यधः स्रंसनं तद्यथा स्यात् कृतमालकः ।।" (शा.) (भा. प्र.) (बाहावा)
भेदन

14. मलादिकमबद्धं च बद्धं वा पिण्डितं मलैः । भित्त्वाऽधः पातयति तद्भेदनं कटुकी यथा ।।"
रेचन

15. दोषहरणमधोभागं विरेचनसंज्ञकम् । (च. क. १)
सलीलपृथ्वात्मकत्वात् अधोभागप्रभावात् तच्चौषधमधःप्रवर्तते ।। (च. क. १५)
विपक्वं यदपक्वं वा मलानि द्रवतां नयेत् ।
रेचयत्यपि तज्ज्ञेयं रेचनं त्रिवृतायथा ।। (शा.)

तत्रोष्णतीक्ष्णसूक्ष्मव्यवायिविकाशीन्यौषधानि... अध:प्रवर्तते ।।" (च. क. १)

विरेंचनद्रव्याणि पृथिव्यम्बुगुणभूयिष्ठानि, पृथिव्यापो गुर्व्य: ता गुरुत्वादधो गच्छन्ति तस्माद्विरेचनमधोगुणभूयिष्ठमानात् ।" (सु. सू. ४१)

गुरुत्वं चेह प्रभावविशेषाधिष्ठित त्रिवृतादि समवेतं ग्राह्य न तु गुरुत्वामात्रम्, अन्यथा मत्स्यपिष्टान्नसूरादीनां विरेचकत्वं स्यात्" । (च. द.)

काचिदास्वादमात्रेण काचिद्गन्धेन भेदयेत् । काचित् स्पर्शेन दृष्ट्या वा चतुर्धा भेदयेच्छिवा ।" (भा. प्र.)

स्त्रोतोविशुद्धीन्द्रियसम्प्रसादो लघुत्वमूर्जोग्निरनामयत्वम् । प्राप्तिश्च विट्पित्तकफानिलानां सम्यग्विरिक्तस्य भवेत् क्रमेण ।।" (च. सि. १)

'An ideal purgative should not have any other effect except on the intestines.

16. श्लिष्टान् कफादिकान् दोषानुन्मूलयति यद् बलात् । छेदनं तद्यथा क्षारा: मरिचानि शिलाजतु ।" (शा.)

द्रव्याणि हि अम्ल-लवण-कटूनि शारीरक्लेदादीनि छिन्दन्ति ।" (ग.)

17. रसादि धातु व वातादि दोष यांचे शोषण करुन पातळ करतात ती लेखन-जसा मध. लिख्यते शस्त्रेण इव (अ. हृदय. सू. २३)

लेखनम् ईषत् चर्मविदारणं घर्षणेन । तस्मै हितम् लेखनीयम् (सू. स. ४६) टीका.

धातून् मलान्वा देहस्य विशोष्योल्लेखयेत् च यत् ।
लेखनं तद्यथा क्षौद्रं नीरमुष्णं वचा यवा: ।। (शा. सं.)

लेखनमनिलभूयिष्ठम् । (सु. सू. अ. ४१) लेखनम् कफमेदसो: (डल्हण)

18. पुरीषस्य अतिसरत: संग्रहणं संग्रह: तत्र हितं पुरीषसंग्रहणीयम् (यो.)

पक्वामग्राहकत्वेन द्विविधं हि संग्राहकम् । तत्र यत् ग्रहण्यामामं संपाच्य वह्निं कृत्वा तत्रस्थं द्रवं च शोषयित्वा संग्रहण करोति तदुष्णग्राहकं ज्ञेयम्, यद् द्रव्यमतीसारादौ पक्वमलदिकं संस्तभ्य संग्रहं करोति तच्छितसंग्राहकं ज्ञेयम्, एतदग्निभूयिष्ठम् । (आ.) १दीपनं पाचनं यत् स्यादुष्णत्वाद् द्रवशोषकम् । ग्राहि तच्च यथा शुण्ठी जीरकं गजपिप्पली ।।" (शा.)

लवणतीक्ष्णोष्णेभ्योऽन्यत् सांग्राहिकं तत् पार्थिववायव्यम् ।" (र. वै.)

सांग्राहिकमनिलगुणभूयिष्ठम् । अनिलस्य शोषणात्मकत्वात् ।" (सु. सू. ४१)

रौक्ष्यात् शैत्यात् कषायत्वात् लघुपाकाच्च यद् भवेत् ।
वातकृत् स्तम्भनं तत् स्याद्यथा वत्सकटुण्टुकौ ।। (शा.)

19. स्तंभनं स्तंभयति यद्, गतिमन्तं चलं ध्रुवम् : (च. सू. २२।१२)

स्तंभयति निरुणद्धि । चलं इति किंचित् गतिमत्वम् । गतिमन्तमिति प्रव्यक्त गतिमन्तम् । एतच्चातिसार, शोणितस्त्रुति, विष, दाह, वेदनेषु बोद्धव्यम् । न केवलं वाते गतिमन्तं प्रति, स्तंभकस्य वर्धकस्यात् ।

20. बुद्धिं लुम्पति यद्द्रव्यं मदकारी तदुच्यते । तमोगुणप्रधानंच यथा मद्यं सुरादिकम् । (शा.)

सर्वान् रसान् तीक्ष्णोष्णलघुरूक्षविशदांश्च गुणात मदनीयम् ।
तदाग्नेयं वायव्यम् च । (र. वै. ४-११-१२)

मद्यं हृदयमाविश्य स्वगुणैरोजसो गुणान् । दशभिर्दश संक्षोभ्य चेतो नयति विक्रियाम् ।। लघूष्णतीक्ष्णसूक्ष्माम्लव्यवाय्याशुगमेव च । रूक्षं विकाशि विशदं मद्यं दशगुणं स्मृतम् ।

गुरु शीतं मृदुश्लक्ष्णं बहलं मधुरं स्थिरम् । प्रसन्नं पिच्छिलं स्निग्धमोजो दशगुणं स्मृतम् ।।

गुरुत्वं लाघवाच्छैत्यमौष्ण्यादम्लस्वभावत: । माधुर्य मार्दवं तैक्ष्ण्यात्, प्रसादं चाशुभावनात् ।।
रौक्ष्यात् स्नेहं व्यवायित्वात् स्थिरत्वं श्लक्ष्णतामपि । विकासिभावात् पैच्छिल्यं वैशद्यात् सान्द्रतां तथा ।
सौक्ष्म्यान्मद्यं निहन्त्येवमोजस: स्वगुणैर्गुणान् । सत्त्वं तदाश्रयं चाशु संक्षोभ्य जनयेन्मदम् ।। (च. चि. २४)
बुद्धिस्मृतिप्रीतिकर: सुखश्च पानान्ननिद्रारतिवर्धनश्च । संपाठ्यगीतस्वरवर्धनश्च प्रोक्तोऽतिरम्य: प्रथमो मदो हि ।।" (मा. नि.)

'In small doses, it produces a feeling of mental & physical wellbeing. Imagination becomes brighter, feeling elevated, intellect clearer, Senses more acute, bodily activity more predominant and some of the lower appetites sharpened.' (R. Ghosh)

9अव्यक्तबुद्धिस्मृतिवाग्विचेष्ट: सोन्मत्तलीलाकृतिरप्रशान्त: । आलस्यनिद्राभिहतो मुहुश्च मध्येन मत्त: पुरुषो मदेन ।। गच्छेदगम्यान्न गुरुंश्च मन्येत् खादेदभक्ष्याणि च नष्टसंज्ञ: । ब्रूयाच्च गुह्यानि हृदि स्थितानि मदे तृतीये पुरुषोऽस्वतन्त्र: । चतुर्थे तु मदे मूढो भग्नदार्विव निष्क्रिय: । कार्याकार्यविभागज्ञो मृतादप्यपरो मत: ।। (मा. नि.)
ऊप Law of primary stimulation & Subsequent depression.

9ओजस्यविहते पूर्वो हृदि च प्रतिबोधिते । मध्यमो विहतेऽल्पे च विहते तूत्तमो मद: ।।

Binz and his followers maintain that it first stimulates the nerve cells in the central nervous system and subsequently depresses them. The other view is that of Schmiedeberg. He holds that alcohol acts as a narcotic from the very commencement and the symptoms of stimulation are the effect of the depressant action on certain higher cerebral functions which normally exert a controlling influence. (R. Ghosh)

प्रधानावरमध्यानां रुक्मणां व्यक्तिदर्शक: । यथाग्निरेवं सत्त्वानां मद्यं प्रकृतिदर्शकम् ।।" (च. चि. २४) तस्मात् प्रथमद्वितीयतृतीयमदा: सत्त्वरजस्तमोभूयिष्ठानां क्रमेण भवन्ति । 9(मधुकोष) 9चिरेण श्लैष्मिके पूंसि पानतो जायते मद: । अचिराद्वातिके द्रष्ट: पैत्तिकेशीघ्रमेव तु ।।" (सू. सू. ४५)

21. प्रकर्षेण मथितुं स्त्रोतोभ्यो दोषसंचयं निर्हर्त्तुं शीलं यस्य तत् प्रमाथि ।"
निजवीर्येण यद् द्रव्यं स्त्रोतोभ्यो दोषसंचयम् ।
निरस्यति प्रमाथि स्यात्, तद्यथा मरिचं वचा ।।" (शा.)

22. अभिष्यन्दयति अवरुणद्धि क्लेदयति च स्त्रोतांसि इति अभिष्यन्दि ।"
अभिष्यन्दि दोषधातुमलस्त्रोतसां, क्लेदप्राप्तिजननम ।" (ड.)
पैच्छिल्याद् गौरवाद् द्रव्यं रुद् ध्वा रसवहा: सिरा: ।
धत्ते यद् गौरवं तत् स्यादभिष्यन्दि यथा दधि ।।" (शा.)

23. व्यवायी चाखिलं देहं व्याप्य पाकाय कल्प्यते ।" (सु.)
पूर्वं व्याप्याखिलं कायं तत: पाकं च गच्छति ।
व्यवायि तद्यथा भंगा फेनञ्चाहिसमुद् भवम् ।।" (शा.)

24. विकासी विकसन्नेव धातुबन्धान् विमोक्षयेत् ।"
सन्धिबन्धाँश्च शिथिलान् करोति हि विकासि तत् ।
विश्लिष्यौजश्च धातुभ्यो यथा क्रमुककोद्रवौ ।।" (शा.)

CHAPTER ELEVEN
MORPHOLOGY AND PROPERTIES

Various classes (gana) of medicinal plants

Ayurveda has divided plants in different classes depending upon their morphology, properties, actions, families, practical uses and similarities .

Among these some classes are as follows:-

Classes in which the roots of the plants are used -

Dashamoola- (bruhatpanchamoola and laghupanchamoola together form dashamoola) Dashamoola consists of ten roots of the plants viz. Aegle marmelos, Gmelina arboria, Premna integrifolia, Stereospermum suaveolens, Oroxylum indicum and Solanum xanthocarpum, solanum indicum, Desmodium gangeticum, Ureria picta, Tribulus terrestris.

The trees of bruhatpanchamoola are bigger in size.

This class of trees is laghu, bitter, astringent, little sweet, having pungent vipak and ushna veerya. It alleviates kapha and vata and improves appetite.

The trees of laghupanchamoola are smaller in size (shrubs). (They are described as a panchagana in Raj nighantu).

This class of trees is astringent, bitter, sweet, laghu and warm. It is a tonic, having an astringent, antipyretic and antiasthamatic propeties. It is lithotrypsic and alleviates vata and pitta.

Properties of dashamoola - It is tridoshaghna. It is useful in asthma, cough, headache, swelling, pyrexia, abdominal distension, costochondrial pains and distaste.

Dashamoola stands first in the drugs which alleviate vata and swelling. Use of dashamoolakwath or dashamoolarishta for basti (intra rectal administration of medicinal drugs) has a good action.

Kantakapanchamoola - (Class of five roots having thorns on their trees) Carissa congesta, Barleria prionitis, Tribulus terrestris, Asparagus racemosus and Zizyhpus sativus are called as Kantakapanchamoola because they bear thorns.

Properties - Alleviates kapha, haemorrhagic disorders, swelling, urinary disorders and sperm (semen) disorders.

(It is an experienced fact that these plants mainly have kapha alleviating activity).

Vallipanchamoola (Class of roots of five creepers) - Puerraria tuberosa, Hemidesmus indicus, Cryptolepis buchanana, Tinospora cordifolia and Momordia charentia are called as vallipanchamoola (valli = creeper).

The properties of this class are the same as kantakapanchamoola.

Trunapanchamoolaa (class of roots of five grasses) - Desmostachya pipinata, Saccharam spontaneum, Devanal, Darbha and Kandekshu are known as trunapanchamoola. (According to some Acharyas trunapanchamoola contains Desmostachya bipinala, Saccharum spontaneum, Saccharum officinarium, darbha and sugarcane).

As they are all grasses, they are called as trunapanchamoola.

Properties - Diuretic, alleviates pitta, cures dysuria and haemorrhagic disorders.

Madhyamapanchamoola - It consists of plants namely Sida cordifolia, Boerhavia diffusa, Ricinus communis, Gymnema sylvestrus and Phascolus mungo.

Properties - Alleviates kapha and vata. It is warm and laxative. It does not aggravate pitta.

Jeevanapanchamoola - It contains Asparagus racemosus, kakoli, Corchorus fascicularis, jivak and rushabhak. It is beneficial to eyes. It is aphrodisiac and alleviates vata and pitta.

Class of plants of which bark is used

Panchavalkala - Ficus bengalensis, Ficus racemosus, Ficus religiosa, Nevelia papulnea and Calamus tenuis are known as panchavalkala. These plants have latex.

Properties: It has astringent property and is very good in wound healing.

Plants which have latex (ksheer)

Ksheerivruksha - All the above 5 trees are known as ksheerivruksha.

Properties - Same as above.

Class of plants of which leaves are used

Panchpallava - Amra, jambu, mahalung, kawath and bilva. Leaves of these trees are used. (These leaves have specific odour and they are astringent).

Properties - These are used in conditions where actions of odour is expected.

Group of plants of which fruits are used

Triphala - Three fruits namely Terminalia chebula, Terminalia belerica and Emblica officinalis, in equal quantities are called as triphala. Some vaidyas say that these fruits should be measured in numbers like 1 fruit of Terminalia chebula, 2 of Terminalia belerica and 4 of Emblica officinalis should be taken. But this method also contributes same proportions. All three fruits of triphala should

Dhatus, like doshas, are present everywhere in the body including the skin. Ulcers in the mouth heal quickly and therefore this skin should be considered as rakta-dhatu-pradhan.

be used in a dried form. They are also called as kashayatriphala as these fruits are astringent to taste (kashaya = astringent).

Properties - Mainly astringent, rest 5 tastes are anurasa. Vipak - madhur (sweet), veerya - ushna (hot), triphala alleviates all the 3 doshas (haritaki - vataghna + bibheetaka - kaphaghna and amalaki - pittaghna). But being an astringent, triphala is effective in alleviating kapha and pitta. It is a mild laxative, improves digestion, acts on mansa dhatu, alleviates eye disorders, urinary disorders, blood disorders, dermatoses, vishamajwara and distaste. Ash of triphala is also effective in dermatoses and wounds. Being a good detoxifying and alleviating drug, it has a great importance in Ayurveda. Triphala is the best rasayana (rejuvenating drug). Because of its efficacy, it is also called as vara, uttama and shreshtha.

Trikatu - mixture of 3 pungent drugs namely Zingiber officinalis, Piper logum and Piper nigrum is called as tri-katu. (katu = pungent) (It is also called as vyosh).

Properties - Taste pungent, vipak - katu (pungent), ushna (hot) veerya, hence alleviates vata and kapha. It is used in asthma, cough, gulma, urinary disorders, obesity, meda disorders, filariasis and chronic rhinitis. Being diaphoretic, it stimulates the skin and is used in dermatoses.

It acts on respiratory, digestive and circulatory systems and medovaha srotas.

Trimada - Embelia ribes, Cyperus rotundus and Plumbago zeylanica = trimada. This class acts on digestive system.

Chaturushan - Ushan means hot (pungent). Zingiber officinalis, Piper nigrum, Piper longum (trikatu) + root of Piper longum = chaturushan.

Panchakola - Piper longum and its root, Piper officinarum, Plumbago zeylanica and Zingiber officinalis = Panchakola (Kola = Piper longum. Group in which Piper longum is mentioned first is called panchakola) or mixture of drugs taken in the same quantity ie. kola (1/2 karsha) is called as panchakola. Since all these five drugs are pungent (ushna), it is also called as 'panchoshna' (पंचोष्ण).

Shadooshana - Shadooshana is formed by adding Piper nigrum to panchakola. Because of unctuousness and madhur vipak of Piper longum and Zingiber officinalis, panchakola is also unctuous. But addition of Piper nigrum reduces its unctuousness and makes it more teekshna. Thus shadooshana becomes dry (ruksha) and also becomes more hot (ushna). It has an antidotal property by prabhav.

Properties - Useful in disorders induced by kapha and vata both and also in respiratory disorders.

Chaturbeeja - Powders of Trigonella foenum graecum, Lepidium sativum, Carum carvi and Trachispermum amami.

Properties - Alleviates vata by ushna veerya and useful in vata disorders, lateral chest pain,

In a mango fruit, the rasas change from kashaya to amla and madhur respectively. Through these changes prithvi mahabhoota remains unchanged and therefore mango is the bests parthiv dravya.

lumbar pain, indigestion, colicky pain and flatulence.

Jeevaniya Gana - जीवन्ती काकोल्यौ..... (वा.सू. अ. १५) - Harinkhuri, kakoli, ksheerakakoli, meda, mahameda, mudgaparni, mashaparni, jeevak, rushabhak and yashtimadhu.

Properites - Rejuvenating and restorative.

Amlapanchaka (Group of 5 sour drugs) - Amlavetas, jambeer, mahalunga(Citrus medica), naring (Citrus reticulata) and lemon are called amlapanchaka.

Rajnighantu has described different amlapanchaka as follows.

1) Badri (Ziziphus sativus), dalimb (Punica granatum), amsul (Garcinia indica), chuka (Rumex vesicarius) and amlavetas (Garcinia pedunculata).

2) Jambeer, narang (Citrus reticulata), amlavetas (Garcinia pedunculata), chincha (Temarindus indica) and mahalunga (Citrus medica).

Properties - Best appetizer, reduces excessive thirst.

Mahapanchavisha - Shrungik, kalkuta, mustak (Strychnos nux-vomica), vatsanabh (Aconitum ferox) and saktuk together form panchamahavisha.

Upavisha - Latex of ark (Calotripis procera), latex of nivdung (Euphorbia nerifolia), kalalavi (Gloriosa superba), kanher (Narium indicum), gunja (Abrus precatorius), aphoo (Papever somnifera) and dhatura (Dhattura stramonium) are seven upavisha.

Ashtavarga - Mixture of 8 drugs namely jeevak, rushabhak, meda, mahameda, kakoli, kshirakakoli, ruddhi and vruddhi form ashtavarga.

Properties - Rasa and vipak- madhur, sheeta veerya and guru hence it is aphrodisiac and tonic. It is restorative, helps in reunion of fractures, increases strength, helps in raktapitta, acts as a febrifuge and alleviates vata-pitta. It acts as a rasayana on mansa, meda, asthi and shukra dhatus.

Trijat - Mixture of tvak (Cinamonum zeylonica), laghu ela (Elletaria cardamomum) and tamalpatra (Cinnamomum tamal) forms trijat. (Jat = fragrance).

Properties - It has action on respiratory and digestive system.

Chaturjat - Chaturjat is formed by mixing of tvak (Cinamonum zeylonica), ela (Elletaria cardamomum), tamalpatra (Cinnamomum tamal) and nagkesar (Mesua ferrea).

Properties - Trijat and chaturjat both the groups are ruksha, teekshna, laghu and ushna veerya. They alleviate kapha and vata, aggravate pitta, improve appetite, enhance complexion and have an antidotal property. Because of their fragrance, they destroy bad breath and help to cleanse

Man has the capacity to excrete wastes through various apertures. Likewise, plants must also have excretory apertures.

the mouth. (त्रिजात + नागकेसर = चर्तुजात)

Panchatikta - Stalk of guduchi (Tinospora cordifolia), bark of neem (Azadirachta indica), leaves of vasa (Adhatoda vasica), whole plant of kantakari (Solanum xanthocarpum) and leaves of parval (Trichosanthes dioica) are collectively called panchatikta.

Properties - Deepan, febrifuge, alleviates raktapitta and cough.

Ksheerashtaka - Milk of cow, buffalo, sheep, goat, horse, elephant and woman are called as ksheerashtaka.

Mutrashtaka - Urine of animals namely sheep, goat, cow, buffalo, elephant, camel, horse and donkey is called as mutrashtaka.

Pittapanchaka - Bile of 5 animals viz fish, cow (or bull), horse, human being and peacock is called as pittapanchaka.

Lavanapanchaka - Saindhava, souvarchal, bidlon, samudra and sambarmeeth.

Kshardwaya - Sajjikshar and yavakshar.

Ksharashtaka - Kshar of palash (Butea frondosa), vajri (cactus), apamarg (Achyranthes aspera), chincha (Temarindus indica), ark (Calotropis procera), stalk of till (Sesamum indicum) and yavakshar + sajjikshar are collectively called ksharashtaka.

(The properties of the substances formed by combination of various substances are very difficult to determine because it is not as simple as solving a mathematical problem.)

A list useful for the study of medicinal plants

Vagbhattacharya has really done tremendous service to those who practice only Ayurvedic medicine. Vagbhattacharya must have foreseen the level of intellect of future generations and at the same time he must have also anticipated lack of hardwork in successive generations. He wrote his whole scripture in the form of aphorisms keeping his readers in mind, avoided highly philosophical discussions and made it as simple as possible through systematic classification. While saying this, I do not wish to under-rate scholars like Charaka and Sushruta, but Vagbhattacharya structured his scripture taking into consideration the changes of that era and the social set-up of the sixth century. Until recently, there were many vaidyas who memorised the whole scripture. Taking all this into consideration, he made this subject very easy for not only students but also other curious people by classifying all the available dravyas into various categories like audbhid, pranij, khanij etc. The same dravyas were then described as medicinal dravyas in the Chikitsa sthana. Thus, he has done a great service to vaidyas as well as students.

In the 40th chapter of Uttartantra, Vagbhatta has proposed an elaborate thought to decide which dravya should be used after arriving at a provisional or a confirmed diagnosis, but at the same

One wonders as to whether the idea of transplantation of body organs originated by observing grafting of plants.

time, he has also devoted the full 15th chapter of Sutra sthana to proper selection of dravyas. This is an advantage for all the students of Ayurveda. The list of dravyas should be refered to for selection only after one obtains a general idea of the doshas, dhatus, malas, samprapti and awastha. For this, he formed thirty- three groups which included almost all the conditions. He also provided the flexibility to all vaidyas to delete whichever dravya was unnecessary, use any dravyas which was found necessary and to substitute any unavailable dravya with another similar dravya.

These can be classified in the following manner. In this classification, due consideration has been given to the symptoms, diseases, dosha-dhatu-malas and srotas.

1) **Generalised bodyache** (rasagat) - vidaryadigana

2) **Loss of appetite** (rasagat) - guduchyadi, varanadi

3) **Burning sensation** (internal) - anjanadi

4) **Distaste** (rasagat) - patoladi, surasadi, shyamadi

5) **Internal abscess** - (doshas from rakta upto asthi) varanadi

6) **Calculus** (urinary system) - ushakadi, vellantaradi, mushkakadi,

7) **Diarrhoea** (caused by ama) (antarmarga, pureesh) - vachadi.

8) **Diarrhoea** (pakvamala, koshtha) - priyangwadi, ambashthadi, nyagrodadhi, rodhradi.

9) **Piles** (7th layer of skin, loss of appetite) - mushkakadi, vatsakadi,

10) **Urustambha** (shakhagat vata, kapha & meda) - varanadi, vachadi

11) **Urdhvashwas** (pran, rasa, udan) - vidaryadi

12) **Kapha** (from other parts) - arkadi, asanadi, aragwadhadi, ushakadi, guduchyadi, mushkakadi, patoladi, mustadi, vatsakadi, varanadi, vachadi, rodhradi, shyamadi, surasadi.

13) **Kapha and pitta** (in combination) - anjanadi

14) **Pruritus** (shakhagat kapha) - aragwadhadi, eladi

15) **Cough** (pran, udan, respiratory organs) - vidaryadi, surasadi

16) **Jaundice** (srotas (channels) of rakta & pitta) - patoladi

17) **Helminthiasis** (kapha, intestine) - asanadi, arkadi, surasadi,

18) **Dermatoses** (seven dushyas including kapha) - patoladi, aragwadhadi, asanadi, arkadi.

The individuals having vata, pitta and kapha prakriti or diseases should worship gods who are offered Aegle marmelos, Cynodon dactylon and Ocimum sanctum.

19) **Koth** (rasagat kapha) - eladi.

20) **Gulma** (vata aggravation) - vidaryadi, varanadi, ushakadi, mushkakadi, vatsakadi, shyamadi

21) **Vomiting** (gastric irritation) - anjanadi, guduchyadi, aragwadhadi.

22) **Pyrexia** (rasa, pitta, sweda) - sarivadi, patoladi, guduchyadi, aragwadhadi, vatsakadi.

23) **Polydysia** (kloma, vata, pitta) - sarivadi, parushakadi, guduchyadi, nyagrodhadi.

24) **Tushti** (rasa, mind, heart) - padmakadi, jeevaniya

25) **Burning Sensation** (ushna pitta) - sarivadi, guduchyadi, nyagrodhadi.

26) **Nasya** (above jatru) - velladi

27) **Anaemia** (alparakta, alpameda, dhatushaithilya) - asanadi, mushkakadi.

28) **Pitta** (sarvamargag) - durvadi, nyagrodhadi, sarivadi, shaliparni, prushniparni, kamal,bhadramotha, anjanadi, patoladi, guduchyadi, priyangwadi, ambashtadi.

29) **Chronic rhinitis** (tridosha, urdhwamarg) - vatasakadi

30) **Pimples / Boils** - eladi

31) **Anabolic** (mansagami) - padmakadi, jeevaniya

32) **Rhinitis** (aggravation of vata) - surasadi

33) **Prameha** (meda, mansa, kleda, mutra, basti, drava kapha) - parushakadi, aragwadhadi, asanadi.

34) **For basti** - madankutajadi

35) **For weight gain** (mansa) - vidaryadi

36) **Malapachana** (all) - mustadi

37) **Urine sugar** - vellantaradi

38) **Renal calculi** - ushakadi, vellantaradi, mushkakadi

39) **Dysuria** - parushakadi, ushakadi, vellantaradi, shyamadi,

40) **Oliguria** - vellantaradi

41) **Obesity** (meda, kapha) - asanadi, varanadi, ushakadi, rodhradi, nyagrodhadi, arkadi, surasadi, mushkakadi, vatasakadi, vachadi.

Sushrutacharya did not divide the year into seasons on the basis of Hindu calender. Rather, it was divided on climatic conditions.

42) **Vaginal disorders** - rodhradi, mustadi, nyagrodhadi.

43) **Raktagami** - jeevaniya, padmakadi.

44) **Haemorrhagic disorders** - sarivadi, nyagrodhadi

45) **Emetic** (stomach, kapha, pitta) - madanadi.

46) **Complexion enhancer** (rakta) - rodhradi, eladi

47) **Vata disorders** - bhadradarvadi, veertaradi, vellantaradi, vatasakadi, vidaryadi, parushakadi.

48) **Vata, pitta** - vidaryadi, padmakadi, jeevaniya.

49) **Vata-kapha** - eladi

50) **Purgative** (pitta) - nikumbhadi

51) **Poison** - anjanadi, patoladi, aragwadhadi, rodhradi, arkadi, eladi, shyamadi

52) **Aphrodisiac** - padmakadi, jeevaniya.

53) **Ulcers** (infective) - aragwadhadi, arkadi, surasadi

54) **Wound healing** -priyangwadi, ambashthadi, nyagrodhadi

55) **Headache** (rakta) - varanadi

56) **Pain** (colicky) - vatasakadi

57) **Pthysis** (mansa) - vidaryadi

58) **Asthma** - surasadi

59) **Leucoderma** (skin) - asanadi

60) **Shukranashan** - mushkakadi

61) **Sandhaniya** - priyangwadi, ambashthadi, nyagrodhadi (rasa), vachadi, mustadi

62) **Purifying lactation** (rasa) - vachadi, mustadi

63) **Galactogogue** (rasa) - padmakadi, jeevaniya

64) **Cardiotonic** (rasa, rakta, marma) - vidaryadi.

The remedies mentioned above possess gamitva on the srotasas which are vitiated by the respective diseases. Their vibrations are generated directly or through a chain of events.

As we are ignorant about the man who is getting treated, in the same manner, we are ignorant about the medicine.

CHAPTER TWELVE
NOMENCLATURE AND SYNONYMS OF DRAVYAS

The derivation of synonyms

It is essential to obtain complete knowledge about the food or medicinal dravyas made up of panchmahabhootas. Charakcharya mentions three facets for this purpose, namely - name, appearance and properties.[1] The first aspect is name and /or synonyms. One dravya carries many names, differently mentioned in the regional languages. Charakacharya also insists that one acquire the knowledge of plants from the shepherd, hunter, nomadic tribes etc. Even today, all these sources of the names, appearance and properties of plants enrich the science of dravyaguna. This is however, not sufficient.

In earlier times, modern scientific methodology was not available for the identification of a dravya. During that period there was only one method. Each plant had many synonyms. Therefore the plant fulfilling the meanings of maximum synonyms was decided upon without any doubt. For example, the identity of Achyranthes aspera (apamarga), also known as shikhari, kharamanjari, kinihi, adhahshalya, shaikhirika, pratyakpushpee and mayurak, can be confirmed after studying all the synonyms attributed to it.

There is a definite basis for these synonyms. Once the method of attributing these synonyms is understood, it becomes easy to recognise the plants. Synonyms of the plants were based on their structure, source, habitat, season, properties and actions, customs, organs, routine use, perception by the senses and historical importance.

The details are as follows -

Names and synonyms of the plants

Shape - Chhatra, karnikar, chaturangul, deerghaphala, gokshur, trivrutta, dronapushpi, danti, karshaphala, kana, shalparni, prushniparni, anshumati, adhahshalya, anantmoola, vishanika, saptachakra, aksha, chakralakshana, sharapunkha, shunyamadhya, sanvarta, utkantaka, kundalini, kutil, kurchasheershak, kshudra jambu, golmaricha, granthil, triputa, trikonaphala, deerghavrunt, netropamaphala, prasarani, mrudangaphala, trikantak, akashvalli, tilpushpak, ajashrungi, atibrihatphala, adhahpushpi, panchangul, kandaguduchi.

Terrestrial and aquatic - Jalaj, dhanvayas, haimavatee, kutaj, pashanbhed, upkulya, ambuja, kamal, akashvel, vrikshadani, ambuvasini, ambhoruha, aranyakarpasi, girij, giriparpat, jalakumbhi, jalajbrahmi, nadisarja, neerbhrahmi, pankeruha, bhuiringani, bhumyamalaki, vriksharuha etc.

Habitat - Vaidehi, dravidi, nepali, saurashtri, turushka, balhik, paraseek, yavani, kababchinee, chopchinee, kambojee, kashmari, kalinga, khorasani, ajawan, gujrati, marathi, dweepantarvacha,nepalidhaniya, parseek vacha, marubhuruha, malayavacha, magdhi, upkulya,

If we grow a tree like teak, in exchange it gives us approximately 15 lacs 70 thousand rupees in the form of dravyagunakarma (Dr. Das).

kumari.

Taste - Patramla, tikta, katvi, amlika, kashaya, amalaparni, pancharasa, rason, kiratatikta, madhuyashthi, ambuti, atimadhuram, amlavetas, ushna, kadunimba, kadujeere, kadubhopala, kadukavitha, tiktak, tiktashak, gudashakari, swaduphala, swadukantak, swadukanda, swaduparni.

Smell - Ashwagandha, vidarigandha,ugragandha, vitkhadir, gandhaprasarani, ajagandhika, kushthagandhini, gandhaphali, gandhamarjar, gandhapushpa, gandhapriyangu, gandhabola, gandhadhya, ghrandukhada, teekshnagandha, padmagandhi, patalagandhi, putikaranja, putiphali, hridyagandha, ajagandha.

Appearance - Peetmula, peetyuthika, peetshala, peetvriksha, peelanagkeshar, krishna, peeta, peetdaru, peetdugdha, peetpushpa, raktachandan, kapila, raktaniryas, rajvriksha, jyotishmati, haridra, agnishikha, angarvriksha, kanchanakshiri, swarnakshiri, kaladana, kalikhajuri, kalabola, kalakasturi, kalimiri, krishnabeeja, krishnavrunta, krishnasara, krishnaguru, shahjeera, saptarangi, sitchhatra, safedahaldi, safedamusali, safedajeera, chitrapatra, nagavalli, tamrapushpi, tamrapallav, dhumrapatra, neeli, pandurdrum, haridruh, hemadugdhika, agnishikha, angarvriksha, karnikar.

Touch - Dusparsha, khajkuhili, namaskari, himahva

Sound - Khatkhati

Leaf - Saptaparna, anghriparna, apatra, amlapatrika, asipatra, uttampatrak, udumbarparni, asitparni, ksharpatra, kharpatra, tamrapallav, tilparni, triparni, darvipatra, patraddhya, parnabeeja, parnayavani, pruthakparni, bahuptra, balapatra, bhadraparni, madhuparni, snigdhapatra, surabhichhada, sukshmapatra, hingupatri, madhucchada, mahapatra, mashaparni, mriducchada, yugmaptra, rampatri, vishamacchada, lomashparni, variparni, shatapatri, shalaparni, shurpaparni, sahastrapatra, karkashacchada, tailaparna.

Flower - Samlapushpa, suchipushpa, sthirapushpa, kritamala, naktamala, swarnat, tilpushpak, shatapushpa, shankhapushpi, adhahpushpi, kumbhipushpi, kharamanjiri, gudapushpa, tilpushpi, neelpushpa, prasthapushpa, pratyakpushpa, mridupushpa, raktapushpa, lohitpushpak, vakrapushpa, vrittapushpa etc.

Fruits - Anshumataphala, atibruhatphala, atmagupta, avartaphala, karshaphala, erandphala, kantakiphala, krishnaphala, granthiphala, pruthushimbi, tulaphala, deerghaphala, drudhaphala, pindaphala, brihatphala, mahaphala, raktaphala, rekhaphala, sthirphala etc.

Historical names - Bodhidruma, arjuna, indravaruni, indrayava, indragopa, indrayani, ishwari, ishwarmula, aindree, kuberakshi, gandharvahasta, gopakanya, gopi, chhotachand, chandrashur, shashankrekha, chandrika, tapaswini, tapodhana, devkanchan, devdangari, devtada, devdar, devdhup, devanala, naradhindi, brahmavriksha, bheemsenikapur, shakradruh, seetaphala, ramphala, somarajee, harasingar etc.

Just as in sthoola sharir, in the finest molecules of sukshma sharir, there are koshthas, shakhas and madhyam margas - one should consider these.

Therapeutic description - Kushthaghni, putrada, vyadhighat, ashmaghna, ashmantak, ashmabhit, kasamarda, kasari, kushthavairi, gandari, dadrughna, vishvabheshaj, shvitrabheshaj, krumighna, aragvadha.

Disease producing - Arushkar, rechani, kalalavi, kalidruma, kupeelu, keshahantri.

Health promoting - Abhaya, arogyashimbi, avyatha, vayastha, pranada, vyadhighat.

Body parts - Asthishrunkhala, asthisamhari, amashayaphala, kesharuha, kesharanjan, dantacchada, dantashatha, dantashodhan, panchangul, chaturangul, pittapapada, mukhapriya, pleehaghna, pleehashatru, mansarohini, shishubhaishajya, hadjodi, anganapriya, yoshitpriya.

Resembling animals - Mayurshikha, hansapadi, hansaraj, shikhigreeva, neel kantha, gavajban, gojivha, goroohan, gostani, golomi, gavakshi, godanti, vyaghranakhi, vaghati, vyaghrapuccha, mahishaksha, dhorgunja, ajamoda, chhagantri, ajagandha, ajabala, ajavayan, ajashringi, meshalochan, medhashingi, ashwakarna, ashwagandha, ashwamarak, ghodavaj, vajidanta, hayamar, ghunapriya, ghunavallabha, ahiphena, nagbala, khadyanag, nagdaman, shukanasa, kinshuk, shukpriya, nagkeshar, sarpagandha, nakuli, pashumehankarika, pishachkarpas, vatsadani, dukkarkanda, kapikacchu, kapeetan, kokilakshak, keetmari, bharadwaji, alarka, gandhamarjar, bidalaksha, matsyashakala, manduki, undirkani, bedaki, edagaj, gajpippali, gajvajipriya, gajakarni, krimija, kaktundi, kaknasa, kakmachi, kaktinduk, kawli, sinhasya, sinhamukhi, shrugalvinna, kuleervishanika.

Calotropis procera (arka) is named after sun, Plumbago zeylanica (chitraka) is named after agni (fire), Cyperus rotundus (nagarmotha) is named after clouds while Nelumbo nucifera (kamal) is named after water.

The popular vernacular names of many plants are distorted versions of their original sanskrit names. Nomenclature of plants is a subject of study and knowledge as well as of entertainment. Every name is meaningful and points to some aspects of properties and morphology of the plant. Similarly, a single name can indicate three or four different plants e.g. amruta which indicates Tinospora cordifolia, Papaver somniferum as well as Terminalia chebula.

This confusion can be overcome only by accepting the modern method of standardisation which is universal because it is based on appearance and on histological characteristics. This method is useful in ascertaining the name and appearance of the plants. Rajnighantukar was aware of this fact and that is why he stressed the importance of the word peefleefuebiewë(classification). Synonyms are not sufficient to ascertain the appearance thus leading to confusion. Therefore the classification based on histological description of a plant must be accepted. It is very important to classify and name a dravya or a plant by some method which is universally accepted. It will certainly not be detrimental, but on the contrary it will help to enrich Ayurveda. Charakacharya has already described the triplet of name, appearance and properties for classification. The first two i.e. name and appearance along with inclusion of synonyms described in Ayurveda for dravyas will enrich this ancient science. The gunas of dravyas can be studied by Ayurvedic method independently.

In place of a single dravya, if there is a combination of many dravyas, then not only the dravyas change but consequently rasa, veerya and vipak also change.

Ecology

Ayurveda has classified land into anoop (marshy), jangal (arid) and sadharan (intermediate between anoop and jangal).

Appearance and properties of plants are affected by the nature of the land. Therefore ecology is an important factor and has its own significance.

Anoopdesha - This kind of land consists of more water, more vegetation, less heat and mild windy air. Diseases are prevalent in this type of land and therefore it is considered to be bad. People of this region have kapha or kaphavata predominant in their constitution. Also watery or marshy vegetation grows abundantly with large leaves and short stature.

Jangaldesha - This type of land consists of less water, less vegetation, less rainfall with bright sunshine and strong wind. The constitution of the people in this region is predominantly vata-pitta. Tall plants like catechu and babool having small leaves with astringent property are found in abundance. Healthwise, the region is better since less diseases occur endemically.

Sadharandesha - In this region, the characters of anoop and jangaldesha are in a mixed proportion. Considering doshas, the constitution is average and health is also maintained in a better state.

Optimal timing for usage

There is a limitation for the development of every food and medicinal plant. Time consideration is important for plants. Any plant unless fully grown and completely developed, does not acquire its attributes of properties and actions. Properties and actions mentioned in the books are those of the mature plants. Immature plants, if used, do not show the desired effects. Some drugs mature in summer, some in winter and rest in the rainy season. Flowering and fruiting makes the plant rich in its properties.

Latex of a plant should be collected before sunrise. Milky juice of cactus is never collected before the plant is two to three years old. Consideration of time for such collection methods is important. To observe the effect of a drug on the body, every second, minute, hour, morning, afternoon, evening, month, year etc. are considered. Similarly in the patient, various stages of digestion like aam, semidigestion, full digestion, prerigor stage, pyretic stage etc. are also important.

Drugs - their collection and preservation

Ayurveda has considered that all the drugs are made up of five elements (ie. panchamahabhootas).

Substanaces of any use, medicinal or dietary, are intimately related to the type of land in which they are produced. Therefore, due consideration should be given to the type of land ie. soil. Land, which ultimately determines the guna-karmas of dravyas produced in it, is classified into five types.

Among the three and half lacs plants identified, only two thousand plants are medicinal plants and out of these, fifteen hundred are in Konkan area (Sawant).

Though soil is panchamahabhautik, its composition in relation to individual mahabhootas varies at different places hence the change in properties and actions.

Parthiv - This type of soil containing stones is hard, black, with tall trees and grass.

Aapya - This soil is clayey, cold, containing water source, white in colour, grassy and soft to touch.

Tejas - This soil is of different colours, full of small stones, brownish white coloured and grassy.

Vayaveeya - Dry, ash coloured, trees scattered, dry, hollow and grassy.

Akasheeya - This soil is soft but uneven, water tasteless, trees of useless varieties, large mountains, and blackish colour.

Soil and water are responsible for the formation of rasas just as panchamahabootas form various dravyas. Herbs, shrubs and climbers continously ingest water. Water is devoid of rasa but it is expressed in climbers and plants because of contact with the soil. Therefore soil and environment become important factors while considering the dravyas.

As all the medicinal dravyas from various sources are related to soil, its study for fertility and usefulness becomes essential.

Infertile land - Uneven pits, deep trenches, collection of dirty and waste water, heaps of ant hills, funeral places, temples and desert land are indicative of infertile land.

Fertile land - Land having even surface, saltless, near pond or lake, where grass grows, soft, black, white or red colour, without cultivation, containing only medicinal plants and no other vegetation, jangal and sadharan land is considered to be fertile.

The possibility of undergound gold, silver, iron or copper can be judged by the habitat and growth of plants in that region. It is also rational to think that the same gunas aquired from the metals into the plants would be useful as medicine. The presence of Ficus racemosa tree indicates an underground water source. (Discovery of Varahamihir is useful in this direction.)

Which drugs should be preserved?

Drugs need preservation for future use in treatment. They should be easily available. A drug used as medicine should not come in contact with bacteria, insects, poison, instruments, smoke, sunshine, air, fire and water. Plants with deep and thick roots, fulfilling the essential properties of rasa, guna, colour, smell and proportion and plants grown in favourable season are suitable for proper preservation and treatment of diseases.

In India, the Himalayas lie towards the north and there is a belief that moon, which is the guardian of the north, is the ruler of plant kingdom. Therefore, plants grown in the Himalayas and in

Mere touch of Gloriosa superba by a woman immediately after her delivery helps to expel placenta due to induction of uterine contractions.

the northern region are considered of the best quality and their use is advocated.

The use of Tinospora cordifolia, Asparagus racemosus and Herpestis moniera are advocated in fresh form and therefore should not be preserved.

Honey, Piper longum and Embelia ribes should be used after preserving these for one year. This time is required for their maximum efficacy.

Method of drug preservation

For collecting the plants grown in suitable soil as mentioned above, a person should pluck or uproot the plant after a bath wearing white clothes, mind stabilised by reciting shlokas, praying to gods, Ashwinikumaras, cow, brahmin and faithfully facing the north or east direction. East indicates vitalising the plant energy through the sun and north is the symbol of the moon, the ruler of plants. Similarly, regarding time, pushya nakshatra, ashwin nakshatra and mriga nakshatra are considered to be superior. Moon being the ruler of pushya and mriga nakshatra, it (moon) transfers its properties into the plant during these nakshatras. Ashwini nakshatra is considered because Ashwinikumars are the rulers of this nakshatra. This must be related to aptopadesha (experience and advice of ancestors, the former generation). (Modern science is trying to co-relate this with the help of experiments).

'The Secret Life of Plants' written by Peter Topkins and Cristopher Bird is a very valuable book. Some of the chapters are worth studying, like grasping senses of the plants, uses of plants, ants sensing the human mind, hormonal life of plants, plants and electromagnets, force fields, humans and plants, plant and human aura, similarity in chemical composition of soil, humans and plants, effects of the mind on panchamahabhootas etc. The book is recommended for its overall study on the scientific background of plant biology. Anyone going to pluck a plant should have a dialogue with the plant on the previous day. The book also solves the mystery of their expression of anger, needs, satiety etc.

Just as man is controlled by cosmos, plants are also under the influence of the cosmos. Therefore the study of environment for their preservation is essential. Plants collected in the rainy season always tend to perish, therefore rainy season is unsuitable for preservation. Also perennial plants are immature in their rasas during rainy season. Generally, some are plucked at the end of winter and some at the end of autumn since they are fully enriched with their rasas.

Specific period of preservation

While preserving the plant, its useful parts should also be given due importance. Generally, the part or the specific portion which is considered for use, must grow to full maturity. Charakacharya, from his experiences, has mentioned different periods for preserving specific useful parts.

According to Raj nighantu - Tuber - hemant; root - shishir; flower - vasant; leaves - greeshma and panchang - sharad.

According to some other acharyas: root - pravrutt; leaves - varsha; bark - sharad; latex -

Two types of opposite vibrations are produced by the proximity of persons whom you like and dislike. In the proximity of plants why should not such vibrations be produced?

hemant; juice - vasant and fruit - greeshma.

Useful parts		Period
Branches	:	Rainy season or autumn (time for full growth of a plant)
Leaves	:	Rainy season or autumn (in between the flowering and fruiting of the plant).
Root	:	Summer or winter (shedding of old leaves and the appearance of the new ones.)
Bark Tuber Latex	:	End of summer or the beginning of winter. Latex of Calotropis procera to be collected at the beginning of summer
Sar (Juice)	:	End of winter.
Flower Fruit	:	Blossom and fruiting period of the specific plants.

Veerya in drug procurement

Above mentioned seasonal view may not be useful while considering veerya. Instead of considering specific parts in specific season for drug collection, due importance should be given to its veerya. Sheeta veerya drugs which possess madhur, snigdha and sheeta gunas should be collected during visarga kala while ushna veerya drugs which posssess tikta, ruksha and ushna properties must be collected in adan kala.

Consideration of karma in drug procurement

Similar to veerya, consideration of the action of a drug is also important. To bring about effective purgation, the drug must be collected from the soil containing prithvi and jala mahabhootas which have a tendency to move downwards. Similarly, for emesis, the drug should be collected from soil predominantly containing agni and vayu mahabhootas which tend to move upwards. Drug acting for both the purposes (e.g. deodangari) must be collected from the soil containing akash mahabhoota so that the expected action is achieved.

Sharangdhar mentions that for emetic and purgative action, the drug should be collected at the end of vasant ritu and for rest of the actions, in the sharad ritu, but the best period is when they are enriched with their rasas.

Collection of dietary items

Food contains different parts of plants like fruit, tuber, seed, panchang etc. Sushruta has laid down the following guidelines -

Taking up and giving up, these two functions occur in body and mind. The pair of "prana-apan" has this responsibility.

Fruits - Only ripe (not raw or over ripe) fruits are collected. The exception is Aegle marmelos which is collected in a raw form which is very effective (therefore called shalatu). Fruits, which are diseased, insect affected, untimely grown, affected by fire or cold or artificially ripened are not to be collected.

Vegetables - Over ripe, worms and insect affected, spoilt, grown in dirty soil, untimely, tasteless and dried vegetables should not be collected (exception is radish). Vegetables which are soft, mature, unspoilt, grown in proper season and soil and are wet, are advocated for consumption.

Kanda (Tuber) -Tubers which are raw, untimely grown, old, diseased and eaten by insects should be discarded. They should be well nourished, timely grown, and pest free.

Cereals - Cereals which are affected by too much heat or cold, fire, poisonous gases, insect affected, wet, grown in unsuitable soil, untimely, with other cereals and valueless should be discarded and those of suitable quality must be collected.

Collection of drugs of animal origin

Similar consideration must be given to the collection of drugs of animal origin. Animals from whom blood, hair or nails are to be collected, must be fully grown. (These animals mature at 1/4th the age of the total life span of the species. This span varies with different species.) Similarly, milk, urine etc. of animals should be collected after complete digestion of their food.

Preservation of drugs

After collection of the drug as mentioned above, preservation and protection is equally important. Otherwise the drugs once spoiled cannot be used in treatment. For this reason, the drugs in the store room must be protected from wet soil, dust, water, fire, smoke, dirt, vapours, rats, cockroaches, ants, flies etc. Even the containers like vessels, jars, drums etc. must be such that they will not affect the rasa, properties and actions of the drugs.

Efficacy of sheeta veerya drugs increases if kept in cold storage or refrigerator. At least it will not decrease. In olden days, such medicines were kept in earthen pots, coconut kernel, covering of hard fruits and brass vessels. But now many varieties of containers are available where it can be protected in a better way.

Storage of medicines

Sushruta has mentioned in the 37th chapter of Sutra sthana of a store house for the protection of medicinal drugs. Store house should be clean and open towards north or east for better ventilation. An open north side helps to provide light but prevents direct sunshine. Besides these natural provisions, fragrant flowers, latex of sal tree, light, offerings, spray of insecticides etc. should be provided to prevent bacterial growth. Store house should be equipped with cloth bags of best quality and earthen pots made of suitable soil. It should also have wooden drums, racks, cupboard, and kegs where rain water is prevented from entering. Store house should be adequately ventilated and special

The best (or ideal) medicine is that which gives sound health and the best doctor is the one who gives relief from the disease.

provision be made to prevent the entry of mice, rats, cockroaches, lizards, scorpions, ants, etc. An underground store house is more safe.

Every container for storing the medicines must be properly labelled as to name, place of origin, date of manufacture of drug and have a proper lid. Poisonous medicines must be kept in a separate cupboard and container labelled as poison in red ink. Dry, solid medicines are kept on the upper shelves and the liquids on the lower shelves. Medicine without batch numbers or labels should be discarded.

Potency period of the drug

The main aim of collection and preservation of the drug is to maintain its potency by conserving its properties and actions. Even the best selected and protected medicine loses its effectiveness after a certain period. Generally they are potent for one year. Therefore a proper label giving the date of manufacture, batch number and the expiry date must be attached.

The successful preservation of drugs depends on air, changing seasons, container and packaging. Then the potency of a drug will be preserved for a longer period. Sunshine, humid air, rainy season, torn or open container immediately depotentiate the drug, making it ineffective.

Preservaton of fresh and dried drug specimens

Different methods are followed for preserving dry and green plants. This is useful for identification.

Leaves of the plant in intact condition must be pressed between two sheets of blotting paper to absorb humidity. Then they must be stuck or stitched to the paper, treated with liquid hydrogen-perchloride or dipped in gelatine and then dried. This process helps preservation for a longer period.

Better than this method is the preparation of megaslides. It maintains the natural colour, appearance and shape of the specimen and hence it is more suitable.

This process is as follows :-

Method of preserving the specimen of plants in natural state

(Dr. Mrs.Shyamalatai Chitale's Technique)

(1) Branch of a tree or a creeper bearing leaves and flowers or small sprout with the primary root is collected and immediately dipped for 5 minutes in the mixture mentioned below. If the flowers and leaves are too delicate for the mixture then the sample must be sprinkled with the mixture and then spread on blotting paper for 1-2 hours under pressure. The mixture is prepared by 5 to 10 gms. of tannin powder dissolved in 500 ml of water, boiled and filtered and preserved in glass or stainless steel container or jar with a tight lid.

(2) 10 gm. of camphor and 10 gm. of menthol are mixed with equal quantity of castor oil and kerosene to make up to one litre. Camphor and menthol take 10-15 minutes to dissolve uniformly in the mixture. The solution should be applied to a paper with the help of a brush and then spread over the sample. Another paper is kept on the sample after spreading it with the mixture. Then the sample is wrapped between the two papers. A hot iron is used to dry the sample by pressing the upper paper which is removed repeatedly to test the dryness of the sample. Then it is transfered between the cloth fold and again a hot iron press is used to absorb the remaining moisture by the cloth. Left over solution makes the sealing of the sample in a polythene bag, difficult.

(3) A sample prepared in the manner described above is sealed in a polythene bag. For the process, a sample is kept between two polythene sheets of required thickness and then transferred between the folds of the cloth bag. A hot iron press is applied over the cloth. The two polythene papers stick together because of the pressure and heat applied. While sealing the polythene bag, it is repeatedly observed that excess of heat is prevented which may burn or wrinkle the polythene bags. Practice, experience and a use of proper hot press makes the sealing optimum.

Principles of this method and its advantages

(a) Tannic acid is the best preservative of the colour, even then, excess of acid may change the colour. For example, the colour of Hibiscus rosa sinensis changes from red to violet. Many times citric acid is used along with tannic acid to preserve the red colour. Application of lemon juice over the hibiscus flower for 3-4 minutes induces dehydration and preserves the red colour of the flower.

(b) Pressure and artificial heat of the hot press dehydrates the sample rapidly . Infiltration of this oily mixture helps to preserve and protect the colour of the plants. Oily mixture also makes the sample transparent for examination of the internal structures as well as protect it from insects and fungus.

(c) Oil mixture makes the sample soft and elastic. Sealed polythene bag protects it from becoming friable and also makes it easier to observe the sample from both, dorsal and ventral surfaces. This transparent sample can be better studied under the microscope. Overall, it helps to identify the sample in an easy way.

(By Courtesy of Dr. Sau. Shyamalatai Chitale)

Chitale technique is the best modern preservative method to study plants. Even then the old method of preservation should be known and was as follows :-

Collected fresh and wet leaves after cleaning and drying were kept between two sheets of blotting paper under pressure in a frame. Humidity is absorbed by the blotting paper and the required aeration is given by opening the press intermittently. Wet paper is also changed frequently.

By this process, the sample dries. Subsequently it can be glued or tied to drawing paper.

In the ancient science of Ayurveda, prasanuprasas, vyaprajokti, vyangokti etc. are used liberally.

Before this process, it is treated with a solution of 1:1000 hydrogen perchloride to protect it from insects, mites and fungus.

In this method, even after following all the precautions, the natural colour fades and gets spoiled by air after some days. Rainy season is not suitable for preservation by this method as no precaution can prevent fungal growth in this season. Best season is between October and June.

The process of preservation of fresh plants

Green wet plants dipped in 5-10% formalin in an air tight jar remains for many years in the original form which can be used for identification of the plant. For medicinal use, these plants are incorporated in formulations which are based on honey, oil or ghee. Fruits and vegetables are preserved in air-tight jars. Wet plants can be preserved in polythene bags for a long duration (needs scientific research).

While preserving fresh powders or tablets, the old ones must be discarded completely to prevent the danger of using non-effective drugs. Wet and fresh vegetables can be preserved for 7-8 days in air-tight plastic bags.

Method of measuresments

Etymology of the word 'maan' - The method by which a substance is weighed or measured is called maan ie. weights and measures.

The knowledge of weights and measures is useful for two reasons -

(1)Weights and measures are essential for the mixing of different drugs in a definite ratio. (2) In the treatment of a patient, maintenance of health and relief of suffering, the prescribing of medicine needs detailed consideration of a patient's constitution, age, sex, weight, stage of disease, strength, dushya, time or duration (kala), country, tolerance, agni, acceptability, diet etc. Achievement of both or either is impossible without the knowledge of weights and measures.

In ancient literature, three methods of measurements are mentioned :-

1) Pautavmaan - Measures of weights - Medicines are suitable for weighing.

2) Druvayamaan - Solids or liquids having volume are measured by this method.

3) Payyamaan - Measure of length - Substances having length, breadth, height and depth are measured by this method.

In this modern period, decimal method in terms of metre, litre, gram and kilogram is used commercially.[2] Eventhough, the knowledge of ancient method will help to study these concepts for comparison.

Charaka has not included human urine in the classification of eight types of urine eventhough it has been found to be very effective. What is the reason behind it?

Comparative study of the ancient and modern methods

Measure of weight

Sushruta method

1 Dhanyamasha	=	1/2 ratti.
12 Dhanyamasha (Medium size black gram.)	=	1 Suvarnamasha (6 ratti = 1 aana)
16 Suvarnamasha	=	1 Suvarnakarsha = 96 Ratti - 1 Tola.
11 Nishpav (Medium size beans)	=	1 Dharana.
2 1/2 Dharana	=	1 Karsha = 1 Tola.
4 Karsha	=	1 Pal = 4 Tolas
4 Pal	=	1 Kudav = 16 Tolas.
4 Kudav	=	1 Prastha = 64 Tolas.
4 Prastha	=	1 Aadhak = 256 Tolas = 3 Sher 16 Tolas.
4 Aadhak[3]	=	1 Drona = 12 Sher 64 Tolas.
100 Pal[4]	=	1 Tula = 400 Tolas = 5 Sher
20 Tula	=	1 Bhar = 100 Sher.

This measurement scale is for dry drugs. Wet drugs are taken in double the quantity with the exception of the usual freshly used drugs like Tinospora cordifolia, Holarrhena antidysentrica Adhatoda vasika, Benincasa hispid, Withania somnifera, Barleria prionitis, Viola odorata and Paederi foetida.

In measurement of length according to Charakacharya, the smallest particle seen in sun rays entering through the small hole in the windowpane is called vanshi or dhwanshi. This is considered as one unit.

6 Vanshi	=	1 Marichi
6 Marichi	=	1 Sarshapa
8 Sarshapa	=	1 Tandul
2 Tandul	=	1 Dhanyamasha
2 Dhanyamasha	=	1 Yava = 1/2 Ratti.
4 Yava	=	1 Andika (2 Ratti)

Altogether fifty-one types (classes) of dravyas are used e.g. 19 animal (jangam)), 18 flowering and fruiting plants (audbhid) and 14 - inorgnic (parthiv).

4 Andika	=	1 Mashak (8 Ratti)
3 Mashak	=	1 Shana (24 Ratti = 1/4th Tola)
2 Shana[5]	=	1 Kola (48 Ratti = 1/2 Tola)
2 Kola	=	1 Karsha (96 Ratti = 1 Tola)
2 Karsha	=	1 Shukti (2 Tolas)
2 Shukti	=	1 Pala (4 Tolas)
2 Pala	=	1 Prasrut (8 Tolas)
2 Prasrut	=	1 Kudav (16 Tolas)
2 Kudav	=	1 Manika (32 Tolas)
2 Manika	=	1 Prastha (64 Tolas)
2 Prastha	=	1 Aadhak (256 Tolas = 3 Sher 16 Tolas)
4 Aadhak	=	1 Drona (1024 Tolas = 12 Sher 64 Tolas)
2 Drona	=	1 Shurpa (2048 Tolas = 25 Sher 48 Tolas)
2 Shurpa	=	1 Khari (4096 Tolas = 51 Sher 16 Tolas)
32 Shurpa	=	1 Vaha (65536 Tolas = 819 Sher 16 Tolas)

Measurment of weight according to Sharangadhar (Magadhamaan) is done taking 'parmanu' as the unit. Charaka has a smaller unit than Sushruta while Sharangadhar has the smallest unit.

30 Molecules	=	1 Vanshi
6 Vanshi	=	1 Marichi
6 Marichi	=	1 Rajika
3 Rajika	=	1 Sarshap
8 Sarshap	=	1 Yava
4 Yava	=	1 Gunja (Ratti)
6 Ratti	=	1 Mashak
4 Mashak	=	1 Shana (1/4th Tola)
2 Shana	=	1 Karsha (1 Tola)
2 Shukti	=	1 Pala (4 Tolas)
2 Pala	=	1 Prasruti (8 Tolas)
2 Prasruti	=	1 Kudav (16 Tolas)
2 Kudav	=	1 Manika (= Sharav = 32 Tolas)
2 Sharav	=	1 Prastha (64 Tolas)
4 Prasthak	=	1 Aadhak (256 Tolas = 3 Sher 16 Tolas)
4 Aadhak	=	1 Drona (1024 Tolas = 12 Sher 64 Tolas)
2 Drona	=	1 Shurpa (2048 Tolas = 25 Sher 48 Tolas)
2 Shurpa	=	1 Droni (4096 Tolas = 51 Sher 16 Tolas)
4 Droni	=	1 Khari (16384 Tolas = 204 Sher 64 Tolas)
2000 Pala	=	1Bhar (8000 Tolas = 100 Sher)

There are three types of dravyas to be considered; 1) Doshaprashaman - for treatment 2) Dhatupradushan - promoting disease and 3) Swasthavritta karak - imparting sound health.

Sharangadhar's tabulation in multiples of four

4 Masha	=	1 Tank (Shana)		
4 Tank (Shana)	=	1 Aksha (Pichuh,Panital, Suvarna, Kavalgrah, Karsha, Bidalpadak, Tinduk, Panimanika)		
4 Aksha (Karsha)	=	1 Bilva	=	4 Tolas
4 Bilva	=	1 Kudav	=	16 Tolas
4 Kudav	=	1 Prastha	=	64 Tolas
4 Prastha	=	1 Aadhak	=	256 Tolas
4 Aadhak	=	1 Rashi (Drona)	=	1024 Tolas
4 Rashi (Drona)	=	1 Droni	=	4096 Tolas
4 Droni	=	1 Khari	=	16384 Tolas

(Pala, Prakuncha, Mushti, Amra, Chaturthika are the five synonyms of Bilva).

Magadha and Kalinga measures - They are designated so because of their use in these territtories. Sharangadhar's tabulation, given above, already follows the Magadha measures given above. Kalinga measure is as follows :-

12 Gaur Sarshap	=	1 Yav
2 Yav	=	1 Gunja
3 Gunja	=	1 Wal
8 Gunja	=	1 Masha
4 Masha	=	1 Shana
6 Masha	=	1 Gaddyana
10 Masha	=	1 Karsha
4 Karsha	=	1 Pala
4 Pala	=	1 Kudav

Measures used thereafter were similar to Magadha system, mainly because Magadha was the capital and therefore important.

Regularly available cereals were used as units in common practice. During this period,there was no standard unit. Just as three barley corn = 1 inch was used as a unit for measuring length and we have accepted that,similarly, the unit of that era must have been widely accepted.

Sharangadhar's tabulation for liquid measures

To measure liquids, a container made of china clay, bamboo or metal and 4 fingers in height, length and breadth was used. The equivalent quantity of liquid dravya was called as 1 Kudav.

1 Kudav	=	16 tolas.
1 Pav	=	1 1/4 Kudav ; 1/2 Sher = 1 1/2 Sharav.

As not two persons are alike, there is no patent medicine in Ayurveda and if at all it is there, then it is of no value.

Comparison of measures described by Charaka - Sushruta - Sharangadhar

Charaka - 8 Ratti	=	1 Masa.
Sushruta - 6 Ratti	=	1 Masa.
Sharangdhar - 6 Ratti	=	1 Masa.

However all the three consider 24 Ratti = 1 Shana or 1/4th Tola.

Because according to Charaka 3 Masa	=	1 Shana
Sushruta 4 Masa	=	1 Shana
Sharangdhar 4 Masa	=	1 Shana.

But according to all the three 96 Ratti = 1 Karsha.

As according to Charaka 12 Masa	= 1 Karsha	=	(12 x 8 = 96 Ratti)
Sushruta - 16 Masa	= 1 Karsha	=	(16 x 6 = 96 Ratti)
Sharangdhar - 16 Masa	= 1 Karsha	=	(16 x 6 = 96 Ratti)

Kola is also the same in all the three measurement systems ie. 48 Ratti or 1/2 Tola. Further steps are similar in all the three.

Till the period of Sushruta the minute measurements were not in practice and therefore not in use. But the use of metals in chemical preparations made it essential to use minute measures, hence the mention of these in the later scripts is seen.

Commonly used table (Indian Measures & Weights)

8 Gunja	=	1 Masa
12 Masa	=	1 Tola (180 Grains)
5 Tolas	=	1 Chhataka = 2.056 Ounce
4 Chhatak	=	1 Pavsher
4 Pavsher	=	1 Sher = 2.2/35 pound
40 Sher	=	1 Mana (821/7 pound)
20 Mana	=	1 Khandi

Measures of capacity and volume according to Ayurveda

When two phalanges of the index finger are immersed in a liquid and taken out, it will form a drop which is called a Bindu. The following table follows Bindu as a unit.

8 Bindu	=	1 Shana
32 Bindu	=	1 Shukti
64 Bindu	=	1 Panishukti

(Currently, these measures are not in practice).

Prakruti which is made up of combination of mahabhootas (having dravya, guna and karma) and prakruti which is made up with the help of satva, raja and tama are not identical too.

English measures of weight

1 Grain	=	1 Wheat (1/2 Gunja (Ratti) approx.)
4371/2 gr.	=	1 Ounce
16 Ounces	=	1 Pound
14 Pounds	=	1 Stone
28 Pounds	=	1 Quarter
4 Quarter	=	1 Hundred weight
20 Hundred weights	=	1 Ton

Metric System

1 Gram	=	15.431 Grains
1 Decigram	=	1/10 Gram.
1 Centrigram	=	1/100 Gram. = 0.154 Grain.
1 Milligram	=	1/1000 Gram. = 0.015 Grain
1 Kilogram	=	1000 Gram. = 2.2046 Pound
1 Grain	=	0.0648 Gram.
1 Ounce	=	28.350 Gram.
1 Pound	=	0.4536 Kg.
1 Hundred weight	=	50.8 Kg.
1 Ton	=	1016.0 Kg.
1 Milligram	=	0.015 Grain
1 Centigram	=	0.154 Grain
1 Gram	=	15. 431 Grains.
1 Kilogram	=	2.2046 Pounds = 35.29 Ounces
1 Quintal	=	1.968 Hundred weight (cwt)
1 Tonne	=	0.984 Ton.
1 Gunja	=	2 3/16 Grains.
1000 Grm.	=	1 Kg.
2.204 Pounds	=	1 Kg. (Precise)
2. 2046 Pounds	=	1 Kg. (More precise)
1 Kilogram	=	2.2 Pounds (Lbs) 2.2046 Pounds = 35.29 Oz. (Ounces)
1 Gram.	=	15.43 Grains
1 Milligram	=	0.001 Gram.
1 Gamma or Microgram	=	0.001 Mgm.
1 Microgm.	=	0.000001 Gram, 1 Oz = 28.35 Gram
1 Pound (Lbs)	=	16 Oz. = 453.59 Gram.
1 Grain	=	0.0648 Gram = 64.8 Mgm.

(Lb hints at the zodiac sign of Libra)

It is true that no two persons are totally identical. God should be praised for this. Or is it his inability to make identical persons?

Comparative study of systems

2 1/4 Pound	=	1 Kilo
1 Pound	=	453 Grams = 0.4535 Kg.
8 Oz.	=	226 Grams
1 Oz.	=	28 Grams (28.35 Grams)
1/2 Oz.	=	14 Grams (14.175 Grams)
100 Grains	=	6.5 Grams
1/8th Oz.	=	3.5 Grams
20 Grains	=	1.3 Grams
10 Grains	=	0.65 Grams
5 Grains	=	0.325 Grams
3 Grains	=	0.2 Grams
2 Grains	=	0.13 Grams
1 1/2 Grain	=	0.1 Gram.
1 Grain	=	0.065 Gram. = 0.0648 Gram.
3/4th Grain	=	0.48 Gram.
1/2 Grain	=	0.032 Gram.
1/3rd Grain	=	0.02 Gram.
1/4th Grain	=	0.016 Gram.
1/10th Grain	=	6.5 Mgm.
1/12th Grain	=	5.0 Mgm.
1/16th Grain	=	4.0 Mgm.
1/32th Grain	=	2.0 Mgm.
1/64th Grain	=	1.0 Mgm.
1/100th Grain	=	0.65 Mgm.
1/200th Grain	=	0.3 Mgm.
1/250th Grain	=	0.25 Mgm.
1/300 Grain	=	0.2 Mgm.
1/400th Grain	=	0.15 Mgm.
1/500th Grain	=	0.125 Mgm.

English system for liquid measures (Imperial system)

1 Drop	=	1 Minim
60 Minims	=	1 Fluid Drachm
8 Fluid Drachm	=	1 Fluid Ounce.
16 Fluid Ounce	=	1 Fluid Pound.
20 Fluid Ounce	=	1 Pint
8 Pint	=	1 Gallon
4 Gill	=	1 Pint

Snigdha and ruksha are two ends. However, there is no dividing line between these two.

2 Pint	=	1 Quarter
4 Quarters	=	1 Gallon
8 Gallon	=	1 Bushel
1 Gill	=	1.4 Decilitres.
1 Pint	=	20 Oz. = 568.25 Ml. = 0.5682 Ltr.= 0.57 Ltr.
1 Quarter	=	1.136 Litres.
1 Gallon	=	4.546 Ltr.
1 Bushell	=	36. 37 Ltr.
1 Centilitres	=	0.07 Gill
1 Litre	=	1000 Ml. = 61.027 Cubic Inches (35.196 Fluid Ounces)
1 Hectolitre	=	2.75 Bushells.

Metric System

1 Ml.	=	16.7^{O}C of 1 Gm. distilled water.
1 Dl.	=	16.7^{O}C of 10 Gm. distilled water.
1 C. Ltr.	=	16.7^{O}C of 100 Gm. distilled water.
1 Litre	=	16.7^{O}C of 1000 Gm. distilled water.

British measures of weight

16 Dram	=	1 Ounce
16 Ounces	=	1 Pound
14 Ponds	=	1 Stone
2 Stones	=	1 Quart
1 Litre	=	1000 Millilitres = 61. 027 Cubic Inches = 35. 196 Liquid Ounces.
1Gallon	=	4.546 Litres
1 Cubic Centimetre or Millitre	=	16.9 Minims
1 Pint	=	20 Ounces = 568.25 Millilitres = 0.5682 Litre.
1 Liquid Ounce	=	28.41 Millilitres
1 Minim	=	0.059 Millilitres
100 Ginins Water	=	109.71 Drops (62° F)

In the universe, three main functions occur day and night; the representatives of these functions are vata, pitta and kapha.

Comparison of Imperial and Metric system

Imperial		Metric
1 Gallon	=	4.5 Litres.ss
1 Pint (20 fluid ounces)	=	568 Ml.
12 Fluid Ounce	=	340 Ml.
8 Fluid Ounce	=	225 Ml.
1 Fluid Ounce (480 Minims)	=	28.5 Ml
360 Minims.	=	21 Ml.
240 Minims.	=	16 Ml.
180 Minims.	=	12 Ml.
120 Minims.	=	8 Ml.
90 Minims.	=	6 Ml.
60 Minims.	=	4 Ml.
20 Minims.	=	1.25 Ml.
15 Minims.	=	1 Ml.
8 Minims.	=	0.5 Ml.
5 Minims.	=	0.3 Ml.
3 Minims.	=	0.2 Ml.
2 Minims.	=	0.12 Ml.
1 1/2 Minims.	=	0.1 Ml.
1 Minims.	=	0.06 Ml.
1/2 Minims.	=	0.03 Ml.
1/4 Minims.	=	0.015 Ml.

Indian Measures of Length

1 Finger breadth	=	3/4 inches = Area occupied by four Yava.
12 Finger breadth	=	1 extended palm breadth = 9 inches (approx.)
21 Finger breadth	=	1 Aratni = 16 1/2 inches (approx.)
2 Extended palm breadth	=	1 extended arm = 18 inches
4 Extended arms breadth	=	1 Vyay = 6ft.

British Measures of length

1 Tenth	=	1/10 Inch
12 Inches	=	1 Foot
3 Feet	=	1 Yard
220 Yard	=	1 Furlong
8 Furlong	=	1 Mile (1760 Yards or 5280 Feet)

Though the mind is made up of extremely subtle components, its malfunctioning is manifested through the body.

Imperial system

1 Metre	=	39.37 Inches.
1 Decimetre	=	1/10 Mtr.
1 Cm.	=	1/100 Mtr.
1 Mm.	=	1/1000 Mtr.
1 Km.	=	1000 Mtr.
8 Km.	=	5 Miles (approx.)
1 Inch.	=	0.0254 Mtr. = 25.4 Mm.

Comparison of British and Metric Measures

1 Foot	=	0.3048 Metres.
1 Yard	=	0.91439 Mtr.
1 Millimetre	=	0.0394 Inches.
1 Cm.	=	0.3937 Inches
1 Mt.	=	39.3708 Inches
1 Km.	=	1093.63 Yrds.
1 Km.	=	0.6214 Miles.
1 Inch	=	2.54 Cm.
1 Inch.	=	25.4 Cm.
1 Mm.	=	1/1000 Mtr.
1 Micron	=	0.001 Mm. = 0.00004 Inch (average).

Measures of Area

2.47106 Acre	=	1 Hector
1 Hector.	=	2 1/2 Acre (approx.)

	Measures in text	Decimal system	Approximate decimal
1.	1/8 Gunja	15.19 Mgm	15 Mgm.
2.	1/4 Gunja	30.38 Mgm	30 Mgm.
3.	1/2 Gunja	60.75 Mgm	60 Mgm.
4.	1 Gunja (Ratti)	121.50 Mgm	120 Mgm
5.	2 Gunja	243.00 Mgm	250 Mgm.
6.	4 Gunja	486.00 Mgm	500 Mgm
7.	8 Gunja = 1 Masa	972.00 Mgm	1 Gm
8.	2 Masa	1.944 Gm	2 Gm
9.	3 Masa	2.92 Gm	3 Gm
10.	4 Masa	3.83 Gm	4 Gm
11.	6 Masa	5.83 Gm	6 Gm
12.	12 Masa = 1 Tola	11.66 Gm	12 Gm
13.	2 Tola	23.33 Gm	24 Gm

Even if the leg or the toe is amputated, the pain of leg or toe lasts in one's mind.

14.	2 1/2 Tolas	29.16 Gm	36 Gm
15.	4 Tolas = 1 Pala	46.66 Gm	48 Gm
16.	8 Tolas = 2 Pala	93.22 Gm	96 Gm
17.	80 Tolas = 1 Sher	933.00 Gm	1000 Gm

Comparative measures of Ounce

1 Dram	=	3.685 Ml	=	3.5 Ml
2 Dram	=	7.29 Ml	=	7 Ml
4 Dram - 1/2 oz.	=	14.58 Ml	=	15 Ml
8 Dram - 1 oz.	=	29.16 Ml	=	30 Ml
2 Ooz.	=	58.32 Ml	=	60 Ml
4 Oz.	=	116.64 Ml	=	120 Ml

Liquid

40 Tolas = 1 Lb.
16 Oz = 1 Lb.
2 1/2 Tolas = 1 Oz

Weight and Measures

1 Micron (μ)	=	0.001 Mm - 0.00004 Inch.
1 Kilogram	=	2.2 Lb - 35.29 Oz.
1 Gm.	=	15.43 Grains
1 Mgm.	=	0.001 Gm.
1 Gamma (Y) or microgram (μg)	=	0.001 Mgm.
1 Ugm	=	0.000001 Gm.
1 Oz.	=	28.35 Gms.
1 Lb.	=	16. Oz. = 453.59 Gm.
1 Gr	=	0.0648 Gm. = 64.8 Mgm.
1 Litre (lit)	=	1000 Ml = 61.027 Cu.Inch. = 1.76 Pints = 35.196 Fl.Oz.
1 Cc or 1 Ml	=	16.9 Minims.
1 Pint	=	20 Ozs. = 568.25 Ml = 0.5682 Lt.
1 Fl.oz.	=	28.41 Ml. = 16 Drams.
1 Minims.	=	0.059 Ml.
1 Km.	=	0.6214 Miles.
1 In.	=	2.54 Cm. = 25.4 Mm.
1 Cm.	=	0.393 Inches
1 Mm	=	1/1000 Metre
100 Grains Water	=	101.71 drops at 62°F temp.

Unless Yama-Niyama are observed, Yoga is not complete. In the same manner, without observing sadvrutta, Ayurveda is not complete.

1 Galon	=	4.546 Litres.
1 Lb. x 0.4539	=	1 Kilogram
1 Kgm ÷ 2.204	=	1 Lb.

Weight

16 Dramm.	=	1 Ounce.
16 Oz.	=	1 Lb.
14 Lb.	=	1 Stone
8 Stones	=	1 Hundered Weight (cwt)
12 Masas	=	1 Tola
5 Tolas	=	1 Chatak = 2.056 Ounce
16 Chatak	=	1 Sher = 2.056 Lbs
40 Sher	=	1 Mana = 82 1/7 Lbs

Conversion of Metric system

Length and Distance

1 Inch	= 25.4 Mm.	1 Mm	=	0.03937 Inches
1 Inch	= 2.54 Cm.	1 Cm.	=	0.3937 Inches
1 Foot	= 0.305 Metre	1 Mt.	=	3.281 Feet
1 Yard	= 0.9144 Metre	1 Mt.	=	1.094 Yard
1 Mile	= 1.609 Km.	1 Km.	=	0.6214 Miles.

Square area Measures

1 Sq.Inch.	= 6.452 Sq. Cm.	1 Sq.Mt.	= 0.155 Inch.
1 Sq. Ft.	= 0.093 Sq. Mt.	1 Sq.Mt.	= 10.764 Sq.Ft.
1 Sq.Yard	= 0.836 Sq. Mt.	1 Sq.Mt.	= 1.196 Sq. Yd.
1 Sq. Acre	= 0.405 Hect.	1 Hect.	= 2.471 Acres.
1 Sq. Mile	= 2.58999 Sq. K. Mt.	1 Sq.K.Mt.	= 0.3861 Sq. Miles

Cubic Area

1 Cu. Inch.	= 16.387 Cu.Cm.	1 Cu.Cm.	= 0.061 Cu.Inch
		1 Cu.Mt.	= 35.315 Cu.Ft.
1 Cu.Foot	= 0.028 Sq.Mt.	1 Cu.Mt.	= 1.308 Cu.Yard

"तिलोद्भ तैलम्" Til taila does not unnecessarily increase or decrease the body mass. Rather, it maintains the body mass at an optimum level.

References -

1. न नामज्ञानमात्रेण, रूपज्ञानेन वा पुनः ।
ओषधीनां परां प्राप्तिं कच्छिद्वेदितुमर्हति ।।
औषधं अनभिज्ञातं नामरूपगुणैस्त्रिभिः ।। (च. सू. २ अ. १.१२१-१२५)
2. एकं दहं शतं चैव सहस्त्रं अयुतं तथा । लक्षं च नियुतं चैव कोटिः अर्बुदमेवच । वृन्दः खर्वो निखर्वश्च शंकुः पद्मश्च सागरः । अंत्यो मध्यः परार्धश्च दशवृद्ध्या यथाक्रमम् ।। भारतीय दशमान पद्धति । (एकापुढे सतरा पूज्ये) अंक लिहिण्याची पद्धति –
अंक लिहिण्याची पद्धति खरोष्टी आहे. अंकानां वामतो गतिः । उजवीकडून डावीकडे लिहीत जाणे (देवनागरी आदि पद्धति ब्राह्मी आहेत, डावीकडून उजवीकडे.)
3. शाणं पाणितलं मुष्टिः कुडवं प्रस्थमाढकम् ।
द्रोणं वहं च क्रमशो विजानीयात् चतुर्गुणम् ।। वा. क. ६/२२)
4. तुला पलशतं, तानि विंशतिः भार उच्यते ।। वा. क. ६/२८
5. द्वौशाणो वटकः कोलं बदरं द्रंक्षणश्चतौ ।
अक्षं पिचुः पाणितलं सुवर्णं कवलग्रहः ।
कर्षोबिडालपदकं तिंदुकः पाणिमानिका ।
अक्ष, पिचु आदि अपरपर्याय आहेत. वा. क. ६/२५/२६.

CHAPTER THIRTEEN
VARIOUS IMPURITIES IN DRAVYAS

Impurities in dravyas and their purification

The word 'impurity of matter' is relative as far as human health is concerned. To use matter for a particular action, some unwanted properties have to be removed and some incorporated in it. Removal of unwanted properties from matter is done by purification. If left unpurified, it produces harmful effects on the body. In some substances, these properties are so strong that the action of pacifying the doshas and creating their equilibrium and establishing harmony does occur but at the same time it produces harmful effects on dhatus like rasa and rakta which are the basic infrastructure of the body. Therefore such toxic substances have to be especially 'purified'.

Also, in case of dravyas like Semecarpus anacardium, Plumbago zeylaniacum and mineral substances, purification is imperative and essential.

These impurities can be broadly classified in to three groups.

(1) Physical (2) Chemical (3) Natural.

(1) Physical - Substances collected from their source are usually contaminated with sand, mud etc. Even afterwards, if not protected properly, the substances may get mixed up with unwanted materials. Dishonesty of the proprietor selling them commercially also plays an important role. Original substances can be adulterated in this process. All these extraneous, unwanted materials are called as mala or physical impurities.

(2) Chemical - When mineral substances are mined, many unwanted metalic substances are also collected with them. These are called as 'vahnidosh', also known as chemical impurities.

(3) Natural - Toxic substances like poisons, though chemically and physically pure, do have very destructive effects on the body. Thus, it is essential that such properties should be either nullified or reduced. Such impurities are called natural impurities.

The meaning of the word 'shodhan' (purification) is to be taken in this context. Removal of the extranious matter and unwanted properties and converting the matter for safe use in preparations is called purification. The main aim of purification process is this - an efficacious safe use.

Common methods of purification

Objectives of purification are already mentioned above. These objectives can be achieved through various methods. Many different methods can be applied for various substances as per requirements.

Described below are some of them -

Vata Kalakaleeya adhyaya, which is the twelth chapter of Sutra sthana of Charaka Samhita, alone is sufficient to explain the philosophy of tridoshas.

1) Washing - Extraneous substances like sand, mud and other physical impurities can be removed in this way.

2) Sifting - Substances such as foodgrains are sifted through a sieve of meshes of different pore sizes. Gravel, mud, sand etc. can be easily removed this way.

3) Elutration - Substances soluble in water can be separated by this method. Such substances are mixed with enough water. Insoluble extraneous matter later precipitates at the bottom. The solution is then filtered off.

(4) Evapouration - The filtered solution is heated (or exposed to sunlight), so that water evapourates and dry pure matter can be collected.

(5) Percolation - The (liquid) matter is separated from impurities with the help of percolation. It is another way of filtration.

(6) Maceration - Substances soluble in alcohol can be separated thus. Insoluble impurities settle down at the bottom and can be filtered off.

(7) Dialysis - It consists of separating colloidal parts of the mixture form crystalloid parts through parchment floating on the water surface.

(8) Despumation - When liquids of organic nature are boiled, a froathy substance is formed which floats on the surface. Most of the impurities are in that frothy substance. Removal of that substance purifies the original liquid substantially.

(9) Decolouration - To separate active principles from substances, the colouring agents from the substances have to be removed. For this, first the substance may have to be treated with charcoal.

(10) Steaming - Few substances are cooked in liquids like cow's urine or juices of various plants using dolayantra. This is called as 'swedan'. This is mostly useful in removing all the three types of impurities.

(11) Trituration - Trituration done with mortar and pestle is useful in removing chemical and natural impurities. The following reference substantiates the statement.

पुटे पुटे विधातव्यं मर्दनं दृढवत्तरम ।।

–रसेंद्रचूडामणि

During trituration friction and pressure are applied simultaneously and both are syner gistic to each other. Both actions are important. During trituration the particle size of the substance is reduced, increasing and enhancing its properties. Trituration is supposed to create heat during the procedure which helps purifying the substance.

-In this universe, both, material and immaterial substances exist. But it is difficult to demonstrate the immaterial, as it cannot be perceived by the senses.

Churning is also a type of trituration in which semisolid substances like curds are churned so as to form a homogenous thick solution. Thus curds are converted into butter milk with churning. Chakradatta, in his commentary on Charaka's Viman sthana, says, "Curds may cause oedema whereas buttermilk is used in treatment of oedema."

Trituration of any substance is carried out in small quantities. The process is influenced by the following factors (i) force (ii) friction (iii) pressure (iv) velocity (v) weight (of the pestle) (vi) heat (vii) time and (viii) air. As a combined effect of all these, many impurities or unwanted properties are reduced and the drug becomes effective. For example, in the preparation of a drug called Chausashti Pimpali, Piper longum is triturated for 64 hrs. continuously. Triturating continuously makes it not only fine (सूक्ष्म) but an active principle called 'piperine'is separated due to this process. The process is also called as dinamization.

Similarly, fruits of Terminalia chebula, when chewed in mouth (which is a sort of trituration) and then ingested, increase appetite. Husks of the grains of rice are similarly removed in a mill. Drugs like aspirin are microfined so that they get absorbed quickly and their side effects due to late absorption are avoided.

(12) Moorchhan - Trituration with specific dravyas

When a substance is triturated with specific dravyas in such a way that its original appearance is completely changed, the process is known as moorchhan. It is one of the series of processes mentioned for purification of mercury.

(13) Nirvapan -

When a substance (usually a metal or metalic compound) is heated or melted and then immediately immersed in specific liquid substances, physical or chemical changes are brought about which are useful in purifying the original substance. This is called nirvapan.

(14) Sublimation -

This method is useful in those solid substances which on heating are converted into gaseous state e.g. - mercury, sulphur etc.

Purification

Following are the plants or plant derivatives which are used only after purification.

(i) Tubers - Gloriosa superba, Aconitum ferox, Allium sativum (garlic), Asparagus racemosa, Amorphophallus companulatus.

(ii) Stems - Euphorbia antigorum.

(iii) Latex - Opium, Garderia gummifora, Euphorbia antigorum, Aloe barbadensis, Asafoetida.

One of the reasons why mankind must have invented te concept of rebirth is that it prompts one to do good deeds in the present life. Ayurveda has accepted the concept of rebirth.

(iv) **Gum** - Commiphora mukul.

(v) **Leaves** - Cannabis sativa.

(vi) **Fruits** - Areca catechu, Piper longum, Aegle marmelos, Semecarpus anacardium, Piper nigrum etc.

(vii) **Flowers** - Cannabis sativa.

(viii) **Seeds** - Achyranthes aspera, Plantago ovata, Cirtulus colocypthis, Ricinus communis, Pongamia glabra, Mucuna pruriens, Gossypium herbaceum, Strychnos nuxvomica, Luffa acutangulata, Abrus precatorius, Croton tiglium, Cuminum cyminum, Picrorrhiza kurroa, Sesamum indicum, Luffa echinata, Balliospermum montanum, Datura stramonium, Azadirachta indica, Butea monospermia, Trichosanthes dioica, Cassia fistula, Borassica juncea, Cirtrus medica, Argyria speciosa, Moringo pteriosperma, Caesalpinia crista.

(ix) **Roots** - Nerium indicum odorum, Plumbago zeylanica, Argyria speciosa.

(x) **Exudates** - Garcinia morella (or Indian Gamboge) Camphor, Honey etc.

Knowledge of artificial substances and adulterants

Properties of medicinal substances described in books are of original natural material, but often, due to the scarcity of such substances, these are adulterated. While adulterating, care is taken so that size, colour, odour, weight, taste etc. are similar to that of the original natural substance. Requirements and idea of the consumer about the substance is also considered before adulterants are mixed. Such adulteration is many a times observed in Aconitum ferox, Plumbago rosae, gallstones of cow, Terminalia chebula, musk, saffron, Cuminum cyminum, honey, jaggary etc.

(1) **Terminalia chebula fruits** - Fruits of this plant are supposed to be ideal when they are quite big and heavy. Tough convering of the fruit is skillfully stuck over a mudball to make good quality 'survari' hirda.

(2) **Gall stones of cow (gorochan)** - A small sized gall stone is dipped in a solution of turmeric powder and then dried. Many such layers are thus formed resembling the original substance and is sold commercially as such.

(3) **Musk** - Black earth powder, oil and musk when taken together and mixed thoroughly, artificial musk is formed. It is often sold in pouches made up of deer's skin.

(4) **Cuminum cyminium seeds** - These are of two types - (i) whitish and (2) black. The black is imported from Iran and being such is not easily available. The white variety is coloured black and sold as black variety (shahajeera).

(5) **Jaggery** - During transportation of sugar, some amount is wasted always by way of spilling over. It is scrubbed from the floor, mixed with water to separate the sugary part, coloured and

One of the problems with learned teachers is that they are unable to impart (teach) knowledge to others. (Should we still call them teachers?)

moulded to form artificial jaggery.

Given below is a description of some original substances, their characteristics and possible adulterants.

(6) **Aconitum heterophyllum** - The roots are very britle. If broken, four to five black spots can be observed on the broken surface. It is tapering towards distal end and it is very bitter to taste.

Adulterants - Roots of Asparagus racemosa or such roots which are tapering towards the ends, are sweetish to taste and hard to break.

(7) **Morphine** - It is bitter in taste with peculiar odour.

Adulterants - Black earth, oil etc.

(8) **Root of Sausaria lappa** - It is usually zig-zag, twisted, about a finger long, heavy, grey coloured, with vertical striations and heavy.

Adulterants - Mud and cowdung are usually mixed with the roots. By immersing in water, these can be removed.

(9) **Roots of Hemidesmus indicus** - It has a sweetish odour.
Adulterants - Thin sticks, roots of coconut tree are mixed.

(10) **Seeds of Coleus amboinicus**- It has specific fragrance and is granular. It is mixed with dust, mud etc.

(11) **Seeds of Piper cubeda** - Seeds when broken in mouth, immediately produce a tingling sensation. If air is sucked at the same time, cool sensation can be experienced. It has lot of frangrance.

Similar looking seeds of gulabakshi (four o'clock flower) are mixed usually for adulteration. However, they are lighter with no characteristic properties.

(12) **Gum of Commiphora mukul**- It has specific fragrance. Gum of shallaki (Boswellia serrata) is mixed.

(13) **Kathalya gond** - Usually mixed with gum of kandol (Trichosanthes bracteata).

(14) **Extract of Acacia catechu (white)** - It produces astringent effect on teeth and gums. It is not brittle by itself. Pieces of chalk or clay are mixed for adulteration.

(15) **Scrapings of skin of fruits of Mallotus phillipinensis** - It does not mix with water. If ignited, burns readily. It is soft and gives out bright yellow colour if rubbed on wet paper.

It is usually adulterated with brick powder. The adulterant sinks to the bottom if spread over water whereas the original substance floats.

Shodhan dravyas bring about their actions. The act of shodhan (purification) is a reaction of the body to shodhan dravyas. Naturally, one requires good physical and mental health to sustain it.

(16) **Picrorrhiza kurroa roots -** A substance known as 'kadu' is mixed for adulteration. Roots of coconut palm are also used for the purpose.

(17) **Crocus sativus (saffron) -** It is soft, easily colours water and has a specific fragrance. Almost dissolves in water. Usually hairy portions of androecium-gynaecium of sunflower are mixed in the original saffron. The adulterant material, Carthamus tinctorium, is lighter than the original saffron. Small paper strips or petals of yellow chrysanthamum, can also be mixed. They do not dissolve in water.

(18) **Resin of Tinospora cordifolia -** If examined under microscope, the grains of starch having a specific shape can be seen.

Substances like potato, starch, powdered banana and other substances of starch origin are mixed. As both substances give bluish black colour when treated with iodine, it (the adulterant) cannot be separated or distinguished from the original one.

(19) **Roots of Plumbago zeylanicum -** It is definitely hot in taste, produces tingling sensation in the mouth. If its paste is applied on the skin, it immediately produces inflammatory reaction in the form of red colouration and bullae formation. Roots have vertical striations.

Many times roots of Acacia indica are mixed with the original. But strong astringent taste of this adulterant can differentiate it from the original.

(20) **Latex of Euphorbia antigorum and Calotropis procera -** Solution of slaked lime (Calcium hydroxide) is mixed.

(21) **Cinnamomum zeylonica -** This is used in the form of thin bark of the tree. It has specific fragrance and is hot to taste. Thin barks of similar appearance can be mixed for adulteration.

(22) **Piper longum -** Natural and original fruits are comparatively hard to break. If broken, a typical wheel-like configuration can be seen. At the centre of this wheel is a small reddish brown grain of seed which is also hard and hot to taste.

Fruits of similar appearance like fruits of Piper betle are mixed. But they are rather flat, soft and without internal lumen.

(23) **Roots of Piper longum -** They are blackish white in colour, wrinkled and with tapering ends.

Sticks of other creepers or sticks of Piper longum itself are mixed as roots. But these can be distinguished from the original because their ends appear similar as they are cut from their stems.

(24) **Aconitum ferox -** This tuber is thicker at one end and tapers down at the other end. It is about four fingers in length, often heavy and curved. Its outer surface is greyish. If cut transversely, it shows white pulp like a sweet potato.

Human beings, animals and trees have similar mechanisms of dosha-dhatu-malas. Therefore the sceince of treatment was advised for all of them.

It is adulterated with small wooden pieces and roots of Asparagus adscendens. These are lighter in weight and do not show properties of the original substance.

(25) Gum of Acacia arabica - It is white in colour. The gum of other plants like Acacia catechu, Moringa oleifera are mixed. The gum of the latter is red coloured.

(26) Honey - Few drops of honey without adulteration, if sprinkled on fire, burn without producing any sound, because the water content in honey is almost nil. A wick soaked in honey can burn like one soaked in oil or ghee without producing any sound. The semisolid consistency of honey becomes liquid when heated. Therefore, if a drop of honey is rubbed between fingers, it liquifies. Honey usually has air bubbles in it which gives it a specific external appearance. The taste of honey depends on flowers from which it is collected. Still, generally it is sweet and astringent.

While burning, it does not give out a bad odour. It has a specific sweetish odour, but one cannot smell it for prolonged time. The original odour of honey is so strong, it can be superimposed on strong smelling substances like castor oil or cod-liver oil.

Honey is usually adulterated with syrups of jaggery and sugar. As these syrups contain substantial amounts of water, if at all it burns, it produces lot of crackling sound. External appearance of such adulterated honey also changes. Taste of adulterated honey is only sweet. There is no trace of astringence in it. If such honey is burned, it produces characteristic odour of burnt sugar.

(27) Leaves of Cassia angustifolia (Indian senna) - Usually adulterated with leaves of bhuitaravdi.

(28) Seeds of Piper nigrum - Cortex of the seed is rough externally and coarse. It is round in shape. The seeds of 4 o'clock flower (gulabakshi) and seeds of Embelia ribes (vavding) are mixed in this substance for adulteration.

Both these seeds, though black in colour, have smooth external surfaces. The seeds of 4 o'clock flower are oval rather than perfectly round.

(29) Menthol - True menthol is not soluble in water. Gratings of ammonium chloride are mixed in the original substance. It can be easily removed by dissolving it in water.

(30) Seeds of Fumaria parviflora - Seeds of Vitex negundo are mixed. Many people consider these seeds as seeds of Vitex negundo.

(31) Bark of Tecomella undulata - Bark of jamun trees (Eugenia jambolinum) are mixed.

(32) Shweta rohida - Bark of white variety of the above plant is often adulterated with bark of khurchafa.

(33) Cardamom seeds -These seeds are adulterated with the fruits of Alpinia galanga.

For obtaining the permission of cutting trees, one must be obliged to perform the duty of growing trees and taking carc of thom.

(34) Alpinia galanga - Roots of Piper betle are usually mixed.

(35) Swertia chirata - Adulterated with Andrographis paniculata.

(36) Glycerrhiza glabra - Yashtimadhu - Indian Liquorice is adulterated with roots of Abrus precatorius.

(37) Mesua ferra - Red buds of surangi.

(38) Mesua ferra (black) - Buds of undani.

(39) Wagatea spicata - It is bitter,wrinkled,starchy and light in weight.

It is mixed with bhuikohla or roots of Wagatea spicata itself. Both these are fibrous, smooth, hard and heavy.

(40) Arsenic oxide - Pieces of tiles or crockery are mixed.

(41) Arsenic trisulphide - Pivdi.

(42) Balliospermum montanum - Roots of red variety of Ricinus communis.

Original dravyas and their substitutes

When particular medicinal substances are specifically mentioned, they must be used. There should not be any substitute. Use of pure authentic substitutes instead of adulterated original substances is becoming the order of the day now-a-days. It is a wrong practice altogether.

For example, to advertise that a particular formula contains ashtavarga without using it actually is to deceive. It is cheating. To say that it contains representatives of ashtavarga will be more correct. But still, representative substitutes are substitutes only !

Some Representatives (That means open adulteration)

1)	Instead of jivak, rushabhak	-	Pueraria tuberosa.(Bhavprakash)
2)	Kakoli, ksheerkakoli	-	Withania somnifera.
3)	Meda, mahameda	-	Asparagus racemosus.
4)	Ruddhi, vruddhi	-	Dioscoria bulbifera
5)	Garcinia pedunculata	-	Pumex vescicarus.
6)	Aconitum heterophyllum	-	Cyperus rotundus.
7)	Ajwala	-	Ocimum sanctum.
8)	Sugarcane (Sachham officinarum)	-	Arundo donax.

-Proper understanding of the etymologies of various sanskrit synonyms of medicinl plants will help in their standardisation.

9)	Trachi spermum	-	Carum roxburghianum
10)	Nelumbo nucifera	-	Kamalaksha.
11)	Musk	-	Piper cubeda, Jasmine grundi florum or Jasminum officinarum, flowers or leaves.
12)	Kali musli and shweta musli	-	Asparagus adscendens.
13)	Aquillaria agallococha	-	Cedrus deodar
14)	Premanon integrifolia	-	White Premanon integrifolia
15)	Camphor	-	Fragrant Cyperus acariosus.
16)	Desmostachya bipinnata	-	Soccnarum spontaneum.
17)	Crystaline sugar	-	Powdered sugar.
18)	The starch of Tinospora cordifolia	-	Any other (starchy) material triturated with juice of Tinospora cordifolia.
19)	Pumex vesicarious	-	Roots of Piper longum.
20)	Sandal wood (Santalum album)	-	Veteveria zizonoides.
21)	Ptreocarpus santalinus	-	Santalum album.
22)	Plumbago zeylanica	-	Baliospermum montanium or alkaloids of Achyranthes aspera.
23)	Chuka	-	Lemon or lime juice.
24)	Nardostachys jatamansi	-	Mankand
25)	Myristica fragrans leaves	-	Fruits of Myristica and cloves
26)	Seeds of Cuminum cyminum	-	Shahjeera
27)	Glycerrhiza glabra	-	Woodfordia floribunda.
28)	Dioscorides bulbiferasativa	-	Bulb of chambharavli

The gunakarmas of dravyas are the yardsticks by which they are deemed as dietary, medicinal or toxic dravyas.

29) Valerian Wallichi - Sausserea lappa.

30) Taxus baccata - Swarnalata

31) Thuner - Sausserea lappa.

32) Berberis aristata - Curcuma longa.

33) Vitis venifera fruits - Fruits of Gemlina arborea or flowers of Madhuka indica.

34) Mesua ferra - Nymphea stellata.

35) Vitex negundo - Ocimum sanctum leaves.

36) Blue lotus - White lotus.

37) Alhaji mourorum - Alhaji mourorum pseudo.

38) Solanum xanthocarpum - Mayurshikha

39) Boerhavia diffusa - White punarnava

40) Ipomia racemosa - Roots of castor.

41) Mimusops elengi - Blue lotus.

42) Mimusops elengi Bark - Bark of Acacia arabica.

43) Faniculum vulgare - Anethum sova.

44) Seeds of Psoralea corylifolia. - Seeds of Cacia tora.

45) Semecarpus anacardium - Nadi bhallatak

46) Clerodendron serratum - Abies webbejana or Solanum xanthocarpum

47) Pueraria tuberosa - Asparagus racemosus.

48) Honey - Old Jaggery.

49) Clematis tiloba - Rubia cordifolia.

50) Rasanjan - Berberis aristata.

51) Phaseolous trilobus - Phaseolous mungo.

Unviable plants like tulsi which yield neither flowers nor fruits and shade are considered worthy of daily worship! Great ideals indeed!

52)	Pluchea lanceolata	-	Alpinia galanga.
53)	Solanum xanthocarpum	-	Solanum indicum.
54)	Vitiveriaz	-	Black vitiveriaz
55)	Fruits of Gmelina arborid	-	Flowers of Madhuka indica.
56)	Desmodium gangeticum	-	Ureria picta.
57)	Fruits of Terminalia chebula	-	Unripe fruits of Terminalia chebula or Rhus succedania.

Various medicinal substances are mainly of two types - primary and secondary. Substitutes may be permissible or tolerable if used instead of these secondary medicinal dravyas. But to use substitutes for primary or main substances is totally wrong and unpardonable.

(Just like the case of substances of plant origin, adulteration of food material and minerals is also common now-a-days. The people doing adulteration are mentally so prepared for it, that they even prepare important drugs like chyavanprash using red pumpkin instead of fruits of Emblica officinalis. How one can expect results from such preparations? The preparations are not at fault.)

Extraordinary global materia medica

In ancient times also, our ancestors were keen to identify and standardize the substances mentioned in the materia medica. This is so clear if one goes through various 'Nighantu' specially prepared for compilation of identification norms of dravyas. 'Nighantu' means a sort or dictionary. But the scope of Nighantu was not restricted to offer only synonyms. If we consider only the points from which each substance mentioned in the nighantu is considered, we will be astonished to realise the work done by our ancestors as being beyond praise.

These points are :-

(1) properties (2) colour (3) appearance (4) odour (5) feel (6) tastes (7) similarities (8) life cycle (9) place of origin or occurance (10) description of stages of growth (11) diseases on which it acts (12) effects on body humors (13) its action on various body systems (14) description of its roots, stem, bark, leaves, fruits, flowers, seeds etc. (15) description of soil and temperatures in which it grows freely (16) its gender (17) its usefulness from point of view of other creatures (18) to whom it will be useful and so on and so forth.

To study the etymology of synonyms of plants and their derivatives is altogether a different subject for study. To study Latin and botanical names, families of the plants etc. is alright, but it is my earnest wish that not only Ayurvedic physicians but other scholars should also be involved in this subject. Many of them have not even tried. It is necessary to have atleast a basic knowledge of Latin to understand nomenclature and terminology of modern medicine and botany. It is essential to know Sanskrit for this study. If such a knowledgable person tries the etymology of synonyms, he will defi-

Substances used for preparing diet or medicines should have favourable properties and actions in addition to favourable physical properties.

nitely unveil much knowledge which will be so very useful for 'Standardization' of the drugs, about which we are so concerned. Various names were given to plant substances, many a times in tens or fifteen, not because our ancestors had nothing more to do on their hands but only to pinpoint and to standardize a particular substance, which had so many descriptive names. It only shows a very critical and deep study they have made about each substance. For example, following is the list of substances with the number of descriptive synonyms they have given -

1.	Emblica officinalis	43
2.	Mangifera indica	72
3.	Aconitum heterophyllum	26
4.	Carum roxburghianum	37
5.	Sida shinasa, Sida cordifolia	21
6.	Withania somnifera	40
7.	Terminalia chebula	33
8.	Terminalia bellerica	30
9.	Tinospora cordifolia	40
10.	Premna integrifolia	25
11.	Gmelina arboria	35
12.	Oroxylum indicum	38
13.	Tribulus terrestris	23
14.	Desmodium gangeticum	44
15.	Leptadenia reticulata	32
16.	Kakoli	24
17.	Alhaji mourorum	30
18.	Croton tiglium	20
19.	Cirtulus colocynthis	50
20.	Picrorrhiza kurroa	33
21.	Adhatoda vasica	23
22.	Achyranthes aspera	30
23.	Balantshep	26

If after going through all these many synonyms one cannot pinpoint or identify a plant, then one should doubt one's intelligence; of course this study is not for examinations, but for knowledge and science. It is meant for those scientists who have respect for all sciences. If once, botanical name according to modern Botany is fixed, its synonyms with proper meaning can be added as a supplement and thus a worldwide 'materia medica' can be definitely prepared.

An unintelligent person will not be able to even read Charaka Samhita, leave aside comprehending it! But it is certain that its understanding increases intelligence.

CHAPTER FOURTEEN
THERAPEUTIC CONSIDERATIONS

तदेव युक्तं भैषज्यं च. सू. १/१३४

A medicinal substance is the one which helps to restore and maintain health.

Charakarcharya has described four attributes of best medicinal dravya.

1. Bahuta (Availability) - The dravya must be available in sufficient quantity.

2. Yogyata (Suitability) - The dravya must be suitably effective according to the condition and status of the disease and the tolerability of the patient.

3. Anekvidh kalpana (Multiple formulations) - Different preparations of the same dravya, such as juice, decoction, pulp, infusion, tablets etc. must be possible. One should be able to prepare the medicine considering the taste of the patient, choice and the pathophysiological state of the disease.

4. Sampat (Enrichment) - The dravya must possess all the qualities like rasa, veeryadi gunas as well as deepanadi actions. Older dravya becomes ineffective as it loses its gunas and karmas. Therefore it is advisable to use fresh medicinal plants as they are equipped with their gunas and karmas. Ghee, jaggery, honey, cereals, Piper longum and Embelia ribes are exceptions to this rule and should be used when old.[1]

Use of different parts of medicinal plants

Medicinal plants do not contain all the essential effective properties equally distributed in all the components, therefore it is advisable to use that specific part of the plant which is full of effective medicinal qualities.

Dravya

↓ ↓

Plant origin [2]

Root, bark, trunk, gum, resin, juice, latex, fruits, flowers, tender leaves, leaves, tubers, ash, oil, spikes, buds.

Animal origin[3]

Honey, milk, curd, buttermilk, ghee, bile, fat, marrow, blood, muscle, urine, faeces, skin, semen, bones, tendon, horns, hair, nails, hood, etc.

As mentioned above, different dravyas of plant origin and animal origin are used

There is no doubt that Ayurveda will bestow fame and honour on any practitioner who follows its teachings in spirit and in practice.

internally or externally in different conditions as medicine :

Root - Dashmoola.

Bark - Terminalia arjuna, Azadirachta indica.

Trunk - Sandal wood.

Gum - Asafoetida, Commiphora mukul.

Stalk - Lotus.

Juice - Barassus flabellifera, Palm tree (juice oozed out of wounded spathe of palm) or juice extracted by crushing the leaves by hand or machine.

Tender leaves - Mango, Eugenia jambolana.

Leaves - Taxus baccata, Adathoda vasica, Vitex negundo.

Salts - Achyranthes aspera, Butea frondosa, barley, lotus.

Latex - Calotropis procera, cactus.

Fruits - Terminalia chebula, Terminalia bellerica, Emblica officinalis.

Flowers - Butea frondosa, Calotropis procera, rose.

Ash - Calotropis procera, Semecarpus anacardium, triphala

Oil - Ricinus communis, Seasamum indicum, Terminalia bellerica.

Spikes - Savar.

Tubers - Allium sativum, Curcuma longa, Zingiber officinalis.

Areal roots - Ficus bengalensis.

When no specific part is mentioned in the texts, roots are used. If root is thick, then its skin is used but if thin, then the whole root is used.

Compatibility of dravyas

In treatment, many dravyas have to be used in combinations. When two or more dravyas are mixed, it is called combination. Combination is done to increase the efficacy of the drug, to reduce the toxicity or to enhance the action on a particular tissue or organ. All combinations are not beneficial to health; some may be harmful too. A number of times, they are incompatible and harmful to health. But even such incompatible combinations are sometimes used in treatment, especially in certain purification procedures.

Ayurveda recommends maintenance of unctuousness not only in the digestive system but also in all the minute apertures and systems of the body.

For example, a mixture of curd, milk, salt and black gram is given as a premedication for vomiting on the previous night. This mixture helps to induce effortless vomiting. Incompatibility is of five types :

1. Quantitative incompatibility - Some dravyas, when mixed in a particular proportion, are incompatible. For example, honey and ghee in equal quantity are incompatible.

2. Physical and chemical incompatibility - Incompatibility in rasa, veerya and vipak of dravyas.

Rasa incompatibility - A combination of salt and milk (which is sweet) is incompatible.

3. Veerya incompatibility - Fish (ushna veerya) + milk (sheeta veerya).

4. Vipak incompatibility - Radish (katu vipak) and milk (madhur vipak).

5. Physiological incompatibility or antagonism - Drugs having physiological opposite actions are antagonist and should not be used in combination. For example, jayapal (puragative) + dhataki (constipative) is an incompatible combination. Similarly, snehan and rukshan are incompatible procedures.

But even such incompatible combinations are sometimes used in treating diseases. For example, niruh basti (ruksha) and anuvasan basti (snigdha) are often used in combination. The treatment of kshaya kasa also involves the use of such combinations. Of course, such combination of drugs are effective only because they are synergestic to each other, e.g. roots of Boerrhavia diffusa (punarnava) are purifier whereas mandur (ferrous oxide) is astringent. But when combined together, they act mutually synergistically. Such combinations may also help to enhance the gamitva of the dravya.

The effects of the above five types of combinations results in the harmful effects in terms of gunas and karmas. Because some components of such combinations either vitiate the doshas, or the other remaining components may supress the doshas so that they become harmful to health. This incompatibility may result in conditions like sterility, blindness, erysepalus, ascites, blebs, schizophrenia, fistula, fainting, flatulence, pharyngitis, anaemia, rheumatism, keloid, skin diseases, duodenitis, swelling, haemorrhagic diathesis, fever, defective siblings or even death. That is why, careful consideration must be given to combinations at the time of treatment as well as during health. (Ashtangsangraha सू. 9, Charaka सू. अ. 26, Sushruta सू. अ. 20, Ashtanghridaya अ.7)

There are certain dravyas which do not actually combine with other dravyas, but still they show harmful effects. Charakacharya has classified them as follows :

1. Desha viruddha - Ruksha, teekshna diet in jangal desha, abhishyandi diet in anoop desha.

2. Kalaviruddha - Consuming cold items in winter and hot items in summer.

3. Agniviruddha - Consuming heavy and unctuous food when there is no appetie or immediately

It is difficult to understand why the 'marmas', which are given so much importance in the Sharir sthana of Ayurvedic texts, are neglected to an equal extent in the remaining sections of the texts.

after food.

4. Matraviruddha - Ghee and honey in equal proportions.

5. Satmyaviruddha - Eating cold items when the body is used to hot items.

6. Doshaviruddha - Ruksha items in diseases of vata, ushna items in diseases of pitta and unctuous items in diseases of kapha.

7. Sanskarviruddha - Peacock's meat roasted on fire produced by burning twigs of castor plant.

8. Veeryaviruddha - Consuming ushna veerya dravyas along with sheeta veerya dravyas e.g. milk + fish, milk + black gram.

9. Koshthaviruddha - Using a mild purgative and that too in a small dose.

10. Avasthaviruddha - Using kapha increasing dravyas in states of drowsiness.

11. Kramviruddha - Eating before the bowels are cleared.

12. Pariharviruddha - Drinking warm water after consuming bhallatak.

13. Upcharviruddha - Drinking cold water after consuming ghee - oil.

14. Pakviruddha - Eating uncooked or overcooked food.

15. Samyogaviruddha - Sour fruits with milk.

16. Hridviruddha - Eating disliked food.

17. Sampatviruddha - Eating stale and tasteless food.

18. Vidhiviruddha - Eating curds while not following the guidelines laid down in the texts.

We may predict the properties and actions of a combination but one can never be 100% sure about his predictions because the properties of a combination cannot be ascertained by arithmatical calculations; unexpected outcome may result. Therefore, it is said that 'मुनिरेव विजानाति द्रव्यसंयोगजं फलम् ।'

Medicinal preparations

Many formulations prepared by combination of different dravyas are mentioned in Ayurveda. These formulations were, in a way, prescriptions of the vaidyas of that era which contained many dravyas. Some of these formulations are named by the principle drug of the formulation e.g. Chitrakadivati, Hingwashtak choorna, Tapyadiloha etc. Some are named Chyavanprash, Agasthiharitaki leha etc. after the name of the person who made the formulation and popularised it.

Some are named due to their resemblance with some other substance e.g. parpati while

An integrated medical practitioner is the one who can sucessfully solve the medical problems of the integrated disciplines.

others are named after their indications e.g. Sheetapitta prabhanjan, Jvaramurari etc.

Some formulations have been named symbolically without a definite etymology in their names e.g. Laxmivilas, Laxminarayan etc.

In such preparations, there are associate drugs to remove the toxicity along with the primary drug. For example, Piper longum in vasavaleha is used to help as an antitussive and ghee is used to overcome the dryness of adulsa and prevent vatavriddhi or supress vatavriddhi if it occurs. Honey overcomes the increase in kapha due to the sweetness of avaleha and supresses cough. Sugar and water help to make it tasty and paste-like. The same can be stated for other preparations. Every formulation has a specific indication. Creating a formulation is an art of medical science. While preparing formulations, the pathogenesis of the diseases and its stages, systemic and local effects, absorption, distribution, degradation and excretion of the drugs and appearance and palatability of the formulations should be kept in mind. Basic concept behind a formulation is to balance the vitiated doshas.

Preparation of a drug must be such that it is suitable to the patient's choice and the pathological stage of the disease.

The preparation has to be multifacted ie. counteracting many diseases at the same time. One has also to take into consideration that it should be available for use in various forms like juice, pulp, decoction, hot and cold infusions, tablets, sneha, asava, arishta etc.

While manufacturing drugs, all these factors are considered and hence in a way, the art of preparing medicines is a cullinary art. This art must be achieved by the physican.

Posology or Dosage

Ayurveda has rightly given due importance to dose and time of drug administration. However, dose of a drug is never fixed as it varies with disease, digestive capacity, strength, age, region, season etc. Desired effect is never achieved by giving less or more dose. Small dose in serious conditions will be ineffective and may result in death of the patient. Therefore dose of the medicine in a treatment is very important.

It must be administered in a proper dose. The following factors must be considered before administration . A single drug, with variation in dose, shows different effects and actions.

Age - Life span is divided into three stages - 1-16 yrs childhood, 17-70 adulthood, 70 onwards old age. A maximum dose can be administered in adulthood ie. between 17-70 years. A minimum dose is used at the two extremes.

Age -	1 month	-	dose 120 mgm.
	2 months	-	dose 250 mgm
	12 months	-	dose 1.5 gm

For treating any patient, even while giving first aid, it is essential to have knowledge, sympathy and practial experience.

Upto 16 years - every year, the dose should be increased by 1 Masa. Thus, at the age of 16 years, the maximum dose is 1 Tola. (A maximum dose is never possible to administer)

From 17-70 years - 12 gms

Thereafter the dose is reduced by 500 mgm each year.

This tabulation is applicable for pulp and powder. The dose of decoctions is considered to be fourtimes that of powder and pulp. Modern experts have also devised certain formulae in this regard. These are as follows :

Young's formula -

$$\text{Dose for a Child} = (\text{Adult dose}) \times \frac{\text{Age}}{\text{Age} + 12}$$

As per this formula, 1 yr child's dose $= \frac{1}{1+12} = 1/13$th of the adult dose (not applicable to morphine and such lethal substances. For such substances, dose should be still smaller) Similar to age, weight of the patient is also one of the criteria for deciding the dose. Such dosage is based on kilograms. Many other factors should also be considered while ascertaining the dose. However, weight is chiefly considered as it provides an objective criteria for assessment.

Cowling's formula

$$\text{Child's dose} = \text{Adult dose} \times \frac{\text{Age} + 1}{24}$$

ie. 1 yrs child's dose $= \frac{1+1}{24} = \frac{2}{24} = \frac{1}{12}$ of adult dose.

Following factors are also considered along with age, while ascertaining the dose.

1. Strength (Bala) - Maximum dose for nondebilitated patients and reduced dose according to debility.

2. Sex - Female patients should be given a smaller dose compared to male patients. Besides, in females, dose should be adjusted according to menstruation as well.

3. Appetite (Agni) - Larger doses are required in patients who have good appetite while lesser doses are required in patients with reduced appetite.

4. Dosha - Dose is increased in proportion to vitiation of doshas and vice versa.

5. Disease - Increased dose is required in serious pathological conditions and lesser dose in ordinary conditions. Drug becomes effective and also tolerable in large doses when specific drug in

Diseases like ascites and dermatosis, which are caused by accumulation of malas, can never be eradicated without persistent purification.

specific disease is administered e.g. large dose of morphine is used as analgesic sedative in liver and renal conditions.

6. Intestine - Large dose is required in constipation and full bowel, whereas smaller dose in empty bowel and mild reactive bowel.

7. Medicine - Smaller dose of highly potent dravyas and larger dose of mildly potent dravyas is required.

8. Constitution - Persons of some constitution show idiosyncrasy to certain drugs. The cause is not ascertained, yet there is definitely an intolerance to certain drugs.

9. Habit - Certain addictive and toxic drugs like morphine, alcohol etc. become ineffective after prolonged use and they require more medicinal dose.

10. Absorption and excretion - A drug which shows quick absorption and delayed excretion remains in the circulation for a longer duration and hence such drugs are given in smaller doses. This the reason why drugs administered by injections or unctuous dravyas administered by matra basti are always given in small doses.

11. Mental condition - If the mental condition of the patient is favourable and he has faith in the person who is treating him then a smaller dose is also effective. This is of prime importance.

12. Climate - Cold and sheeta veerya drugs are useful in places having hot climatic conditions and vice versa.

13. Time - In cold season, ushna veerya drugs should be used and sheeta veerya drugs should be used in hot season.

14. Preparation - Dose also depends on the type of preparation. Thus a smaller dose is required for rasakalpa than choorna and quath.

Anupan

A substance used for mixing the drug at the time of administration or which is given thereafter is called anupan (vehicle). This is necessarily a liquid, e.g. honey, milk, warm water, juice of Ocimum sanctum etc.

Anupan helps the medicine to be transformed into liquid state which, in turn, enhances its obsorption and action. Certain drugs act specifically and effectively when administered with specific anupan.

Anupan is useful for proper and effective action of a drug when the drug is difficult to administer or the drug is destroyed after consumption or a specific action on target cell is desired. Also, it helps to overcome the untoward or toxic effects of the drug. For example, in vata disease, the anupan

If one doesnot have faith in the subject which he teaches and promotes, it is better not to do so.

should be snigdha and ushna, in pitta diseases - madhur and sheeta (cold), in kapha diseases - ruksha and ushna. The anupan in a particular disease can be selected from the dravyas which are included in the regimen of diet for that particular disease. Medicinal effect is then attributed to the combination of the drug and the anupan. e.g. Tapyadiloha which is given along with honey in anaemia. Certain dravyas which are considered harmful in specific diseases, when combined as an anupan with medications, are not only effective but also enhance the action of the medicine. For example, curds is absolutely contraindicated in jaundice as it is abhishyandi. Yet, it is our experience that when calcium hydroxide is given with curds as an anupan, it is always helpful in jaundice. This action of calcium hydroxide is enchanced by yakrut gamitva of curds.

Drugs mixed for trituration could also act as excellent anupan along with the drug used for treatment. The following anupan are used in general - hot or cold water, decoction, alcohol, fruit juice, milk, meat juice, honey, ghee, butter milk, curd, oil, cow's urine etc. Juice of different plants, decoctions and infusions and extracts are also used as anupan. Choice of the anupan is made by considering the medicine, patient and the disease.

Consumption of oil or ghee as medicine must be followed by hot water as anupan. Especially, when food contains vegetable ghee (saturated fats), hot water is the most suitable anupan. Recently, vegetable ghee is used as a substitute for ghee in treatment but the saturated fats of vegetable ghee are harmful to a patient of reduced appetite. A hot anupan helps to overcome this harmful effect to some extent. An anupan of buttermilk is the most effective in preventing as well as treating the symptoms of excess intake of ghee or oil.

Disease		**Anupan**
1. Colic	-	Ghee + asafoetida
2. Chronic fever	-	Honey + Piper longum
3. Vata disease	-	Ghee + garlic
4. Asthma	-	Honey + trikatu
5. Cold (Rigors)	-	Beatle leaf + Piper nigrum
6. Diabetes	-	Triphala + sugar
7. Vomiting	-	Fried rice water.
8. Diarrhoea	-	Kutajavaleha
9. Haemetemesis	-	Adulsavaleha
10. Piles	-	Chitrakamoola
11.Intestinal worms	-	Vidang quath

Lack of sanitation facilities for defecation and urination for the city dwellers is one of the causes of hypertension, heart diseases, gastrointestinal disorders, asthma and aging.

12.Indigestion	-	Warm water
13. Sannipat	-	Honey + ginger juice
14. Fever	-	Decoction of nagaramotha + parpat
15. Duodenitis	-	Butter milk
16.Poison	-	Gold
17. Tuberculosis	-	Milk or mutton soup
18. Anaemia	-	Punarnava
19. Bronchitis	-	Vasa
20. Debilitated patients	-	Alcoholic beverages prepared from cereals
21. Obesity	-	Honey and water

Anupan may be changed according to the disease condition. For example, in haemorrhagic diathesis, goat's milk and sugarcane juice are used as anupan. It is observed that the same medicine with different anupan may be useful in different diseases. Some specific anupan are mentioned in different texts.

Sushruta has laid down the following principle in Sutra sthana regarding administration and choice of the drug -

यस्य देहस्य यत्सात्म्यं यच्चास्याचरितं भवेत् ।
तेन भेषजसंयुक्तं भैषज्यमुपकल्पयेत् ।।.

Proper anupan may not be available at the time of administration of the drug and therefore the drugs for anupan are used at the time of trituration which is also effective but to a lesser extent.

Time of administration

Time of administration is also equally important.
Time of administration of drugs as per Charaka falls into 11 catergories.

1. Early morning (Fasting) - Medicine on empty stomach acts best by retaining its potency which does not get diluted or destroyed. Patients with good strength should be given medicines on empty stomach. Also in kapha diseases and in patients having kapha prakriti, medicines should be given in the morning.

2. Pragbhakta (Premeal) - This is useful for vata diseases and conditions involving the large intenstine.

Vagbhatta says that the occurence of heart disease is associated with witholding ten out of the thirteen natural urges.

3. Madhyabhakta (During meal) - Action of samanvayu starts at the middle of the meal therefore the diseases of the organs related to the field of samanvayu eg. liver, spleen, pancreas, duodenum etc. should be treated by giving the medicine in the madhyabhakta kala. Similarly in diseases of pitta and agni also, medicines should be administered in the same kala. Since the medicine gets mixed with food particles, it is most useful in removing the obstruction of srotas.

4. Pashchadbhakta (Post lunch) -This period is related to the action of vyan vayu and therefore useful in heart diseases. Medicines given in this period act on the upper half of the trunk and on kapha diseases. It is best suited for administering rasayana dravyas.

5. Pashchadbhakta (Post dinner) - This period is related to the action of udan vayu and therefore conditions like cough, breathlessness, bronchitis etc. are best treated by administering medicines in this period. At night, during rest, the blood circulation is predominantly in the trunk which enhances the effect of the drug.

6. Muhurmuhuh (Frequently) - Conditions of bouts or attacks like asthma, bronchitis, cough, hiccough, vomiting, thirst etc. need medicines very frequently to overcome / control the attack. Generation of vibrations of the medicine acting on the disease condition is required to counteract the attack.

7. Samudga (Adjacent to meal) - It is useful in diseases of vyan and apan vayu as well as in conditions involving upper and lower part of the trunk. It is also useful in hiccough, tremors and epilepsy. The food must be light to digest so as to be superseded by medicine.

8. Samabhakta (Along with meal) - This is used to make the food tasty. Sour and tasty drugs are mixed during cooking for this purpose. Children and debilitated as well as reluctant patients may be administered medicines in this way. It is useful for generalised disease conditions because the medicine which is treated with the cooked food, easily spreads throughout the body.

9. Sagras (With every morsel) - Useful in diseases of pran vayu. Specially deepan (appetiser) and aphordisiac drugs in the form of paste, tablets etc. are administered in this way. The concept of pran vayu is concerned with the act of swallowing.

10. Grasantar (In between two morsels) - This period is also concerned with the act of swallowing which is controlled by pran vayu. Drugs given in this period also act on disorders of pran vayu.

11. Nisha (Before sleep) - Drugs are administered in this period for treating diseases of the supraclavicular organs. The restorvative activity going on during sleep is enhanced by drugs given in this period.

According to some texts (Ashtangsangraha), emesis and fumigation should be done at night since the srotasas of the koshtha are blocked at night thereby allowing the drug to act on the upper part of the body.

The fear of diseases doesnot bother one who follows healthy regimens of dinacharya, ratricharya, rutucharya, swasthaniyam and sadvrutta.

In Ashtangsangraha, one more time of administration is mentioned which is called as anantarabhakta. In this, drug is administered after the lunch gets completely digested and once the drug is digested, dinner is taken. This is effective in patients with strong agni and diseases of vyan vayu.

The periods mentioned above are also related to the action of different vayus since vayu is responsible for movement and makes the medicine reach the tissues and organs. Pitta and kapha are considered as secondary since vayu only carries them all over the body. Diseases produced by various vayus can be treated by administering drugs in their respective periods.

Sharangdhar has summarised these eleven periods into five types viz.

1. Early morning 2) Lunch time 3) Dinner time 4) Frequent 5) Night time.

1. Early morning - Medicines useful for inducing emesis and purgation should be given in early morning. Charakacharya's abhakta kala corresponds to this period.

2. Lunch time - All periods related to pre and post lunch periods are included in this category.

3. Dinner time - Periods of administration which are with morsel , between two morsels etc. are included in this category.

4. Frequently - Conditions of periodical attacks like asthma and hiccough, show good response to this time of administration.

5. Night - Useful for the diseases of supracavicular region. Classification done by Vriddha Vagbhatta and Charaka is included in these five types.

Even though the specificity between different vayus and administration of drugs is observed, yet for optimum benefits the following description will be useful wherein specific timings for administering specific drugs have been given -

1. Mineral acids should be used before meals.

2. Salts and acids should be used after food to dilute them. Iron which causes irritation of the stomach, should be administered immediately after food. Blood tonics should be administered 1 hour after meal.

3. Antacids are given in the morning on empty stomach.

4. Appetisers should be given before meal.

5. Disgestive medicines should be given after food.

6. Intestinal digestive medicine should be given 1-2 hours after meal as the food reaches the intenstine

It is extremely important to have correct knowledge of dosage of even those drugs which are used for external application.

at this time.

7. Fats, cod liver oil etc. should be given after food. Similarly, formulations containing arsenic, iron etc. should only be given after food.

8.Strong cathartic puragatives (Mag. sulph., Castor oil) should be given in the morning during pitta kala and mild laxatives at night.

9. Drugs related to menstrual cycles should be given 1 week before menstruation.

10. Drugs used for inducing sleep should be given half an hour before bed time.

Besides these periods, alterations can be made depending on the necessity and the availability of the medicine to be administered. Broadly, morning, afternoon and evening periods are considered according to kapha, pitta and vata respectively but it cannot be considered as absolutely scientific. Just as in case of purifying procedures, the periods of administration of shaman (ameliorating) drugs should not be missed.

Channels of administration

According to Charaka, drugs which are used for purification can be classified into two classes viz. (1) for internal purification and (2) for external purification. The ways or channels of administration of such purifying drugs are similar to the drugs which are used to establish a state of equilibrium of doshas in the body without removing them out of the body. The site of aggravation of the doshas and the site of the disease, influence and decide the different ways of administration of drugs. For purification purposes, 'the nearest way out' can be considered as the basic principle. And therefore various excretory outlets of the body can be used to administer medications. There are 2 eyes, 2 ears, 1 anus, 1 urethra, 1 vagina and 1 mouth in a human body which form 10 big openings. In addition to these openings, there is the skin which covers almost all the area of human body with its millions of small openings. All such body orifices can be used to administer drugs.

(1) Mouth cavity

(A) Can be used for local afflictions. It is commonly used for gargles, dental fillings, external massage etc.

(B) It can also be used for administration of drugs which act as appetizers, digestives, emetics, purgatives etc.

(C) Procedures which are useful on the respiratory tract like inhalation of steam or medicinal smoke are administered through mouth.

(D) The mouth cavity can also be used in administration of drugs which act systemically all over the body. Drugs administered through this route are digested and then assimilated through intestines to act on all systems of the body.

By dedicating one year to each disease, W.H.O. gives the world an opportunity to think about it in detail.

(2) Nostrils

(A) A famous statement from the classics says, "Nostrils are doors to the head". Afflictions of supraclavicular parts of the body like diseases of eyes, nose, throat etc. can be treated using this route of administration. It can also be used to treat local diseases of nose.

(B) Drugs acting on lungs and other respiratory organs can be administered through nostrils in the form of inhalations of vapours and other gases. Anaesthetic drugs are good examples of this type.

(C) This route is also used to administer such drastic treatments like shirovirechan. Also this route is specifically to be used in 'punsavana' - a ritual to be carried out in the first trimester of pregnancy to have a child of the desired gender. This route is also used when oral route cannot be used for some reasons.

(3) Eyes - This route is mostly used for local ailments. The drugs can be applied in the form of fomentation, drops, intraconjunctival applications etc.

In few systemic conditions like unconsciousness and also to induce sleep, many a times medicines are administered in the eyes.

(4) Ears - For various ear diseases like ear discharge, otalgia, polyps etc., medicines are administered locally in the ears. Oil instillation is also used to induce sleep.

(5) Anus - Various medicated enemas can be given through this route. It is used not only for local but general diseases also.

(6) Urethra - Drugs can be instilled through this route in urinary bladder. Such drugs are offen in the form of medicated oils, decoctions or suppositories.

(7) Vagina - Medicated swabs, uterine suppositories, douches are used for medication through this route. Fumigation with smoke of medicated materials can also be applied. Abortions are also carried out using this route.

(8) Skin - The routes of administration of drugs mentioned above are obvious and are considerably large in size. There are still infinite ways to administer drugs in the form of the minute pores of the skin. Oil massage, steam baths, anointing, fomentation, powder massage, baths etc. are ways in which medicines can be administered in the body. Treatment of skin ulcers, incisions, scraping, cauterization, branding etc. are achieved through the skin . Treatment by acupuncture is carried out through skin only.

To produce acute pruritus using powder of Mucuna pruriens, to insert medicines in nail beds using needles, or to insert medicines directly into the blood through an incision on the scalp, is done through the skin. Similarly, various routes of administration mentioned in modern pharmacology like subcutaneous, intradermal, intramuscular, intravenous, intra-arterial, intrathecal (lumbar puncture) are through skin. Therefore skin is a vast route since it covers all the external area of our body.

While treating diseases of the senses, one should carefully consider the status of the mahabhoota which constitutes that sense as well as the sense organ.

Inoculation of small pox vaccine into the skin by taking a small superficial incision with a lancet is another example of this route. Tattooing with medicines is also another form of using this route. In using this route, various stages of body doshas and their conditions may not be useful directly. However, these conditions ought to be considered while deciding the contraindications. For example, oil massage is contraindicated in samadosha or tub bath is contraindicated immediately after food.

While using injections as a route of administration, care must be taken that body pH value must remain in equilibrium. Otherwise there is a strong possibility of lysis of the local tissues like muscle, fascia and skin resulting in abscess formation. pH value of every organ of the body is different. The pH value of drug should be equal to the pH of that organ so as to avoid such untoward effects. pH value of seven is taken as neutral. As this value decreases, the substance becomes more and more acidic. e.g. pH value of 1.5 is strongly acidic and 6.5 is mildly acidic.

In any diseased condition, at least one or more excretory organs of the body are affected. Therefore drugs can be administered through organs of excretion also. It has been mentioned in the classical texts e.g. in fever, loose motions etc.

When it is not possible to use the oral route, e.g. in cases of deep coma, the drugs are directly inserted into the body by puncturing the nail beds of the patient. Similarly in the seventh stage of treatment of poisoning, drugs are advised to be given directly into the blood by incising the scalp area superficially. Therefore these can also be considered as routes of administration of drugs.

Prescription writing

Separate paper is to be used for prescription for each individual. One should not prescribe medicines for two or more individuals on the same paper as it sure will create confusion amongst the patients.

Prescriptions should be written only after examining the patient thoroughly and after reaching a definite conclusion about the diagnosis of the disease. Its proper treatment consisting of drugs acting on affected doshas, drugs acting on the disease or drugs acting in both ways should be written. Tolerance of the patient must be considered at this stage. One must be very careful while prescribing drugs to infants, the elderly and pregnant women. Medicines prescribed to children should be mild, also either astringent or sweet to taste. It should be administered with either milk or honey. Their drugs should be of optimum nature; not too fatty or sour and should be digested easily. When toxic substances or poisons have to be used, extra care is needed.

For infants who are breastfed, medicines can be given to their mothers (so that they will be excreted in the milk and hence reach the child easily) or it can be applied in the form of ointment over the nipple. There are many drugs which are excreted in the milk. Such drugs become palatable to the infant for easy action on the body.

It is imperative to consider the elderly from the point of view of their body, its strength etc. Their tolerance to a particular substance or drug is almost known to them by previous experience.

All the symptoms of vitiation of srotasas are basically caused by obstruction to the flow of their contents. These symptoms are similar to the symptoms of vitiation of all the doshas.

Their temperament should also be considered.

In cases of female patients, the menstrual period, pregnancy, postpoartum period, menopause - all these points must be taken into account.

Prescription writing may differ from individual to individual. However, there must be some order or some method to which one should adhere.

It should begin with name, age, detailed address and diagnosis with main symptoms of the patient. Then treatment should be written down. In this part of the prescription, name of the main drug should be written first along with its dose. Instruction to the compounder/ chemist about packing the drugs should be given neatly. Instructions about way of administration, anupan in which the drug should be taken, when it is to be taken etc. should come next. If more than one drug are to be given, it should be clearly mentioned in the prescription.

If the drug is to be tapered off, this point should also be mentioned. Period for which the drug is to be taken must be mentioned.

Other general instructions for the patients about diet, behaviour, other do's and don't's may also be written on the prescription clearly so that the compounder can instruct the patient accordingly. Every prescription must have the signature and name of the doctor with date.

Following is an example of a typical prescription.

Name of the Patient	:	Mr. Vishnu Mahadeo Gogte, Age 72 years. Madhu Sanchaya, Tilak Path, Nasik -422 001 Phone 2377.
Diagnosis	:	Fatigue due to heavy work and Vataja Kasa (Apatarpanjanya)
Treatment	:	1) Complete Rest. 2) Balatail massage. 3) Bath with Dashamoola Quath. 4) Chyavanprashavaleha. Every morning 2 teaspoonfuls, add Sitopaladi

References -

1. बहुता तत्र योग्यत्वं अनेकविधकल्पना ।
संपत् चेतितुष्कोऽयं द्रव्याणां गुणसंग्रह: । (च. सू.)
बहुकल्पं बहुगुणं संपन्न योग्यमौषधम् । (वा. सू. अ. १)

2. मूलत्वग् सारनिर्यासनालस्वरसपल्लवा: । क्षारा: क्षीरं, फलं, पुष्पं, भस्मतैलानि कण्टका: । पत्राणि शुंगा: कंदाश्च प्ररोहाश्चौद् भिदो गण: ।। (च. सू. अ. १-७३)

3. मधूनि गोरसा: पित्तं वसा मज्जासृगामिषं । विण्मूत्रचमरितोऽस्थिस्नायुशृंगनखाखुरा: । जंगमेभ्य: प्रयुज्यन्ते केशलोमानि रोचना: ।। (च. सू. अ. १/६८-६९)
तत्र स्थावरेभ्य: त्वक् पत्र पुष्प फल मूल कंद निर्यासस्वरसादय: । जंगमेभ्यश्चर्मनखरोमरुधिरादय: । (सु. सू. अ. १/३१)

CHAPTER FIFTEEN

BRIEF HISTORY OF DRAVYAGUNASHASTRA

Vedanta Ayurveda

It is debated whether the vedas are human or divine compilations from times immemorial. However all accept their existence. Mention of the use of medicinal plants is found in all the four vedas namely Rgveda, Yajurveda, Samveda and Atharvaveda. Ayurveda, which is a text on the preventive and curative aspects of diseases is a part of Atharvaveda. A text which describes the origin of life and provides knowledge about life, happiness and sorrow, benefits and losses, life span, how to maintain health, how to treat diseases and regain healthy state, is called Ayurveda.

Rgveda - It is believed to be written between 4500 and 1600 B. C. In Rgveda, medicine is appreciated as is a mother. Very few plants useful for treatment are mentioned. It says that one who possesses a variety of medicinal plants should be called as vaidya. The word 'bheshaj' as well as terms related to disease and medicine are repeatedly found in the Rgveda. Water is considered as the best medicine (1-23-20 and 10-137-68). The word 'tridhatu' is mentioned and the use of pippali is also found.

Yajurveda - A reference is found regarding diseases like shleshma, piles, cough, measles and anaemia.

Samveda - This is specific to music or singing. Experiments are quoted for reviving an unconscious person by singing sutras from Samveda.

Atharvaveda - It is full of management of diseases. It includes treatment by medicine as well as by other means like mantra, tantra etc. 125 dravyas like Achyranthes aspera, Terminalia arjuna, Piper longum, Commiphora mukul etc. are mentioned in Atharvaveda. The chief or principal sutra volume of Atharvaveda is kaushiksutra (400 to 300 B.C.). Reference on the use of decoctions of plants, use of leeches, turmeric and use of honey in management of wounds is found.

The word 'atharva' is used for medicine by Gopatha Brahmins. Four types of treatments namely atharvani, angirasi, daivi and manushi are mentioned in Atharvaveda. Manushi treatment refers to the use of plants. Angirasveda is also called Bhaishajyaveda. There is also a mention of vata, pitta and kapha in Atharvaveda (A.V.6-109-3). Atharvaveda is the last among the vedas and is closely related to Ayurveda. The concept of pran is common to all four types of treatments.

There are 260 plants mentioned in the vedas out of which 130 plants are synonymous to those mentioned in Ayurveda. Charaka mentions less than 500, Sushruta 385, Kautilya 330, Babar manuscripts 400 and Dhanvantari Nighantu 324. Ayurvedic Dravyaguna contains 666 plants. The vedas describe 500 to 600 mantras in relation to diseases while forty diseases are mentioned. Treatment by dravyas of plant origin is given more emphasis than by animal sources. The principle of 'Similia

To maintain health, it is essential to counteract the vibrations of harmtul gunas by producing vibrations of beneficial gunas.

similibus" was observed (मज्जा मज्ज्ञा भवतु॥ मज्जा मज्ज्ञा संधीयताम् चर्मणा चर्म रोहतु ॥ (अ. वे. काण्ड ४ सू. 22).

Time of collection of plants, swaras, quath, phanta, mantha etc. are described in Shatpath Brahminic literature.

Description about the actions and uses of plants by Charakacharya seems to be in minute detail. The panchabhautik composition of plants, their rasas, vipak, veerya etc. are classified on the basis of their actions. Though medicinal classification is action based, it is also done on morphological basis in relation to diet. Dietary plants are classified on morphological base in Charaka samhita.

Dietary dravyas are classified into 12 groups depending on their structure and different properties. Diet may comprise of meat of animals, fresh and dried spices and seasonings, liquid diet, cooked food and other dravyas related to diet. Thus there are 12 main groups viz. (1)Shookadhanya (cereals) (2) Shamidhanya (pulses) (3) Mansavarga (meat) (4) Shaakvarga (vegetables) (5) Phalavarga (fruits) (6) Haritvarga (green vegetables). (7)Madyavarga (alcohol or beverages) (8) Jalavarga (water) (9) Gorasvarga - animal origin (cow)(10) Ikshuvarga (sugarcane) (11) Krutannavarga (readymade food) (12) Aharyogivarga (supplementary diets)

Medicinal plants are classified on the basis of their action. Keeping in mind their composition, Charaka has classified dravyas into doshaprashaman, dhatupradushan and swasthahita in the first chapter of Sutra sthana; but action based description of dravyas is found in the fourth chapter.

In this chapter, classification into 50 groups is based on the action on various systems of the body. And as this is more useful in daily life, these 50 groups can be classified as follows :

Medicinal dravyas acting on -

1. Digestive system - deepan, pachan, vamak, virechak, grahi etc.
2. Circulatory system - shonitsthapan.
3. Respiratory system - kasahara, shwashara, chhedan etc.
4. Reproductive system - vrushya, vajikar, prajasthapan, garbhasthapan etc.
5. Urinary system - mutrasangrahaneeya, mutravirajaneeya, mutravirechaneeya etc.
6. Skin - swedopag, swedapnayan, romashatan, romasanjanan, kandughna, kushthaghna etc.
7. Body Temperature - jvarahara
8. Nervous system - medhya, sangnyasthapan, madak etc.
9. Satmikaran - rasayan, balya, bruhan, jeevaneeya etc.

While treating any disease, it is secondary to treat the apparent site of the disease. It is more important and fundamental to treat the vitiated srotasas.

Apart from these groups, certain other groups like mukhashodan, dantashodan, rakshoghna, aparapatan etc. have also been mentioned at appropriate places.

Classification in the Sushruta period

Sushruta period follows after Charaka. In this period, the classification of dravyas took a favourable turn for improvement. Sushruta classified dietary dravyas on structural basis following the same pattern as Charaka. In general, he described dietary class in two chapters (सु. सू. अ. 45 & 46). Liquid dravyas are divided into ten groups while staple food into thirteen groups. It means that the progress of classifying dietary substances into twenty three divisions was achieved during the period of Sushruta.

Liquid substances - Water, milk, curd, buttermilk, ghee, honey, sugarcane juice, alcohol and urine.

Soild substances - Pulses, cereals, meat, fruits, vegetables, flowers, roots, salt, metals and readymade substances.

Sushruta's classification is superior to Charaka's for the following reasons -

1. Charaka mentions cow's product as a single group whereas Sushruta describes four - milk, curd, buttermilk and ghee.
2. Liquid dravya - Oil, alcohol and urine class is totally new in Sushruta's classification.
3. Charaka describes cereals as one group whereas Sushruta mentions two - shali varga and kudhanya varga.
4. Charaka describes vegetable group as only one whereas Sushruta describes it as flowers and tubers, separately.
5. Sushruta mentions salt and minerals separately into two groups.
6. Progressively the use of metals and gems increased, hence Sushruta classified them into two groups.

Sushruta also classified medicinal dravyas based on their actions into 44 types. (Refer to 38 and 39 chapters of Sutra sthana). But instead of naming these groups by their action, they are named after the first medicine in that particular group. Out of 44 types, 37 are of this nature and out of the remaining, four are sanshodhan and three are sanshaman.

Sushruta samhita is predominantly based on surgery. Therefore a mention of surgically important groups like vimlapan, pachan, ropan etc. appears typical of Sushruta. Examples of classification based on prominent plants are vidarigandhadi, aragwadhadi etc. and are further mentioned in samhita as atidesh. Rasayana dravyas are also subdivided into saumya and divaya by Sushruta. Not only this, but even mixed types are also denoted by numerals such as trikatu, triphala, panchamoola and dashamoola. Charaka has also described certain groups by naming them by their parts like

The diet of a woman in the days immediately preceding her conception certainly has an influence on the foetus.

mulini and phalini (मूलीनी, फलिनी) which remained unnoticed. But Sushruta has extensively used such criteria in his classification.

Ashtangsangraha (Vriddha Vagbhatta) - This is a collective volume as the name implies. This volume emerged as a collection from Sushruta, Charaka and other ancient literature. Therefore incorporation of principles of Charaka and Sushruta into this volume is natural. With changing times, it has progressed as well as new thoughts have been incorporated. For this reason, for two chapters of Charaka and Sushruta samhita, Ashtangsangraha requires seven chapters for the same subject. The author of this volume describes chapters on liquid dravyas and dietary dravyas similar to two chapters of Sushruta samhita. These two chapters are further classified into twelve types. The author of Ashtangsangraha has taken into account the views of Charaka and Sushruta. Instead of classifying separately, salt, minerals, metals and gems are all included in the same chapter.

Similarly, out of fifty mahakashaya of Charakacharya, 45 are included in mahakashaya group and remaining five in shodhanadigana. Sushruta has described twenty five groups in the Vividhaganasangraha adhyaya. He has mentioned doshashaman dravyas in chapter 14. Three associated chapters on volatile substances are exclusive of Ashtangsangraha.

A classical tabulation of medicinal plants according to their action is as follows :-

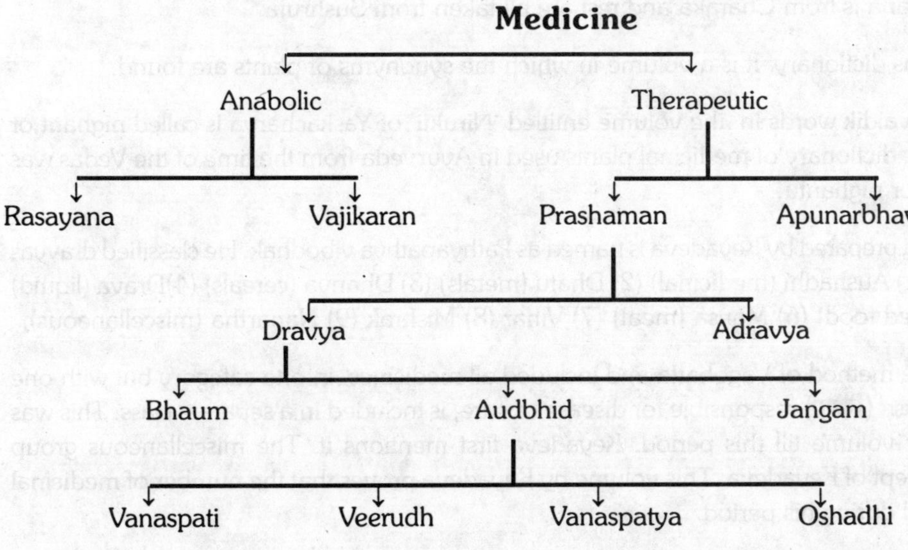

The author of Ashtangsangraha has mentioned many mixed ganas. Triphala, trikatu, panchamoola, trijat, chaturjat, panchakol etc. are described independently. Credit of preparing new mixed ganas goes to Ashtangsangraha because it initiated a new system of mixed ganas.
Vagbhatta has descrbied 155 dravyas in Agrasangraha while Charaka mentions 152. Besides this, Vriddha Vagbhatta puts forth the guiding principles to new vaidyas. The concept of haritakyadi varga has evolved through this thinking. Over all, Ashtangsangraha is not only a treatise about expansion

Eventhough doshas are called the causes of diseases, the fundamental causes are raja and tama (the vies of the mind).

but it also incorporates new concepts which are practically sound. Study of Ashtangsangraha is a must besides the samhitas of Charaka and Sushruta.

Ashtanghridaya - Ashtangsangraha is a large compilation. The concise edition of it is Ashtanghridaya. This was written probably in 3-6 century A. D. Vagbhatta describes fluid dravyas into five groups viz. (1) water (2) milk (3) sugarcane juice (4) oil (5) alcohol. Mutra varga is casually mentioned after alcohol but it is not described as an independent group.

Food dravyas are classified into 7 types :-

(1) Shookadhanya varga (cereals) (2) Shimbidhanya varga (pulses) (3) Krutanna varga (readymade food) (4) Mansa varga (meat) (5)Shaak varga (vegetables) (6) Phala varga (fruits) (7) Aushadhi varga (drugs).

Aushadhi varga includes haritaki, lavana and kshar along with other dravyas of mishra varga like triphala, trikatu etc. We should admire the speciality of Vagbhatta of classifying a separate Aushadhi varga (class) and describing its properties. Vaidyas of later period are his followers. Classification of plants based on action is similar to both Sushruta and Vagbhatta.

33 ganas are mentioned in the shodhanadiganasangraha of chapter 15 of Sutra sthana out of which jeevaneeya gana is from Charaka and rest are all taken from Sushruta.

Nighantu means dictionary. It is a volume in which the synonyms of plants are found.

A collection of vaidik words in the volume entitled 'Nirukti' of Yaskacharya is called nighant or nighantu. Therefore, dictionary of medicinal plants used in Ayurveda from the time of the Vedas was also called nighant or nighantu.

In fact, nighantu prepared by Keyadeva is named as Pathyapathya vibodhak. He classified dravyas into nine types viz (1) Aushadhi (medicinal) (2) Dhatu (metals) (3) Dhanya (cereals) (4)Drava (liquid) (5) Pakvanna (cooked food) (6) Mansa (meat) (7) Vihar (8) Mishrak (9) Nanartha (miscellaneous).

He followed the method of Vagbhatta and included all medicines in one category but with one exception that exercise (विहार) responsible for disease or cure, is included in a separate class. This was not so in any other volume till this period. Keyadeva first mentions it. The miscellaneous group (नानार्थ) is also a concept of Keyadeva. This volume by Keyadeva proves that the number of medicinal plants had increased during his period.

Dhanvantari nighantu

The format of a compilation changes according to the period. Dhanvantari nighantu is a classic example of this.

He formed different classes of medicines and expanded the compilation greatly. He also gave more importance to medicinal dravyas instead of dietary dravyas which was a shift from the format

Plants like sandal and neem have to intially take the support of other plants like creepers.

followed in previously existing nighantus. It appears that this writer of sixth century A. D. was a minister in the court of King Vikramaditya.

Dhanvantari nighantu defines seven groups.

(1) Guduchyadi (2) Shatpushpadi (3) Chandanadi (4) Karaviradi (5) Amradi (6) Suvarnadi (7) Mishrakadi

(Those dravyas which cannot be included into the first six groups are all grouped into a mixed group).

The study of medicine expanded as medicinal classfication became scientifically based during the period of Dhanvantari. Similarly, the number of new medicinal plants increased. Dhanvantari nighantu's attempt at classification of medicinal plants as systematically as possible is considered as pioneering work. Many new dravyas whose actions were found similar, were grouped into one group and this group was named after the prominent dravya of that class. Guduchyadi varga contains the following medicinal plants with similar actions.

(I) Guduchyadi varga - गुडुच्यादिरयं वर्ग: प्रथम परिकिर्तित: । उर्ध्वाधो दोषहरण: सर्वामय विनाशन: ।
(Guduchi by its cholagogue action is used in jaundice). Medicines having rasayana property and उर्ध्वाधो संशोधन: are included into this class - e.g. guduchi, madanphala, danti etc.

(II) Shatpushpadi varga - This includes deepan, balya and mukhashodhan dravyas like mishi, vacha, ela etc.

(III) Chandanadi varga - Chandan, saffron, usheer etc. These dravyas are fragrant.

(IV) Karviradi varga - This includes different types of dravyas. No specific action is observed. Kanher, tulsi, nakuli etc.

(V) Amradi varga- This class includes the plants whose fruits, flowers and bark are used in medicine e.g. mango, jasmine, arjuna etc.

(VI) Suvarnadi varga - It includes metals, wheat, barley and other shamidhanya besides oil, milk, alcohol, meat etc.

(VII) Mishrakadi varga - All remaining dravyas including triphala, trikatu etc.

This volume mentions mercury and refers to the actions and properties of different types of magnets, morphine and khaskhas. It gives an indication of the adaptibility of Ayurveda.

Rajnighantu

This includes more classes. With reference to medicine, 16 classes are described as - guduchyadi,

Dams destroy many plants by submerging them under water. There is no way to cultivate plants on the submerged land.

shatahvadi, parpatadi, pippalyadi, mulakadi, salmalyadi, prabhadradi, karaviradi, amradi, chandanadi, suvarnadi, paniyadi, kshiradi, shalyadi, mansadi and mixed class.

There is lot of similarity between this classification and that of Dhanvantari nighantu. These volumes are not based on similar principles. Some classes (vargas) are based on action and some on property. Since suvarnadi class contains oil, ghee and mansa, it is difficult to understand the basis of classification by either action or property. Previous compilations were action-based, but here, this is not so. Successive authors have omitted the references of Charaka and Sushruta. They all seem to follow Dhanvantanri nighantu and Raj nighantu in their classification of medicines. This author from Kashmir has mentioned more dravyas than the other nighantus of his time.

Madanvinod or Madanpal nighantu

This volume was written in 1374 A. D. by Madanpal and his classification is as follows:

(1) abhayadi (2) shunthyadi (3) karpuradi (4) suvarnadi (5) vatadi (6) phaladi (7) shakadi (8) paniyadi (9) ikshukadi (10) dhanyaguna (11) dhanyakritannadi (12) mansa (13) mishrak (mixed). Nothing is mentioned specifically in the mixed class.

The format of this volume is based on Dhanvantari nighantu. Mandanpal was the King of Kaccha kingdom on the banks of the river Yamuna, north of Delhi. He had studied many nighantus. This book includes dravyas like heroin, morphine, parasikyavani etc.

Bhavprakash nighantu

Bhavmishra in 1596 (i. e. sixteenth century) compiled and completed a volume acceptable to many during the period. This includes 20 classes as (1) haritakyadi (2) karpuradi (3) guducchyadi (4) pushpavarga (5) phalavarga (6) vatadi (7) dhatuvarga (metal) (8) dhanyavarga (grains) (9) shaakvarga (10) varivarga(11) dugdhavarga (milk) (12) dadhivarga (curd) (13) takravarga (buttermilk) (14) lonivarga (butter) (15)ghritvarga (ghee) (16) mootravarga (urine) (17) tailavarga (oil) (18)madhavarga (honey) (19) ikshuvarga (sugarcane) (20) sandhanvarga

Classification of dietary dravyas of Bhavprakash is more relevant and correct. A genuine attempt to make it correct has been made. Haritakyadi varga includes those dravyas whose fruits or roots are used. Karpuradi varga includes dravyas having odours. Guduchyadi varga includes those dravyas whose panchang or roots are used. Vatadi class includes the tall trees. The only shortcoming is that, why are saindhav (rock salt), samudra (sea salt) and bid lavana etc. included into haritakyadi varga ? Is it because of pancharasa ?

Many compilers (nighantukars) followed Bhavprakash. All those who follow the classification of Bhavprakash understandably carry the same defect. Rajvallabh nighantu (1760), Nighantu Sangrah (1815), Nighantu Ratnakar (1924) and Shaligram nighantu (1953) are prepared according to Bhavprakash.

It is observed that Charaka and Sushruta classified dravyas by considering actions and morphology. Thereafter, the writers deviated from this basic principle and classified according to properties of dravyas.

Amarkosha - This is a volume which contains names of dravyas useful for treatment. Classifications of dravyas based on their names is first observed in this compilation.

It was perhaps written in 4th - 5th century. However, the medicinal uses of these dravyas are not mentioned in this book.

Abhidhan Ratnamala - This is also based on names.

Dravyagunasangraha - This can be called as the first nighantu written by Chakrapani - the commentator on Charaka samhita. Like Charaka and Sushruta, the use of grains and meat etc. is found. (Shivdas Senani has commented on this book).

This nighantu is written by considering the classification based on properties and actions described by Charaka, Sushruta and Vagbhatta (11th Century).

Siddhamantra - Vaidya Keshav has written this nighantu. (Bopdeo, his own son, has commented on this). Bopdeo was a scholar in the court of Yadav Kings Mahadeo and Ramchandra of Deogiri. He belongs to the period 1271 to 1309 A. D. Classification of dravyas into vatapittaghna and vatashleshmaghna is observed in this volume.

Other volumes on Dravyaguna appear in the medieval period, out of which some are independent or some are part of other volumes. For example -

1) Ashtang nighantu.

2) Paryayratnamala (Ratnamala) - The author of Madhav Nidan has written this book. (Harun-Al-Rashid translated it into Arabic in 8th century). Many synonyms with different meanings are found in this volume.

To prepare an Ayurveda nighantu, it is essential to know the names, morphology and properties of various plants. Even then, the morphology of plants is the main criterion on which classification is based. The modern concept of classification of plants is based on morphology and is acceptable for the identification of dravyas. As it is universally accepted, it is advantageous in obtaining the desired dravya anywhere in the world. This classfication is mainly based on flower pattern.

List of popular authors who have scientifically written volumes :

1) Arundatta (2) Agnivesha (3) Amarsingh (Amarkosh) (4) Antubhai Vaidya (Vanaspati Parichaya) (5) Agnihotri (Avadhavihari) Bhaishajyakalpanavignyan (6) Apate (Raj nighantu and Dravyaguna nighantu) (7) Aadhamalla (8) Atreya 9) Acharya Yadavs jiitrikamji (10) Apasangikar (Manual of Botany) (11) Ogale (Chikitsa Prabhakar and Bilvadi Vignyan - 20th century (13) Kamat (Medicinal

Although there are seven basic colours (as in a rainbow), forty different shades are seen in the leaves and flowers of plants.

Plants in Dhanvantari nighantu 20th century) (14) Kalidas (Vaidyamanorama) (15) Kashyap (3000-5000 B.C.) (16) Kurtadkar (Dravyagunashastra 20th century) (17) Kumar Krishna (Ayurvedic Aushadhi Nighantu) (18) Krishnanandaji Maharaj, (19) Keyadeo (Keyanighantu) (20) Ashtang Hridaya Kosha (K.M. Vaidya) (21) Keshav (Vaidyavar) Siddhamantra (22) Ganapati Singh (Amba) (23) Gadre R. V. (24) Gajanan Book Depot (Sangrah Aushadhibad, Aushadhi Sangrah etc). (25) Gupta Vanitacharan (Vanaushadhi darpan) (26) Gupta Parvatishankar (27) Gupta Durgaprasad (Gula) (28) Charaka (Charaka Samhita 3000-5000 B.C.) (29) Chakrapani (1040 A.D.) Shabda Chandrika (30) Chandrachandan (Gana Nighantu) (31) Chitre (Abhinavanighantu (32) Krishna Chandra (Vanaspatik Anusandhan Darshika) (33) Chidananda Vinayak Laxman (Gharcha Batva (34) Chobe Dattaram (Abhinav Nighantu) (35) Jayakrishna Indraji (Vanaspati Shastra) (36) Jamnagar (Gulabakunwarba Sanstha) Charaka Sahava Khanda (37) Jangle Hiraman Motilal (Sachitra Rangeet Vanaspati Gunadarsha) (38) Joshi Harprasad Bhaishankar (Sandigdha Dravya Vignyan) (39) Joshi Sundarlal Nathalal (Udbhijja Shastra) (40) Joshi L. N. (Phalahar Chikitsa) (41) Joshi R. V. (Aushadhi Dipika) (42) Joshi Prayagdatta (43) Zandu-Bhatji (1899) Aushadi Sangrah (44) Thakur Balwant Singh (Vanaushadhi darshika) (45) Thakur Daljit Singh (Unani dravyagunavignyan) (46) Thakar Jayakrishna Indraji (Plants of Kutch) (Guj.) 47) Dalhan (comments on Sushruta) 10th century A.D. (48) Trimallabhatta (Dravyagunashatshloki (49) Trivedi Krishnaprasad (50) Trivedi Triveniprasad (51) Trivedi P. Vishwanath (Nighantu Adarsha) (52) Tryambakraj (Vaidya Tryambaki) (53) Damale R. V. (Vanaspati Vichar) (54) Datar A. V. (Vanaspati Swabhav) (55) Dixit Ramsnehi (Drakshe) (56) Dwivedi Vishwanath (Aushadhi Vignyan Shastra. Ayu. Aushadhi Vargikaran (57) Durgaprasad Sharma (Vanaushadhi Shatak) (58) Deo Niranjan (Ayurvediya Dravyagunavignyan) (59) Desai Dr. Waman Ganesh (Aushadi Sangraha 1925) (60) Dhamankar Purushottam Vinayak (Ayurvediya Aushadhikaran Part 1 & 2) (61) Narhari (1400 A.D.) Raj nighantu (62) Navare Krishna Shastri 63) Narayanshastri (Dhanvantariya Nighantu) (64) Nilkanth Mishra (Paryayarnav) (65) Pade S. D. (Vanaushadi Gunadarsha Part 7) Aushadhikriya (Nighantu Shiromani) (66) Patwardhan Maharshi Annasaheb (Sulabh Deshi Aushadhi) (67) Patwardhan Umabai (Aushadhi Sangrah) (68) Patel Ramgopal (69) Pandit Bindumadhav (Gharatil Aushadhi, Aushadhi Bagicha, Batava) (70) Paranjpe G. P. (71) Patil Parshuram (72) Padhye A. B. (73) Pathak Dattaram (Brihannighantu Ratnakar parts 1 to 5) (74) Pathak Kedarnath (Madha) (75) Pande Gangasahay (Bhavprakash Vidyotini tika) (76) Pande Ranjitray (77) Priyavrat Sharma (20th century) Dravyagunavignyan parts 1 to 4) (78) Purandare (Dhanvantariya nighantu and Raj nighantu (79) Puranik (Ayurvediya Aushadhikaran Parts 1 & 2 (80) Phadke G. A. (Aushadhi Shastra parts 1 & 2 Dravyaguna Shastra (81) Balvant Singh (Prarambhik Udbhiji Shastra) (82) Birdwood (Practical Bazar Medicine) (83) Balram (19th century) Atanktimirbhaskar (84) Badodekar S. V. (Nighantusar) (85) Bapalalji Shah (1) Nighantu Adarsha (2) Sanskrit Sahityatil Vanaspati 3) Bheshaj Samhita 4) Prarambhik Udbhijja Shastra 5) Brihattrayitil Vanaspati (86) Bapat Naringrekar - Vanaushadhi Prakash (Lithopress Sachitra) (87) Bambadai Gokuldas Khimji (Vanaushadhi Srushti) (88) Bodas Prashanottar Dravyaguna shastra; Dravyagunarasashastra (20th century) (89) Bopdeo (1271 to 1309 A.D.) Hridaya Deepak (90) Bhavmishra (16th century) Bhavprakash 1596 A. D. (16th century) (91) Bhandari Chandraraj (Vanaushadhi Chandrodaya 10 volumes 1951 to 1957 A. D.) (91) Kathobhatta 1850 (92) Bhojraja (980 A. D. approx.) Nasyane Sammohini Grantha (93) Bhoge R. D. (20th century) Aji baincha Batva Parasatil Aushadhi (94) Madanpal (1374 A.D.) Madanpal Nighantu (95) Mallinath

In the ancient days, debates and symposia were held only among thinkers, philosophers and scholars.

(Abhidhan Ratnamala) (96) Mahendranath Shastri M. K. Dravyagunadarsha sachitra laghu) (97) Mahajan S. D. Medicinal plants in Dhanvantari Nighantu (98) Madhav (700 A.D.) Paryayaratnamala (99) Malaviya Pravasilal Varma (100) Mohammed Abdullah (101) Mishra Baldeoprasad (Ayurveda Chintamani) (102) Mudgal Dravyaratnakar (103) Moreshwar (son of Manik Bhatta) Ahmednagar (1681 A.D. Vaidyamrut) (104) Modak G. G. (Nityopayogi Nivadak Aushadhi) (105) Mantri P. G. (Bharatiya Vanaspati Samuha) (106) Rajvallabh (Samvat 1760), (107) Raje (Vanaspati Shastra Pravesh) (20th century) (108) Ramsushil Singh (Vanaushadhi Nidarshika) (109) Ramnarayan P. (Sanyasiyoki Jadibuttiya) (110) Ramprasad (111) Rugnath Indraji (Nighantu Sangrah) (112) Rupalalji Vaidya (Sachitra Abhinav Butidarpan volume 1 & 2) (113)Laxmipati Dr. A. (20th century) 100 useful aushadhi (Eng) (114) Lale (Kikavikar) Pathyapathyanighantu (115) Lala Shaligram (20th century) Shaligram Nighantu (116) Limaye Sou. (Vrukashavalli Amha) (117) Vagbhatta 600 A. D. Ashtangasangraha, Ashtanghridaya (118) Vangsen (15th century) (119) Vyankteshwar (Dakshinamurty Nighantu) (120) Vrinda (9th century) (121) Vijay rakshit (13th century) (122) Vishwanath Sen (Pathyapathya Nighantu) (123) Vijayacharan Gupta (Vanaushadhi darpan) (124) Vedi Ramesh (Chaulmogra, Suntha...........) (125) Vaidyavatans (126) Vaidya S. L. (Vanaspatichi Kule) (127) Shaligram Nighantu (Samvat 1953) Bhraman. (128) Shastri M. K. Sachitra Laghugunadarsha (129) Sharangdhar (14th century) Sharangdhar Samhita (130) Shah Tribhuvandas Narottam (Sharir and Vaidyak Shashtra) (131) Shivdatta 1677 A. D. Shivprakash (15th Century ?) (132) Shivdas Sen (133) Shukla P. Devidas (134) Shodhal (13th century) Shodhal Nighantu (16th century ?) (135) Sawant Sadashiv Yashwant 20th century (Divya Vanaspati of Maharashtra) (136) Sathe Appashastri 19th & 20th century) Gharghuti aushadhi. (137) Singh R.P.N. (Our trees - Eng. Govt. Publication) (138) Sutariya 20th century Text Book of Systemic Botany (139) Surendra Mohan (Keyadeo Part 1 and 2) (140) Sureshwar Surpal (Shabdapradip) (141) Sushruta (Sushruta Samhita) (142) Hari Sharanananda Swami (Aushadhi guna dharma vignyan) (143) Haraswarup Sharma (Bhaishyajya Sarasangraha) (144) Hakim Maulavi (145) Hirlekar Vaidya, Aushadhivignyan (146) Hemadri (147) Hemchandra Sen (Paryay Muktavali) (148) Hemchandra 1088 to 1172 A. D. Nighantu Shesha (149) Harichand Mehta (Vanaspati Pustika) (150) Aushadhi Nighantu (Gunadeepika) (151) Vaidya Bapalal (Charaka, Sushruta, Vagbhatta, Vanaspati Vivaran Sahakosha, Aushadhi Upyogi Ayurvediya Vanaspati Kosha.) (152) Dr. V. N. Naik (Identification of vanaushadhi) (153) The Secrets life of plants (Peter and Christopher) (154) Joshi Bapu Gangadhar (Nighantu Prakash 1839 A. D.) (155) Garde Dr. R. K. (Sunbaicha Batva 1955) (156) Ku. Vaidya Deshpande (Nasyachikitsa).

Some volumes on plants

(1) Anubhut Yogasar (2) Abhinav Butichitravali (3) Ashtangsangraha (Vagbhatta) (4) Ashtangthidaya (Vagbhatta) (5) Ashtang Nighantu (Vagbhatta) (6) Abhinav Nighantu (7) Ayurvediya Aushadhi Vargikaran (8) Ayurvediya Dravyagunavignyan (9) Amba (10) Atanktimirbhaskar (11) Ayurveda Vignyan (12) Ayurveda Chintamani (13) Aam ke guna (14) Abhidhan Ratnamala (15) Amar Kosh (16) Aushadhikriya (17) Aushadhi Vignyan Shastra (18) Aushadhideepika (19) Aushadhi Parichaya (20) Aushadhi Gnyan (21) Aushadhi Gunaratna (22) Aushadhi Gunadosha (23) Aushadhi Sangraha (24) Aushadhi Shastra (25) Aushadhi Bagicha (26) Aushadhi Gunadharma Vignyan (27)

As with all animals, every plant takes its own time to grow to complete maturity.

Udbhijja Shastra (28) Karanjopyoga (29) Keyadeo (30) Plants of Kutch (31) Kosha Nighantu (32) Guna Nighantu (33) Gunadosha (34) Gul (35) Grihaushadhi darsha (36) Gharguti Aushadhe (37) Gharacha Batva (38) Charaka (39) Chikitsa Prabhakar (40) Chaulmogra (41) Tambakhuguna (42) Tulasi (43) Dashmoola (44) Dakshinamurti Nighantu (45) Dravyagunadarsha (46) Dravyaguna shatshloki (47) Dravyaguna shastra (48) Dravyamuktavali (49) Dravyaguna sangraha (50) Dravyaratnakar (51) Dravyagunavignyan (52) Dravyagunarasashastra (53) Drakshe (grapes) (54) Dhatture ke guna (55) Dhanvantari 1050 A. D. (56) Dhaniya ke guna (57) Nalpak (58) Nam nighantu (59) Nighantu Bhushan (60) Nighantusar (61) Nighantu Shesha (62) Nighantu Shiromani (63) Nighantu Ratnakar 1815 Samvat. (64) Nighantu Sangraha (65) Nighantu Adarsha (66) Nibandha Sangraha (67) Selective medicines of daily use (68) Uses of Neem (69) Nrupa Nighantu (70) Paryayaratnamala (71) Paryayarnav (72) Paryayamuktavali (73) Pathyapathya Nighantu (74) Pathyapathya vivek (75) Palanduguna upyoga (76) Phalahar chikitsa (77) Use of Babhali (78) Brihat Nighantu Ratnakar part 1 to 3 (Chaukhamba series) (79) Medicines of Brihattrayee (80) Bilva mahattva (81) Brihat Nighantu (82) Bhavprakash (83) Bharatiya Vanaspati Sangrah (84) Bharat Varshiya Vanaspati Sangrah (85) Bhartiya Jadibuti (86) Bheshaj samhita (87) Bheshaj manimala (88) Bhaishajya Kalpana Vignyan (89) Bhaishajya Sarsangraha (90) Madanpal Nighantu (91) Uses of Honey (92) Special flora of Maharashtra (93) Uses of chilli (94) Medicinal plants in Dhanvantari Nighantu (95) Unani dravyagunavignyan (96) Raj nighantu (97) Rajvallabh (Samvat 1760) (98) Garlic (99) Vanaspatishastra pravesh (100) Vanaspati swabhav (101) Vanaspati srushti (102) Vanaushadhi Gunadarsh (103) Vanaushadhi Darshika (104) Vanaushadhi Shastra (105) Vanaushadhi darpan (106) Vaidyak Paribhasha pradeep (107) Vanaspatiyan (108) Vanaspati Prabhav (109) Vanaspati vichar (110) Vanaspati swabhav (111) Vanaushadhi prakash (112) Vanaushadhi shatak (113) Vanaspati gunadarsha (114) Vanaspatichi kule (115) Vanaushadhi chandrodaya (116) Vanaspati shastra (117) Vanaushadhi Nidarshika (118) Vagbhatta (119) Vanaspatik Anusandhan darshika (120) Vishwa Nighantu (121) Vishwaprakash (12th century) (122) Vrikshavalli (123) Vaidyamanorama (124) Vaidyamrut (125) Shabdachandrika (126) Shabdapradeep (127) Shaligram Nighantu (128) Shivprakash (129) Sheshraj (130) Shodhhal Nighantu (131) Vanaspati from Sanskrit literature (Guj.) (132) Sachitra Abhinav Buti Darpan (133) Sachitra laghudravya gunadarsh (134) Sachitra vanaspati gunadarsha (135) Sandigdha dravyavignyan (136) Sandigdha nirnaya (137) Sanyasiyoni gupta jadibuti (138) Sankshipta dravyagunavignyan (139) Siddhamantra (140) Siddha Bhaishajya manimala (141) Sushruta (142) Ginger (143) Halayudha (144) Hridaya deepak (145) Kshemkutuhal (146) Materia medica (Kirtikar-Basu 4 vol.) and many other volumes.

Some useful references

Aristotle, Theophratus and Dioscoriodes (Father of Botany) undertook the classification of plants in 370 B. C. Their classification was based on trunk, leaves, seeds etc. and it contained the following groups -

1) Unicotyledons - Dicotyledons

2) Annual rings 3) Hilly plants

Man has to ultimately succumb to the inevitable and the anforeseen. But that is the last resort. Ayurveda has conveyed emphatically that man makes his own destiny.

4) Marshy plants 5) Plants around rivers and lakes

6) Watery plants etc.

Kent, Whers, Whijil have classified agricultural plants as well as medicinal plants.

Diosioridus - born in Asia minor in 64 A.D. discovered many medicinal plants.

Brunfelse (1530 A. D.), **Bauk** (1539 A.D.), **Fuches** (1542 A.D.), **Lobelius** (1576 A.D.), **Glucine**, **Obel** - all these scientists collected and studied medicinal plants.

After this, **William Tunner** wrote the history of herbal plants. Similarly, **Valerin Cordes** (German scientist), **Endrisisalpeen** (Italian scientist) wrote plant histories.

John Jirardes Harbal (1597) did the classification of grasses, plants yielding food grains and tubors.

Kospis Bauhuhin (Swiss) identified 6000 plants and classified them by binomial method.

John (England), in 1704, wrote the history of monocotyledons and dicotyledons namely Historia Planterea.

Torn Fort (1657 to 1708) classified plants on the basis of corolla of the flowers.

Gamerarius (1665 to 1721) classified plants by studying their sex.

Carl Linnaenicus (1735 - the father of taxonomical botany) also classified plants by studying their sex organs. He classified plants depending on single stamen, two stamens or multiple stamen. The Linnaenian Society was established in London to commemorate his conributions.

Existing classification of plants by Antoli De Jusis is based on all the four parts of sex organs. **Dr. Wise** wrote two books in 1845 on surgical methods, a book on nine methods of medicine, three books on medicinal plants, one book on posology, one book on medicinal science and one book on medicine used with metals.

Kathobhatta (1850) - wrote Nighantu Sangraha.

Lisboa J. C. (1884) - wrote a book on useful plants of Bombay Province.

Dimak W. Warden wrote the history of chemical principles of plants in British India.

Pandas C. F. (1901) wrote a book on medicinal and poisonous plants of India.

Dr. A. Laxmipati in 1927 wrote a book on 100 plants. Dr. Kirtikar and Major Basu (Allahabad 1935), Stedman T. L., Dr. Khory, Dr. Ghosh, Dr. Hemchandra Sen, Shri Y. C. Datta, Dr. Chopra (Indigenous drugs), Dr. Nadkarni (Indian Materia Medica), Dr. Vaman Ganesh Desai (Aushadhi Sangrah).

How about considering a man who is happy to see plants growing in his surroundings as healthy and the man who is not, as unhealthy?

S. K. Jain - Medicinal plants (1968) National Book Trust, New Delhi.

Dr. S. P. Adharkar, Gazzettier of Bombay State, Volume General - A, Botany part 1, Medicinal plants, 1953 A. D.

Dr. B. Mukherji - The Indian Pharmaceutical Codex, New Delhi, 1953. **Wealth of India** - Raw Materials, Volume 1 - VII New Delhi 1948 to 1960 (Govt. of India Publiation).

D. K. Kamat and **S. D. Mahajan** - Medicinal plants in Dhanvantari Nighantu (Poona 1971).

Large botanical gardens have been set up in western as well as in other countries. 1) Padua (1545) 2) Pisa (1545) 3) Volga (1567) 4) Oxford (1621) 5)Que (1841). The botanical garden of Calcutta in India with huge banian tree is famous.

Method of naming the plants - This method is called as Binomial method (Bi = two, Nomial = naming). Every plant named by this system has two names out of which the first name belongs to the genus and other to the species. As seen in the following example, L or LINN which comes after these two names indicates the name of the scientist who named that plant.

For example, kuchala (Strychnos nuxvomica).

Strychnos	nuxvomica	Linn
|	|	|
Genus	Species	Scientist.

This method of naming the plants is found very useful in the identification and study of plants.

Universally, all botanists follow this method which uses Latin or Greek terminology. So all over the world it is advantageous to have a uniformly named plant. Many names of scientists are found in this method, giving due credit to the discoverer.

Pharmacognosy

Identification of specific dravyas-

(1) Guduchi : This is a perennial creeper surrounding and spreading on mango or neem tree (कडुनिंब). At different sites the arial roots sprout and hang downwards to enter the soil. After scraping the brown thin skin of the stem, a greenish fleshy part is exposed. The transverse section of the trunk appears like a cartwheel and so it is named as chakralakshana. The thin outer skin is tasteless but the inner fleshy part is bitter to taste. Empty space among the spokes of the central part contains essence (सत्व). If viewed under the microscope, its structure is different from other carbohydrates. Therefore it is easy to differentiate guduchisatva from other carbohydrates. It turns black in contact with iron, so a wooden hammer is used for extraction. Old but wet trunk is used as medicine. End of May is the best season for collection. The outer thin skin is easily removed by scraping as it is very loose.

If the laws prohibiting the cutting of forests are made stringent, it would be a boon for human race.

Guduchi contains carbohydrates, berberine and has a bitter taste.

(2) Manjishtha (Rubia cordifolia) - This creeper spreads over a long distance and bears multiple branches and sub-branches. The trunk is square like that of apamarga and is reddish in colour; (roots are also reddish). The creeper is shapeless and dusty. It grows in a cold climate and in hilly areas like Mahabaleshwar and on the deccan plateau. It bears four leaves in a circle, out of which 2 are small and two big. The stalk is long. Roots measure 2.5 to 5 cm and are slightly thick. The colour is reddish and grey when fresh. On breaking, the inner part is red in colour. Older plant becomes blackish. Taste at the beginning is sweet but later on turns bitter and pungent. Four types are found - (1) Indian (inferior) 2) Nepali 3) Iranian and 4) Afghan - the last one is considered to be superior. Roots of Rubia cordifolia are used for colouring. What is available in the market are the pieces of the trunk and not the roots.

Leaves

(3) Markandika :- The tree is 1/2 to 1 mt. tall.

Leaves - compound.

Leaflet contains 1 to 8 pairs and is 2.5 to 5 cm. long.

Leaves contain glucosides, campharine, anthraquinone (laxative), calcium oxallate, crysophenic acid, cathartic acid and a volatile oil. (Cathartic acid is the main purgative). Two types of leaves of sonamukhi are found.

(1) Trivelli (abundantly grown in South India) and (2) Arabic (Alexandrian - leaves of this type are round, long and blunt). In Indian type, the leaves are found mixed with other leaves. It increases intestinal peristalsis and secretions. This causes diarrhoea with yellow coloured stool, in large quantity and results in griping. It is antihelminthic and vermicidal. Leaves of taravdi are used for adulteration. Senna pods are also used as laxative.

(4) Aloe indica (कुमारी) :- The small variety grows upto 1/2 to 1 mt. tall and is full of leaves which are thick and tapering to a point at the tip. Leaves bear thorns at the margins. Length is 30-50 cms. Leaves are covered with a thin green skin. On breaking, it contains ghee-like sticky pulp. The method of extracting the pulp is to first remove the thorns and cut the leaf horizontally into two halves separating the upper and lower surfaces. Put each half on the wooden plate with the lower surface below. Knife cuts are made, the pulp scraped off from the bottom surface; multiple cuts are made into the pulp and then scraped from the botttom. Repeat the process with the other half. Thus the whole pulp is collected. Prepare the thick satva by boiling and reducing the quantity. This is known as kalabol, kumarisar, musabbar, sahasar, kanyasar, elua, elia, alio, aloe, arabic-sibra, persian-shabyar, Eng. - aloes.

This contains aloin, barbeloin (glycoside), aloemodin, volatile oils etc. Kumari is found at Kanyakumari in abundance. Besides, it is also grown in sandy soil and near the sea shore. Marshy

Vata, having normal dravyagunakarma, is Lord Shiva (Shankar). When it becomes vitiated, it is like Rudra (very troublesome).

and salty land is favourable for its growth. Punjab, Sindh, Kathiawad and coastal areas near Madras are other places of cultivation. Kalabol is prepared at Jaffarabad and in Mysore (known as musambra). Large quantity is imported from Arab countries to Mumbai port. This is known as yamani, mokka and adan alava. Alava coming from Zanzibar is superior. It is golden yellow in colour, harder on the surfaces but soft inside. It has a fragrant aroma. Jaffrabadi is black in colour. It is available in round lumps. It appears like resin on breaking.

Flower

(5) Lavang (Syzygium aromaticum) :- Lavang available in the market are buds. Oil is extracted from fruit. The superior quality is blackish, shining and oil drips on crushing with finger. Marketed Syzygium aromaticum is greyish and rough. The tree is 10-15 mts. tall and evergreen. Outer surface of the flower is orange red and divided into four triangular parts. The first flowering appears after 9 years. Syzygium aromaticum was originally grown in Malaya. Now-a-days it is grown in Sumatra, Malacca, Zanzibar, Penang, Mauritius, Borneo, Brazil, Guana and islands of western part of India.

Composition - Volatile oils 16-20%, karpur 6%, uginine, cariophiline, tannin and gum. Oil contains phenol like uginol 85 to 92%.

(6) Nagkesar (Mesua ferrea) :- It is a beautiful, medium-high tree appearing evergreen. Fragrant flowers of 3-4 cms in diameter grow from the tip of upper bunch of leaves. It contains yellow stamen in clusters. Outer coating of the flower is hard and durable. The tree flowers in summer. Stamens are used in medicine. This is called as nagkesar. Flower is called nagpushpa. Stamen contains two bitter components. Mesua ferrea trees are found in Nepal, eastern parts of Himalaya, Bengal, Assam, South India, Burma, Andaman islands and Konkan coast.

Seeds

(7) Karanja (Pongamia pinnata) :- Tall tree, 8-16 mts. in height, evergreen and bears legumes which are 3-4 cm. long, flat, egg shaped, hard and slightly bent on the dorsal aspect. Every legume contains a single seed measuring 2 1/2 to 3 cm. which contains oil. It grows abundantly in central and south India and Sri Lanka. Whole seed is useful. Seed is covered with reddish brown thin layer. It contains pongamia oil (27%) which is bitter and dark in colour. The latin name is Pongamia pinnata (Linn Merr) while the names in other languages are naktamal, guchchapushpak, ghrutpur, snigdhapatra (glabra), Hindi - dithauro, Bengali - dahar karanj, Telugu - kanagu, Tamil - puggum, Malayali-ponnam,
Kannada - honge, English - Indian beech.

Bark

(8) Banyan tree - This huge widespread tree is known to all. Latin - Ficus bengalensis Linn, Sanskrit - vata, nyagrodha, bahupad, raktaphal, shungi, kshiri, Hindi - bad, Bengali - vat, Punjabi - bod, Marathi and Gujarati - vad, Tamil - ala, Telugu - peddimari, Arabic - kabirul ashjar, Persian -

Sama-prana-prakriya is a concept which teaches us to accept only that which is required for healthy body and mind. Sama-apan-prakriya is a concept where one takes up what is not required.

darkhterish, English - banyan tree.

It bears widespread branches. Bark is whitish, grey and thick. It contains 10% tannin, wax and rubber. It acts as an astringent.

(9) Neem (Azadirachta indica) :- It grows 8-10 mts. high. Lat - Azadirachta indica, Sanskrit - nimba, pichumarda, tiktak, arishta, paribhadra, hinguniryas, Marathi - kadunimba, Tamil - vepa, Punjabi - nimba, Malayali - veppu, Sindhi - nimu, Persian - azad darakhteh hind, Arabic - azad rakhtul hind, English - margosa tree. The trunk is straight and branching in all directions. The bark is blackish, thick and rough. A juice oozes out of the bark like that of palm tree. The bark contains margosine, volatile oil, gum, milky liquid, sugar and astringent substances. Outer skin is pungent but inner side is bitter and brownish and contains 60% pungent substances besides maltose, fructose, gum, pigments, proteids, calcium, potassium, iron, aluminium and carbondioxide.

Latex

(10) Asafoetida :- This is the latex of asafoetida tree. Latin - Ferula foetida, Sanskrit - hinga, jatuk, sahastra-vedhi, balhik, ramath, Guj.- hing, Tamil - perungayam, Tel. - engu, Kannada - yang, Persian - angajad, Arabic - hillit, English - asafoetida.

Perennial tree of 2-3 mt. height. There are two types - white and black - white is scented, is called hira hinga and used in medicine. Black, used in daily cooking, is foetid. Different types are available in the market because of variation in origin, type, preservation and collection.

Process of extraction - Summer is the proper period for the collection of this latex. Just above the roots the skin is peeled off with a knife. The latex (gum) oozes out at the site within 1-2 days, is collected and again the skin is peeled off in the same way. Thus hinga (latex) is collected repeatedly. To protect the site, a stony wall is constructed around the tree. It is preserved in a bag prepared with goat skin. So it is not considered as sacred or pure.

Adulterated hinga is available in the market. It is mixed with wheat and small pieces of stones or sand. Therefore it does not burn completely or dissolve in water ; some residue settles at the bottom.

Tests for purity - When immersed in water, asafoetida should radiate whitish milky lines running towards the bottom. It should dissolve completely and the whole water in the glass should turn milky white. It should burn completely with a match stick. Asafoetida used in medicine should be of good quality, white in colour and having a sharp smell and pungent taste. Purification is done by two processes. Asafoetida is dissolved completely in water and then heated in iron vessel till pulp is formed. Secondly, it is roasted in cow's ghee and is used when dried and becomes rough.

Composition - It contains volatile oil 6-17%, rason oil and allyl persulphide - the specific smell is because of this. Besides, it contains latex 65%, gum 25%, salt and minerals 3-4% and feruallic, mallic, formic and valerianic acids. Roasted asafoetida is used in abdominal diseases whereas raw type is used in lung diseases.

Vata-prakopa means increase in vata-gunas like ruksha. To reduce the production of these gunas is the treatment on vata.

(11) Guggulu (Commiphora mukul) :- Latin - Commiphora (Commi=gum) mukul, Sanskrit - guggul, deodhup, kaushik, pur, mahishaksha, palankash, kumbha, ulukhal, Hindi - gugul, Guj - gugal, Sindhi - gugaru, Kannad - kasthagan, Tamil - gukkulu, Telegu - maishakshi, gumbulu, Arabic - muklul, yahud, Persian - buyen, jahudan, English - gumguggul.

The tree grows 1.5 to 2 mt. high, gum is thick, scented and multicoloured. Burns in fire, melts in sun heat. Hot water turns to white if guggulu is added to it. These are the qualities of good guggulu. Five types of guggulu are described -

1. Krishna (Black) - Useful for humans
2. Neel (Bluish) ⎤
3. Kapish (Brownish) ⎥ Useful for animals.
4. Rakta (Reddish) ⎦
5. Peeta (Yellow) - Useful for humans.

Other five types are described in Unani medicine.

1. Mukle Arjak - Coppery red
2. Mukle Saklavi - Kapish (Brownish)
3. Mukle Hindi - Shyam Varna (Blakish)
4. Mukle Yahud - Yellowish.
5. Mukle Arabi Kapil (Brown)

Two types are available in daily use.

1. Kana - Available in Marwar and its crystals are soft and brownish yellow.
2. Mahashaguggul - Available in Sindh and Kutch. This is greenish yellow in colour.

Characteristics of good quality guggul - One which dissolves completely in water, devoid of mud and sand, unctuous, soft, slimy, sweet smelling, bitter and yellow coloured.

It grows abundantly in Marwar, Arabastan, Africa, Sindh, Kutch, Kathiawad, Assam, Bangladesh, Vidarbha and Mysore province.

It is to be collected in winter, yet its yield is more in the summer due to high temperature.

It contains volatile oils, resins, gums and alkaloids.

Life = vibration, vibration = vata; therefore vata = life. Life full of vibrations is not without vata.

Jangam Dravyas

Honey - Detailed description is available in part IV.

Names of the plants for preparing album

1) Agnimanth 2) Aparajita 3) Apamarg 4) Arka (5) Arjun 6) Ashwagandha 7) Ashok 8) Amalaki 9) Adrak 10) Aragwadh 11) Udumbar 12) Arand 13) Kantakari 14) Kapikacchu 15) Karveer 16) Karanj 17) Kanchnar 18) Kutaj 19) Khadir 20) Guduchi 21) Gokshur 22) Chitrak 23) Chandan 24) Jambu 25) Tulasas 26) Dadim 27) Danti 28) Dhattur 29) Dhayati 30) Nagbala 31) Nimba 32) Nimbuk 33) Nirgundi 34) Palash 35) Punarnava 36) Prushniparni 37) Baladwaya 38) Bakuchi 39) Brahmi 40) Bibhitak 41) Bilva 42) Bruhati 43) Bharangi 44) Bhrungaraj 45) Madanphal 46) Mandukparni 47) Latakaranj 48) Vasa 49) Vidanga 50) Shatpushpa 51) Shatavari 52) Sharpunkha 53) Shalparni 54) Shalmali 55) Shigru 56) Shirish 57) Shounyak 58) Saptaparna 59) Sarivadwaya 60) Haritaki 61) Agasta 62) Adhapushpi 63) Amarvalli 64) Amlika 65) Aristak 66) Asmantale 67) Ashwattha 68) Asthisanharak 69) Akhuparni 70) Ingudi 71) Irimed 72) Katveera 73) Katak 74) Kamal 75) Karamarda 76) Kasir 77) Karpas 78) Kash 79) Kasamarda 80) Krishnabeeja 81) Kokilakshak 82) Kampillak 83) Gunja 84) Chakramarda 85) Chhikkika 86) Jaipal 87) Jati 88) Tagar 89) Tinduk 90) Tilparni 91) Damanak 92) Panas 93) Parnabeej 94) Pateal garudi 95) Parijat 96) Paribhadra 97) Parish 98) Peelu 99) Bakul 100) Babbul 101) Bhumyamalki 102) Madhuk 103) Mayur Shikha 104) Markandeeka 105) Mashparni 106) Mundi 107) Mudgaparni 108) Murva 109) Rohish 110) lajjalu 111) Langali 112) Vrikshadani 113) Vansh 114) Vikankat 115) Shami 116) Shinshape 117) Sleshmatak 118) Swarnakshini 119) Suddab 120) Saireyak 121) Hansaraj 122) Rohitek 123) Shar 124) Veertaru.

Bibliography

1) Dravyagunavignyan (Vd. Priyavrat Sharma Sarvagranth)

2) Aushadhi Sangraha (Dr. Vaman Ganesh Desai)

3) Charaka Samhita

4) Sushruta Samhita

5) Ashtangasangraha

6) Ashtangahridaya

7) Amarkosh

8) Bhavprakash

9) Maharashtratil Divya Vanaspati - (Sawant S.Y.)

10) Madanpal Nighantu

Any one who believes in authentic pramanas is honest. Ayurveda also believes in pratyakshadi praman and that is why it is honest.

11) Dravyagunashastra (Kurtudkar)

12) Ayurvediya Aushadhikaran

13) Vanaushadhi Gunadarsh (Pade)

14) Aushadhishastra (G.A. Phadke)

15) Nighantu Sar (Badodkar)

16) Ayurvedacha Itihas

17) Dravyagunarasashastra (Bodas)

PART II

MEDICINAL PLANTS

INTRODUCTION

The following two parts contain description of commonly used medicinal plants. The Sanskrit name of each plant is given first followed by its binomial nomenclature. The description of each plant is accompanied by its sketch. Wherever possible, classification of the plant as described in Charaka samhita, Sushruta samhitá and Bhavaprakash has been given. This is followed by its kula and family.

An effort has been made to describe the etymology of the family and binomial nomenclature of each plant. Understanding the etymology of binomial nomenclature facilitates identification of plants and hence additional effort has been made to describe it here since it is generally not found in other volumes on medicinal plants. The meanings of certain names provided here are doubtful. Though, errors have been minimised by getting the names verified by experts.

The identity of some plants is also not certain. There are differences in opinions about their names too. Regional names may vary considerably. Not all plants are used everywhere. Understanding the synonyms and verifying them by actually observing the plant will go a long way in helping the student in identification. Teachers should guide them in this.

English name is given below the Latin name followed by Sanskrit synonyms. If a conscious effort is made to study these synonyms and their etymologies then it would certainly enrich our current understanding of identification and standardisation. It is certain that the ancient Ayurvedic scholars undertook the tedious exercise of providing innumerable synonyms to plants only with the aim of facilitating identification and standardisation. In addition, these synonyms provide information about many aspects of the plant like its area of origin, therapeutic uses and effects on dosha, dhatus and malas. Study of binomial nomenclature should be coupled with the study of these synonyms since it will undoubtedly enrich our knowledge. Providing the etymologies of all the Sanskrit synonyms is a task in itself and will require a separate volume.

Varieties of the plant, its habitat and chemical composition have been described after the Sanskrit synonyms. This is followed by properties (gunas), actions (karmas), external uses, effects on various systems in the body, parts used, dose, formulations, srotogamitva and lastly, references about the plant from Ayurvedic texts.

While ascertaining srotogamitva, these references (shlokas) were taken as guidelines. If a dravya is described as mehaghna (anti-diabetic), then it implies that it brings about the desired action by acting (i.e. possessing srotogamitva) on kapha, meda, mansa, kleda, basti and mutra. An antipyretic dravya cannot reduce fever if it does not possess srotogamitva on pitta, rasa and sweda. The study of dravyaguna involves such consideration of every symptom and its pathogenesis.

The Ayurvedic texts used for references are Raj nighantu, Keyadeva nighantu, Madanpal nighantu, Bhavaprakash nighantu, Dravya nighantu, Nrupa nighantu, Gana nighantu, Kosha nighantu, Charaka samhita, Sushruta samhita, Ashtangsangraha, Ashtanghridaya, Bhaishajya Ratnavali, Bangasen, Shodhal samhita etc.

Abbreviations used in the following two parts :

C. - Charaka samhita

S. - Sushruta samhita

Bh. - Bhavaprakash nighantu

Gk. - Greek

(1) AGNIMANTHA

Premna integrifolia Linn.

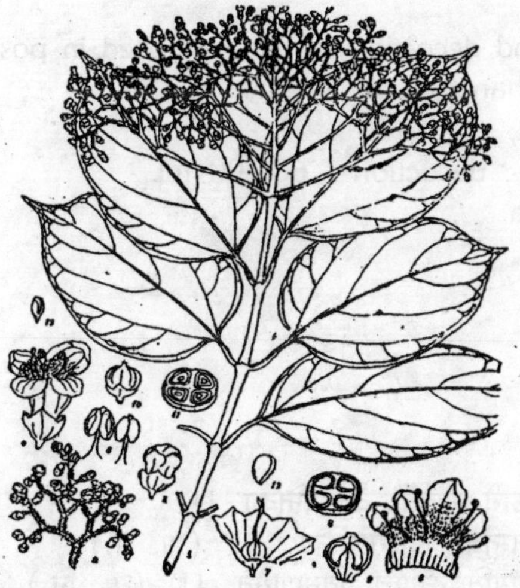

Gana : Shothahar, Sheetprashaman, Anuvasanopag (C.); Brihatpanchamoola, Vatasamshamana, Veeratarvadi, Varunadi (S.)

Kula : Nirgundi kula.

Family : Verbenaceae - with flexible branches.

Latin name : Premna = Premnon (Greek) = a stump, low stature of the species, integri = entire or whole; folia = leaves.

Sanskrit names : Agnimantha (the branches when rubbed against each other, generate fire), Jaya (gains victory over diseases), Shriparna (having beautiful leaves), Ganikarika, Asavarika (grows in groups and promotes health), Vataghni (alleviates vata), Matha, Ketu, Nadeyi.

Botanical Description : The tree grows upto a height of 8 - 10 meters. Bark - smoke coloured. Leaves - opposite, ovate, tapering and soft. Flowers - white, aromatic and in clusters. Fruits - small like coriander fruit. Flowering stage is spring.

Varieties : There are 2 varieties of Agnimantha. 1. Large variety - known as Agnimantha which is described above. 2. Small variety - also known as Ṭarkari [Clerodendron phlomoidis (Linn.)] [Kleros = chance, Dendron = tree (Gk.) phlomoides = resembling phlomis (Jerusalem sage)] 'Jaya, Jayanti, Tarkari, Nadeyi, Vaijayantika' are the Sanskrit names for small variety mentioned in Bhavprakash.

Habitat : Throughout India, mainly in the Gangetic plain , Uttar Pradesh, Bihar and Orissa. Many trees of Agnimantha occur in Ramadas Takali near Nasik (Maharashtra).

Properites :

Guna : ruksha, laghu; **Rasa** : tikta, katu, kashaya, madhur; **Vipak** : katu; **Veerya** : ushna.

Karma : Kaphavatanashak, hence useful in kapha - vata disorders.

External uses : Ushna property helps in clearing obstruction of the channels and acts as anti-inflammatory and analgesic. The paste of the leaves is used for sprains.

Internal uses :

Circulatory system : Best anti-inflammatory drug.

Nervous system : Used in neuralgia and acts as an analgesic; chiefly used in vata disorders.

Digestive system : Its appetizing, digesting and laxative properties are useful in loss of appetite, ama-dosha and constipation.

Respiratory system : It is kaphaghna (alleviates kapha) and acts on diseases caused by obstruction of respiratory system by vitiated kapha e.g. cough, asthma and common cold.

It is not possible to have complete translation of classics like Charaka samhita and that is why a student who reads translations cannot reach the soul of the author.

Urinary system : It has effects on kapha, meda and urinary tract. Therefore useful in urinary disorders especially in chyluria. The decoction of root is used in pyuria.

Skin : Cures skin disorders. Pulp of its root is given orally in the treatment of urticaria, which has potential to check the pathogenesis of urticaria. The juice of leaves in a dose of 15 ml. thrice a day is also useful in urticaria.

Satmikaran : Being a bitter tonic, the juice of leaves and decoction of bark are used in post pyrexial debility and is also useful in anaemia to enhance tissue vitality.

Parts used : Leaves and root bark.

Dosage : Powder - 0.5 - 1 gm.; juice - 15 - 25 ml.; decoction - 60-100 ml.

Formulations : Agnimantha kashaya, Dashamoolaristha.

Srotogamitva :

Dosha : Kaphakshayakarak, vatakshayakarak.

Dhatu : Rakta, meda (anaemia), inflammation.

Mala : Digestive system.

Organs : Respiratory system.

References -

'अग्निमन्थो जयः सास्यात् श्रीपर्णी गणिकारिका । जया जयन्ती तर्कारी नादेयी वैजयन्तिका ।।
अग्निमन्थः श्वयथुनुद् वीर्योष्णः कफवातहृत् । पाण्डुनुत् कटुकस्तिक्तस्तुवरो मधुरोऽग्निदः ।।' (भा. प्र.)
'तर्कारी कटुका तिक्ता तथोष्णाऽनिलपाण्डुनुत् । शोथश्लेष्माग्निमांद्यामविबन्धांश्च विनाशयेत् ।।' (ध. नि.)
'तर्कारी कटुका तिक्ता तुवरा मधुराऽग्निदा । वीर्योष्णा हरते वातकफश्वयथुपाण्डुताः ।।
अग्निमन्थो गुणैस्तद्वद्विशेषाद् वातशोथहा ।' (के. नि.)

(2) AGURU
Aquilaria agallocha

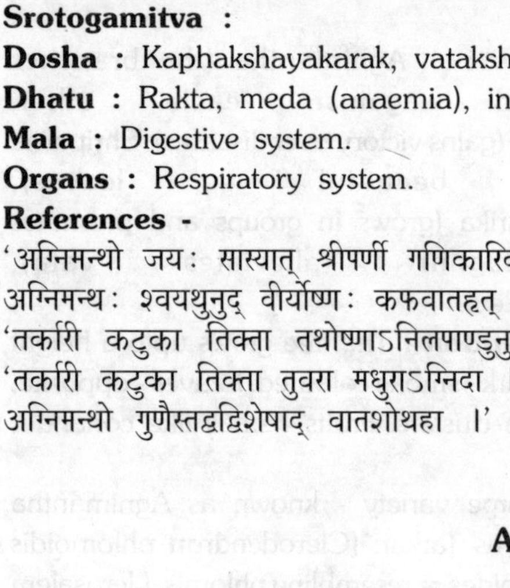

Gana : Sheetaprashaman, Shvashara, Shirovirechak, Tiktaskandha (C.); Eladi, Salsaradi, Shleshmasamshaman (S.)

Kula : Agaru kula.

Family : Thymelaecae - Thyme like foliage and olive like fruits.

Latin name : Aquilaria agallocha (Linn). Aquilaria = pertaining to eagle; agallocha = Agallo-ocha (Greek) = to make exceedingly glorious .

English name : Aloe wood / Eagle wood.

Sanskrit names : Agni, Loha (heavy as iron i.e. loha and black in colour), Krimij, Rajarha, Bhringraj, Agnikashtha, Vanshik, Vanadrum, Puram, Dhupagam, Mallikagandh.

Botanical Description : It is an evergreen tree. The bark is paper thin. (Used for writing as Bhurj patra). The wooden bark is whitish, soft and fragrant on cutting. Inner portion

While classifying the plants, their similar srotogamitva is taken into consideration.

becomes black as the tree grows; and smells like honey. Leaves are thin and leathery, pin headed, 5-7 cm.in length. Flowers are white and in clusters. Fruit is 1-2 cm. in length, as soft as velvet in touch. The tree blossoms in summer and gives fruits in rainy season.
Inner bark of old trees is known as 'aguru'. The black, fragrant heavy type which sinks in water is considered as the best aguru. A kind of small worm grows in old bark, that secretes a type of resin, which gives fragrance to aguru.
Habitat : Eastern Himalaya, Assam, Manipur, Chitgaon, Bhutan, Brahmadesh, Sumatra, Malaysia Dwipkalpa. Krishnaguru is cultivated mainly in Assam (Dahaguru), Gujarat and Kedarnath (Mangalyaguru).
Varieties : Raj Nighantu describes four types as - 1) Krishna (black) 2) Kashth (yellow) 3) Daha 4) Mangalya. The fourth one is the best in quality. Unani system describes three types on the basis of its pattern of sinking in water - Gurki, Samal and Neemgurki. There are different types depending on habitat.
Chemical composition : It contains a volatile oil.
Properties :
Guna : laghu, ruksha, tikshna; **Rasa :** katu, tikta; **Vipak :** katu; **Veerya :** ushna.
Karma : Kaphavatashamak, generally used in kapha-vata disorders.
External uses : The lepa (local application) is stimulant and fragrant. It is antiinflammatory and analgesic. It helps in skin disorders. It is used in static condition (or restricted movements), chronic ulcers and wounds, ringworm, skin diseases and inflammatory and painful condition. It helps in rhuematoid arthritis and osteoarthritis. It also relieves itching in pruritus.
Internal uses :
Nervous system: Nerve stimulant and vatahara in nature. It has been recommended in paralytic condition and vata diseases.
Digestive system : It is a mouth freshner; carminative and appetizer. In bad breath, it is chewed. It is given internally in rheumatoid arthritis, loss of appetite and other digestive ailments.
Circulatory system: It is a stimulant, improves blood circulation. It is used in gout.
Respiratory system : It reduces cough and helps in bronchitis and asthma. 1-2 drops of aguru oil is applied to betel leaves and those leaves are chewed in asthma. Aguru is also used as nasal insufflation (nasya therapy) in kapha disorders.
Urinary system : It relaxes the bladder, helps in preventing bedwetting and polyuria.
Skin : It is used in skin diseases.
Temperature : Because of its cooling effect, it is used in fevers associated with chills, both internally and externally. Oil massage is effective in rigours in fevers.
Satmikaran : Being rejuvenative, used as a tonic. It helps in fatigue and debility.
Parts used : Inner bark and oil.
Dosage : 0.5 to 1.5 gm. of powder; 1-2 drops of oil.
Formulation : Agurvadi oil.
Srotogamitva :
Dosha : Pittavardhak, kaphavataharak.
Dhatu: Rakta (skin diseases), rasa (skin disorders).

If a book is read again, it not only gives rise to many queries but it enables one to understand its shortcomings. However, while teaching it to students, the doubts become clear and one can solve the difficulties.

Mala : Purisha (anthelmintic).
Organs : Ear, eyes.
References -
'अगुरूष्णं कटु त्वच्यं तिक्तं तीक्ष्णं च पित्तलम् । लघु कर्णाक्षिरोगघ्नं शीतवातकफप्रणुत् ।।
कृष्णं गुणाधिकं तत्तु लोहवद् वारिमज्जति । अगुरुप्रभवः स्नेहः कृष्णागुरुसमः स्मृतः ।।' (भा. प्र.)
'रास्नागुरुणि शीतापनयनप्रलेपनानाम् ।' (च. सू. २५-४०)
'अगुरुसारस्नेहास्तिक्तकटुकषाया दुष्टव्रणशोधनाः कृमिकफकुष्ठानिलहराश्च ।' (सु. सू. ४५)
काकतुंडाकृतिः स्निग्धो गुरुश्चैवोत्तमोऽगुरुः । असारपाण्डुरं रूक्षं लघुं चाधममादिशेत् ।।
नादेयं नाप्युपादेयं तित्तिरिपक्षकागुरुः । शाल्मलीकाष्ठसंकाशो नैव ग्राह्यः कदाचन ।।' (भै. र.

(3) AJMODA

Carum roxburghianum Benth.

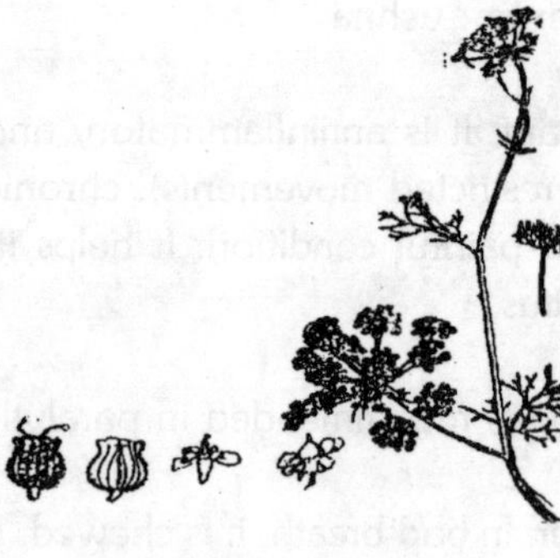

Gana : Shoolaprashaman, Deepaniya (C.) Pippalyadi (S.).
Kula : Shatpushpa kula.
Family : Umbellifereae- Producing an umbel. (Umbel = flowers in cluster in which stalks nearly equal in length spring from common centre and from flat or convex or concave surface as in parsley.
Latin name : Carum roxburghianum (Dc. Sprague); Carum (from caria) - roots as well as seeds are edible; roxburghianum (Benth).
Sanskrit names : Ajmoda (it smells like a goat or goats like it), Kharashva, Karvi, Markati, Shikhimoda, Moodadhya, Ugragandhika, Phalmukhya, Yavani.
Botanical Description : The shrub is small, almost 1/3 to 1 mtr. high. Leaves-winged. Flowers are round, 5-20 in cluster. Seeds- greyish in colour. There are small spots on seeds. It blossoms and gives fruits from rainy season to summer.
Habitat : All over India but more in Maharashtra.
Chemical composition : It contains a volatile oil.
Properties :
Guna : laghu, ruksha, tikshna; **Rasa :** katu, tikta; **Vipak :** katu; **Veerya :** ushna (tikshna).
Dosha : Ajmoda pacifies kapha and vata dosha due to tikshna and ushna properties. It increases pitta dosha. Though useful in kapha-vata disorders, it cannot be used when pitta dosha is equally vitiated.
External uses : Analgesic. It is applied locally in bodyache. The juice of leaves or oil is used in arthritis.
Internal uses :
Digestive system : Carminative, appetizer, analgesic and anthelmintic. It is used in emesis, loss of appetite, hiccoughs, flatulence, stomachache and helminthiasis.
Circulatory system : It acts as cardiac stimulant in cardiac disorders.

Today test-tube baby is not a mere imagination, it is a fact. But successful experiments create various problems.

Respiratory system : Due to its kaphaghna property, it is used in cough (bronchitis), asthma, hiccough in the form of churna (powder) and also in the form of smoke (dhoomapan). Its smoke gives quick relief in cough, hiccough and asthma.
Nervous system : The decoction of roots nourishes brain and gives strength to nerves. But it is contraindicated in epilepsy.
Urinary system : It is used when there is pain in urinary bladder, renal calculi and urinary obstruction. It acts as a diuretic.
Reproductive system : It is a uterine stimulant as well as an aphrodisiac. Therefore it is used in amenorrhoea, dysmenorrhoea and infertility. Though friendly to females, it should not be given in pregnancy.
Satmikaran : It is bitter and nutrient. Therefore used in general debility.
Parts used : Seeds.
Dosage : 5-7 gm. powder.
Formulations : Ajmodadi churna, Ajmodadi Vatak, Agnitundi, Krimikuthar, Kankayanadi gutika, Kapithashtak, Chitrakadi, Narayan, Mahahingvadi, Mahasudarshan, Lavantritrayadi, Vaishvanar, Hingvashtadi Churna, Phalaghrita.
Srotogamitva :
Dosha : Reduces kapha and vata.
Dhatu : Shukra (aphrodisiac).
Mala : Purisha (anti-helminthic).
Organs : Basti (bladder), netra (eyes), hridaya (heart), garbhashay (uterus).
References -
'अजमोदा कटुस्तीक्ष्णा दीपनी कफवातनुत् । उष्णा विदाहिनी हृद्या वृष्या बलकरी लघुः ।।
नेत्रामयकफच्छर्दिहिक्काबस्तिरुजो हरेत् ।' (भा.प्र.)
'अजमोदा तु शूलघ्नी तिक्तोष्णा कफवातजित् । हिक्काध्मानारुचिर्हन्ति कृमिजिद्वह्निदीपनी ।। (ध.नि.)

(4) ATIVISHA

Aconitum heterophyllum Wall.

Gana : Arshoghna, Lekhaneeya, (C.) Pippalyadi, Vachadi, Mustadi (S.)
Kula : Vatasanabha kula.
Family : Ranunculaceae (crow-foot-habitat in swamps of most species).
Latin name : Acontium heterophyllum i.e. aconite with dissimilar leaves.
Sanskrit names : Ativisha (non-piosonous though belonging to poisonous plant family), Shuklakanda, Shishubhaishajya (useful in paediatric diseases), Shrungi, Virupa, Pittadivallabha, Shwetvacha.
Botanical Description : A small plant with height of 1-1.5 mtrs. with straight bark and flat stems, leaves are 5 to 10 cm in length, egg or heart shaped. Lower leaves are big and are divided into five parts whereas upper leaves are small. Flowers are blue or green, with inner most layer largest and like a hood. The fruit has two sections, one from the previous year, and one from the current year. Transverse section is white with 4-5 black spots; good quality fruit tapers towards one end. It is 2.5 to 5 cm in length. If the transverse section does not show 4 -5 black spots one can assume

There is a definite sequence in the appearance of symptoms of any disease. Similarly, there is also a sequence of disappearance of symptoms after treatment.

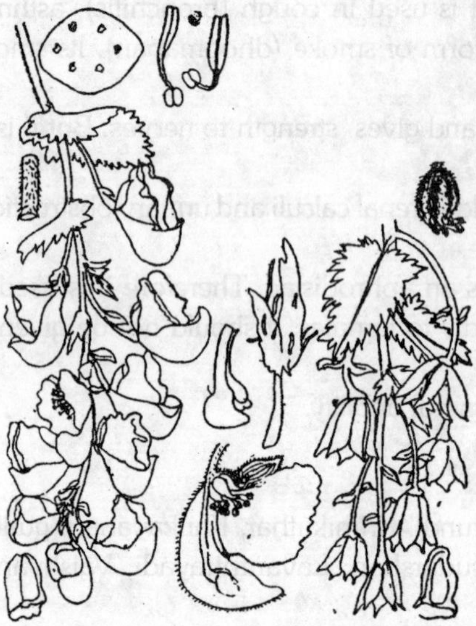

that it is the adulterated form, not the genuine one.
Varieties : Madanvinod has described four varities viz. 1) white 2) yellow 3) red and 4) black. Raj Nighantu has described only three varities i.e. white, red and black. In actual practice, only white variety is available.
Habitat : Found in Himalayas at the height of 2000 to 6000 meters. Also found in Sindh-Kumaon mountain ranges.
Properties :
Guna : laghu; **Rasa :** tikta, ruksha;
Vipak : katu; **Veerya :** ushna.
Karma : Tridoshahara, alleviates kapha and pitta by bitterness.Vata is alleviated by ushna veerya.
Internal uses :
Digestive system : It has appetizing, digestive, astringent, antihaemorrhoidal and anthelmintic properties due to its bitter, pungent and ushna properties. Useful in diarrhoea and dysentery.
Circulatory system : It is a blood purifier, haemostatic and antiinflammatory drug because it alleviates pitta.
Respiratory system : Reduces phlegm and clears airways.
Reproductive system : Purifies milk secretion (lactation) because of its katu property. Aphrodisiac due to ushna property.
Temperature : Febrifuge, useful as a prophylactic in intermittent fever.
Satmikaran : Reduces body weight due to ruksha guna, bitter tonic and antidote for poisons. useful in scorpion bite.
Indications :
Dosha : Diseases induced by all three doshas, but mainly useful in kapha and pitta diseases.
Digestive system : Useful in dyspepsia, indigestion, amadosha, vomiting, fever associated with diarrhoea, diarrhoea, haemorrhoids, helminthiasis. Along with C. sativa and C. calamos it is effective for diarrhoea in children. Appetizing, digestive and astringent activities are carried out in sequence by A. heterophyllum.
Circulatory system : Useful in cold and cough.
Reproductive system : Useful in impotency.
Temperature : Effective in fevers, mainly in periodical fevers. It should be given in a dose of 2-3 gms as a prophylactic treatment for malaria and acts faster if given along with any fragrant drug.
Satmikaran : Useful in post pyrexial debility because it is a bitter tonic. It is an antidote for rat poison.
Specific uses : No medicine is better than A. heterophyllum for paediatric diseases (hence the name 'Shishubhaishajya' - shishu = child and bhaishajya = medicine).
Parts used : Tuber.
Dosage : 0.5 - 2.5 gms, it should be used in the powder form only along with trikatu (ginger,

Just as humans, forests also have three stages of life viz. childhood, youth and senility. Spring is considered as the youth of forests.

black pepper and long pepper) and Achorus calamus.
Formulations : Balasanjeevani churna, Balachaturbhadra, Ativishadi churna.
Side effects : A. heterophyllum in a higher dose of 4 - 5 gms causes dryness of mouth and tremors etc., vata symptoms, hence it is called as ativisha. It is a poison (visha) if given in higher dose (ati), hence the name ativisha.
Purification : Tubers are heated with cowdung and dried in sun, thus they are purified.
Adulteration : Rootstalks of Asparagus racemosus. (These are not bitter and do not have spots inside).
Srotogamitva : Tridosha (it gives yellow colour to stools).
Dhatu : Rasagani (digestion), stanyagami, purifies lactation.
Mala : Purishagami (antidiarrhoeal, astringent).
References -

'विषा त्वतिविषा विश्वा शृंगो प्रतिविषारुणा । शुक्लकन्दा चोपविषा भंगुरा घुणबल्लभा ॥
विषा सोष्णा कटुस्तिक्ता दीपनी पाचनी हरेत् । कफपित्तातिसारामविषकासवमिक्रिमीन् ॥' (भा.प्र.)
त्रिविधातिविषा ज्ञेया शुक्ला कृष्णा तथारुणा । रसवीर्यविपाकेषु निर्विशेषा गुणेऽधिका ॥
अतिविषा शुक्लक्दा ज्ञेया विश्वा च भंगुरा । मृद्धी च शिशुभैषज्या विषरूपा महौषधिः ।-
शोफापहाऽतिसारघ्नी शुक्लकन्दा च सा स्मृता ।' (नि.सं.)
'अतिविषा दीपनीयपाचनीयसंग्राहकसर्वदोषहराणाम् श्रेष्ठा ।' (च.सू. २५)
विषात्रयं त्रिदोषघ्नं पाचनं ग्राहि तिक्तकम् । बालानां सर्वदा पथ्यं वमिशोथविमर्दनम् ॥' (शो.)
'कासज्वरच्छर्दिभिरर्दितानां समाक्षिकां चातिविषां तथैकाम् ।' (शो.)
'घुणाप्रियाऽतिसारघ्नी बालानां रोगनाशिनी ।' (ध.नि.)
'श्यामकन्दा प्रतिविषा विरूपा घुणवल्लभा' (नि.सं.)
'अंकोटस्य त्रयोभागाः भागश्चैकोऽरुणाभवः । तण्डुलोदकसंपीतः सर्वकुक्ष्यामयापहः ॥' (वं.से.)

(5) APARAJITA
Clitoria terneata Linn.

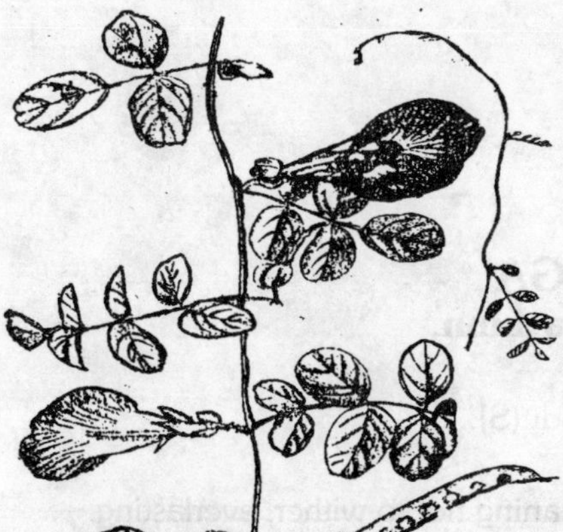

Kula : Aparajita kula.
Family : Papilionaceae-Flowers are butterfly shaped with two open wings.
Latin name : Clitoria (Kleio = to shut), Clitoria = an anatomical organ fancied to exist in flower;
terneata = of the islands of ternate.
English name : Winged leaved clitoria.
Sanskrit names : Gokarnika, Asphota, , Katabhi, Dadhipusphika, Vishantri, Mohanashini, Vishnukranta, Vajikhura.
Botanical Description : It is a perennial creeper with lavender coloured flowers. The flowers are of the same shape of cow's ears. One type has blue and the other has white coloured delicate flowers. The pods are of the

That which passes away continuously and does not return is called youth. Senility, on the other hand, never goes away after arriving.

length of a finger with 4-5 seeds. The pod opens when dried and seeds fall off.
Chemical composition : The seeds contain pale, bitter, saffron coloured resin which is acidic in nature.
Habitat : All over Maharashtra. It is also seen in gardens.
Properties:
Guna : ruksha, laghu; **Rasa :** tikta; **Vipak :** katu; **Veerya :** sheeta.
Karma :
Dosha :Tridoshashamak.
External uses : In otitis with lymphadenitis, the crushed leaves, mixed with saindhav are applied locally. The seeds crushed in honey are applied locally on throat, in tonsilitis. Nasal insufflation of roots is beneficial in headache (especially migraine).
Internal uses :
Respiratory system : The juice of roots along with milk is an expectorant. Root powder is given orally in cervical lymphadenitis.
Digestive system : Seed and root are used in ascites. Seeds are laxative. Shunthi (zingiber) is given to reduce griping pain.
Urinary system : The seeds are diuretic, the root decoction reduces burning of urinary tract. It increases volume of urine.
Reproductive system : Root is used in spermatorrhoea. The decoction of roots is also used in burning of vagina.
Ciruculatory system : The juice of leaves along with juice of zingiber reduce perspiration.
Parts used : Root, seeds, leaves.
Dosage : The powder of roasted seeds - 1.5 to 4 gms.; root powder - 3 to 6 gms.
Srotogamitva :
Dosha : Tridoshaghna.
Dhatu : Majja (brain tonic), rakta, shukra, meda.
Mala : Mutra (diuretic), purisha (laxative), sweda.
References -
श्वेतनीलपुष्पा अपराजिता नामानिगुणाश्च :-
आस्फोता गिरिकर्णी स्यात् विष्णुक्रान्ताऽपराजिता ।
अपराजिते कटू मेध्ये शीते कण्ठ्ये सुदृष्टिदे ।
कुष्ठमूत्रत्रिदोषामशोथव्रणविषापहे ।।

(6) APAMARGA
Achyranthes aspera Linn.

Gana : Shirovirechan, Krimighna, Vamanopag (C.) Arkadi (S).
Kula : Apamarga kula.
Family : Amaranthaceae; Amaranth is a Latin word meaning not to wither, everlasting.
Latin name : Achyranthes -Akanthes = thorn; aspera = rough, with very short stiff or hard points.
English name : Chaff tree.

Chapati becomes light on baking; its lightness depends on how and what it is roasted on.

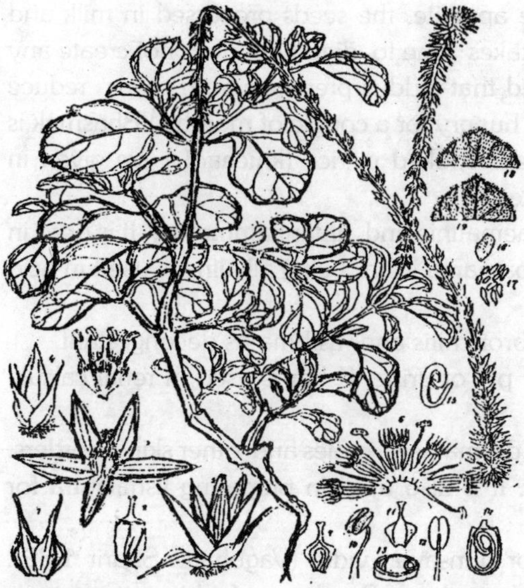

Sanskrit names : Durgraha, Adhashalya (the thorns are in upward direction), Kharmanjri (the inflorescence is tough), Pratyak-pushpi (the flowers are in upward direction in contrast to their usual downward direction), Kinihi (it heals wounds), Markat pippali, Kshavaka (apamarga seeds are used for "nasya" i.e. nasal insufflation), Karkatpippali, Kshudhapamarga (it reduces appetite).

Botanical Description : It is a small herb 0.5 to 1 meters high. The branches are thick at the end. The leaves are small, elliptic or ovate, 6-8 cm. long, 5-8 cm. broad, soft and hairy. The leaves are whitish on the dorsal side. The flowers are greenish white and appear in inflorescence. Fruits - thin, elliptic and greyish. The flowers blossom in winter and seeds disperse in summer.

Varieties : Two varieties viz. 1) White and 2) Red (A. rubrofusco = red dusky).

The branches, leaves, flowers, all organs of red variety are red in colour, hence the name. The branches are thin and quadrangular. Modern scientists describe two varieties-

1. A. Porphystachs (red spikes) = Raj Apamarga - the herb is 1.5 to 2 mtrs. high and leaves are 6 cm to 0.25 mtrs. long.
2. A.argentea - the leaves are silver white in colour.

Habitat : It grows all over India.

Chemical composition : The seeds and pentads (leaves, flowers, fruits, stem and root) contain potassium salts.

Properties :

Guna : laghu, ruksha, tikshna; **Rasa :** katu, tikta; **Vipak :** katu; **Veerya :** ushna.

Karma :

Dosha : Kaphavatashamak, kaphapittasamshodhak. The seeds are used for nasya (nasal insufflation) especially in kapha disorders. Its juice is given in pitta disorders, whereby it reduces acidity. Apamarga is supposed to be the best medicine in gall stones.

External uses : Antiinflammatory, analgesic, antidote, antiseptic, nasal decongestant. Crushed leaves are applied on inflammatory lesions. Its anjan is applied in opthalmic disorders. Juice of leaves is used in wounds. The leaves are crushed and applied on the area of scorpion stings. Oil processed in apamarga kshar is used in earache (otitis). A fine powder of seeds is used for pradhaman nasya (where this powder is blown through small tube into the nose). This reduces heaviness in the head instantly. The salts (kshars) are used in moles and fistula. Crushed seeds are applied locally in bleeding piles. The juice being haemostatic, stops bleeding from wounds.

Digestive system : Carminative, appetizer, antacid and anthelmintic in nature. It is a good remedy for excessive appetite. It is used in emesis, loss of appetite, abdominal pain, indigestion, flatulence,

Panchamahabhootas come alive in chapati while being roasted as it swells up (akash) with hot (agni) air (vayu). Dough is formed of flour (prithvi) and water (jala).

ascites, piles, gall-stones, helminthiasis etc. In excessive appetite, the seeds processed in milk and sugar are given as a food supplement. This preparation takes time to digest but does not create any disorders. Thus, it pacifies hunger as well. (It is believed that laddus prepared from seeds reduce appetite to such and extent that the person does not feel hungry for a couple of months.) Bhasmak is a disease where there is a voracious appetite. The seeds cooked in rice (khichadi) are given in bhasmak for one week. Apamarga kshar is used in ascites.

Circulatory system : It is a blood purifier, it is also a haematinic and antiinflammatory. It is used in anaemia, rheumatoid arthritis, oedema and scrofula. Apamarga kshar being alkaline is used in acid peptic disorders.

Respiratory system : The powder of roots is used in bronchitis and asthma as decongestant.

Urinary system : It is a diuretic and reduces acidic pH of urine. Kshar is used in renal calculi, cystitis and nephritis.

Skin : It is a diaphoretic and yet antipruritic. It is used in dermatoses, moles and other skin disorders. Mole falls off when tied with kshar sutra of apamarga. It is also used in preparing ksharsutra for treating anal fistula.

Reproductive system : Apamarga has been used for punsavan vidhi (Vagbhatta Sharir 1/39). Punsavan vidhi is a procedure to beget an offspring of desired sex. Panchang of white apamarga is crushed and taken internally in pushya nakshatra. Apamrga roots are tied on abdomen for easy and safe delivery.

Temperature : In malaria and typhoid, it is advised that apamarga roots should be tied on arms. This action is said to be due to 'prabhav'. The nasal insufflation of roots reduces fever.

It is a bitter tonic. Black pepper and apamarga root along with water are given to drink in snake poisoning.

Srotogamitva :

Dosha : Alleviates kapha and vata.

Dhatu : Medoghna, raktagami.

Mala : Purisha, useful for eliminating exudates from nose by nasya, urine (lithotripsic).

Organs : Heart, head, liver (cholagogue).

Digestive system : Appetizer, digestive.

References -

'अपामार्ग: सरस्तीक्ष्णो दीपनस्तिक्तक: कटु: । पाचनो रोचनश्छर्दिकफमेदोनिलापह: ।।
निहन्ति हृद्रुजाध्मानकण्डुशूलोदरापची: (भा.प्र.)
'अपामार्गस्तु तिक्तोष्ण: कटुक: कफनाशन: । अर्श: कण्डूदरामघ्नो रक्तहृदग्राहिवान्तिकृत् ।।' (ध.नि.)
प्रत्यक्पुष्पी शिरोविरेचनानां श्रेष्ठा । (च.सू. २५-४०)

(7) ARKA

Calotropis procera R. Br.

Gana : Bhedaneeya, Vamanopaga, Swedopaga (C.), Adhobhagahara, Arkadi (S.)

Kula : Arka kula.

Family : Asclepiadaceae = Swallow wart. God of healing.

A dravya which lacks a rasa automatically leads to a decriment in its guna etc. It is not advisable to use such dravyas.

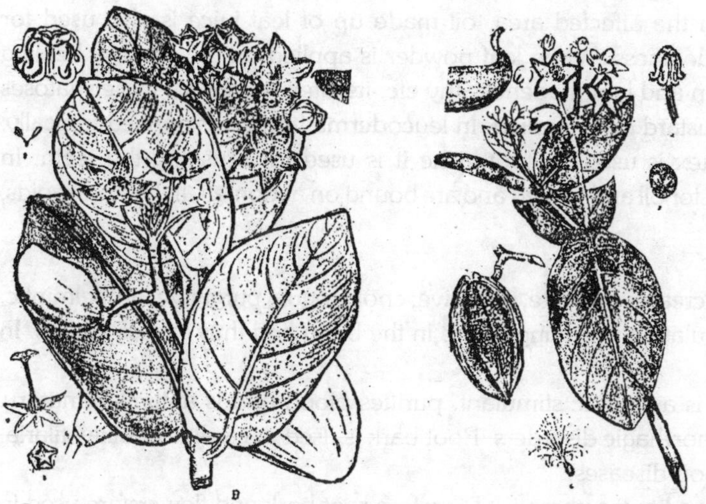

Latin name : Calotropis = (Kalos = beautiful) beautiful corona of the flower; procera = tall.

English name : Madar.

Sanskrit names : Red Calotropis - Toolaphala (cotton containing fruit), Ksheerparna (whole leaf contains latex), Shwetarka, Mandar, Vasuka, Alarka, Raktarka, Arkanama, Arkaparna.

White calotropis - Shuklarka, Tapan, Supushpa, Vrittamallika.

Rajarka - Vasuka, Alarka, Gunaroopa, Viksheer.

Botanical Description : It is a shrub. Its stem is hard having bark with grey striations on it. Leaves - are 10 to 15 cm long and 2.5 to 7.5 cm wide, big and ovoid in shape (like Ficus bengalensis). Upper surface of the leaf is smooth and dorsally it is hairy. Flower stalk grows in the acute angle of leaf and it has many branches. The inflorescence is in a cluster. Flowers are white externally, but internally they are reddish. Fruits- are long, curved and break open on drying. It gets automatically perforated and soft cotton comes out. It has seeds. They are spread everywhere by wind flow. Seeds are small and black in colour. Flowering occurs in spring and fruiting in summer.

Varieties : There are two varieties depending on the colour of the flowers - 1) white and 2) bluish red. The bluish red coloured plant is called as rui. White coloured variety is known as alarka or mandar. The Latin name of mandar is Calotropis gigantia. A big tree of calotropis is known as rajarka. Raja nighantu has described four varieties - 1) Arka 2) Rajarka 3) Shuklarka 4) Shweta mandar.

Habitat : All over India in dry and pungent soil, Srilanka, Afghanistan, Iran and Africa.

Chemical composition : Its root bark has a bitter principle. It has yeast in small amount because of which hot milk curdles immediately (gets solidified). Besides that, it also contains Madar alban, Madar Fluabil, resin and rubber. Some plants of calotropis have sugar-like white gum.

In communities which do not welcome female infants, the child is fed the sugar-like gum and death occurs. (Bha. Pra. Pande and Chunekar).

Properties :

Guna : laghu, ruksha, teekshna; **Rasa :** katu, tikta; **Vipak :** katu; **Veerya :** ushna.

Karma :

Dosha : As it is ushna, it acts as kaphavatashamak. Root bark, latex are used in kaphavataj disorders. As red calotropis flowers are bitter and sweet-due to its rasa it does the function of kaphapitta shaman. Therefore used in kaphapittaj disorders.

External uses : As it is analgesic, antinflammatory, vranashodhan, anti-dermatosis, anti microbial , it is used in elephantitis and rheumatoid arthritis. Conditions in which there is inflammation and pain,

A tree which grows at a height of approximately ten thousand feet above sea level, if planted on the land at sea level, how will it look in its natural form.

leaves are heated and are bound on the affected area, oil made up of leaf juice is also used for massage. This oil is used in otalgia, deafness. When leaf powder is applied on the wound, healing occurs faster. In tumour, inflammation and lymphadenopathy etc. its latex is applied. In dermatoses and other skin diseases its latex + mustard oil is applied. In leucoderma its latex is applied topically. In alopecia and haemorrhoids its latex is used. In toothache it is used for brushing the teeth. In flatulence its leaves are applied with castor oil and heated and are bound on abdomen. In haemorrhoids, the piles are exposed to its smoke.

Internal uses :

Digestive system : It is an emetic, increases appetite, digestive, cholagogue, purgative, anthelmintic. It causes irritation of stomach by stimulating vomiting centre in the brain and thus causes emesis. In anorexia, its latex is used.

Circulatory system : Root bark is a cardiac stimulant, purifies blood and is antiinflammatory. Flowers of red variety is used in haemorrhagic disorders. Root bark is used in cardiac debility, filaria, chancroid ulcers and many other blood diseases.

Respiratory system : Expectorant and anti asthmatic. Therefore root bark and flowers are used in kaphavataj kasa and asthma. Alkaline extract of flowers is useful in many disorders.

Skin : As it is a diphoretic, antidermatosis, therefore it is used in dermatosis. It is a very potent remedy for scabies.

Temperature : Febrifuge and also effective in typhoid. A layer of salt is put on the leaf and is covered with another leaf and then it is kept in a mudpot and is heated. The extract which is obtained is effective in periodical fever.

Satmikaran : It is a bitter tonic and stimulates all the body elements with increase of strength. It is antitoxic. In snake bite, its root sap with black pepper is given as an antidote.

Parts used : Root bark, latex, flowers, leaves, kshar.

Dose : Root bark powder - 1/2 to 3/4 gm; latex -1/4 to 1/2 gm; flowers - 3/4 to 2 gm.

Special formulations : Arka lavan, Arka oil, Arkeshwar, Arkadi churna, Arkakolakandavati, Praval Panchamrit, Sootika bharan, Ekangveer, Mahavatavidhvansa.

Misues : Root bark given in a dose of 2 to 5 gm. causes burning sensation of stomach and vomiting. Milk, ghee and other sheeta, shamak, snigdha and antitoxic substances must be given as antidotes. It is used to control different diseases like vaginal diseases, dermatosis, otalgia, asthma, splenomegaly, ulceration of penis, hernia etc. It is also useful in piles, wounds and stiffness of joints.

Medicines : Its latex is used to give bhavana for making medicines. A greater quantity can be collected before sunrise.

Srotogamitva:

Dosha : Vata, kapha, pitta (emetic and purgative).

Dhatu : Rakta (blood) (spleen).

Mala : Purish (worms); latex is the best purgative and diphoretic.

Organ : Respiratory system (kshar of flower).

References -

क्षीरमर्कस्य विज्ञेयं वमने सविरेचने ।' (च.सू. १)

अर्कद्गं सरं वातकुष्ठकण्डूविषव्रणान् । निहन्ति प्लीहगुल्मार्श:श्लेष्मोदरशकृत्क्रिमीन् ।।

Vibrations and nerve impulses are the characteristics of life. It is a mistake to expect these where there is no life.

अलर्ककुसुमं वृष्यं लघु दीपनपाचनम् । अरोचकप्रसेकार्श: कासश्वासनिवारणम् ।।
रक्तार्कपुष्पं मधुरं सतिक्तं कुष्ठकृमिघ्नं कफनाशनं च ।
अर्शोविषं हन्ति च रक्तपित्त संग्राहि गुल्मे श्वयथौ हितं तत् ।।
क्षीरमर्कस्य तिक्तोष्णं स्निग्धं सलवणं लघु । कुष्ठगुल्मोदरहरं श्रेष्ठमेतदविरेचनम् ।।'' (भा.प्र.)
'अर्कस्तिक्तो भवेदुष्ण: शोधन: परम: स्मृत: । कण्डूव्रणहरो हन्ति जन्तुसन्ततिमुदगताम् ।।' (ध.नि.)
'अर्कस्तु कटुरुष्णश्च वातजिद्दीपनीयक: । शोथव्रणहर: कण्डूकुष्ठकृमिविनाशन: ।।' (रा.नि.)
'मन:शिलाले मरिचानि तैलमार्कपय: कुष्ठहर: प्रदेह: ।' (च.सू. ३-१२)
'सप्तच्छदार्कदुग्धाभ्यां पूरणं क्रिमिदन्तनुत् ।' (च.द.)

(8) ARJUNA

Terminalia arjuna Wight. and Avn.

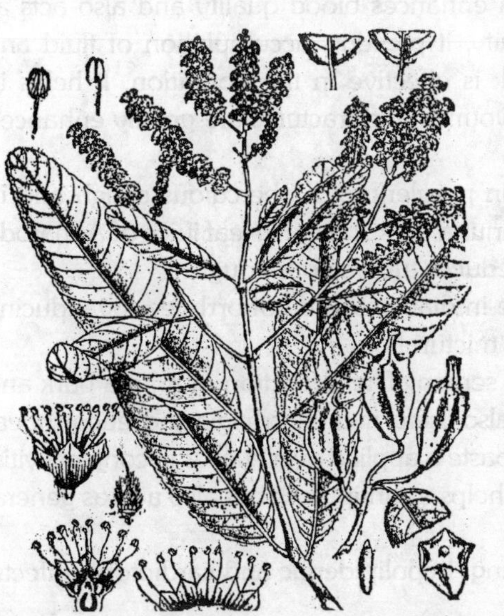

Gana : Kashayaskandha, Udardaprashaman (C.); Nyagrodhadi, Salsaradi (S.)

Kula : Haritaki kula.

Family : Combretaceae (combratum - after butter strub).

Latin name : Terminalia = disposition of leaves of some species towards the end of bracelets. (The plants in this family have 1 small node at the top of the petioles immediately below the leaves on each side); arjuna - arjuna.

English name : Arjuna.

Sanskrit names : Arjuna, Dhawal (pale white bark), Kakubha (spreading branches), Indradu (large tree), Viravriksha, Nadisarja (commonly found near rivers and is similar to sarja [Sal tree - Shorea robusta (Linn)].

All the names of 'Arjuna' mentioned in 'Bhagwadgeeta' are used as synonyms of arjuna plant. Gaura, Kashaya, Shakataksha, Dhurandar, Partha, Dhananjay.

Botanical Description : This is a large tree attaining a height of 20 to 26 mtrs. Trunk - straight, pale white and smooth externally and tender, thick and reddish internally. Leaves - subopposite, similar to guava leaves, 10-15 pairs of leaflets at the end. Leaflets - tongue shaped, 10-15 cm in length and 8-10 cm in breadth. There are small nodes at the top of the petioles immediately below the leaves. Flowers - occur all round white or yellow stalk. Fruit - similar to kamarah - fruit (Averrhoa cavambola Linn.). Flowering stage is in summer whereas fruiting stage is in winter. The bark is shed like snake skin once in an year.

Habitat : In 'Terai' region at the foot of Himalaya, Bengal, Bihar, Madhya Pradesh and Brahma Pradesh.

Chemical composition : The bark contains calcium carbonate 34%, other calcium salts 9% and tannin 16%. Besides, it also contains aluminium, magnesium, organic acid, colouring matter and sugar.

In all diseases, doshas are the real culprits. However, these doshas take refuge in all the three rogmargas (entire body), so those are also culprits.

Properties : Guna : laghu, ruksha; **Vipak :** katu; **Rasa :** kashaya; **Veerya :** sheeta; **Prabhav :** hridya.
Karma : Dosha : Kaphanashak by kashaya, ruksha, laghu properties and pittanashak by sheeta property. It is used in diseases inuced by kapha and pitta.
External uses : It helps in wound healing and joining by astringent property. It is haemostatic. The bark paste is locally applied on wounds, ulcer and specially used in promoting the union of fractures.
Internal uses :
Digestive system : It has astringent property, reduces motility. Being haemostatic it controls bleeding in dysentery and haemorrhoids.
Circulatory system : It is a cardiac tonic. It gives strength to the cardiac muscles and improves cardiac function and rhythm. It reduces cardiac rate. It increases the peripheral resistance by constricting capillaries which leads to rise in blood pressure. Arjuna enhances blood quality and also acts as haemostatic. By virtue of its capillary constricting activity, it prevents accumulation of fluid and thereby reduces oedema. The decoction of bark in milk is effective in this condition. It helps in cardiomegaly. Healing processes in ulcerated, contused wounds and fractures are greatly enhanced by systemic administration of arjuna.
Respiratory system : Its astringent property is useful in purulent and tuberculous cough and in haemoptysis. It reduces heartburn and cough. Powdered arjuna bark soaked in leaf juice of Adhatoda vasika mixed with honey, sugar- candy and cow's ghee reduces tuberculous cough.
Urinary system : By its astringent property it is effective in diabetes and gonorrhoea, by reducing urinary discharges and relieving burning and pain during micturation.
Reproductive system : It prevents early ejaculation of semen. The decoction of arjuna bark and white sandalwood is effective in spermatorrhoea. Arjuna is also useful in menorrhagia and leucorrhoea.
Skin : It is used in skin diseases with pruritus. Externally its paste is applied over eyelids in conjunctivitis.
Temperature : It is febrifuge. In chronic fever it not only helps as antipyretic but also acts as general tonic.
Satmikaran : It is astringent and possesses wound healing, hypolipidemic and cardiotonic effects. Arjuna is the drug of choice in cardiac debility.
Parts used : Leaves and root bark.
Dosages : Decoction in milk - 6 to 12 ml; juice - 12 to14 ml; powder - 1 to 3 ml; decoction in water - 60 to 100 ml.
Processing : Use of its bark as a decoction with milk (ksheerapak) is more effective. Besides, it can be used in the form of juice, decoction in water, powder or as a 'ghrita'. Use of ksheerapak has a dual advantage of reducing dryness inducing property of arjuna and also kapha aggravating property of milk.
Formulations : Kakubhadi churna, Parthadyarishta (Arjunarishta), Arjunaghrita, Pushyanuga churna, Ashwagandharishta, Arvindasava, Devadarvyarishta.
Bark of Arjuna : It is effective on heart, blood vessels and rakta dhatu. It provides nourishment to the heart. It increases relaxation period of the heart and acts as a cardiac tonic. It increases the force of contraction of heart and regulates its rythm. It is a cardiac stimulant.

It is possible to infer upon the actions of those dravyas which act in accordance with their properties. The prabhav of dravyas can be guessed on the basis of their actions.

Blood vessels : It constricts the capillaries, it corrects low blood pressure and tones up the capillaries.
Rakta dhatu : Makes blood components more balanced and increases coagulating property of blood.
Strotogamitva :
Dosha : Kapha, pitta kshayakarak.
Dhatu : Meda (diabetes), rakta (haemoptysis), asthi (promotes union in fractures), shukra (spermatorrhoea).
Mala : Mutra (diabetes).
Organs : Heart, kidney and uterus (in malapresentation of foetus).
Antidote Property : Its acts as cardiac tonic in vatsanabh (Aconitum ferox Linn) poisoning.
References -
ककुभोऽर्जुननामाख्यो नदीसर्जश्च कीर्त्तित: । इन्द्रद्रुर्वीरवृक्षश्च वीरश्च धवल: स्मृत्त: ।।
ककुभ: शीतलो हृद्य: क्षतक्षयविषास्त्रजित् । मेदोमेहव्रणान् हन्ति तुवर: कफपित्तहृत् ।।' (भा.प्र.)
'अर्जुनस्य त्वचा सिद्धं क्षीरं योज्यं हृदामये । सितया पञ्चमूल्या वा बलया मधुकेन वा ।।
घृतेन दुग्धेन गुडाम्भसा वा पिबन्ति चूर्ण ककुभत्वचो ये । हृद्रोगजीर्णज्वररक्तपित्तं हत्वा भवेयुश्चिरजीविनस्ते ।।'(च.द.)
'भग्न: पिबेत्त्वक् पयसाऽर्जुनस्य गोधूमचूर्ण सघृतेन वाथ ।' (च.द.)

(9) ASHWAGANDHA
Withania somnifera Dunal.

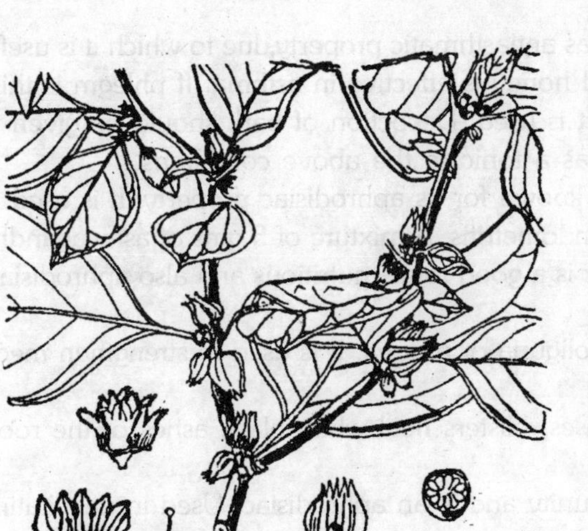

Gana : Balya, Bruhaniya, Madhurskandha (C.)
Kula : Kantakari kula.
Family : Solanaceae (Solamen = comforting) (German botanist).
Latin name : Withania = Withan (scientist); somnifera = sleep producing.
English name : Winter cherry.
Sanskrit names : Balada, Gandhanta, Vajinama, Vajini, Pushtida, Punya, Vataghni, Balya, Hayahya, Vrusha.
Botanical Description: This is a shrub attaining a height of 1-2 mtrs. Branches - distributed in all directions and rounded. Leaves - alternate, 5-10 cms long, rounded and hairy. Flowers - inflorescence in bunch, umbrella erupting from the base of the leaves. Sessile flowers, greenish or lurid yellow cyme. Fruits - small, round, juicy, capsulated, bright red like gunja, that's why it is known as dhorgunja. Seeds - small, slimy and flat. Roots - 1/3 to 1/2 mtr. long and as thick as a finger, grey from outside and white from inside (within). Tender wet roots smell like horse so it is called ashwagandha. (After taking ashwagandha,

What could have happened if physics had invented microscope or X-ray machines during the time of Charaka and Sushruta! What would happen if these sophisticated instruments were not existing today!

it makes the person energetic like horse i.e physically and sexually). Flowering season is sharad ritu (i.e. approximately October - November) and then the plant fruits.

Varieties : There are two varieties viz. 1) Cultivated and 2) Wild. The wild variety is sedative, hallucinative, diuretic and used externally. Cultivated variety is used internally.

Habitat : All over India.

Chemical composition : In the roots of wild variety there is somniferin which is a hallucinogen. Cultivated variety has sugar (sucrose), gum, resin and pigment dyes.

Properties :

Guna : laghu, snigdha; **Rasa :** madhur, kashay, tikta; **Vipak :** madhur; **Veerya :** ushna.

Karma :

Dosha : Kapha vata shamak. It is used in the diseases induced by kapha and vata.

External uses : It reduces oedema and pain, that is why leaves or root paste is applied on enlarged cervical glands or swelling of other glands. In vata diseases and weakness, oil massage is done. The juice of ashwagandha leaves is used as eardrops in ear discharge.

Internal uses :

Nervous system : As it is a sedative and nervine tonic, it helps in atonic nerves, fainting, giddiness and insomnia.

Digestive system : The bark powder is appetizer, carminative and anthelmintic and hence is used in abdominal pain, constipation and worms.

Circulatory system : It has an effect on the heart, purifies the blood and reduces oedema. So it is used for the weakness of heart, blood disorders and oedema. Its decoction is used in rheumatoid arthritis.

Respiratory system : It is an expectorant and has antiasthmatic property,due to which it is useful in cough. Ashwagandha ash along with ghee and honey is effective in asthma. If phlegm is thin, it is used in the form of ash or its alkaline extract is used. Decoction of bark should be given in low dose for cough and asthma. It is also used as a tonic in the above conditions.

Reproductive system : Ashwagandha is well known for its aphrodisiac property. It is used in semen disorders and leucorrhoea caused due to endometritis. A mixture of 5 gms of ashwagandha powder + 10 gms of ghee + 250 ml milk + sugar is a good tonic, nutritious and also aphrodisiac. It completely cures puerperal backache.

Urinary system : It is a diuretic and so used in oliguria or anurea. It is used to strengthen meda dhatu.

Skin : It is used in vitiligo and other skin deseases, blisters heal when black ashes of the roots are applied on them.

Satmikaran : It increases weight, improves immunity and is an aphrodisiac. Used in debilitating diseases and marasmus in children.

Useful parts : Roots, salts, ashes, leaves (roots are boiled in milk).

Dose : Powder 3 to 5 gms., salts and ashes 2 to 3 gms.

Formulations : Ashwagandhadi churna, Ashwagandha rasayana, Ashwagandhaghrut, Ashwagandharishta, Askandpak, Maharasanadi, Sukumarghrut, Saubhagyasunthipak, (Ashwagandha is aphrodisiac).

Every word in Charaka samhita talks to us and tells us volumes. We should listen to it and we should be able to follow it.

Srotogamitva :
Dosha : Vata, kaphashamak
Dhatu : Shukra (aphrodisiac), atishukrala, mansa, meda (nourishing), majja (induces sleep, sedative).
Mala : Mutra (stops burning).
Organs : Genitals (both sexes).
References -

कंदिनी वाजिगंधा स्यात् क्षुपा पर्पोटिवत् फला । वनजा वृत्तपर्णी च कंदो वाजीकरः स्मृतः ।। (शि.)
'अश्वगन्धानिलश्लेष्मशिवत्रशोथक्षयापहा । बल्या रसायनी तिक्ता कषायोष्णातिशुक्ला ।।' (भा.प्र.)
'पीताश्वगंधा पयसार्धमासं घृतेन तैलेन सुखाम्बुना वा ।
कुशस्य पुष्टिं वपुषो विधत्ते बालस्य शस्यस्य यथाम्बुवृष्टिः ।।' (च.द.)
'शिशिरे योऽश्वगंधायाः कन्दचूर्ण पलोन्मितम् । मासमत्ति, समध्वाज्यं सवृद्धोऽपि भवेद्युवा ।। (रा.भा.)
'पादकल्केश्वगंधायाः क्षीरे दशगुणे पचेत् । घृतं पेयं कुमाराणां पुष्टिकृत्बलवर्धनम् ।।' (चे.द.)

(10) ASHOKA
Saraca indica Linn.

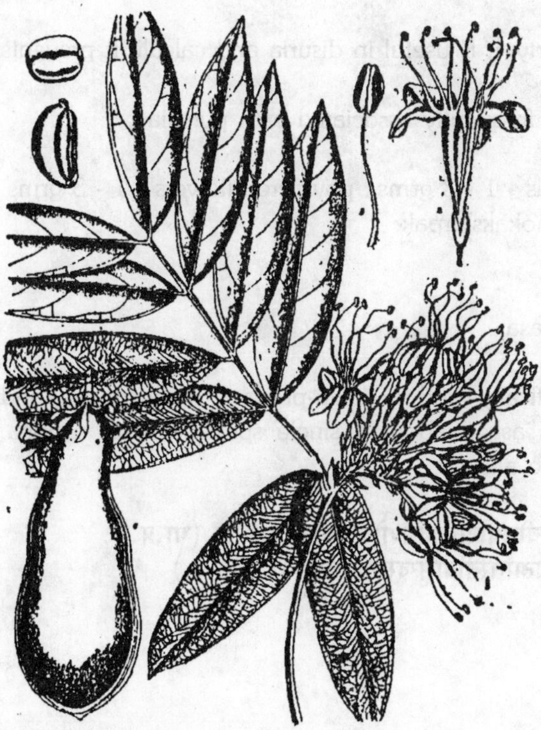

Gana : Kashayaskandha, Vedanasthapan (C.), Rodhradi (S.)
Kula : Shimbi kula (leguminoceae).
Upakula : Pootikaranja (Caesalpinaceae).
Latin name : Saraca indica Linn.
Sanskrit names : Hemapushpa, Kankeli, Shokanash, Karnapurak, Subhag, Smaracivas, Doshahari, Rama, Pallavadru, Raktak, Ragi.
Botanical Description : The ashoka tree resembles mango tree. It grows up to ten mtrs. in height. Even its leaves are similar to those of mango tree (98 to 10 cms long). Its tender leaves are red coloured. Its attractive flowers are arranged in a cluster, and when tender, they are yellow coloured . They gain red colour as they mature. Its pods are flat and eight to twenty-five cms. long. It contains five to six flattened seeds. Flowering occurs in spring and it fruits in winter.
Habitat : The tree is found in abundance in Bengal, South India and Burma. It is also available in plenty at Kanakeshwar near Alibaug, Maharashtra. This is khota (false) ashoka. Khota ashoka, known as Polyalthea longifolia is used as an ornamental tree in gardening.

Youth comes with a promise to go away every moment. But if old age comes, it comes to stay!

Chemical composition : The bark contains an active component, haematoxylin. It also contains tannin and catechin in substantial amount and ferrous compounds in a smaller quantity.

Properties :

Guna : laghu, ruksha; **Rasa:** kashaya, tikta; **Vipak:** katu; **Veerya** : sheeta.

Karma : Kaphapittashamak, hence useful in disorders induced by kapha and pitta.

External uses : The bark has analgesic and antidotal properties. Hence its paste is used in pains and poisoning for local application.

Internal uses :

Nervous system : It has a tranquillizing effect on the nerves and therefore is used in painful vata disorders.

Digestive system : Due to its astringent, anthelmintic and antidyspeptic properties, it is useful in diarrhoea, dysentery, helminthiasis and dipsia.

Circulatory system : It has haemostatic, blood purifying and antioedematous effects. Hence it is used in diseases of the blood and oedema. Its flowers are used in haemoptysis and internal bleeding.

Reproductive system : It strengthens the muscles of the uteres and reduces uterine discharge and pain in the uterus and so it is useful in menorrhagia, leucorrhoea and dysmenorrhoea. Since the decoction of the bark acts as a tonic for the endometrium of the uterus, it is useful in many diseases of the uterus.

Urinary system : By virtue of its diuretic property, it is useful in disuria and calculi. It prevents the formation of a calculus.

Temparature : It reduces the burning sensation frequently associated with pyrexia.

Parts used : Bark, seeds and flowers.

Dose : Bark (for decoction) - 10 - 20 grms.; seeds - 1 - 3 grms.; powdered flowers - 1 - 3 grms.

Formulations : Ashokarishta, Ashokaghrita, Ashokakshirpak,

Srotogamitva :

Dosha : Kapha, pitta kshayakarak.

Dhatus : Rakta (haemostasis), meda, mansa, rasa.

Mala : Purisha (astringent), mutra (diuretic).

Organ : Uterus (in menorrhagia). Ashoka is specifically used for rakta-pradara (menorrhagia) and hence it is called a friend of women. If one is asked about a single special use of ashoka, undoubtedly, "pradaradi stree roga" would be the answer.

References -

अशोक: शीतलस्तिक्तो ग्रीही वर्ण्य: कषायक: । शोषापचीतृषादाहकृमिशोथविषास्त्रजित् ।। (भा.प्र.)
'अशोकवल्कलक्वाथशृतं दुग्धं सुशीतलतम् । यथाबलं पिबेत्प्रातस्तीव्रासृग्दरनाशनम् ।।' (च.द.)
'अशोकस्य त्वचा रक्तप्रदरस्य विनाशिनी ।' (शो.)

Just like food and sleep, sex is the essential third pillar of life. It is necessary to be generous about sex. Complete celebacy is only possible to sages.

(11) AHIFEN

Papaver somniferum Linn.

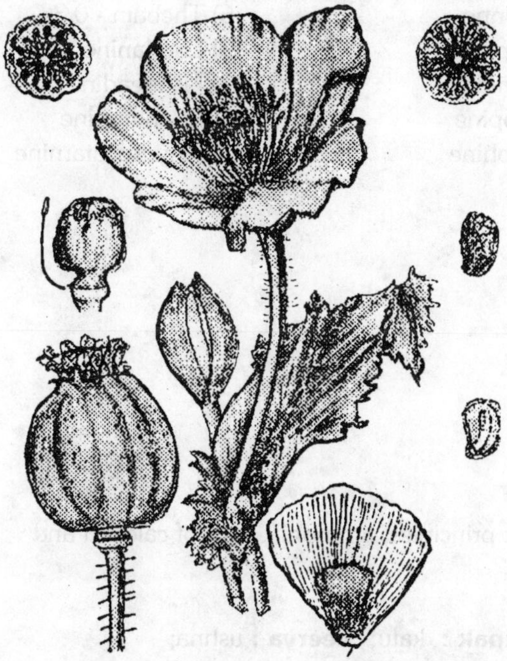

Kula : Ahifen kula.
Family : Papaveraceae (Gk Papa = milky juice - poppy).
Varga : Upavisha.
Latin name : Papaver somniferum (Linn). (somni = sleep, fera = producing).
English name : Opium.
Sanskrit names : Aaphook, Ahifen, Aphan, Niphen, Nagaphen, Rasodbhootam, Khaskhasrasa.
Botanical Description : The tree is 1 to 1.5 mtrs. high. Stalk is green in colour, tender, hairy and snigdha. Root are subtle and medium. Leaves are long and wide, alternately arranged with serrated margins. Flowers are white, red or black in colour. The fruit has the size of pomegranate fruit having different cells, small size, and it gets ruptured on its own. It is called as doda. This fruit shell is called as poshta. Seeds are white or black in colour, unctuous and sweet. They are called as poppy seeds (poshta dana or khaskhas.) Aphoo is the latex of this fruit. The raw fruit is incised in the evening and on the next day, early in the morning, the latex is scratched and dried. This is morphine.
Varieties : According to the flowers, it is of 3 varieties.
1) Khaskhas White - Its flower is yellowish white and seed is white.
2) Khaskhas Mansoor - Both flower and seed are red in colour.
3) Khaskhas black - Both flower and seeds are black or blue.
There are four varieties according to flowers mentioned in Nighantu :
1) White 2) Yellow 3) Black 4) Chitra
According to action, four varieties have been described :
1) Jaran 2) Maran 3) Dharan 4) Saran
Modern science has classified it by names of the countries of origin -
1) Turkey 2) European 3) Persian 4) Indian.
Turkish opium is used most frequently.
Habitat : In the countries of the northern temperate zone, Asia minor, Persia, China, Nepal, Burma, India. In India also especially Uttar Pradesh, Bihar, Bengal, Vindhya Pradesh, Malva, Assam. Morphine is widely used illegally.
Chemical composition : It has 29 different active principles amongst which morphine (5.2%), codeine (0.3-4%), thebaine (0.3%) and narcotine (2 to 7%) are the main principles.

All types of vata, pitta and kapha are present in every minute constituent of the body. "ते व्यापिनः" means the same.

CHEMICAL COMPOSITION

1) PRIMARY ALKALOIDS

1) Morphine - 5-21%	2) Coderine - 0.3-4%	3) Narcottine- 2-0%
4) Nardin	5) Papaverine	6) Thebain - 0.3%
7) Pseudomorphine	8) Cryptopine	9) Laudanine
10) Laudanoisine	11) Meconidine	12) Rhoeadine
13) Codamine	14) Nascopine	15) Lanthopine
16) Xanthaline	17) Protophine	18) Hydrocatarnine

2) SECONDARY ALKALOIDS

1) Apomorphine	1) Thebamine
2) Oxydimorphine	2) Porphyroxine
3) Apocodeine	3) Catarnine
4) Desoxycodeine	4) Rhosadenine

3) NEUTRAL PRINCIPLE

1) Opionin 2) Meconin 3) Meconoidin.

4) ORGANIC ACIDS

1) Lactic acid 2) Meconic acid.

Water - 16%, resin, glucose, fat, volatile oil, aromatic principles, ammonia, salts of calcium and magnesium.

Properties :

Guna : sookshma, ruksha; **Rasa :** tikta, kashaya; **Vipak :** katu; **Veerya :** ushna;

Prabhav : madak (intoxicating in nature).

Karma :

Dosha : As it is ushna veerya, kapha vata shamak and vitiates pitta, intake of higher dose induces ojahakshaya and vatavriddhi and produces delirium. Since it is toxic, death may also occur. It is useful in kapha vata disorders.

External uses : As it is ushna, it acts as an analgesic and antiinflammatory. It is used in inflammation of joints, pleuritis and in inflammation of many parts of body, as single drug or mixed with any other liquid mixture for external applicaton. In pain in the eyes, conjuctivits, otalgia-its application or aashchotan is done.

Its suppository is used in haemorrhoids, fissures and other rectal disorders. Its enema is used in perianal pain.

Internal uses :

Nervous system : As it is vyavayee, vikashi, intoxicating and ushna, it alleviates vata. Therefore it acts as an analgesic, sedative and anticonvulsant.

As it stimulates vomiting centre in the brain, vagus nerve and centres of contraction of pupils, it is useful in abdominal colic, renal colic, sciatica and parshvashool. It is effective in pain induced insomnia. As it is anticonvulsant, it is used in epilepsy, spasm, Parkinson's disease (kampa vata), dhanustambha (tetany) and in strychnine poisoning.

Digestive system : As it is ruksha and kashay, it reduces salivation, lowers appetite and acts as an

Heart is the facilitator of the functions of prana, mind, life, vata and rasa dhatu. If it stops functioning, everything will stop. This is the biggest secret of life.

astringent. Due to its astringent action, excessive quantity of urine, sweat, breastmilk and also bile are reduced. It also reduces blood sugar.

The special property of morphine is to reduce pain. It induces constipation by contracting abdominal muscles, stomach and intestines. Due to these properties, it is used in abdominal colic, gastritis, diarrhoea, initial stages of cholera to reduce delirium, it acts as a sedative, haemostatic and constipative. Due to all these properties, it is also useful in 'enteric fever'. Its functions are seen from mouth upto the anus.

Circulatory system : Though it reduces the heart rate, it increases the strength of the heart. It also acts as haemostatic, hence is used in bleeding disorders, mainly internal. Being cardiotonic, it is useful in cardiac asthma and in cardiac pain.

Respiratory system : It is a depressant of the respiratory system. As it is ushna, it is kaphanashak and antiasthmatic. It is useful in cough caused by vata and kapha, whooping cough, pleuritis, rhinitis and asthma.

Urinary system : Normally the quantity of urine dose not get reduced but sometimes it causes retention of urine. It helps in reducing urine sugar in diabetes. It is useful in ikshumeha.

Reproductive system : As it is ruksha, kashay, vyavayee and vikasi, it reduces all the dhatus and impotency occurs. But due to aphoo, shukra stambhan occurs. It does not produce shukra immediately. It is useful in those men in whom shukra skhalan occurs immediately (premature ejaculation). It immediately reduces pain after delivery or abortion.

Skin : As it is ushna, it acts as diaphoretic and is useful in sheetajanya effects.

Temperature : As it is bitter and diphoretic, it is used as an antipyretic and especially in fever associated with chills when often other medicines are not effective.

It is useful in pyrexia in filaria.

Eyes : It constricts the pupils and increases the intraoccular pressure.

Absorption and excretion : In the stomach its slow absorption occurs, but its absorption occurs faster in the intestine. It is excreted 90% through urine and its remaining 10% is excreted through stool, breastmilk, gastric juice and sweat. As it is excreted through breastmilk, its effects occurs also in the sucking babies. It is absorbed through placenta also, so effects occur in the foetus in the womb. Ordinarily, in 6 hours morphine is excreted through the body. 75% of the morphine is excreted through urine in 24 hours.

Useful parts : Fruit pulp.

Dose : 1/4 to 1 gunja, stimulant in small dose, in high dose it acts as depressant and is fatal.

Formulations : Ahiphenasav, Nidrodayavati, Karpoor rasa, Dugdhavati.

Contraindications :

1) In pneumonitis, chhinna shwas.
2) Meningitis, pyrexia` and in brain haemorrhage due to exertion.
3) In intestinal weakness and gastric weakness and in their relaxation state.
4) In serious kidney diseases especially in uremia.
5) Children and old people.
6) If in chronic diseases, morphine is given for treatment, by its continuous intake the person is addicted.

Ayurveda has used the word 'pushti' for healthy nourishment and the word 'sthoulya' is used for obesity (which is pathologic).

To be remembered about morphine:

It is a poison, by its improper intake, death may occur, so -

1) In children its effects occur immediately, so it should not be used. But if it is necessary, then one should use a very little quantity.

2) Its disastrous effect is more likely to occur in females than in males. Especially in pregnant women and post partum women, extra precautions must be taken.

3) Prakruti : A person of vata prakruti cannot tolerate it. If it is given in a little higher dose, there are symptoms like insomnia (Dravyagunavignyan, Priyavrat Sharma), delirium, giddiness, vomiting, depression etc.

4) Habitual : It can be become an addiction. For addicts and habitual users, it should be given in higher quantity.

5) Diseases : In highly painful diseases morphine should be given in higher dose. But in the diseases of lungs, heart, kidney, and brain it should be used carefully.

6) Formulation: Dravyas which are given with opium should not be harmful to dhatus or mala. (Dhatu shoshan or mala shoshan should not occur.)

Opium poisoning :

1) Tandra (Drowsiness), sleep, sanyas (unconscious state of mind), depression, dyspnoea and even death may be caused due to opium poisoning.

First pupils become pinpointed, but few minutes before death they dilate. Normally within 4 to 6 hours depression is seen followed by death in 6 to 12 hours.

Death due to opium intake is not troublesome for a dying person.

Treatment :

1) Shodhan - Vomiting is induced by water of sapindus or mustard paste with hotwater. Stomach tube is used to wash the stomach continuously till the aspirated water becomes clear.

2) Use of antidotes - Sapindus, hingu (asafoetida), Emblica officinalis, Ricinus communis, saraki (cotton seeds), banana juice, dronapushpi, ghee, tobacco, tejapatra, Azadiracta indica, vasanvel etc. are the antidotes of opium. They are used continously.

3) Stimulants and cardiotonics - To decrease cardiac depression, black coffee without milk is given. Besides that, makaradhvaja, kastoori, jundabedastar, jadvar, jaharmohara etc. are given with honey.

Note : Till the toxic effects are present, patient should not be allowed to sleep. By sleep its toxic effects increase.

Purification of opium :

It is dossolved in water, rinsed and boiled at a lower temperature. Dried opium, when impregnated with juice of ginger for 21 times, becomes purified. Such opium is used for medicinal purposes.

Period of collection and preservation - January / February.

Other Information : Seeds of opium are called as khaskhas. It is madhur in rasa, balya and virilizer. The properties of shell of fruit are same like that of opium. It is available in the market. It is not described in Charaka, Sushruta, Vagbhatta, but in Raj Nighantu and Bhavaprakash its description is available. It had been used for the first time in 3rd century in Asia Minor. Then Arabs used it and later popularised it in India and Iran. Opium is a majjagami dravya. It acts first on majja dhatu. It reduces fluidity in the body but sweat, urine and breastmilk are not reduced.

Why is til oil called the best medicine? Because it decreases krushata (debility) and sthoulya (obesity) both. It is a wonderful drug.

Srotogamitva :
Vyavayi -spreads all over the body.
Dosha : Kaphaghna, vitiates vata-pitta, acts on kaphavahasrotas and vatavahasrotas.
Dhatu : Rakta, acts on majja, shukra (useful in impotency).
Mala : Urine, purisha (reduces motility).
Organ : Respiratory system.
References -
'तिलभेदः खसतिलः खाखसश्चापि संस्मृतः । स्यात् खाखसफलोदभूतं वल्कलं शीतलं लघु ।।
ग्राहि तिक्तं कषायं च वातकृत् कफकासहृत् । धातूनां शोषकं रूक्षं मदकृद्वाग्विवर्धनम् ।।
मुहुर्मोहकर रुच्यं सेवनात् पुंस्त्वनाशनम् ।'
उक्तं खसफलक्षीरमाफूकमहिफेनकम् । आफूकं शोषणं ग्राहि श्लेष्मघ्नं वातपित्तलम् ।।' (भा.प्र.)
'खस्खसः सूक्ष्मबीजः स्यात्सुबीजः सूक्ष्मतंडुलः । खस्खसोमधुरः पाकेकान्तिवीर्यबलप्रदः' (रा.नि.)

(12) AMALAKI
Emblica officinalis Gaertn.

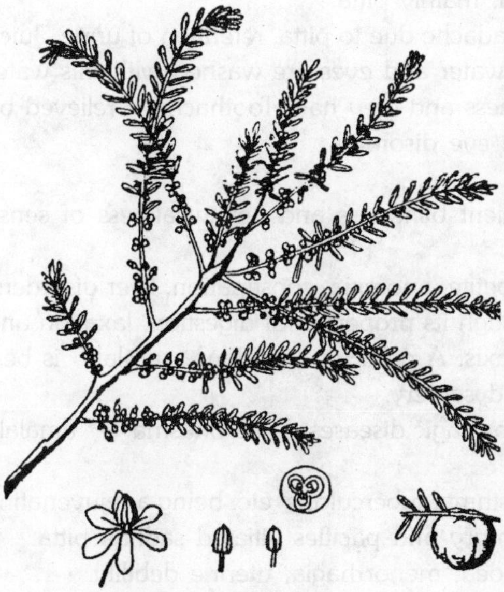

Gana : Vayahsthapan, Virechanopag (C.), Triphala, Parushakadi (S.)
Kula : Eranda kula (Euphorbiaceae).
Family : Euphorbiaceae (Spurge); Euphortous - physician to king Juba of Mauretania.
Latin name : Emblica = from Sanskrit Amlika; sour (juice of the fruit) old generic name; officinalis - sold in shops, of service to man.
Englsih name : Emblic Myrobalan.
Sanskrit names : Shriphala, Dhatrika, Amruta, Sheeta, Gayatrei, Vrushya, Rochani, Tishyaphala, Pancharasa, Kayastha.
Botanical Description : Middle sized tree 8 to 10 mtrs. high. Bark - whitish, thin. Its wood is strong and red. Leaves - having the appearance of tamarind leaves but more thin and small. Long petioles. Flowers - stalk is long. Flowers are small and yellow, flowering in autumn. Fruits - round and greenish yellow. Six striations with seeds. Banaras awala is of the best quality. It weighs 5 tolas. No remnant fibres after eating is a test for quality.
Varieties : 2 varieties 1) Cultivated large, soft and fleshy, 2) Wild - small, hard.
Habitat : All over India.
Properties :
Guna : laghu, ruksha, sheeta; **Rasa :** pancharasa (except salt taste - Charaka); **Vipak :** madhur; **Veerya :** sheeta (atisheeta).

That which is favourable to body, mind, senses and intelligence is called satmya.

Karma :

Dosha - Tridoshahara. Vatanashak by sour taste. Pittanashak by madhur taste and sheeta property and kaphanashak by ruksha property and kashay taste. So this drug is tridoshaghna but mainly pittanashak.

External uses : Refrigerant, hair tonic, complexion enhancer.

Internal uses : Strengthens nervous system, bone marrow and sense organs.

Digestive system : It improves taste and appetite, curative, antacid, biliousness. Small dose causes constipation while large dose is laxative.

Circulatory system : Cardiac tonic and haemostatic.

Respiratory system : Reduces cough.

Reproductive system : Aphrodisiac and helps in conception.

Urinary system : Useful in diabetes though it is a diuretic.

Skin : Useful in skin diseases (Manibhadrayog) (Vag. Chi. 19/31).

Temperature : Antipyretic, refrigerant.

Satimakran : Rasayani - (Chyavanprashadi kalp - Charaka).

Uses :

Doshas : It is used in diseases induced by tridosha, mainly pitta.

External uses : Paste is applied locally in burning, headache due to pitta, retention of urine. Juice is used in eye disorders. Fruits are kept overnight in water and eyes are washed with this water in the morning. Hair wash by amala is done in baldness and grey hair. Toothache is relieved by chewing fruit skin. Leaf juice is used as eye drops in eye disorders.

Internal uses :

Nervous system : Strengthens bone marrow, incipient blindness and any weakness of sense organs.

Digestive system : It acts in loss of taste, loss of appetite, anorexia, constipation, liver disorders, acid peptic diseases, eructations, ascites and piles through its properties of digestion, laxation and rasayan. Its juice is given in haematemesis and epistaxis. A paste of chandan + amlaki is best in pittaj vomiting. Leaf juice useful in haemorrhagic dysentery.

Circulatory system : Useful in heart diseases, haemorrhagic diseases. Loha bhasma + amalaki kalp is best in anaemia.

Respiratory system : Used in diseases like cough, asthma, tuberculosis etc. being a rejuvenating agent. Amlaki is a good brain tonic. It improves memory and pacifies vitiated sadhak pitta.

Reproductive system : It is useful in spermatorrhoea, menorrhagia, uterine debility.

Urinary system : Fresh amla juice is used in dysuria and pittaj prameha. Bark and leaves are also useful.

Skin : In skin diseases and erysipelas, it is given internally for longer period.

Temperature : Useful in chronic fever, thirst, burning sensation etc.

Satmikaran : Rasayan, rejuvenator.

Parts used : Fruit, leafjuice, seeds, (useful in acidity).

Dosages : Fruit juice -12 ml.; powder - 3 to 6 gm. Being a dietary product, large dose is harmless.

Kruratva and mardava of koshtha is not only related to koshtha but it is also related to microconstituents of the body.

Contraindication : Don't use amlaki and sour fruits at night or before sleeping as they weaken the tooth and also lead to pharyngitis.

Formulations : Chyavanprash, Bramharasayan, Dhatriloha, Amrutprash, Amalaki rasayan, Chandan amalaki chatan (best in vomiting due to acidity).

Terminalia chebula (haritaki) and amalaki have same properties. In haemorrhagic diseases and prameha, amalaki is used more than haritaki. In haemorrhagic diseases, amalaki is given as a laxative.

Srotogamitva :

Dosha : Pitta, kapha, vata-nashak, pittashamak though sour.

Dhatus : Rakta (haemorrhagic disease, jaundice), meda - prameha, shukra - aphrodisiac, all dhatus - rasayan (rejuvenating) especially muscles.

Mala : Purisha (laxative). Fresh fruit is laxative and dry is constipative. Vit. C does not perish even if amla is boiled because of tannin. Amla doesn't contain salt.

Organs : Eyes, spleen, liver, lungs.

References -

'हरीतकीसमं धात्रीफलं किन्तु विशेषत: । रक्तपित्तप्रमेहघ्नं परं वृष्यं रसायनम् ।।' (भा.प्र.)

'विद्यादामलके सर्वान् रसान् लवणवर्जितान् ।' (च.सू.२७)

'तान् गुणांस्तानि कर्माणि विद्यादामलकीष्वपि । यान्युक्तानि हरीतक्या वीर्यस्य तु विपर्यय: ।।' (च.चि. ३.)

'अम्ल समुधरं तिक्तं कषायं कटुकं सरम् । चक्षुष्यं सर्वदोषघ्नं वृष्यमामलकीफलम् ।
हन्ति वातं तदम्लत्वात्पित्तं माधुर्यशैत्यत: । कफ रूक्षकषायत्वत्फलेभ्योऽभ्यधिकं च यत ।।' (सु.सू. ४६)

'कटुमधुरकषायं किंचिदम्लं कफघ्नम् । रुचिकरमतिशीत हन्ति पित्तास्रतापम् ।
श्रमवमनविबन्धाध्मानविष्टम्भदोषप्रशमनममृताभं चामलक्या: फलं स्यात् ।।' (रा.नि.)

(13) ARAGVĀDHA

Cassia fistula Linn.

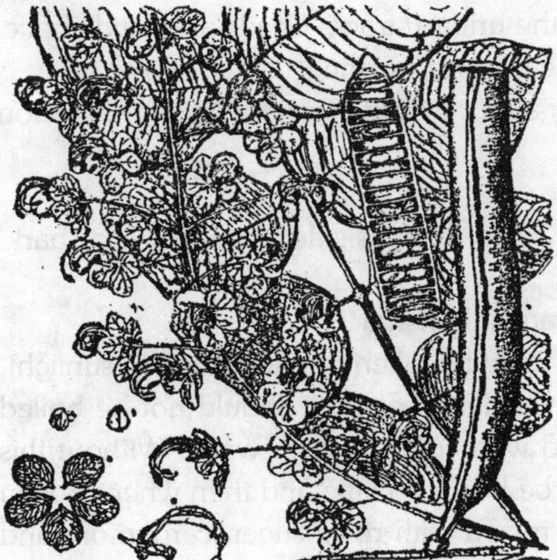

Gana : Kushthaghna, Kandughna, Virechana, Tiktaskandha (C.); Aragvadhadi, Shyamadi, Adhobhagahar (S.)

Kula : Shimbi kula (leguminosae).

Upakula : Pootikaranja upakula (Caesalpinioideae).

Family : Caesalpinioid - after the name of a celebrated Italian botanist.

Latin name : Cassia = kasia (Greek) from a Heebrew word - name of plant; fistula = tube, pipe or reedlike; (Old name = laburnum = Aragvadha).

English name : Drumstick or purging cassia.

Sanskrit names : Aragvadha, Arogyashimbi, Svarnat, Karna, Dirghaful, Rajvriksha (beautiful tree), Shampak, Chaturangul, Arevat (laxative), Krutaned, Suvarnak (nice colour), Kandughna.

Like in mind, the function of uha (intake) and apoha (giving up) also occur in the body. Pran-apana is the pair responsible for it.

Botanical Description : Medium sized tree, 8 - 10 mtrs. high. Stem - straight, bark is smooth and greenish grey or light red. Leaves - compound, 0.33 mtrs. in length having 8 to 16 pairs of leaflets on it. Flowers - yellow, grow in branches having fragrance. There are 5 petals and 10 androceum, 3 big and 3 small. Flower stalk - oblong. Fruits - 0.33 to 1 mtr. in length, 2.5 cms. in width, hard with narrow ends. Unripe pod is green and ripe is black. Pulp is black. There are septa inside the pod. Seeds - many, smooth, flat and grey seeds are present between two septa. Dry pod gives a sound on shaking.

Chemical composition : Pulp - glucose 60%, glutin, pectin, dyes, calcium oxalate, minerals, gum and water.

Habitat : All over India.

Properties :

Guna : guru, snigdha; **Rasa :** madhur, tikta; **Vipak :** madhur; **Veerya :** sheeta.

Karma : Vatashaman by madhur, snigdha properties, pittashaman by sheeta veerya. It is purgative so used in kapha and pitta sanshodhan. In vatapitta disorders it is used as sanshaman and in pittakapha disorders used as sanshodhan.

External uses : It is antiinflammatory, analgesic. The pulp and leaf paste are used in nodular oedema, gout, rheumatoid arthritis etc. The decoction is used for gargling in diseases of oral cavity and throat. Leaf paste is used in skin disease and itching.

Internal uses :

Nervous system : It is analgesic by vatahar property, so useful in vata diseases.

Digestive system : It is bitter so improves taste. It is a liver stimulant and purgative by snigdha property. It is a mild purgative drug and is useful in constipation and jaundice.

Circulatory system : It is cardioprotective, antiinflammatory, purifies blood so useful in heart disease, haemorrhagic disorders, gout and swellings.

Respiratory system : As it is madhur, snigdha, removes kapha and soothes internal organs by mridu property, in dry cough and dyspnoea flower's avaleha is given.

Urinary system : Diuretic by sheeta property. It soothes the urinary tract. Seeds are antidiabetic.

Skin : Kushthaghna and refrigerant, so used in skin disease and burning.

Temperature : It is antipyretic, so used in fever and purgation. Its bitter taste works in digestion and is pittashamak. Bark of root is used in fever.

Parts used : Pulp, root bark, flowers and leaves.

Dosages : Pulp - 10 to 20 gms.; pulp for purgation - 20 to 40 gms.; decoction of root bark - 2 to 4 mls.; flowers - 5 to 10 gms.

Formulation : Aragvadhadi taila, Aragvadhadi leha, Aragvadharishta.

Ripe pods should be kept in sand for 30 days. Then they should be taken out and dried in sunlight. After drying the pulp from the fruit should be taken out in a clean vessel. It should not be boiled as then the properties are lost. So the pulp should be used with cold or warm water. Without this procedure, the pulp might get spoilt. The old pods have to be heated a little and then when broken the pulp can be extracted with a spoon. The pulp can be mixed with milk, sugar, cardamom and a good drink can be made. It can be used as a laxative.

The pathogenesis of doshakshayaj diseases, which is simple and can be grasped easily, has become very rare.

Srotogamitva :
Dosha : Pitta, kapha.
Dhatu : Rakta (liver stimulant).
Mala : Purgative.
References -
'आरग्वधो राजवृक्षः शम्पाकश्चतुरंगुलः । आरेवतो व्याधिघातः कृतमालः सुवर्णकः ।।
कर्णिकारो दीर्घफलः स्वर्णाङ्गः स्वर्णभूषणः । आरग्वधो गुरुः स्वादुः शीतलः स्रंसनो मृदुः ।
ज्वरहृद्रोगपित्तास्रवातोदावर्त्तशूलनुत् । तत्फलं स्रंसनं रुच्यं कोष्ठपित्तकफापहम्।।
ज्वरे तु सततं पथ्यं कोष्ठशुद्धिकरं परम् ।' (भा.प्र.)
'चतुरंगुलो मृदुविरेचनानां (श्रेष्ठः) (च.सू. २५)
'ज्वरहृद्रोगवातासृगुदावर्त्तादिरोगिषु । राजवृक्षोऽधिकं पथ्यो मृदुर्मधुरशीतलः ।।
बाले वृद्धे क्षते क्षीणे सुकुमारे च मानवे । योज्यो मृद्वनपायित्वाद्विशेषाच्चतुरंगुलः ।।' (च.क.८)

(14) ARDRAK
Zinziber officinale Roscoe.

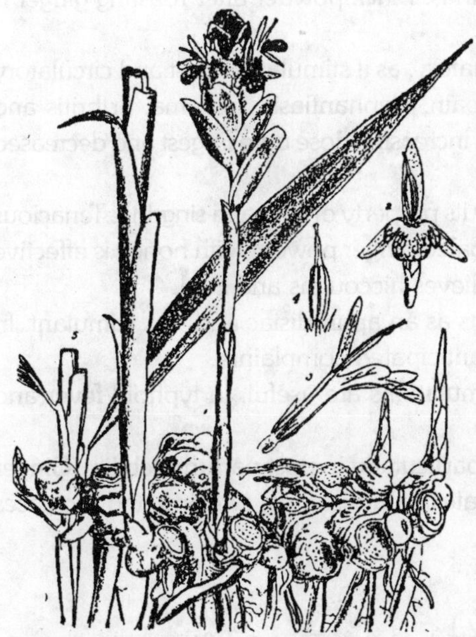

Gana : Truptighna, Arshoghna, Deepaniya, Shoolaprashaman, Trushnanigrahan (C.); Pippalyadi, Trikatu (S.); Panchakola, Shadushan (Bh.)
Kula : Haridra kula.
Family : Scitaminaceae (food stuff and condiments) Ginger- Zingibar (Shrungber).
Latin name : officinale = sold in shops or used in medicine or in the arts.
English name : Fresh ginger/ Dry ginger- when skin of the fresh ginger rhizome is peeled off and then dried it is called as dry ginger.
Sanskrit names : Shunthi, Vishva, Nagar, Vishvabheshaj, Vishvoushadha, Katugranthi, Katubhadra, Katushan, Sauparna.
Botanical Description : Plants grow up to 1 to 1.5 mtr. high. Leaves are 13-30 cms. long, broad and tapering at the top. Stalk of the flower is 5 to 8 cms.long, stamens are dark voilet coloured.
Varieties : According to habitat and processing, there are many varieties. Dry ginger is smoky in colour. White coloured ginger (ardranagar- kaiyadev) is found in South India which is used in practice-peeled rhizome boiled in milk and dired is called 'Dudhiyasuntha'.
Chemical composition : 1/5% yellow volatile oil, gingerol, gingerin (pungent resin), carbohydrates, oil and resin is found just under the skin. Gingerol does not evapourates with oil.
Habitat : Hot and damp climate like Madras, Kerala, Kochin , Bengal, and Punjab.

The thought of "avrutta" dose not even cross the mind of modern generation of Ayurvedic practitioners, though it is discussed in detail in ancient scriptures.

Properties : Guna : laghu, singdha (fresh ginger is ruksha, tikshna and guru); **Rasa :** katu; **Veerya :** ushna; **Vipak :** madhur.

Karma : Being katu, snigdha and ushna, it is useful in kaphavata diseases.

External uses : By its sheetprashaman, anti inflammatory and analgesic properties, it is used as local application in swollen joints and rheumatoid arthritis. It helps to reduce cold and stiffness. Ginger powder + oil is used for massage to reduce chills. Paste prepared in water or milk is useful in infantile cold and swelling. Dry ginger powder is rubbed on the skin in excessive swelling and hypothermia.

Internal uses :

Nervous system : It is the best medicine for all vata disorders. Ginger stimulates nerves, improves impulse transmission and relieves pain.

Digestive system : Ginger is an excellent appetizer, antisatiety, digestive, antiflatulent, antihaemorrhoidal and antispasmodic. It helps in alleviating vatakapha and pitta. Being appetizer, ginger along with salt is given before meals.

Due to these properties, ginger is used in anorexia, nausea, vomiting, loss of appetite, indigestion, flatulence, abdominal pain, jaundice and piles. Putpak of ginger powder dipped in castor oil and wrapped in castor leaves is very useful in rheumatoid arthritis. Black powder after roasting ginger is antiflatulent.

Circulatory system : It purifies blood and is antiinflammatory, as it stimulates heart and circulatory system. Therefore it is useful in cardiac debility, cardiac pain, elephantiasis, oedema, arthritis and urticaria. In oedema, ginger with equal quantity of jaggery in increasing dose upto largest and decreased to the orginal is useful as rasayan.

Respiratory system : It is kaphaghna and antiasthmatic by its property of tikta and singdha. Tenacious sputum of pharyngitis is relieved by chewing ginger. Charcoaled ginger powder with honey is effective in asthmatic bronchitis. Licking ginger juice with honey relieves hiccoughs and cold.

Reproductive system : Due to madhur vipak, ginger acts as an aphrodisiac and sex stimulant. In puerperium, saubhagyashunthipak is useful in almost all anticipated complaints.

Temperature : In fever with chills, ginger containing formulations are useful. In typhoid fever and innumerable conditions, ginger juice is used as adjuvant.

Satmikaran : Shuntipak is useful in general debility and particularly in post partum debility. Ginger keeps digestive and respiratory system healthy. It ameliorates vata diseases, swelling and increases the strength.

Useful parts : Rhizomes.

Doses : Ginger juice 2-4 cc.; powder .75 to 1.5 gm.

Formulations : Ardrakhanda, Panchasama churna, Samasharka churna, Saubhagyashunthipak, Vyoshadighrut. Many drugs are triturated in ginger juice.

Contraindications : Ginger being ushna and tikshna, it should not be used in anaemia, dysuria, bleeding disorders, ulcer, pyrexia, and in summer season and autumn.

Srotogamitva :

Dosha : Kaphavataghna.

Dhatu : Rasa (amapachan), shukra (aphordisiac), rakta (alleviates urticaria), dhatvagnivardhan.

To be a successful Vaidya, one must read "Dasbodh" which is a book based on experience.

Mala : Purisha (constipative).
Organs : Heart, internal and external routes.
Gudardrak vardhaman yog is useful in internal and external oedema. By its kledpachak and agni dipti properties, it reduces swelling.
References -
'शुण्ठी रुच्यामवातघ्नी पाचनी कटुका लघुः । स्निग्धोष्णा मधुरा पाके कफवातविबंधनुत् ।।
वृष्या स्वर्या वमिश्वासशूलकासहृदामयान् । हन्ति श्लीपदशोफार्शआनाहोदरमारुतान् ।।'
'आर्द्रिका भेदन गुर्वी तीक्ष्णोष्णा दीपनी मता । कटुका मधुरा पाके रूक्षा वातकफापहा ।।
ये गुणाः कथिताः शुण्ठ्यां तेऽपि सन्त्यार्द्रकेऽखिलाः ।.....
भोजनाग्रे सदा पथ्यं लवणार्द्रकभक्षणम् । अग्निसंदीपनं रुच्यं जिह्वाकण्ठविशोधनम् ।।
कुष्ठे पाण्डवामये कृच्छ्रे रक्तपित्ते व्रणे ज्वरे । दाहे निदाघशरदोर्नैव पूजितमार्द्रकम् ।।' (भा.प्र.)
'नागरं कफवातघ्नं विपाके मधुरं कटु । वृष्योष्णं रोचनं हृद्यं सस्नेहं लघु दीपनम् ।।
कफानिलहरं स्वर्यं विबन्धानाहशूलनुत् । कटुष्णं रोचनं हृद्यं वृष्यं चैवार्द्रकं स्मृतम् ।। (सु.सू. ४६)
'रोचनं दीपनं वृष्यमार्द्रकं विश्वभेषजम् । वातश्लेष्मविबन्धेषु रसस्तस्योपदिश्यते ।।' (च.सू. २७)
'शुण्ठीगोक्षुरकक्वाथः प्रातः प्रातर्निषेवितः । सामे वाते कटीशूले पाचनो रुग्विनाशनः ।।' (वृन्द.)
'नागरं वा पिबेदुष्णं कषायं चाग्निवर्धनम् । कासश्वासानिलहरं शूलहृद्रोगनाशनम् ।।' (वृन्द)
'आर्द्रकस्य रसः पेयः पुराणगुडसंयुतः शीतपित्तापहः श्रेष्ठो वह्निमांद्यविनाशनः ।। (भा.प्र.)
'अतिसारसंहरणमग्निहितं ग्रहणीविकारगुदकीलहरम् ।
जठरार्तिशोफगररुकशमनं सुमहौषधं जयति तक्रयुतम् ।।' (शो.)

(15) INDRAVARUNI

Citrulus colocynthis Schrad.

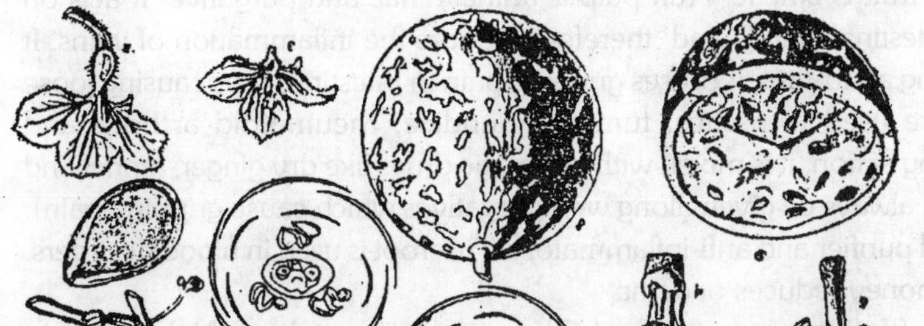

Gana : Virechan, Mulini (C.); Adhobhagahar, Shyamadi (S.)
Kula: Koshataki kula.
Family : Cucurbitaceae (guord-large fleshy fruit on trailing or climbing plants).
Latin name : Citrulus = citrus family ?; colocynthis = bitter apple, gourd, plant with bitter pulped fruit.
English name : Bitter cucumber.
Sanskrit names : Indravaruni, Aindri, Chitra (fruit is striped), Vishaghni, Peetpushpi, Indravalli, Varuni, Balakpriya, Amruta, Vishvalli, Suravanini, Sthanukarni, Dhanushreni, Suryahava, Manisambhava, Chandri, Tulsi.

Human heart is a naturally selfish organ right from conception. It is seen in its anatomy that it first takes its own nutrition.

Botanical Description : The herb is a creeper. It is rough and hairy. The leaves are ovate, serrated and similar to leaves of watermellon. They are 5 to 7 cm. in length. Flowers arise from the same stalk. Flowers are yellowish and bell shaped. Fruits - 5 to 7 cm. in diameter, smooth with stripes on it; they are greenish when raw, seeds are greyish black. Flowers and fruits come in winter.

Types : There are many types out of which two are more useful.

1) Indravaruni-also called as indrayan. The fruit is small and becomes yellow when ripe.

2) Vishala-It is also called as indravana. It is similar to cucumber and hence the names mrigadani, mrigervaru. The Latin name is Trichosanthes palmita. The flowers are white and ripe fruits are big and beautiful. The pulp of fruits is dark green. Fruits are called as "crow's mango" in western coast of Maharashtra especially in Konkan. They are put on doors as decoration. The fruit looks like a red ball in a Billiards game.

Chemical composition : Pulp of fruit contains colocynthin. It has glucoside 14%, resin, colosynthetin, pectin, gum, salts (11%), seeds contain 17% stable oil.

Habitat : All over India, but manily, Kerala, Madhya Pradesh and North-West India.

Properties :

Guna : laghu, ruksha, tikshna; **Rasa :** tikta; **Vipak :** katu; **Veerya :** ushna.

Karma :

Dosha : It ameliorates kapha and pitta. So used in the kapha-pitta disorders.

External use : The roots are anti-inflammatory and antiseptic. The oil of seeds is a hair tonic that nourishes the scalp and is an antidote. It is used locally in abscess. The juice is applied on wounds. The oil is used in snake venom and scorpion poisoning. It is also used in baldness, premature greying of hair.

Internal uses :

Digestive system : The skin of fruit is emetic. Fruit pulp is anthelmintic and purgative. It acts on liver and intestine. It stimulates intestinal glands and therefore reduces the inflammation of veins. It increases the acidic secretion. Being an irritant, it causes gripping pain in intestines thus causing loose motions. Fruit pulp and root are used in ascites, tumour, jaundice, rheumatoid arthritis and helminthiasis. To reduce its gripping action, it is mixed with aromatic drugs like dry ginger, fennel and hen-bane (Aromatic drugs should always be given along with purgatives which cause gripping pain).

Circulatory system : It is a blood purifier and anti-inflammatory. The root is used in blood disorders. Fruit juice mixed with sugar and honey reduces oedema.

Respiratory system : The skin of fruit is an expectorant. The root is given in bronchial asthma in children.

Reproductive system : The root has oxytocin-like action and hence contracts uterus. Therefore used in dysmenorrhoea and painful labour where it is inserted in the vagina.

Urinary system : It is hypoglycaemic, therefore used in diabetes.

Temperature : It is used in fever being antipyretic.

Satmikaran : If given in small dose it acts as a tonic. The powder of root is given in small amount and for a long duration in post-pyretic weakness, anaemia.

Parts used : Fruit and root.

Dosage : Fruit powder -1/4 to 1/2 gm; juice of roots- 6 to 12 cc; powder of roots -1 to 3 grms.

Amongst five types of vayus, prana vayu is the most important, that is why it is said "प्राणोरक्ष्य : चतुर्भ्योऽपि". No other vayu has regulating procedure like pranayam which regulates prana vayu.

Formulations : Narayan churna, Pleehodaradi churna.
Contraindications : Pregnancy, children, colitis.
Srotogamitva :
Dosha : Pitta, kapha-hara.
Dhatu : Rakta (jaundice), meda (diabetes).
Mala : Purisha (purgative), sarvamala shodhan (ascites).
Kesha : Ranjan (hair dye).
Organs : Liver (jaundice), uterus (abortifacient), spleen.
References -
'ऐन्द्रीन्द्रवारुणी चित्रा गवाक्षीच गवादनी । वारुणी च पराशुक्ला सा विशाला महाफला ।।
श्वेतपुष्पा मृगाक्षी च मृगैर्वारुमृगादनी । गवादनीद्वयं तिक्तं पाके कटु सरं लघु।।
वीर्योष्णं कामलापित्तकफप्लीहोदरापहम् । श्वासकासापहं कुष्ठगुल्मग्रन्थिव्रणप्रणुत् ।।
प्रमेहमूढगर्भामगंडामयविषापहम् ।' (भा.प्र.)
'इन्द्रवारुणिकाऽत्युष्णा रेचनी कटुका तथा । कृमिश्लेष्मव्रणान् हन्ति हन्ति सर्वोदराण्यपि ।।' (ध.नि.)
'मूलं गवाक्ष्याः । स्मरमन्दिरस्थं पुष्पावरोधस्य वधं करोति ।
अभर्तृकाणां व्यभिचारिणीनां योगोऽयमेव द्रुतगर्भपाते ।।' (वै.जी.)
'इन्द्रवारुणिकाबीजतैलेनाभ्यङ्गमाचरेत् ।प्रत्यहं तेन कालाग्निसन्निभाः कुन्तला अलम् ।।' (शा.)

(16) UDUMBAR
Ficus racemosa Linn.

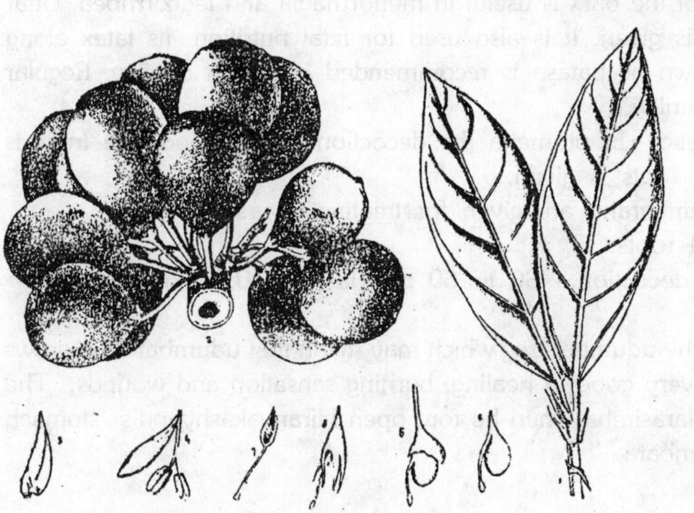

Gana : Mutrasangrahniya, Kashayskandha(C.); Nyagrodhadi (S.), Kshirivriksha, Panchavalkal (Bh.)
Kula : Vata kula.
Family : Urticacae (sting like) a nettle whip with nettles = to restore feeling (?)
Latin name : Ficus (old name used by Horace, Cicero and others); racemosa - having inforescence with a long undivided axis or glomerata compactly clustered into a round heap or head.
English name : Cluster fig, country fig.

Sanskrit names : Udumbara, Jantuphala, Hemdugdhaka, Kshirvriksha, Sadaphala, Kalaskandha, Yagnyayoga, Sheetvalka, Phalasambadha, Yagnyasara, Panibhuk.
Botanical Description : The tree is 10-14 mtrs. tall. Gives shade perennially, bark is reddish and smoky, leaves are 7-10 cms. long with tapering tips, having three veins. Fruits are green

A combination of dry ginger and jaggery acts as agnideepak i.e. it increases appetite. Dry ginger itself or only jaggery is not useful for this purpose.

when raw and red when ripe. The tree flowers in spring and bears fruits in monsoon. Fruits have small worms within them.

Chemical composition : Tree contains tannins, wax, rubber and ash which contains silica and phosphoric acid.

Habitat : All over India.

Guna : guru, ruksha; **Rasa :** kashaya, madhur; **Vipak :** katu; **Veerya :** sheeta.

Karma :

Dosha : Kaphapittashamak, used in kaphapitta disorders.

External uses : Reduces oedema - its latex is used as liniment for swelling and pain. For wound healing its raw stem is used in the form of liniment. A thick decoction of bark is applied locally for stomatitis. Topical use reduces burning sensation. Extract of bark is used as mouthwash and gargling in pharyngitis and stomatitis (udumbarsar).

Internal uses :

Digestive system : Agnisadak and astringent. Ripe fruits are anthelmintic. Because of the astringent property, decoction of bark is given in dysentery and diarrhoea associated with bleeding per rectum and sprue or raw fruits are given as cooked vegetables. The latex with sugar is used for infantile diarrhoea and teething problems. In case of bhasmak roga, the powder of bark is given with human milk and water. Fruit juice is given for hiccups.

Circulatory system : Udumbar is raktagami, so bark and fruits are used in haemorrhagic disorders. Half a leaf is given with betel leaves for treating jaundice.

Reproductive system : Decoction of the bark is useful in menorrhagia and leucorrhoea. Uttar basti (vaginal douche) of decoction is given. It is also used for fetal nutrition. Its latex along with sugar or sugar preparation known as batasa is recommended in sperm debility. Regular consumption of ripe fruits causes sterility.

Urinary system : It is an antidiuretic. In prameha the decoction of bark and ripe fruits is given. In diabetes, juice of fruits or roots is given.

Temperature : Ripe fruits being refrigerant, are given for treating fevers.

Parts used : Bark, fruit, latex and roots.

Dosage : Powder - 1.5 to 3gms.; decoction - 30 to 60 ml.; latex - 10 to 20 drops.

Formulation : Udumbarsar.

It is believed that water is found near the udumbar tree which may mean that udumbar tree grows near a water source. Ripe fruits are very good in healing, burning sensation and wounds. The burning sensation on the fingers of Narasimha when he tore open Hiranyakashyapu's stomach was ameliorated by the fruits of udumbara.

Srotogamitva :

Dosha : Alleviates pitta and kapha.

Dhatu : Acts on raktadhatu, enhances complexion, helps in wound healing and cures haemorrhagic disorders, varnya, vrana ropan, raktapittaghna.

Mala : Ripe fruit - purisha - mild laxative; raw fruit - astringent.

Organs : Digestive system - supresses appetite, uterus.

*जीर्णज्वरे... शस्यते गुडपिप्पली... **means a combination of guda-pippali acts on the factors responsible for chronic fever.***

References -
'उदुम्बर: क्षीरवृक्षो हेमदुग्ध: सदाफल: । अपुष्पफलसंबद्धो यज्ञांग: शीतवल्कल: ।।
कृमिवृक्षो जन्तुफलो मशकी जघनेफल: । पुष्पशून्य: शीतफल: पवित्र: सुप्रतिष्ठित: ।।'
'उदुम्बरो हिमो रूक्षो गुरु: पित्तकफास्रजित् । मधुरस्तुवरो वर्ण्यो व्रणशोधनरोपण: ।।' (भा.प्र.)
'औदुम्बरं कषायं स्यात् पक्वं तु मधुरं हिमम् । कृमिकृत् रक्तपित्तघ्नं मूर्च्छादाहतृषापहम् ।।' (ध.नि.)
उदुम्बरक्वाथयुतं सिताढ्यं सुगंधशालिप्रभवं सितं च ।
या पिष्टमश्नाति न गर्भपातपीडामसौ विन्दति जातु नारी ।।' (शो.)
'नारीस्तन्येन संयुक्तां पिबेदौदुम्बरीं त्वचम् । आभ्यां वा पायसं सिद्धं दद्यादत्यग्निशान्तये ।।' (च.चि. १९)

(17) USHEERAM

Andropogon muricatus Retz.

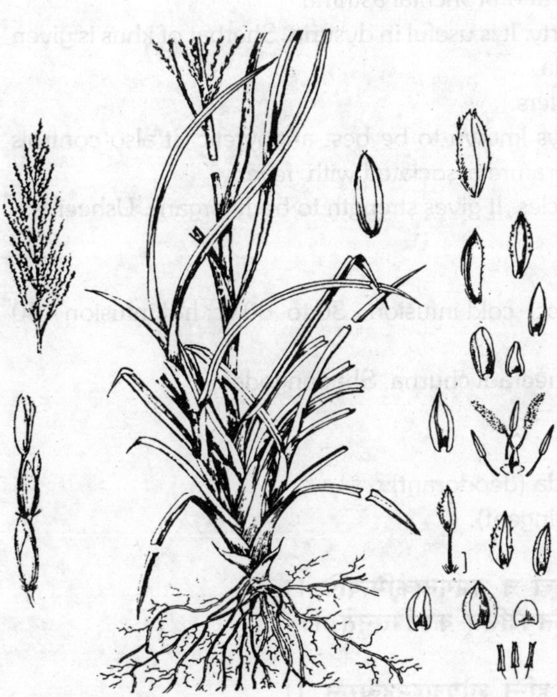

Gana : Varnya, Stanyajanan, Chardinigrahan, Dahaprashaman, Tiktaskandha (C.); Sarivadi, Pittasamshaman (S.)

Kula : Yava kula.

Family : Gramineae (Grass family).

Latin name : Andropogon (Ader=man, pogon=beard); muricatus (covered with sharp, short points, prickles or small spikes).

English name : Khuskhus grass or vetiveria, zizanoides.

Sanskrit names : Usheer, Samagandhak, Javavasa, Haripriya, Varitara, Shishir, Nalad, Bahumulak, Veernayak.

Botanical Description : Usheer is aromatic, a type of grass with stem 1 to 1.5 mtrs. high. Leaves- 25-50 cm., straight. The stalk of flowers is 10-30 cm. long. It flowers in rainy season and fruits thereafter.

Chemical composition : It contains a volatile oil, resin, dyes, calcium carbonate, ferrous oxide and starch.

Habitat : South India, Bengal, Rajasthan, Chota Nagpur, in watery, shrubby and marshy land.

Properties :

Guna : ruksha, laghu; **Rasa :** tikta, madhur; **Vipak :** katu; **Veerya :** sheeta.

Karma :

Dosha : Kaphashamak (due to tikta, ruksha and laghu properties). Pittashamak (due to sheet veerya). Useful in kaphapittaj disorders.

External use : A thin layer of usheer is cool, refrigerant, deodorant and reduces perspiration (Charaka).

In ancient Ayurvedic practice, gold was used liberally as it is a potent antitoxic agent. As gold has become scarce, our bodies are full of toxic substances.

The mat curtains made up of usheer are used in hot summer to reduce temperature by wetting the mat periodically.

Internal use :

Nervous system : It gives strength to the brain and nerves. It is useful in unconsciousness vertigo and brain disorders.

Digestive system : It gives strength to the stomach. It reduces gastric secretion and hence is useful in acid-peptic disease. It is a carminative, appetizer, antidipsetic, antiemetic and astringent. It is useful in loss of appetite, indigestion, anorexia, diarrhoea and fever. Fruit of bilva and usheer are given in amoebic dysentery.

Circulatory system : It is a blood purifier because of tikta rasa. It reduces extra water from blood. It is haemostatic and cardioprotective. It is useful in epistaxis. It is used internally as well as externally in diaphoresis.

Respiratory system : It is used in cough, hiccups and bronchial asthma.

Urinary system : It is diuretic due to sheeta property. It is useful in dysuria. Sherbat of khus is given in summer to avoid burning micturation and dysuria.

Skin : It is a deodorant, hence useful in skin disorders.

Temperature : It is antipyretic, tikta rasa is always known to be best antipyretic. It also controls diaphoresis. It is useful in burning, thirst and temperature associated with fever.

Satmikaran : Tika rasa reduces flabbiness of muscles. It gives strength to body organs. Usheer is an antidote and also useful in tuberculosis.

Parts used : Root.

Dosage : Powder - 3 to 6 gms; extract - 10 to 20 cc; cold infusion - 30 to 60 cc; hot infusion - 40 to 80 cc.

Formulations : Usheerasav, Usheeradi kwath, Usheeradi churna, Shadangodak.

Srotogamitva :

Dosha : Reduces kapha and pitta.

Dhatu : Rasa (antipyretic), rakta (in epistaxis), meda (deodorant).

Mala : Sweda (reduces perspiration), purisha (astringent).

References -

'वीरणस्य तु मूलं स्यादुशीरं नलदं च तत् । अमृणालं च सेव्यं च समगन्धकमित्यपि ।।
उशीरं पाचनं शीतं स्तम्भनं लघुतिक्तकम् । मधुरं ज्वरहृद्वान्तिमदजित् कफपित्तनुत् ।।
तृष्णास्त्रविषवीसर्पदाहकृच्छ्रव्रणापहम् ।' (भा.प्र.)
'उशीरं शीतलं रूक्षं स्वादुतिक्तं हिमं लघु । पाचनं स्तम्भनं हन्ति शोषदाहमदज्वरान् ।।
तृष्णास्त्रविषदौर्गन्ध्यकृच्छ्रकुष्ठवमिव्रणान् ।' (कै.नि.)
लामज्जकोशीरं दाहत्वग्दोषस्वेदापनयनप्रलेपनानाम् ।' (च.सू. २५)
'मुस्तपर्पटकोशीरचन्दनोदीच्यानागरैः । शृतशीतं जलं देयं पिपासाज्वरशान्तये ।। (च.चि.३)
'उशीरकालीयकलोध्रपद्मकप्रियंगुकाकटफलशंखगैरिकाः ।
पृथक् पृथक् चन्दनतुल्यभागिकाः सशर्करास्तण्डुलधावनाप्लुताः ।।
रक्तं सपित्तं तमकं पिपासां दाहं च पीताः शमयन्ति सद्यः ।' (च.चि. ४.७३)

Ayurveda not only makes one free of diseases but it also helps one to attain mukti (salvation) from vicious circle of life.

(18) ERAND
Ricinus communis

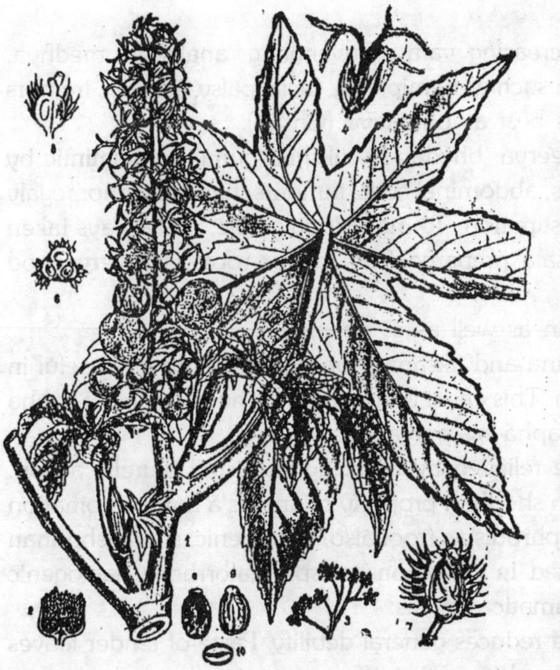

Gana : Bhedniya, Swedopag, Angamardaprashaman, Madhurskandha (C.); Vidarigandhadi, Adhobhagahar, Vatasanshaman (S.)

Kula : Erand kula.

Family : Euphrobiaceae (after the name of Euphorbus, a physician to king Juba).

Latin name : Ricinus - a little tick - resemblance of seeds thereto; communis - common.

English name : Castor plant.

Sanskrit names : **White erand** - Erand, Gandharvahasta, Panchagjul, Vatari, Chitra, **Red erand-** Vyaghra, Hastikarna, Nagakarna, Karaparna, Vyaghrakar.

Botanical Description : Shrub growing 2-3 mts high. Leaves-green or brown, broad, interrupted, pointed like five fingers. Stalk-10-30 cms. long. Flower stalk - thick and branching. Flower - unisexual male flower, 0.75 cms. in circumference, many stamens. Ovary is tricornuated, flat. Fruits - soft spike and bifid. Seeds - elongate, shiny, fleshy, smoky, blackish, bear white streaks and dots. Roots-thick, tapering with secondary and tertiary roots.

Varieties : According to colour (i) White - subtyped as (a) small - roots and oil from seed is used in medicine (b) big or large - leaves are used (ii) Red - oil is used which is more sharp in action. According to longevity : 1. annual and 2. perennial whose fruits and seeds are large and contain more oil.

Chemical composition : Stable oil 45%, slimy substance, sugar, white juice, and salt 10%, seeds contain toxic element called ricin. This dissolves in alcohol. Ricin contains ricin oil, palmitin, sterine. Oil obtained is clean, light, yellowish and without much smell but slightly pungent.

Habitat : All over India, Tamilnadu, Bengal, Maharashtra. It is cultivated at the periphery or border of the fields.

Guna : guru, snigdha, tikshna, sukshma; **Rasa** : madhur, katu, kashaya; **Vipak** : madhur; **Veerya** : ushna; **Prabhav** : purgative.

Karma :

Dosha: It is vatakaphashamak and pittavardhak by its property of ushna veerya. But madhur rasa decreases pitta. Therefore it is used in vatakapha diseases. In paittik condition, it is used as purgative.

External uses : It alleviates vata, swelling and pain, therefore it is used in conditions like backache, sciatica, chest pain, cardiac pain, rheumatic pain, neuralgia, kushtha, uraemia, mastitis, flatulence,

To practice Ayurveda, it is not enough to have knowledge of only Ayurveda. One should be aware of different allied sciences too.

laryngitis. Warm leaves or oil is locally applied. Carbon particles prepared by castor oil flame mixed with cow ghee and camphor is used to cure conjunctivitis. Foreign bodies are removed by this oil drop. Massaging is done by applying oil to gymnastic bar.

Internal uses :

Nervous system : Due to its properties of decreasing vata, rejuvenating, analgesic, medhya, relieving bodyache it is used in diseases due to vata such as hemiplegia, facial palsy, sciatica, tremors as well as headache and bodyache. Castor oil is best as purgative (Ch.Su).

Digestive system : It is deepan being ushna veerya, bhedan by tikshna guna, anthelmintic by its property of snigdha. Therefore it is used in ascites, abdominal colic, tumours, hepatosplenomegaly and piles. Oil taken at breakfast cures chronic constipation. To make it palatable, it is always taken by preparing emulsion with hot tea. Black masala prepared from castor roots is a very good carminative.

Circulatory system : It is useful in cardiac pain as well as in oedema.

Respiratory system : It is kaphaghna by its ushna and tikshna property, therefore it is useful in bronchitis and asthma with predominance of kapha. This effect is attributed to the presence of kapha in stomach while castor oil effectively removes kapha by purgation.

Urinary system : Dysuria and bladder pain are relieved by reducing pain and diuretic action.

Reproductive system : Aphrodisiac together with shodhan property of drug is a rare combination which is found in castor oil. It is madhur, snigdha, aphrodisiac (root also), lactogenic, shukrashodhan (tikshna) and uterine shodhan. Therefore it is used in conditions of spermatorrhoea, lactogenic disorders and vaginal disorders. It is best in rheumatic arthritis.

Satmikaran : Balya and antiageing, antidote and reduces general debility. Paste of tender leaves prepared in water is given in snakebite. Its emetic and purgative effect removes the snake poison from the body. (Paste is locally applied at the site of snake bite). This action can also be seen in aconite and opium poisioning. Juice of castor leaves is given in jaundice where bile is drained into the intestine.

Skin : In skin diseases it is given for shodhan.

Temperature : When kapha pitta doshas are in the lower part of intestine (or colon), purgative property of castor oil helps to relieve the fever.

Rasadhatu : Castor oil is excreted through breast milk in lactating women. Castor oil massage and castor leaves applied locally act as galactagogue. It reduces excessive thirst and acts as an appetiser.

Parts used : Root, leaves, seed and oil (best castor oil is prepared in France and Italy).

Doses : Root paste - 3-6 gms; leaf paste 10-20 gms; seeds - 2 to 6; oil - 20-50 cc. (according to the patient's intestinal response. Risin may lead to death.)

Formulations : Erandipak, Erandmuladi kadha, Erand-Saptak-kashaya.

Srotogamitva :

Dosha : Vata-kapha-pitta.

Dhatu : Shukra root (aphrodisiac), rasa (beneficial to skin), rakta (complexion), raktaprakopan, vayasthapan (rasayan), majja (promotes intellect), hepatosplemomegaly, lactogenic.

In Rajayakshma, mansa, strength and agni should be protected. All malas which depend on mansa should also be protected.

Mala : Oil-purisha (purgative), shodhan and helminthiasis.
Organ : Lower half of body (bladder pain, headache), joints (amavata).
References -
'एरण्डमूलं वृष्यवातहराणाम् ।' (च.)
'लघुभिन्नशकृत्तिक्तं लांगलक्युरुबूकयो: (शाकम्) ।' (च.)
'एरण्डतैलं मधुरमुष्णं तीक्ष्णं कटुकषायानुरसं सूक्ष्मं स्त्रोतोविशोधनं त्वच्यं वृष्यं मधुरविपाकं वय:स्थापनं योनिशुक्रविशोधनमारोग्यमेधाकान्तिस्मृतिबलकरं वातकफहरमधोभागदोषहरं च ।(सू.सू. ४६)
आमवातरूपीं गजेंद्राला एरंडेल हे सिंहाप्रमाणे मारक आहे.

(19) ELA
Elettaria cardemomum Maton.

Gana : Katukaskandha, Shwasahara, Angamarda, Shirovirechan (C.); Eladi (S.)

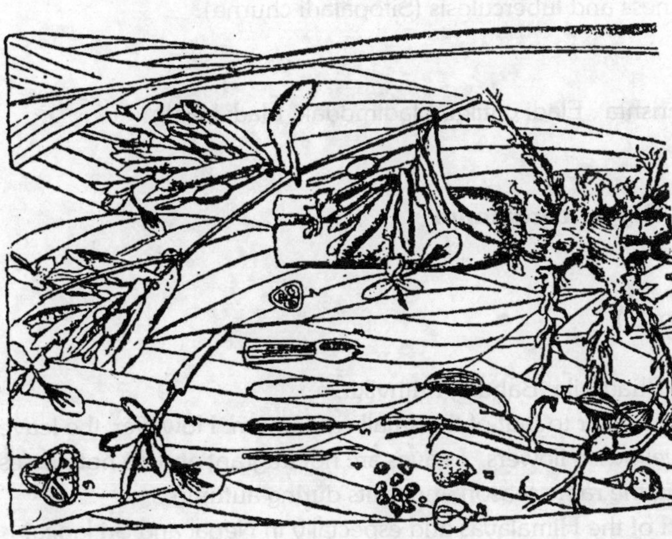

Kula : Haridra kula.

Family : Scitaminaceae (often used as spices).

Latin name : Elettaria = Elacetar - derived from Malyalam; cardamomum - kardamon - amomon cress = pungent (due to pungency of seeds); amomum - A= without; momos = impurity; amomus = without impurity (The plants belonging to this family are narrow, stiff and tapering from a broad base to a fine point.)

English name : Malabar cardmum.

Sanskrit names : Chandrabhaga, Ela, Bahulgandha, Nishkuti, Gandhaphalika, Bahula, Dravidodbhava, Korangi, Triputi.

Small Cardamum

Botanical Description : Trunk - root stalk woody or fleshy and branching. Leaves - subsessile, 20 - 40 cms. long 2.5 to 5 cms. broad and fragrant. Flowers - are many, have long stalks. Fruits - are many; within the fruits there are several black seeds with pungent odour.

Varieties : There are several varieties. 1) Madhara - (those which are ready in Feb -March); 2) Kanti - (those which are ready in Oct- Nov); 3) Neel - black and long variety.

Habitat : Gujarat, Mysore, Coorg, Kerala, Srilanka and Brahmadesh.

Chemical Composition : Seeds contain 10% stable oil, 5% volatile oil, 3% potchlor, 3% starch, Mucin 2%, yellow colouring matter and bhasma 6 - 10%. This bhasma contains manganese.

Mansa dhatu continuously replenishes malas to be excreted through many channels of the body.

Properties :
Guna : laghu, ruksha; **Rasa :** katu, madhur; **Vipak :** madhur; **Veerya :** sheeta.
Karma : Tridoshahara. Kaphanashak (due to laghu, ruksha and katu), vata nashak (due to madhur vipak), pitta nashak (due to sheeta veerya).
External uses : The oil of cardamum seeds is useful in the treatment of toothache.
Internal uses :
Digestive system : It is a mouth freshener, deodorant and antidipsetic. Seeds and oil are appetizer, digestive and laxative. A whole cardamum burnt in charcoal is a good carminative. It is useful in oral disorders, abdominal pain and piles . Antiemetic [but Vagbhatta includes it in emetic class].
Circulatory system : Useful in general weakness.
Respiratory system : Because of its expectorant property, it is used in cough, asthma and other respiratory disorders. It ameliorates dyspnoeic attack in pertusis.
Urinary system : Seeds are diuertic, useful in dysuria.
Temperature : Useful in burning sensation.
Satmikaran : Useful in general weakness and tuberculosis (Sitopaladi churna).
Parts used : Fruits (cardamum).
Dosages : 0.5 to 1 gm.
Formulations : Eladi churna, Eladyarishta , Eladi gutika, Eladimodak, Eladi kwath.

Bigger cardamum

Kula : Haridra kula.
Family : Scitaminaceae.
Latin name: Amomum subulatum (Roxb.)
English name : Bigger cardamum.
Sanskrit names : Bruhadela, Sthula, Bhadraila, Bahula, Prithvika.
Botanical Description : The trunk is similar to that of the small cardamum. However, the leaves are larger - subsessile and oblong with yellowish flowers. Leaves are not fragrant and do not possess a distinct odour. Flowers blossom during the rainy season and fruits during autumn.
Habitat : It is found in the eastern part of the Himalayas and especially in Nepal and Sri lanka.
Chemical composition : The seeds have essential oil and abundant amount of cyaniol.
Properties :
Guna : laghu , ruksha; **Rasa :** katu, tikta; **Vipak :** katu; **Veerya :** ushna.
Karma :
Dosha : Tridoshashamak, so used in diseases due to tridosha.
External uses : Deodorant, analgesic, cures skin diseases and has wound healing property. The decoction is used for gargling in oral and ear disorders. Application of paste relieves headache and pruritic disorders.
Internal uses :
Nervous system : Useful in painful vata disorders.
Digestive system : Being appetizer, digestive, cholagogue and carminative, it is used in anorexia,

nausea, vomiting, thirst, loss of appetite, colic, liver disorders and piles.
Circulatory system : Cardiotonic, hence used in cardiac debility.
Respiratory system : Expectorant, hence useful in cough and asthma.
Urinary system : Useful in dysuria, as it is a diuretic.
Skin : Used in skin disorders.
Temperature : Febrifuge and refrigerant.
Satmikaran : Useful in weakness and poisoning.
Parts use : Fruits.
Dosages : 0.5 to 1 gm.
Srotogamitva :
Dosha : Tridosha.
Dhatu : Raktagami.
Mala : Mutra (dysuria).
Organs : Head, urinary bladder and heart.
References -
स्थूला च कटुका पाके रसे चानलकृल्लघुः । रूक्षोष्णा श्ले,मपित्तास्रकण्डूश्वासतृषापहा ।।
हृल्लासविषबस्त्यास्यशिरोरुग्वमिकासनुत् ।' (भा.प्र.)
भद्रैला कटुका पाके रसे पित्ताग्निकृल्लघुः । रूक्षोष्णा रोचनी श्वासकासवातास्रपित्तहा ।।
हन्ति हृल्लासतृटकण्डूशिरोबस्त्यास्यरुग्वमीः ।' (कै.नि.)
'रसे तु कटुका शीता लघ्वी वातहरी मता । एला सूक्ष्मा कफश्वासकासार्शोमूत्रकृच्छ्रहृत् ।।' (भा.प्र.)
'सूक्ष्मैला मूत्रकृच्छ्रघ्नी श्वासकासक्षये हिता । सूक्ष्मैला शीतला स्वाद्वी हृद्या रोचनदीपनी ।।' (ध.नि.)
'सूक्ष्मैला मूत्रकृच्छ्रार्शः श्वासकासक्षये हिता ।' (शो.)
'सूक्ष्मैलामागधीमूलं प्रलीढं सर्पिषा सह । नाशयत्याशु हृद्रोगं गुल्मानपि विशेषतः ।।'

(20) KATUKA

Picrorrhiza kurroa Royle ex Benth.

Gana : Bhedaniya, Lekhaniya, Stanyashodhan, Tiktaskandha (C.) Patoladi, Pippalyadi , Mustadi (S.)
Kula : Tikta kula.
Family : Scrophulariceae (fig wort family) like scrophula (latin scurfy).
Latin name : Picrorrhiza - palmented root (?)
English name : Hellebore.
Sanskrit names : Katuka, Tikta, Katurohini, Chakrangi, Matsyapitta, Shataparva, Krushnabheda, Krushna, Aamghni, Viprangi, Mahaushadhi.
Botanical Description : Roots are like raddish. Trunk hard. Leaves serrated, 5-10 cm. long with rounded tip. Flowers stalk - hard, pointing upwards and with flowers in cluster or bunches. Root - of a finger's thickness, 15-25 cm. long.
Commercial kutaki is available in the form of 2.5 to 5 cm. long pieces with reddish brown colour, having thin covering and circular markings inside. It breaks easily with black colour inside. Summer is the flowering and fruiting season.

Charaka samhita has described a list of foods which are to be eaten daily, some that have to be eaten sometimes and some food items which are never to be eaten (Charaka Sutra 5/9 12).

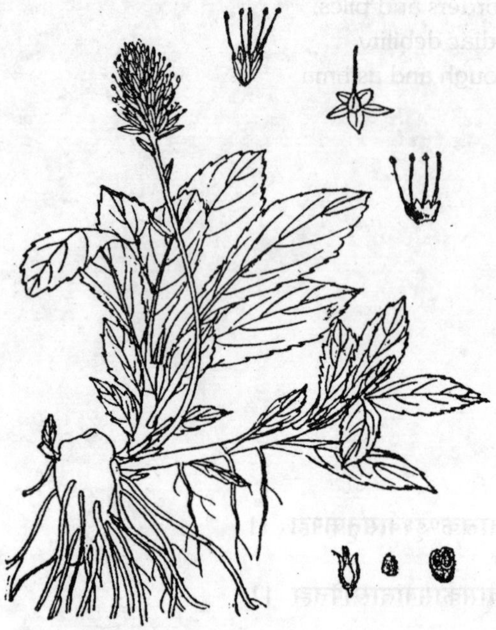

Habitat : Grows in the Himalayas from Kashmir to Sikkim at the height of 2 to 4 thousand mtrs.

Chemical composition : Roots contain picrorrhizin (a bitter ingredient) 15%, cathartic acid 9%, also glucose, wax etc.

Properties :

Guna : ruksha, laghu; **Rasa :** tikta; . **Vipak :** katu; **Veerya :** sheeta.

Karma :

Dosha : Kaphapittashodhak so useful in kaphapittaj diseases.

Internal uses :

Digestive system : Bitter to taste, if given in small dose it stimulates taste buds and increases appetite, liver stimulant and cholagogue. In excess amount acts as a purgative. It is also anthelmintic. In small doses it is useful in conditions like loss of appetite, liver disorders and jaundice which are due to obstruction in biliary passages. In constipation, flatulence and ascites, it acts as a purgative if given in large dose.

When given in congestive cardiac failure it causes a watery diarrhoea. This reduces the circulatory hydrostatic pressure on the heart and thereby the workload on it. It is an appetizer, purgative and vermifuge and hence is useful in abdominal diseases.

Circulatory system : It is pittavahasrotogami and raktavahasrotogami. It reduces heart rate and palpitations. It increases the heart strength and blood pressure. By purifying blood it reduces inflammation. It reduces pulse rate which is similar to the action of digitalis. In heart disease kutaki and glycyrrhiza in equal quality with sugar, is prescribed. It is used in jaundice and anaemia.

Respiratory system : As it acts on the rakta dhatu, it reduces pulmonary disorders. Being an expectorant, it alleviates cough and dyspnoea.

Urinary system : It acts as a diuretic in diabetes.

Skin : It reduces burning and pruritus induced by improper secretion and excretion of bile. It reduces kapha and pitta dosha in blood. It is used in many skin disorders.

Temperature : Useful in fever, pittashodhan and increases flow of bile, reduces burning in fever. Rigors in malarial fever are suppressed with kutaki shodhan in 3 gm. dose.

Adulteration : Bitter plants and sometimes roots of coconut are used.

Satmikaran : Rasayani in small dose, acts as scraping (lekhan) in large dose. It is a boon to physician by this dual action.

Parts used : Root.

Doses : 0.75 to 1 gm. (minimum) 3 to 6 gm. (purgative and chronic fever).

Formulations : Arogyavardhani (50% kutaki), Katukadyavaleha, Tiktadiquath, Tiktadighrut.

Charaka and many other rishis used to perform Agnihotra which conserved external agni but besides this, they also used to conserve sharir agni as well as agni of the mind.

Srotogamitva :
Dosha : Kaphapitta.
Dhatu : Rasa (fever), rakta (skin disorders), meda (meha), raktadahaghna (acts on liver and spleen).
Mala : Purisha (cathartic), anthelmintic and appetizer.
Organ : Heart.
Respiratory tract : Asthma, cough. (It removes bitterness of mouth though it is bitter itself. This is attributed to its action on pitta).
References -
'कटवी तु कटुका तिक्ता कृष्णभेदा कटंभरा । अशोका मत्स्यशकला चक्रांगी शकुलादनी ।।
मत्स्यपित्ता काण्डरुहा रोहिणी कटुरोहिणी । कटुका कटुका पाके तिक्ता रुक्षा हिमा लघुः ।।
भेदनी दीपनी हृद्या कफपित्तज्वरापहा । प्रमेहश्वासकासास्रदाहकुष्ठकृमिप्रणुत् ।।' (भा.प्र.)
'कटुका पित्तजित्तिक्ता कटुः शीतास्रदाहजित् ।
बलासारोचकान् हन्ति विषमज्वरनाशिनी ।।' (ध.नि.)
'मम द्वयं विस्मयमातनोति तिक्ताकषायो मुखतिक्तताघ्नः ।' (वै.जी.) (हा विशेष आहे.)

(21) KANTAKARI
Solanum xanthocarpum

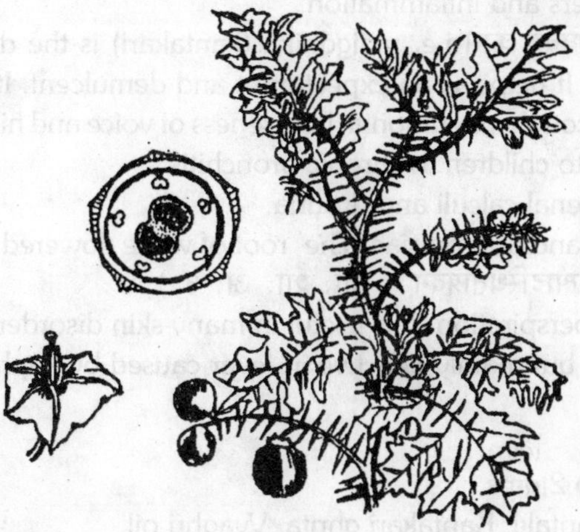

Gana : Kasahara, Kanthya, Hikkanigrahana, Shothahara, Sheetapittaprashaman, Angmardaprashaman (C.), Brihatyadi, Varunadi, Laghupanchamool (S.)
Kula : Kantakri kula.
Family : Solanaceae (night shade).
Latin name : Solanum (night shade); xantho - carpum (xantho = yellow, carpum = fruit).
English name : Wild egg plant.
Sanskrit name : Kantakari, Dusparsha, Vyaghri, Nidigdhika, Bahukanta, Kantalika, Dhavani, Bahugudakuli, Vartaki, Sprushi, Rashtriki.
Botanical Description : It is a thorny shrub of almost 0.75 to 1.25 metres height and glossy green in colour. The leaves are 10 to 13 cm. long and 5-7 cm. wide. They have thorns on the dorsal aspect. Flowers-blue coloured. Fruits -round, small and thorny. They are green with white streaks when raw and turn yellow (xantho) on ripening. The flowering season is summer.
Varieties : There are 2 varities, one with blue flowers and other with white. The blue flowered plant is available freely whereas white one is rare. The white flowered 'ringni' is used as laxmana. The flowers and plant itself being white in colour, it has been named as chandrapushpa, durlabha, shwetalaxmana.

It should be constantly born in mind that human body and mind can become slaves of habits.

Habitat : Bengal, Assam, Punjab, Southern India.
Chemical composition : It contains an alkaloid 'solenin', potassium chloride, potassium nitrate, iron and organic acids. Fruit contains solenocarpin.
Properties :
Guna : laghu, ruksha; **Rasa :** tikta, katu; **Vipak :** katu; **Veerya :** ushna.
Karma :
Dosha : Kaphavatashamak due to ushna veerya.
External use : It is analgesic, antiinflammatory and has antibacterial properties. Therefore its fumes are inhaled in dental caries, dental pain and piles. (It is said that this type of fumigation with kantakari destroys the bacteria in teeth).
Internal use :
Nervous system : It is used a neurological disorders like epilepsy and convulsions as a stimulant due to its irritant property. The juice droplets are put in nose, which helps in stimulating nerves (Sangnya prabodhana). It pacifies vata due to ushna guna. Its local application helps in bodyache and arthritis.
Digestive system : Being katu, tikta and ushna, it can be used as an appetizer and carminative. Its irritant nature helps in purgation and in dewormification. It is used in loss of appetite, constipation and helminthiasis. Fumes and powder of seeds is used in dental aches.
Circulatory system : It is cardio-stimulant, blood purifier and anti-inflammatory. Therefore is used in cardiac disorders, skin disorders, blood disorders and inflammation.
Respiratory system : As the sutra goes- निदिग्घिका कासे i.e. nidigdhika (kantakari) is the drug of choice on cough. It helps in vataj type of cough. It helps as an expectorant and demulcent. It stops hiccups and also helps in asthma, chronic rhinitis, cough, pneumonia, hoarseness of voice and hiccups. Powdered S. xanthocarpum with honey is given to children in chronic bronchitis.
Urinary system : Its diuretic property helps in renal calculi and dysuria.
Reproductive system : The seeds are oxytosic and aphrodisiac. The root of white flowered ringni is used in punsavan vidhi (पयसा लक्ष्मणामूलं पुत्रोत्पादस्थितीप्रदम । (वा. शा. अ. १)
Skin : Being ushna (hot) in nature, it increases perspiration. It is useful in many skin disorders.
Temperature : Febriguge because of bitterness, but mainly effective in fever caused by kapha and vata.
Parts used : Panchang (whole plant).
Dosages : Decoction- 60-100 ml.; powder - 1 to 2 gms.
Formulations : Nidigdhikadi kadha, Vyaghri haritaki, Kantakari ghrita, Vyaghri oil.
S. xanthocarpum is one of the constituents of laghu panchamool and dashamool. The plants in laghupanchmool are small. This plant is included is dashmool, which is a class of antipyretic and anti-inflammatory plants. This itself shows the importance of the plant.
Srotogamitva :
Dosha : Pittavardhak, reduces kapha and vata.
Dhatu : Shukra (fruit increases mobility of sperms and ejaculation), meda (hara), garbha karini.
Mala : Purisha (purgative), bhedan (in renal calculi and dysuria), diaphoretic.
Organs : Lungs (cough, whooping cough).

A vaidya should have memory, knowledge of causes of diseases, experiential knowledge, self control and courage to face any emergency that may occur.

References -

'कण्टकारी सरा तिक्ता कटुका दीपनी लघुः । रुक्षोष्णा पाचनी कासश्वासज्वरकफानिलान् ।।
निहन्ति पीनसं पार्श्वपीडाकृमिहृदामयान् । तस्याः फलं कटु रसे पाके च कटुकं भवेत् ।।
शुक्रस्य रेचनं भेदि तिक्तं पित्ताग्निकृल्लघु । हन्यात् कफमरुत्कण्डूकासमेदः कृमिज्वरान् ।।
तद्वत् प्रोक्ता सिता क्षुद्रा विशेषाद् गर्भकारिणी ।' (भा.प्र.) (पांढरी रिंगणी लक्ष्मणा)
'कण्टकारीरसे सिद्धो मुदगयूषः सुसंस्कृतः । सगौरामलकः साम्लः सर्वकासभिषग्जितम् ।।' (च.चि. २२)
'सम्यग् विपक्वं द्विगुणेन सर्पिर्निदिग्धिकायाः स्वरसेन
चैतत् ।
श्वासाग्निसादस्वरभेदभिन्नान् निहन्त्युदीर्णानपि पञ्चकासान् ।' (सु.)
'व्याघ्रीकुसुमसंजातकेसरैरवलेहिकाम् । जगध्वापि चिरतो जातं शिशोः कासं व्यपोहति ।। (वंसगेन)
'निदिग्धिकाञ्चामलकप्रमाणां हिंग्वर्धयुक्तां मधुना सुयुक्ताम् ।
लिहेन्नरः श्वासनिपीडितो हि श्वासं जयत्येव बलात् त्र्यहेण ।।' (सु.उ.५१)
'...बृहतीद्वयञ्च । आलोड्य दध्ना मधुरेण पेयं दिनानि सप्ताश्मरिभेदनाय ।।' (च.चि. २६)
'निदिग्धिकारसो वापि सक्षौद्रः कृच्छ्रनाशनः ।।' (शोढल.)
निदिग्धिका कासे । (वा.उ.)

(22) KAPIKACHHU

Mucuna pruriens Bak.

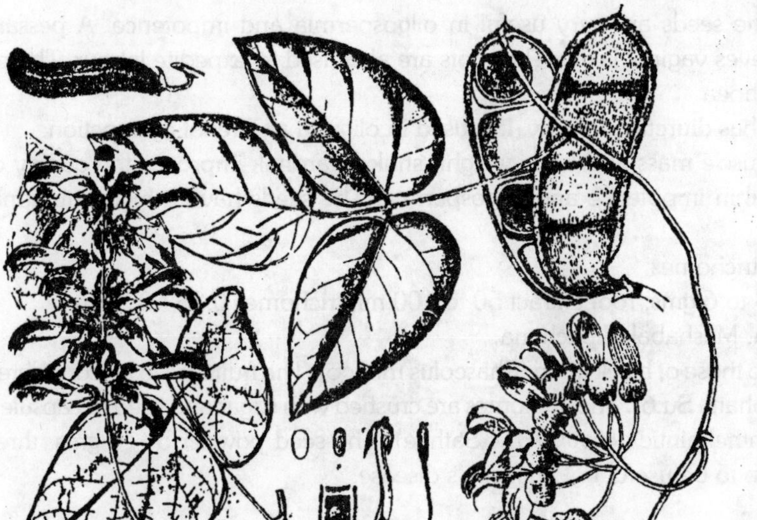

Gana : Balya, Madhurskandha (C.); Vidarigandhadi, Vatashaman (S.)
Kula : Shimbi kula.
Family : Leguminosae (Legumine = pulse).
Latin name : Mucuna - as called in Brazil; pruriens = prurita - producing itching or irritable sensation when touched.
English name : Cowhage plant.
Sanskrit names : Atmagupta (well protected because of the pruritic trichome of the legume), Kapikachhu (one starts itching like a monkey - Kapi), Markati (hair covering like monkeys), Pravrushayana (grows in the rainy season), Kandura, Swayamgupta, Durabhigraha, Tikshna, Romalu, Visharoma, Romavalli.

Botanical Description : It is a creeper. Leaves - are 7 to 13 cms. long, trifoliate and with fine hairs

A surgeon should have the vision of an eagle, heart of a lion and delicate fingers like a lady to achieve surgical skills.

on the surface. Flowers- the stalk of the flower is bent, 15-30 cms. long. There are 2.5 to 4 cms. long purple, eggplant- coloured violet flowers on the stalk. Fruits - these legumes are 5 - 7 cms long, slightly curved (like tamarind), with abundant trichomes on the surface. These hairs, on touch, cause intense itching, burning and erythematous swelling of the skin. Each legume has 5 to 6 flat, black-yellow or white seeds with black opening. The creeper grows during monsoon. Flowering stage is from November to January, followed by fruiting. The tender legumes are eaten as vegetables and pickles.
Habitat : All over India. More in the tropical regions.
Chemical composition : The seed contains L-dopa, proteins, oil and a trace of manganese. The trichomes contain 5 - HT and an enzyme - protease - mucunain. Several alkaloids have been isolated.
Properties :
Guna : guru, snigdha; **Rasa :** madhaur , tikta; **Vipak :** madhur; **Veerya :** ushna.
Karma : Tridosha shamak - useful in diseases caused by tridosha.
Internal uses :
Nervous system : The roots and seeds are tonic for the neurons. The root is useful in hemiparesis and facial palsy. The seed - powder is useful in Parkinson's disease.
Digestive system : The trichomes on the legumes are anthelmintic for roundworm. Trichomes 0.25 - 0.5 gm. are given mixed with butter, jaggery or honey. Next day a laxative is given. The round worms are killed and expelled out.
Reproductive system : The seeds are very useful in oilgospermia and impotence. A pessary soaked in the root extract relieves vaginal laxity. The roots are also used to expedite labour. The oil from seeds is useful in leucorrhoea.
Urinary System : The root has diuretic property. It is used in oliguria and renal dysfunction.
Satmikaran : It promotes muscle mass and body-weight; shukrawardhak-improves the quality of semen. Hence it is very useful in impotence and oligospermia. The seeds have a high nutritional property.
Parts used : Seed, root and trichomes.
Dosage : The seed powder 3 to 6 gms; root extract 50 to 100 ml; trichomes 0.25 - 0.5 gm.
Formulations : Vanarigutika, Mashabaladipachana.
Seeds have properties similar to those of black gram (Phaseolus mungo). The fruits are to be considered equivalent to black gram (Vagbhatta Su.6). The trichomes are crushed with sugar and filled in capsules. It has been shown to have anthelmintic activity (B.V. Sathye). The seed powder 5- 10 gms. three times in a day has been shown to be useful in Parkinson's disease.
Srotogamitva :
Dosha : Tridoshasrotogami.
Dhatu : Shukra (aphrodisiac), mansa - meda (brimhana), raktagami.
Mala : Purisha (sara).
Beeja : Vatashaman.
Dosha: Vatashaman.
Dhatu : Shukra (an aphrodisiac, promoting ejaculation).
Its guna karma are like black gram.

A surgeon who is brave, acts promptly, employs sharp instruments and has no sweat or tremors, will be very successful.

References -

'कपि कच्छुर्भृशं वृष्या मधुरा बृंहणी गुरुः । तिक्ता वातहरी बल्या कफपित्तास्त्रनाशिनी ।।
तद्बीजं वातशमनं स्मृतं वाजीकरं परम् ।' (भा.प्र.)
'कपिकच्छुभवं मूलं क्वाथयेत् विधिना भिषक् । योनिः संकीर्णतां याति क्वाथेनानेन धारयेत् ।। (भा.प्र.)

(23) KARKATASHRINGI

Rhus succedania Linn.

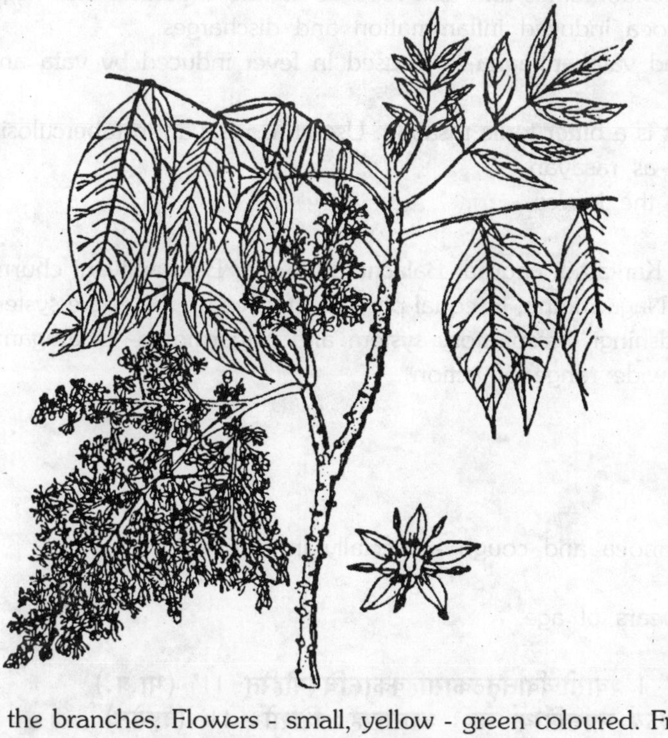

Guna : Kasahar, Hikkanigrahan (C.); Kakolyadi (S.)
Kula : Amra kula.
Family : Anacardiaceae (Anacardium = cashew nut).
Latin name : Rhous - name of the plant used by Theophretus; succedania - used as a substitute.
Sanskrit names : Shrungi, Kuleershrungi, Ghosha, Chandra, Kalinga, Vakra, Vanajamardhaja, Kulira, Karkata, Karkataki, Ajashrungi, Arthachampika.
Botanical Description : The tree is known as kakkar in Hindi. (Kakad and kakkar are synonyms). It is 8 to 10 mtrs. high. Bark - grey in colour. Leaflets - 5 to 13 cm. long and 2.5 to 7 c.m. broad. Leaves - are 15 to 20 cm. long and arising from the tip of the branches. Flowers - small, yellow - green coloured. Fruit - is small, flat and thin. Flowering occurs in January-February followed by fruiting in March.
Typical type of worms make horn shaped cocoons on the branches and leaves. These cocoons are called as kakadshingi. They make these cocoons by sucking juice from the leaves. Kakadshingi is 1 to 3 cm. long, 1 to 2 cm. narrow, grey in colour, hollow, light and soft.
Habitat : Himalyan slopes, Kumaon, Nepal, Assam, Bengal.
Chemical composition : It has 60% tanin and 1.21% volatile oil. (Fresh hirda, maiphal also has tannins in large quantities.)
Karma :
Dosha : Ushnaveerya, so kaphavatanashak and therefore useful in kaphavataj disorders.
External use : It is applied on swelling (edema). In pyorrhoea, gargles of decoction is useful. Powder is applied on both fresh and chronic wounds.

In the commentary on the 33rd shloka of chapter 2 of Charaka samhita, a condition called "raudhirmada" is described. Is it caused due to hypertesion?

Internal use :

Digestive system : Being ushna, it is an appetizer, carminative and astringent in nature, thus useful and effective in anorexia, dipsia and diarrhoea, dysentry. Mainly effective in children's diseases.

Respiratory system : Because of its bitter and pungent taste it is an expectorant and kaphaghna. Helps in hiccoughs, cough and dyspnoea. It acts as an expectorant and prevents, further productive cough and strengthens the respiratory membrane (inner lining of the surface). It is also effective in pharyngitis and sore throat.

Reproductive system : It alleviates endometritis and also reduces uterine exudates; thus helps in healing. It also alleviates gonorrhoea induced inflammation and discharges.

Temperature : Being a febrifuge and vatakaphagna, it is used in fever induced by vata and kapha.

Satmikaran : Being bitter and hot, it is a bitter tonic rasayan. Useful as rasayan in tuberculosis. In Kashmir, the fruits are also used as rasayan.

Parts used : Hornlike cocoons on the leaves.

Dosage : 0.75 gm to 1.5 gms.

Formulations : Shrungyadi churna, Karkatadi churna, Balachaturbhadra, Balasanjivani churna (Mixture of Ativisha, Kakadshingi and Nagarmotha, in equal parts is effective on the entire system of the child. Ativisha-digestive, Kakadshingi - respiratory system and Nagarmotha- Dhatugami. Therefore Balasanjivani churna has wide range of action).

Srotogamitva :

Dosha : Kaphaghna, vatashamak.

Dhatu : Rasayani - rasa (fever).

Mala : Purisha - constipative.

Srotas : Respiratory system - (dyspnoea and cough - specially in children).
Uterus (endometrium).
Age - children upto 3-4 years of age.

References -

'शृंगी कषाया तिक्तोष्णा कफवातक्षयज्वरान् । श्वासोर्ध्ववाततृटकासहिक्कारुचिवमीहरेत् ।।' (भा.प्र.)

'कुलीरशृङ्गचूर्णञ्च मूलकस्य फलं तथा । युक्तोऽयं मधुसर्पिभ्यां लेहः श्वासापहः शिशोः ।।' (वङ्गसेन)

(24) KARPOOR
Cinamomum camphora

Kula : Karpoor kula.

Family : Lauraceae (Lauraceae cherry, with laurelike leaves).

Latin name : Cinamomum = from Arabic name kinamon; camphora = from Arabic name kufur and karpoor.

English name : Camphor.

Sanskrit names : Ghanasar, Shashank, Chandra, Himavaluka, Shila, Gaur, Tushar, Mihika,

Strength of the srotas of various body constituents is the investment of a doctor. He who forgets these will never be successful.

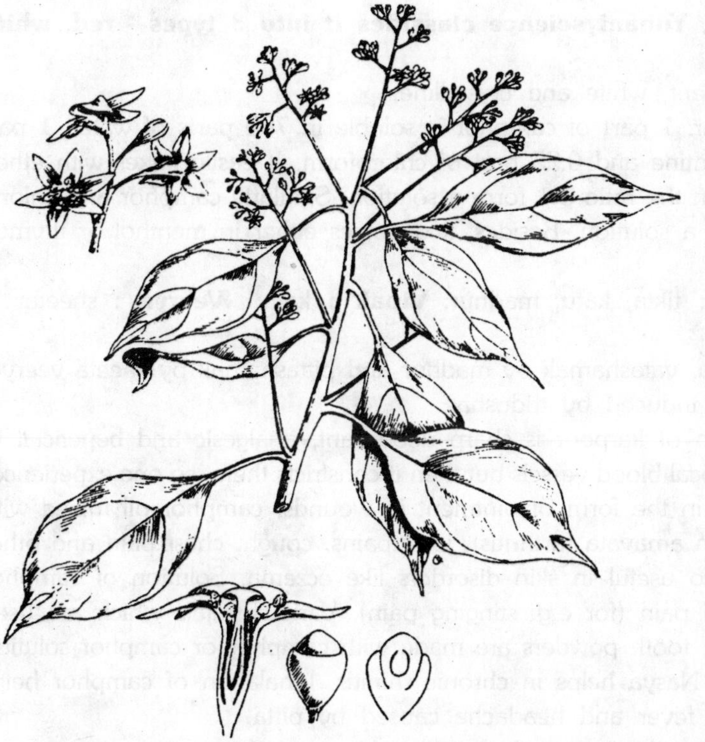

Sphatik, Sphatikopam, Bhasma, Tarusar, Chandrabhasma.

Botanical Description : Tree is 12 to 13 mtrs. high, ever green. Bark - externally rough and internally slimy. Leaves - resemble cinamon leaves. Flowers - green, yellow. Fruits - grow in bunches like beans. Tree smells like camphor. Flowering season is spring and fruiting occurs in premonsoon season. 4 to 5 kg. camphor is obtained from one tree.

Varities : Depeding on the country of origin, production and colour, it is of various types.

Depending on the country, it is of 3 types -

1) Bhimseni - It is known as Borneo or Sumatra camphor, as it is widely available in these islands. The tree belongs to Dipterocarpae family. Its latin name is Dryobalanops aromatica. This tree grows very high and if the bark is cut, latex comes out and forms camphor. The oil derived from it is camphor oil.

2) Japanese - Also known as Chini camphor. It is Cinamomum camphora in Latin which is described here.

3) Indian - Found in Dehradun, Calcutta, Nilgiri. The tree resembles tulsi tree and has a strong odour to the leaves. It is called as 'kapoor tulsi'. It belongs to labiatae family and is called Ocimum kilimands charicum in Latin.

(2) Nighantukars have described 2 types of camphors - Pakwa and other apakwa.

Pakwa - means artificially prepared, procedure of which is as follows : root, bark and branches are cut into small pieces. Keep them in the container having (little) water. Cover the container with a cloth and sieve the above through the cloth so that water and the root, bark and branches will not come in direct contact. By this process camphor gets collected in the lid. Take it out and purify by evaporation. This is an artificial camphor. It is clear and crystalline. It has strong odour. Specific gravity is 0.995. (It floats in water). It gets burnt by heat and gets evapourated.

Natural camphor does not require above method. It sinks in water. Natural camphor is better than artificial one. Now-a-days artificial camphor (synthetic) is prepared by chemical method.

While doing panchakarma or shodhan, one should never forget that these should be done without harming the body.

(3) Depending on the colour, Yunani science classifies it into 3 types - red, white and natural.

Description - it is translucent, white and crystalline.

Odour - typical strong odour. 1 part of camphor is soluble in 700 parts of water, 1 part of alcohol, 1.5 part of terpentine and 0.25 part of chloroform. It easily mixes with ether. Camphor and carbolic acid in the ratio 3:1 form a solution. Similarly camphor and chloral hydrate in same ratio form a solution. Besides, it dissolves either in menthol or thymol.

Properties :

Guna : laghu, tikshna; **Rasa :** tikta, katu, madhur; **Vipak :** katu; **Veerya :** sheeta.

Karma :

Dosha : Kaphanashak by tikta, vatashamak by madhur and pittashamak by sheeta veerya. Thus it is useful in the diseases induced by tridoshas.

External use : Local application of karpoor is sharp deodorant, analgesic and beneficial to the eyes. Initially it stimulates the local blood vessels but then it constricts them, so one experiences a feeling of cold. It can be used in the form of ointment in wounds; camphor oil mixed with various oils is used for massage in amavata (arthritis), joint pains, cough, chest pain and other diseases like pneumonia. It is also useful in skin disorders like eczema. Solution of camphor and pepermint etc. helps in local pain (for e.g. stinging pain). Various kajals which are used in eye disorders contain camphor; tooth powders are made with camphor or camphor solution is used in pyorrhoea, toothache. Nasya helps in chronic rhinitis. Inhalation of camphor helps too. Paste made in milk relieves fever and headache caused by pitta.
Various balms used in headaches contain camphor.

Internal use :

Nervous system : In a low dose it is a brain tonic and an analgesic. When administered it causes an initial excitation but then acts as a sedative, thus relieving convulsions. Camphor is used as a respiratory stimulant. It is also used in impairment of brain function, vata disorders, hysteria and convulsions.

Digestive system : Being fragrant, it relieves bad breath. In the mouth it first feels cold then warm. It increases salivation and improves taste. Also improves appetite and digestion by stimulating digestive glands in the stomach. Being vermicidal, it is used in helmenthiasis. Higher doses cause nausea and vomiting. It is used in various oral disorders. In addition to diarrhoea, colitis, cholera, it is also used in renal diseases.
(Amritadhara - camphor, Asmantara - thymol).

Circulatory system : Cardiac stimulant and protective. It is a vasoconstrictor so it increases the blood pressure. It regularises the heart rate in cardiac arrythmia or bradycardia. It dilates the subcutaneous vessels, so it is used as a cardiac tonic in cardiac hypertrophy and sannipat jwar i. e. fever caused by all the three doshas.

Respiratory system : It increases the blood circulation in the mucus membrane of the respiratory system and is an expectorant; thus it acts as a demulcent.

Urinary system : As it is excreted through urinary tract, it increases the volume of urine. Being a diuretic and antiseptic, camphor is used in dysuria and gonorrhoea.

Shirovirechan, vaman, virechan, asthapan and asravisruti are the five shodhanas. There is a difference between panchakarma and panchashodhan.

Reproductive system : Aphrodisiac in lower dose but higher dose causes the reverse action. It should be given in a lower dose in infertility. Paste is applied on the breast or it is given orally in galactorrhoea.

Skin : It is used in burning of skin and skin diseases. Ointment of camphor and sulphur is used in scabies.

Temperature : Due to its diaphoretic property, it is used either internally or externally in fever. To alleviate thirst induced by fever, camphor is put in drinking water.

Satmikaran : It has a scraping action by laghu and tikshna gunas. It is also an antidote. It is used in lipid disorders and various toxicities either external or internal.

Excretion : Skin, lungs and urinary tract.

Parts used : Exudate.

Dosage : 0.25 to 0.5 gm.

Formulation : Karpoor rasa, Karpoorasav, Amritadhara, Amritabindu, Karpooradivati.

Mode of administration : It is given in milk with sugar, these being the best anupanas of camphor. Excess camphor develops pain in abdomen, nausea, vomiting, giddiness, blindness, convulsions, cyanosis, urine retention, coma and death too. Camphor taken for many days causes weakness and anaemia.

In the toxicity of camphor, emesis, stomach wash and purgation should be given. Then stimulants like kasturi, amber etc. are given.

Srotogamitva :

Dosha : Kaphaghna,pittashamak.

Dhatu : Shukra (aphrodisiac), medoghna, majja (brain tonic).

Mala : Purisha (anthelmintic).

Organs : Eyes.

Antidote.

References -

'पुंसि क्लीबे च कर्पूरो हिमाह्वो हिमबालुकः । घनसारश्चन्द्रसंज्ञो हिमनामापि सः स्मृतः ।।
कर्पूरः शीतलो वृष्यः चक्षुष्यो लेखनो लघुः । सुरभिर्मधुरस्तिक्तः कफपित्तविषापहः ।।
दाहतृष्णास्यवैरस्यमेदोदौर्गन्ध्यनाशनः । कपूरो द्विविधः प्रोक्तः पक्वापक्वप्रभेदतः ।।
पक्वात् कर्पूरतः प्राहुरपक्वं गुणवत्तरम् ।
चीनसंज्ञस्तु कर्पूरः कफक्षयकरः स्मृतः । कुष्ठकण्डूवमिहरस्तथा तिक्तरसश्च सः ।।' (भा.प्र.)
'कर्पूरं कटुतिक्तं च मधुरं शिशिरं विदुः । तृण्मेदोविषदोषघ्नं चक्षुष्यं मदकारकम् ।।' (ध.नि.)
'चीनकः कटुकस्तिक्तो हृद्यः शीतः कफापहः । कण्ठदोषहरो मेध्यः पाचनः कृमिशानः ।।' (रा.नि.)
'धार्याण्यास्येन वैशद्यरुचिसौगन्ध्यमिच्छता ।... कर्पूरनिर्यास... । (च.सू. ५)
'स्वच्छं भृङ्गारपत्रं लघुतरविशदं तोलने तिक्तकं चेत्,
स्वादे शैत्यं सुहृद्यं बहलपरिमलामोदसौरभ्यदायि ।
निःस्नेहं दार्ढ्यपत्रं शुभतरमिति चेद्राजयोग्यं प्रशस्तं,
कर्पूरं चान्यथथा चेदबहुतरमशने स्फोटदायि व्रणाय ।।' (रा.नि.)

In Charaka samhita it is mentioned that only an insane person asks as to (1) how many teeth a crow has? (2) what is the weight of the testis of sheep and (3) donkey has how many hair?

(25) KARANJA
Pongamia glabra Linn.

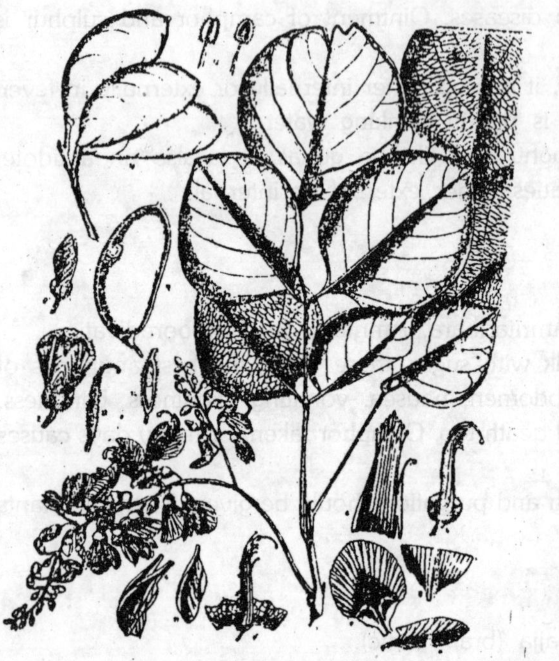

Gana : Kandughna, Virechan, Katuskandha, Tiktaskandha, (C.); Aragwadhadi, Varunadi, Arkadi, Shyamadi, Shirovirechan, Kaphasamshaman. (S.)
Kula : Shimbi kula.
Family : Leguminosae.
Latin name : Pongamia (from Tamil name pungam, from Malayalam name ponnam); glabra (having shiny leaves) smooth, hairless.
English name : Indian beech (Pongamia pinnata - compound leaf with pinnate (leaflet) arranged on either side of the rachis).
Sanskrit names : Karanja, Naktamal (blooming at night), Guchchhapushpa, Ghrutpur (thick oil like ghee comes out from seeds), Snigdhapatra, Prakirya, Chirbilva, Putiparna, Vruddhaphal, Rochan.
Botanical Description : Medium sized tree i. e. 8-16 mts. high. Leaves - slimy, smooth and green in colour. Leaflets - 5-7 in number, 5 to 10 cm. long, having branches and sub-branches. From it 1.25 cm. long, blue flowers arise. Androecium - total 17, tenth one lies in the centre of the flower. Fruit - 4 to 5 cm. long, flat, oval, very hard and concave on the dorsal surface. Seeds - one in each fruit having a length of 1.25 to 4 cm. and containing oil. Flowering is in spring, then fruiting starts.
Varities : Nighantus have described four varities, they are 1) Karanja 2) Putikaranja 3) Chirbilva and 4) Karanji. Tree and organs of karanji are similar but smaller than karanja.
Habitat : Grows by the road side very easily. Found in central and South India, Sri Lanka .
Chemical composition : Seeds contain 27% bitter and dark (sherry) coloured fixed oil (pongamia oil). Bark contains bitter alkaloid, resin, mucilage and sugar.
Properties :
Guna : laghu, tikshna; **Rasa** : tikta, katu, kashaya; **Vipak** : katu; **Veerya** : ushna.
Karma :
Dosha : Kaphavataprashamak by ushna veerya. It is used in diseases induced by kapha and vata.
External use : Bark, leaves and seeds are antiseptic, antipruritic and analgesic. Oil derived from the seeds has antiparasitic, wound healing and analgesic properties. Powder of the seeds

Charaka samhita has 120 chapters i.e. 1) 30 chapters on Sutra 2) 8 on Nidan 3) 8 on Viman 4) 8 on Sharir 5) 12 on Indriya 6) 30 on Chikitsa 7) 12 on Kalpa and 8) 12 on Siddhi.

is used for nasya. Also useful in various skin diseases and wounds. Oil is used for massage in vata disorders. Poultice of leaves removes the bacteria from wounds. Paste of flowers is applied in alopecia. Hot leaves are also used. Paste of leaves is useful in wound healing.

Internal uses :

Digestive system : Being katu and tikta, it improves appetite and digestion. It is purgative, anthelmintic and liver tonic due to ushna and tikshna properties. Leaves and bark are used in loss of appetite, digestive disorders, constipation, helminthiasis, and haemorrhoids. Oil derived from the seeds is given orally in helminthiasis..

Circulatory system : Being bitter, it enhances blood flow and its ushna guna reduces swellings. This effect is also augmented by its action on blood circulation. Effective also in rheumatoid arthritic swelling.

Respiratory system : Being kaphaghna, kasahara, it is used in cough; especially in whooping cough, powdered seeds in water are used. A necklace of the pods are put round the neck in children as a preventive measure for whooping cough.

Urinary system : Useful in urinary disorders as it reduces the quantity of urine by pungent and hot nature. Flowers are used in ikshumeha.

Reproductive system : Its ushna and tikta guna makes it keep the uterus in good condition.

Skin : Kushthaghna, effective in all skin disorders. Karanja oil is the best treatment for fatty ulcers of skin.

Parts used : Bark, leaves, flowers and seeds.

Dosages : Juice of bark or leaves - 6-12 ml; juice of flowers - 6-12 ml; powder of the seeds - 1-3 gm.

Formulations : Karanjadi churna, Karanjadya ghrit, Karanjadi tailam.

Srotogamitva :

Dosha : Kaphaghna, vataghna. **Leaves :** Kapha, vataghna.

Dhatu : Meda, rakta (spleen), pleeha, medogami.

Mala : Purisha.

Internal pathway : Deepan, pachan.

References -

'करञ्जो नक्तमालः स्यान्नक्ताह्लो गुच्छपुष्पकः । घृतपूरः स्निग्धपत्रः प्रकीर्या पुष्पमञ्जरी ।।
करञ्जः कटुकः पाके रसे तिक्तकषायकः । कटुको गुणतस्तीक्ष्णो वीर्योष्णो विनियच्छति ।।
बलासपित्तकुष्ठार्शोमेहोदरव्रणक्रिमीन् । तत्पत्रं कटुकं पाके रसे दीपनपाचनम् ।।
कफवातापहं शाफविषार्शः कृमिकुष्ठजित् ।' (कै.नि.)

'करञ्जः कटुकस्तीक्ष्णो वीर्योष्णो योनिदोषहृत् । कुष्ठोदावर्त्तगुल्मार्शोव्रणक्रिमिकफापहा ।।
तत्पत्रं कफवातार्शः कृमिशोथहरं परम् । भेदनं कटुकं पाके वीर्योष्णं पित्तलं लघु ।।
तत्फलं कफवातघ्नं मेहार्शः कृमिकुष्ठजित् ।' (भा.प्र.)

'करञ्जश्चोष्णतिक्तः स्यात् कफपित्तास्रदोषजित् । व्रणप्लीहकृमीन् हन्ति भूतघ्नो योनिरोगहा ।। (ध.नि.)

'करञ्ज... फलं जन्तुप्रमेहजित् । रूक्षोष्णं कटुकं पाके लघुवातकफापहम् ।। (सु.सू. ४६)

'करञ्ज...तैलानि तीक्ष्णानि लघून्युष्णवीर्याणि कटूनि कटुविपाकानि सराण्यनिलकफकृमि कुष्ठप्रमेहशिरोरोगहराणि च ।' (सु.सू. ४५)

The second chapter of Sutra sthana of Charaka samhita describes internal purification and the third describes external purification.

(26) KARAVEER

Nerium indicum Mill.

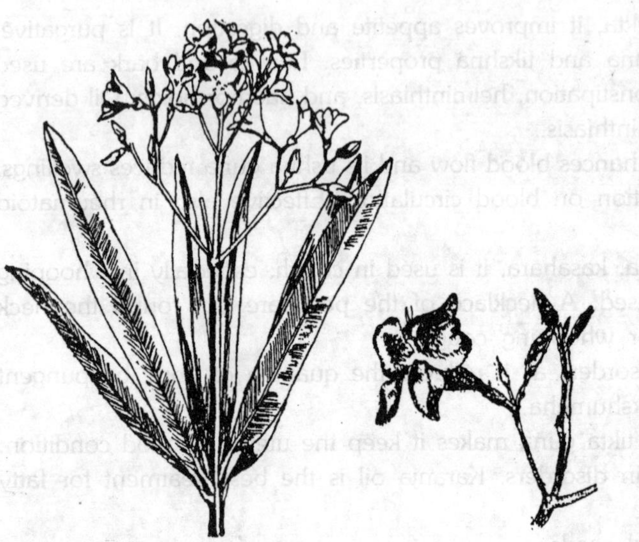

Gana : Tiktaskandha, Kushthaghna (C.); Lakshadi, Shirovirechana dravya (S.)

Kula : Kutaja kula.

Family : Apocyanaceae (harmful to dogs, horses?).

Latine name : Nerium = humid, Neras = moist, grows in moisture; indicum = of India, odorom = sweet smelling.

English name : Rose Berry (Spurge).

Sanskrit name : Attach the word 'maar' to the names of horse in Sanskrit i. e. Hayamaar, Ashwamaar, Vajimaar etc. Mahaveer, Hayaghna, Shatakunda, Ashwarodhak, Ashwaghna, Haripriya, Ashwamohak. Red - Raktaprasav, Bhutahari, Ganeshakusum.

Botanical Description : Tree is usually 3 to 4 mtrs. high. Root and stem produce branches and sub-branches, so that makes the tree thickly trellised one. Leaves - in threes, 10-15 cm long, linear lanceolate and tapering at the end. On scraping the leaves and bark, milky juice comes out. Flowers-fragrant, white, red, yellow and blue. Fruit - round or oval in shape. Flowers come in the premonsoon or monsoon season and fruits come in the winter.

Varieties : They are of four varities depending on the colour of flowers - 1) White 2) Yellow 3) Red and 4) Blue or Black. Blue and black varities are very rare. Fruits of white, red and black Nerium are 11 to 15 cm. long. Yellow Nerium has round or oblong fruits.

Habitat : Afghanistan and India upto 1800 mtrs. Found in gardens.

Chemical composition : It is a poisonous drug. It contains two powerful cardiotoxic principles; of them neriodorin is insoluble in water and other neriodorine is soluble in water. Besides, it also contains glucoside, rosaginine, an essential oil, a crystalline principle like digitalin, nereine, tannic acid and wax. Leaves contain an alkaloid oleandrine, glucoside, pseudoqurarine, nereine and neriantine.

Properties :

Guna : laghu, ruksha, tikshna; **Vipak** : katu; **Rasa** : katu, tikta, kashaya; **Veerya** : ushna.

Karma :

Dosha : Kaphavatashamak, so used in kapha vata disorders.

External use : It cures skin disorders, cleanses and heals wounds and reduces swelling. The

Charaka in the Sutra sthana, has dedicated four chapters each to medicine, health, basic principles, formulations, diseases, treatment planning and diet. Two chapters have been dedicated to prana and oja.

application of root paste is helpful in skin disorders, cancer, ulcers and ringworm infection. Leaf juice is put in the eyes in eye disorders. (Care must be taken as it is a poisonous plant).

Internal use :

Digestive system : Stimulant of appetite and useful in loss of appetite, digestive disorders and constipation.

Circulatory system : In a low dose it provides energy to the heart. But in higher dose, it is lethal to the heart. Nerium is a blood purifier. It is useful in oedema, weakness and dyspnoea induced due to cardiac debility.

Urinary system : It increases the blood flow in the kidneys, thus increasing the urine quantity and flow. It is used in dysuria and stones.

Skin : Diaphoretic and useful in clearing skin infection. It can be used in very chronic skin diseases.

Temperature : Febrifuge, mainly episodic fever. The action of 1 ratti (ie. 120 mg.) of the bark of yellow nerium is same as 15 ratti of the bark of Cinchona. In malaria, after the temperature comes to normal, only 1/2 ratti kanher ghan satva helps by preventing the reccurence of fever. But it should not be given on an empty stomach.

Satmikaran : It is a powerful poison, this should be kept in mind.

Higher dose : Causes toxicity, feeble pulse, cardiac arrest, respiratory arrest and then leads to death.

Antidote : After stomach wash, cow's ghee should be given.

Parts used : Roots, bark of the root.

Dosage : 1/8 to 1 ratti.

Formulation : Karveeradya taila.

Srotogamitva :

Dosha : Kaphaghna, pittavardhak.

Dhatu : Raktagami, rasa (febrifuge).

Mala : Purisha (worms).

It is better to avoid internal use of this plant.

References -

'करवीरोऽगुलिपत्रः स्यात् श्वेतो रक्तश्च पीतकः । तथा पाटलपुष्पश्च गुणैस्तुल्यश्चतुर्विधः ।। (शि.)

'करवीरद्वयं तिक्तं कषायं कटुकं च तत् । व्रणलाघवकृन्नेकोपकुष्ठव्रणापहम् ।।
वीर्योष्णं कृमिकण्डुघ्नं भक्षितं विषवन्मतम् ।' (भा.प्र.)

'करवीरः कटुस्तिक्तो वीर्ये चोष्णो ज्वरापहः । चक्षुष्यः कुष्ठकण्डूघ्नः प्रलेपादविषमन्यथा ।।' (ध.नि.)

(27) KANCHANAR

Bauhinia variegata

Gana : Vamanopag (C.), Urdhwabhaghara, Kashay (S.)

Kula : Shimbi kula.

Upkula : Putikaranja.

Family : Leguminosae.

Charakacharya has advised that panchakarma should not be initiated in any patient, unless the doshas are mobilised by snehan and swedan.

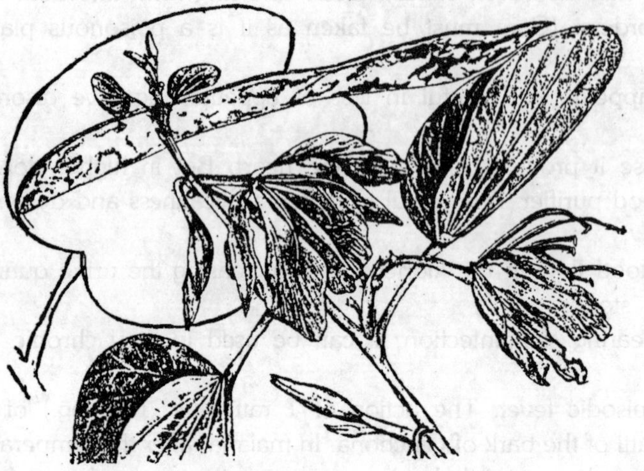

Latin name : Bauhinia (In memory of the two famous French Botanist brothers of the 16th century John and Casper Bauhin); variegata = variegated with patches of different colours.

Sanskrit names : Kanchnar, Pakari, Kovidar, Dalak, Chanari, Peetpushpa, Girij, Yugmaputra, Mahapushpa.

Botanical Description : It is a medium sized tree growing straight. The bark is rough. Flowers are white, yellow or red in colour. Each pod contains 10 - 15 hard seeds. Flowering occurs in spring and in rainy season, pods are seen.

Varieties : Depending on the colour of the flower, it is classified into 3 types- 1) white 2) red and 3) yellow. The trees with white and red flowers are of same height but trees with yellow variety are taller. Trees with orange flowers are called kovidar.

Habitat : Everywhere in India. Found in mountain ranges.

Chemical composition : The bark contains tannin, sugar and gum.

Guna : ruksha, laghu; **Rasa :** kashay; **Vipak :** katu; **Veerya :** sheeta; **Prabhav :** gandmala nashak.

Karma:

Dosha : Kaphashamak by ruksha, laghu and tikta properties. It is pittashamak because of sheeta veerya and therefore it is used in kapha pitta diseases.

External uses : It helps in wound cleaning and healing , it cures skin disorders and inflammations. Decoction is used for washing wounds and skin disorders. The bark ground in a paste is useful in lymphadenitis. Decoction made from its bark, pods of babool (Acacia) tree and flowers of pomegranate is used for gargles in oral disorders. Decoction is used for fomentation in rectal prolapse.

Internal uses :

Digestive system : It has astringent and anthelmintic properties but it causes vomiting in excess dose. Being sweet, flowers are mild laxative. Astringent property is useful in diarrhoea, dysentery, rectal prolapse, haemorrhoids and helminthiasis. It enhances emetic action when used in conjunction with emetic drugs. Gulkand prepared from the flowers is used in constipation, while dried buds are used in haemorrhoids.

Circulatory system : It acts as haemostatic and reduces the inflammation of the lymph nodes (lymphadenitis). It is effective in haemorrhagic disorders. (Paste of bark, roots and flowers is used).

Respiratory system : Used in cough (kaphaghna).

Vaidya gets success by skillful planning and planning, in turn, depends on dose and timing. So consequently, the success of vaidya depends on dose and time.

Urinary system : Controls polyurea in diabetes.
Reproductive system : In menorrhagia, it acts as a haemostatic by astringent property.
Skin : Used in skin diseases. Mixture of kanchanar bark, rice water, and ginger is effective in osteoporosis (asthikshaya).
Satmikaran : Because of ruksha property, it is fat reducing. Used in lipid disorders.
Parts used : Leaves, root bark and flowers.
Dosages : Powder 3-5 gm; decoction 40-80 ml; juice of flowers 10-20 ml.
Formulations : Kanchanar guggul, Kanchanaradi kwath, Kanchan gutika.
Srotogomitva :
Dosa : Kaphaghna, pittaghna.
Dhatu : Rakta, meda (lymphadenitis), menorrhagia, haemorrhagic disorders.
Mala : Purisha (stops diarrhoea and prolapse).
References -
'काञ्चनारो हिमोग्राही तुवरः श्लेष्मपित्तहृत् । कृमिकुष्ठगुदभ्रंशगण्डमालाव्रणापहः ।।
कोविदारोऽपि तद्वत् स्यात् तयोः पुष्पं लघु स्मृतम् । रूक्षं संग्राहि पित्तास्रप्रदरक्षयकासनुत् ।। (भा.प्र.)
'कोविदारपुष्पाणि मधुराणि मधुरविपाकानि रक्तपित्तहराणि च ।' (सु.सू. ४६)
'कोविदारस्य.... । पुष्पं ग्राहि प्रशस्तं च रक्तपित्ते विशेषतः ।।' (च.सू.२७)

(28) KIRATATIKTA
Swertia chirata Buch-Ham.

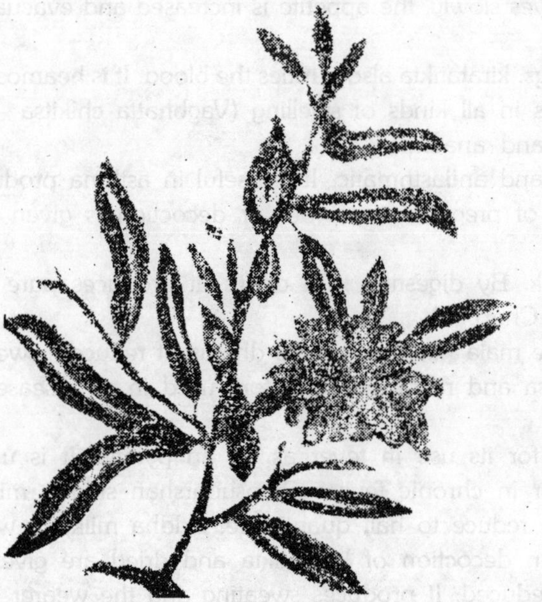

Gana : Tiktaskandha, Stanyashodhan, Trishnanigarahan (C.); Aragvadhadi (S.)
Kula : Bhoonimba kula.
Family : Gentianaceae (king of Illyria first identified the porperties and actions of this family, so it was named accordingly).
Latin name : Swertia (the name has been given in the memory of E. Swert - a Dutch botanist. One more meaning of Swertia is that it grows in hilly tracks); chirata = kirata.
English name : Chiretta.
Sanskrit names : Kiratikta, Kairat, Ramsenak, Naditikta, Jwarantak, Nidrani, Anaryatikta, Katutikta.
Botanical Description : This small plant is 0.75 to 1 mtr. high, with slightly thick trunk, round shaped but quandrangular at the top. Leaves - unequal of 5-8 cm. length, 1-2 cm. wide and pointed at the tip. Stalk of flowers

- many in number. Branches and sub - branches bear small flowers of green and yellow colour at the top. Seeds - very thin. It flowers and bears fruits in winter. As soon as it flowers, the plant is taken out of earth and allowed to dry.

Varieties : Though many varieties are found, Bhavprakash has divided it in two ie. 1) bitter and 2) semibitter. The semibitter is called sweet chiratta in comparison to the variety which is more bitter.

Habitat : It grows in the Himalayan range from Kashmir to Bhutan ie. 1.5 to 3 thousand mtrs. height. It is specially grown in Nepal. It is also found in central and south India.

Chemical composition : A bitter substance named ophelic acid, yellow glycoside (chiratin), resin, gum, pottash, carbonate, phosphate, lime and magnesium are the constituents. It does not contain tannin.

Properties :

Guna : laghu, ruksha; **Rasa :** tikta; **Vipak :** katu; **Veerya :** sheeta.

Karma :

Dosha : It is kaphapittashamak and therefore it is useful in diseases due to kapha pitta.

External uses : Its decoction is used to clean discharging wounds. Persons suffering from generalised itching are asked to take bath with its decoction (kwath).

Internal uses :

Digestive system : Increasses appetite, relieves thirst, helps in amapachan, cholagogue, laxative, anthelmintic, therefore kiratatikta is useful for loss of appetite and dyspepsia. Similarly the decoction (kadha) or powder of kiratatikta can be given in thirst due to ama, dysfunction of liver, constipation and worms. With this, digestive system improves slowly, the appetite is increased and evacuation of faeces improves.

Circulatory system : Like all other bitter drugs, kiratatikta also purifies the blood. It is heamostatic and antiphlogestic. The use of this is famous in all kinds of swelling (Vagbhatta chikitsa - 17/38) It is useful in bleeding piles, jaundice and anaemia.

Respiratory system : It is an expectorant and antiasthmatic. It is useful in asthma produced by obstruction of air passage. In vomiting of pregnancy, powder or decoction is given with honey.

Reproductive system : Purifies breast milk. By digesting rasa dhatu, it produces pure and easily digestible milk (Vagbhatta uttartantra Chap. 2).

Skin : Helps in skin diseases by reducing the mala (kled) of all the dhatus. It reduces swelling due to inflammation. It improves agni of rasa and rakta and therefore used in all diseases of skin and pruritus.

Temperature : Kiratatikta is more famous for its use in fever as an antipyretic. It is useful in malarial fever. In post febrile weakness or in chronic fever, mahasudarshan siddha milk is used (powder is boiled in milk and water to reduce to half quantity ie. siddha milk). It works wonderfully well. Children's clothes dipped in decoction of kiratatikta and dried are given to children to wear so that the temperature is reduced. It produces sweating and the wearer feels relieved. Enlargement of spleen is also reduced with this.

Satmikaran : Kiratatikta is bitter, nutritious and increases strength. Weakness after indigestion and fever is reduced with this. It is the best rasayan in post febrile conditions where siddha milk is used.

Useful parts : Whole plant.

Doses : Decoction 60 - 100 ml; powder- 2 - 6 gms.

Formulations : Mahasudarshan churna, Kiratadi kwath, Medoyogsharkara, Kiratadi taila.

Srotogamitva :

Dosha : It reduces kapha pitta.

Dhatu : Rakta (swelling), rasa - improves agni.

Mala : Purisha (laxative).

Organs : Strengthens stomach, rectum (piles).

References -

'किरातः सारको रूक्षः शीतलस्तिक्तको लघुः । सन्निपातज्वरश्वासकपित्तास्रदाहनुत् ।।
कासशोथतृषाकुष्ठज्वरव्रणकृमिप्रणुत् ।' (भा.प्र.)
'किरातको रसे तिक्तः सरः शीतो लघुस्तथा । श्लेष्मपित्तास्रशोफार्शः कासतृष्णाज्वरापहः ।।' (ध.नि.)

(29) KUTAJA
Holarrhena antidysenterica

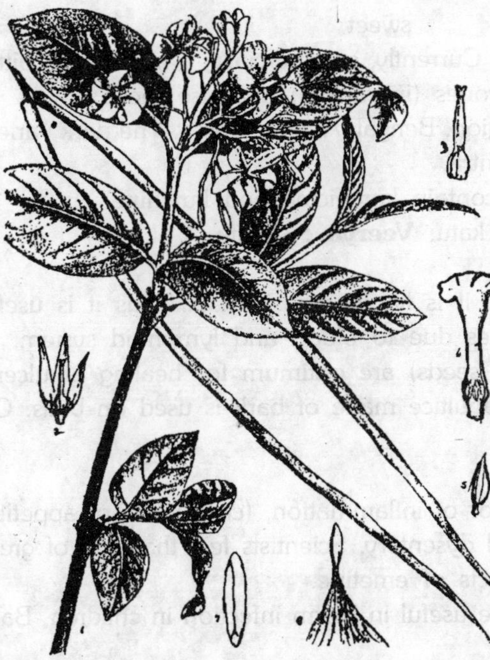

Gana : Arshoghna, Kandughna, Stanyashodhana, Asthapanopaga, Vamana (C.), Aragvadhadi Pippalyadi, Haridradi, Brihatyadi, Lakshadi, Urdhwabhagahara (Vamana) (S.)

Kula: Kutaja kula.

Family : Apocyanaceae (away from dogs) Apo from; kyons - dog, Dog's bane (poison to dogs) Bane = it is poisonous to dogs.

Latin name : Holarrhena - Holos =whole; Arrhen = (Greek) male = whole male = entire anther; antidysenterica = against dysentery, antidote for it.

English name : Kurchi.

Sanskrit names : Kutaja, Shakra, Vatsaka, Girimallika, Kalinga, Pravishya, Shakrapadaka, Varatika, Yavaphala, Mahagandha, Koti, Shatrubhuruha.

Botanical Description : The tree is 7-9 metres tall. The bark is pale or brownish in colour. The inner wood is pale and soft. Leaves - 10-30 cms. long and 3-5 cms. wide. They appear similar to those of kadamba - always green and shiny. They are 10-16 in pairs with prominent veins on them. Flowers - white, fragrant, similar to jasmine flowers, 2.5 - 3.75 cms. in length. Fruits - two pods arise on the same stalk.

They are long and hard, 20-40 cms. in length, and thin.
They exude a grainy white substance, in white spots. The pods contain seeds embedded in soft cottonlike material. The pods burst spontaneously and the seeds are dispersed with the help of the feathery cotton-like substance.
The plant flowers in the rainy season and fruits in cold weather.
Habitat : Throughout India but mainly in the jungles of Saharanpur.
Varieties : Charakacharya mentions two varieties 1) male kutaja and 2) female kutaja.
Male kutaja - Stem, bark - white. Female kutaja - stem, bark - dark.
Male kutaja - Large pods, reddish flowers and small leaves.
Female kutaja - Small pods, pink flowers and small leaves.

Modern classification of varieties of kutaja :

	White	Black
1.	Bark - smoky brown	dark (black) bark
2.	Leaves - white on drying	black on drying
3.	Flowers - white, small, slightly fragrant	strongly scented
4.	Pods - arranged in pairs but partly seperate	grow in pairs joined at origin
5.	Seeds - bitter (indrayava)	sweet

The white bark and bitter seeds are more beneficial. Currently, commercially, a mixture of bitter and sweet seeds is sold. Still, separate the bitter ones (indrayava) and use these.
Habitat : White variety occurs in the Himalayan region, Bengal, Assam, Orissa. The dark variety is found more often in South India and Maharashtra.
Chemical composition : The bark and seeds contain kurchicine and kurchine.
Guna : ruksha; **Rasa :** tikta, kashaya; **Vipak :** katu; **Veerya :** sheeta.
Karma :
Dosha : Being ruksha, tikta, kashaya and sheeta, it is kapha-pittashamak. Thus it is useful in many diseases of kapha and pitta and diseases due to blood and lymphoid system.
External use : Stem, bark and indrayava (bitter seeds) are optimum for healing of ulcers. A decoction of these helps in ulcer treatment. A poultice made of bark is used on boils. On exuding ulcers, a dressing of indrayava is used.
Internal use :
Digestive system : Vatashaman, deepan, inhibitor of inflammation, (cures) loss of appetite, pittasarak and parasiticidal. Useful in diarrhoea and dysentery. Scientists feel that it is of great use in amoebiasis without the long term side effects of emetine.
The total alkaloids of the tender pods and leaves are useful in worm infection in children. Bark is most effective in jaundice.
Circulatory system : Useful in bleeding disorders.
Reproductive system : Removes muscular weakness and tones up vaginal tissues after delivery.
Fevers : Antipyretic, specially in fevers of lymphatic or blood origin. Therapeutic in typhoid,

One sprinkles water around a dinner plate to keep the dust from flying around. Chitrahuti is a symbol of sacrifice.

when given as decoction with kalinga.
Satmikaran : Due to its tissue healing properties, it is useful in weakness.
Parts used : Stem, bark, seeds (indrayava; kalinga).
Dose : For decoction of seeds - 0.5 to 1.00 gm.
Formulations : Kutajarishta, Kutajavaleha, Kutajaghanavati, Kutajasharkarakalp, Kutajashtaka kwath.
Stem bark is most effective in diarrhoea and dysentery. Mixed and ingested with butter milk, it has very good action. There are no side effects even in pregnant women. Bark is digestive and helps circulation.
Srotogamitva :
Dosha : Lessens kapha and pitta.
Dhatu : Rakta (raktapitta, kushtha), rasa.
Mala : Purisha (dysentery, diarrhoea), sangrahi.
Organs : Grahani, amashay, rectum.
References -
'शिंबिफल: श्वेतपुष्प: कटुजो दीर्घपत्रक: ।'(शि.)
'कुटज: कटुको रुक्षो दीपनस्तुवरो हिम: । अर्शोतिसारपित्तास्त्रकफतृष्णामकुष्ठजित् ।' (भा.प्र.)
'इन्द्रयवं त्रिदोषघ्नं सग्राहि कटु शीतलम् । ज्वरातिसाररक्तार्श: कॉमिवीसर्पकुष्ठनुत् ।।
दीपनं गुदकीलास्त्रवातास्त्रश्लेष्मशूलजित् ।' (भा.प्र.)
'रक्तपित्तकफघ्नस्तु सुकुमारेष्वनत्यय: । हृद्रोगज्वरवातासृगवीसर्पादिषु शस्यते ।।' (च.क.५)
'कुटजत्वकश्लेष्मपित्तरक्तसांग्राहिकोपशोषणानाम् । (च.सू.२५)

(30) KUPEELU
Strychnos nux-vomica Linn.

Kula : Karaskara kula.
Family : Loganiaceae (Logan - name of a scientist).
Latin name : Strychnos - having poisonous properties; nux = nut; vomica = which causes vomiting.
English name : Nux vomica.
Sanskrit names : Kuchala, Karaskara, Kupeelu, Vishatinduka, Kunchvruksha, Kakatinduka, Kalapeelu, Kulaka, Markatatinduka.
Botanical Description : The tree is 12-16 mtrs. high. Branches - thin but strong. Bark- thin soft, grey in colour. Interior substance of the stem looks white on breaking but becomes pale yellow after some time. Leaves - glabrous and having slight odour. Leaf stalk - thick, leaves are 5-9 cm. long. Flower - small, greenish-white smelling like turmeric. Androceium - five in number. Ovary is divided into 2 parts. Fruit - ovoid like guava, ripe fruit is yellow, fruit shell is very hard. Fruit pulp is tender, white and very bitter. Seed - each fruit has 2-5 seeds having a breadth of 2 cm. and thickness 0.5 mm. Seed is big, round like button, concave on one side and convex on the outer side, soft, covered with striations. It is hard and whitish dusky in colour. The tree bears flowers in spring and fruits in winter.
Habitat : It is a wild tree. In India, it appears in the forests of torrid zone. Mainly Chennai, Kerala,

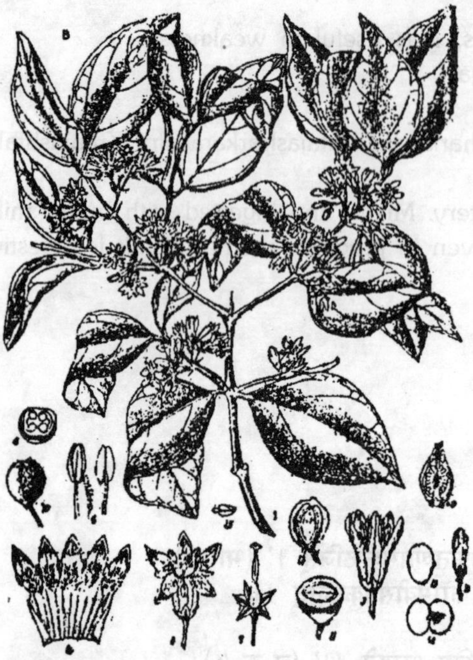

Konkan, Orissa and Sri lanka.

Chemical composition : Nux vomica fruit is available in India. It contains 2.6 to 3% alkaloids. It contains 1.25 to 1.5 % strychnine. Besides, it also contains brucin, bomisine, loganine, glucoside, protid (11%), bile principle, oil, gum, white sugar (6%), wax, phosphate and ash.

Brucin is a major component of fresh bark (3.1%). Leaf and wood contain less quantity.

Properties :

Guna : ruksha, laghu, tikshna; **Rasa** : tikta, katu; **Vipak** : katu; **Veerya** : ushna.

Karma :

Dosha : Kaphaghna by tikta, katu and ruksha properties, vataghna by ushna property. Impure or purified seeds in excess dose leads to ojakshay (poison and ojas have opposite properties) and convulsions by vitiating vata. Purified and low dose of Nux vomica doesn't cause convulsions. It is effective in many disorders induced by kapha and vata.

External uses : Vatashamak, it alleviates pain, oedma and is an analgesic. It is used for external application in rheumatoid arthritis, osteoarthritis. An application of Nux vomica seeds with turmeric cures oozing and foul smelling ulcers. This paste is also effective in ulcers with toxic symptoms. The pulp of the leaves in the form of poultice is very useful in oozing ulcers.

Internal uses :

Central nervous system : It alleviates vata and pain and because of its sharpness, it stimulates and strengthens nerves. Useful in vata disorders like neuralgia, facial palsy, hemiplegia, insomnia. Excess dose leads to intoxication and convulsions.

Digestive system : Being bitter and pungent, it is a good appetizer, digestive and astringent. Useful in abdominal pain by ushna and vata alleviating property. It is used in loss of appetite, gastric inflammation, amadosha, colitis, piles and parasitic infection. It is the best medicine for gastric laxity and spasm.

Circulatory system : Being ushna and tikshna, it is a cardiac stimulant and hypertensive. It alleviates oedema caused by kapha. Useful in disorders like cardiac laxity.

Respiratory system : Being pungent and bitter, it is kaphaghna and alleviates cough. It is also useful in inflammations of lungs.

Urinary system : Dribbling of the urine due to atonicity of bladder is corrected by it. It is an effective medicine for nocturia in children and adults.

Reproductive system : It is an aphrodisiac. It cures premature ejaculation and impotency.

Satmikaran : It is an excellent rasayan. It cures the laxity of body tissue. It is a good medicine for the

Philosophers claim that there is a very subtle difference between extreme intelligence and madness. This may be seen in people having an I.Q. above 160.

elderly complaining of loss of appetite, insomnia and laxity of body.
Skin : Nux-vomica is useful in dermatoses, pruritus and excess perspiration.
Temperature : Nux-vomica is effective in fever with shivering and periodical fever. It reduces shivering and rigours.
Parts used : Inner hard, button like purified seed.
Dosage : 1/2 to 1 ratti (1-2 grain).
Formulations : Agnitundi, Vishamushti, Navajeevan, Vajravati, Krumimudgar.
Toxic effets : Impure or excess dose of nux-vomica causes convulsions and causes symptoms similar to tentanus. These symptoms appear within 10 to 20 minutes after its oral administration and leads to death by asphyxia.
Antidote : As soon as toxic symptoms appear, give stomach wash and give cow's ghee along with cow's milk. Use antidotes like opium, belladona, camphor, ganja and tobacco.
Purification of seeds : Seeds of nux-vomica are soaked in cow's urine for 7 days. Then outer covering is removed and the seeds are cooked with cow's milk. Then they are fried in cow's ghee. (This nux vomica is used in medicines). These roasted seeds have specific savour. (In hoarseness of voice caused by excessive talking, tobacco addiction induced blindness, nocturia in children, impotency caused by excess sexual intercourse and old age, dysponea and morning sickness in pregnant women, purified nux-vomica (seed) ground in a fine powder should be used along with milk and sugar.
Now-a-days modern treatment has changed widely but about 2 decades ago, modern doctors used 'tincture nux vomica' in their prescription. Nux vomica is a Latin name which means 'nut which causes vomiting'.
Srotogamitva :
Dosha : Alleviates vata, kapha.
Dhatu : Rakta (cures dermatoses).
Mala : Purisha (antihaemorrhoids), mutra (antidiuretic).
Organs : Stomach (tonic), rectum (piles).
References -
'कारस्कर: कटूष्णश्च, तिक्त: कुष्ठविनाशन: ।
वातामयास्त्रकण्डूर्तिकफामार्शोव्रणापह: ।। (रा.नि.)

(31) KUMARI
Aloe vera

Kula : Rasona kula.
Family : Liliaceae.
Latin name : Aloe = (Alloch Arabic through alos Gk); vera - indica.
English name : Indian aloe.
Sanskrit names : Kumari, Ghritakumari, Gruhakanya, Deerghapatrika, Ajara,Veera, Taruni, Rama, Kapila, Sthaldala, Mata, Mandala, Akshayakaraka, Atipittala.
Botanical Description : Its shrubs are 30-60 cms. high. Leaves - thick, filled with juice, 3 to 4 fingres in circumference and 1 to 2 ft. in length. The margins of the leaves have spikes.

Any medical practitioner, of any discipline, should study along with medicine, fundamental principles and the practical applications of his discipline.

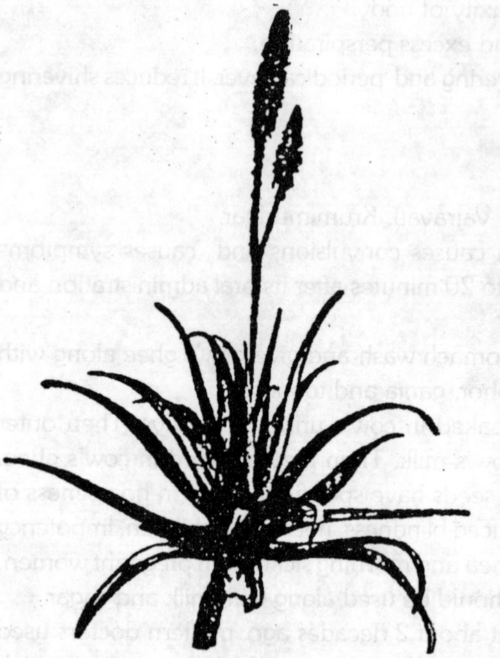

Leaves contain a thick and mucilagenous juice. Once the shrub becomes old, a straight stalk emerges from its centre which bears red flowers in cluster. The plant flowers and fruits at the end of winter.

The solid gum obtained after boiling the juice of kumari is called alia bol, kala bol, kumarisar, musabbar etc. It is called aloes in English. It appears that kala bol was not used in the earlier period because none of the nighantus mention the properties of kala bol.

Varieties : Kala bol is available in four varities- 1) Sacrotine - imported from Zanziber and ports of the Red sea, 2) Arabian, 3) Jaffarabadi and 4) Maisuri. Just like asafoetida, kala bol is also packed in sacks made from the skin of goats and sheep. The quality of kumari differs in different regions and seasons affect its quality as well.

Habitat : Kumari is predominantly found in Africa, Arabia and India. In India it is abundantly seen in the south. Its name may be related to the name of a place called Kanyakumari.

Chemical composition : Korphad has aloin, barbaloin as crystalline glucosides, aloe amodine, resins and water soluble substances.

Properties :

Guna : snigdha, pichchil; **Rasa** : bitter, sweet; **Vipak** : katu; **Veerya** : sheeta.

Prabhav : bhedan.

Kala Bol : laghu, ruksha, tikshna and ushna.

Karma :

Dosha : Useful in diseases caused by all the three doshas.

External use : Poultice - antiinflammatory, can be applied on inflammed parts. Kala bol powder can be applied on small wounds. A warm paste of kumari juice with turmeric churna can be applied over swollen, painful and enlarged spleen. Juice can be used in the eyes for conjunctivitis. In headaches and eye problems, the pulp can be applied locally. The juice is refrigerant.

Internal use :

Digestive system : In small doses, kumari has deepan, pachan, bhedan and uttejak properties. In large doses, it is virechaka and krumighna.

It increases the secretions of small intestine and promotes the peristalsis of large intestine. Since its action is slow, the laxative effect is observed after 10 -12 hours. If taken in excess quantity, rational action is not observed but ill effects in the form of gripping, constipation and sometimes bleeding is observed. In moderate quantity, stools are observed to be soft and solid and dark coloured. There is increased congestion in the anal region due to con- sumption of kumari. Very often it may result in formation of piles. Juice of kumari is useful in loss of appetite, ascites, tumour, liver and spleen enlargement and abdominal colic. It is laxative, antiflatulent and anthelmintic.

Cardiovascular system : It is yakritgami, raktavahasrotogami and is useful in purification of blood and affections of liver. It is used in splenomegaly in combination with haridra.

Urogenital system : It is a known diuretic. By virtue of being snigdha and pichchil, it promotes the secretion of semen and acts as an aphrodisiac. Being ushna, it increases the flow of blood to the uterus and promotes contraction as a result of which it leads to uterine bleeding. Hence kala bol is used locally for treatment of amenorrhoea.

Skin : Useful in common conditions of skin, it promotes hair growth.

Temperature : It is useful in chronic fevers.

Satmikaran : Kumari juice or kala bol can be used as a restorative in generalised weakness. It is a tonic. The juice is anabolic and increases strength.

Parts used : Leaves, juice from leaves, kala bol.

Dosages : Juice of leaves - 2 to 4 spoons; kala bol - 1 to 4 ratti.

Formulations : Kumari asava, Kumaripak etc.

Excretion : Kumari is excreted through breast milk and small amounts through urine.

Absorption : If kala bol is applied over fresh skin wounds, it can result in absorption and hence result in loose motions.

Administration : For purgation, if kumari is used along with kshar or scented herbs, there is no colicky pain. For good menstrual flow, kala bol can be started 7 days before periods.

Srotogamitva :

Dosha : Vata reducing, kapha reducing, pittasarak.

Dhatu : Rasayani, mansa (bruhani), shukra (vrushya), rakta (jaundice), rasa (febrifuge), meda (granthihar).

Mala : Purisha (bhedak), artavajanak.

Prabhav : Has antidotal properties.

Organs : Eyes, uterus.

References -

'कुमारी क्षारभूदेशे पंक्तिकन्ददला बला । विस्तारी बाढकन्दिनी विशाला पिच्छसंभृता ।।
ध्वजाभमध्यदण्डा सारुणराजियुता पृथुः ।' (शि.द.)

'कुमारी गृहकन्या च कन्या घृतकुमारिका । कुमारी भेदनी शीता तिक्ता नेत्र्या रसायनी ।।
मधुरा बुंहणी बल्या वृष्या वातविषप्रणुत् । गुल्मप्लीहयकृदवृद्धिकफज्वरहरी हरेत् ।।
ग्रन्थ्यग्निदग्धविस्फोटपित्तरक्तत्वगामयान् ।' (भा.प्र.)

'गृहकन्या हिमा तिक्ता मदगन्धिः कफापहा । पित्तकासविषश्वासकुष्ठघ्नी च रसायनी ।।' (रा.नि.)

वीरास्त्राव: सहासार: कुमारीरसम्भव: सहासारोऽग्निजनन: पित्तनिर्हरणो मत: ।।
बलकृद्रेचन: पुष्पजननो गर्भपातन: । विटसङ्गे कृमिरोगे च संन्यासेऽपस्मृतौ तथा ।।
लुप्ते रजसि नारीणां शीतपित्ते शिरोरुजि ज्वरे श्लेष्मोदभवे प्लीह्नि मन्देऽग्नौ च प्रयुज्यते ।।
अर्शसस्तं न सेवेत नान्तर्वत्नी न पुष्पिणी । न चासृग्दरिणी नापि यकृदवृक्कादिरोगवान् ।।' (आ.वि.)

Every medical practitioner must know his own limitations and his strengths.

(32) KUSHTHAM

Saussurea luppa

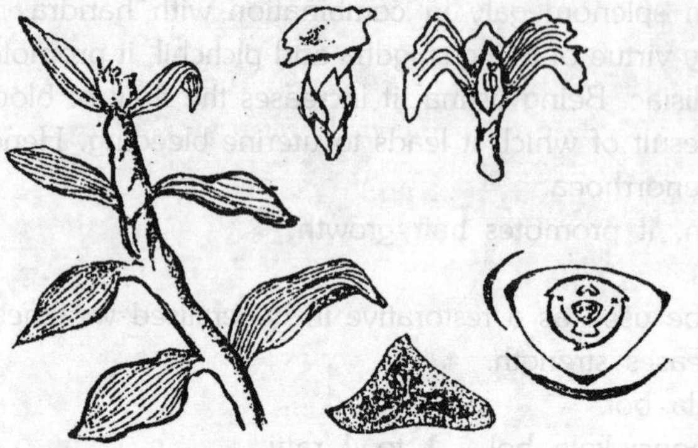

Gana : Shukrashodhan, Lekhaneeya, Asthapanopag (C.); Eladi (S.)
Kula : Bhringaraj kula.
Family : Compositae (in which the so called flower is ahead of many flowers).
Latin name : Saussurea = covered with tufts of prickles; luppa = lappa (Hopuke in forem C.B. Clarke, Hop = spring)
English name : Costus (from kuṣhtha ?)
Sanskrit names : Yapya, Brahmateertha, Pushkarasya, Shwasari, Padmateertha, Pushkarsagar, Shoolahara, Punyasagar, Moolaveer.

Botanical Description : The shrub is 2 to 3 mtrs. high and found in watery places. Trunk - solid and of the thickness of little finger. Leaves - large, heart shaped and the stalk is 0.5 to 1 mtr. long. Flowers - round and violet in colour. Seeds - small and curved. Roots - thick, perinneal and fresh shoots emerge from these roots every year. Flowers and fruits appear in autumn. Collection of roots must be done during fruit bearing season. Roots 8 to 15 cms. long, 1.5 to 4 cms. thick, carrot shaped, cracked on one side, white internally and brown-black externally. The roots have a strong fragrance. In China they are used for aromatic smoke.

Habitat : Kashmir.

Chemical composition : Roots contain 1.5 % aromatic oil, glucoside, saussurin salt, resin, tannin, inulin 18 %, stable oil, nitrate, glucose etc. Leaves do not contain aromatic oil. On incinerating, roots yield 3.5 % ash. It contains a large quantity of manganese.

Properties :

Guna : laghu, rukhsa, tikshna; **Rasa** : tikta, katu, madhur; **Vipak** : katu; **Veerya** : ushna.

Karma :

Dosha : Kapha, vatasrotogami, reduces kaphavata and hence used in many vatakapha diseases.

External uses : Removes foul smell, antibacterial, analgesic, varnya, kushthaghna, therefore used in chronic ulcers, headache, toothache, synovitis, rheumatoid arthritis, dermatitis as a poultice or fumigation. It is applied locally in alopecia. Oil is used for massaging the gums.

Internal uses :

Nervous system : Used in vata diseases, especially in epilepsy since it is vatahara and antiepileptic.

Digestive system : Appetizer, digestive and carminative. It is used in loss of appetite, indigestion, ascites, colicky pain, diarrhoea and cholera.

Circulatory system : Raktashodhan, shothaghna, stimulant, therefore used in vatarakta, visarpa, rheumatism, oedema and weakness of the heart. In rheumatoid arthritis, caster oil + kushtha is given orally.

As human body has originated from the universe, those rules which apply to universe must also apply to human body.

Respiratory system : Kaphaghna, expectorant and hence used in cough, asthma, pleurisy, hiccups and dyspnoea.

Reproductive system : Uterine stimulant, enhances ovulation, breast milk, improves semen quality, aphrodisiac and therefore used in amenorrhoea, dysmenorrhoea and as a uterine tonic in post partum conditions. It is a galactogogue. It acts as an aphrodisiac by improving semen quality. It produces stimulant action on the reproductive organs of both sexes when given along with turmeric, honey and ghee.

Urinary system : It is mutravahasrotogami and therefore used as a diuretic in renal diseases.

Skin : Increases sweating, kushthaghna, therefore used in skin diseases. It improves blood circulation and complexion of the skin (therefore called kushtha ?).

Temperature : It is a febrifuge and therefore useful in vata kapha fevers.

Satmikaran : Used as rasayan in debility.

Parts used : Root.

Doses : 0.25 to 1.25 gm.

Formulation : Kushthadi churna, kwath and taila.

Adulteration : On breaking, its sticky material should not get separated. Cowdung, mud and similar substances are mixed in it for adulteration. The smell of kushtha is so strong that it masks the smell of the adulterants and it becomes difficult to differentiate them from the original substance. The roots of rasna are also mixed for adulteration. (Kushtha is used for fumigation in China. It is also used for preservation of clothes.)

Srotogamitva :

Dosha : Vatakaphaghna.

Dhatu : Shukra (stimulant), rakta (visapra, vatarakta, kushtha).

Mala : Diuretic.

Organ : Pranvahasrotas.

(It is a good idea to try kushtha for rasayan therapy.)

References -

'कुष्ठमुष्णं कटु स्वादु शुक्रलं तिक्तकं लघु । हन्ति वातास्रवीसर्पकासकुष्ठमरुत्कफान् ।।' (भा.प्र.)
'कुष्ठं वातकफश्वासकासहिक्काज्वरापहम् ।' (रा.व.नि.)
'कुष्ठं वातहराभ्यंगोपयोगिनाम् ।' (च.सू.२५)
'यः कुष्ठचूर्ण रजनीविरामे मध्वाज्यसंमिश्रितमत्ति नित्यम् ।
स मत्तमातंगबलः सुगन्धिर्वाग्मी चिंरायुश्च भवेन्मनुष्यः ।।' (रा.मा.)

(33) KUSHMAND

Benincasa hispida Thum.

Gana : Valliphala.

Kula : Koshataki kula.

Family : Cucurbitaceae (Lat. cucurbita = gourd, large fleshy fruit).

Latin name : Benincasa = of Benin; hispida = hispid = thickly covered with long stiff bristly hairs.

English name : White pumpkin, white gourd melon.

Each footnote of mine is thought-provoking. I hope, when all footnotes are compiled together, they make entire Ayurveda.

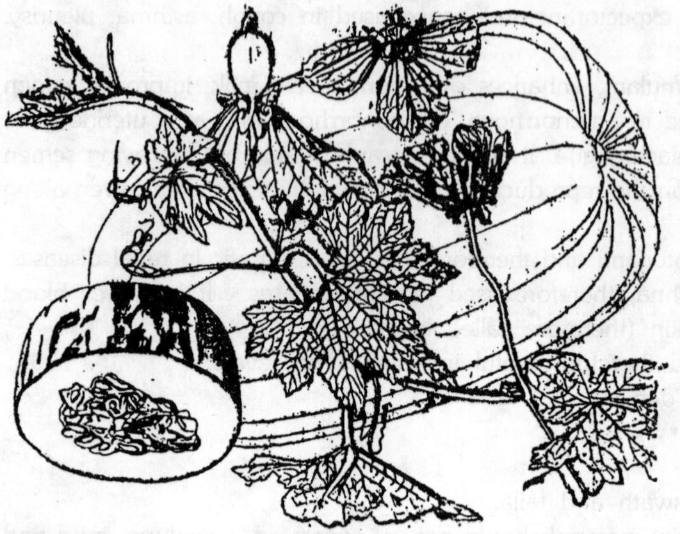

Sanskrit names : Karkotika, Kushmandi, Suphala, Kumbhaphala, Kshirphala, Kushmandaki, Karkati, Mahaphala, Pushpaphala (bearing flowers and fruits simultaneously), Peetpushpa, Valliphala, Somaka (sheeta veerya).

Botanical Description : Creeper grows annually. Leaves - 10-15 cm. in diameter, hard, white coloured, thickly covered with stiff bristly hairs. Flower - stalk of male flower is 10 cm. while that of female is 30 cm. Fruit - size of a large egg bearing white bristly hairs. Seed - flat, white, flowering in winter and fruits ripen in summer and are viable for 1 year.

Variety : One more variety is called Cucurbita moschata.

Habitat : All over India.

Chemical composition : Cucurbitine, bitter resin, myosine, viteline, starch and salts. Seed contains stable oil. Fruit contains 96% water.

Properties :

Guna : laghu, snigdha; **Rasa :** madhur; **Vipak :** madhur; **Veerya :** sheeta; **Prabhav :** medhya.

Karma :

Dosha : Being madhur and snigdha, it acts as vata shamak and madhur, sheeta gunas make it pittashamak.

External use : Local application of fruit pulp ameliorates burning sensation. The juice of the leaves is applied in burns.

Internal use :

Nervous system : It acts as a brain tonic as well as improves memory. It acts as a tranquiliser and therefore useful in schizophrenia, debility and memory loss.

Digestive system : By its property of madhur and snigdha, it acts a laxative and also alleviates thirst. It is especially useful in tapeworm. 2 - 4 tolas of seed pulp is given followed by a purgative to act as a helmenthicide. Seed oil is also used for this condition in a dose of 10-25 gm. Laxative and coagulative property helps in bleeding piles. Salts are used in abdominal colic.

Circulatory system : It is a cardiac stimulant and ameliorates raktapitta (haematemesis) by its properties of madhur, snigdha and sheeta. Its vasoconstrictive effect stops bleeding in any part. It is a very useful medicine in cardiac debility, haematemesis and chest pain.

Respiratory system : Being madhur and snigdha it is useful in cachexia, tuberculosis, bronchial asthma, cough, fever and epigastric burning. Haemoptysis is reduced when given along with mauktik bhasma.

Agnihotra has good effects on the enviroment of plants and therefore trees grow well, they bloom and bear fruits and flowers (Shri Tambade, Nasik).

Urinary system : Sheeta veerya property shows a stimulating effect on urine formation. Therefore fruit pulp and seeds are used in nephritis, anuresis and renal calculi.
Reproductive system : It is used in loss of libido as madhur and snighdha gunas make it spermatogenic.
Skin and temperature : Syrup of seeds and sweets prepared from the fruits are used in summer to relieve burning sensation and fever. It is also used in burning of chronic fever.
Satmikaran : Since it is madhur and snigdha, it acts as a restorative and anabolic. Hence it is used in generalised debility and weakness. The juice of the fruit is used in mercury poisoning. Overuse of kushmand results in kapha vata diseases. In such diseases, a mixture of salt, Piper nigrum and shatapushpa may be given.
Useful parts : Fruits, fruit juice, seeds, oil of seeds, leaves. (Fruits are used after preserving them for an year).
Dose : Fruit juice - 60 to 120 ml.; seed powder 3 to 6 gms; oil - 6 to 12 ml.; leaves - for external use.
Formulations : Kushmandpak, Kushmandkhand, Kushmand churna, Kushmandgud, Kalyanak Ghrut.
Substitute : White gourd.
Misconceptions (Beliefs) : There are certain misconceptions associated with this plant like hair turn white on touching after handling the fruit. Another misconception - if the creeper bears plenty and excessive fruits, it may cause the death of a person in the family which grows that creeper. Gourd is used instead of animals in yagnya for sacrifice. Two types of sweets prepared from kushmand are available at Agra and Mathura.
Srotogamitva :
Dosha : Ameliorates vata and pitta, vitiates kapha.
Dhatu : Mansa and meda, rakta, majja, shukra (aprodisiac).
Mala : Urine (calculi, aneuresis, diabetes).

(34) KRISHNAJEERAK
Carum carvi Linn.

Kula : Shatapushpa kula.
Family : Umbelifereae (umbel = flower; ferae=bearing. Flower heads of all species are umbels = flower clustered uniformly).
Latin name : Carum (caria = where it was discovered. Roots as well as seeds are edible); carvi (Linn) caraway (Arab original - Karawia)
English name : Black cumin.
Sanskrit names : Krishna, Bhedini, Ruchya, Jeeraka, Sugandha, Kanajeer, Krishnajaji, Hridya, Kalajeerak, Krishnajeerak.
Botanical Description : Shrub grows 0.75 mtr to 1 mtr. in height. Leaves-serrated margin, oblong. Flower- umbrella type, seed-blackish, smaller, thinner and scented than white variety. (The marketed variety is adulterated by coloured seeds of plants like carrot but they do not have that specific odour.)
Habitat : Kashmir, Gadhwal, Border states, Afghanistan, Iran.

Seasons should be identified by the flowers that bloom during that particular season and not by a calender.

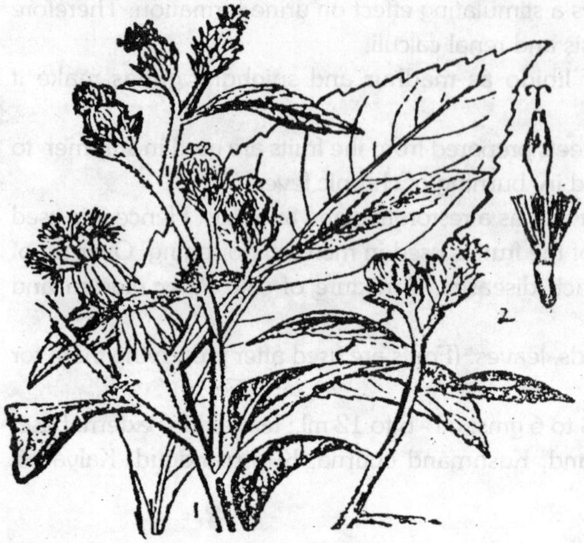

Chemical composition : Contains volatile oil which gives the specific scent to black cumin.

Properties :

Guna : laghu, ruksha; **Vipak :** katu; **Rasa :** katu; **Veerya :** ushna.

Karma :

Dosha : Its ushna property alleviates kapha and vata diseases .

Digestive system : It is deodorant, improves taste, appetite and digestion, constipative and antiflatulent, therefore useful in bad breath, anorexia, vomiting, loss of appetite, diarrhoea, indigestion, flatuence and dysentery (duodenitis).

Circulatory system : Cardiotonic and antiinflammatory, therefore useful in cardiac debility and anasarca (oedema).

Reproductive system : It is used in post partum conditions to improve uterine involution and breast milk secretion.

Temperature : It is used in chronic fever to improve appetite, digestion, absorption, reduce fever and acts as a tonic.

Parts used : Seeds.

Dose : 5-15 gms. oil is used in medicine as scent. Decoction is used in pediatric medicine as an antiflatulent.

Srotogamitva :

Dosha : Vitiates pitta and ameliorates kapha.

Dhatu : Majja , rasa (antipyretic), shukra (aphrodisiac).

Mala : Stool (antidiarrhoeal).

Organ : Uterus, eyes, stomach (antiemetic).

References -

'जीरकत्रितयं रूक्षं कटूष्णं दीपनं लघु । संग्राहि पित्तलं मेध्यं गर्भाशयविशुद्धिकृत् ।।
ज्वरघ्नं पाचनं वृष्यं बल्यं रुच्यं कफापहम् । चक्षुष्यं पवनाध्मानगुल्मच्छर्द्यतिसारहृत् ।।' (भा.प्र.)
'जरणा कटुरुष्णा च कफशोफनिकृन्तनी । रुच्या जीर्णज्वरघ्नी च चक्षुष्या ग्राहिणी परा ।।' (ध.नि.)

(35) KHADIR
Acasia catechu Willd.

Gana : Kushthaghna, Kashayskandh (C.) Salsaradigana (S.)

Kula : Shimbi - Leguminoseae.

Family : Babbul (Mimosoideae) sensitivity of the leaves.

Planting trees around the house should be done much before it is built. A house takes an year to build but it takes nearly 10 years for trees to grow.

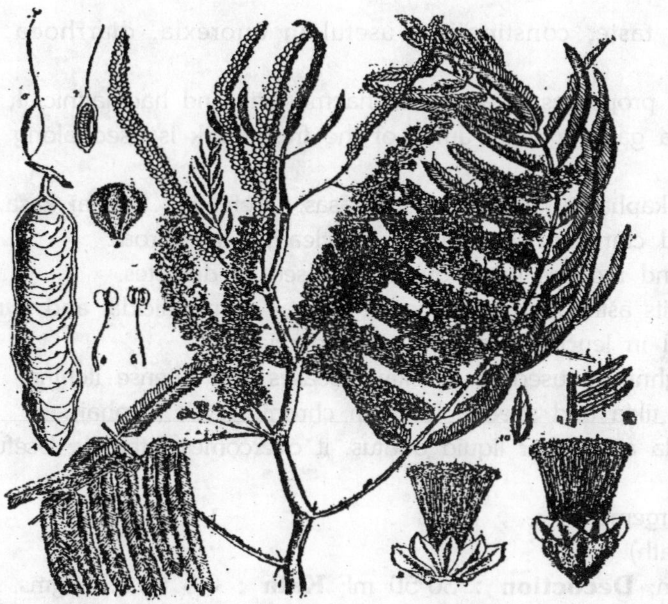

Latin Name : Acasia spines - gum tree; catechu = kachu (Kannad) (Willd).

White khadir - Acasia ferrucinea (Dc.), Somavalka, Kadar, Gayatri.

Vitkhadir - Acasia farniciana (Willd), Arimeda.

English name : Catechu tree.

Sanskrit names : Balpatra, Kantaki, Dantadhavan, Kushthari, Bahushalya, Bahusar, Medhya, Kushthaghna, Irimed.

Botanical Description : This is a medium sized tree. Trunk - rough, spiny, yellowish from outside and reddish from inside. Leaves - compound, 8-10 cms. long, 30-50 leaflets are seen in pairs. Flowers small, yellow, having three petals. Fruit-legume - 5 to 10 cms. long, thin, slightly smoky in colour and shining, contains 5-8 round seeds. Bears leaves in summer, flowers in rainy season and legumes in autumn.

Habitat : In Himalayas at the height of 5000 ft. and dry climate.

Chemical composition : 35% catechu, 57% catechin.

Khadirsar - 5 types

1. White.
2. Blackish brown - Externally blackish brown, soft and easily breakable. Used in medicine.
3. Brown - Used for chewing in betal leaves.
4. Black - Not good for consumption, of bad quality.
5. Vitkhadir - Arimeda or Irimeda. Foul smelling like stools or fats.

Properties :

Guna : laghu, ruksha; **Rasa :** tikta, kashaya; **Vipak :** katu; **Veerya :** sheeta;
Prabhav : kushthaghna.

Karma : Kaphapittashamak by tikta, kashaya rasa and sheeta veerya and therefore used in kaphapitta diseases.

External uses : Stambhan and kushthaghna. Being astringent and haemostatic, powder is used in wound healing and in dental conditions.

Gargling is useful in cough and hoarseness of voice. In leprosy, bathing with the decoction of khadir is advised. Used for oral hygiene and pharyngeal ulcers.

In memory of the sixteen sanskars of a human being, if we grow atleast one tree for every sanskar, our forests will be very prosperous.

Internal uses:

Digestive system : Improves taste, constipative, useful in anorexia, diarrhoea and intestinal parasites.

Circulatory system : Due to its properties, it acts as a haemostatic and haematinic. It also reduces oedema. Khadir acts as a galactogouge. Juice of the fresh bark is used along with asafoetida in haemoptysis.

Respiratory system : Reduces kapha by tikta, kashaya rasas. Useful in kaphaj kasa. A lozenge prepared from khadir and cinnamonum is used for clearing the throat.

Urinary system : Kaphaghna and reduces urine output so used in diabetes.

Reproductive system : Due to its astringent properties, it acts as a spermicidal and is used as a uterine tonic. It is also used in leucorrhoea and menorrhagia.

Skin : Kushthaghna and kandughna so used in all skin diseases and intense itching.

Temperature : Antipyretic being tikta and sheeta. Used in chronic fever (kaphaj).

Satmikaran : By reducing meda and other liquid dhatus, it overcomes lethargy. Useful in hyperlipidaemia.

Spleen : Useful in spleenic enlargement.

Parts used : Bark and resin (kath).

Dosage : Bark powder - 1.5 gm; **Decoction** : 30-50 ml; **Kath** : 0.5 to 0.75 gms.

Formulations : Khadirarishta, Khadiradi quath, Khadirashtak, Khadiradivati, Irimedadi taila. (Kath is prepared by boiling the branches of khadir in water and then solidifying it. People doing this business are called Katkari)

Srotogamitva :

Dosha : Reduces pitta, kapha.

Dhatu : Rakta, meda (anaemia), shukra.

Mala : Urine.

Prabhav : Kushthaghna.

References -

खदिरो रक्तसारश्च गायत्री दन्तधावनः । कण्टकी बालपत्रश्च बहुशल्यश्च यज्ञियः ।।
खदिरः शीतलो दन्त्यः कण्डुकासारुचिप्रणुत् । तिक्तः कषायो मेदोघ्नः कृमिमेहज्वरव्रणान् ।।
श्वित्रशोथामपित्तास्रपाण्डुकुष्ठकफान् हरेत् ।' (भा.प्र.)
'खदिरस्तु रसे तिक्तः शीतपित्तकफापहः । पाचनः कुष्ठकासास्रशोथककण्डूव्रणापहः ।।' (रा.नि.)
'खदिरः कृमिकुष्ठघ्नः कफरेतोविशोषणः ।' (ध.नि.)
'खदिरः कुष्ठघ्नानाम् ।' (च.सू. २५)
'शनैर्मेहिन खदिरकषायम् ।' (सु.चि. ११)
'दिदृक्षुरन्तं कुष्ठस्य खदिरं कुष्ठपीडितः । सर्वथैव प्रयुञ्जीत स्नानपानाशनादिषु ।।' (सु.चि. ९)
'यथा सर्वाणि कुष्ठानि हतः खदिरबीजकौ । तथैवार्शांसि सर्वाणि वृक्षकारुष्करौ हतः ।।' (सु.चि. ६)

Human body is examined by touching different parts of the body. Similarly, plants should be examined by touching its leaves, flowers and fruits.

(36) GUGGULU

Commiphora mukul Hook ex stocks.

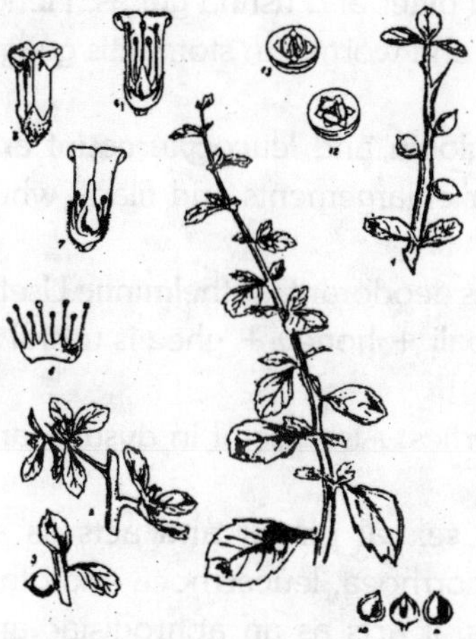

Gana : Eladi (S.) Vedanasthapan.
Family : Byrseraceae of Bursera family named after Burser.
Latin name: Commiphora (phore = bearer); mukul (Arabic).
English name : Gum - Guggul, Indian bedellium.
Sanskrit names : Guggul (protects from diseases), Deodhoop, Mahishaksha (seen blakish like buffallo's eyes), Palankash (pal-flesh), Kashi (scraping - reduces fat in obese person), Kumbha Deveshta, Rakshouha, Jatayu.
Botanical Description : Tree - 1.5 - 2 mtrs high. Leaves - similar to Melia azadirachta leaves,composite , leaflets sessile to subsessile. Flowers- brownish, five petals. Fruits - pulpy, round and red coloured. Gum - (gum resin) thick, scented, multicoloured, burnt on fire, liquefies in sun heat. When dissolved in water, it turns milky white. Guggul tree is small and thorny.
Varieties : Five varieties based on colour.
1. Mahishaksha - (Mhashya guggul) black, for human use, 2. Mahaneed - blue, 3. Kumud - white, 4. Padma - brown, for animal use, 5. Kanak - (Kanaguggul) - yellow, for human use.
Two varieties of guggul are sold commercially; 1. Kana guggul - it is found in marwar, greenish yellow, soft and grannular, 2. Bhaisa (Mhasha) guggul - is found in Sindh and Kutch, greenish yellow but brittle and soft. Medicinal guggul is known as kanaguggul.
Identification test for purity : Pure guggul is singdha, soft, sticky with sweet smell, bitter taste, yellowish tinge, soluble in water, not contaminated with mud or sand. Any variety other than these qualities should be considered as impure. Potency lasts for twenty years.
Habitat : Marwar, Sindh, Kutch, Mysore, Assam, East Bengal, Arabia and Africa.
Collection : In summer, due to heat of the sun, gum of guggul melts and oozes from the tree and gets solidified in winter when it is to be collected.
Chemical composition : Contains essential oil, resin, gum, and bitter principle.
Properties :
Guna : laghu, tikshna, snigdha, pichchil, sukshma and sara; **Rasa :** tikta, katu, madhur, kashaya; **Vipak :** katu; **Veerya :** ushna; **Parbhav :** tridoshahara.
Dosha : Vataghna by madhur, ushna, snigdha and pichchil; pittaghna - by kashaya and madhur rasa; kaphaghna by tikta, katu and tikshna; thus guggul is useful in disorders induced by tridosha.
External uses : Anti inflammatory, analgesic, cleaning of wound and healing due to antibacterial action . Paste of guggul is locally applied in rheumatoid arthritis, cervical lymphadenitis, skin diseases, piles etc. It reduces foul smell and swelling of wound. Its vapours are useful as deodorant and disinfectant in the house. Gargling is useful in pyorrhoea and dental disorders.
Internal uses :
Nervous system : Vatashamak, analgesic, nervine tonic, so guggul is useful in neuralgia, rheumatoid

In archeological excavations, it is discovered that the organic matter in bones is destroyed and they become porous. The same process may be taking place in osteoporosis.

arthritis, sciatica, facial paralysis, hemiplegia and gout etc. It is well known and popular medicine for vata disorders. Triphala + guggul is a popular medicine given internally in wounds.

Digestive system : It is an appetizer by pungent and bitterness; laxative by snigdha, pichchila,sara and tikshna; liver stimulant, antihaemorrhoidal and anthelmintic by bitter and ushna gunas. Hence guggul is useful in loss of appetite, constipation, liver diseases, piles and worms. In stomatitis guggul kept in the mouth helps in wound healing.

Circulatory system : It is a cardiac tonic. It increases haemoglobin and leucocyte count and enhances blood quality. It helps in oedema, lynphadenitis, glandur enlargements and filaria when given for a longer period.

Respiratory system : Expectorant being snigdha and pichchila. It is deodorant, anthelmintic.Useful in chronic cough and chronic asthma. Preparation of guggul +pippali + honey + ghee is useful in kapha disorders.

Urinary system : Lithotryptic due to tikshna and diuretic properties. Also useful in dysuria and gonorrhoea.

Reproductive system : Guggul is ushna, tikshna, increases sexual power and acts as an emmenagogue. It is also useful in oligosperima, impotency, dysmenorrhoea, leucorrhoea and other gynaecological diseases. Due to snigdha and pichchila properties, it acts as an aphrodisiac and antiinfertility.

Satmikaran : Guggul works on all tissues of body and is effective in rejuvenating body tissues and increasing strength. Fresh guggul is useful in weakness and loss of weight, but on becoming old, is useful in diabetes and obesity. It is also a good rasayan in obesity and diseases of vatakapha. It also helps in digestion of oil and ghee.

Skin : Effective in dermatoses, enhances complexion and useful in many skin diseases.

Temperature : Sheetaprashamak by ushna property, its vapours are useful in typhoid.

Parts used : Gumresin (guggul is purified by boiling in cow's milk in dolayantra.)

Dosage : 0.5 to 1.5 gms. (ghee is used as anupan).

Formulations : It has been used in plenty of formulations. Formulations like gokshuradi, yograj, mahayogaraj, saptavinshati, kaishor, chandraprabha vati etc.

Avoid sour food, concentrated alcohol, indigestion, sexual intercourse, exercises, roaming in sun light and anger.

Caution : In Ayurveda it is mentioned that guggul is very useful, still one has to be careful about injudicious use of it. The dose should be adequate. Misuse of guggul leads to pathological changes in liver and lungs while excess dose causes vertigo, dryness of mouth, impotency, loss of weight, and dryness of skin. Guggul should not be used in patients with above complaints.

Treatment : Saffron is used as an antidote.

Substitute : In absence of guggul Commiphora myrrh is used.

Srotogamitva :

Dosha : Kaphaghna, vataghna, pittashodhak and tridoshaghna.

Dhatu : Mansa, meda (brihan - increases body weight), asthi - promotes union of fractures, shukra - promotes fertility, rasayan - old -medokarshan.

To maintain good health, one must have (1) rochan (2) deepan (3) pachan (4) sangrahan and (5) utsarjan, in that order.

Mala : Purisha, mutra (in renal stone).
Organs : Madhyam marg.
Black guggul : Rakta and pittagami.
Yellow guggul : Kapha and pittagami.
White guggul : Vata and pittagami.
Potency of guggul lasts for twenty years, so guggul has been used in many fromulations in combination with other drugs.

References -
'सुगंधि: सुलघु: सूक्ष्मस्तीक्ष्णोष्ण: कटुकोरस: । कटुपाक: सरो हृद्योगुग्गुल: स्निग्धपिच्छिल: ।
स नवो बृंहणो वृष्य: पुराणस्त्वतिलेखन: । तैक्ष्ण्यौष्ण्यात कफवातघ्न: सरत्वान्मलपित्तनुत् ।
सौगन्ध्यात् पूतिकोष्ठघ्न: सौक्ष्म्याच्चानलदीपन: ।' (सु.)
'गुग्गुलुर्देवधूपश्च जटायु: कौशिक: पुर: । कुम्भोलूखलकं क्लीबे महिषाक्ष: पलंकष: ।।
महिषाक्षो महानील: कुमुद: पदम इत्यपि । हिरण्य: पञ्चमो ज्ञेयो गुग्गुलो: पञ्च जातय: ।
भृङ्गाञ्जनसवर्णस्तु महिषाक्ष इति स्मृत: । महानीलस्तु विज्ञेय: स्वनामसमलक्षण: ।।
कुमुद: कुमुदाभ: स्यात् पद्मो माणिक्यसंनिभ: । हिरण्याख्यस्तु हेमाभ: पञ्चानां लिंगमीरितम् ।
महिषाक्षो महानीलो गजेन्द्राणां हितावुभौ । हयानां कुमुद: पद्म: स्वस्त्यारोग्यकरौ परौ ।
विशेषेण मनुष्यानां कनक: परिकीर्तित: । कदाचिन्महिषाक्षश्च मत: कैश्चिन्नृणामपि ।।
गुग्गुलुर्विशदस्तिक्तो वीर्योष्ण: पित्तल: सर: । कषाय: कटुक: पाके कटुरूक्षो लघु: पर: ।।
मग्नसन्धानकृदवृष्य: सूक्ष्म: स्वर्यो रसायन: । दीपन: पिच्छिलो बल्य: कफवातव्रणापची: ।।
मेदोमेहाश्मवातांश्च क्लेदकुष्ठाश्ममारुतान् । पिडकाग्रन्तिर्शोफाशोगंडमालाकृमीञ्जयेत् ।।
माधुर्याच्छमयेद्वातं कषायत्वाच्च पित्तहा । तिक्तत्वात् कफजित्तेन गुग्गुल: सर्वदोषहा ।।
स नवो बृहणो वृष्य: पुराणस्त्वतिलेखन: । स्निग्ध: काञ्चनसंकाश: पक्वजम्बूफलोपम: ।।
नूतनो गुग्गुलु: प्रोक्त: सुगन्धिर्यस्तु पिच्छिल: । शुष्को दुर्गन्धिकश्चैव त्यक्तप्रकृतिवर्णक: ।।
पुराण: स तु विज्ञेयो गुग्गुलुर्वीर्यवर्जित: ।
अम्लं तीक्ष्णमजीर्णं च व्यवायं श्रममातपम् । मद्य रोषं त्यजेत् सम्यग् गुणार्थी पुरसेवक: ।।' (भा.प्र.)
मरुभूमिषु जायन्ते प्रायश: पुरपादपा: । भानोर्मयूखै: सन्तप्ता: ग्रीष्मे मुञ्चन्ति गुग्गुलुम हिमान्विते हेमन्ते च विधिना तं समाहरेत् ।'
आतपैस्तेविलीयन्तेक्षिप्ताश्चाग्नौज्वलन्तिहि । स्वभावविशदा: स्निग्धा: स्वामोदा: कण्ठशोधना: ।।
सर्वे समानवीर्यास्ते सर्वे रसगुणै: समा: । आस्वादे तिक्तकटुका: कषाया: स्वादव: परम् ।।'
'कृष्ण: शोणितपित्ते च श्लेष्मपित्ते च पिंगल: । वातपित्ते तथा श्वेतो गुग्गुल: शस्यते परम् ।। (क.नि.)
वन्हौ ज्वलन्ति तपने विलयं प्रयान्ति, क्लिद्यन्ति कोष्णसलिले पयसा समाना: ।
ग्राह्या: शुभा: परिहरेच्चिरकालजातानङ्गारवर्णसमपूयविगन्धवर्णान् ।।' (प्रयोगामृत)

(37) GUDUCHI

Tinospora cordifolia Willd Meirs.

Gana :Vayasthapan, Dahaprashaman, Trushnanigrahan, Stanyashodhan, Truptighna (C.), Guduchyadi, Patoladi, Aragwadhadi, Kakolyadi, Vallipanchamool (S.)
Kula : Guduchi kula.
Family : Menispermaceae - meni = moon , sperm = seed; moonlike seed.

Dose of a medicine should be either increased or decreased in conjunction with increased or decreased rasaprudhan diet.

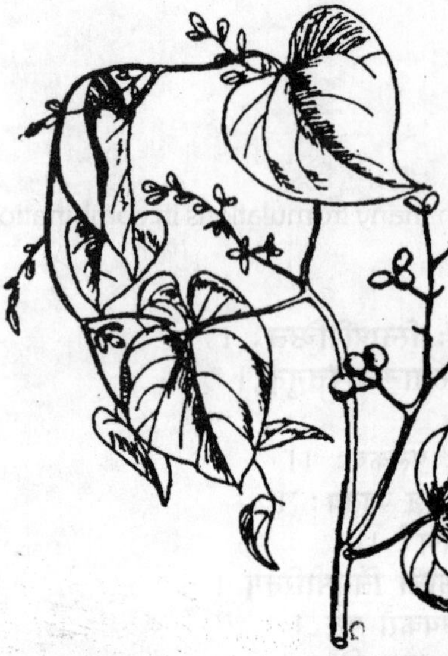

Latin name : Tinospora cordium. The plant stitches like a bow with the seeds curved around the intruder endocarp and the heart shaped leaves at the base.

Sanskrit names : Guduchi (one which protects the body), Madhuparnika, Chhinnodbhava, Amruta, Vishalya, Chakralakshana, Tandrika, Jvaranashi.

Botanical Description : It is a long lasting creeper climbing over the trees like mango, neem etc. The stem is covered by transparent layer and can be peeled off. It has many tentacles hanging down. Leaves - heart shaped, individualized, pointed at the tip and slimy. Flowers- small yellow flowers appearing in clusters. Fruits - bean shaped, appearing red on ripening and flourish in cold and moderate climate.

Varieties : Padmaguduchi and Kandaguduchi (has large tri-fissured leaves with number of buds on the stem - hence the name Kanda).

Habitat : All over India.

Properties : **Guna** : laghu, singdha; **Rasa** : tikta, kashay; **Vipak** : madhur; **Veerya** : ushna; **Prabhav** : vishaghna.

Karma : Tridoshashamak and pittasarak.

External uses : Antiseptic and analgesic. Guduchyadi oil is used in common skin conditions and gout.

Internal uses :

Digestive system : Controls emesis and thirst, appetizer, digestive, eristaltic, anthelmintic and antacid.

Circulatory system : Cardiotonic, haemopoetic and acts specifically on vata - rakta.

Respiratory system : Anti-inflammatory and anti-secretory action is observed.

Reproductive system : Aphrodisiac.

Urinary system : Anti-diabetic, promotive.

Skin : Useful in number of common skin infections (should be used along with guggulu, haridra neem, khadir and amla).

Temperature : Antipyretic, specially effective in chronic fevers.

Satmikaran : It is known to be a good restorative - tikta, balya, rasayani.

Usage : In tridoshas, ghee + guduchi - vatashamak; sugar + guduchi - pittashamak; honey + gudduchi - kaphashamak.

Indications :

External : Guduchi oil is used for massage in dermatoses, gout etc.

There is a tremendous difference between growing a tree and cutting it. Cutting does not take more than five minutes but to grow a tree even fifty years are sometimes not enough.

Internal :
Digestive system : Useful in thirst, vomiting, loss of appetite, abdominal pain, liver disorders, jaundice, acid-peptic disorder, dysentery, sprue and worms. It increases appetite.
Circulatory system : Raktavahasrotogami. Guduchi satva is effective in cardiac debility, blood disorders, rheumatoid arthritis, splenomegaly, gout and anaemia.
Respiratory system : Useful in cough.
Reproductive system : Aphrodisiac being shukragami, snigdha and madhur vipak.
Urinary system : Effective in prameha, mainly in diabetes and disorders of urinary bladder.
Skin : It is used in skin disorders like dermatoses and erysepalas etc. It is also useful in syphillitic ulcer.
Temperature : Juice of guduchi is used in chronic fever and typhoid fever. It reduces burning, normalises temperature, improves appetite and increases the strength.
Satmikaran : Useful in weakness and pthisis and good rasayan for all seven dhatus.
Part used : Bark.
Dosage : Decoction - 60 -100 ml.; powder - 1-3 gms; satva - 3/4 - 2 gms.
Formulations : Guduchyadi churna, Guduchyadi kwath, Guduci loha, Amrutarishta, Guduchi Taila.
Srotogamitva :
Dosha : Tridosha.
Dhatu : Rakta, meda, dravdhatu, shukra (aphrodisiac), rasayani.
Mala : Mutra.
Organs : Liver, kidney and spleen.
References -
'गुडूची कटुका तिक्ता स्वादुपाका रसायनी । संग्राहिणी कषायोष्णा लघ्वी बल्याग्निदीपनी ।।
दीषत्रयामतृङ्दाहमेहकासांश्च पाण्डुताम् । कामलाकुष्ठवातास्त्रज्वरकृमिवमीहरित् ।।' (भा.प्र.)
'अमृता साग्राहिक-वातहर-दीपनीय-श्लेष्मशोणितविबन्धप्रशमनानाम् ।' (च.सू.२५)
ज्ञेया गुडूची गुरुरुष्णवीर्या तिक्ता कषाया ज्वरनाशिनी च ।
दाहार्त्तितृष्णावमिरक्तवातप्रमेहपाण्डुभ्रमहारिणी च ।।' (रा.नि)
'कन्दोद्भवा गुडूची च कटूष्णा सनिपातहा । विषघ्नी ज्वरभूतघ्नी वलीपलितनाशिनी ।।' (ध.नि.)
'अमृतायाः शतं चूर्णं वाससा परिशोधितम् । पृथक् षोडशभागाः स्युः गुडमाक्षिकसर्पिषाम् ।।
यथाग्निः भक्षयदेतन्नरो हितमिताशनः । नास्य कश्चिद् भवेद् व्याधिः न जरा पलितं न च ।।' (भा.प्र.)

(38) GOKSHUR
Tribulus terrestris Linn.

Gana : Mutravirechan, Shothahar, Krimighna, Anuvasanopag, Vidarigandhadi, Veertarvadi, Laghupachamoola (C.), Kantakpanchamola, Vatashmaribhedan (S.)
Kula : Gokshur kula.
Family : Zygophyllaceae (yokeleaf) (zygo = bones of human face yoke), phyllus = leaves.
Latin name : Tribulus = having three sides; terrestris = of the ground.
English name : Small Caltrops.

Trees do not live for themselves. They do not smell their own flowers, eat their own fruits or enjoy their own shade.

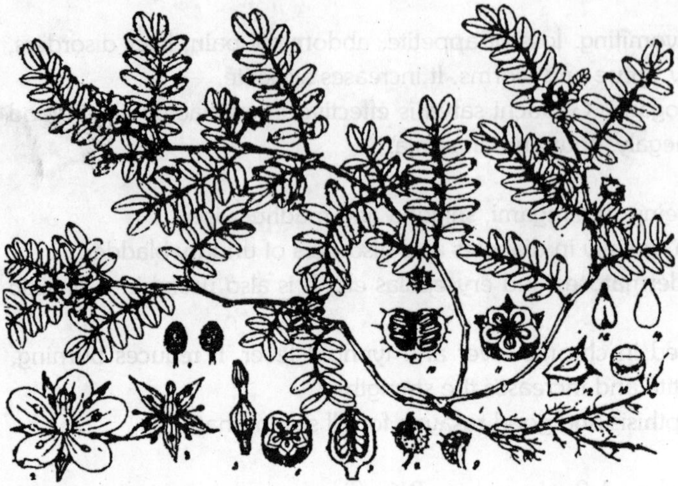

Sanskrit names : Gokshur (Go=organ, kshurati =damaging - causing damage to organs), Gokantak (Go = sticks to leg of cow while grazing), Swadanshthra (like dog's teeth), Trikantak, Vanasharungat, Chanadroom , Kshurak, Palankasha, Kantaphal, Bhakshyatak, Kantaki.

Botanical Description : Shrub spreads on land with 0.5-1 mtr. of height. Branches spread from all the sides. Leaves -like that of gram plant. Flowers- small, yellow coloured with five petals. Fruits - slightly pentagonal having 2-3 sharp thorns. Seeds- many, contain scented oil. Roots - 10-13 cms. long, smoky with slightly strong smell and sweet. Flowering occurs in autumn followed by fruiting.

Varieties : Two 1. Bruhat(large) - Pedaliaceae family, Pedalium murex, having large leaves and fruits; 2. Laghu (small) - which is described above.

Habitat : All over India, specially North and South India.

Properties :

Guna : guru, snigdha; **Rasa :** madhur; **Veerya :** sheeta; **Vipak :** madhur.

Karma :

Dosha : Vatapittakaphashamak.

External use : Leaves are tied on wounds.

Internal uses :

Nervous system : Analgesic and vatashamak. Therefore used in neural debility, painful conditions and vata disorders.

Digestive system : Stomachic, astringent, anthelmintic, but laxative in large dose. Therefore it is used in low appetite, piles and helminthiasis.

Circulatory system : It is a cardiotonic, antiinflammatory and helps in haemorrhagic disorders.It is used in heart diseases. Fruit juice is useful in amoebiasis and splenomegaly.

Respriatory system : Expectorant, therefore used in cough and asthma.

Reproductive system : It is an aphrodisiac and helps in conception, useful in preventing abortion, vaginal disorders, impotency and post-natal discharges.

Urinary system : Diuretic, dissolves calculi and amorphous calculi. Therefore useful in urinary calcúli, dysuria and cystitis. Fresh leaves dipped in water make it slimy, this water is used for medicinal purposes.

Satmikaran : Useful in debility.

Parts used : Fruit, root, pentad.

Doses : Fruit powder - 2.5 to 5gms., decoction - 60 to 100 ml.

To cultivate healthy forests, it is essentail to cut old trees. It is like sharir shodhan (panchakarma) done for good health.

Formulations : Gokshuradichurna, Gokshuradi-avaleha, Gokshuradi guggul, Gokshuradi kwath, Dashmoolarista (ingredient of dashmool).

Srotogamitva :

Dosha : Tridoshashamak.

Dhatu : Shukra (aphrodisiac), mansa-meda, raktagami (spleen).

Mala : Mutra (dysuria, calculi).

Organ : Urinary bladder, heart, urinary tract, intestine.

Note : Gokshur is very effective in dysuria.

References -

'गोक्षुरः शीतलः स्वादुर्बलकृद्वस्तिशोधनः । मधुरो दीपनो वृष्यः पुष्टिदश्चाश्मरीहर. ।।
प्रमेहश्वासकासार्शः कृच्छ्रहृद्रोगवातनुत् ।' (भा.प्र.)
'गोक्षुरको मूत्रकृच्छ्रानिलहराणाम् ।' (च.सू. २५)
'त्रिकण्टस्य बीजानां चूर्ण माक्षिकसंयुतम् । अविक्षीरेण सप्ताहमश्मरीभेदनं पिबेत् ।।' (सु.चि. ७)
चूर्ण श्वदंष्ट्राफलवाजिगन्धाविनिर्मितं माक्षिकसंप्रयुक्तम् ।
क्षीरेण सार्धं परिपीयमानं शोथं च कासं च निहन्ति पुंसाम् ।' (रा.मा.)

(39) GANDHAPRASARANI
Paederia foetida Linn.

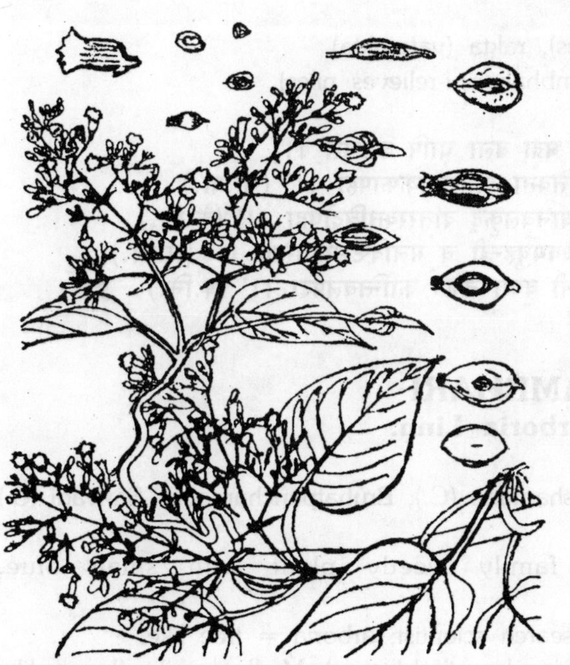

Kula : Manjishtha kula.

Family : Rubiaceae - Rubus = red-dye, a family for the edible products, dyes and drugs.

Latin name : Paederia = rank odour of all the parts when bruised; foetida = bad smell.

English name : Chinese flower plant.

Sanskrit names : Prasarani, Sarani, Bhadraparni, Rajabala, Pratanini, Bhadra, Bala, Katambhara.

Botanical Description : It is a long creeper. Leaves - grow on alternate side of the stem at regular intervals. Flowers - bluish, red, having 6 petals. Fruit - having feather-like shape, yellow coloured, round and 1 cm long. Seeds - small. Flowering season is at the end of monsoon and autumn and fruiting starts in winter.

Habitat : Marshy land, eastern Himalayas upto 3000 mts. and also Nepal, Assam, Bengal. (It should be collected in autumn. It becomes ineffective after drying).

Chemical composition : It contains a volatile oil having an offensive odour and two alkaloids, alpha paederine and beta paedirine.

"Vitamin A" deficiency can be cured by leaves of drumsticks (Moringa oleifera).

Properties :
Guna : guru, sara; **Rasa** : tikta; **Vipak** : katu; **Veerya** : ushna.
Karma :
Dosha : Kaphavatanashak by ushna veerya. Also pittasarak. Useful in disorders induced by kapha and vata.
External use : Analgesic, anti-inflammatory. Therefore it is used in all the vata disorders. It is the best medicine for it.
Internal use :
Digestive system : It is an antiflatulent and mild laxative. So it is used in abdominal pain, flatulence and constipation with hard stool. Cooked leaves or the warm paste of leaves is given in abdominal pain.
Circulatory system : It purifies the blood by its tikta rasa and alleviates vata by its ushna veerya. Therefore it is used in vatarakta.
Reproductive system : Aphrodisiac by guru property. So used in infertility.
Satmikaran : Bitter tonic, mainly used as a tonic in vata disorders and fever.
Parts used : Roots and leaves.
Dosage : Juice 1 to 2 tsp.; decoction 100 ml.
Formulations : Prasarini taila, Prasarini leha.
Srotogamitva :
Dosha : Tridoshaghni.
Dhatu : Shukra (aphrodisiac), asthi (bones), rakta (vatarakta).
Mala : Purisha (mild laxative), (malavishtambhaharini-relieves piles).
References -
'प्रसारिणी राजबला भद्रपर्णी प्रतानिनी । सरणी सारणी भद्रा बला चापि कटंभरा ।।
प्रसारिणी गुरुर्वृष्या बलसंधानकृत्सरा । वीर्योष्णा वातकृत्तिक्ता वातरक्तकफापहा ।।' (भा.प्रा.)
प्रसारिणी सरा तिक्ता वीर्योष्णा शुक्रला गुरुः । वर्णसन्धानबलकृद् वातररक्तत्रिदोषहा ।।' (कै.नि.)
'प्रसारिणी गुरूष्णा च तिक्ता वातविनाशिनी । अर्शः श्वयथुहन्त्री च मलविष्टम्भहारिणी ।।' (रा.नि.)
'प्रसारिणी गुरुस्तिक्ता सरा सन्धानकृन्मता । त्रिदोषशमनी वृष्या तेजः कान्तिबलप्रदा ।।' (ध.नि.)
संग्रहकाल - 'समूलपत्रामुत्पाट्य शरत्काले प्रसारिणीम् ।'

(40) GAMBHARI
Gmelina arboria Linn.

Gana : Shothahara, Virechanopaga, Dahaprashamana (C.); Bruhatpanchamoola, Sarivadi (S.)
Kula : Nirgundi kula.
Family : Verbenaceae. The vervain family weedy plant with small blue, white, purple flowers.
Latin name : Gamelina = name of the research scientist; arboria = tree like.
Sanskrit names : Mahabhava, Shriparni (having beautiful leaves), Madhuparnika (honey like sweet taste of the leaves), Kashmari, Pita-rohini (having yellow flowers), Kashmiri (as it grows in Kashmir), Bhadraparni, Madhurasa, Gopabhadra.

Combination of blue and yellow makes green colour. Matured leaves and fruits become yellow. Does that mean that the blue colour is removed from them ?

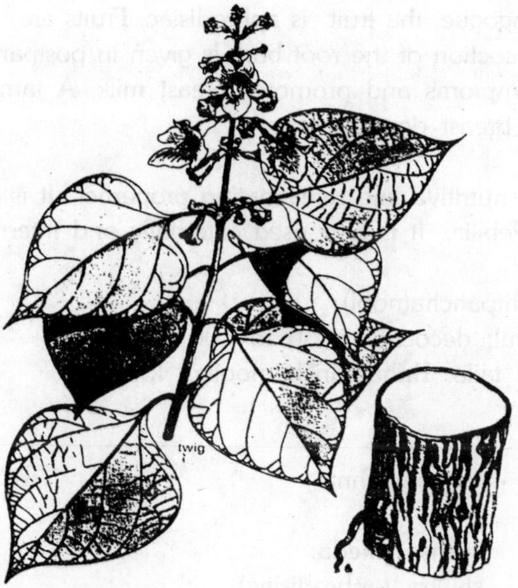

Botanical Description : Large tree of height 13 to 20 mts. Bark is white. Leaves - long and broad. Petiole - long like pippal leaf, 7cm long. Leaves are heart shaped, having thin and sharp ends. Flowers - yellow and resemble vasa flowers. Fruit - oval shaped like bakul fruits. They are yellow having sweet, astringent taste and odour. If the tree is on the river bank and if it falls in water, it spreads fragrance all over. Seeds - each fruit has 2 to 3 seeds. The tree flowers in spring while fruits in summer.

Habitat : The tree grows in the hilly areas of the Himalayas, Nilgiri and also on the eastern and western coast of India.

Chemical composition : Its root contains a thick yellow oil, resin, an alkaloid and benzoic acid. Fruit contains butyric and tartaric acid, an alkaloid, sugar, resin and astringent component in less quantity.

Properties :

Guna : guru; **Rasa** : madhur, tikta, kashaya; **Vipak** : madhur; **Veerya** : ushna but ripe fruit is sheeta veerya.

Dosha : Tridoshashamak, pittashamak by kashaya, tikta and vatakaphanashak by ushna veerya. Therefore useful in the disorders caused by all the three doshas.

External uses : Because of cooling and soothing actions, the leaves relieve burning and pain. In such cases, leaves are tied to the affected part. Paste of the leaves is applied over the forehead in case of headache caused by fever.

Internal uses :

Central Nervous system : It is used in vertigo, brain debility and vata disorders. It is also a brain tonic.

Digestive system : Fruit - relieves excessive thirst; root - aperient, improves appetite and digestion, so used in diarrhoea, constipation and haemorrhoids.

Circulatory system : The bark of the root is used internally in oedema due to any cause, as it is relieves oedema. Its ripe fruit is cardiotonic. Its juice is useful in cardiac disorders and the mixture of roots of gambhari + gunja leaves + yashtimadhu + sugar with milk is a good galactogogue.

Respiratory system : Ripe fruit is a nutritive tonic, so useful in tuberculosis and cachexia.

Urinary system : Fruits and leaves are diuretic. The juice is given in dysuria, gonorrhoea and cystitis. In such cases if the juice is given along with cow's milk and sugar, it increases urination, relieves pain and swelling.

Under the guise of religion, almost all rituals are planned to benefit physical and mental health.

Reproductive system : Besides being a galactagogue, the fruit is aphrodisiac. Fruits are used in semen debility and to prevent miscarriage. Decoction of the root bark is given in postpartum disorders. It relieves uteritis, fever and other symptoms and promotes breast milk. A tampon of oil derived from gambhari juice is kept for breast development.
Temperature : Relieves fever and burning.
Satmikaran : The bark is a bitter tonic having nutritive and rejuvenating properties. It is also an antidote. The bark is used in post pyrexial debility. It is also used externally and internally in scorpion and snake bite.
Parts used : Root and fruit (one of the brihatpanchamool).
Dosage : Juice of the root bark 12 to 20 ml; decoction - 50 to 100 ml.
Formulations : Shriparnyadi kwath, Shriparni taila, Brihatpanchamooladi kwath.
Srotogamitva :

	Root	**Fruit**
Dosha :	Pittavataghna, Kaphavardhak.	Vatapittaghna
Dhatu :	Majja (brain tonic)	Mansa, meda, shukra (aphrodisiac), majja (brain tonic)
Mala :	Purisha (cathartic)	Rakta, hair tonic.

References -
'काश्मरी तुवरा तिक्ता वीर्योष्णा मधुरा गुरु: । दीपनी पाचनी मेध्या भेदनी भ्रमशोथजित् ।।
दोषतृष्णामशुलार्शोविषदाहरज्वरापहा । तत्फलं बृंहणं वृष्यं गुरु केश्यं रसायनम् ।।
वातपित्ततृषारक्तक्षयमूत्रविबन्धनुत् । स्वादु पाके हिमं स्निग्धं तुवराम्लं विशुद्धिकृत् ।।
हृदयाद् दाहतृषावातरक्तपित्तक्षतयान् ।' (भा.प्र.)
हृद्यं मूत्रविबन्धघ्नं पित्तासृग्वातनाशनम् । केश्यं रसायनं मेध्यं काश्मर्यं फ्रलमुच्यते ।।' (सु.सू. ४६)
'काश्मर्यफलं रक्तसांग्राहिकरक्तपित्तप्रशमनानाम् ।' (च.सू. २५)
... 'काश्मर्यतैलानि मधुरकरषायणि कफपित्तप्रशमनानि ।' (सु.सू. ४५)

(41) CHANDANA
Santalum alba Linn.

Gana : Dahaprashaman, Angamardaprashaman, Trishnanigrahan, Varnya, Kandooghna, Vishaghna, Tiktaskandha (C.); Salasaradi, Patoladi, Sarivadi, Priyangwadi, Guduchyadi, Pittasamshaman (S.)
Kula : Chandana kula.
Family : Santalacae; Santal = derived from the word chandana, from that 'sandalwood'.
Latin name : Santalum - from Greek word Santalon. Chandana -Sanskrit name - Gladening aroma and medicinal properties; alba = white.
English name : Sandalwood.
Sanskrit names : Shrikanda, Gandhasara, Chandradyuti, Shwetachandana, Sheetala, Sarvapriya, Rajayogya.
Botanical Description : Evergreen tree, 12-14 mtrs. high. Bark is dusty black externally while

Previously nobody thought of pollution caused by industrial revolution. It has now become imperative to think about pollution and formulate a plan to deal with it.

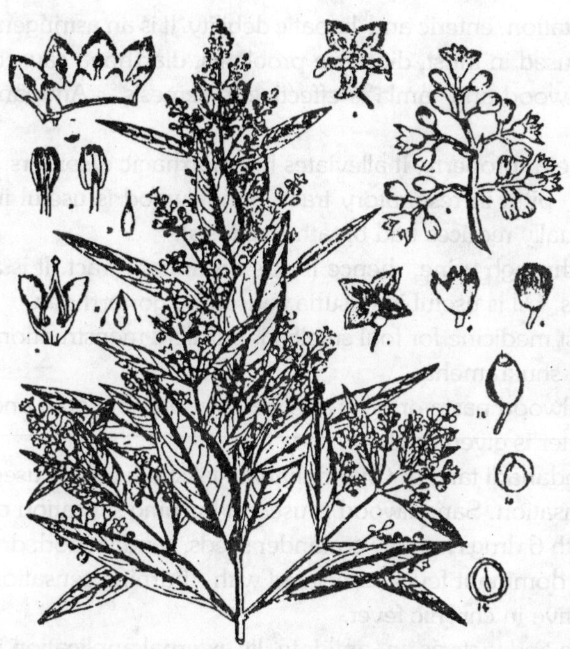

reddish within. Bark has vertical striations. The heart of the wood is white and odourless externally but inner part is greyish yellow, aromatic and hard, contains oil. Leaves - 2.5 to 5 cms. long, oval, green with tapering ends. Flowers - have yellowish shade and are brinjal coloured. Fruit - round having diameter 1 cm. Ripe fruit is black. Its leaves, bark and flowers are odourless. The tree bears flowers from rainy season till winter and then fruiting occurs. Fruits are called as 'chandana charoli'. The tree takes 50 years for complete growth. Young tree doesn't have aroma.

Varieties : Some people call outer heart of the wood as 'white sandalwood' and inner heart as 'yellow sandalwood'. There are 7 varieties described in Raj Nighantu according to region and fragrance.

Habitat : Originally sandalwood trees grew widely in Karnataka, Kurg and Kerala. The tree also grows very well in stony parts of mountains and more oil is derived from it. In Maharashtra, many trees are found in the gardens. Mainly Persian society cultivates these trees more. The fire temples of Parsis are always kept alighted with holy-fire of sandalwood. But these are of low quality.

Chemical composition : 3 to 6% volatile oil is derived from the heartwood and roots. Roots contain comparatively more oil. 125 gm of oil can be derived from 20 kgs. of sandalwood. This oil is yellow, thick, having fragrance, bitter and pungent. Sandalwood oil contains 90% santalol.

Pieces of margosa wood perfumed with sandalwood are sold in the market. But since it is cheap, people buy it. 'Malaygiri' sandalwood of best quality is available in the fire temples of Parsis. Sandalwood oil is available in small jars of aluminium. To test good quality of sandalwood - it is bitter to taste and becomes yellow after rubbing. The wood is white and hard externally and red after pricking. The best is which has strong scent. Malayagiri sandalwood is the best sandalwood.

Properties :

Guna : laghu, ruksha; **Rasa :** tikta, madhur; **Vipak :** katu; **Veerya :** sheeta.

Karma :

Dosha : Pittashamak, kaphashamak. Useful in disorders induced by pitta and kapha.

External uses : The (thin) paste is refrigerant, deodorant, complexion enhancer and cures skin disorders. It is used in burning sensation of different organs, erysipelas, dermatoses caused by pitta, discolouration of skin. It is used as deodorant in diaphoresis. Sandalwood oil is used in ear discharges. It acts as a deodorant and heals the wounds.

Central nervous system : It is beneficial to brain and pleases the mind. It is useful in mental irritability, mental debility and brain impairment.

Every physician must recognize his own limitations. If a disease can be cured by surgery, he should advise it.

Digestive system : It alleviates thirst, gastric irritation, enteric and hepatic debility. It is an astringent and vermicide. Because of these activities, it is used in thirst, digestive problems, diarrhoea caused by pitta, dysentery and worms. A lick of sandalwood and amla is effective in emesis. Anupan-honey.
Circulatory system : It is a cardiotonic by sheeta property. It alleviates haemorrhagic disorders.
Respiratory system : It alleviates kapha and pitta in respiratory tract. Sandalwood is useful in hemoptysis and purulent expectoration. It gradually reduces bad breath (halitosis).
Urinary system : Sandalwood oil is excreted through urine, hence it acts on urinary tract. It is a mutragami dravya. Useful in dysuria and cystitis. Oil is useful in dysuria caused by gonorrhoea.
Reproductive system : Sandalwood is the best medicine for foul smelling, purulent menstruation. It is also used in menorrhagia, leucorrhoea and shukrameha.
Skin : It cures dermatoses and pruritus. Sandalwood paste or oil is applied over burning area and pruritus caused due to eczema. Sandalwood water is given orally.
Temperature : Febrifuge and refrigerant. Chandanadi taila or Chandanabala-lakshadi taila is used for massage in fever associated with burning sensation. Sandalwood is used in burning sensation of internal organs. Shadangodaka (water boiled with 6 drugs namely coriander seeds, sandalwood, dry ginger, parpat, khas and ambu) is given in pitta dominant fever associated with burning sensation and thirst. A thin paste of sandalwood is effective in chronic fever.
Satmikaran : It alleviates generalised bodyache and acts as an antidote. Its external application is used in swelling caused due to poison or vitiated pitta. It can be given orally.
Parts used : Heartwood, oil.
Dosage : Powder- 2 to5 gms; oil - 5 to 20 drops.
Formulations : Chandanadi churna, Chandanadi vati, Chandanasava, Chandanabala-lakshadi taila.
Srotogamitva :
Dosha : Pittakaphaghna (burning-pitta).
Dhatu : Rakta medagami, rakta (haemorrhagic disorders).
Mala : Mutramargagami.
Organs : Urinary bladder, urinary system, skin - (refrigerant).
References -
'चन्दनं दुर्गन्धहरदाहनिर्वापणलेपनानाम् ।' (च.सू. २५)
'चन्दनं शीतलं रूक्षं तिक्तमाल्हादनं लघु । श्रमशोषविषश्लेष्मतृष्णापित्तास्रदाहनुत् ।।' (भा.प्र.)

(42) CHANGERI

Oxalis corniculata Linn.

Kula : Changeri kula.
Family : Geraniaceae - of geranian family, (Geranium = green house and border), (geranose - crane cranis = bill).
Latin name : Oxalis = source of oxalic acid; corniculata - corni = horn, having hornlike appendages.

Plants can efficiently provide four basic necessities of human beings viz. food, clothes, shelter and health.

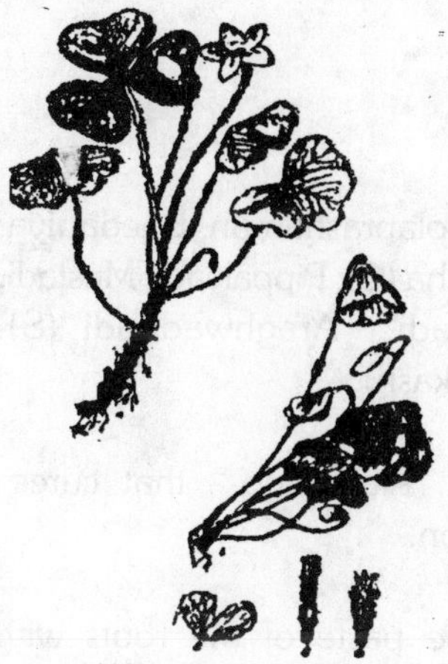

English name : Indian Sorrel.
Sanskrit names : Changeri, Amlaparnika, Triparni.
Botanical Description : It is a small shrub growing in moisture and petioles are long. It has three conjugated leaves. Flower - small, yellow. Fruit - oval. Seeds -are many. Flowering and fruiting occur in autumn.
Varities : It has one smaller variety which is called as 'triparni' or tinpatiya. It has smaller leaves.
Habitat : All over India.
Chemical composition : It contains potassium and oxalic acid.
Properties :
Guna : laghu, ruksha; **Rasa** : amla, kashay; **Vipak** : amla;
Veerya : ushna.
Karma :
Dosha : Kaphavatashamak and pittavardhak by ushnaveerya (?), so it is useful in kaphavata disorders (sheeta veerya- according to some of the texts).
External uses : Analgesic, antiinflammatory, denudate. Its local application helps in inflammation, headache, moles and eye disorders.
Internal uses :
Nervous system : Juice is given in alcoholism.
Digestive system : It improves the taste and appetite. It is also liver stimulant and astringent therefore useful in distaste, anorexia, haemorrhoids, dysentery, rectal prolapse. Curry of the leaves improves appetite. Leaves boiled in butter milk are used in dysentery.
Circulatory system : Cardiotonic and haemostatic. It is vasoconstrictor because of astringent property. It is effective in heart diseases and bleeding disorders.
Temperature : Ushna veerya but cool to touch and also febrifuge.
Satmikaran : Antidote for intoxicants, mainly dhattura seeds.
Parts used : Whole plant.
Dose : Juice 2 to 3 teaspoons.
Formulation : Changeri ghrita.
Srotogamitva :
Dosha : Alleviates kapha and vata and vitiates pitta (by ushna veerya).
Dhatu : Raktavardhak, snayugami, meda - useful in rectal prolapse and strengthens muscles.
Mala : Purisha (constipative).
Organs : Liver (stimulant) intestines.
References -
'चांगेरी दीपनी रुच्या रुक्षोष्णा कफवातनुत् । पित्तलाम्ला ग्रहण्यर्शः कुष्ठातीसारनाशिनी ।। (भा.प्र.)
'दीपनी चोष्णवीर्या च ग्राहिणी कफमारुते । प्रशस्यतेऽम्लचांगेरी ग्रहण्यर्शोहिता च सा ।। (च.सू. २७)
'ग्रहण्यर्शोविकारघ्नी साम्ला वातकफेहिता । उष्णा किञ्चित् कषाया च चांगेरी चाग्निदीपनी ।। (सु.सू. ४६)

To heal the wounds in human body, there is no dhatu except blood. Similarly, plants have latex and gum which serves the same purpose.

(43) CHITRAK
Plumbago zeylanica

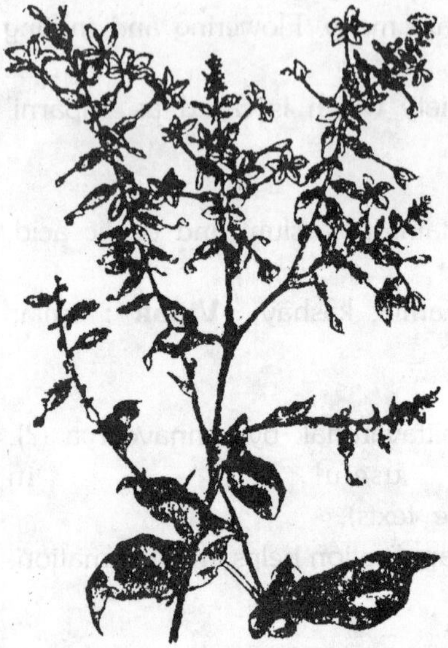

Gana : Deepaniya, Truptighna,Shoolaprashaman, Bhedaniya, Arshoghna, Lekhaniya, Katukaskandha (C); Pippalyadi, Mustadi, Amalakyadi, Mushkakadi, Varunadi, Araghwadhadi (S). Panchakol, Shadushan (Bhavaprakash).

Kula : Chitrak kula.

Latin name : Plumbum = lead. Plumbago - that cures lead palsy; zeylanica = of ceylon.

English name : Leadwart.

Sanskrit names : Chitrak (if the paste of the roots with water is applied on the skin, blisters appear within few minutes and become red in colour after bursting. Any colour on another one = chitra.), Agni (chitrak has all the synonyms of fire), Shardul, Chitrapali, Krushnanudahan, Vyal, Jyoti, Palak, Anal, Darun, Vahni.

Botanical Description : Long living herb, 1 to 2.5 mtrs. high. Stem - thin, round, nodular and delicate having vertical striations on it. Leaves -oval shaped resembling bilva leaves, 10 cm. long and 4 cm. broad. Stalk of flowers - 10 to 20 cm. long, having many branches. Fruits - legumes, oval shaped with cover. It is sticky to touch. Seeds - each fruit has one oval seed. Roots - finger like thick, like shatavari, red from outside but white inside but one can bend them easily. Roots are pungent to taste. Flowering season is winter followed by fruiting after a month.

Varities : Depending on the flowers, it is of 4 varities - 1) White 2) Yellow 3) Red 4) Black. White and red chitrak are being used widely in practice. Red chitrak is more potent but is rare.

Habitat : White chitrak - Bengal, Uttar Pradesh, South India, Srilanka. Red Chitrak - Hills, Sikkim, Kuchabihar.

Chemical composition : Pungent, having yellow and irritant principle called as plumbagin, 91%. Active principle does not dissolve in cold water. In boiling water or alcohol it dissolves easily. So cold water should not be used for formulations.

Properties :

Guna : tikshna, laghu, ruksha; **Vipak** : katu; **Rasa** : katu, tikta; **Veerya :** ushna (excessive).

Karma :

Dosha : Being ushna-tikshna, it is vata kaphashamak but pittavardhak. Useful in various disorders induced by kapha and vata.

External uses : Being irritant and hot, it developes blisters and has scraping action. Its paste causes blisters resulting in discolouration. So it is called as chitrak (chitra= two colours). In skin disorders like filariasis, oedema, vitiligo etc., paste causes blisters thus relieving vitiated doshas. Paste is applied in arthritis.

Internal uses :

Central nervous system : Stimulant in low dose but sedative in higher dose. Useful in nerve weakness and vata disorders.

Digestive system : Due to its pungent, hot properties, it acts as an appetiser, digestive, but anstringent and anthelmintic. Therefore, it is useful in anorexia, indigestion, abdominal pain, liver disorders, sprue, haemorrhoids and worms. Mainly effective in non-bleeding piles.

Chitrak enhances the circulation of gastric mucus membrane, thus helps in digestion and absorption. Non-bleeding piles are caused by vata and kapha.

Circulatory system : Chitrak vitiates pitta and reduces oedema, so it is useful in oedema, liver and spleen disorders and proctitis.

Respiratory system : It is effective in chronic rhinitis and cough.

Reproductive system : It causes uterine contraction, cures menstrual disorders and post partum disorders. It is also used internally and externally in impotency.

Skin : Diaphoretic, useful in skin disorders (vitiligo etc.) 15 to 45 drops of alcoholic extract of chitrak acts as a potent diaphoretic. Application of small quantity of chitrak is used in abscess.

Temperature : Febrifuge. It is used in chronic fever (kapha) and malaria. It improves liver function, digestion and helps in splenomegaly. Chitrak is the best medicine for diseases like haemorrhoids, which are caused by abnormality of agni.

Satmikaran : Acts as a bitter tonic in low dose. It is helpful in post pyrexial debility (kaphaj).

Parts used : Root bark (use fresh).

Dosage : 0.5 to 1gm. High dose causes burning and intoxication. (To be used cautiously).

Formulations : Chitrakadi gutika, Chitrakharitaki, Chitrak ghrit, Chitrakadi churna, Trimad churna (Chitrak, vavding and nagarmotha in equal quantity.)

Improper use of chitrak causes toxicity. Higher dose of it creates irritant and intoxicant effects. It causes burning of tongue, throat, stomach and all over the body, nausea, vomiting, diarrhoea, dysuria, burning micturtion. Pulse becomes feeble and skin becomes wrinkled and cold. If given in pregnancy, it causes irritation of pelvic organs which leads to abortion.

There is a tradition of keeping chitrak root in the vagina for abortion. This causes bleeding from uterus. Uterus gets contracted and abortion occurs within 3-6 hrs.

(Quacks use chitrak roots for abortion but many a times it causes death of the mother as well as the foetus.)

Treatment for excessive dose - cold, unctuous and non-irritant substances like cow's ghee should be used.

Chitrak is added to milk while boiling it and later on curds and buttermilk is prepared from that milk. Such buttermilk is an excellent remedy for non-bleeding piles produced by vata and kapha.

Srotogamitva :

Dosha : Alleviates vata, kapha and eliminates pitta (gives yellow colour to the stools).

Dhatu : Rakta, meda (vitiligo).

A medical practitioner must not only take care of plants but forests too.

Mala : Purisha (astringent), chitrak gives yellow colour to the stools when taken orally.
Organs : Liver, duodenum, rectum, spleen, uterus. (Haemorrhoids - chitrak is the best rasayan for all disorders caused due to improper function of the agni.)
References -
‘चित्रक: कटुक: पाके वह्निकृत् पाचनो लघु: । रूक्षोष्णो ग्रहणीकुष्ठशोथार्थ: कृमिकासनुत् ।।
वातश्लेष्महरो ग्राही वातार्श: श्लेष्मपित्तहत् ।’ (भा.प्र.)
‘चित्रकोऽग्निसम: पाके कटुक: कफशोफजित् । वातोदरार्शोग्रहणीकृमिपाण्डुविनाशन: ।। (ध.नि.)
‘चित्रकमूलं दीपनीयपाचनीयगुदशोथार्थ: शूलहराणाम् ।’ (च.सू.२५)
‘यथास्वं चित्रक: पुष्पै: ज्ञेय: पीतसितासितै: यथोत्तरं स गुणवान् विधिना च रसायनम् ।।
छायाशुष्कं ततो मूलं मांसं चूर्णीकृतं लिहन् । सर्पिषा मधुसर्पिर्भ्यां पिबन् वा पयसा यति: ।।
छायाशुष्कं ततो मूलं मांसं चूर्णीकृतं लिहन् । सर्पिषा मधुसर्पिर्भ्यां पिबन् वा पयसा यति: ।।
अम्भसा वा हितान्नाशी शतं जीवति नीरुज: । मेधावी बलवान् कान्तो वपुष्मान् दीप्तपावक: ।।
तैलेन लीढो मासेन वातान् हन्ति सुदुस्तरान् । मूत्रेण शिवत्रकुष्ठानि पीतस्तक्रेण पायुजान् ।। (वा.उ. ३९)

(44) JATAMANSI

Nordostachys jatamansi Dc.

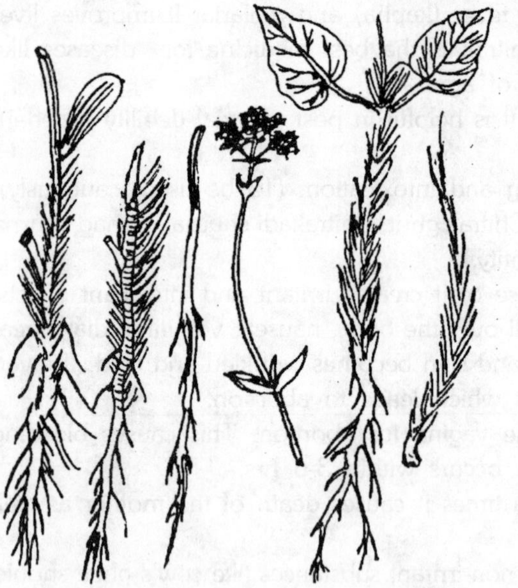

Gana : Sangnyasthapan.
Kula : Mansi kula.
Family : Valerianaceae. 'To be strong' in Latin. It has powerful medicinal properties. Valerius Pubicola is said to have been the first man to make use of it as a medicine.
Latin name : Nort = Valerina celtica, stachys = spiked.
English name : Valeman.
Sanskrit names : Jatamansi (shaggy, having thick hairy roots or matted hair like plant which destroys flesh loving ghosts), Bhutajata (with matted hair like ghost), Sulomasha (very shaggy/hairy), Nalada (giving fragrance), Jatila, Keshini, Jata, Hinstra, Mansini.
Botanical Description : This herb is 0.5 - 1m high. Roots - shaggy with fragrance. Rhizomes resemble pig hair. Leaves - thin, long, 15 - 17 cm long and 3 cm broad. Flowers - pink and grow in cluster. Fruit - shaggy.
Habitat : Grows at a height of 2000 - 6000 mtrs. in watery land like Kashmir, Nepal. It also grows in South Himalayas where snow covered peaks supply moisture.
Chemical composition : It contains mainly 1% volatile oil, greenish yellow in colour. It floats on water, evapourates in the air and has camphor like smell, bitter-spicy taste. Also

Vrikshayurveda has reported many amazing experiments about the growth of leaves, flowers and fruits of plants. This would be an ideal subject for the department of research in agriculture.

contains resin 6%, camphor and gum etc. The extract of the plant named Valerina officinalis is used in modern medicine. Jatamansi has a smell like tagar. It also contains an active substance called jatamansin with a strong smell.

Properties :

Guna : laghu, tikshna, snigdha; **Rasa** : tikta, kashaya, madhur; **Vipak** : katu; **Veerya** : sheeta.

Prabhav : Bhutaghna, manasrogaghna.

Karma :

Dosha : Vatashamak by snigdha; pittashamak by sheeta, tikta, kashaya, madhur; kaphashamak by tikta and tikshna. Ultimately it is tridoshashamak but specially kapha-pittanashak.

External Uses : Paste is used in burning of skin. It improves the complexion and is antipyretic. Paste is also used in inflammation and pain. Paste is effective in many skin disorders. Its fine powder is used in excessive sweating and reducing foul smell of sweat.

Internal Uses : Jatamansi acts on digestive, circulatory, urinary, nervous, skin and also reproductive system i.e. on all systems of the body.

Nervous system : Jatamansi mainly acts on this system. It is a brain and health tonic. It is best used in convulsions and pain, in epilepsy, hysteria, syncope etc.so it is called as bhutaghna or rakshoghna. In these disorders, the bulbous root, flowers, are also used. As a brain tonic, it is used in loss of memory. For headache, jatamansi is one of the best medicines and is also a sedative.

Digestive system : It is an appetizer, digestive, laxative, cholagogue, useful in pregnancy. It is an analgesic and laxative and has vataprashaman karma. Because of this karmas, jatamansi is used in loss of appetite, abdominal distension, abdominal pain and amoebiasis. Also useful in liver enlargement and jaundice by cholagogue action.

Circulatory system : It is a cardiac depressant and hypotensive drug. Jatamansi is the best medicine for anasarca and hypertension.

Respiratory system : Effective in cough and dyspnoea by bitterness.

Urinary system : It stimulates the kidneys and increases micturition, so effective in dysuria and cystitis.

Reproductive system : It is useful in infertility, dysmenorrhoea and uterine inflammation.

Skin : Effective in various skin disorders and erysipelas; the oil is used in alopecia. Jatamansi oil is famous in South India.

Satmikaran : It is a tonic, so useful in weakness.

Temperature : Bitter, antipyretic, relieves burning, effective in sannipat jwar (fever with delirium). Reduces fever, gives strength and relieves burning.

Precaution : Higher dose of jatamansi causes hyperemesis, griping pain, dysentery and inflammation of the kidney (nephritis).

Parts used : Roots - dose 1 - 3 gm should be used (fresh).

Formulations : Mansyadi kwath, Rakshoghna ghrit, Sarvoushadhisnan.

Srotogamitva:

Dosha :Tridosha.

Every small or big plant expects our affectionate look and touch like we would give to our own children.

Dhatu : Majja (brain tonic), rakta (improves the complexion, used in burning, erysipelas, and skin diseases).
Mala : Sweat.
Organ : Brain.
Prabhav : Antidote.
References -
'जटामांसी भूतजटा जटिला च तपस्विनी । मांसी तिक्ता कषाया च मेध्याकान्तिबलप्रदा ।।
स्वाद्वी हिमा त्रिदोषास्रदाहवीसर्पकुष्ठनुत् ।।' (भा.प्र.)
'सुरभिस्तु जटामांसी कषाया कटुशीतला । कफहृदभूतदाहघ्नी पित्तघ्नी मोदकान्तिकृत् ।।' (रा.नि.)
'जटामांसी तु तुवरा शीतला कान्तिकारका । बल्या कटवी स्वादुतिक्ता कफान्तर्दाहपित्तहा ।।
विसर्पकुष्ठत्वग्दोषभूतबाधाज्वरापहा । दाहं त्रिदोषं वातं च रक्तदोषं विषं हरेत् ।।' (नि.स.)

(45) JATIPHALAM
Myristica fragrans Houtt.

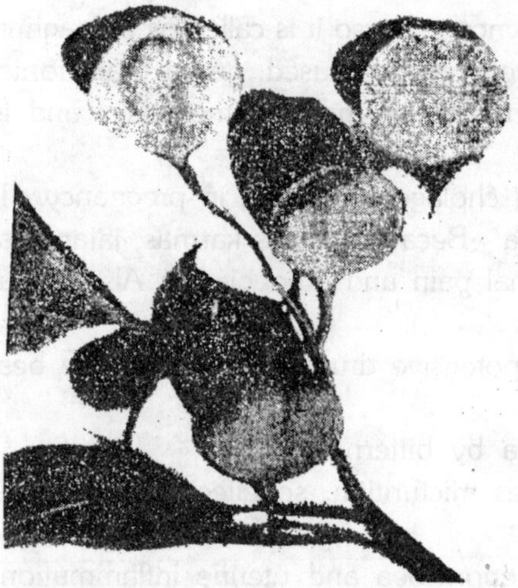

Kula : Jatiphala kula.
Family : Myristicaceae- belonging to the family having fragrance similar like myrrh - sweet perfumed (myrrh = a fragrant drug).
Latin Name : Myristica = sweet perfumed.
English name : Nutmeg.
Sanskrit names : Jatiphala (fragrant fruit), Jatikosha (having fragrant lobules), Malatiphala, Shalooka, Majjasar, Putha, Sumanphala, Soumanaphala, Jatija.
Botanical Description : A lofty tree with slender branches. Leaves - like jamun leaves but small, coriaceous having fragrance. Dorsal side of the leaf is dark green while ventrally it is pale yellow. Flowers - small, fragrant, yellow in colour. Fruit - ovoid (3-8 cm.) resembling a small betelnut. Fruit is a drupe surrounded by arillus and flesh. Rind - pale yellow and thick. Its hard outer shell is yellow. On drying, it becomes coral coloured. It is called as mace (jatipatri / jaipatri). A seed with hard shell which is enclosed in this mace is called as nutmeg (jaiphala). The kernel is used in medicine and food (for fragrance). When fruit becomes ripe, it ruptures on its own and mace is removed and the nutmeg is collected. Flowering stage is after the rainy season and fruiting stage is after that.
Varieties : It has another variety which is without smell. It is known as 'raiphal' and its thin covering is called as 'raipatri'.
Habitat : The Malay peninsula, Penang, Srilanka and Southern India.
Chemical composition : It contains 2.8% volatile oil. It also contains a stable oil, protein, fats, starch, slimy mucilage principle and alkaloid. Jaipatri has 8.17% volatile oil, resin, fats, sucrose and

If we provide all the needs of plants and give them love and affection, then plants of any country would grow anywhere in the world.

slimy mucilage principle. Stable oil in nutmeg is known as butter of nutmeg. It contains myristin, myristic acid and an essential oil. Mace has yellow aromatic oil having fragrance like nutmeg, which contains macin.

Properties :

Guna : laghu, snigdha, tikshna; **Rasa :** katu, tikta, kashaya; **Vipak :** katu; **Veerya :** ushna.

Karma :

Dosha : Being both fragrant and hot, it is used in disorders induced by vata and kapha.

External uses : Analgesic, stimulant and deodorant. Its paste is used in headache, arthralgia. Ointment is used as deodorant and an analgesic in skin diseases. Its oil is used for massage in cases of cold and skin laxity. In impotency, nutmeg oil is applied on the penis and then betel leaves are tied over it. Its powder is applied on foul smelling wounds. In case of common cold and fever of children, nutmeg oil is applied on the forehead. Nutmeg and dry ginger power in water alleviate headache due to common cold. In diarrhoea, powder is applied on the umbilicus.

Central nervous system : It is analgesic, anticonvulsant and vatashamak. Excessive dose is intoxicant. The actions of camphor and nutmeg on brain are similar. It is useful in insomnia. It also alleviates vata disorders like pain, convulsions etc.

Digestive system : Nutmeg reduces bad breath temporarily. It improves the taste. It is a stimulant, an appetizer, digestive, liver stimulant, carminative, astringent and anthelmintic. Hence it is used along with other medicines in anorexia, indigestion, liver disorders, diarrhoea, colitis and helminthiasis. It reduces the foul smell and blackness of stools. Nutmeg is given in excessive thirst and emesis. In cholera, water boiled with nutmeg is used (after cooling).

Circulatory system : Low dose acts as a circulatory stimulant.

Respiratory system : Being an expectorant and kaphaghna, it helps in chronic rhinitis, cough, dyspnoea, hiccoughs.

Reproductive system : Being an aphrodisiac and stimulant of menstruation, it is used in impotency and premature ejaculation. It is also used in dysmenorrhoea.

Temperature : Nutmeg is used when fever and diarrhoea occur simultaneously.

Satmikaran : Nutmeg is used as a tonic in post diarrhoeal weakness and post- sprue debility.

Part used : Nutmeg, mace.

Dosage : 5 to 10 mg.; oil 7 to 15 drops (be cautious as higher dose is injurious).

Formulations : Jatiphaladi churna, Jatiphaladiguti. Mace is more easily palatable, complexion enhancer, analgesic than nutmeg, though properties of both are similar.

Srotogamitva :

Dosha : Kaphavataghna.

Dhatu : Ashti, mansa, shukra (aphrodisiac).

Mala : Purisha (astringent), foetid smell scavenger, anthelmintic.

Organ : Heart.

References -

'जातिफलं जातिकोषं मालतीफलमित्यपि । जातिफलं रसे तिक्तं तीक्ष्णोष्णं रोचनं लघु ।।
कटुकं दीपनं ग्राहि स्वर्य श्लेष्मानिलापहम् । निहन्ति मुखवैरस्यं मलदौर्गन्ध्यकृष्णताः ।।
कृमिकासवमिश्वासशोषपीनसहृद्रुजः ।' (भा.प्र.)

If every small and big tree receives our love as we would give to our children, then they will yield the best flowers and fruits (Shri Tambade Nasik).

'जातिफलस्य त्वक् प्रोक्ता जातिपत्री भिषग्वरैः । जातिपत्री लघुः स्वादुः कटूष्णा रुचिवर्णकृत् ।।
कफकासवमिश्वासतृष्णाकृमिविषापहा ।' (भा.प्र.)
'जातिकोशोऽथ कर्पूरं जातिकटुकयोः फलम् ।... तिक्तं कटु कफापहम् ।।
लघु तृष्णापहं वक्त्रक्लेददौर्गन्ध्यनाशनम् ।' (सु.सू. ४६)
'तैलं जातिफलोदभूतं समुत्तेजनमग्निदम् । जीर्णातिसारशमनमाध्मानाक्षेपशूलनुत् ।।
आमवातहरं बल्यं दन्तवेष्टव्रणार्तिनुत् ।' (आ.सं.)

(46) JEERAK

Cuminum cyminum Linn.

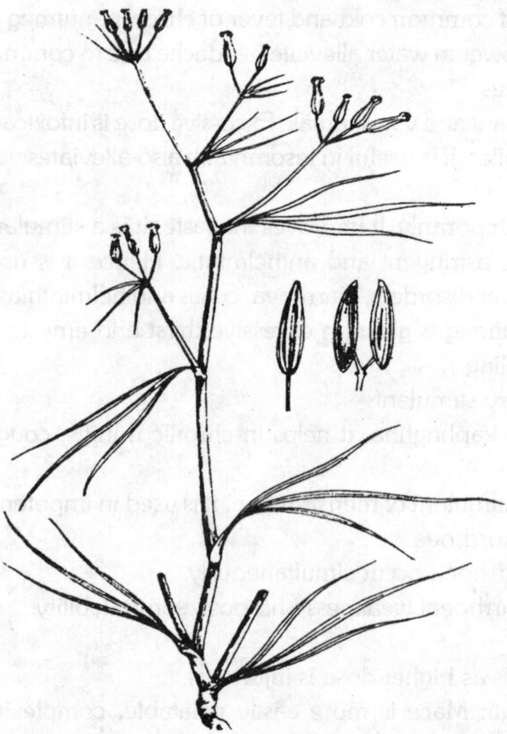

Gana : Shoolaprashaman, Shirovirechana (C.); Pippalyadi (S.)
Kula : Shatapushpa kula.
Family : Umbelliferae.
Latin name : Cuminum (Gk-Kyminor) provides the culinary (fit for cooking).
English name : Cumin seed.
Sanskrit names : Jaran (helps in digestion), Deerghajeerak, Ajaji, Kanavha, Kanajeerna, Deepya, Sitajaji, Shuklajaji, Deerghak.
Botanical Description : A small plant 0.33 to mtr. high resembling fennel plant. Leaves - small, flowers - white in colour, fruit - cylindrical, white, grey in colour. The plant bears flowers and fruits at the end of winter season.
Habitat : All over India, but more in Rajasthan and Punjab. Also in Asia minor and Persia.
Chemical composition : It contains 3.5 to 5.2% volatile oil called as thymene, because of which it has peculiar taste and fragrance.
Properties :
Guna : laghu, ruksha; **Rasa** : katu;
Veerya : ushna; **Vipak** : katu.
Karma : Vatakaphashamak and pittavardhak by ushna property. Useful in disorders caused by kapha and vata.
External uses : The paste is an antiinflammatory and an analgesic, hence it is applied in painful oedema. Useful in skin diseases, in depigmentation. The paste is used in kachhu and pama (types of scabies). Decoction of cumin seeds is used for cleansing in skin disorders. Paste also helps in haemorrhoids and pain due to scorpion sting.
Chewing of cumin seeds is useful in stomatitis and pharyngitis by alleviating the inflammation and soreness. This action is done by the cumin oil.

If a plant is taken care of and provided all its needs, then any plant can gow in any country.

Internal use :

Digestive system : Being palatable, appetizer, digestant, carminative, analgesic, astringent and anthelmintic, it is used in disorders caused by distrubance in agni like anorexia, emesis, loss of appetite, indigestion, flatulence, pain in abdomen, sprue and haemorrhoids etc. Powder of roasted jeerak with honey is given for licking. Hiccups are relieved by smoking cigarette made with ghee and cumin seeds.

Circulatory system : It is a stimulant and blood purifier. It is useful in cardiac and blood disorders.

Urinary system : Diuretic. Cumin seed powder along with sugar is given in renal colic, gonorrhoea and calculi. Juice made in water is also useful.

Reproductive system : It alleviates the inflammation of uterus. It is also a galactagogue and aphrodisiac. It is used in leucorrhoea. Jaggery and cumin seed powder is used as a galactagogue. Jeerak is used for post-partum women as it is a galactagogue, improves lactation and gives strength.

Skin : It is used in most of the skin disorders.

Temperature : Febrifuge. In acute and chronic fever, particularly in vata dominant fever, it is very useful.

Satmikaran : It acts as a rasayan being a bitter tonic.

Parts used : Seed

Dosage : 3 to 6 mg.

Formulation : Jeerakadi modaka, Jeerakadi churna, Jeerakadya taila, Jeerakadyarishta.

Srotogamitva :

Dosha : Vatavardhak, pittavardhak, shleshmaghna.

Dhatu : Rakta (blood disorders).

Rasa : Galactagogue.

Organ : Eyes, uterus.

(Gulmaghna though it increases vata.)

Prabhav : For scorpion sting, paste of cumin seeds + ghee + saindhav is applied topically.

References -

'जीरकं कटुकं रूक्षं वातकृद्दीपनं परम् । गुल्माध्मानातिसारघ्नं ग्रहणीकृमिहृत् परम् ।। (ध.नि.)

'तीक्ष्णोष्णं कटुकं पाके रुच्यं पित्ताग्निवर्धनम् । कटु श्लेष्मानिलहरं गन्धाढ्यं जीरकद्वयम् ।। (सु.सू. ४६)

'शुभ्रजीरं कटु ग्राहि पाचनं दीपनं लघु । किञ्चिदुष्णं च मधुरं चक्षुष्यं रुचिकृन्मतम् ।।
गर्भाशयशुद्धिकरं रूक्षं बल्यं सुगन्धिकम् । तिक्त वमिक्षयाध्मानवातं कुष्ठं विषं ज्वरम् ।
अरोचकं रक्तदोषं अतिसारं कृमींस्तथा । पित्तं च गुल्मरोगं च नाशयेदिति कीर्तितम् ।। (नि.र.)

'अजाजी गुडसंयुक्ता विषमज्वरनाशिनी । अग्निसादं जयेत् सम्यग् वातरोगांश्च नाशयेत्' ।। (च.द.)

'जीरकस्य कृतः कल्को घृतसैन्धवसंयुतः । सुखोष्णो वृश्चिकार्त्तानां सुखलेपो व्यथापहः' ।। (च.द.)

(47) JYOTISHMATI
Celastrus paniculata

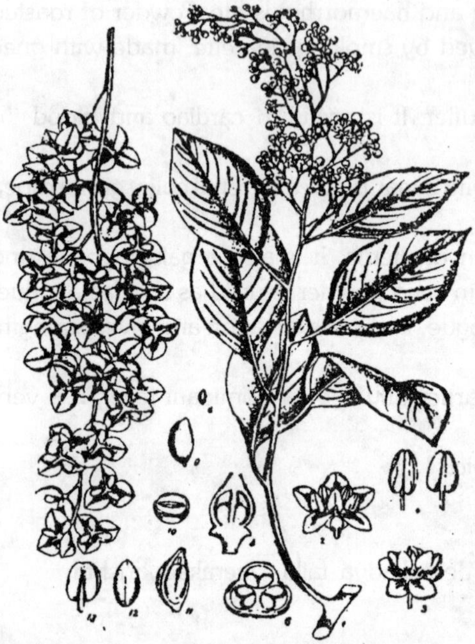

Gana : Shirovirechan (C., S.), Adhobhaghar.
Kula : Jyotishmati kula.
Family : Celastraceae (Staff tree family).
Latin name : Celastrus-Privet, a bushy evergreen shrub; paniculata - having an inflorance, the axis of which is divided into branches bearing two or more flowers.
English name : Staff tree.
Sanskrit names : Jyotishmati (because of medhya property, stalk bears white spots), Kakandaki (fruit similar to crows egg), Peetataila (extract of yellow oil), Vega (grows very fast), Swarnalata, Kshipra, Medhya, Matida, Saraswati, Vrusha.
Botanical description : Vertically growing large netted creeper attaining a large height. Leaves - egg shaped, tapering with serrated edges. Flowers - greenish, sweet taste, inflorance in summer. Fruits - round like pea, yellow and tripartite. Each of the parts contains saffron coloured, triangular single seed, fruiting in rainy season. Stalk - soft, fibrillar, white spotted (dots) which are clearly visible in young creeper. It bears shining, reddish yellow bunches of fruits, thus called as jyotishmati.
Habitat : All over India but specially in hilly areas like Punjab, Kashmir. Creeper grows on the tall trees upto the top in hilly area.
Chemical composition - Seeds contain 62.2% oil which is thick, reddish yellow coloured, bitter and having smell. Besides, it also contains bitter resin, 5% salts. Oil is extracted by two methods.
1) In oil mills by crushing seeds - oil is yellow in colour.
2) Patal yantra - oil is blackish in colour and contains kriosotes. Application of heat in this process could be responsible for the black colour.
Guna : tikshna, sthir, sara; **Rasa** : katu, tikta; **Vipak** : katu; **Veerya** : ushna; **Prabhav** : medhya.
Dosha : Vataprashamak by snighdha and ushna; kaphashamak by katu, tikta and ushna. Therefore jyotishmati is used in vatakapha diseases.
External use : Oil massage is vatanashak, vedanashamak and stimulant. Because of these properties, it is used in paralysis, backache, Bell's palsy, arthritis and sciatica. Stimulant property helps in loss of libido. Betel leaves impregnated with its oil are tied on penis. It is also useful in adenitis, cervical lymphadenopathy, tuberculosis, adenitis because of ushna veerya.

The sail of a ship is made from the tenacious wood of kanchan.

Internal use :

Nervous system : Improves memory by medhya guna. Ushna property enhances grasping power. Cow's ghee and jyotishmati oil mixture is used as a memory enhancer. Morphine addiction can be counteracted by daily consumption of 60 ml. of leaf juice of jyotishmati. It is a medha rasayani.

Digestive system : Being an appetizer by katu, tikta and ushna guna, it is used in loss of appetite. Snigdha and ushna gunas improve peristalsis and are therefore useful in overcoming constipation and abdominal distension (flatulence).

Circulatory system : Ushna guna stimulates heart, improves cardiac output. Therefore useful in bradycardia and oedema. Black oil of jyotishmati is useful in beriberi. Yellow oil is used in osteoarthritis (external use).

Respiratory system : It is used for nasya by its property of katu, ushna, kaphaghna and shirovirechak, also useful in asthma and bronchitis.

Urinary system : By increasing the renal circulation due to ushna it acts as a diuretic. Therefore it is used in dysuria due to excessive cold.

Reproductive system : Aphrodisiac and emmenagogue. It is used in infertility (impotency). Black oil with milk is given for internal use. Leaves fried in ghee are used as vegetable in dysmenorrhoea.

Skin : Diaphoretic and cures skin disorders. It is used as antipruritic.

Temperature : By katu and tikta property which is amapachak and diaphoretic, it is used as antipyretic. Within 2-3 hrs. it reduces fever by promoting sweating.

Parts used : Leaves, seeds and oil (old Ayurvedic physicians were using jyotishmati oil - malakangoni taila - on large scale because of its specific mode of action).

It is seen that intelligence promoting drugs are usually agnivardhak and this agni is sadhakagni. (Sadhak is one of the types of pitta). A person of pitta prakruti has sharp agni. He/she feels more thirsty and more hungry. Pitta prakruti people are intelligent.

Srotogamitva :

Dosha : Kaphavataghna (oil) , pitta and agni vardhak.

Dhatu : Majja, rasa (emmenagogue).

Mala : Purisha (sara), sweda (10-20 drops).

Its best action is seen on the nervous system.

Organ : Stomach (emetic).

Doses : Seed - 5 to 15; oil - 1 to 10 drops.

References -

'पक्वरक्तफला गुच्छा पीततैला च वर्तुला । पंक्तिपत्रा रक्तबीजाऽणुपुष्पा वनजा स्मृता ।।' (शि.)

'ज्योतिष्मती कटुस्तिक्ता सरा कफसमीरजित् । अत्युष्णा वामनी तीक्ष्णा वह्निबुद्धिमतिप्रदा ।।' (भा.प्र.)

'कटु ज्योतिष्मतीतैलं तिक्तोष्णं वातनाशनम् । पित्तसंतापनं मेधाप्रज्ञाबुद्धिविवर्धनम् ।। (रा.नि.)

'सकाञ्चिकं... भृष्टं ज्योतिष्मतीदलम् । प्राश्य वनितात्वार्तवं लभेत् ।।' (च.द.)

Since the wood of parish is elastic, it is used in horse carraiges.

(48) JAMBU

Eugenia jambolana

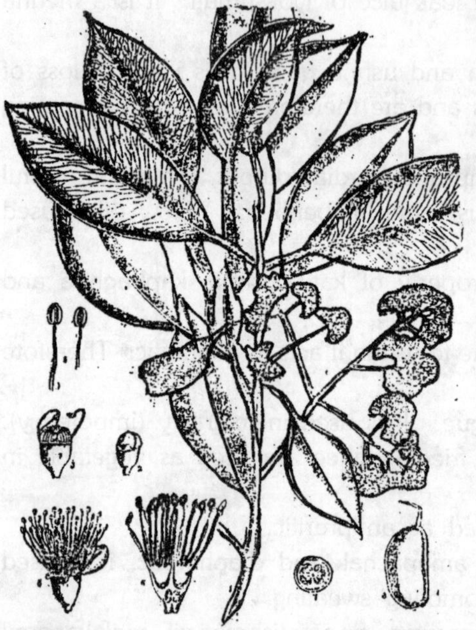

Gana : Mutrasangrahaniya, Purisha-virajaniya, Chhardinigrahana (C.) Nyagrodhadi (S.), Panchapallav (Bh.)

Kula : Lavanga kula.

Family : Myrtaceae (having perfume) - (Greek Myron = Perfume).

Latin name : Eugenia - after the name of the prince Eugene of Savoy, patron of botany; jambolana - derived from Sanskrit word Jambu.

English name : Jambul, Black berry.

Botanical Description : Big evergreen tree with leaves 8 to 15 cms long and 5 to 6 cms. wide. Flowers - white and golden. Fruits - 2 to 3.5 cms. ovoid. Raw jambul is green while ripe fruit is purple/red and fully ripe fruit is dark blue in colour. Seed is small. The tree bears flowers in spring while fruits at the end of summer and beginning of the rainy season.

Varieties : Various varieties. The main varieties are Rajajambu, Kshudrajambu, Nadijambu (Kak jambu), Bhumijambu and Gulabjambu. The description given above is of Rajajambu. Kshudrajambu is also known as Kashtajambu. The fruits are smaller in size and having less flesh. Nadijambu (Kakjambu) is a wild variety and it grows near jungle or gutter. The tree of Bhumijambu is round and small. It has pea sized seeds. Gulabjambu is a foreign fruit. It grows in Brahmadesh and Bengal. It is seedless, round and pearl coloured, fruit has a rose like perfume. This is one of the varieties of Rajajambu. Rajajambu is the best quality.

Habitat : All over India.

Chemical composition : Seed contains a glucoside - jamboline, ellagic acid, yellow essential oil, chlorophyl, resin, gallic acid, albumin etc. Bark has 12% gum.

Properties :

Guna : laghu, ruksha; **Vipak** : madhur; **Rasa** : kashaya, madhur, amla; **Veerya** : sheeta.

Karma :

Dosha : Kaphashamak by ruksha and astringent and pittashamak by sheeta and astringent, strongly vatavardhak by ruksha, sheeta and astringent properties. Jambul is effective in kapha-pitta disorders.

External uses : Astringent, refrigerant and cures skin disorders. The bark powder is sprinkled in bleeding disorders and wounds. Fruit pulp mixed with sesame oil is applied in burning condition. In sannipat jwar (fever caused by all the three doshas) associated with burning and delirium, a piece of cloth soaked in the above mixture is kept on the forehead. The oil boiled with the leaves is used for application in chanchroid and syphilitic ulcers.

It has been experienced that refracted light from a prism affects the growth of leaves, flowers and fruits of a plant (Naik, pune).

Internal uses :

Digestive system : Its fruit is an appetizer, digestive and liver stimulant. Impairment of liver function associated with diabetes is improved by seed powder. It is also an astringent. Leaves are antiemetic while bark is astringent. Excessive use of fruits causes constipation. The fruits and fruit juice are effective in disorders like loss of appetite, indigestion, pain and dysentery. Jambul fruit powder + bark powder + leaf juice is very effective in chronic diarrhoea and dysentery. Leaves are given for relieving emesis. In tooth and throat pain, gargling with decoction of bark helps. Leaf juice + goat's milk is useful in infantile diarrhoea.

Circulatory system : Haemostatic. Leaf juice is used in haemorrhagic disorders. Jambul seeds are used in menorrhagia and diarrhoea with bleeding per rectum.

Urinary system : The fruit and seed powder along with milk when administered helps in glucose metabolism in the liver, due to which blood and urine sugar levels become low causing hypoglycemia. Fruit and seed powder are the best medicines in ikshumeha and udakameha. Fruit juice is also useful in prameha.

Parts used : Fruit, seed, bark and leaves.

Dosage : Juice 12 to 25 ml.; powder 1 to 3 gms.

Formulations : Jambadyataila, Panchapallavayoga, Jambvarishta.

Crushed leaves kept with iron particles for 6 months, give good quality of iron bhasma.(A nail hammered in the stem of jambu tree gets brittle within one year.)

Srotogamitva :

Dosha : Kaphapittaghna, vatavardhak.

Dhatu : Meda and majja (diabetes mellitus).

Mala : Mutra, purisha (astringent).

Jambu is the topmost vatavardhak medicine.

References -

'जम्बू: संग्राहिणी रूक्षा कफपित्तास्त्रदाहजित् ।' (भा.प्र.)

'जाम्बवं कफपित्तघ्नं ग्राहि वातकरं परम् ।' (च.सू. २७)

'अत्यर्थवातलं ग्राहि जाम्बवं कफपित्तजित् (सु.सू. ४६)

'जाम्बवं वातजननानाम् ।' (च.सू. २५)

'ग्राही कषायस्तन्मज्जा विशेषान्मधुमेहहा ।' (नि.र.)

'जम्बू: कषायमधुरा श्रमपित्तदाहकंठार्त्तिशोषशमनी कृमिदोषहन्त्री ।
श्वासातिसारकफकासविनाशिनी च विष्टम्भिनी भवति रोचनपाचनी च ।'' (रा.नि.)

(49) TALISPATRAM

Abies webbiana Lindle.

Gana : Shirovirechak (S.)

Kula : Devdaru kula.

Family : Conifereae (having cones).

Latin name : Abies = fur tree; webbiana = after the name of Barker Web, a naturalist and a traveller.

In some countries, there was death penalty for killing a man and cutting a tree. The value of man and tree was the same for them.

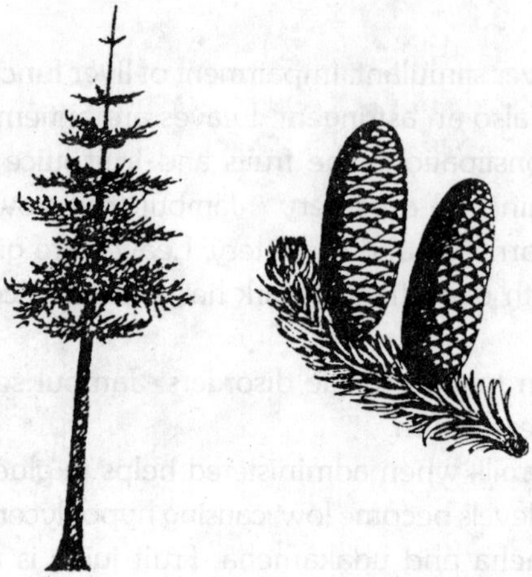

English name : Silver fur.
Sanskrit names : Talees, Patradhya (evergreen plant), Dhatripatra (leaves resemble amla leaves), Talispatra, Shukodara, Arkavedha, Karipatra, Neelambar, Granthikapatra.
Botanical Description : Evergreen tree having a height of 50 to 70 mtrs. Circumference of the stem measures approximately 10 mtrs. Tender branches are thin, greyish, hairy and are bent downwards. Leaves - 2.5 to 5 cms. in length, 4 cms. in breadth and crooked at the tip. They are smooth and dark dorsally while ventral side is dusky with central vein. Fruit - elongated, 15 cms in length and violet or blue in colour. Seeds are feathery with 1.5 to 3 cms. of length.

Varieties : Three varieties of drugs having name `talisapatra' are available in the market.

1) Abies webbiana
Plant described above

2) Rhedodendron anthopogon.
It is famous in Nepal.

3) Taxus baccata
Used in Rajaputana, Maharashtra and Gujarat. It is known as Thuner.
It is a poisonous plant.

Habitat : Kumaon hills, Bhutan, Afghanistan, Baluchistan.
Chemical composition : It contains an alkaloid - taxine and a volatile oil.
Properties :
Guna : laghu, tikshna; **Rasa** : tikta; **Vipak** : madhur; **Veerya** : ushna.
Karma :
Dosha : Ushnaveerya, vatakaphanashak. Useful in various vatakapha disorders.
External uses : It is an analgesic and is applied in headache.
Internal uses :
Digestive system : It is bitter and ushna. Being an appetizer and carminative, it is used in anorexia, flatulence and loss of appetite.
Respiratory system : Bitter, pungent and tikshna. Effective in cough, asthma, hoarseness of voice and tuberculosis.
Urinary system : It has diuretic property. It alleviates oedema caused by kapha.
Temperature : Febrifuge (vata kapha). It regularizes the temperature, acts as an expectorant, alleviates chest pain.
Satmikaran : It has madhur vipak, though it is tikshna and ushna. Hence it is a tonic and used in tuberculosis and general debility.
Parts used : Leaves.
Dosage : Powder 4 to 8 mgs.
Formulations : Talisadi churna, Talisadi vati.

Plants give leaves, flowers, fruits and shade to others. They do not enjoy any of these things for temselves. They lead a life of an ideal donor.

Srotogamitva :
Dosha : Vatakaphaghna.
Dhatu : Srotorodhanashak.
Mala : Purisha.
Organ : Stomach.
References -
'तालीसयुक्तं पत्राढ्यं धात्रीपत्रं च तत् स्मृतम् । तालीसं लघु तीक्ष्णोष्णं श्वासकासकफानिलान् ।
निहन्त्यरुचिगुल्मामवह्निमान्द्यक्षयामयान् ।' (भा.प्र.)
'तालीसपन्नं तिक्तोष्णं मधुरं कफवातनुत् ।
कासहिक्काक्षयश्वासच्छर्दिदोषविनाशकृत् ।।' (रा.नि.)

(50) TRIVRUT

Operculina ipomoea Linn.

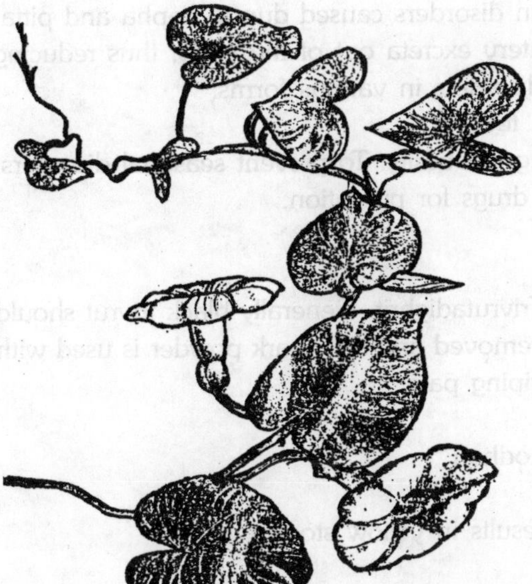

Gana : Bhedaniya (C.); Adhobhagahara (S.)
Kula : Trivrut kula.
Family : Convolvulaceae (Entwing).
Latin name : Operculina = opening by a lid.
English name : Turpeth.
Sanskrit names : Red - Kalindi, Triputa, Tamrapushpika, Kasanashika, Rechani, Rasayani, Koshafala.
Black - (Shyam) Trivrut, Malavika, Shyama, Keshadhifala, Kalakeshi.
Botanical Description : It is a creeper. Stem - erect, triangular and hairy. Leaves are of various shapes, some are oval and some are triangular. Flowers - white, bell-shaped. Fruit - 2.5cm. long, round or oval. Seed - black. Each fruit has 4 seeds. Root thick, red white in colour. White latex comes out on scratching. Roots are available in the market. Flowering is in rainy season while fruiting season is winter.

Varieties : Charaka has mentioned two varieties.

(1) White
Root is red-white, mild laxative,
Less harmful than black variety.
Useful in children, weak patients,
aged patients and patients having mrudu koshtha.

(2) Black
Root is black, strong purgative and is used in patients having krura koshtha.

Habitat : All over India.

Even though tall buildings are built, their beauty lies in the green gardens and lawns surrounding them.

Chemical composition : Root bark contains terpethene which causes purgation. Besides this, it has resin, yellow coloured principle, albumin, starch, lignanine, iron and some salts.

Properties :

Guna : laghu, ruksha, tikshna; **Rasa :** katu, tikta, madhur, kashay; **Vipak :** katu; **Veerya :** ushna.

Karma :

Dosha : Pittashamak by kashay, tikta and madhur, kaphanashak and vatavardhak by ruksha. It is used for elimination of doshas from anus in kaphapitta disorders.

Internal uses :

Digestive system : It has cathartic and purgative actions. It is the best drug for mild laxation. It has similar properties to Jalap. This drug causes yellow coloured loose motions with mild griping pain. It has been mentioned that it is used for purification in various enteric diseases due to its kaphapitta and malashodhan actions. Useful as purgative in many diseases viz. chronic flatulence, constipation, haemorrhoids, jaundice, gout, rheumatoid arthritis, cough, asthma and oedema. Mixture of trivrut and triphala is used for piles.

Circulatory system : It is used for purgation in skin disorders caused due to kapha and pitta, erysepelas, spleen enlargement. Trivrut eliminates watery excreta out of the body, thus reducing oedema. It is used as a purgative in haemorrhagic disorders in various forms.

Temperature : Root powder with honey is given in fever.

Satmikaran : Used for fat metabolism and curretting in obesity. To prevent seasonal disorders, trivrut is used as a main drug with other supportive drugs for purgation.

Parts used : Root bark, dry roots and stem.

Dosage : 10 to 30 mg (Root powder 4 gms.)

Formulations : Trivrutadi churna, Trivrutadigutika, Trivrutadighrit. Generally black trivrut should not be used. Central part of the root of red trivrut is removed and only bark powder is used with dry ginger, fennel or saindhav, sugar etc. to avoid griping pain.

Srotogamitva :

Dosha : Vatavardhan, pittashodhan, shleshmashodhan.

Dhatu : Rasa (fever), rakta (spleen, anaemia).

Mala : Purisha (purgation, purgation of pitta results in yellow stools.)

Organs : Intestine.

Trivrut stands first in the diseases where purgation is indicated. It will be beneficial to Ayurvedic practitioners if they start using trivrut again.

(त्रिव-न्मूलं विरेचने श्रेष्ठम् - वा. कल्प अ. १/ १)

References -

'श्वेता त्रिवृद्रेचनी स्यात् स्वादुरुष्णा समीरकृत् । रूक्षा पित्तज्वरश्लेष्मपित्तशोथोदरापहा ।।'
'श्यामा त्रिवृत्ततो हीनगुणा तीव्रविरेचनी । मूर्च्छादाहमदभ्रान्तिकण्टोत्कर्षणकारिणी ।।' (भा.प्र.)
'त्रिवृदुष्णा कटुस्तिक्ता रूक्षा स्वाद्वी विरेचनी। कषाया कटुका पाके वातला कफपित्तहा ।।'
'ज्वरशोफोदरप्लीहपाण्डुव्रणविनाशिनी ।' (कै.नि.)

Karanj (Pongamia glabra) is named as Nakta (night) mala (flower). To understand its meaning, one should go under this tree in early morning.

'त्रिवृता कटुरुष्णा च कृमिश्लेष्मोदरज्वरान् ।
शोफपाण्डवामयप्लीहान् हन्ति श्रेष्ठा विरेचने ।।' (ध.नि.)
'त्रिवृत् सुखविरेचनानाम् ।' (च.सू. २५)
'विरेचने त्रिवृन्मूलं श्रेष्ठमाहुर्विरेचने ।' (च.क. ७)
'कषाया मधुरा रूक्षा विपाके कटुका च सा । कफपित्तप्रशमनी रौक्ष्याच्चानिलकोपनी ।।
सेदानीमौषधैर्युक्ता वातपित्तकफापहैः । कल्पवैशेष्यमासाद्य सर्वरोगहरा भवेत् ।।
मूलं तु द्विविधं तस्याः श्यामं चारुणमेव च । तयोर्मुख्यतरं विद्धि मूलं यदरुणप्रभम् ।।
सुकुमारे शिशौ वृद्धे मृदुकोष्ठे च तच्छुभम् । मोहयेदाशुकारित्वाच्छ्यामा कण्ठं क्षिणोत्यपि ।।
तैक्ष्ण्यात् कर्षति हृत्कण्ठमाशुदोषं हरत्यपि । शस्यते बहुदोषाणां क्रूरकोष्ठाश्च ये नराः ।।
गुणवत्यां तयोर्भूमौ जातं मूलं समुद्धरेत् । उपोष्य प्रयतः शुक्लवासाः समाहितः ।।
गम्भीरानुगतं श्लक्ष्णमतिर्यग्विसृतं च यत् । तदविपाट्योद्धरेद् गर्भ त्वचं शुष्कां निधापयेत् ।।' (च.क.७)

(51) TULSI

Ocimum sanctum Linn.

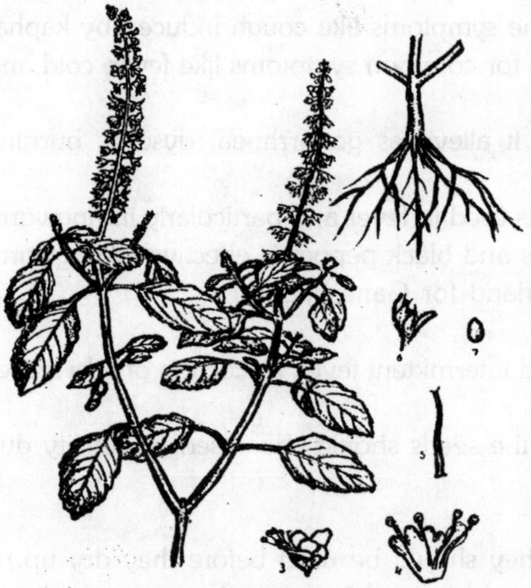

Gana : Surasadi (S.) (V.)
Kula : Tulsi kula.
Family : Labiateae. Mint family, herbs or shrubs yielding fragrant volatile oils.
Labious = large lipped.
Latin name : Ocimum - derived from Greek work okimon. Theophratus named this plant. Ozo (Gk.) means smell; sanctum - holy. Used for religious purpose, (Sanctus = sacred, chaste).
English name : Holy Basil.
Sanskrit names : Tulsi, Vrinda, Swarasa, Bhutaghni, Gouri (white tulsi), Manjari, Apetarakshasi (small insects remain away from it?), Shoolaghni, Shyama (black tulsi).
Botanical Description : A shrub of height 0.5 to o.75m. Leaves - are 3 cm. long, round having strong odour. Flowers - inflorescence 12 to 14 cms. long. Seed - small, pale black or red. It bears flowers and fruits (seeds) in winter.
Varieties : Grossly 2 varieties, 1) White and 2) Black.
White tulsi bears white branches and leaves, while black variety bears black leaves. Black tulsi is more potent than white one. Besides these varities, there is one more variety ie. wild tulsi. This plant is bigger and bears big leaves. One more variety is camphor tulsi from which camphor is derived.
Habitat : All over India, in front of many houses, temples and in gardens.
Chemical composition : It contains pale yellow-green essential oil which becomes crystalline over a period. It is called as basil camphor.

Delicate green leaves announce the arrival of spring. Despite the abundance of green and delicate leaves, the water content of the soil is less. Why is it so?

Properties :
Guna : laghu, ruksha; **Rasa** : katu, tikta; **Vipak** : katu; **Veerya** : ushna
(Seeds - snigdha, pichchila and sheeta).
Karma :
Dosha : Kaphavatashamak and pittavardhak. Useful in kapha-vata disorders.
External uses : Because of its insecticidal, deodorant, stimulant, vatahara and oedema relieving actions, the paste of the leaves is useful in chronic ulcers, oedema and pain.
Scrubbing of the juice on the skin improves the intradermal circulation. Juice is also used as eardrops in earache.
Internal uses :
Digestive system : Being an appetizer, digestive, laxative and anthelmintic, it is used in anorexia, emesis, abdominal pain and helminthiasis. Tulsi seeds are soaked in water and slimy kheer is prepared from it which is given in dysentery. Tulsi leaves should be chewed in pyorrhoea.
Circulatory system : Since it is a cardiac stimulant, blood purifier and antiinflammatory, it is used in cardiac debility, vatakapha disorders of blood and inflammations.
Respiratory system : Tulsi has a main action on respiratory system. When tulsi leaves are given with honey, they act as an expectorant and alleviate the symptoms like cough induced by kapha, dyspnoea and fever. Tulsi is a very good home remedy for common symptoms like fever, cold and cough.
Urinary system : Tulsi seed (tukumrai) is diuretic. It alleviates gonorrhoea, dysuria, burning micturation, cystitis, calculi and also urethritis.
Skin : Diaphoretic, effective in skin diseases. Hence it is used in fever and particularly in ringworm infection, eczema and scabies. The paste of tulsi leaves and black pepper is effective in ringworm infection (It is worn with red hibiscus flowers in a garland for Ganeshpooja).
(गजकर्णाय नमः तुलसीपत्रं समर्पयामि । Ganeshpooja).
Temperature : Febrifuge. Useful in fever with chills and intermittent fever. Decoction of tulsi leaves is also useful in chronic fever.
Satmikaran : Seed is a tonic. Kheer prepared from the seeds should be used in debility due to pittadosha.
Parts used : Leaves, root and seeds.
(Leaves become less potent after a few days hence they should be used before they dry up.)
Dosage : Juice 10 to 20 ml.; seed 1 to 2 tsf. (Mostly tulsi is used for trituration or as anupan)
Formulations : Tulsi leaves are being used for trituration in preparing many Ayurvedic formulations. (It may act as a preservative).
Srotogamitva :
Dosha : Pittavardhak, kaphavatashamak (reducing foul smell of sputum).
Dhatu : Rakta (skin disorders), fat metabolism.
Mala : Mutra (dysuria), diaphoretic, mala (foetid smell scavenger).
Organs : Heart, respiratory system.

Many plants have innumerable synonyms. If they are studied carefully, they will throw light on their overall gunakarmas.

References -

'तुलसी कटुका तिक्ता हृद्योष्णा दाहपित्तकृत् । दीपनी कुष्ठकृच्छ्रास्रपार्श्वरुककफवातजित् ।।' (भा.प्र.)
'हिक्काकासविषश्वासपार्श्वशूलविनाशनः । पित्तकृत् कफवातघ्नः सुरसः समुदाहृतः ।।' (च.सू. २७)
'कफानिलविषश्वासकासदौर्गन्ध्यनाशनः । पित्तकृत् पार्श्वशूलघ्नः सुरसः समुदाहृतः ।।' (सु.सू. ४६)

(52) TUVARAKA

Hydnocarpus laurifolia Demst Sleumer.

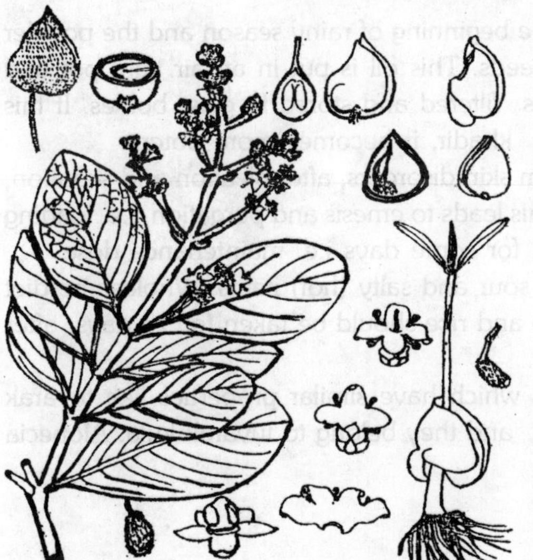

Kula : Tuvaraka kula (वृक्षास्तुवरा नाम पश्चिमार्णव).
Family : Flacourticeae (Flacourt is a scientist's name); (Tropical evergreen trees and shrubs).
Latin name : Hydno - carpus = fruit; laurifolia = leaves like laurel, glossy leaved shrubs. Bay trees; leaves of laurel are emblem of victory or merits.
Sanskrit names :Tuvarak, Katukapittha (bitter pulp), Kunthavairy.
Botanical Description : Tree is 13-16 mtrs. high. Leaves - 10 to 12 cms. long and 7 to 10 cms. broad. They are smooth but stiff and have serrated margins. Flowers - white, appear in cluster. Fruits - round, small, apple shaped, hairy. Seeds - many, yellow coloured resembling almond.
Habitat : Available in Southern India, Western mountains, Southern Konkan, Kerala and Srilanka.
Chemical composition : Seeds contain 44% stable oil, chawlmogric acid, hydnocarpic acid and paemitic acid in less quantity.
Properties :
Guna : laghu, tikshna, snigdha; **Rasa** : tikta, katu, kashaya; **Vipak** : katu; **Veerya** : ushna.
Karma :
Dosha : Kaphavatashamak by ushna property. Useful in kapha-vata disorders.
External uses : Tuvarak is the best medicine for skin disorders, as it alleviates skin diseases(chief action), it has also antipruritic, antiparasitic, cleaning and healing of wounds and curative properties. Oil is used for local application in skin disorders. Effective in tuberculoid lymphadenopathy, fistula and bone ulcers. Aslo useful in rheumatoid arthritis, gout in which pain is the chief complaint. Bhasma prepared from the fruit pulp is used as an anjana which has curative action.
Internal uses :
Nervous system: Analgesic by ushna property, because of which it is used in neuralgia, rheumatoid arthritis and gout for relieving pain.
Digestive system : Useful in ascites and helmithiasis. Emetic, purgative and anthelmintic by ushna and tikshna properties.

Eventhough it is advised that meat should be eaten for body building, it should be remembered that an elephant is totally vegetarian and has a big and healthy body.

Circulatory system : Blood purifier. Effective in blood disorders.
Urinary system : Useful in urinary disorders, because it is bitter, pungent and astringent.
Skin : As it cures skin disorders and pruritus, oil or powder is used in these disorders.
Parts used : Seeds, seed oil (Butter or milk cream as anupan).
Dosage : Powder of the seeds - 1 to 3 mg.; oil - 8 ml for emesis and purgation, 5 to 10 drops for oral administration but can be increased upto 30 to 60 drops. Oil is used along with butter, ghee or milk cream.
Formulation : Tuvarakadi taila.
Method of collection : Ripe fruits are collected in the beginning of rainy season and the powder of the dry seeds is made. Oil is derived from these seeds. This oil is put in an air tight pot and is buried in the stock of grains for 15 days. Then it is filtered and stored in glass bottles. If this oil is boiled along with three spoons of decoction of khadir, it becomes more potent.
Mode of administration :- In a patient suffering from skin disorders, after oleation and sedation, 10 ml. (i.e. 3 teaspoons)of oil should be given orally. This leads to emesis and purgation. i.e. loading dose. But after that only 1ml. of oil should be taken for some days i.e. maintenance dose.
During this period : Unwholesome diet - pungent, sour and salty (hot) items. Wholesome diet - milk, ghee, sweet fruits should be used. Moong soup and rice should be taken for 15 days after withdrawl of the drug.
Additional information : There are 2 more plants which have similar properties like tuvarak namely Gaino-cordia-ororata and Hydnocarpus kurzai and they belong to tuvarak kula. Alopecia is relieved by massage of tuvarak oil and lime water.
Srotogamitva :
Dosha : Kapha srotas (fluid absorbant).
Dhatu : Rakta, meda, majja, snayu.
Mala : Mutra.
Organ : Eyes - ointment is useful in various eye disorders.
References -
पञ्चकर्मगुणातीतं श्रद्धावन्तं जिजीविषुम् । योगेनानेन मतिमान साधयेदपि कुष्ठिनम् ।।
वृक्षास्तुवरका येः स्यु पश्चिमार्णवभूमिषु ।...
भिन्नस्वरं रक्तनेत्रं विशीर्णं कृमिभक्षितम् । अनेनाशु प्रयोगेण साधयेत् कुष्ठिनं नरम् ।।
शोधयन्ति नरं पीता मज्जानस्तस्य मात्रया । महावीर्यस्तुवरकः कुष्ठमेहापहः परः ।।
सान्तर्धूमस्तस्य मज्जा तु दग्धः क्षिप्तस्तैले सैन्धवं चाञ्जनं च ।
पैल्लं हन्यादर्मनक्तान्ध्यकाचान्नीली रोगं तैमिरं चाञ्जनेन ।। (सु.चि. १४)

(53) TEJOVHA
Zantho-xylon alatum Roxb.

Gana : Tiktaskandha, Shirovirechana (C.)
Kula : Jambir kula.
Family : Rutaceae (ruta = rue street, rus = flow).
Latin name : Zantho = yellow, xylon = wood; alatum = having wings.

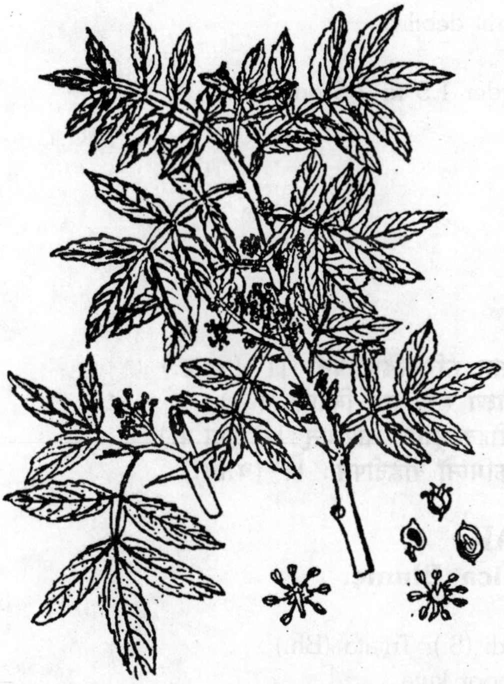

English name : Toothache tree.
Sanskrit names : Herb - Tejaswini, Tejovati (because of tikshna guna); Fruit - Tumbaru, Tumbul.
Botanical Description : It is a thorny herb. Leaves are 3 to 15 cms. long. Leaflet 2.5 to 6 cms. long with serrated margins. Flower - very small, 0.25 to 0.5 cms. long. Fruit - hollow like big coriander seed but sometimes lustrous. Externally fruit has tiny oily glands and has thin septum internally. Flowering season is rainy season and fruiting season is autumn.
Varieties : It has another variety which grows in south and is called as tirfal or chirfal.
(Latin - Xanthoxyline retetsa). Chirfal is relatively bigger than tumbaru.
Habitat : In Himalayas, Jammu, Bhutan at the height of 2 to 3 thousand mtrs.
Chemical composition : Bark contains berberin like principle.
Properties :
Guna : laghu, ruksha, tikshna; **Rasa** : katu, tikta; **Vipak** : katu; **Veerya** : ushna.
Karma :
Dosha : Kaphavatashamak and pittavardhak, hence useful in disorders induced by kapha and vata.
External uses : It is antiparasitic, stimulant and prevents necrosis. Its powder is used for dusting on wounds. Local application is used in headache and heaviness of head. Juice is used for gargling in oral, dental and throat disorders. Powder can also be applied. (Toothache tree-useful in toothache).
Internal uses :
Nervous system : Vatahara and nervine stimulant, hence useful in vata disorders (paralysis and rheumatoid arthritis.)
Digestive system : Being an appetizer, digestive, liver stimulant and anthelmintic, fruit is chewed and kept in mouth for brushing in dental diseases. Tejovha is used in anorexia, diarrhoea, liver and spleen enlargement and haemorrhoids.
Circulatory system : Because of tikshna, ushna and cardiac stimulant properties, it is used in heart diseases caused by kapha.
Respiratory system : Useful in asthma and cough as it is kaphaghna.
Urinary system : Being diuretic, it is used in dysuria caused by kapha.
Skin : Diaphoretic and cures skin disorders, hence useful in skin diseases.
Temperature : Febrifuge, useful in fever caused due to vatakapha - reduces temperature by diaphoretic action.

For increasing muscle mass, eating meat of carnivorous animals is advised. But it is interesting to note that these carnivorous animals ultimately survive on herbivorous animals.

Satmikaran : Bitter tonic, useful as a tonic in general debility.
Parts used : Fruit and bark.
Dosage : Fruit powder 0.5 to 0.75gm.; bark powder 1.5 to 2.5 gms.
Formulation : Tumbru-adi churna.
Srotogamitva :
Dosha : Vataghna, kaphaghna.
Dhatu : Rakta (liver, spleen).
Mala : Mutra (diuretic).
Organ : Digestive and respiratory system.
References -
'तेजस्विनी कफश्वासकासास्यामयवातहृत । पाचन्युष्णा कटुस्तिक्ता रुचिवह्निप्रदीपनी ।।' (भा.प्र.)
'तुम्बरु कथितं तिक्तं कटु पाकेऽपि तत्कटु । रूक्षोष्णं दीपनं तीक्ष्णं रुच्यं लघु विदाहि च ।।
'वातश्लेष्माक्षिकर्णोष्ठशिरोरुग्गुरुताकृमीन् । कुष्ठशूलरुचिश्वासप्लीहकृच्छ्राणि नाशयेत् ।।' (भा.प्र.)
'तुम्बरुः कटुतीक्ष्णोष्णः कफमारुतशूलजित् । अपतन्त्रोदराध्मानकृमिघ्नो वह्निदीपनः ।।' (ध.नि.)

(54) TWAK

Cinamonum zeylonica Blume.

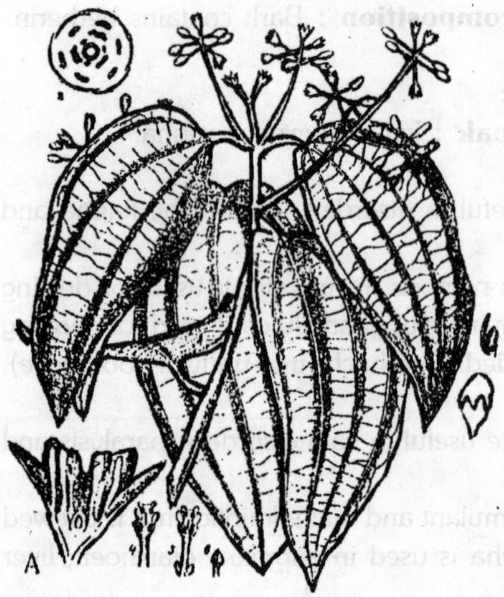
A

Gana : Eladi (S.); Trijata (Bh.)
Kula : Karpoor kula.
Family : Lauraceae - (glossy leaves) laurus - bay tree (laurels of the classic. Sacred to Apollo, with which poets, triumphant generals and even ancestral busts were crowned).
Latin name : Cinnamomum = Gk. Kinnomonon, from Arabic Kinamon, colour bright, brown, mixed with yellow and red.
English name : Cinnamon.
Sanskrit names : Twak (bark of the tree), Utkat, Tanutwak, Valkala, Shakala (bark), Saihala (from Sinhal island), Vanya, Surasa, Bahugandha, Mukhashodhya, Hridya.
Botanical Description : Medium sized tree having pale red and 16 cms. thick bark. Inner portion of it is red coloured; leaves - like leather and hairy. They have shiny dorsal aspect with 3 to 5 veins on them. Flowers - dusky colured. Fruits - violet and 12 cms. long. The tree bears flowers and fruits in spring.
Varieties :
1) Chinese - imported from China and Singapore.
2) Sinhali - imported from Srilanka. It is very thin and sweet.
3) Indian - The trees of Cinamon grow at the height of 1.25 to 2 thousand mtrs. in Himalayas, which are called as Cinemomum tamala. It is very thick and becomes soft if ground in water.

A reference in Raghuvansham gives evidence of plant conservation. Even in dense forest, one adopts a tree for protection !

The leaf is called as tejapatra or tamalapatra and dry fruit is called as black nagakesar. Practically, Chinese and Sinhali are known as Cinnamon while Indian variety is Taja. But 'Sinhali' is the best as it has sweet perfume and is sweet in taste.

Habitat : The main source of cinnamon is Srilanka. Also grows in Brahmadesha, China, Southern India and Himalayas.

Chemical composition : It contains 2% volatile oil which is called as oil of cinnamon. It also contains cinneric acid, resin, tannin, sugar, starch, mucilage and ash. Like bark, oil is also derived from leaves and root. Leaf oil is dark in colour and has clove-like aroma. Root oil is yellow coloured and water insoluble.

Properties :

Guna : laghu, ruksha, tikshna; **Rasa** : katu, tikta, madhur; **Vipak** : katu; **Veerya** : ushna.

Karma :

Dosha : Vatakaphanashak and pittavardhak by ushna. But sweet cinnamon is pittashamak. It is used in disorders induced by kapha - vata.

External use : It is stimulant and analgesic. It is used for mouth wash in bad breath and keeps teeth healthy. This is done by chewing of cinnamon. Chewing of cinnamon helps in nausea. The paste is applied in skin diseases like moles and skin tags etc. It is applied locally in headache and also in inflammation. In dental cavity, cotton wool soaked in 1-2 drops of cinnamon oil relieves pain. In a chancre, oil or paste is locally applied on penis. Cinnamon oil relieves pain and inflammation caused due to scorpion bite. It is also used for cleaning and healing of tuberculoid ulcer.

Internal uses :

Nervous system : Cinnamon is used in neural debility and paralysis.

Digestive system : It is an appetizer, digestive, carminative, liver stimulant and astringent by bitter, pungent and ushna properties. Hence it is useful in anorexia, amadosha, abdominal pain and haemorrhoids. Its antiprotozoal action is seen in enteric fever.

Circulatory system : It is a cardiostimulant, blood purifier and promotes white blood count. Therefore, it is used in cardiac debility and blood disorders caused due to bacterial infection.

Respiratory system : It is an expectorant and antitubercular drug. Cineremic acid seems to have an antitubercular property. It acts as a haemostat, ulcer healer and foul smell scavenger in lungs.

Urinary system : Its ushna and tikshna properties stimulate the bladder and act as a diuretic. Effective in disorders induced by kapha and meda.

Reproductive system : It has oxytocic and aphrodisiac properties. Hence it is useful in amenorrhea and infertility. Ashoka + cinnamon is used in uterine laxity.

Fever : It reduces intestinal foetid smell in enteric fever. Oil is also used.

Parts used : Bark, oil and leaves.

Dosages : Bark powder and leaves powder - 0.33 to 1gm.; oil 2 to 5 drops.

Formulation : Sitopaladi churna.

('Chini' word in dalchini is due to its sources from China and Brahmadesha).

We do not grow trees only because they give us flowers, fruits and shade. What do we get from tulsi ?

Srotogamitva :
Dosha : Pittavardhak, kaphavataghna.
Dhatu : Rasa, meda, shukra (aphrodisiac), rakta (complexion enhancer), artava (emmenagogue).
Organs : Heart, urinary bladder and stomach.
References -
'त्वचं लघूष्णं कटुकं स्वादु तिक्तं च रूक्षकम् । पित्तलं कफवातघ्नं कण्ड् वामारुचिनाशनम् ।।
हृद्वस्तिरोगवातार्शः कृमिपीनसकासजित् ।'
'त्वक् स्वाद्वी तु तनुत्वक् स्यात्तथा दारुसिता मता ।
उक्ता दारुसिता स्वाद्वी तिक्ता चानिलपित्तहृत् ।।
सुरभिः शुक्ला वर्ण्या मुखशोषतृषापहा ।' (भा.प्र.)
'पत्रकं मधुरं किञ्चित्तीक्ष्णोष्णं पिच्छिलं लघु । निहन्ति कफवातार्शोहृल्लासारुचिपीनसान् ।।' (भा.प्र.)
'वह्निमान्द्यानिलहरमाध्मानाक्षेपनाशनम् । वान्त्युत्केशप्रशमनं संग्राहि दशनार्त्तिहृत् ।।
त्वाचं तैलं रजः रजः स्त्रावि तोये क्षिप्तं निमज्जति ।' (आ.सं.)

(55) DADIM

Punica granatum Linn.

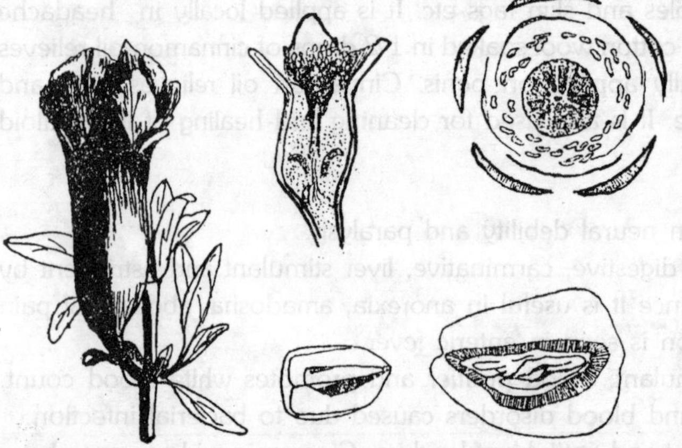

Gana : Hridya, Chhardinigraha (C.), Parushakadi (S.)
Family : Punicaceae.
Latin name : Punica (Lat) = pertaining to Carthage - Cartheginian apple; granatum = filled with seeds.
English name : Pomegranate.
Sanskrit names : Lohitapushpaka, Suphala, Rochan, Shukavallabha, Sunil, Raktakusum, Shukapriya, Dashanabeej, Raktapushpa, Pindapushpa, Dalima.
Botanical Description : The shrub is 3-5 mtrs. high. The stem bark is red externally and yellow internally. Leaves 5-7 cms long, 3cms broad, with tapering ends. Flowers - red in colour. Fruits -round with a diameter of 5 cms., containing many seeds. The tree has two gender-types - one gets only male flowers, and has reddish leaves. The other has both male and female flowers.
Types : On the basis of rasa, experts have classified three types - madhur (sweet), madhuramla (sweet and sour) and amla (sour).Commercially, many types are available in different parts of the world. `Seedless' Kabuli pomegranates are renowned, Muscat pomegranates with white seeds are of a high quality.
Habitat : Africa, Afghanistan (Kabul) and Iran are the main countries of origin. Now a days all varieties of pomegranate grow in India. Kabuli and Quetta pomegranates are considered the most superior variety.

The life-styles of a Yogi and a Vaidya have to be totally identical. There is not much of a difference between Ayurveda and Yoga.

Chemical composition : The stem bark and fruit rind contain 22-25 % tannin. The root bark has punicotannic acid 20-25%. There is a subtle substance in the root called pelletierine. The fruit contains 15% fructose.

Guna : laghu, snigdha; **Rasa :** madhur, kashaya, amla; **Vipak :** madhur of madhur, amla of amla; **Veerya :** anushna.

Karma : Sweet fruit tridoshaghna, pittashaman by sweet and astringent tastes and kaphavatashaman by ushna veerya. Sweet-sour fruit is slightly pittakar by its sourness. Sour fruits - kaphavatashamak but pittaprakopak. Sweet fruits are used in disorders induced by all three doshas while sour fruit is used in kapha-vata disorders.

External uses :
Due to its astringent nature the decoction of the bark is used in throat disorders and oral disorders as a gargle and also in ulcers. In epistaxis, nasal drops of the juice of the fruit are very effective.

Internal uses:

Nervous system : The fruit acts as a brain tonic. It acts on mental debility and associated disorders.

Digestive system : The fruit is an appetite stimulant, increases desire for foods, inhibits thirst, and acts as an astringent. The juice of the fruit and decoction of the root bark are strong vermifuges (hook worm). It is also used on tape worm. In a disinclinication to eat, weak apptite, amoebiasis, dipsia, acidpeptic disorder and such pitta disorders, and also diarrhoea, loose motions, it is extremely useful. In worm infestation 10-20 ml. of the rootbark decoction is given on an empty stomach followed by a laxative next day. The worms, killed by the decoction, are expelled immediately (vermicidal).

Circulatory system : The fruit is cordiotonic and haemostatic. It is useful in blood disorders like anemia and bleeding disorders. In nose bleeds, the decoction of the fruit rind should be given as a nasal insuffulation (nasya). Seeds should be used in acid peptic disease.

Respiratory system : Being astringent, the bud ameliorates kapha. The fruit acts as an expectorant. In infantile kapha disorders, the fruit is ground in goat's milk and is given as a licking agent. The flowers are useful in cough induced by vata and pitta. It acts as an expectorant and reduces the dryness in the respiratory tract. Nasal insuffulation of ghee processed with pomegranate flowers, saffron and sugar is an effective remedy for chronic rhinitis.

Urinary system : Pomegranate is a diuretic and hence useful in urinary disorders.

Reproductive system : As it promotes semen, it is used in seminal debility. The decoction of fruit rind is used for uttarbasti in vaginal discharges.

Temperature : Being an antipyretic, it is a useful diuretic food in fevers. It reduces the fever and its associated symptoms thus enhancing the strength of patient.

Satmikaran : Pomegranate is a useful food even in health. Due to its strengthening (tonic) properties, pomegranate juice is used in all ordinary weaknesses.

Parts used : Fruits, rind of the fruit, root, root bark.

Dose : Fruit juice - 2-5 tolas; rind decoction - 4-8 tolas.

Formulations : Dadimachatursama, Dadimashtaka, Dadimadichurna, Dadimadighrita, Dadimadya taila, Dadimavaleha.

Various treatments are available for humans for weight loss, fever, pthisis and infertility. In the same manner, treatments are available for plants too.

Take a whole promegranate and remove a small part of its rind. In that opening fill opium, the size of one green gram seed. Replace the rind and slowly roast it and extract the juice. This medicine is very effective in ama, amarakta and diarrhoea.

Srotogamitva :

Dosha : Tridoshaghna.

Dhatu : Shukra (shukrala), rakta, rasa (antipyretic), majja (brain tonic).

Mala : Purisha (astringent).

Organs : Breast, ear.

References -

'दाडिमः करको दन्तबीजो लोहितपुष्पकः । तत्फलं त्रिविधं स्वादु स्वाद्वम्लं केवलाम्लकम् ।।
तत्तु स्वादु त्रिदोषघ्नं तृङ्दाहज्वरनाशनम् । हृत्कण्ठमुखरोगघ्नं तर्पणं शुक्रलं लघु ।।
कषायानुरसं ग्राहि स्निग्धं मेधाबलप्रदम् । स्वाद्वम्लं दीपनं रुच्यं किञ्चित्पित्तकरं लघु ।।
अम्लं तु पित्तजनकमामवातकफापहम् ।' (भा.प्र.)
'अम्लं कषायमधुरं वातघ्नं ग्राहि दीपनम् । स्निग्धोष्णं दाडिमं हृद्यं कफपित्ताविरोधि च ।।
रूक्षाम्लं दाडिमं यत्तु तत् पित्तानिलकोपनम् । मधुरं पित्तनुत्तेषां तद्धि दाडिममुत्तमम् ।।' (च.सू.)
'कषायानुरसं तेषां दाडिमं नातिपित्तलम् । दीपनीयं रुचिकरं हृद्यं वर्चोविबन्धनम् ।।
द्विविधं तत्तु विज्ञेयं मधुरं चाम्लमेव च । त्रिदोषघ्नं तु मधुरमम्लं वातकफापहम् ।।' (सु.सू. ४६)
'विपाचितं दाडिमकल्कयुक्तं तैलं भवेत् सर्पषसम्भवं यत् ।
अभ्यंजनात्तत् कुरुते नितान्तमुच्चैः स्तनौ वृद्धियुतौ च कर्णो ।।' (रा.मा.)

(56) DARUHARIDRA

Berberis aristata De.

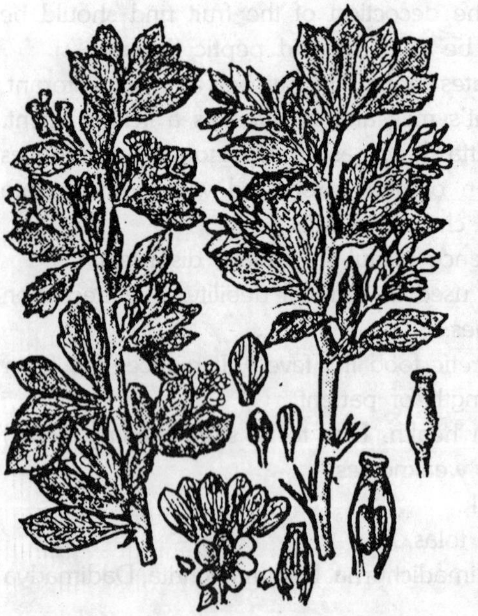

Gana : Arshoghna, Kandughna, Lekhaniya, (C.) Haridradi, Mustadi, Lakshadi (S.)

Kula : Daruharidra kula.

Family : Berberidae (from Berberys = Arabic name).

Latin name : Berberis = belonging to the Berberis family and aristata = furnished with an elongated projecting bristle, in connection with the costa (rib).

English name : Indian berbery.

Sanskrit names : Daruharidra (having yellow coloured wood like turmeric), Darvi, Katankateri, Peetika, Sthiraraga, Kamini, Peetachandan, Hemakanta, Peetak, Haridru, Nisha.

Botanical Description : Evergreen shrub having height 1.25 to 3 mtrs. The leaves are strong with fine whorled venation, straight, but with dentate or corrugated margins. Inflorescence 5 to 8 cms long, with large yellow coloured flowers. The fruits are bluish purple and small (called zarishka in yunani). Flowers bloom in the spring and

A man requires to take help of panchang (a Hindu calender) to identify spring but a cuckoo identifies spring by looking at the panchang (the five parts) of plants.

fruits in the winter. The stem is ash coloured from outside but is dark yellow coloured inside. Rasanjan (rasot) is prepared from the chemical or juice of the chitra variety of daruharidra.
Types : There are 12/13 types, the important ones being Berberis aristata, Berberis chitra, and Berberis lycium.
Habitat : Himalaya, Parasnath, Nilgiri and Nepal at the height of 0.75 to 4.25 thousand mtrs.
Guna : laghu, ruksha; **Rasa** : tikta, kashay; **Vipak** : katu; **Veerya** : ushna.
Fruit is sweet and sour, and sheeta veerya.
Karma :
Dosha : Kaphapittahara, the fruit is pittashamak, hence used in diseases originating from kapha - pitta.
External uses : Shothaghna or reduces inflammation or oedema, removes pain, cures and heals ulcers, also used for eye diseases. Hence in severe conjunctivitis, the paste is applied around the eyes and 250 mg rasanjan mixed with 20 ml. of rosewater is used as eyedrops (or can be applied on eyelids). This fluid can also be applied in the ears in earache or ear discharge. In diseases of the mouth and throat, rasanjan is used for gargling. Rasanjan can be used to wash wounds or its paste can be applied on ulcers. Chancroid ulcers, goitre, fistula, erysipelas and other diseases are treated by the application of the paste. Vaginal discharges are treated by the douche prepared from berberis. Puerperal diseases are treated by the application of rasanjan on perianal wounds.
Inernal uses :
Digestive system : Appetiser, liver stimulant, cholagogue but astringent. A larger dose is laxative. The fruit is very tasty and antidipsetic. Because of these actions, daruharidra is a superior medicine in agnimandya, dysentery, jaundice and other liver disorders. The tablet of rasanjan prepared in radish juice is useful in bleeding piles. It is also effctive in diarrhoea. Daruharidra formulation gives excellent results in cholera.
Circulatory system : Blood purifier and haemostatic agent. Daruharidra decoction is given in syphilis and other sexual diseases. Hematemesis, malena and menorrhagia respond only to rasanjan or coagulant preparations + rasanjan. Reduces pus. Daruharidra acts on rakta dhatu. Because of daruharidra, the inactive forms of malarial parasite in the spleen come out in the blood stream and this is very useful for the diagnostic test for malarial parasite by peripheral smear.
Respiratory system : It is useful in the treatment of cough being kaphaghna.
Reproductive system : Useful in uterine inflammations and vaginal discharges.
Skin : Diaphoretic, useful in diseases of the skin like pruritus, boils etc. Daruharidra decoction is useful in cleansing wounds. Rasanjan + honey is used externally in puerperal diseases. It is specially useful in ulcer. The decoction is used for gargling in stomatitis.
Temperature : Febrifuge and diaphoretic and is a prophylactic treatment for typhoid, hence it is useful in common fever and also in chronic fever. It causes sweating, is antipyretic and is useful in recurrent malaria. When malarial parasites hide in the liver, quinine is not effective but daruharidra is very effective. After administering a mild laxative, 1 gm. of rasanjan is dissolved in water and given 3 to 4 times in a day. Then the patient is covered with thick clothes and

blankets and made to sleep. After a while the patient will feel thirsty but should not be given water. After an hour there will be sweating. The sweat should be wiped clean. Warm milk or sage kheer should be given orally. This preserves and increases the patient's strength. The fever is reduced and there is reduction in hepatosplenomegaly.

Satmikaran : It is bitter and strengthening, hence useful in general debility.

Parts used : Roots, stem and fruit.

Dosage : Juice of root 10 to 20 ml.; decoction - 50 to 100 ml.; rasanjan - 1/4 to 1/2 gms; fruit - 1 gm. in malaria (total) 5 to 10 mg. as a stimulant for heart but larger dose can lead to cardiac depression.

Adulteration : Daruharidra is adulterated with shoots of plants like samudrashosha after boiling them in decoction of turmeric. The shoots of real daruharidra are elastic and do not lose their yellow colour even after boiling.

Formulations : Darvyadikwath, Darvyadileha, Darvyaditaila.

Rasanjanshuddhi : Rasanjan available in the market should be purified by mixing in four parts of hot water and subsequent straining. Then it should be cooked on fire after mixing with milk or should be dehydrated by exposure to sunlight.

Srotogamitva :

Dosha : Reduces kapha.

Dhatu : Meda, rasayan, raktagami.

Mala : Mutra - purisha - sweda.

Organs : Eyes, liver, spleen and skin.

References -

'तिक्ता दारुहरिद्रा स्याद्रूक्षोष्णा व्रणमेहनुत् । कर्णनेत्रमुखोदभूतां रुजंकण्डूं च शोषयेत् ।।' (ध.नि.)

'दार्वीक्वाथसमं क्षीरं पादं पक्त्वा यदा घनम् । तदा रसाञ्जनं ख्यातं नेत्रयोः परमं हितम् ।।
रसाञ्जनं कटु श्लेष्मविषनेत्रविकारनुत् । उष्णं रसायनं तिक्तं छेदनं व्रणदोषकृत् ।। (भा.प्र.)
तोयेऽत्युष्णे परिक्षिप्य द्रवीकुर्याद्रसाञ्जनम् । वाससा स्त्रावयित्वा च पयसा मिश्रयेत् पुनः ।।
मन्दाग्निना पचेद्वापि शोषयेत् सूर्यरश्मिना । एवं विशोधितं तार्क्ष्यशैलं कर्मसु योजयेत् ।।' (स्व.)

(57) DEVADARU

Cedrus deodar Roxb - Loud.

Gana : Stanyashodhana, Anuvasanopaga, Katukashkandha (C.); Vatasamshaman (S.)

Kula : Devdaru kula.

Family : Conifereae.

Latin name : Cedrus = Latin. Cedar tree, wood having aromatic like cedar. Arabic origin of the name Kedron or Kedree = power, majestic appearance of these trees; deodar = Sanskrit name (Roxb-Loud).

English name : Deodar.

Sanskrit names : Deodaru (Himalaya is God's country where this tree is grown), Bhadradaru (good fragrant wood), Daru, Suradaru, Snigdhadaru, Shambhava, Bhootahari, Bhavdaru, Suravha, Indradu, Snehavriksha.

One who does not practice panchashuddhi or panchakarma either on himself or on his patient is only half a doctor.

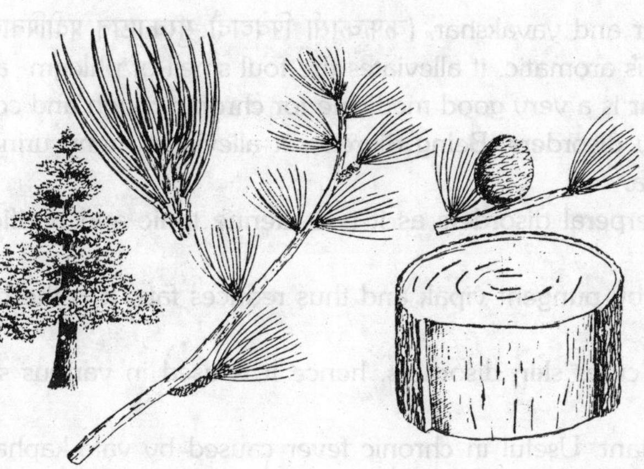

Botanical Description : Big tree of height 85 meters. Stem - big erect having circumference 12 meters. Bark - thick and cracked. Leaves - are green, elongated with tapering ends. Flowers - green, yellow and appear in clusters. Fruit - ripe fruit is black having seed 1 cm. long. The tree bears new fruits in October, which ripe within a year. Deodar tree has a long life having life span of 600 years. (Life span of Sequoia tree in California is 3000 years).

Types:

DEVADARU

Snigdhadaru	Kashthadaru
It has thick and oily wood and available in the market in the name of 'Dhoopa'	Ashoka tree is known as Kashthadaru. The leaves of this tree are used for festive occasions. Its latin name is Polyalthia longifolia, Anonaceae family and Sitafala Kula.

Habitat : At the height of 2000 to 3000 meters in Himalayas.

Chemical composition : It contains dark coloured oil and resin.

Properties :

Guna : laghu, snigdha; **Rasa :** tikta, katu; **Vipak :** katu; **Veerya :** ushna.

Karma :

Dosha : Kaphashamak by tikta, katu and ushna, vatashamak by snigdha and ushna properties. Useful in disorders induced by kapha - vata.

External uses : Inflammation is relieved by its local application. Useful in skin disorders, helminthiasis and ulcers. Its local application and oil are used in arthritis. Its oil (terpentine) is a very good wound cleaner and healer. Application of oil destroys bacteria from infected wounds. It is also useful in oral and nasal disorders and other wounds. It removes the foul smell of wounds. Fomentation of hot water and oil relieves flatulence.

Internal uses :

Central nervous system : Deodar is the topmost in the analgesics, hence it is used in chronic inflammatory arthritis, osteoarthritis, sciatic neuralgia and painful conditions like headache.

Digestive system : Due to pungent and bitterness it is an appetizer, digestant, laxative and also effective in destroying the cause factors of worms.

Circulatory system : As it is ushna, bitter and pungent, it is a cardiostimulant, blood purifier and alleviates swelling. Oil is useful in mumps, filaria and chancre.

Respiratory system : It is an expectorant by snigdha, pungent, bitter properties. In cough caused by kapha, oil is given along with dry ginger and yavakshar. (कफकासी पिबेदादौ सुरकाष्ठात् प्रदीपितात् ।) Because it acts on the respiratory tract and is aromatic, it alleviates the foul smell of phlegm and hiccoughs caused due to vata-kapha. Deodar is a very good medicine for chronic cough and cold.

Urinary system : It is effective in urinary disorders. Being diuretic, it alleviates many urinary disorders. Useful in dysuria and gonorrhoea.

Reproductive system : It is used in puerperal disorders as it is a uterine tonic and purifies breast milk.

Satmikaran : Deodar has curating action by pungent vipak and thus reduces fats. It is the best medicine in obesity.

Skin : It has diaphoretic property and it cures skin disorders, hence it is used in various skin diseases.

Temperature : It is diaphoretic and digestant. Useful in chronic fever caused by vata-kapha.

Parts used : Inner substance of wood and oil.

Dosage : Powder - 1 to 3 gm.; oil - 20 to 40 drops.

Formulations : Deodarvadi kwath, Deodarvyadi churna, Rasnadi kwath, Deodarvyarishta

Srotogamitva :

Dosha : Kaphaghna, vataghna.

Dhatu : Rakta, meda (mumps) (filariasis), rasa.

Mala : Purisha - mutra - diuretic.

Organs : Respiratory system, uterus.

References -

'देवदारुलघु स्निग्धं तिक्तोष्णं कटुपाकि च । विबन्धाध्मानशोथामतन्द्राहिक्काज्वरास्रजित् ।। प्रमेहपीनसश्लेष्मकासकण्डूसमीरनुत् ।।' (भा.प्र.)

'देवदार्वनिलं हन्ति स्निग्धोष्णं श्लेष्मपाकतः ।' (ध.नि.)

'देवदारुस्नेहास्तिक्तकटुकषाया दुष्टव्रणशोधनाः कृमिकफकुष्टानिलहराश्च ।' (सु.सू. ४५)

'दशमूलस्य वा क्वाथमथवा देवदारुणः । तृषितो मदिरां वापि हिक्काश्वासी पिबेन्नरः ।।' (च.चि. १७)

(58) DRONAPUSHPI

Leucos cephalotus Spreng.

Gana : Tulsi kula.

Family : Labiatae.

Latin name : Leucas = or leucos = white flowers of all the species.; cephalotus = kepale = head - in heads as of flowers.

Sanskrit names : Dronapushpi (having drona-shaped flowers (drona=a vessel made of leaves), Drona, Falepushpa (flowers on fruit).

Botanical Description : It is a shrub having a life-span of one year and which grows in rainy season. Stem - is 0.5 to 1 m., rectangular and hairy. Leaves - are 5 to 8 cm. long and 1.25 cm. wide. Leaves are hairy having serrated margins. Flowers - white - appear in clusters having circumference 2.5 to 5 cm. 2-3 leaves grow on the top of the cluster (In villages, the phrase 'leaves on flowers` must be derived from Dronapushpi). Flowers are drona-shaped (cup or bucket).

During treatment, functions of vitiated vayu are to be decreased and at the same time, precaution must be taken that physiological functions of vayu are produced.

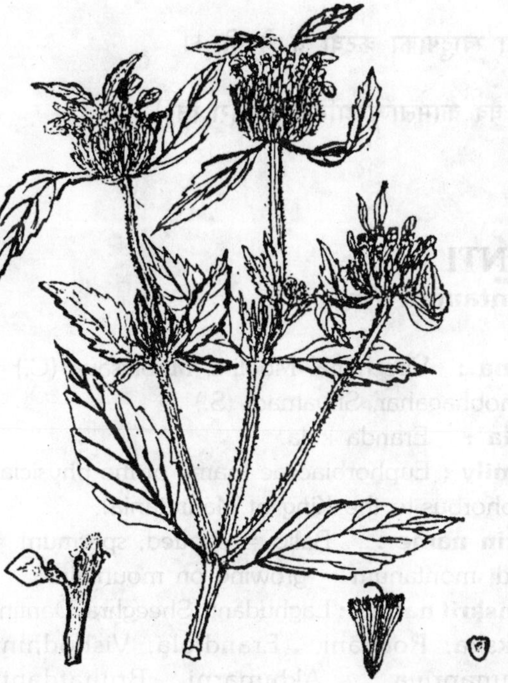

Flowering season is winter, while in summer the plant dries off.

Habitat : At the height of 1.25 thousand meters in Himalayas. All over India and Srilanka.

Chemical composition : Flower has an aromatic oil and alkaloids.

Properties :

Guna : guru, ruksha, tikshna; **Rasa :** madhur, katu, lavana; **Vipak :** madhur; **Veerya :** ushna.

Karma :

Dosha : Kaphavatashamak, pittashodhan. It is used for alleviation in disorders induced by kapha-vata, while for elimination in pitta disorders.

External use : It is an expectorant, antiparasitic and antidote. Its juice is used as nasal drops in cold and headache. Decoction is used for cleaning wounds. Juice is applied locally on snake bite. It is used as an eye-ointment in jaundice.

Internal use :

Digestive system : Being an appetizer, carminative, laxative and antiparasitic, its juice is used in flatulence, abdominal pain, constipation, icterus and worms - juice is used as an eye-ointment in jaundice.

Circulatory system : Blood purifier, alleviates oedema, hence useful in blood disorders and oedema. Juice is used as nasal drops in headache due to cold.

Respiratory system : It is an expectorant. Its decoction or hot infusion is useful in cold, cough and dyspnoea.

Reproductive system : Being an emmenagogue, it is used in amenorrhoea and dysmenorrhoea.

Skin : Useful in skin disorders. It eliminates vitiated doshas from the skin by its diaphoretic action. Juice is used for massage in pruritus.

Temperature : Febrifuge (because of its diaphoretic property), mainly in typhoid and fever induced by vata-kapha.

Satmikaran : Antidote, effective in snake bite.

Parts used : Panchanga (all parts), leaves, flowers.

Dosage : 5 to 10 mg.

Dronapushpi is a stimulant.

Srotogamitva :

Dosha : Vitiates vata and pitta, alleviates kapha.

Dhatu : Amadhatu (digestive), rakta (jaundice), rasa (fever).

Mala : Purisha (cathartic) (anti parasitic), sweda (fever).

Organs : Respiratory system (asthma).

Treatment means stopping health-threatening channels and activating health-promoting channels.

References -
'द्रोणपुष्पी गुरुः स्वादू रूक्षोष्णावातपित्तकृत् । सतीक्ष्णा लवणा स्वादुपाका कटवी च भेदनी ।।
कफामकामलाशोषतमकश्वासजन्तुजित् ।' (भा.प्र.)
'द्रोणपुष्पी कटुः सोष्णा रुच्या वातकफापहा । अग्निमांद्यहरा चैव कामलाज्वरहारिणी ।। (रा.नि.)
'द्रोणपुष्पीरसो वापि निहन्ति विषमज्वरान् ।' (भा.प्र.)
'अंजने कामलार्त्तानां द्रोणपुष्पीरसो हितः ।' (वृन्द.)

(59) DANTI

Baliospermun montanum Arg.

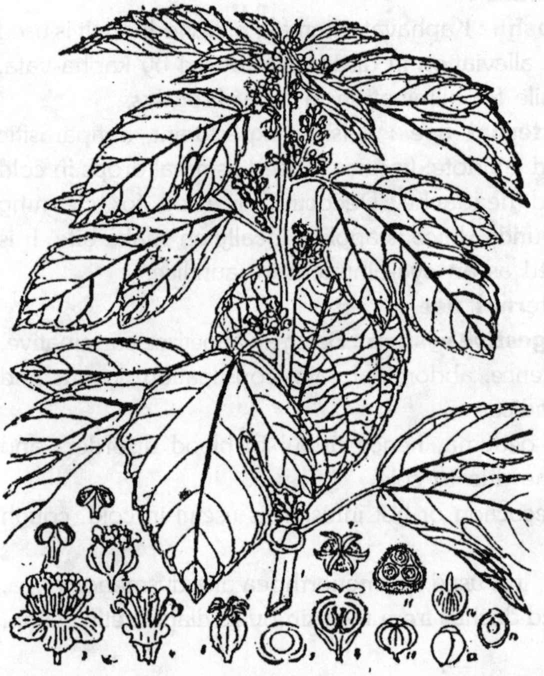

Gana : Virechana, Moolini, Moolasava (C.) Adhobhagahar, Shyamadi (S.)
Kula : Eranda kula.
Family : Euphorbiaceae (name of the physician Euphorbus-to the King of Mauretania).
Latin name : Balio = spotted, spermum = seed; montanum = growing on mountains.
Sanskrit names : Laghudanti, Sheeghra, Dantini, Ruksha, Rochani, Erandfala, Vishodhini, Ghunapriya, Akhuparni, Bruhatdanti, Bhishagbhadra, Dravanti, Visha.
Botanical Description : A small tree of hight 1-2 mtrs. Leaves - have different shapes and sizes from bottom to the top. New leaves are 15 to 30 cm. long while upper leaves are 5 to 8 cm. in length. Lower leaves are broad. Flowers - homogenous pale green. Androecium is bigger as compared to the stalk. Fruit - 1.5 to 2.5 cm., divided in to 3 compartments having 3 coloured seeds. Flowering season is spring. Growth of danti needs the shades of other trees.

Varities : It is of 2 varieties.
1) Laghudanti (It is known as danti).
2) Bruhatdanti (it is known as dravanti). Above described plant is danti.

One more plant named Nagadanti is described (Puner from Bengal - Croton oblongifolia-Roxb).
Habitat : It mainly grows in Bengal, Bihar, Southern India and Brahmadesha.
Chemical composition : Roots contain resin and starch, seeds contain oil.
Properties :
Guna : guru, ruksha, tikshna; **Rasa :** katu; **Vipak :** katu; **Veerya :** ushna.
Prabhav : virechaka, ashukari, vikashi.

Karma :
Dosha : Eliminates kapha - pitta, hence useful in kapha-pitta disorders where elimination is necessary.
External use : The paste of roots and seeds is used in oedema and pain. The root paste is applied on painful oedema and haemorrhoids. Seed oil is used for massage in vata disorders.
Internal use :
Digestive system : Being an appetizer, liver stimulant, cholagogue and laxative, it is used in anorexia, haemorrhoids and helminthiasis.
Circulatory system : It is a blood purifier, raktagami. It reduces oedema by its eliminative action. Useful for elimination of doshas in jaundice.
Respiratory system : Decoction of the leaves is used in dyspnoea.
Urinary system : Useful in calculi.
Skin : As it is diaphoretic, it cures skin disorders by eliminating doshas.
Temperature : Useful in fever with constipation.
Satmikaran : It has an antidote action though vikasi is the property of poison.
Parts used : Leaves, roots, seed.
Dosage : Root powder 1 to 3 mg.; seed 1/2 to 1 ratti (1ratti = 125 mg.); decoction of leaves 40 to 80 ml.
Formulations : Dantyarishta, Dantyadi churna, Dantiharitaki, Granthibhedana lepa (Some formulations are also described in Kalpa sthana of Vagbhatta and Charaka samhita.)
Processing : Danti causes griping pain in abdomen and nausea. So aromatic drugs like dry ginger, fennel etc. should be used along with it.
Method of collection : Take the root of danti-dravanti which is stiff like an elephant tooth, thick, blackish red in colour, add long pepper and honey and make a paste. Then cover it with kushas (a particular type of grass) and give putapak. Then make it dry by keeping it in sunlight or by heating it on a stove. This process reduces the vikasi action of danti-dravanti.
Higher dose causes intoxication. Antidote is sweet and unctuous drugs, sugar, water, milk and ghee.
Adulteration : mixing red castor roots.
Srotogamitva :
Dosha : Alleviates kapha, pitta, vitiates vata.
Dhatu : Rakta (skin disorders, rubefacient).
Mala : Purisha (drastic purgative), mutra (calculifragous).
Prabhav : Anthelmintic, antidote, vikasi, ashukari.
Organs : Rectum, lower parts of the body.
References -
'दन्तीद्वयं सरं पाके रसे च कटु दीपनम् । गुदांकुराश्मशूलार्शः कण्डूकुष्ठविदाहनुत् ।।
तीक्ष्णोष्णं हन्ति पित्तास्रकफशोथोदरकृमीन् ।' (भा.प्र.)
'तीक्ष्णोष्णान्याशुकारीणि विकाशीनि गुरूणि च ।
विलाययन्ति दोषौ द्वौ मारुतं कोपयन्ति च ।।' (च.क. १२)
'तयोर्मूलानि संगृह्य स्थिराणि बहलानि च । हस्तिदन्तप्रकाराणि श्यावताम्राणि बुद्धिमान् ।।

All treatments should strengthen and stabilize prana. It should not weaken or destabilize it.

पिप्पलीमधुलिप्तानि स्वेदयेत् मृत्कुशान्तरे । शोषयेदातपेऽग्न्यर्कों हतो ह्येषां विकाशिताम् ।। (च.क. १२)
'दन्तीद्रवन्तीस्नेहास्तिक्तकटुकषाया: अधोभागदोषहरा कृमिकुष्ठकफानिलहरा: दुष्ट-व्रणशोधनाश्च ।' (सु.सू. ४५)

(60) DHATTURA

Dhattura stramonium

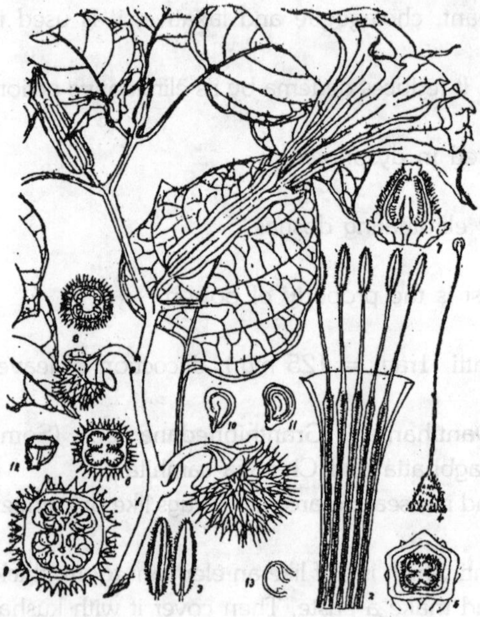

Kula : Dhattura kula.

Family : Atropaceae (Atra = black).

Latin name : Dhattura = from sanskrit word; stramonium = inclined to madness. (straminis - straw coloured).

English name : Thorn apple.

Sanskrit names : Dhoorta, Unmatta, Kanaka, Kharjughna, Khala, Kantafala, Matta, Madakar, Matula, Mahamohi, Matula, Shivapriya.

Botanical Description : It is of 3 varities - white, black and rajadhotra (5 varities according to some others).

Chemical composition : Leaves contain a principle similar to that found in henbane.

Properties :

Rasa : kashaya, madhura, tikta; **Vipak** : katu; **Veerya** : ushna; **Prabhav** : madakari.

Karma:

Dosha : Both vatashamak and vatakar actions are seen depending on the dosages.

Varieties :

Rajadhattur : Grows in Kashmir, Gadhwal and Nepal. Seed is black, kidney-shaped and flat. Leaves are hairy. Flowers are white. It has 4 compartments.

(White) Shwetadhattura : Flowers are white, completely hairy plant. Fruits are elongated with thorns on them and leaves are big. Seeds are brown and flat. Fruit ruptures irregularly.

(Black) Krishnadhattura : Same as shweta variety but without hair on it. Stalk is pale blue-veins of leaves are pale black. Externally, flowers are purple-black. Fruits have flat thorns on them instead of elongated. Seed is brown, flat. Used for medicinal purpose. Fruit ruptures irregularly.

External use : Leaf juice is applied in alopecia and inflammation. It alleviates pain. The paste of turmeric with juice of dhattura leaves is used in mastitis. In mastitis with galactorrhoea, hot fomentation of leaves is effective.

Internal use :

Central nervous system : It is an intoxicant.

Respiratory system : Fomentation of the leaves and seeds is useful in asthma.

Reproductive system : Seeds are useful as aphrodisiac in some patients.

Health and disease are known by their symptoms. Symptoms are induced by karmas. Karmas are the functions of gunas. So the philosophy of gunas is superior.

Digestive system : Formulations of dhattura seeds are used in enteric pains. Formulations like sutashekhar are useful in pain induced by pitta.
Temperature : In fever with rigors, dhattura seeds in curds are given before rigors start. It alleviates rigors and also post pyrexial burning sensation and bodyache.
Antidote : Mixture of shwetapunarnava 1/2 tola i. e. 5 gms. and datura root 4 gunja (500 mg) in cold water or milk should be given in rabies.
Parts used : Leaves, seed, root (seeds are purified by processing in dolayantra along with cow's milk). Seeds are kept in cow's urine for a week for purification.
Formulation: Kanaksundar.
Dosage : Seed powder 0.5 to 1mg,; leaf powder 0.5 to 1.5 mg.; for smoking 0.33 to 1 gm.
Srotogamitva :
Dosha : Vatavardhak, shleshmaghna.
Dhatu : Rasa (fever), rakta (skin diseases), majja.
Mala : Lice scavenger.
Organ : Brain.
References -
धत्तूरो मदवर्णाग्निवातकृत् ज्वरकुष्ठनुत् ।
कषायो मधुरस्तिक्तो यूकालिक्षाविनाशकः ।
उष्णो गुरुर्व्रणश्लेष्मकण्डुक्रिमिविषापहः ।। (भा.प्र.)

(61) DHATAKI
Woodfordia floribunda Kurz.

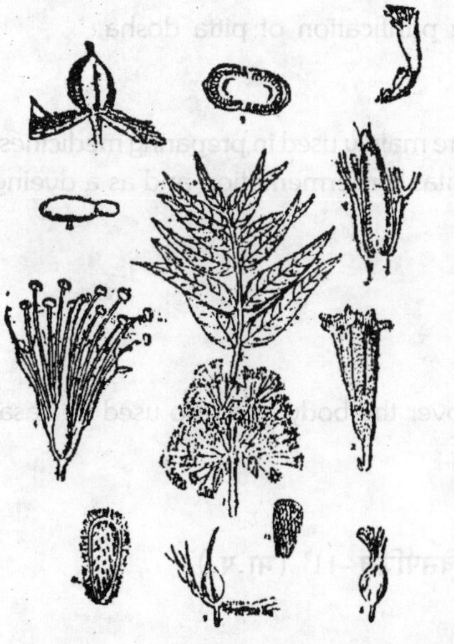

Gana : Purishasangrahaniya, Mutravirajaniya, Sandhaniya (C.), Priyangwadi, Ambashthadi (S.)
Kula : Madayantika kula (Dhayati kula).
Family : Lythraceae (loose strife) luthrum = from Gk. Luthron = black blood (colour of the flowers).
Latin name : Woodfordia = J. Woodford - botanist; floribunda = flowers appear in clusters or fructicosa = shrubby.
English name : Downy grislea.
Sanskrit name : Dhataki, Vahnipushpi, Tamrapushpi, Dahani, Parvati, Kumuda, Guchhapushpa, Madani, Pramadani.
Botanical Description : A shrub with many branches. Leaves - sessile, resemble pomengranate leaves, 5 to 10 cm long, stalkless. The leaf is hairy from beneath because of which it looks whitish. Flowers- shiny, red coloured. Seed - is grey and slimy. The plant bears flowers in winter and fruits in rainy season. Leaves and new branches have black spots on them.

Habitat : All over India, mainly on hilly regions.
Chemical composition : Flower contains 2% tanin.
Properties :
Guna: laghu, ruksha ; **Rasa:** kashaya, katu; **Vipak:** katu; **Veerya:** sheeta.
Karma :
Dosha : Kaphapittanashak. Useful in disorders induced by kapha, pitta.
External uses : Being refrigerant, haemostatic, wound healer, powdered flower is sprinkled externally over bleeds and wounds. Powdered flower is rubbed over gums to prevent teething problems and the juice is used for massage in headache induced by pitta.
Internal uses :
Digestive system : It has astringent properties useful in chronic diarrhoea and dysentery. Powdered flower is useful in haemorrhoids.
Circulatory system : It has binding and alleviating property, hence useful in bleeding disorders. Powder of the flowers is used in heart diseases.
Urinary system : Vitiation of pitta leads to discolouration of urine like dark yellow, red and blue. The flowers cure such disorders and also used in prameha caused by pitta.
Reproductive system : Useful in per vaginal discharges. In menorrhagia or leucorrhoea, it is given either with rice water or honey or in the form of jam.
Skin : Kushthaghna, used in erysipelas and other skin disorders.
Temperature : Febrifuge - mainly fever caused by pitta dosha. In Konkan region, patient suffering from pittajwar (fever caused by pitta dosha) is asked to hold sesame oil in his mouth and juice of these leaves is applied on the head. This procedure changes the colour of oil to yellow and then the oil should be spitted out. Again fresh oil is held in the mouth. This procedure is done twice or thrice till oil retains its original colour which indicates the purification of pitta dosha.
Parts used : Flowers, leaves.
Dosage : Powder 1 to 3 gms.
Formulations : Dhatakyadi churna, Dhatakyaditaila. Flowers are mainly used in preparing medicines. These flowers are used in making nearly 95% asavas and arishtas for fermentation and as a dyeing agent.
Srotogamitva :
Dosha : Alleviates pitta.
Dhatu : Rakta (haemostat) (erysipelas), majja (narcotic).
Mala : Purisha (astringent) (antidiarrhoeal).
Prabhav : In snake-bite, leaf juice is given orally, rubbed all over the body and also used as nasal drops. This is considered an infallible treatment in Konkan.
References -
'धातुकी दाडिमीपत्रा रक्तपुष्पा च मादिनी । (शि.)
धातकी कटुका शीता मदकृत्तुवरा लघुः । तृष्णातीसारपित्तास्रविषक्रिमिविसर्पजित् ।।' (भा.प्र.)
'प्रवाहिकातिसारघ्नी विसर्पव्रणनाशिनी ।' (रा.नि.)
'धातकीकुसुमं शीतं रक्तपित्तातिसारजित् ।' (रा.व.)

In the chapter called Mashaparneeya Adhyaya of Charaka samhita, it is not mentioned as to how many days the leaves of mashaparni are give to a cow to make it mashaparna bhrita. It will at least take a month.

(62) DHANYAKAM

Coriandrum sativum Linn.

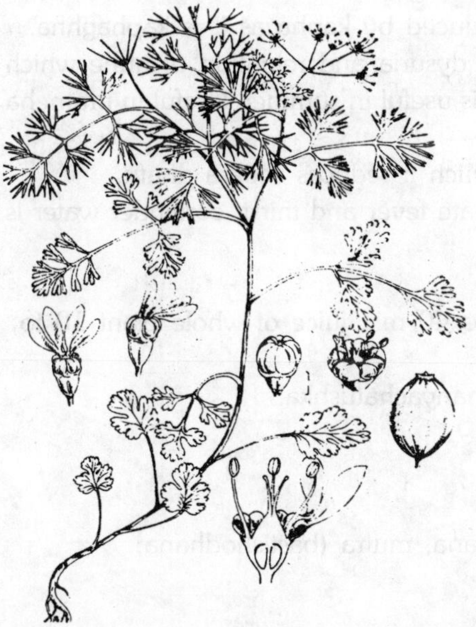

Gana : Trishnanigrahana, Sheetaprashamana (C.) Guduchyadi (S.)
Kula : Mandookaparni kula.
Family : Umbelliferae.
Latin name : Coriandrum - corys = helmet, andrum = antheres; sativum = because it is being cultivated.
English name : Coriander.
Sanskrit names : Dhanyaka, Chhatra (umbrella-shaped flowers), Vitunnaka, Chhatradhanya, Sugandhi, Sukshmapatra, Haridgandha, Hridya, Veshna.
Botanical Description : A small herb having many branches and sub-branches. New leaves are oval but arial leaves are elongated. Flowers - white, having slightly brinjal like shade. Fruits - round, divided into 2 parts. The herb bears flowers and seeds at the end of winter.
Types : 2 types - rural and wild.
Habitat : All over India.
Chemical composition : Green coriander contains 84% water. Seeds contain 1% volatile oil, 13% stable oil, 13% resin, astringent principle, malic acid and alkaloids, coriander oil contains coriandrol, jirenyol and vebriniol.
Properties :
Guna : laghu, snigdha; **Rasa :** kashaya, tikta, madhur; **Vipak :** madhur; **Veerya :** ushna.
Karma :
Dosha : Tridoshahar, snigdha, ushna=vatashaman; kashaya, tikta, madhur = pittashaman; tikta, katu and ushna = kaphashaman. Green coriander being cold is pittashamak. Coriander is used in many diseases induced by all the 3 doshas.
External use : Local application of coriander seeds alleviates swelling and pains. Paste of green coriander has very good action on headache caused by pitta. Externally, powdered green coriander alleviates burning sensation and pain in diseases like inflammation caused by pitta, erysipelas and lymphadenopathy. Decoction of green coriander is useful in stomatitis. In epistaxis, nasal drops of green coriander acts as a haemostat and thus stops bleeding. In conjunctivitis, either juice or decoction of green coriander is put in eyes. The paste of dry coriander is used in headache.
Internal use :
Central nervous system : Tonic for majjadhatu. Only pulp from coverless coriander should be taken and boiled with milk. This milk cures vertigo, syncope and memory loss.
Digestive system : Being antidypsetic, appetizer, digestive, astringent, liver stimulant and anthelmintic, cold or hot infusion is used in fever related thirst. Repeated administration of coriander water is

Fattening medicines (American food) are given to animals like cow or bull fifteen days before they are slaughtered for eating purpose.

effective in distaste, emesis, anorexia, indigestion, dysentery, diarrhoea abdominal pain, piles and helminthiasis.

Circulatory system : Green coriander is effective in bleeding disorders.

Respiratory system : Useful in cough and dyspnoea induced by kapha as it is kaphaghna.

Urinary system : It is the best diuretic. It is effective in dysuria and retention of urine which commonly occurs in summer season. Thandai of coriander is useful in summer. Useful in prameha caused by pitta.

Reproductive system : It is an astringent because of which it reduces shukra dhatu.

Temperature : Febrifuge and refrigerant. In fever, to alleviate fever and thirst, coriander water is given repeatedly.

Parts used : Seeds and whole plant.

Dosage : Seed powder 2 to 4 mg.; cold infusion 20 to 40 ml.; juice of whole plant 10 to 20 ml.

Formulations : Dhanyakadi Hima, Dhanyapanchaka, Dhanyachatushka.

Srotogamitva :

Dosha : Tridoshashamak.

Dhatu : Shukra, rasa (fever).

Mala : Mutra (diuretic), purisha (astringent), srotovishodhana, mutra (bastishodhana).

Organs : Eyes, heart.

References -

**'धान्यकं तुवरं स्निग्धमवृष्यं मूत्रलं लघु । तिक्तं कटुकमुष्णं च दीपनं पाचनं स्मृतम् ।।
ज्वरघ्नं रोचनं ग्राहि स्वादुपाकि त्रिदोषनुत् । तृष्णादाहवमिश्वासकासामार्श कृमिप्रणुत् ।।
आर्द्र तु तदगुणं स्वादु विशेषात् पित्तनाशि तत् ।' (भा.प्र.)
'धान्यकं कासतृड्छर्दिज्वरहच्चक्षुषो हितम् । कषायं तिक्तमधुरं हृद्यं रोचनदीपनम् ।।' (ध.नि.)
'धान्यतुम्बरु । रोचनं दीपनं वातकफदौर्गन्ध्यनाशनम् ।।' (च.सू.२७)
'भक्ष्यव्यञ्जनभोज्येषु विविधेष्ववचारिता । आर्द्रा कुस्तुम्बरी कुर्यात् स्वादुसौगन्ध्यहृद्यताम् ।। (सु.सू. ४६)
'प्रातः सशर्करः पेयो हिमो धान्यकसंभवः । अन्तर्दाहं तथा तृष्णां जयेत् स्त्रोतोविशोधनः ।।' (भा.प्र.)
'धान्यनागरसिद्धं तु तोयं दद्यात् विचक्षणः । आमाजीर्णप्रशमनं शूलघ्नं बस्तिशोधनम् ।।' (बं.से.)
धान्यं शर्करया युक्तं तण्डुलोदकसंयुतम् । पानमेतत् प्रदातव्यं कासश्वासापहं शिशोः ।।' (ब.से.)**

(63) NAGKESAR
Mesua ferrea Benth + hook.

Gana : Eladi, Sugandhivarga, Priyangvadi, Anjanadi (S.) Chaturjat (Bhavaprakash) (संकेसर चतुर्जातम्)

Kula : Nagakesar kula.

Family : Guttifereae (guttetus = marked with drops or spots of different colours).

Latin name : Mesua = After the name of two Arab scientists 8th - 9th century; ferrea = rust coloured.

English name : Iron Wood tree, Cobra's saffron.

Sanskrit names : Kinjalka, Champeya, Nagakinjalka, Kanchan, Suvarna, Rukma, Nagapushpa, Ahipushpa, Mahapushpa, Hemapushpaka, Gaja.

Science is related to lifelessness. It is necessary to establish a link between life and lifelessness for the use of science in our lives.

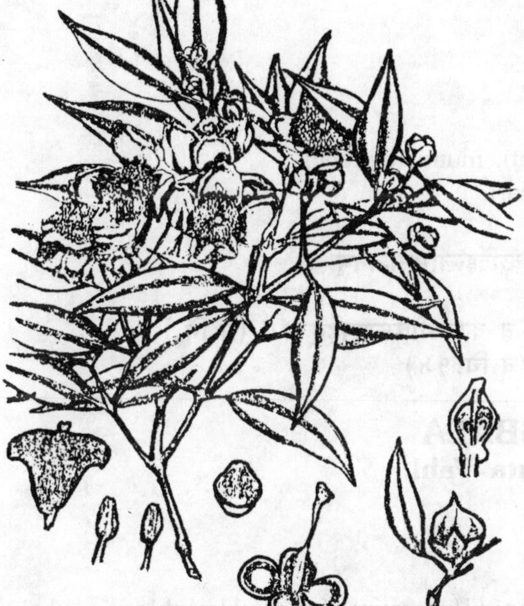

Botanical Description : Evergreen medium sized, beautiful tree. Bark - reddish, pale yellow-green gum comes out from the bark. Leaves - 5 to 15 cm. long, 4 to 7 cm. broad, tapering at both ends.
Habitat : Mainly Nepal, Eastern Himalayas, Bengal, Assam, Konkan, Kerala, Andaman and Brahmadesha upto 1.65 thousand mtrs. from the sea level.
Chemical composition : Raw fruit contains oily resin and also yellow and fragrant oil. Seeds also contain thick oil. Saffron contains 2 bitter principles.
Properties :
Guna : laghu and ruksha; **Rasa** : kashaya, tikta; **Vipak** : katu; **Veerya** : slightly ushna.
Karma :
Dosha : Kaphapittashamak, so useful in disorders induced by kapha - pitta.
External uses : Seed oil is analgesic. Saffron is deodorant, antidiaphoretic and stimulant. Hence seed oil is used in inflammatory arthritis for massage and saffron is used in foul smelling, excessive perspiration and wounds. It is locally applied over penis in impotency (due to its stimulant action). Nagkesar mixed with shatadhouta ghee is applied on burning palms and soles.
Internal uses :
Central nervous system : Being brain tonic it is useful in brain debility and hysteria.
Digestive system : It is an appetizer, mainly digestive, antidipsetic, antiemetic, antihaemorrhoid, astringent and vermicide, hence it is used in anorexia, distaste, dipsia, emesis, worms, bleeding piles, dysentery. It acts as a haemostatic in bleeding piles. It should be given as a single drug.
Circulatory system : Being cardiac tonic and haemostatic, it is used in cardiac debility, rakta pitta, and blood disorders.
Respiratory system : It is used in cough induced by kapha, dyspnoea and hiccougs as it alleviates kapha.
Reproductive system : It is used as an aphrodisiac and as a haemostatic in menorrhagia.
Urinary system : Diuretic, hence useful in retention of urine.
Skin : Kushthaghna. It is used in skin disorders, erysipelas.
Temperature : Febrifuge. Useful in fever.
Satmikaran : It is used as a tonic and antidote.
Parts used : Stemens.
Dosage : 1 to 2 gms.
(Nagkesar which is available as a spice in the market is not original nagkesar)
Bark of the tree and sugar is used to induce diaphoresis while decoction of flowers helps in reducing

A man who misuses either science or weapons doesnot realise the good of the society. It requires a spiritual mind for their judicious use.

diaphoresis. Also useful in bleeding piles and burning of palms and soles. Oil should be used for massage in inflammatory arthritis.

Srotogamitva :

Dosha : Kapha, pitta (alleviation).

Dhatu : Rakta, majja, shukra (aphrodisiac).

Mala : Sweda (antidiaphoretic), purisha (astringent), mutra (diuretic).

Special action : Bleeding piles (butter + nagkesar).

References -

'नागपुष्पं कषायोष्णं रूक्षं लघ्वामपाचनम् । ज्वरकण्डूतृषास्वेदच्छर्दिहृल्लासनाशनम् ।।
दौर्गन्ध्यकुष्ठवीसर्पकफपित्तविषापहम् ।' (भा.प्र.)
'नागकेशरमल्पोष्णं लघु तिक्तं कफापहम् । बस्तिवातामयघ्नं च कण्ठशीर्षरुजापहम् ।।' (रा.नि.)
केशरनवनीतशर्कराभ्यासात् । अर्शांस्यपयान्ति रक्तानि ।।' (च.चि.१४)

(64) NAGBALA

Grewia hirsuta Vahl.

Kula : Parushaka kula.

Family : Tiliaceae (Tilia, lime tree family).

Latin name : Grewia (Nahemiah Grew M.D.Botanist, (anatomy of vegetables); hirsuta = hairy.

Sanskrit names : Nagabala, Mahabala, Kharagandha, Chatuhfala, Mahoday, Mahapatra, Arishta, Devadanda, Gangeruki, Khandari, Shasha.

Botanical Description : A small shrub 13 to 18 cm. high having long life-span. Leaves - 5 to 8 cm. long, tapering at both the ends, hairy and with serrated margines. Flowers - 2/3 flowers grow from the base of the leaf which are yellow internally and pink from outside. Fruit - small, yellow, divided into four compartments and breaks when becomes ripe. Ripe fruits are sweet and tasty. They are called as 'shikari mewa'. Each fruit has 5 to 6 seeds. The shrub bears flowers and fruits in autumn and winter.

Habitat : It grows in tropical countries, but also grows in stony and hilly regions. Abundant in Bihar, Vindhyapradesh, Rajasthan and Konkan.

Properties :

Guna : guru, snigdha, pichchila; **Rasa** : madhur, kashaya.; **Vipak** : madhur; **Veerya** : sheeta.

Karma :

Dosha : Vatapittashamak, hence useful in disorders induced by vata-pitta.

External use : It has haemostatic, analgesic and wound healing properties. Paste of either root or leaves is used in bleeding disorders and wounds.

Internal use :

Central nervous system : Being a nervine and brain tonic, it is useful in nerve debility, loss of memory and vata disorders.

Digestive system : Unctuous, antacid and laxative. Useful in acid-peptic disorder and constipation.

Science is a necessity. There is no second opinion about it. But the thought as to who should use it, when and for what purpose, is very important.

Circulatory system : Being an expectorant, it is effective in cough, dyspnoea, bronchiectasis, tuberculosis and hoarseness of voice. (पिबेन्नागबलामूलस्यार्धकर्षादिवर्धितम् ।। वा. चि. 3/117 - 120)
Reproductive system : Aphrodisiac and useful in semen debility, menorrhagia, abortions.
Urinary system : Being diuretic, it is used in retention of urine, dysuria and gonorrhoea.
Temperature : Refrigerant and febrifuge. Useful in fevers.
Satmikaran : Being a tonic it is useful in general debility and muscle wasting.
Parts used : Root bark.
Dosage : Decoction 2 to 4 ounce; root bark powder 1 to 3 gms.
Srotogamitva :
Dosha : Vata, pitta (alleviation).
Dhatu : Tonic for all dhatus.
Mala : Purisha (astringent, diuretic).
References -
'स्निग्धा रुच्या बल्या वृष्या ग्राहिणी वातपित्तजित् । तद्वन्नागबलाऽत्यर्थकृच्छ्रक्षीणे क्षतेहिता ।। (रा.व.)
'....नागबलामूलानि... पयसा मधुसर्पिर्भ्यां वा संयोज्य भक्षयेत् । जीर्णे च क्षीरसर्पिर्भ्यां शालिषष्टिकमश्नीयात् । संवत्सरप्रयोगात् अस्य वर्षशतमजरमायुस्तिष्ठति इति समानं पूर्वेण ।' (च.चि.१)
'पिबेन्नागबलामूलस्यार्धकर्षविवर्धनम् । पलं क्षीरयुतं मासं क्षीरवृत्तिरनन्नभुक् ।।
एषः प्रयोगः पुष्ट्यायुर्बलारोग्यकरः परः ।' (वा.चि. ३-११७)
'रसोनयोगं विधिवत् क्षयार्त्तः क्षीरेण वा नाबलाप्रयोगाम् ।' (सु.उ. ४१)
'चूर्णं नागबलायास्तु घृतमाक्षिकमिश्रितम् । प्रलिह्यात् प्रातरुत्थाय क्षयव्याधिनिवारणम् ।।' (शो.)
'मूलं नागबलायास्तु चूर्णं दुग्धेन पाययेत् । हृद्रोगश्वासकासघ्नम्...' (च.द.)

(65) NIMBA
Azadirachta indica Linn.

Gana : Kandughna, Vaman, Tiktaskandh (C.); Aragvadhadi, Guduchyadi, Lakshadi (S.)
Kula : Nimba kula.
Family : Meliaceae (Meli-honey) bead tree (Latin) Plants of melia.
Latin name : Azadirachta (Persian name meaning best great tree); indica (of or from India)
English name : Margosa tree.
Sanskrit names : Nimba, Pichumarda (pichu = leprosy, that which cures leprosy), Hinguniryas, Sarvatobhadra, Sheeta, Peetsarak, Arishtaphal, Jeshtamalak, Yavaneshta, Neta, Shukpriya, Subhadra, Krimighna.
Botanical Description : Tree measuring 8-10 mts in height. Trunk straight with branches in all directions. Bark is thick, black, rough from which secretion (neem ki tadi - latex) is obtained. Leaves compound, equidistant, eye shaped, 6 to 14, paired, foliated, bilateral on the stalk. Flowers - small, white, scented. Fruit - green and hard, on ripening it turns yellow and soft. The native term for such fruits is `nimboli'. Fruit contains sweet, slightly pungent and sticky pulp and a single seed. Oil is extracted from the seed. Leaves fall in winter, and in autumn new redish tender leaves appear first followed by flowering and then fruiting at the beginning of rainy season.

During the period of Charaka, many medical sciences existed. These are present today and they will be there in the future too. But Ayurveda has to have healthy competition with them.

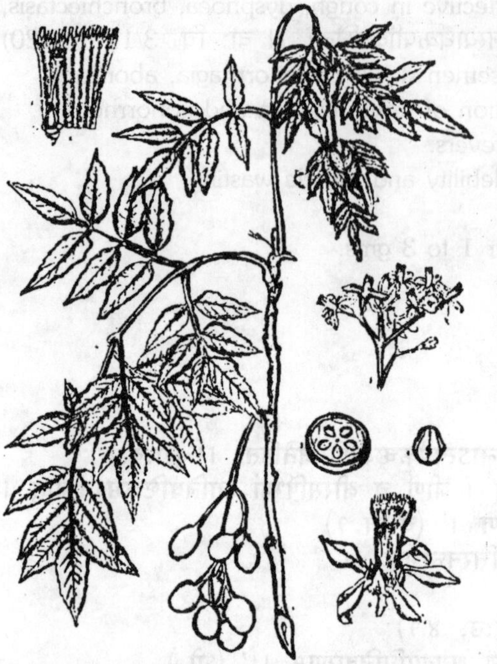

Habitat : All over India. Does not grow and survive in heavy rainfall area (more than 75 inches of rain).

Chemical composition : External skin astringent but internal is pungent. Bark contains a bitter resin called margosin. It also contains volatile oil, gum, white secretion, sugar and astringent element. Seed contains 40% stable oil and traces of sulphur.

Guna: laghu; **Rasa** : tikta, kashay;

Vipak : katu; **Veerya :** sheeta.

Karma :

Dosha : Kaphashamak and pittashamak by tikta property, therefore it is useful in diseases induced by kapha and pitta.

External uses : Leaves and bark are antimicrobial, vranapachan, vranashodhan, removes foul smell, reduces burning sensation and itching. Seed oil - wound healing, antileprotic, analgesic, therefore it is used in abscess, lymphadenitis, ulcer (lepa with crushed leaves is applied.). In pruritus hot water bath with decoction of neem leaves is given; neem oil is also applied as massage. Chronic T.B. lymphadenitis and fistulae are treated by wicks dipped in neem oil. In joint swelling and inflammatory arthritis, massage is useful. Application of ground seed is done to control lice or other microbes on the scalp. Nimba tail nasya is used in psoriasis and baldness. Neem leaves are rubbed all over to reduce burning. Poultice of leaves is tied over abscess.

Internal uses :

Digestive system : By its astringent and bitter property it improves taste and is constipative. Fruit is purgative. Leaves are anthelmintic and stimulant of liver functions. Its bark decoction with honey is useful in jaundice, anorexia, vomiting, dysentery, intestinal worms, liver diseases. Ointment prepared from seeds is applied in piles. Fruits are useful in constipation.

Respiratory system : Its property of tikta reduces the kapha from respiratory passage. Leaves are more useful in excessive mucous secretion. Bark decoction is used in chronic cough. 30-60 cc of liquid collected from the trunk is given in T.B. and leprosy.

Urinary system : It is effective in kaphapittaj prameha (diabetes).

Reproductive system : Its seed is uterine stimulant. Seed powder is used in dysmenorrhoea and puerperium. Continuous use of leaves leads to a decrease in the dhatus of the body especially shukra. The juice of the leaves should be given immediately after delivery to postpartum women as it is a uterine tonic. Since it is excreted in human milk, it is useful in preventing cough and skin diseases in infants (so it is called as balant nimba).

Skin : It is useful in all skin conditions especially in burning sensation.

Satmikaran : In general debility, young leaves and gum is useful. The concept behind chewing nimba leaves on Marathi New Year is to prevent kapha diseases. Nimba madya (watery discharge from nimba) is useful in ematiation and T.B. Nimba is best rasayan in medorog (fat disorders). The juice of the leaves is very useful in syphilis.

Temperature : Antipyretic, amapachak and prevents intermittent fever. Also useful in chronic kaphajwar and malarial fever.

Eyes : Tender leaves and flowers are useful in many skin disorders.

Useful parts : Flowers, leaves, bark, seed and oil.

Dose : Bark powder 1-2 gms; leaf juice - 12-14 cc; oil - 4 -10 drops

Formulations : Nimbadichurna, Nimbarishta, Nimbaharidra.

Neem is exclusively found in India. Does not survive where the rainfall is more than 75 inches.

Srotogamitva :

Dosha : Kaphaghna, pittaghna, vatavardhak.

Dhatu : Rakta, meda, leaves - shukra.

Mala : Reduces urine, purisha (constipation).

Organ : Stomach - eye.

References -

'निम्बः स्यात् पिचुमर्दश्च पिचुमन्दश्च तिक्तकः । अरिष्टः पारिभद्रश्च हिंगुनिर्यास इत्यापि ।।
निम्बः शीतो लघुर्ग्राही कटुस्तिक्तोऽग्निवातकृत् । अहृद्यः श्रमतृट्कासज्वरारुचिकृमिप्रणुत् ।।
व्रणपित्तकफच्छर्दिकुष्ठहल्लासमेहनुत् । निम्बपत्रं स्मृतं नेत्र्यं कृमिपित्तविषप्रणुत् ।।
वातलं कटुपाकं च सर्वारोचककुष्ठनुत् । नैम्बं फलं रसे तिक्तं पाके तु कटुभेदनम् ।।
स्निग्धं लघूष्णं कुष्ठघ्नं गुल्मार्शःकृमिमेहनुत् ।' (भा.प्र.)
'निम्बस्तिक्तरसः शीतो लघुः श्लेष्मास्रपित्तनुत् । कण्डूकुष्ठव्रणान् हन्ति लेपाहारादिशीलितः ।।
अपक्वं पाचयेच्छोथं व्रणं पक्वं विशोधयेत् ।' (ध.नि.)
'निम्बस्तिक्तः कटुः पाके लघुः शीतोऽग्निवातकृत । ग्राही हृद्यो जयेत्पित्तकफमेहज्वरकृमीन् ।।
कुष्ठकासारुचिच्छर्दिहल्लासश्वयथुव्रणान् । ग्राहि प्रवालं निम्बस्य रक्तपित्तकफकृमीन् ।।
कुष्ठघ्नं वातजननं नेत्ररोगानं विनाशयेत् । तद्वत्पत्राणि निम्बस्य व्रणघ्नानि विशेषतः ।।
शलाका निम्बपत्रस्य कासश्वासविनाशिनी । कृमिघ्ना तु वरिष्ठा स्यात् कुष्ठज्वरविनाशिनी ।।
चक्षुष्यं निम्बपुष्पं च कृमिपित्तविषप्रणुत् । वातलं कटुपाकं स्यात् सर्वारोचकनाशनम् ।।
फलं तिक्तरसं पाके कटुकं भेदनं लघु । अरूक्षमुष्णं कुष्ठघ्नं गुल्मार्शः कृमिमेहनुत् ।।
निम्बस्य पक्वं मधुरं सतिक्तं स्निग्धं फलं शोणितपित्तरोगे ।
कफे प्रशस्तं नयनामयघ्नं क्षतक्षयघ्नं गुरु पिच्छिलं च ।।'
निम्बबीजस्य मज्जा च कृमिकुष्ठविशोधनिः ।' (कै.नि.)
'निम्ब... फलतैलानि तीक्ष्णानि लघून्युष्णवीर्याणि कटूनि कटुविपाकानि
सराण्यनिलकपकृमिकुष्ठशिरोरोगापहराणि चेति ।' (सु.सु. ४५)
'निम्बस्य तैलं प्रकृतिस्थमेव नस्तो निषिक्तं विधिना यथावत् ।
मासेन गोक्षीरभुजो नरस्य यवाग्रभूतं पलितं निहन्ति ।। (भै.र.)

New horizons of Ayurveda can be unravelled by a deep study of the subject. However, a sincere effort in this direction is needed.

(66) NIMBUKA
Citrus acida

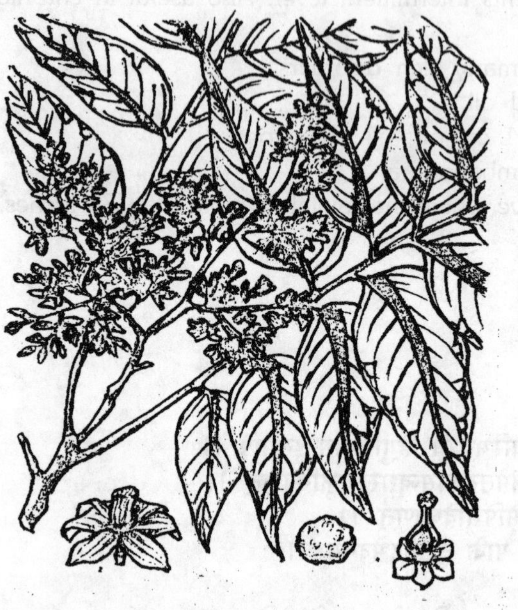

Kula : Jambeer.
Family : Rutaceae (Rus family) (Rus = Ruta).
Latin name : Citrus = lemon, 'Citron' named village in Judea; acida = acidus = sour.
English name : Lime.
Sanskrit names : Nimbooka, Amlajambeera, Vahni, Deepya, Shodhana, Vahnibeeja, Amlasara, Dantaghata, Rochana, Jantumari, Rajnimbooka. Lime is not mentioned in ancient literature.
Botanical Description : Leaves - small, fruit - round and small. Tree 3 to 4 mtrs. high. The peel of the fruit is thin like paper, hence it is known as kagdi limboo. (kagad = paper).
Varieties : One of the varieties has ovoid fruit.
Habitat : All over India, specially in Himalaya Pradesh, Brahmadesh, Bengal, Assam and Maharashtra.
Chemical composition : Fruit juice contains 7 to 10% citric acid, phosphoric acid, malic acid, citrate, sugar, mucin and alkaloids. Its peel contains a volatile oil and hesperidin.
Properties :
Guna : laghu; **Rasa** : amla; **Vipak** : madhur; **Veerya** : anushna.
Karma :
Dosha : Kaphavatashamak by anushna veerya and pittashamak by madhur vipak. Thus it has tridoshaghna action. Hence it is used widely.
Internal use :
Digestive system : Being an antidipsetic, palatable, appetizer, digestant, laxative and collagogue, it is useful in dipsia, emesis, distaste, anorexia, indigestion, constipation, abdominal distension and liver disorders. Pickle of the peel is a good digestant and appetizer.
Circulatory system : As it is a cardiac tonic, antihaemorrhagic and blood purifier, it is used in blood disorders like heart diseases. Peel oil is used in diseases like chicken pox, measles and small pox to smoothen the skin.
Respiratory system : It is an expectorant, hence though it is sour it is used in cough induced by vata and kapha. Lime juice is put in nose in epistaxis.
Urinary system : Diuretic and reduces uric acid. Mixture of lime juice and yavakshar reduces dysuria and uric acid.
Skin : Being diaphoretic, it is used in various skin disorders.

Temperature : Febrifuge, lime in many ways is useful in fever and burning sensations.
Parts used : Fruit.
Dosage : Juice 6 to 12 ml.
Srotogamitva :
Dosha : Alleviates vata, collagogue.
Dhatu : Majja (tonic for eyes), rakta (best medicine for haemorrhagic disorders).
Mala : Mutragami (reduces uric acid), diaphoretic.
Organs : Eyes, alimentary system, stomach, liver.
Oil is used in drinks.
References
'निम्बूफलं प्रथितमम्लरसं कदुष्णं गुल्मामवातहरमग्निविवृद्धिकारि ।
चक्षुष्यमेतदथ कासकफार्त्तिकण्ठविच्छर्दिहारि परिपक्वमतीव रुच्यम् ।।' (रा.नि.)

(67) NIRGUDI
Vitex negundo Linn.

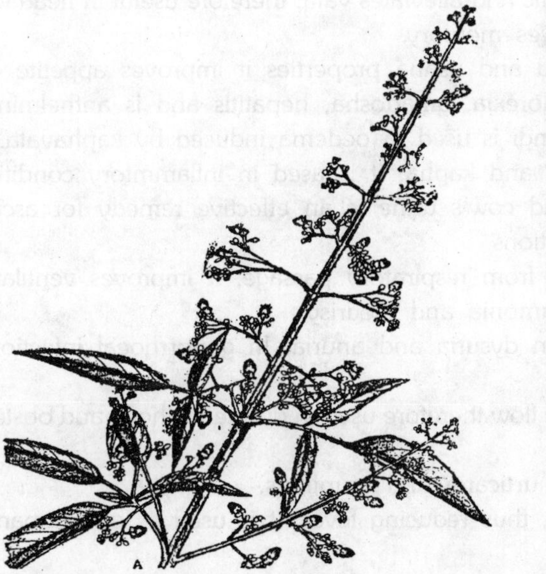

A

Gana : Vishaghna, Krumighna (C.) Surasadi (S.)
Kula : Nirgudi kula.
Family : Verbenacea (Vervein Verhena family); vitex family is named by Pliny; branches of the tree from this family are elastic in nature.
Latin name : Vitex - chaste tree; nigundo (from nirgundi). Trifolia (tri = three, folia = leaves). Because it is trifoliate, it can be used in place of bel leaves for worshiping God.
English name : Three or five leaved chaste.
Sanskrit names : Nirgundi (protects body from diseases), Sinduvarak (white flowers), Shefali, Suvaha (blue flowers), Bhutkeshi, Neelsinduk, Pushpaneelak, Sheetbhiru, Vanak.
Botanical Description : It is a shrub of 3-4 mt. height. Leaves - some are serrated and some have even margin, slimmy. Each stalk is tri or penta foliated. Leaves are 2.5 - 12 cm x 1-4 cm in dimension (trifoliated nirgundi is used instead of bel leaves). Leaves, on crushing, give a typical smell. Flowers - small, in clusters, blue coloured are four in number. Ovary is divided into 2-4 compartments. Fruits - round, become black when ripe. Bark - is bluish grey in colour.
Habitat : All over India, grows in jungles as well as in garden. According to some acharyas, serrated variety is more potent.

As many circles as one sees on the stem of a horizontally cut, full grown, mature tree, is the age of that tree in years.

Chemical composition : Leaves contain volatile essential oil and resin. Fruit contains acidic resin, astringent.

Properties :

Guna : laghu, ruksha; **Rasa :** tikta, katu, kashaya; **Vipak :** katu; **Veerya :** ushna.

Karma :

Dosha : Vatakaphashamak, hence it is used in the disorders caused by vata and kapha.

External uses : Best analgesic, antiinflammatory, antibacterial, cleaning and healing wounds, hair tonic. Heated nirgundi leaves are tied over the affected part (or poultice) in headache, scrotal swelling, synovitis, arthritic pain and rheumatic arthritis. Decoction prepared from leaves is used for tub bath in endometritis, colitis and orchitis. In these conditions it reduces the obstruction of blood and amakapha, increases perspiration, reduces oedema and also relieves pain. Gargles with decoction of leaves is useful in pharyngitis, stomatitis, difficulty in deglutation and inflammation. Smoke of dry leaves is useful in headache, sinusitis and common cold. Nirgundi oil is best in wounds for cleaning, antiinfective and to remove foul smell. Oil is also useful in baldness. Nirgundi is also called a upnah vriksha.

Interal uses :

Nervous system : It is an analgesic, brain tonic and alleviates vata, therefore useful in headache, sciatica, rheumatic arthritis, synovitis, improves memory.

Digestive system : Since it has tikta, katu and ushna properties it improves appetite and digestion. It is useful in loss of appetite, anorexia, amadosha, hepatitis and is anthelmintic.

Circulatory system : White flowered nirgundi is used in oedema induced by kaphavata. As it acts on the raktadhatu and alleviates vata and kapha, it is used in inflammtory conditions of liver and spleen. Mixture of leaf juice and cow's urine is an effective remedy for ascites. Nirgundi is useful in all inflammatory conditions.

Respiratory system : By removing kapha from respiratory passage, it improves ventilation therefore used in kapha kasa, asthma, pneumonia and pleurisy.

Urinary system : Diuretic, hence useful in dysuria and anuria. In gonorrhoeal infection it helps in passing urine smoothly.

Reproductive system : It improves menstrual flow therefore used in dysmenorrhoea and obstetric conditions.

Skin : Valuable medicine in skin diseases, urticaria and eruptions.

Temperature : It helps in digestion of ama, thus reducing fever. It is used as an anupan or a main drug in typhoid and malaria fever.

Medovahasrotas : Decoction is used as a nasya in cervical lymphadenopathy and topical application of leaves also helps.

Eyes - Leaf juice is installed in conjunctivitis. Surma is prepared from seeds.

Ears - Nirgudi oil is useful (leaves + oil) in reducing pain, oozing, inflammation and fungal infection of ear.

Satmikaran : Every part of the body is stimulated, therefore it acts as a rasayan in body. The combination of sheelajit + nirgudi is best rasayan.

Parts used : Leaves, root, seeds, panchang. Tree with serrated leaf type is preferable.

Plant fossils have supplied botanical science with invaluable and massive knowledge.

Doses : Juice of leaves 10-20 ml.; root powder 1-3 gm; seed powder - 6-12 ratti.
Formulations : Nirgudikalpa, Nirguditail, Nirgudighrit.
In large doses it vitiates pitta and therefore causes pitta disorders. Antidote - Latex of Acacia arabica.
Due to strong (pungent) odour, it is used as a mosquito and bed bug repellent. Also prevents insect growth in stored food grains (insecticidal). A parasitic plant grows on nirgundi in rainy season which is useful in mahakushtha. Also effective in guneaworm infestation.
Srotogamitva :
Dosha : Vatashleshmaghna.
Dhatu : Rakta (skin disorders, pruritus, splenomegaly), meda (leucorrhoea), asthi (infected wounds, apachi, toothache).
Mala : Hair (hair tonic), purisha (parasites).
Organs : Eye, respiratory system, uterus, pelvis.
Antidote property.
References -
'सिन्दुबार: श्वेतपुष्प: सिन्दुक: सिन्दुवारक: । नीलपुष्पी तु निर्गुण्डी शेफाली सुवहा च सा ।।
सिन्धुक: स्मृतिदस्तिक्त: कषाय: कटुको लघु: । केश्यो नेत्रहितो हन्ति शूलशोथाममारूतान् ।।
कृमिकुष्ठारुचिश्लेष्मव्रणान्नीला हि तद्विधा । सिन्दुवारदलं जन्तुवातश्लेष्महरं लघु ।।' (भा.प्र.)
'निर्गुण्डी कटुतिक्तोष्णा कृमिकुष्ठरुजापहा । वातश्लेष्मप्रशमनी प्लीहगुल्मारुचिर्जयेत् ।।' (ध.नि.)
'सिन्दुवार: कटुस्तिक्त: कफवातक्षयापह: । कुष्ठकण्डूर्तिशमन: लहृत् काससिद्धिद: ।।
कटूष्णा नीलनिर्गुण्डी तिक्ता रूक्षा च कासजित् । श्लेष्मशोफसमीरार्तिप्रदराध्मानहारिणी ।।' (रा.नि.)
'समूलफलपत्राया: निर्गुण्ड्या: स्वरसै: घृतम् । सिद्धं पीत्वा क्षयक्षीणो निर्व्याधि: भाति देववत् ।। (चक्र)
'समूलपत्रां निर्गुण्डीं पीडयित्वा रसेन तु । तेन सिद्धं समं तैलं नाडीदुष्टव्रणापहम् ।।
हितं पामापचीनान्तु पानाभ्यञ्जननावनै: । विविधेषु च स्फोटेषु तथा सर्वव्रणेषु च ।।' (चक्र.)
'एरण्डतैलं निर्गुण्डीस्वरसे च पृथक् पृथक् । पीत्वा कटिप्रदेशस्थं वातं जित्वा सुखी भवेत् ।।' (वैद्यमनोरमा)
तोडगा: -'प्राचीगतं पाण्डुरसिन्धुवारमूलं शिशूनां गलके निबद्धम् ।
करोति दन्तोभ्दववेदनाया: नि:संशयं मामामकाण्डमेव ।।' (राजमार्तण्ड)

(68) PATOL
Trichosanthes dioica Roxb.

Gana : Triptighna, Trishnanigrahan (C.); Patoladi, Aragwadhadi (S.)
Kula : Koshataki kula.
Family : Cucurbitaceae - creeper which gives big fruit.
Latin name : Trichosanthes (Thrixa = hair, santhes = flower) hairy stem and flowers; dioica = (Gk.) Dioaecious from Dic = two, oikos = houses. Male flowers on one tree (creeper) and female on another.
English name : Serpant gourd.
Sanskrit names : Patol, Tikta, Rajifal, Rajey, Kushtha, Amritfal, Kasbhanjan, Katuphala, Nagamrit, Kasamardan, Kushthaghni.
Botanical Description : It is a long seasonal creeper. Root arises from each node of the

Plants have provided all essential things for development of mankind (e.g. food, water, shelter, wealth, protection etc.)

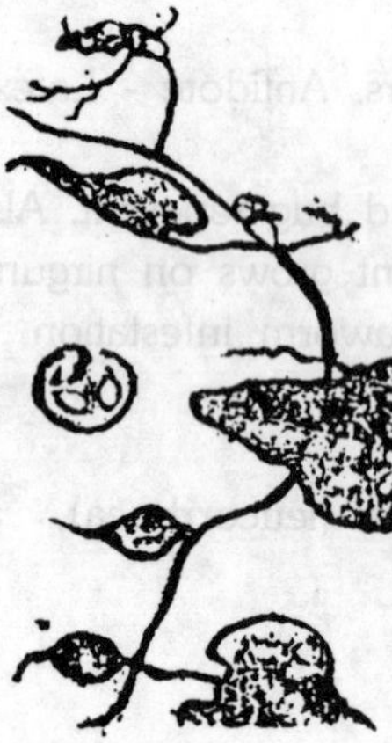

branch. Leaves - heart shaped with rough surface, 7-10 cm long, 5 cm broad having both the ends pointed. Flower - monosexual, white in colour. Fruit - oval shaped, narrow, pointed at both the ends, 5-8 cm long and marked with 5 strips. Unripe fruit is whitish green and ripe fruit is yellowish red in colour.

Varieties : It is of 2 varieties - cultivated (sweet) and wild (bitter). Fruits of cultivated variety are sweet (parval) which is used as a vegetable and wild variety is used in medicine. Each part of the plant is bitter. Bitter parval grows on its own in the jungles.

Habitat : Mainly on the fertile land of the Ganga basal.

Properties :

Guna : laghu, ruksha; **Rasa** : tikta; **Vipak** : katu; **Veerya** : ushna.

Karma :

Dosha : Tridoshashamak, hence it is used in the disorders where all the three doshas are vitiated.

External uses : Root paste is used in headache as it is ananalgesic, hair strengthening, helps in wound cleansing and healing. Leaf juice is applied over wounds and alopecia areata.

Internal uses :

Digestive system : It improves the taste of mouth, appetite and also digestion. It is antidipsetic, cholagogue, improves peristalsis, laxative and anthelmintic. Higher dose causes vomiting and diarrhoea (purgation). It is used in anorexia, loss of appetite, liver disorders, jaundice, ascites, piles and helminthiasis. Leaf juice induces emesis.

Circulatory system : Patol is blood purifier and antiinflammatory, so it is useful in blood disorders and inflammations. Used in jaundice, as it is purgative.

Respiratory system : Kaphaghna. Useful in cough caused by kaphadosha. The whole plant strengthens the chest.

Skin : Kushtaghna. Effective in skin diseases with pruritus.

Temperature : Febrifuge. It is used in `pittajwar', typhoid, chronic fever. Also useful in `rasagat, raktagat and mansagat jwar'.

Satmikaran : Useful in weakness and has an antidote property.

Parts used : Whole plant.

Dosages : Juice 10 -20 ml; decoction 60 - 100 ml.

Formulations : Patoladi kwath, Patholadya churna. Different properties are present in the different parts of the same plant. The best example of it is patol.

Patol leaves - pittaghna; stalk - kaphaghna; fruit - tridoshaghna; root - purgative.

Patol leaves are used in rasagat, raktagat, mansagat jwar (Charaka - Jwar chikitsa).

Srotogamitva :

Dosha : Reduces kapha and pitta.

Dhatu : Shukra (aphrodisiac), rakta (complexion enchancer).

Plants have contributed a lot to literature. There are many proverbs and riddles using the names of plants.

Mala : Purisha (purgative).
Prabhav : Though bitter, it is aphrodisiac and tridoshaghna.
References -
'कफपित्तहरं वर्ण्यमुष्णं तिक्तमवातलम् । पटोलं कटुकं पाके वृष्यं रोचनदीपनम् ।।' (सु.सू. ४६)
'पटोलं कटुकं तिक्तमुष्णं पित्ताविरोधि च । कफासृक्कण्डकुष्ठानि ज्वरदाहौ च नाशयेत् ।।' (ध.नि.)
'पटोलस्य भवेन्मूलं विरेचनकरं सुखात् । नालं श्लेष्महरं पत्र पित्तहारि फलं पुनः ।।
दोषत्रयहरं प्रोक्त तद्वत्तिक्तपटोलिका ।' (भा.प्र.)
'पटोलपत्रं पित्तघ्नं नाडी तस्य कफापहा । फलं तस्य त्रिदोषघ्नं मूलं तस्य चिरेचनम् ।।'(रा.व.)

(69) PALASHA

Butea monosperma Lam-Kutze.

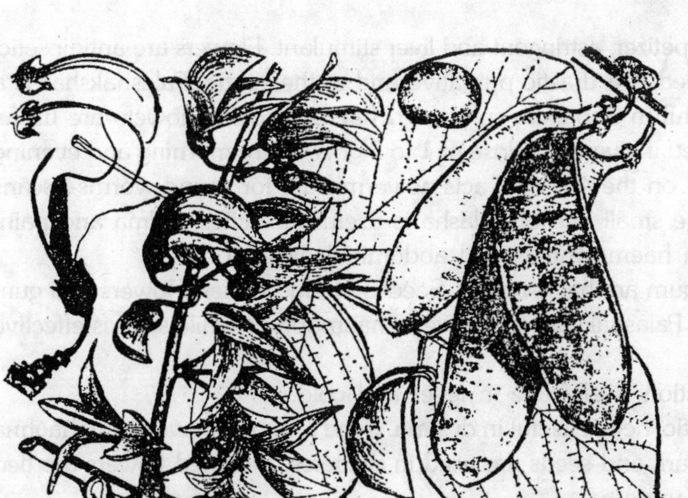

Guna : Rodhradi, Mushkakadi, Ambashthadi, Nyagrodhadi (S.).
Kula : Shimbi kula.
Upakula : Aparajita kula.
Family : Leguminoceae (Legumin = pulse).
Sub-family : Papilionaceae.
Latin name : Butea = named after John Earl of Bute, Patron of Botany; mono = one; sperma = seed. Earlier name was Butea frondosa, frondosa = leafy. Palasha is famous for its leaves. Palishin = any tree with leaves (Lam-Kutze).
English name : Bustard teak.
Sanskrit names : Palasha (pala = flesh, like flesh or blood), Kimshuka (flowers resemble the beak of parrot), Raktapushpaka, Ksharashreshtha, Brahmavruksha (palasha = demon), Samidwara, Triparna (everywhere palash has only three leaves), Vakrapushpa, Trivrunta.
Botanical Description : Tree grows 13 to 16 mtrs. high. Stem is crooked with torn bark. Leaves - 10 to 15 cm. long (palasha has three leaves). Flowers - beautiful, red coloured, grow in spring. It has pale yellow streak, from which dark saffron colour is derived. Legume - 12 to 20 cm. long, 2 cm broad and contains flattened, round, reddish black seeds. Gum oozes from the cracked bark, which is known as Butea gum or Bengal kino. Flowers bloom in spring and then the tree bears fruits. In summer, the blossomed tree is very attractive. Saffron colour of the flowers is used for Rangapanchami, which is known as kimshuka.
Habitat : Entire India and Brahmadesh.
Chemical composition : Bark and gum contain kino and tannic acid, 50% gallic acid. Seeds contain 18% stable oil, which is called as kino oil.

Properties :
Guna : laghu, snigdha; **Rasa :** katu, tikta, kashaya; **Vipak :** katu; **Vipak of flowers -** madhur; **Veerya** : sheeta; **Palashpapadi - Veerya** = ushna.
Karma :
Dosha : Kaphavatashamak. Flowers kaphapitta-shamak. Hence palasha is used in disorders induced by kapha and vata while flowers in disorders induced by kapha and pitta.
External uses : Flowers, bark and gum are astringent. Seed is curative. Leaves alleviate pain and swelling. In retention of urine, warm flowers and leaves are tied over umbilicus and lower abdomen. Decoction of the bark is used for washing wounds, piles and vaginal discharges. Paste of the seeds is useful in skin disorders, oedema and eye diseases. Oil is used for massage in rheumatism. Rubbed seed is applied over scorpion sting. Warm leaves are tied over abscesses.
Internal uses :
Digestive system : Palasha is an appetizer, astringent and liver stimulant. Flowers are antidipsetic, gum is an antacid and astringent. Seed is a drastic purgative and anthelmintic. Palashakshar is a good laxative. Bark decoction is useful in anorexia, sprue and haemorrhoids. Flowers are useful in dipsia and diarrhoea. Powdered seed if given in a dose of 1 to 3 gms. every morning and evening for 3 consecutive days and castor oil on the 4th day, acts as vermicidal for round worms-Ascaris lumbricoidis. Kshar prepared from the small tree of palasha is useful in ascites, gulma and pain. Juice of leaves + flowers is given in haemorrhoids and abdominal distension.
Circulatory system : Flowers and gum are haemostatic. Seed is blood purifier. Flowers and gum are useful in haemorrhagic disorders. Palashakshar is effctive in haemoptysis while seed is effective in vatarakta.
Respiratory system : Bark decoction is effective in fever and cold.
Urinary system : Flowers are diuretic, hence useful in dysuria. Seed and bark have pramehaghna property, hence juice of the leaves, bark and seeds are used in diabetes. Steamed flowers are tied over lower abdomen in retention of urine.
Reproductive system : Gum is aphrodisiac. Seed is stimulant and flowers are astringent. Gum is given orally in sperm debility. Decoction of flowers is useful in vaginal discharges.
Skin : Flowers and seeds are kushthaghna. Flowers and seeds are given orally in various skin disorders. Gum is used in tuberculosis related diaphoresis.
Temperature : Flowers are used as febrifuge and refrigerant.
Satmikaran : Gum is given orally in general debility. Because of this property, amalaki rasayan is prepared by treating it with steam obtained from a decoction of stems of palasha. Skin, flowers and seeds are used in bone fractures. Seeds are good antidote. The whole plant of palasha is used in preparing rasayan (tonic).
Parts used : Bark, flowers, leaf, gum and seeds.
Dosage : Bark decoction 50 to 100 ml.; leaf juice 10 to 20 ml.; flowers 3 to 10 gms. Gum - 1/2 to 1 gms. Seed powder - 1 to 8 gms. (for worms 1/2 to 1gms.)
Formulations : Palashabeejadi churna, Palasha ksharaghrit.
Srotogamitva :
Flowers - Dosha : Vatavardhak, kaphapittashamak.

There are 13 types of plants e.g. water plants, plants that grow on soil, climbers, creepers, plants that shed leaves etc. This is their peculiarity.

Fruit - Vatakaphashamak.
Dhatu : Raktagami, meda-asthi (joining property, rejuvenator, aphordisiac).
Mala : Urine formation (white palasha is memory enhancer).
Organ : Digestive system (sprue, piles, worms).
References -

'पलाशपादपः सिद्धस्त्रिदलः शिशिरे क्षयः । कृष्णवृन्तोज्वलद्रक्तपुष्पश्च तिक्तबीजकः ।
एकबीजायता शिम्बी त्रिपर्णश्च समिद्धवान् । गुणैः सर्वे समा ज्ञेयाः सितो विज्ञानदः परः ।।' (शि.)
पलाशो दीपनो वृष्यः सरोष्णो व्रणगुल्मजित् । भग्नसंधानकृद्दोषग्रहण्यर्शः कृमीन् हरेत् ।।
कषायः कटुकस्तिक्तः स्निग्धो गुदजरोगजित् । तत्पुष्पं स्वादु पाके तु कटु तिक्तं कषायकम् ।।
वातलं कफपित्तास्रकृच्छ्रजित् ग्राहि शीतलम् । तृड्दाहशमकं वातरक्तकुष्ठहरं परम् ।।
फलं लघूष्णं मेदार्शः कृमिवातकफापहम् । विपाके कटुकं रूक्षं कुष्ठगुल्मोदरप्रणुत् ।।' (भा.प्र.)
क्षारश्रेष्ठः कृमिघ्नश्च संग्राही दीपनः परः । प्लीहगुल्मग्रहण्यर्शोवातश्लेष्मविनाशनः ।।
किंशुकस्यापि कुसुमं सुगंधि मधुरं च तत् । बीजं तु कटुकं स्निग्धमुष्णं कृमिबलासजित् ।।' (ध.नि.)
'पलाशतैलानि मधुरकषायाणि कफपित्तप्रशमनानि ।' (सु.सू. ४५)
'किंशुकं कफपित्तघ्नम्' (सु.सू. ४६)
'पलाशबीजानि विडंगयुक्तान्युन्मिश्रितान्यामलकीफलानाम्
रसेन मध्वाज्ययुतानि पीत्वा वृद्धोऽपि मासात्तरुणत्वमेति ।।' (रा.मा.)

(70) PATALA
Stereospermum suaveolens

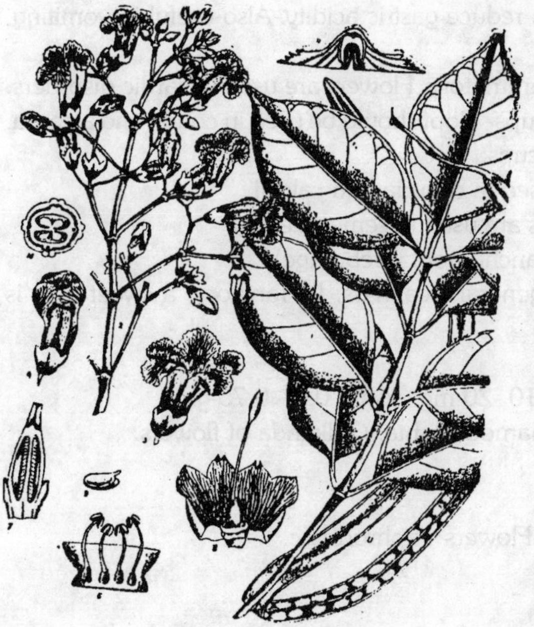

Gana : Shothahara (dashamoola) (C.) Bruhatpanchamoola, Adhobhagahara, Aragwadhadi (S.)
Kula : Shyonak kula.
Family : Bignoniaceae (Abbe Bignon - In the memory of librarian of 5 th Louis) Bignonia = flowers looks like trumpet.
Latin name : Stero = stiff; spermum = seed - seeds usually embedded in notches in the septum of capsule; suaveolens = sweet scented.
Sanskrit names : Patala (patal = red, red coloured flowers), Krishnavrunta (having black stalk), Madhudooti (madhu = spring), Allivallabha (honeybee and black bee get attracted towards it because of fragrance and honey in the flowers), Tamrapushpi, Kuberakshi, Amogha (useful medicine).
Botanical Descripition : A huge tree of height 10-20 mtrs. Stem - smoke coloured externally with black spots on it and pale yellow internally. Leaves -

There is a choice of twenty types of places where plants could grow e.g. farm land, dry, land, marshy land, seashores, fences, hills, waste-filled land, road sides, shades etc.

compound, 30-40 cms. long, wing- shaped. Leaflet -17- 20 cm. long and 8-10 cm broad. Flower- yellow, red and sweet scented. Water becomes fragrant if flowers are dipped in it . Fruit - 40 cm long and 1 cm broad, hairy, surrounded by four stripes. It contains 10-12 seeds. They are 3-5 cm. long. Flowering stage is summer and fruiting stage is winter.

Varieties: There are 2 varities described in Bhavapraksha - one having red flowers and the other having white flowers. Ghantapatala, Kashthapatala and Mushak are the synonyms for white flowered patala which is mentioned in Bhavaprakash. Some nighantu writers describe one more variety having yellow flowers.

Habitat: In india - Bihar, Bengal, Terai regions of Himalaya and Konkan.

Chemical composition : The flower contains albumin, sugar, mucilage and wax.

Properties :

Guna : laghu, ruksha; **Rasa:** tikta, kashaya; **Vipak :** katu; **Veerya :** ushna (slightly) but its flowers and fruits are kashaya, madhur and sheeta .

Karma :

Dosha : Laghu = kapha alleviation, tikta, kashaya = pitta alleviation and ushna veerya = vata alleviation. Bark alleviates kapha and vata while flowers alleviate vata and pitta. Hence different parts are used depending upon the aggravated doshas.

External uses : It has analgesic and wound healing properties, leaves ground in a paste are applied over the wound. Paste of the seeds is applied in migraine.

Internal uses :

Nervous system : Analgesic. It is effective in painful conditions of vata disorders.

Digestive system : It improves the taste. It is antidyspeptic, astringent and a liver stimulant. Hot infusion of the bark is given in acid-peptic disease to reduce gastric acidity. Also useful in vomiting, diarrhoea and piles.

Circulatory system : Bark and flowers are antiinflammatory. Flowers are used in cardic disorders.

Respiratory system : Kaphaghna and reduces hiccups. Root should be used in cough and asthma. Powdered flowers are given to lick with honey in hiccups.

Urinary system : Being a diuretic, patalakshar is used in dysuria and calculi.

Reproductive system : Being aphrodisiac, flowers are used in semen deblity.

Temperature : Febrifuge and refrigerant. (Bruhatpanchamool is febrifuge).

Satmikaran : Gulkand of flowers is effective in general weakness. In Tanjaoor, a sweet dish is prepared from the flowers and is used as a tonic.

Parts used : Root bark, flowers and kshar.

Dosage : Bark powder 0.25 - 1.5 gm.; flower juice 10 -20 mg.; kshar 0.5 - 0.75 gms.

Formulation : Bruhatpanchamooladi kadha, Dashamoolarishta, Gulkanda of flowers.

Srotogamitva :

Dosha : Tridoshaghna.

Dhatu : Rakta (acid peptic disorder, inflammation); Flowers - aphrodisiac.

Mala : Purisha (astringent), piles, vomiting.

Organs : Antarmarga.

Although "Gorakh chinch" has a very big stem, in comparison its branches are very small.

References -

'पाटली पाटलामोघा मधुदूती फलेरुहा । कृष्णवृन्ता कुबेराक्षी काचस्थाल्यलिवल्लभा ।।
ताम्रपुष्पी च कथिता परा स्यात् पाटला सिता । मुष्कको मोक्षको घण्टापाटलिः काष्ठपाटला ।।
पाटला तुवरा तिक्ताऽनुष्णा दोषत्रयापहा । अरुचिश्वासशोथार्थश्छर्दिहिक्कातृषाहरी ।।
पुष्पं कषायं मधुरं हिमं हृद्यं कफास्त्रनुत् । पित्तातिसारहृत् कण्ठ्यं फलं हिक्कास्त्रपित्तहृत् ।।' (भा.प्र.)
'पटोलपाटलाक्वाथो धान्यनागरकान्वितः । जलेन सहितः प्रोक्तश्चाम्लपित्तनिवारणः ।।' (च.द.)

(71) PATHA

Cissempelus pareira Linn.

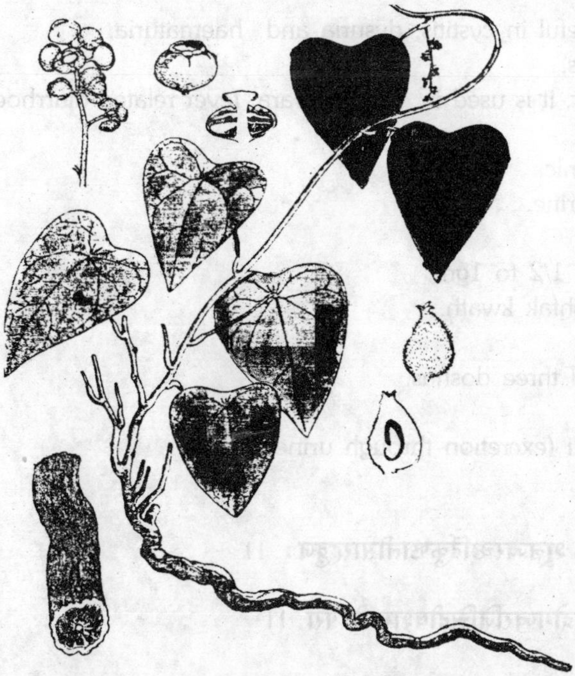

Gana : Stanyashodhana, Jwarahara, Sandhaniya (C.) Aragwadhadi, Pippalyadi, Bruhatyadi, Patoladi, Ambashthadi, Mustadi (S.)

Kula : Guduchi kula.

Family : Menispermaceae (like guduchi); (Moon seed - shape of the seed is like moon). ('Mene' = moon) = climbing evergreen.

Latin name : Cissesmpelus = Ciss (Kissos) = Ivy; Ampeloc = Vine (Resembling ivy in rambling habit and vine; pareira = Chondrodenron tomentosum (hairy); for which this plant was mistaken Latin = Cocculus Hirsutus (Linn).

English name : Velvet leaf.

Sanskrit names : Patha, Ambashtha, Pracheena, Shreyasi, Ekashtheela, Deepani, Varatiktata, Tiktapushpa, Devi, Ateesaranashani.

Botanical Description : Creeper. Leaves - oblong or heart shaped, 2.5 to 10 cm. long and 2.5 to 3.75 cm. narrow. Leaf stalk is 5 to 10 cm. long. Leaves and branches - smooth having white hair on it. Flowers - homosexual, pale yellow coloured. Seeds - crooked; flowers blossom in rainy season.

Varieties : It has another variety called as Rajapatha (Cyclea peltata). It has big leaves.

Habitat : From Sindh and Punjab upto Srilanka.

Properties :

Guna : laghu, tikshna; **Rasa** : tikta; **Vipak** : katu; **Veerya** : ushna.

Karma :

Dosha : Tridoshashamak, specially kaphavatashamak hence used in disorders induced by all three doshas and vata-kapha.

The stems of teakwood, babool, sandlewood and anjan are heavy. But Gvayakam officinale weighs 1386 kg. in one sq. meter.

External uses : Being wound healer, antidote and kushthaghna, paste of leaves and root is used in fistula, pruritus, skin disorders and snake poison. Juice or powdered roots are used as a nasya in ardhavabhedak.
Internal uses :
Digestive system : Being an appetizer, digestive, laxative, astringent and anthelmintic, it is useful in anorexia, indigestion,abdominal pain, diarrhoea and dysentery.
Criculatory system : It is a blood purifier and has antiinflammatory property, so it is used in blood disorders, heart disorders and inflammation.
Respiratory system : Being an expectorant, it is used in cough and dyspnoea.
Reproductive system : Since it purifies breast milk it is used in various disorders of breast milk secretion.
Urinary system : Potent diuretic, hence useful in cystitis, dysuria and haematuria.
Skin : Kushthaghna. Useful in skin disorders.
Temperture : Being febrifuge and refrigerant, it is used in sheeta jwara, fever related diarrhoea and burning disorders.
Satmikaran : Antidote and tonic - bitter tonic.
Excretion : This drug is excreted through urine.
Parts used : Root.
Dosage : Decoction 50 to 100 ml.; powder 1/2 to 1gm.
Formulation : Gangadhara churna, Kutajashtak kwath.
Srotogamitva :
Dosha : Alleviates vata, kapha, alleviates all three doshas.
Dhatu : Rasa, rakta, stanyagami.
Mala : Purisha (astringent), mutramargagami (excretion through urine) .
Organs : Heart, stomach.
References -
'पाठोष्णा कटुका तीक्ष्णा वातश्लेष्महरी लघुः । हन्ति शूलज्वरच्छर्दिकुष्ठातीसारहृद्रुजः ।।
दाहकण्डूविषश्वासकृमिगुल्मगरव्रणान् ।' (भा.प्र.)
'पाठा तिक्तरसा बल्या विषघ्नी कुष्ठकण्डुनुत् । छर्दिहृद्रोगज्वरजित्त्रिदोषशमनी परा ।।
पाठातिसारशूलघ्नी कफपित्तज्वरापहा ।' (ध.नि.)
पाठा...शाकं...विद्याद्ग्राहि त्रिदोषघ्नम् ।' (च.सू. २७)

(72) PARASIK YAVANI

Hyocymus reticulata Linn.

Kula : Kantakari kula.
Family : Solanaceae (Lat. Solanum = comforting) Many species have sedative qualities.
Latin name : Hyocyamus - Hyos = of a hog, cyomos = bane = poison; poisonous to hogs and man; reticulata = nerves forming a network, projecting a little above the surface.
English name : Hen bane.
Sanskrit names : Khurasani yavani, Yavahva, Yavanika, Parasik, Yavani, Teevra, Turuska, Madakari.
Botanical Description : A shrub but bigger than ajawayan. Trunk - thick and hairy. Leaves -

Scientists caim that the tree Drakaina drade on the Canary island lives for 6000 years. Can Savar compete with it?

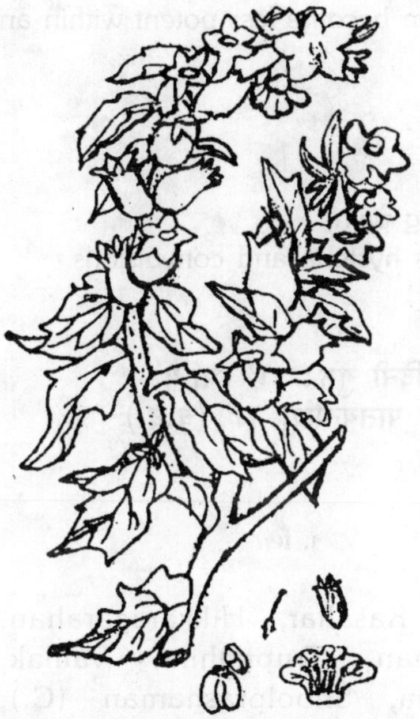

like guldowdy, big, elongated and hairy with serrated margins and blackish green in colour. Flowers - like pomegranate flowers but central and peripheral petals are reddish. Seed - bigger than that of ajawayan, kidney-shaped, dusky white. The plant bears flowers in the month of July and August.

Varieties : According to the colour of the flower, there are three varieties - white, red and black.

Habitat : This plant grows at the height of 3 to 4 meters from the coast. Grows in Himalaya, Kashmir, Ghadwal, Kumaon, also in Europe, Siberia, Asia minor, Khurasan, Baluchistan.

Chemical composition : Seed contains 1/4 stable oil. Leaves and seeds contain hyoscyamine and hyoscine.

Properties :

Guna : guru, ruksha; **Rasa :** tikta, kuta, kashaya; **Vipak :** katu; **Veerya :** ushna; **Prabhav :** madak.

Its properties are like ajawayan and is also a digestive, palatable, astringent and heavy.

Karma :

Dosha : Kaphavatashamak by ushna veerya and hence useful in diseases caused due to kapha-vata. It is pittavardhak.

External uses : Being ushna, it alleviates swelling and pain. Paste is applied over mastitis, orchitis, haemorrhoids and arthralgia. It is used for dhoopan in toothache.

Internal uses :

Central nervous system : It is useful in hysteria, meningitis, insomnia, pain and delirium. This plant is anticonvulsant.

Digestive system : It is pungent and bitter. It acts as an appetizer. It is a carminative just like khurasani ajawayan. It is also digestive, astringent, vermicide and analgesic. Therefore, it is used in abdominal pain, abdominal distension, gulma and also for alleviating pain caused by worms.

Circulatory system : Low dose causes action on heart, which increases the resting period of heart and thus strengthens the heart. Its astringent property has haemostatic action.

Respiratory system : Being ushna it acts as an expectorant and relieves dyspnoea.

Urinary system : It has sedative action on urinary system, hence it reduces renal and ureteric colic. Besides it is used in cystitis, calculi and hastimeha.

Reproductive system : Useful in dysmenorrhoea, vaginal discharges and irregular menstruation.

Parts used : Seed, leaves.

Dosage : Leaf powder 1.5 to 3 gms.; seeds 0.5 to 3 gms. (be careful because excess dose is harmful).

Formulations : Khorasani asava, Parashiyadi churna (In excess dose it leads to certain symptoms viz giddiness, laryngitis, hysteria, coma. Body becomes pale and weak. In such condition, give immediate stomach wash. Give either cow's or goat's milk. Pure honey is used to reduce other symptoms. Opium and poppy seeds are used as a substitute for H. reticulata. Actions of

As a snake sheds its skin, likewise some trees like arjun shed off their bark and get rejuvented. Is this a rasayana for them?

hyoscyamine and atropin are similar. (Seeds of khurasni ajawayan become less potent within an year). Black parasik yavani is more poisonous.

Srotogamitva :

Dosha : Vataghna, kaphaghna, pittavardhak.

Dhatu : Majja.

Mala : Purisha (astringent), vermicide, pachani (reduces gripping pain).

Organs : Brain and intestine (analgesic and sedative), alleviates hysteria and convulsions.

References -

'यवानी यावनी रुक्षा ग्राहिणी मोहिनी कटु:।' (रा.नि.)

'पारसीकयवानी तु यवानीसदृशा गुणे: । विशेषात् पाचनी रुच्या ग्राहिणी मादिनी गुरु: ।।' (भा.प्र.)

'पारसीकयवानिका पीता पर्युषितवारिणा प्रात: । गुडपूर्वा कृमिजातं कोष्ठगतं पातयत्याशु ।।' (च.द.)

(73) PIPPALI

Piper longum Linn.

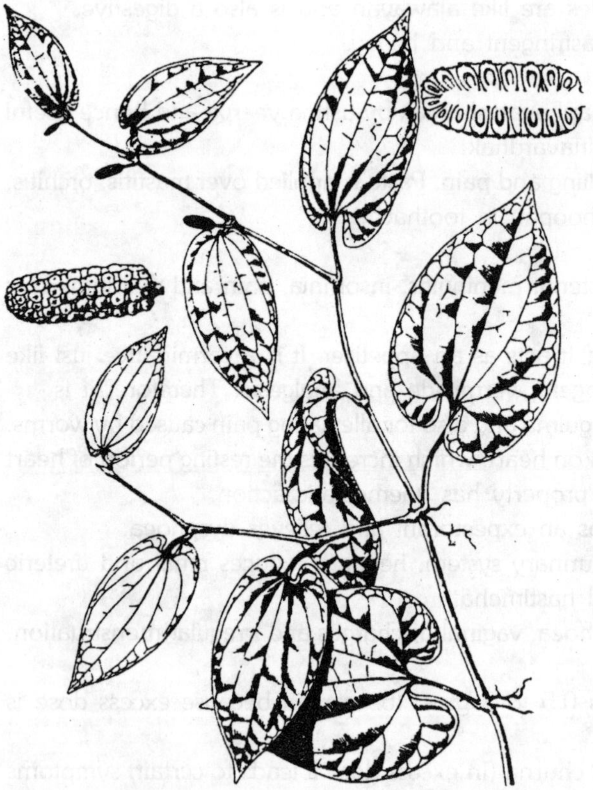

Gana : Kasahar, Hikkanigarahan, Shirovirechan, Truptighna, Vamak, Deepaneeya, Shoolprashaman (C.), Pippalyadi, Oordhvabhagahar, Shirovirechan. (S.)

Kula : Pippali kula.

Family : Piperaceae (Derived from repto = to digest).

Greek : Pepperi. **Latin** : Piper, Pepper. It has digestive stimulating quality.

Latin name : Piper (according to meaning of pepper), peperi (Greek), or pippal (derived from Sanskrit names); longum = long.

English name : Long pepper.

Sanskrit names : Pippali, Magadhi (from Magadh), Krishna (black), Vaidehi (from Videh - north Bihar), Chapala (giving instant action), Kana (having kan or grains), Ushna (hot), Upkoolya (grows near water), Krukara, Katubija, Korangee.

Botanical Description : It is a creeper which spreads on the ground or climbs up nearby trees for support. Leaves 5 to 6 cms long, resemble betel leaves and has 5 veins. They are bitter to taste. Flowers - unisexual. Fruits long, reddish on ripening and turn black when dried. It flowers during rainy season and gives fruits during autumn.

The sun has many names like Mitra, Ravi, Bhanu, Kham, Hiranyagarbha, Aditya, Savita etc. Callotropis procera can be given all these names.

Varieties : There are 4 varieties of Piper longum.

1. **Pippali** - Which is found in Indian places like Magadh, Videha etc.
2. **Gajpippali** - It is an ambiguous drug. Many people call Chavaka's fruit as gajpippali चविकाया: फलं प्राज्ञै: कथिता गजपिप्पली)
3. **Saimhalee** -This variety is imported from Sri lanka, Singapore and other foreign countries. (Jahaaji pippali is the synonym for it.)
4. **Vanpippali** - Grows in the jungles. It grows in abudance in Bengal. But it is small, slender, thin and less tikshna.

This pippali is now to be imported. The big ones should be Saimhalee and the small ones should be from Bengal. The pippali from Paanveli is available under the name of Paan pippali.

Habitat : P. longum is grown chiefly in the following places - Bengal, Bihar, Assam, Travancore, Nepal, Bhutan, Terai region of the Himalayas, islands of Phillipines, Malaysia, Singapore. It is cultivated in Bangladesh.

Chemical composition : Resin, volatile oil, starch, gum, fatty oil, inorganic matter and resin piperine 1-2%.

Properties :

Guna : laghu, snigdha, tikshna; **Rasa** : katu; **Vipak** : madhur; **Veerya:** anushnasheeta (not warm, cooling).

When the fruits of pippali are wet and raw, they are guru, sweet and sheeta veerya.

Karma :

Dosha : Katu - kaphashamak, snigdha - vatashamak, when fresh it is sweet and sheeta and thus is vatakaphavardhak and pittashamak. Disorders related to kapha and vata are the main uses of shushk (dry) pippali.

External uses : It increases blood flow when applied locally. Therefore it is used in swelling accompanied with pain.

Internal uses :

Nervous system : P. longum is a brain tonic and alleviates vata. It is useful in weakness of the brain (majjagami) and vata disorders.

Digestive system : P. longum is an appetizer, truptighna by pungent taste; carminative, analgesic and mild laxative by snigdha and ushna properties. As it is tikshna and acts on the rakta dhatu, it helps in reducing hepatomegaly and splenomegaly. It acts as a vermicide by pungent, tikshna and ushna properties. Long pepper is effective in the disorders which are caused by vibandha and vitiated vata-kapha doshas viz. anorexia, loss of appetite, indigestion, gulma, colic, piles, liver disorders and ascites.

Circulatory system : This is the main action field of long pepper. Being pungent and madhur vipaki, it acts on the rakta dhatu, enhances rakta dhatvagni and rakta dhatu. Therefore, it is used to treat anaemia and various blood disorders. Long pepper is a good rejuvenator for rakta dhatu and regulates the functions of liver and spleen. Long pepper in increasing dose is a boon for chronic fever, typhoid, agnimandya and splenomegaly. Though pungent, dry ginger and long pepper are the only two drugs which are used in bleeding (because of madhur vipak).

Respiratory system : Long pepper is an excellent medicine for cough caused due to kapha

For various reasons, agni has different names. The shrub Chitraka is addressed by all these names.

dosha, asthma and hiccoughs. It acts as an expectorant and prevents the production of mala kapha. It purifies all dhatus. It is used as a tonic in tuberculosis. As it rejuvenates rakta dhatu, it strengthens the lungs.

Urinary system : In diabetes mellitus it reduces ama stage of kapha, meda and mutra (urine), also stabilizes meda.

Reproductive system : Pippali is the only ushna and tikshna dravya which acts as an aphrodisiac (by virtue of madhur vipak). It reduces seminal debility and acts as a rejuvenator. Useful in dysmenorrhoea and painful labour by its action of rasa pachan.

Skin : Long pepper is a rejuvenator of rasa and rakta dhatu and is useful in skin disorders.

Temperature : It is the best medicine for typhoid and chronic fever. Mixture of long pepper and jaggery is useful in chronic fever, but long pepper in increasing dose is the final remedy for it. This remedy is also effective in remittent fever, fever occurring in anupdesha and fever due to tuberculosis.

Satmikaran : In rasayan therapy, pippali is given for a fixed period of time by increasing one or three or five pippali each day. During this period the patient should be allowed to eat only milk and rice.

Useful parts : Fruit.

Dose : Powder - 5-10 gm; can be used in any dose for rasayan therapy. It should not be taken in excess except for rasayan therapy. In excess dose, it works as pramathi. (Salt, pippali and kshar should not be taken in excess as they vitiate all the three doshas in excess dose. This should be always remembered when long pepper is used.)

Formulations : Gudpippali, Vardhamanpippali, Pippalyasar, Chavsasthipippali.

Srotogamitva :

Dosha : Vataghna, kaphaghna, pittavirodhi.

Dhatu : Rakta (liver spleen enlargement), skin disorders, meda, shukra (aphrodisiac), rasayani, majja (brain tonic, sciatica).

Mala : Purisha (purgative).

Organ : Respiratory system (asthma, cough).

References -

'अथ पिप्पलिकावल्लि: नागवल्लीदला मृदु: ।' (शि.)
'पिप्पली मागधी कृष्णा वैदेही चपला कणा । उपकुल्योषणाशौण्डी कोला स्यात्तीक्ष्णतण्डुला ।।
पिप्पली दीपनी वृष्या स्वादुपाका रसायनी । अनुष्णा कटुका स्निग्धा वातश्लेष्महरी लघु: ।।
पिप्पली रेचनी हन्ती वातश्लेष्मोदरज्वरान् । कुष्ठप्रमेहगुल्मार्श: प्लीहशूलाममारुतान् ।।
आर्द्रा कफप्रदा स्निग्धा शीतला मधुरा गुरु: पित्तप्रशमनी सा तु शुष्का पित्तप्रकोपनी ।।
पिप्पली मधुसंयुक्ता मेद:कफविनाशिनी । श्वासकासज्वरहरी वृष्या मेध्याग्निवर्धनी ।।
जीर्णज्वरेऽग्निमांद्ये च शस्यते गुडपिप्पली कासाजीर्णारुचिश्वासहृत्पाण्डुकृमिरोगनुत् ।।'
दीपनं पिप्पलीमूलं कटूष्णं पाचनं लघु । रूक्षं पित्तकरं भेदि कफवातोदरापहम् ।।
आनाहप्लीहगुल्मघ्नं कृमिश्वासक्षयापहम् ।' (भा.प्र.)
श्लेष्मला मधुरा चार्द्रागुर्वी स्निग्धा च पिप्पली । सा शुष्का कफवातघ्नी कटूष्णा वृष्यसंमता ।। (च.सू.२७)
तेषां गुर्वी स्वादुशीता पिप्पल्यार्द्रा कफावहा ।
शुष्का कफानिलघ्नी सा वृष्या पित्ताविरोधिनी ।।' (सु.स. ४६)

In Bhagwad Geeta, Arjuna has ten or more names. The tree Arjuna is known by all these names.

'शृतं पयः शर्करा च पिप्पल्यो मधुसर्पिषी । पञ्चसारमिदं पेयं मथितं विषमज्वरे ।।' (सु.उ. ३९)
'गोमूत्रैरण्डतैलाभ्यां कृष्णाचूर्णं पिबेन्नरः । दीर्घकालोत्थितां हन्ति गृध्रसीं कफवातजाम् ।।' (भा.प्र.)
'क्वाथेन कल्केन च पिप्पलीनां सिद्धं घृतं माक्षिकसंप्रयुक्तम् ।
क्षीरानुपानं विनिहन्त्यवश्यं शूलं प्रवृद्धं परिणामसंज्ञम् ।।' (वंगसेन)
'पिप्पल्यो हि कटुकाः सत्यो मधुरविपाकाः गुर्व्यो नात्यर्थं स्निग्धोष्णाः प्रक्लेदिन्यो भेषजाभिमताश्च, ताः सद्यः शुभाशुभकारिण्यो भवन्ति, आपातभद्राः प्रयोगसमसादगुण्यात्; दोषसंचयानुबन्धाः सततमुपयुज्यमानाः हि गुरुप्रक्लेदित्वाच्छलेष्माणमुत्क्लेशयति, औषण्यात् पित्तं, न च वातप्रशमनायोपकल्पतेऽल्पस्नेहोष्णभावात् । योगवाहिन्यस्तु खलु भवन्ति; तस्मात् पिप्पलीर्नात्युपयुञ्जीत ।' (च.वि.(१/१६)
दशादि दशकैर्वृद्धाः पिप्पलीर्द्विपिचूंस्तिलान् । पीत्वा क्षीरेण लभते बलं देहहुताशयोः ।। (वा.चि. ८/६२)

(74) PUNARNAVA

Boerhavia diffusa Linn.

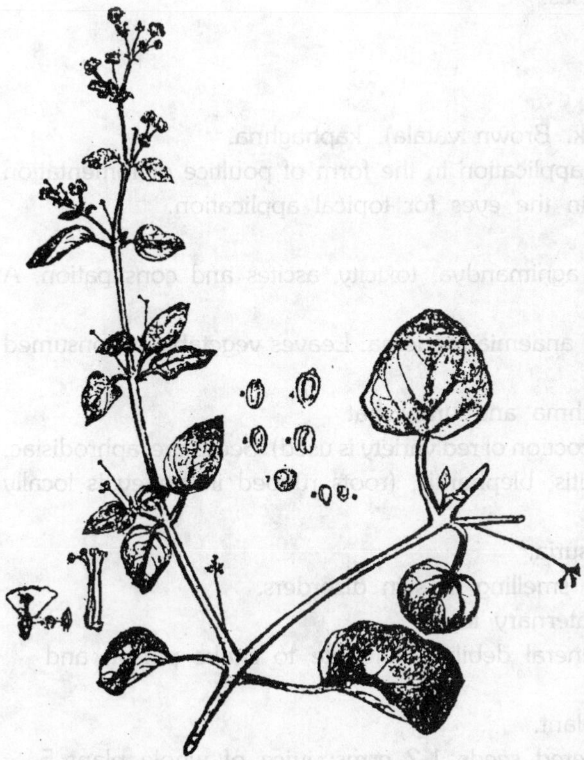

Gana : Vayahsthapan, Kasahar, Svedopag, Anuvasanopag (C.); Vidarigandhadi (S.)

Kula : Punarnava kula.

Family : Nyctaginaceae (Nyx = night, blooming at night). Flowers open at four o'clock in the evening and fall off at the break of day.

Latin name : Boerrhavia (name of a discoverer); diffusa = which spreads or widely spreading. Its roots are found spread on the ground spanning on an area of about 4-5 mts.

English name : Spreading hogweed.

Sanskrit names : (White) - Punarnava, Vishakh, Kshudrapatra, Raktavrintak.
(Red) - Raktavarsha, Shophaghni, Raktapushpika, Piksvara, Vishaghni, Praavrishenya, Sarini,
(Blue) - Neela, Shyama, Krishna.

Botanical Description: Perennial creeper 0.75 to 1 mt in length, sometimes grows upto 4 mts. in rainy seasons and dries in summer. Leaves - 2.5 to 4 cm long, fleshy, with soft hairs, at distance and whitish ventrally. Flowers - small, white coloured. Fruits - 1 cm long, round or circular, containing seeds like cow's beans. Root - thick, twisted on drying. Leaves arising on the opposite sides are unequal in size.

Varieties : Two (1) brown (2) white. Brown variety is longer than white and is easily available. Blue variety is mentioned in Rajnighantu.

Habitat : All over India.

Nerium oleander is a poison for a horse. Therefore all Sanskrit synonyms for this plant are derived by adding the suffix "ceej" (to kill) to the synonyms of horse.

Properties :
Guna : katu; **Vipak :** katu; **Veerya :** sheeta.
Karma : Tridoshahar, pittaghna by madhur, tikta and astringent, kapha-vata shamak by ushna veerya. Red variety is vatavardhak and pittashamak by sheeta veerya.
External uses : Lekhan or antiinflammatory.
Internal uses :
Digestive system : Deepan, anuloman, purgative but emetic in large dose.
Circulatory system : Cardiac tonic, increases blood, accelerates heart rate and acts as an hypertensive.
Respiratory system : Cures cough, antianaemic (Punarnava mandur is used in anaemia).
Reproductive system : Seeds are aphrodisiac.
Urinary system : Diuretic by increasing renal blood flow.
Skin : Diaphoretic and useful in skin diseases.
Temperature : Antipyretic.
Satmikaran : Rasayan and antidode.
Karma :
Dosha : Tridoshaghna, (White - vatashamak, Brown vatala), kaphaghna.
External uses : Punarnava is used for local application in the form of poultice or fomentation in oedema. The juice of its leaves is used in the eyes for topical application.
Internal uses :
Digestive system : It is given internally in agnimandya, toxicity, ascites and constipation. A dose of 3 gms is used to induce vomiting.
Circulatary system : Useful in heart disease, anaemia, oedema. Leaves vegetable is consumed to reduce oedema. 'पुनर्नवा च शोथघ्नी'
Respiratory system : Useful in cough, asthma and urahkshat.
Reproductive system : Menorrhagia, (root decoction of red variety is used). Seeds are aphrodisiac.
Eye diseases : Cataract, chronic conjunctivitis, blepharitis, (roots rubbed in honey is locally applied).
Urinary system : Acts as a diuretic in dysuria.
Skin : Useful in reducing swelling and foul smelling in skin disorders.
Temperature : Antipyretic, especially in quaternary fever.
Satmikaran : As a rasayan therapy in general debility. Antidote to snake poison and rat bite (used internally).
Parts used : Roots, seeds, leaves, whole plant.
Dosage : Decoction of roots 5-10ml; powdered seeds 1-2 grms; juice of whole plant 5-10 ml.
Formulations : Punarnavashtak, Punarnavasav, Punarnavambu, Purnarnavadi mandur.
Srotogamitva :
Dosha : Vatakaphaghna (red variety increases vata).
Dhatu : Rakta - meda (anaemia), rakta (useful in bleeding disorders and urakshat), jaundice.

In the study of dravyaguna, three types of knowledge matters viz. names of the plants, their morphology and properties.

Mala : Mutragami.
Organs : Heart, respiratory tract.
(Hogweed vegetable - mainly used to reduce oedema).
Shothaghni is the synonym for both the varieties.

References -

'कटु: कषायानुरसा पाण्डुघ्नी दीपनी परा । शोफानिलगरश्लेषम्हरी बध्नोदरप्रणुत् ।।' (भा.प्र.)
'पुनर्नवारुणा तिक्ता कटुपाका हिमा लघुः । वातला ग्राहिणी श्लेष्मपित्तरक्तविनाशिनी ।। (भा.प्र.)
'पुनर्नवा भवेदुष्णा तिक्ता रूक्षा कफापहा । सशोथपांडुहृद्रोगकासोरःक्षतशूलनुत् ।।' (ध.नि.)
'वर्षाभूर्मधुरा तिक्ता कषाय कटुका सरा । क्षारोष्णा दीपनी रूक्षा शोफानिलकफायहा ।।
हृद्या रुच्या जयेदर्शोव्रणपाण्डुगरोदरम् ।' (कै.नि.)
'उष्णानि स्वादुतिक्तानि वातप्रशमनानि च । तेषु पौनर्नवं शाकं विशेषाच्छोथनाशनम् ।।' (सु.सू. ४६)
'पुनर्नवस्यार्धपलं नवस्य पिष्टं पिबेद्यः पयसार्धमासम् ।
मासद्वयं तत्त्रिगुणं समां वा जीर्णोऽपि भूयः स पुनर्नवः स्यात् ।।' (यो.र.)

(75) PUSHKARMOOLA

Inula racemosa Hook-F.

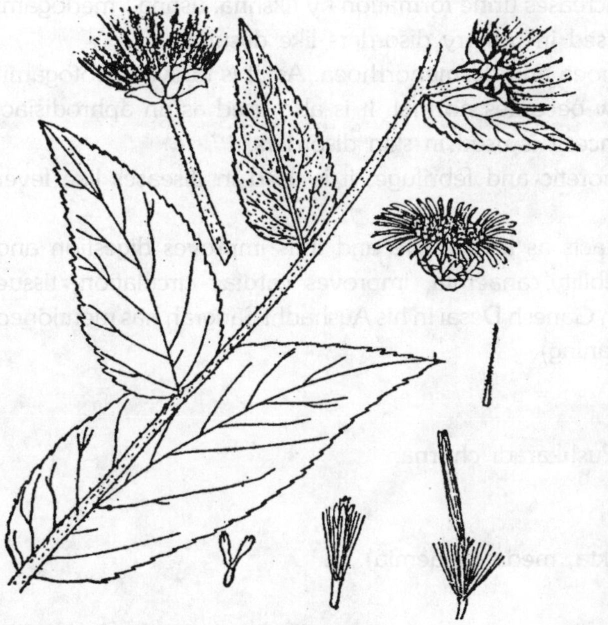

Gana : Shwasahara, Hikkanigrahana (C.); (Shwasahara gana is Hikkanigrahana).
Kula : Bhrungaraja kula.
Family : Compositeae. Compound with two or more parts forming a whole. A flower made up of several florets in one head.
Latin name : Inula = this is an ancient name which might be a misnomer of Belenium (fleabane poison); racemosa = having racemose pattern, having an inflorescence with a long undivided axis.
Sanskrit names : Poushkara, Haimavati, Shwetavacha, Kashmir, Kushthabheda, Kasari, Shwasari, Shoolahara, Sugandhika.
Botanical Description : This plant resembles the plant of kushtha.
Habitat : It grows at the height of 2.25 thousand m. in Kashmir.

Chemical composition : It contains a volatile oil, bitter principle and benzoic acid.
Properties :
Guna : laghu, tikshna; **Rasa** : tikta, katu; **Vipak** : katu; **Veerya** : ushna.
Karma :
Dosha : Vatakaphanashak by ushna veerya. It is useful in disorders induced by vata - kapha.

Initially, the practical knowledge of the use of plants was obtained from cowherds, shepherds, stable-boys and avairy keepers.

External uses: It is an antifungal, it cures pus formation, swelling and pain. Its powder is sprinkled over tuberculoid ulcers or its paste is applied. It is used in painful swelling. (पुष्करमूलं हिक्काश्वासकासपार्श्वशूलहराणाम श्रेष्ठम् । च. सू.२५/३९)
Local application of paste is effective in lateral chest pain by which swelling and pain are relieved.

Internal uses :

Central Nervous system : It stimulates brain and nervous system (majjagami), hence it is useful in cerebral impairment and vata disorders.

Digestive system : Being pungent, bitter and ushna, it is a good appetizer, digestive and deflatulent. It is used in anorexia, indigestion and flatulence.

Circulatory system : Cardiac stimulant and blood purifier, hence useful in cardic debility and blood disorders. It is the best medicine for cardiac asthma.

Respiratory system : It acts as an expectorant by pungent, bitter and ushna properties. Thus it clears the airways and alleviates cough, dyspnoea and hiccoughs. It is effective in chronic cough, hiccoughs, dyspnoea and pleurisy. In these diseases, it alleviates doshas by killing bacteria and relieves fever and pain.

Urinary system : Stimulates kidneys and increases urine formation by tikshna, ushna, medogami and kaphagami properties. Therefore it is used in urinary disorders like dysuria.

Reproductive system : Useful in amenorrhoea and dysmenorrhoea. As it is rajovahasrotogami, it reduces pain during menstruation and flow becomes normal. It is also used as an aphrodisiac.

Skin : It is a diaphoretic though bitter, hence it is used in skin disorders.

Temperature : Being ama digestive, diaphoretic and febrifuge, it is used in diseases like fever caused by vata-kapha and cold.

Satmikaran : Bitterness of pushkarmoola acts as a digestive and thus improves digestion and strengthens all dhatus. Useful in genral debility, anaemia, improves cardiac circulation, tissue metabolism and relieves weakness. (Dr. Vaman Ganesh Desai in his Aushadhi Sangrah has mentioned the word katupoushtik which has same meaning).

Parts used : Root.

Dosage : 0.25 to 0.75 gm.

Formulations : Pushkarmooladi churna, Pushkaradi churna.

Srotogamitva :

Dosha : Vatakaphaghna.

Dhatu : Rasa (fever, lateral chest pain), rakta, meda (anaemia).

Mala : Diuretic.

Organs : Lateral chest (analgesic).

References -

'उक्तं पुष्करमूलं तु पौष्करं पुष्करं च तत् । पद्मपत्रं च काश्मीरं कुष्टभदमिमं जगुः ।।
पौष्करं कटुकं तिक्तमुष्णं वातकफज्वरान् । हन्ति कासारुचिश्वासान् विशेषात् पार्श्वशूलनुत् ।। (भा.प्र.)
'पुष्करं कटु तिक्तोष्णं कफवातज्वरापहम् । श्वासारोचककासघ्नं शोफघ्नं पाण्डुनाशनम् ।।' (रा.नि.)
'पुष्करमूलं हिक्काश्वासकासपार्श्वशूलहराणाम् श्रेष्ठम् ।' (च.सू. २५)
'तिक्तं पुष्करमूलं च कटूष्णं कफवातजित् । ज्वरारोचककासघ्नं शोफार्दितविनाशनम् ।।

Man took the art of painting to its pinnacle, but he got basic inspiration and support by drawing leaves, flowers, inflorescences and creepers.

श्वासोर्ध्ववातपाण्डुघ्नं हिक्कादोषनिवारणम् ।' (ध.नि.)
'चूर्ण पुष्करजं लिह्यात् माक्षिकेण समायुतम् । हृच्छूलश्वासकासघ्नं क्षयहिक्कानिवारणम् ।।' (भै.र.)

(76) PRUSHNIPARNI

Ureria picta Desv.

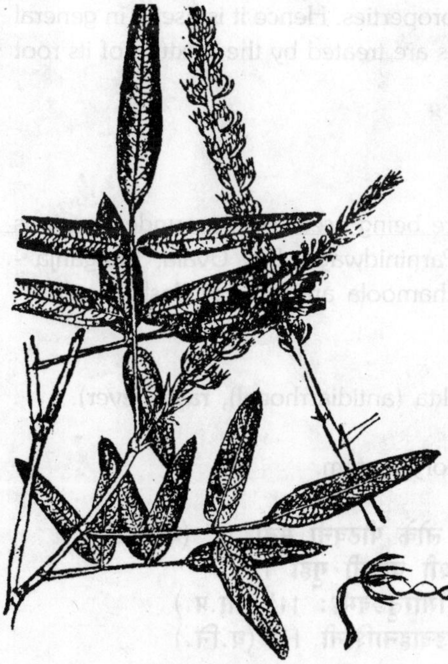

Gana : Angamardaprashamana, Sandhaneeya, Shothahara, Madhuraskandha (C.); Vidarigandhadi, Haridradi, Laghupanchamoola (S.) (The plants in laghu panchamoola are small while those in brihatpanchamoola are big).

Kula : Shimbi kula.

Upakula : Aparajita kula.

Family : Leguminosae.

Sub-family : Papillionaceae - like butterfly.

Latin name : Ureria = (Ouru) (Gk.) tail (the bracts and inflorescence); picta = painted with different colours in streaks of unequal intensity.

Sanskrit names : Kalashi, Dhamani, Mekhala, Shrugali, Deerghaparni, Kroshthukmekhala, Upachitra, Snigdhaparni, Vedavahni.

Botanical Description : The tree is 0.75 to 1.5 mt. high. Leaves - compound, having different shapes, with round base and elongated tapering end. Leaflets - 8 cm. long, having white coloured veins on it. Flowers - tiny, red-blue grow in inflorescense. Fruit - after growing fruits, the inflorescence resembles the tail of a fox. Seeds - kidney-shaped, yellow, 1 to 12 in number. The plant bears flowers in rainy season and seeds in autumn.

Varieties : Many trees are being used under the name of prushniparni like shaliparni, of which Uraria laqapoides and Uraria hamosa are the main plants.

Habitat : All over India in sandy regions and in barren land.

Properties :

Guna : laghu, snigdha; **Rasa** : madhur, tikta;. **Vipak** : madhur; **Veerya** : ushna.

Karma :

Dosha : Tridoshashamak, hence used in disorders caused by all the three doshas.

Internal uses :

Central nervous system : As it is a nervine tonic and alleviates vata dosha, it is used in vata disorders.

Digestive system : Being an appetizer, antidipsetic, deflatulent and astringent, it is used in dipsia, flatulence, diarrhoea, bleeding piles and sprue. Stomatitis is treated by local application of the paste of seeds and honey.

The roots, bark, resin, pulp, gum, stem, sap, leaves, alkaline extract, latex, fruits,flowers, bhasmas, oil, thorns and rhizomes of various plants are used in the preparation of medicines.

Circulatory system : Cardiac tonic, haemostatic and reduces oedema, hence useful in heart diseases, blood disorders, vatarakta and oedema.
Respiratory system : Expectorant. Useful in cough and dyspnoea.
Reproductive system : Aphrodisiac, useful in seminal debility.
Urinary system : Diuretic, therefore effective in dysuria.
Temperature : Febrifuge and refrigerant, hence it is used in fever and burning sensation.
Satmikaran : Tonic, it has binding, analgesic and antidote properties. Hence it is useful in general debility, malaise and bodyache, snake poison. Bone fractures are treated by the mixture of its root decoction and meat soup.
Parts used : Whole plant, root.
Dosage : Decoction 10-20 ml.
Formulation : Dashamoolarishta.
Both the plants, Desmodium gangetium and Ureria picta are being used together under various names viz. Shaliparni - Prushniparni, Amshumatidwaya, Parninidwaya, Pav Uvala, Ranganja - Ranbhal, Salvan- Pithvan. They are included in laghupanchamoola and thus in dashamoola.
Srotogamitva :
Dosha : Tridoshashamak.
Dhatu : Shukra (aphrodisiac), asthi (binding property), rakta (antidiarrhoeal), rasa (fever).
Mala : Purisha (laxative).
Organs : Madhyam marga, duodenum (deepani), respiratory system.
References -
'क्षुपा सशिंबा सत्पन्ना वर्षान्ते च भवेत्तु सा । कटुस्वाद्वणुबीजा स्यात् लोके पीठवनी मता ।।' (क.नि.)
पृश्निपर्णी पृथकपर्णी चित्रपर्ण्यघ्रिपर्णिका । क्रोष्टुविन्ना सिंहपुच्छी कलशी धावनी गृहा ।।
पुश्निपर्णी त्रिदोषघ्नी वृष्योष्णा मधुरा सरा । हन्ति दाहज्वरश्वासरक्तातीसारतृङवमी: ।।' (भा.प्र.)
'पृश्निपर्णी रसे स्वादुर्लघूष्णाऽस्त्रत्रिदोषजित् । कासश्वासप्रशमनी ज्वरतृङदाहनाशिनी ।।' (ध.नि.)
'पृश्निपर्णी सांग्राहिक - वातहर-दीपनीय-वृष्याणाम् श्रेष्ठा ।' (च.सू.अ. २५)
'मूलं शृगालविन्नाया: पीत्वा मांसरसेन तु ।
चूर्णीकृत्य त्रिसप्ताहादस्थिभग्नमपोहति ।।' (भा.प्र.)

(77) BALADWAYA
Sida cordifolia Linn.

Gana: Balya, Brumhaniya, Prajasthapana, Madhuraskandha (C.), Vatasamshamana(S.).
Kula : Karpas kula.
Family : Malvaceae (Gk.); Malva=mallow, word used by Cicero; Malakos = softening.
Latin name : Sida = (Gk.) old name for water lily used by Theophratus; cordifolia = cordi = heart shaped, folia = leaves.
English name : Country mallow.
Sanskrit names : **Bala** - Odanika, Bhadra, Samanga, Baladhya, Vatika, Sanasa, Mahasamanga, Kharayashtika, Sheetapaki, Veeryabala.

Palm, coconut, umber, neem and green grass grow in close proximity of each other; these are the plants which grow on marshy land and water is always found in the vicinity of these plants.

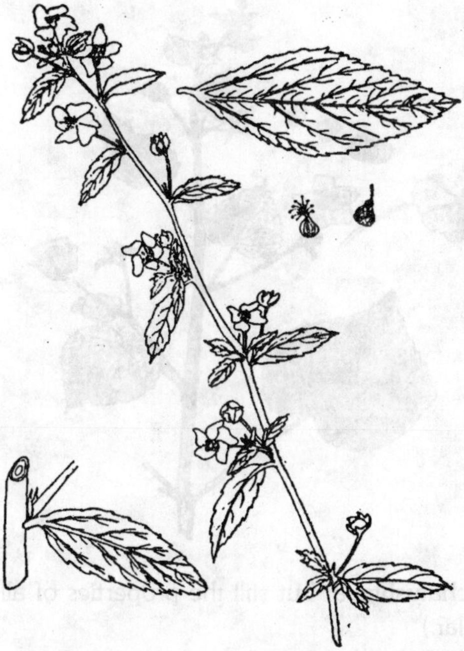

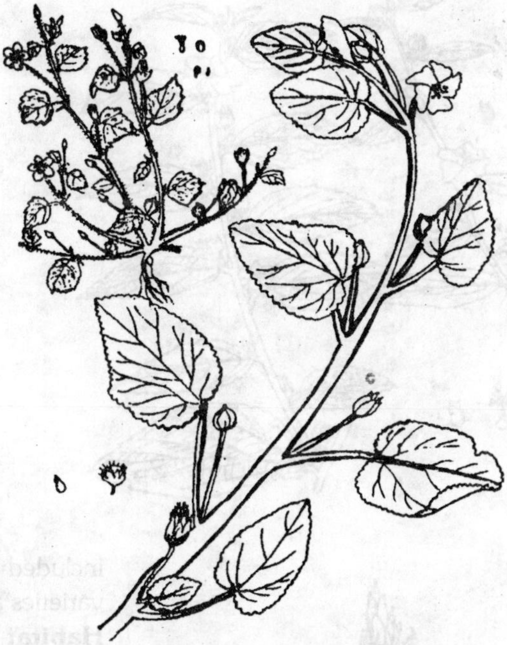

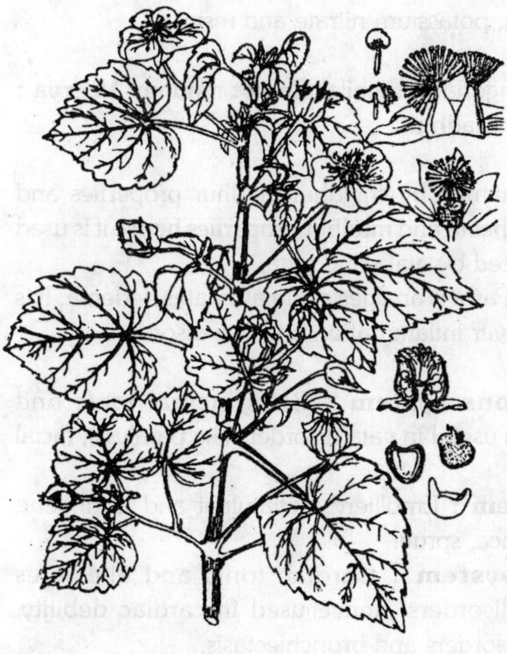

Mahabala - Mahabala, Jyeshthabala, Katambhara, Kesarika, Kesharuha, Sahadevi, Prasarani, Peetapushpi, Vatyayani, Cheerapushpi, Prasadani.

Botanical Description : A small shrub of height 5 to 10 cm. Root and trunk are strong hence it is called as 'bala'. Leaves - alternate, 2.5 to 5 cm. long, 5 cm. broad, ciliate, round, having 7-9 veins on it and serrated margin. Flowers - yellow in colour and originate from the angle of the leaf stalk. Flowers have 5 petals and 5 sepals. Fruits-like moonga, divided into 5 parts. Seeds - small, dusky black and look like peas. The seeds are called as beejabanda. The plant bears flowers and fruits at the end of rainy season.

Varieties : There are 4 varieties as described in Nighantu, which are known as 'balachatushtaya'- 1) Bala 2) Atibala 3) Mahabala 4) Nagabala.

According to morden classiffication, 4 plants come under the name of bala, namely Sida cordifolia, Sida shinosa, Sida acuta and Sida humilis. (Even today, there is no agreement amongst Vaidyas about the plants

A stick of shisav, when ignited, gives light for a long time. It is used like a torch in villages.

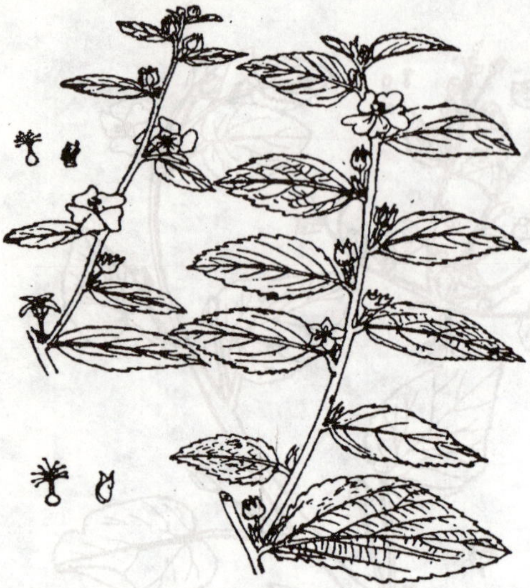

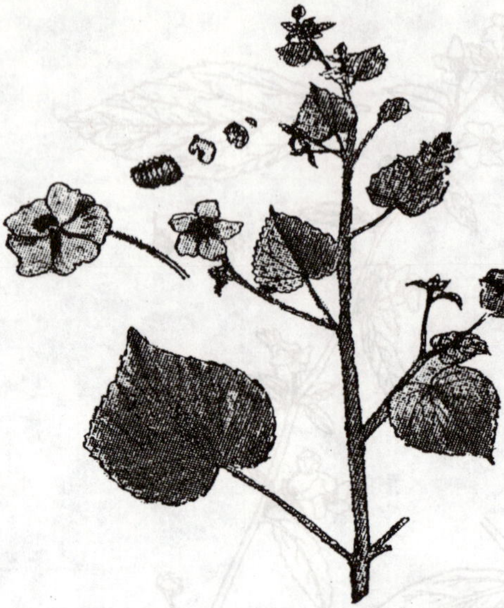

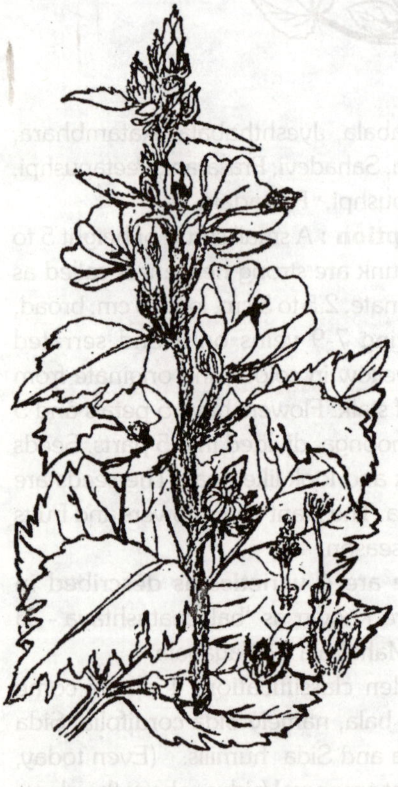

included in balachatushtaya, but still the properties of all 4 varieties are similar.)

Habitat : All over India and Srilanka.

Chemical composition : Major components of seeds are alkaloids. Alkaloid contains mainly ephedrine. It also contains fatty acid, mucin, potassium nitrate and resin.

Properties :

Guna : guru, singdha, pichchila; **Rasa :** madhur; **Veerya :** sheeta; **Vipak :** madhur.

Karma :

Dosha : Vatashaman by snigdha, madhur properties and pittashamak by sheeta and madhur properties hence it is used in diseases induced by vata and pitta.

External use : Paste is analgesic and alleviates oedema. It is locally applied over inflammation and eye disorders.

Internal use :

Central nervous system : Being neural tonic and vatashamak, it is useful in vata disorders like paralysis, facial palsy etc.

Digestive system : Emollient, deflatulent and astringent. Useful in flatulence, sprue.

Circulatory system : Cardiac tonic and alleviates haemorrhagic disorders, hence used in cardiac debility, haemorrhagic disorders and bronchiectasis.

The leaves of Sulfium lasiniatum always point in the north-south direction like the needle in magnetic compass.

Reproductive system : Aphrodisiac and useful in spermatorrhoea.
Urinary system : Diuretic, so useful in dysuria.
Temperature : Useful in fever being a febrifuge.
Satmikaran : Being tonic, it is helpful in general debility, tuberculosis and undernourishment.
Parts used : Root, seeds and leaves.
Dosage : Juice 3 to 6 tsf; powder 1-3 mg.
Formulations : Baladi kwath, Baladya ghrita, Baladyarishta, Chandanabalalakshadi taila.
Srotogamitva :
Dosha : Alleviates vata, pitta.
Dhatu : Rakta, mansa, shukra, oja (enhancer).
Mala : Purisha (astringent).

ATIBALA

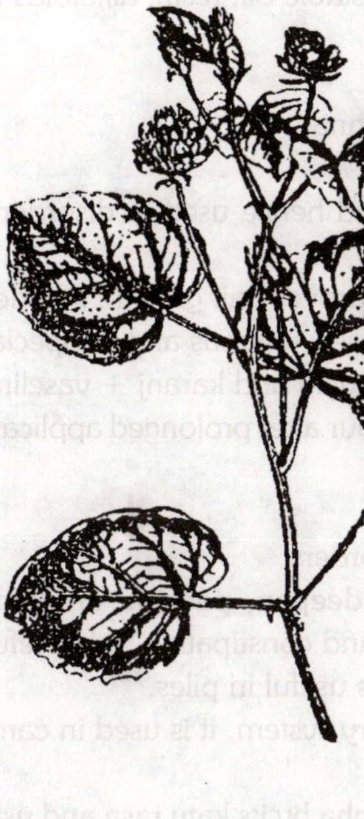

Gana : Balya, Brumhaniya, Madhuraskandha (C.); Vatasamshamana, Madhura gana (S.)
Kula : Karpas kula.
Famiy : Malvaceae.
Latin Name : Abutilon indicum (Linn).
Sanskrit names : Atibala, Kankatika, Rushyaprokta.
Botanical description : Shrub of height 1.25 to 2 mtrs. Leaves - serrated, soft, ciliate. Flowers -yellow, the tube of the androecium is elongated and gynaecium are 15 or more in number. Fruit - round but surrounded by spikes on all sides. Seeds - 15-20 in number, dusky black and called as 'beejabanda'.
Varieties : It is of 2 varieties - 1) small and 2) big = Abutilon hirtum. The shrub of the latter variety is bigger. Its branches and petioles have elongated cilia.
Habitat : All over India and Srilanka.
Chemical composition : Same as bala.
Properties : Same as bala.

References -
'बलाचतुष्टयं शीतं मधुरं बलकान्तिकृत् । स्निग्धं ग्राहि समीरास्रपित्तास्रक्षतनाशनम् ।।' (भा.प्र.)
'बला संग्राहिक-बल्य-वातहराणाम् ।' (च.सू.२५)
'बला स्निग्धा हिमा स्वादुर्वृष्या बल्या त्रिदोषनुत् ।
रक्तपित्तं क्षयं हन्ति बलौजोवर्धयत्यपि ।।' (ध.नि.)

Eventhough leaves of brahmarakshas and banana trees are big, the leaves of Amazon-waterlily are considred to be the biggest in the world.

(78) BAKUCHI
Psoralea corylifolia Linn.

Kula : Shimbi kula.
Upakula : Pappilionaceae (Butterfly like).
Family : Leguminosae.
Latin name : Psoralea - plants with rough surface due to glandular dots or warts.; corylifolia - korus (Gk) helmet, calcine covering of the nut.
English name : Purple fleabane.
Sanskrit names : Somarekha, Shashanklekha, Somaragi, Chandralekha, Bakuchi, Somavalli, Yendavi, Twakdoshaghni
Botanical Description : Seasonal plant 0.5 to 1.5 mt. in height. Trunk straight and branches are strong and elastic. Leaves - 2.5 to 8 cm. long, round or heart shaped, border is undulate. Flowers - yellow, blue 1-30 flowers in branches appear on a long stalk. Fruits - blackish in bundles. Seeds - black, small, tender and give a peculiar scent on rubbing in fingers or hand.
Habitat : India and Sri lanka. Predominantly found in Assam and Uttar Pradesh.
Chemical composition : It contains a volatile yellow oil 20.15 %, stable oil, resin, alkaloids (7.5 %), albumin, sugar, manganese and vermonine.
Properties :
Guna : laghu, ruksha; **Rasa :** katu, tikta; **Vipak :** katu; **Veerya :** ushna.
Karma :
Dosha : Since it has ushna veerya, it acts as kaphavata shaman and hence used in disorders of kaphavata.
External uses : It is useful in skin diseases for wound healing and improves hair growth. Powdered bakuchi or oil prepared from it is used locally in leucoderma, dermatoses, wounds and alopecia. A mixture of bakuchi, karanj and lime juice is used in eczema. Oil of bakuchi and karanj + vaseline is used in chronic skin diseases. White spots of leucoderma turn red in colour after prolonged application of bakuchi.
Internal uses :
Nervous system : Since it is a nervine tonic, it is useful in vata disorders.
Digestive system : By its katu and ushna properties it acts as deepan, pachan, anuloman, anthelmintic and liver stimulant. Hence it is used in indigestion, ama and constipation. It is useful in all types of worms especially round worms. Being a liver stimulant it is useful in piles.
Circulatory system : Since it stimulates the heart and the circulatory system, it is used in cardiac failure and oedema produced by it .
Respiratory system : Used in cough and asthma since it reduces kapha by its katu rasa and ushna veerya.
Urinary system : Useful in diabetes.
Reproductive system : Since it is a stimulant and an aphrodisiac, it is used in impotency.
Skin : Diaphoretic and kusthaghna. Its oil has a specific irritant action on the skin and mucous membrane. On applying the oil on leucoderma, the skin becomes reddish and occassionally blisters may occur. But it does not create any alterations in the normal colour of the skin. The oil acts in

Leaves of touch-me-not close by mere touch or even by breeze. Therefore it is called lajjalu (shying plant).

leucoderma by activating the melanoblastic cells of the skin. It is useful in all skin diseases. In leucoderma, the oil must be so applied that it only produces a change in colour and not blisters. All commercially available preparations for leucoderma contain bakuchi.

Temperature : Febrifuge, used in chronic fever.

Satmikaran : It is a bitter tonic and hence used in anaemia and post-pyrexial debility.

Parts used : Seeds, oil.

Dose : Powder - 1 to 3 gms. ; for worms - 4 to 6 gms.

Purification : The seeds of bakuchi are purified by keeping them in cow's urine or juice of ardrak for seven days.

Srotogamitva : Bakuchi seeds -

Dosha : Kaphanashak; Seeds - pittavardhan, kaphavatashaman.

Dhatu : Rakta, meda ,tvachagami.

Mala : Anthelmintic, hair (asthi, majja).

Special action : Bakuchi is the best medicine for leucoderma.

" So far as is known P. corylifolia is the only drug that has a dual action i. e. action on both Rouget's cell and the melanoblastic cells of the skin. In leucoderma the melanoblastic cells are not functioning properly and their stimulation by the oil leads them to form and exdue pigment which gradually diffuses into decolourised areas!

The oil Bavachi (oil psoralea) changes white skin, grey hair, rough, scaly, disocloured skin, nails, hairs, etc. to normal colour within 3 months and that it is well tried and prescribed by eminent doctor N. C. Basu, School of tropical medicine, Calcutta. In morden medicine too, the compound "psoraler" is applied on the vitiligenous area, which is then exposed to sunlight.

References -

'बाकुची कटुतिक्तोष्णा कृमिकुष्ठकफापहा । त्वग्दोषविषकण्डूर्तिश्वित्रप्रशमनी परा ।।' (रा.नि.)

'तत्फलं पित्तलं कुष्ठकफानिलहरं कटु । केश्यं त्वच्यंवमिश्वासकासशोथामपाण्डुनुत् ।।' (भा.प्र.)

(79) BRAHMI

Herpestis moniera H. B.K.

Kula : Brahmi kula.

Family : Scrophulariaceae (Figwort family) natural order of lobiate herbs.

Latin name : Herpestis = creeping; moniera - moni = necklace.

Sanskrit names : Brahmi, Sarasvati, Mahaushadhi, Swayambhuvi, Madukamala, Matsyakshi, Medhya, Satyavati, Smarani.

Habitat : The plant grows on the edges of streams, hence it is found near water trenches etc.

Botanical Description : A fleshy creeper. Leaves - reniform, having small spots, 6 x2.5 mms in size. Flowers- purplish white or pinkish. Brahmi has 5 to 7 leaves in a bunch, while Ipomoea reniformis has 2 to 3 leaves. The leaves of brahmi are soft and thick, while the leaves of Ipomoea reniformis are hollow having shape of rat ears. These are the differences between Brahmi and I. reniformis.

Chemical composition : It contains an alkaloid which is known as brahmine.

The circumference of a cyprus tree is 34 meters i.e. nearly 132 feet. Even a car can come and go through its stem.

Properties :
Rasa : tikta, kashaya; **Vipak** : madhur; **Veerya** : sheeta; **Prabhav** : apasmar, unmada nashak.
External uses : In rheumatoid arthitis, the fresh juice of brahmi is applied to the inflammed joints, which helps in relieving pain.
Internal uses :
Nervous system : Brahmi is a valuable plant for brain and entire nervous system. Mania and epilepsy are two conditions which require brahmi. It also helps in depression and mental retardation, by enchanching intelligence.
Digestive system : Brahmi is slightly astringent and hence useful in diarrheoa due to vitiated vata. Brahmi may suppress appetite, hence deepan medicines should be given along with it.
Respiratory system : Specially in children, for cold and cough, 1 teaspoonful of brahmi- juice is given to induce vomiting and gives relief. When hoarseness of voice results from excessive talking, pills made from the leaves of brahmi, vasa, pippali, haritaki and vacha are chewed which gives relief.
Cardiovascular system : In small doses, it has cardo-tonic property. It leads to an increase in blood pressure.
Urinary system : Diuretic.
Temperature : In Srilanka, brahmi is used for fever.
Satmikaran : Brahmi is a brain tonic. It enhances memory, intelligence and longevity.
Parts used : Juice of leaves, leaves (volatile oils evaporate when heated).
Dosage : Leaf juice - 2 teaspoonful; leaf powder - .125 to 1.0 gm.
Formulations : Brahmi prash; Saraswatarishta, Brahmighruta, Brahmitaila.
Srotogamitva :
Dosha : Vataghna, pittaghna, kaphaghna, tridoshanashak (sadhakapittagami).
Dhatu : Meda (demulcent), strengthens all seven dhatus (anaemia, urinary disorders).
Mala : Urine (diuretic), keshya (hair growth).
Prabhava : Antidote.
References -
ब्राह्मी हिमा सरा तिक्ता लघुर्मेध्याच शीतला ।
कषाया मधुरा स्वादुपाकाऽऽयुष्या रसायनी ।
स्वर्या स्मृतिप्रदा कुष्ठपाण्डुमेहास्त्रकासिजत् ।
विषशोथ ज्वरहरी (तद्वत् मंडूकपर्णिनी ।)

(80) BIBHEETAKA
Terminalia belerica Roxb.

Gana : Jwarahar, Virechanopag (C.); Triphala, Mustadi (S.)
Family : Combretaceae (caffer butter shrub).
Latin name : Terminalia (derived from terminus) producing from the extremity (end leaves terminal in position); belerica (from the word "beley" which is the arabic name for bibheetaka). The leaves of the Terminalia family have small nodules at the base, one on each side.
Sanskrit names: Bibheetaka (regular use eliminates fear of disease), Karshaphala (the weight of

Though for the practical applications, Ayurveda limits itself to panchamahabhootas, yet for understanding the philosophy of Ayurveda, one has to go up to avyakta.

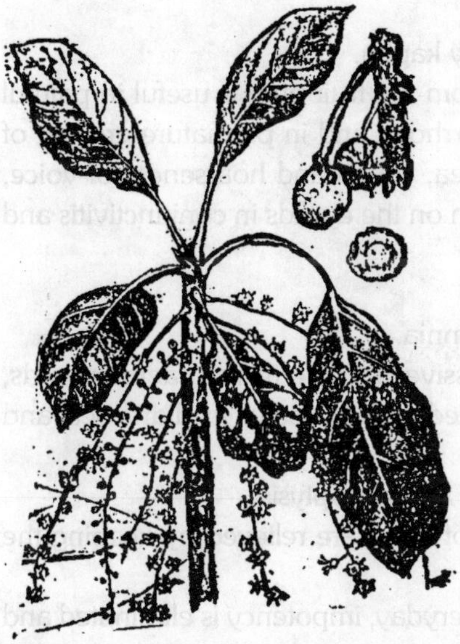

the fruit is one tola), Aksha (the seeds are used in a game of gambling), Kalidrum (gambling under bibheetaka tree definitely results in a qurrel), Telpushpak, Bhootawas (animals take shelter in its shade), Kalivruksha, Romaharsha, Kalind.

Botanical Description : The tree grows upto a height of 16 to 32 mtrs. The bark is brownish in colour. The wood of the trunk is hard. The leaves resemble those of banyan tree and are 8 to 16 cms. in length. The leaves may be long or circular. At the base of the leaves, where the lamina ends, there are two small nodules. Flowers are very small and yellow. There are five small and five large stamens. Fruits are round in shape, brownish and hairy. Each fruit contains one seed. The tree flowers in the summer and fruits in the winter. The fruits ripen in the spring. The seed pulp is sweet to taste but it produces mild intoxication.

Varieties : Depending on the size of the fruits, it is classified into, having small fruits and having large fruits.

Habitat : It is predominantly found in India, Burma and hilly areas.

Properties :

Guna : ruksha, laghu; **Rasa :** kashaya; **Vipak :** madhur; **Veerya :** ushna.

Karma :

Dosha : It is kaphaghna because of its ruksha, laghu, kashaya guna; pittaghna by kashaya and madhur rasa and vatashamak by ushna guna. Thus bibheetaka is tridoshanashak, but mainly kaphanashak (Haritaki is vatanashak, amalaki is pittanashak and bibheetaka is kaphanashak = triphala is tridoshanashak).

External uses : Antiinflammatory, analgesic, haemostatic and gives black colour to the skin and hair. Oil is a hair tonic.

Internal uses :

Nervous system : The pulp is intoxicant and analgesic (the regular synonym of bibheetaka means tandra - a state of mind between sleep and unconciousness. This may be due to the action of bibheetaka on majja dhatu.)

Digestive system : Being ushna, it is deepan, laxative and anthelmintic. Half ripe fruit is purgative and ripe fruit is astrigent. It is anti-emtic and reduces excessive thirst.

Circulatory system : It is used as a blood coagulant due to its astringent property.

Respiratory system : It helps in asthma and cough by reducing the inflammation of the bronchi.

Reproductive system : The pulp is an aphrodisiac.

Temperature : Febrifuge.

Satmikaran : Rasa, rakta, mansa and medogami, dhatuvardhak because of its madhur vipak.

Eyes : Dried bibheetaka is good for the eyes. Bibheetaka + honey is used for local application in eye diseases.

The Ayurvedic philosophy of tritva (triune nature) is related to satva, rajas and tama. The term dosha is related to guna.

Indications :

Dosha : Tridoshaghna but is more useful in diseases caused by kapha.

External uses : An application of the fruit or oil extracted from the fruit pulp is useful in painful inflammatory conditions. The oil is used in skin diseases, leucorrhoea and in premature greying of hair. The rind of fruit is kept in the mouth for relieving dyspnoea, cough and hoarseness of voice, since it acts as mucolytic. The powder is used for local application on the eyelids in conjunctivitis and also acts as haemostatic in fresh wounds.

Internal uses :

Nervous system : The pulp is used in vata disorders and insomnia.

Digestive system : Useful in indigestion, flatulence, excessive thirst, emesis, haemorrhoids, helmenthiasis. Half ripe fruit relieves constipation whereas dried fruit is useful in diarrhoea and dysentery.

Circulatory system : Useful in internal bleeding. More useful in haemoptysis.

Respiratory system : Cold, cough, asthma and hoarseness of voice are relieved by keeping the rind of the fruit in the mouth.

Reproductive system : By consuming the pulp of one seed everyday, impotency is eliminated and libido is improved.

Parts used : Fruit.

Doses : Powder - 0.75 to 1.5 gms.

Formulations : Bibheetaka taila, Triphala churna, Phalatrikadi kwath, Lavangadi vati, Baibheetaki sura.

Srotogamitva :

Dosha : Tridosha.

Dhatu : Majja (intoxication),rakta (haemostatic), shukra (aphrodisiac), rasa - mansagami.

Mala : Purisha (laxative), hair tonic (bibheetaka majja taila).

Organs : Eyes, respiratory system.

References -

'बिभीतकं स्वादुपाकं कषायं कफपित्तनुत् । उष्णवीर्यं हिमस्पर्शं भेदनं कासनाशनम् ।
रूक्षं नेत्रहितं केश्यं कृमिवैस्वर्यनाशनम् । ब्रिभीतमज्जा तृटछर्दिकफवातहरी लघुः ।।
कषाया मदकृच्चाथ धात्रीमज्जापि तदगुणा' (भा.प्र.)
'रसासृङ्मांसमेदोजान् दोषान् हन्ति बिभीतकम् । स्वरभेदकफोत्क्लेदपित्तरोगविनाशनम् ।।' (च.सू. २७)
'भेदनं लघु रूक्षोष्णं वैस्वर्यकृमिनाशनम् । चक्षुष्यं स्वादुपाक्याक्षं कषायं कफपित्तजित् ।।'
'बैभीतको मदकरः कफमारुतनाशनम् ।' (सु.सू.४६)

(81) BILVA

Aegle marmelos Corr.

Gana : Shothahara, Arshoghna, Asthapanopaga, Anuvasanopaga (C.); Bruhatpanchmoola, Varunadi, Ambashthadi (S).

Kula : Nimbooka kula.

Family : Rutaceae - from Ruta, from Ruomal = to preserve, medicinal properties preserved.

One has not to forget that the human body is of the universe and from the universe and it has to be returned gratefully back to the universe.

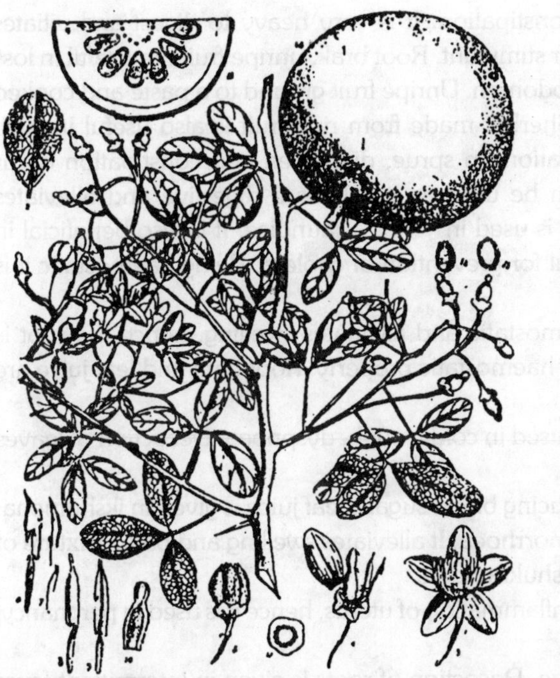

Latin name : Aegle = goat - one of the hesperides daughters of the evening Golden apple; marmelos = Portuguse word meaning acid pearshaped fruit.

English name : Bengal Quince.

Sanskrit names : Bilva, Shalatu (Shalat means unripe. This name is derived as unripe fruit is used), Shalya (having thorns), Hridyagandha (odour of leaves and fruits), Shivadruma (God Shankar likes bilva), Karkata, Trishikha (having 3 leaves), Shaivapatra, Duraroha (one cannot climb on the tree because of thorns).

Botanical Description : Bel tree is 8 to 10 meters high. Leaves - compound, trilaminal, having odour. Flowers - white, having 4-5 petals. The ovary is large and central part of it is stiff like wood. Fruits - large, round and rigid. It has 8-15 compartments. Seed - small, rigid, many in number. The tree bears flowers in the month of May while fruits after 10-14 months (So the tree is called as sadafala). In summer leaves fall off.

Varieties : It is of 2 varieties, wild and enphrated. Fruit of wild variety is small and has thorns on it while that of the other variety is big and has comparatively less thorns .

Habitat : All over India. This tree is cultivated in many gradens. These trees are seen mainly near temples, as bel leaves are required for pooja and found in Bengal, Bihar, Central and Southern India and Brahmadesh.

Chemical composition : Fruit pulp contains mucilage, pectin, sugar, tannin, volatile oil, gum, bitter principle and 2% ash. It contains an active principle known as marmelocin. Fresh leaves contain an essential oil. Seeds contain oil which is laxative. Roots, leaves and bark contain an astringent principle.

Properties :

Guna : ruksha, laghu; **Rasa :** kashaya, tikta; **Veerya :** ushna; **Vipak :** katu.

Karma :

Dosha : Kaphashamak by ruksha, laghu, kashaya and bitter and vatashamak by ushna property.

External uses : In conjunctivitis, leaf juice is put in the eyes and paste of leaves is applied over the eyelids. In disease conditions like swelling, pain in the ribs, leaves are used for fomentation. Leaf alleviates oedema and pain.

Internal uses :

Nervous system : Bel root tranquilises the nerves hence it is used in vatadisorders, insomnia, epilepsy and hysteria.

Digestive system : Unripe fruit is an appetizer, digestant and astringent. Ripe fruit is astringent and

Initially the plants were identified on the basis of the etymology of their synonyms. This will continue in the future too. The seventy-two synonyms of mango will leave no doubt as to its identification.

a sweet, mild laxative. An excess dose causes constipation. It is very heavy to digest and vitiates doshas, gives bad odour to flatus. Leaf juice is liver stimulant. Root brak, unripe fruit are useful in loss of appetite, diarrhoea, dysentery, sprue, pain in abdomen. Unripe fruit ground to a paste and cooked with sugar is very beneficial in bleeding piles. Sherbat made from ripe fruit is also useful in such conditions. Again an excess dose causes constipation. In sprue, diarrhoea and constipation occur simultaneously. So sherbat of ripe fruit pulp can be used as it acts as a digestive and alleviates diarrhoea. Mixture of leaf juice and black pepper is used in jaundice. It is also beneficial in constipation. Both ripe and unripe fruits are useful for prevention of cholera. Being haemostatic it is also used in haemorrhoids.

Circulatory system : It is a cardiac tonic, haemostatic and alleviates swelling, hence the root is used in cardiac debility and palpitations. Fruit has haemostatic property. Root bark and leaf juice are used to alleviate oedema.

Respiratory system : It is kaphashamak hence used in cold, cough, dyspnoea. Decoction of leaves is given for cold.

Urinary system : Juice of bel leaves helps in reducing blood sugar. Leaf juice is given in ikshumeha. Mixture of fresh fruit pulp and kankol is used in gonorrhoea. It alleviates swelling and pain. Mixture of bark juice and sweet cumin seeds is beneficial in shukrameha.

Reproductive system : Bilva root alleviates the inflammation of uterus, hence it is used in pergnancy, leucorrhoea and puerperal disorders.

Temperature : Bilva root and leaves are febrifuge. Decoction of roots is given in intermittent fever while leaf juice can be given in all types of fever.

Satmikaran : Bel is a bitter tonic. Its root and leaves have an anabolic effect on all body tissues. Since the ripe fruit is sweet to taste, it also acts as a tonic.

Parts used : Root, root bark, leaves, both ripe and unripe fruit. Half ripe fruit is used for making murabbha (a sweet preserve - jam), ripe fruit for sherbat and root and root bark for preparing Dashmool kadha etc.

Dosage : Powder 0.75 - 2 gms.; juice - 10 - 20 ml.

Formulations : Bilvamooladi gutika.

Aduleteration : Bel fruit pulp is adulterated by adding kapittha fruit pulp. Bel fruit pulp has cavities unlike kapittha.

Main action : Roots are useful in vata disorders, fruit in disorders of internal channel. Bel, durva and tulsi are used in vata, pitta and kapha disorders respectively.

Srotogamitva :

Dosha : Vitiates pitta, alleviates kapha, vata.

Dhatu : Meda, majja, rakta (astringent, hypoglycemic), rasa.

Mala : Purisha - mutra (astringent), (leaves are antidiuretic).

System : Digestive system, reproductive system (uterus).

References -

बिल्वः शाण्डिल्यशैलूषौ मालूरश्रीफलावपि । गन्धगर्भः कण्टकी च सदाफलः ।।
श्रीफलस्तुवरस्तिक्तो ग्राही रुक्षोऽग्निपित्तकृत् । वातश्लेष्महरो बल्यो लघुरुष्णश्च पाचनः ।।' (भा.प्र.)
'कफानिलहरं तीक्ष्णं स्निग्धं संग्राहिदीपनम् । कटुतिक्तकषायोष्णं बालं बिल्वमुदाहतम् ।।

The effect of drayva on the body and mind are brought about by the dynamic vibrations of rasa, veerya, vipak, guna and prabhav. Rasa etc are the diverse vibrators.

विद्यात्तदेव सं पक्वं मधुरानुरसं गुरु । विदाहि विष्टम्भकरं दोषकृतं पूतिमारुतम् ।। (सु.सू. ४६)
'बिल्वं सांग्राहिकदीपनीयवातकफप्रशमनानाम् श्रेष्ठम् ।' (च.सू.अ. २५)
'बिल्वमज्जाभवं तैलमुष्णं वातहरं परम् ।' (कै.ना.)

(82) BRUHATI

Solanum indicum Linn.

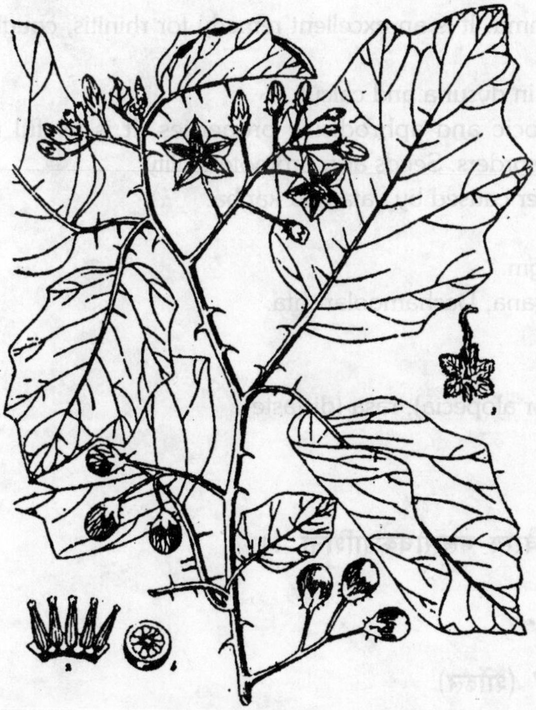

Gana : Kanthya, Hikkanigrahana, Shothahara, Angamaradaprashamana (C); Bruhatyadi, Laghupanchamoola (S).

Kula : Kantakari kula.

Family : Solanaceae = (After the name of a german Botanist). (Solanum = comforting) Many species have sedative qualities.

Latin name : Solanum = German Botanist; indicum = Indian.

Sanskrit names : Bruhati, Mahati, Bahupatri, Kantatanu, Dorali, Dushpradharsha, Mahavartakini, Mahoshri, Sinhi.

Botanical Description : Tree is 0.75 - 2 meters high. It has crooked and flattened thorns on its trunk and leaves with many branches and sub-branches. Leaves - 7-15 cms. long, 0.5-1.5 cms. wide, wing shaped with thorns. Flowers - blue. Fruits - unripe fruit is green with white striations on it. Ripe fruit becomes yellow. Fresh fruit is bitter to taste, which disappears on drying.

Varieties : Like ringni, bruhati is of 2 varieties, according to flowers - blue or white. White bruhati is big with big leaves, white fruit.The latin name is Solanum torvum Swartz. (Torvus= of wild, fierce appearance).

Habitat : Mainly Punjab, Bengal and Southern India but all over India.

Chemical composition : Its root and fruit contain wax, fatty acids and alkaloids namely, solanine and solanidine.

Properties :

Guna : laghu, ruksha, tikshna; **Rasa :** katu, tikta; **Vipak :** katu; **Veerya :** ushna.

Karma :

Dosha : Being ushna veerya and kaphavatanashak, it is used in disorders induced by kapha and vata.

External uses : Since it is an analgesic, antipruritic, hair-tonic and stimulant, it is used for local application. A vaginal suppository made from bruhati, daruharidra and haridra is used in itching.

Instead of using minerals in the form of bhasma, the plants containing those minerals should better be used.

Fumigation with this mixture also helps. Powdered seeds are applied on the genitalia in impotency. In unconsciousness, the powder of the seeds is administered nasally.

Internal uses :

Digestive system : It is ushna veerya, deepan, pachan, astringent and anthelmintic. It is therefore used in indigestion, colic, anorexia and worm infestation. In vomiting, juice of the fruits + cow's ghee+ honey is given.

Circulatory system : Since it is a cardiac tonic, blood purifier and diuretic, it is used in cardiac failure, oedema and blood disorders.

Respiratory system : It reduces cough and asthma. It is an excellent remedy for rhinitis, cough, asthma, soar throat and hiccups.

Urinary system : Since it is a diuretic, it is used in dysuria and calculi.

Reproductive system : Its seeds have oxytocic and aphrodisiac properties. It is useful in ammenorrhoea, dysmenorrhoea and puerperal disorders. Seeds also promote virility.

Temperature : Febrifuge. Hence it is used in fever caused by vata and kapha.

Parts used : Root, seed, fruit.

Dosage : Decoction 40 - 80 ml.; powder 0.5 - 1 gm.

Formulations : Bruhatyadi kwath, Bruhatyadi gana, Dashamoolarishta.

Srotogamitva :

Dosha : Alleviates kapha, vata

Dhatu : Rakta, skin (upadhatu of rakta - paste for alopecia), rasa (distaste).

Mala : Purisha (astringent), (digestive).

Organs : Heart, brain.

References -

'बृहती ग्राहिणी हृद्या पाचनी कफवातहृत् । कटुतिक्तास्यवैरस्य मलारोचकनाशिनी ।।
उष्णा कुष्ठज्वरश्वासशूलकासाग्निमान्द्यजित् ।' (भा.प्र.)
'इन्द्रलुप्तापहो लेपो मधुना बृहतीरसः ।' (शोढल)
एकं बृहत्याः फलपिप्पलीकं शुण्ठीयुतं चूर्णमिदं प्रशस्तम् ।
प्रध्मापयेत् घ्राणपुटे विसंज्ञः चेष्टां करोति क्षवथुप्रबुद्धः ।।' (शोढल)

(83) BHALLATAKA

Semecarpus anacardium Linn.

Class : Kushthaghna, Deepaniya, Mootrasangrahaniya (C.); Nyagrodhadi, Mustadi (S.)

Kula : Amra kula.

Family : Anacardiaceae (Ana = like, cardium = heart).

Latin Name : Semecarpus = Simeion = marking, tracing names, carpus = carpos (Gk.) = nut. Black juice of the nut used for marking or tracing designs upon cloth; anacardium = heart like .

English name : Marking nut (used for tracing marking on cloth).

Sanskrit names : Bhallataka (sharp like spear), Agnimukha (mouth of the fruit-Godambi- looks red like fire), Arushkara (induces blisters), Anala (fire), Krimighna, Bhallata.

Botanical Description : The tree is 7 - 10 mtrs. high. Trunk bark - grey, smoke coloured, but juice

Just like human beings, plants too can be categorized as per dosha, dhatu, mala and psychic prakruti. As for example, milk would be described as of kapha, rasa, mutra or satwa-prakruti.

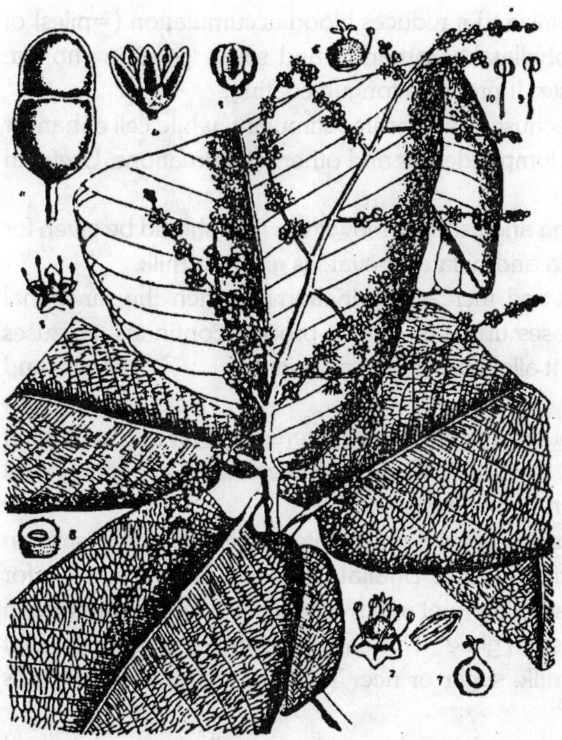

is black in colour. Leaves - develop from the tip of the branches, 7-10 cm. long, having dorsal surface ciliated, broad at the tip and have 15 - 25 stiff veins on it. The leaves fall off in the spring. Flowers - yellow and homosexual. Male and female flowers occur on different trees. Flower stalk - elongated. Fruit - 3-4 cm. long, heart shaped. Uripe fruit is green while ripe fruit is shiny black. Fruit juice is white, on exposure to air it becomes black like blood. Juice of ripe fruit is thick like honey and is black. Fruit has cap-like structure on it. It is red and can be eaten when ripe. Like almond, fruit has a kernel which is called as 'Godambi'. Flowering stage is summer and fruiting occurs in autumn. Marking nut which sinks in water should be used for medicinal purposes. The oil which is derived from burning the nut is called 'shevate'.

Habitat : Throughout India, mainly torrid zone and the foot of Himalaya, Bihar, Bengal, Orissa, Assam.

Chemical composition : The fruit contains 32% vesicating oil.

Properties :

Guna : laghu, snigdha, tikshna, ushna; **Rasa :** madhur, kashaya; **Vipak :** madhur; **Veerya :** ushna (think of bhallataka first in disorders induced by vata & kapha & agnimandya).

Karma :

Dosha : Kaphavatashamak by ushna and tikshna properties but it is pittasanshodhak, useful in many diseases caused by vata and kapha. Also useful in disorders caused by pitta for pitta elimination.

External uses : It induces blisters and is antidotal. In snake bite, incisions are taken on the snake bite region and juice of bhallataka is applied on it. Haemorrhoids become dry and fall off by an incense of bhallataka. (Dry haemorrhoids are caused by vata and kapha). If it is applied over vagina it causes abortion. This nut is applied or cauterisation with the seed is done over pain caused by any injury. It relieves pain.

Internal uses :

Nervous system : Useful in weakness of brain and nerves, epilepsy, sciatic neuralgia, rheumatoid arthritis and hemiplegia.

Digestive system : It is used in gastrontestinal disorders by its actions like appetizer, digestant, purgative, liver stimulant and anthelmintic. Useful in loss of appetite, digestive disorders, constipation, abdominal distension, gulma, ascites, sprue, piles and various types of worms. Shevate is the best remedy for intestinal colic. 10-25 drops of this oil are mixed with sugar and given to the patient. Mainly useful in hookworm. It is an effective medicine for piles because it improves the blood circulation in the liver and that reduces the pressure on the veins and it reduces blood accumulation (=piles) of rectal veins and thus dries the piles. Mixture of bhallataka, tamarind and salt is good in cholera. Tamarind and salt along with the nut improves taste. It prevents tongue coating.

Circulatory system : Useful in cardiac debility because it is a cardiac stimulant, white cell enhancer and alleviates swelling. It has stimulating action on lymphadenitis and other inflammations. Useful in glands of plague.

Respiratory system : Expectorant. Useful in cough and asthma. Flowers in milk should be given for asthma. In cough caused by relaxation of the uvula and palate, shevate is given in milk.

Urinary system : Initially it stimulates kidneys and increases urination but then the functional capacity of the kidneys is reduced and this decreases urination. If this process continues, it causes haematuria. It is used in urinary disorders because it alleviates kapha and vata. shevate and sandalwood oil is useful in gonorrhoea.

Reproductive system : It promotes virility, stimulates penile nerves, hence it is an aphrodisiac. It stimulates uterus by its hot and sharp properties. It is used in seminal weakness, impotency and dysmenorrhoea. For this Godambi should be eaten in winter season.

Skin : It is excreted through the skin. It is a diaphoretic, alleviates dermatoses. Its oral administration causes pruritus and erythema on the mucous membrane. Bhallataka is the best medicine for dermatoses, vitiligo, vatarakta. Shevate +milk is useful on joint inflammation. A needle is inserted in a fruit of bhallataka and is heated over a wick dipped in ghee. This causes oozing of oil from the fruit with a crackling sound. Allow this oil to drop in milk, sugar or rice. These oil drops are known as shevate of bhallataka.

Temperature : Diaphoretic and febrifuge. Specially useful in chronic fever. It alleviates spleen and liver enlargement, loss of appetite which are caused by chronic fever, relieves fever and gives strength.

Satmikaran : It improves agni of each dhatu and also acts as a tonic and rejuvenator. Useful in general debility. The tablet made by bhallaṭaka, haritaki, black cumin seeds and jaggery is used in spleen disorders.

Parts used : Fruit, oil, godambi.

Dosage : Fruit powder 3-6 Masa; oil - 10-20 drops (give 2 masa oil for worms and give laxation after 2 hours). The fruits of bhallataka can be given in a gradually increasing dose regimen. The author has seen a patient who was given 21 fruits of bhallatak at a time by a reputed vaidya.

Formulations : Amritabhallataka, Bhallataka Taila, Bhallataka Khseerapak, Bhallataka Vardhaman prayoga, Bhallataka Kshar, Kalyanaka Kshar, Tiladi Modak.

Usually it causes small blisters, with burning and oozing. For these symptoms, coconut oil and sesamum oil or the albumen of coconut and sesamum seeds should be used.

Method of purification : Take out the bhallataka fruit along with the stalk and keep it in the powder of bricks for a period of one week. Clean and wash thouroughly by rubbing it, then boil it with milk. This purifies bhallataka; impure bhallataka acts as a toxin, hence it should not be used without purifying. Small children, pregnant women, older people, persons having pittaprakruti, patients having tendency to bleed, and those who are allergic to bhallataka should not take bhallataka. It is important for a vaidya to know the contraindications rather than the indications of bhallataka.

Restrictions : While taking bhallataka avoid drugs and activities which vitiate pitta. They should

The natare of Ayurveda, as propagated by Charaka, Sushruta and Vagbhatta period has changed since the time of Nagarjuna. Today it has changed much more.

avoid hot, pugent, sour and salty food items, sitting near fire, hanging or sitting in sunlight. They should also avoid 8 K's - Kalinger (water melon), Karle (bitter gourd), Kela (banana), Kakamachi (Solanum nigrum), Kardai (safflower), Karkoti, Kohla (Beninease hispida) and Kakdi (cucumber). The 8 K's should be avoided while taking any rasayan.

One who is taking bhallataka - should eat milk-rice, ghee-rice, sugar, sesamum oil and coconut oil. Ghee should be applied on the inner side of the mouth before taking bhallataka, so that it protects from the unwanted side effects. Bhallataka is injurious to outer layer of the mouth and not inner layer.

Adverse effects to bhallataka : Impure or pure bhallataka if taken in excess dose, causes pruritus and burning sensation of anus and tip of the penis, excessive perspiration, thirst and reduced red or dusky urination. In such conditions, one should stop taking bhallataka and should start pitta alleviating drugs like doorvadigana, sarivadigana. In conditions like burning sensation or pruritus and swelling of skin, sesamum oil, coconut oil, ghee or resin ointment should be applied locally. In 3-4 days the above symptoms subside. The above should be kept handy before starting bhallataka treatment.

Srotogamitva :

Dosha : Alleviates vata, kapha and eliminates pitta.

Dhatu : Shukra (aphrodisiac), majja (beneficial to brain), rasa (vitiligo).

Mala : Purisha (astringent), mutra (astringent), increases agni, diaphoretic.

Organs : Liver, spleen.

Chief action : Cures haemorrhoids (useful for breaking the samprapti of haemorrhoids).

References -

'भल्लातकं त्रिषु प्रोक्तमरुष्कोऽरुष्करोऽग्निकः । तथैवाग्निमुखो भल्ली वीरवृक्षश्च शोफकृत् ।।
भल्लातकफलं पक्वं स्वादुपाकरसं लघु । कषायपाचनम् स्निग्धं तीक्ष्णोष्णं छेदि भेदनम् ।।
मेध्यं वह्निकरं हन्ति कफवातव्रणोदरम् । कुष्ठार्शोग्रहणीशुल्मशोथानाहज्वरकृमीन् ।।
तन्मज्जा मधुरा वृष्या बृंहणी वातपित्तहा । वृन्तमारुकरं स्वादू पित्तघ्नं केश्यमग्निकृत् ।।
भल्लातकः कषायोष्णः शुक्रलो मधुरो लघुः । वातश्लेश्मोदरानाहकुष्ठार्शोग्रहणीगदान् ।।
हन्ति गुल्मज्वरश्वित्रवह्निमान्द्यकृमिव्रणान् ।। (भा.प्र.)
भल्लातकानि तीक्ष्णानि पाकीन्यग्निसमानि च । भवन्त्यमृतकल्पानि प्रयुक्तानि यथाविधि ।।
कफजो न स रोगोऽस्ति न विबन्धोऽस्ति कश्चन । यं न भल्लातकं हन्याच्छीघ्रं मेघाग्निवर्धनम् ।। (च.चि.१)
यथा कृष्ठानि सर्वाणि हतः खदिरबीजकौ । तथैव अर्शासि सर्वाणि वृक्षकारुकष्रौ हतः ।। (सु.चि. ६/१९)

(84) BHANGA
Canabis sativa Linn.

Kula : Bhanga kula.

Family : Cannabinaceae (canus = whitish grey).

Latin name : Canabis = whitish grey, cana - with a white greyish tinge; sativa = cultivated.

English name : Indian Hemp.

Sanskrit names : Bhanga (which causes insanity), Matulani, Madani (intoxicating), Shivapriya, Vijaya, Jaya, Ganja (Ganja is prepared from one of its varieties), Veerapatra, Chapala, Ananda, Harshani, Mohini.

(This plant has not been described by Charaka, Sushruta and Vagbhatta but has been

As two exactly opposite feelings like peace and anger coexist in a single human being, in the same way dravyas may also contain two opposite gunas.

described Bhavaprakash and others).

Botanical Description : A herb of height 2.5 mts. having life span of an year. Branches-thin and tender. Leaves-resemble Margosa leaves. They are alternate, having 3-7 leaflets arising from each leafstalk. Flowers-small and appear in clusters. Fruit-small, round and granular.

Bhang - Ganja - Charas (Difference)

(i) Bhang	**(ii) Ganja**	**(iii) Charas**
Tender branch having leaves and seeds is called as Bhang	Female cluster flower containing resin is called as Ganja	A substance resembling resin derived from this plant is known as Charas.

Habitat : This plant is found in India, Iran, Iraq and Egypt. In India, mostly it is found in Bihar, Bengal and Uttar Pradesh. Its cultivation is controlled by the government. It is a crime to have this plant in any private farm and garden.

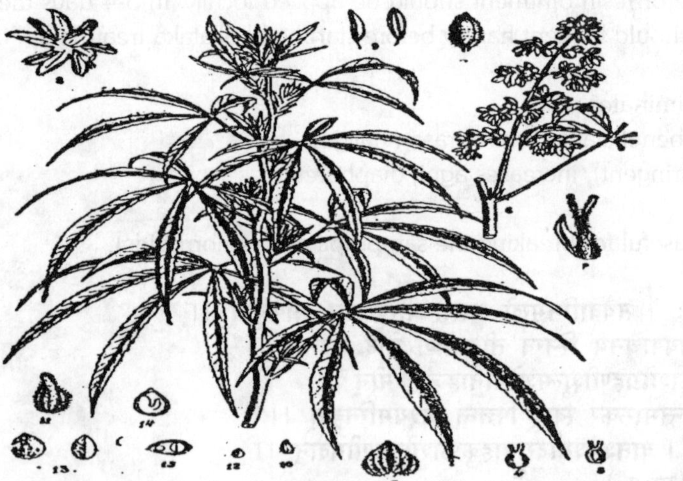

Chemical composition : It contains resin (charas), canabinone, volatile oil, gum, fats, sugar, wax and potassium nitrate.

Properties :

Guna : laghu, tikshna, ruksha; **Rasa** : tikta; **Vipak** : katu; **Veerya** : ushna;

Prabhava : madaka.

Karma :

Dosha : Vatakaphaghna and pittavardhak by ushna property. Useful in disorders induced by vata and kapha.

External uses : Bhanga ground in a paste has a diaphoretic and analgesic action and can also be used for fumigation in piles and other rectal disorders. The ash of ganja is applied over prolapsed rectum and it is then pushed in. Leaf juice destroys external worms. Bhanga is the best appetizer, painkiller, kaphaghna, astringent, digestant and pittavardhak (vitiating pitta) drug.

Internal uses :

Central nervous system : Brain is the main field of action of bhanga. A famous intoxicating drug, bhanga makes the person cheerful initially but then he loses his control and becomes delirious. Being analgesic, it is used in painful conditions like headache, migraine. As its proper dose alleviates vata dosha, it also alleviates pains. Being a narcotic, it is useful in insomnia, less sleep and in pain, apatanak by anticonvulsant property, insomnia (vata dominant), less sleep (pitta- dominant) and excessive sleep (kapha -dominant).

Digestive system : Bhanga is a good appetizer but besides, it is digestant, astringent and cholagogue and has alleviating action in intestines. Because of these properties, bhanga is the best medicine for loss of appetite, diarrhoea, dysentery, sprue, pain in liver and abdomen and haemorrhoids. Bhanga

The disease factors influence particular dosha, dhatu or malas which get affected during the genesis of the disease and the latter have to be acted upon by therapeutic substances.

increases appetite so much that a person does not get satisfied even after eating too much and he eats much more than his usual quantity (once experienced). Bhanga is effective in many digestive disorders.

Circulatory system : Primary stage of intoxication leads to increased pulse rate and stimulates heart. But then pulse rate slows down. Astringent taste has haemostatic property, hence it is useful in conditions of bleeding from any organ.

Respiratory system : Its oral administration increases the respiration initially. It reduces the spasm of respiratory muscles and alleviates dyspnoea. Since it reduces the spasm of respiratory muscles, it is used in asthma and whooping cough.

Urinary system : Bhanga promotes urination and also formation of urine. It alleviates the pain in kidneys. It cures anuria which is caused by the spasm of urinary bladder.

Reproductive system : Useful in impotency and premature ejaculation. Being oxytocic, it is used in dysmenorrhoea and painful labour.

Skin : Bhanga produces anaesthesia of the nerves of the skin and hence it is used as an analgesic.

Satmikaran : Being vyavayi and vikasi, though it makes the person cheerful initially, finally it results in ojashoshan and develops the symptoms of ojakshaya.

Dosage : Bhang 1-2 ratti; ganja -1/2 to 1 ratti; charas - 1/4 ratti.

Parts used : Bhang, ganja, charas (Be cautious, as one can get addicted to it.)

Formulations : Jatiphaladi, Vijayadi, Madananda Modak, Kumari Asav No.3.

Purification : It should be purified before use. It is a toxic drug. It is boiled in cow's milk for 1 prahar (2.5 hrs) using 'dolayantra'. Then it is washed with water, dried and roasted with cow's ghee on low flame.

Toxic effects : Excess dose leads to toxic symptoms. After oral administration, within 1/2 an hour, symptoms occur. (Ganja smoking shows immediate symptoms). The toxic effects of bhanga occur in 2 stages. In primary stage, it leads to 1) vertigo 2) laughing 3) incoherent speech 4) delirium 5) tingling sensation in skin 6) numbness in skin 7) feeling laxity and 8) drowsiness. In this condition, the person sometimes becomes violent. After drowsiness, patient enters into secondary stage. In this stage, the intoxication becomes more severe and the person passes into a stage of deep sleep. Generally, this does not cause death of the patient. But if it occurs, it is caused by respiratory arrest.

Many people are addicted to bhanga. Though it improves appetite and digestion, its addiction causes loss of appetite and also leads to certain chronic effects like insomnia, loss of sexual desire, memory loss, tremors and hysteria.

Effect of bhanga toxin : Mainly on eye sight and brain.

Antidote : Stomach wash, to drink cow's ghee, strychnine injection are antidotes on bhanga poison.

Srotogamitva :

Dosha : Alleviates vata and kapha and vitiates pitta.

Dhatu : Majja (intoxicating), shukra (aphrodisiac), ganja is a strong aphrodisiac.

Mala : Purisha (astringent).

Digestive system : Digestant.

Organ : Brain, mind - loss of sense, intoxicating.

If the genesis of jvara is based on pitta, rasa and swedadushti, how can one neglect them while considering the treatment?

References -
'भंगा गंजा मातुलानी मादनी विजया जया । भंगा कफहरी तिक्ता ग्राहिणी पाचनी लघुः ।।
तीक्ष्णोष्णा पित्तला मोहमदवाग्वह्निवर्धनी ।' (भा.प्र.)
भंगा तु दीपनी रुच्या ग्राणी पाचनी लघुः । निद्रापित्तप्रदोष्णा च कामदा कफवातजित् ।।' (शो.)
'भंगा भंगकरी मतेः रतिपतेरत्यादरं कारिणी,
प्रौढत्वान्न समासमेषु विभवप्रद्योतहृत् संगमे ।
तीक्ष्णोष्णा मदमोहपित्तशमनी वाग्वर्द्धनी ग्राहिणी,
तिक्ता श्लेष्महरा लघुश्च कथिता सन्दीपनी पाचनी ।। (रा.नि.)

(85) BHARNGI

Clerondendron serratum Spreng.

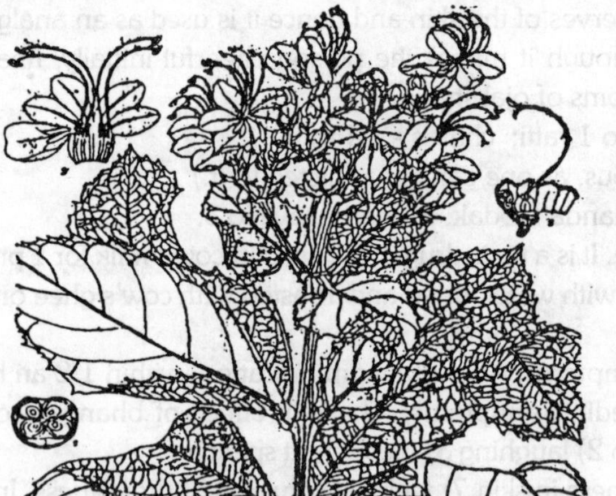

Gana : Pippalyadi (S.)
Kula : Nirgundi kula.
Family : Verbenaceae (Which has pliable branches ?)
Latin name : Clerodendron = cleros = chance, said to be owing to the uncertainty of the medicinal property; dendron = tree; serratum = serrat- having saw toothed margins of the leaves.
There are 2 more varieties of bharngi namely Premna herbacea and Clerondendron siphonanthus.
Sanskrit names : Brahmanyashtika, Kharashaka (rough leaves), Padma (flowers like lotus flowers), Gardhabashaka, Barbaraka, Shukramala, Kasaghni, Bhargakagrani, Mahagardhabagandhika, Bhangura.
Botanical description : A small shurb 2-3 meters high, devoid of branches. Leaves - 10-13 cm. long and 8 cm. broad, rough and pointed. Flowers - grow on the tip of the shrub, appear in a cluster which is blue in colour and fragrant. In jungle, the plant looks delightful when it blooms with flowers. It is therefore called as bharanga. Fruits- round, ripe fruits are purple. Root- thick and nodular. 2-3 leaves grow on each of this nodule. The plant bears flowers in summer and fruits in rainy season.
Habitat : Tarai region of Himalaya, specially Nepal, Kumaon, Bengal, Bihar, Western and Southern India.
Chemical composition : Its thick root contains starch, resin, fats and an alkaloid.
Properties :
Guna : laghu, ruksha; **Rasa** : katu, tikta, kashaya; **Vipak:** katu ; **Veerya:** ushna.

Ayurveda teaches us that whenever we mention dosha, dhatu, mala, we should visualise their srotas.

Karma :

Dosha : Ushna, kaphavatashamak, hence useful in disorders induced by vata and kapha. (Psychosomatic system - Sushruta in Uttar tantra has mentioned the use of Bharngi wine on epilepsy).

External uses : Bharngi is raktagami, vitiates blood and removes the obstruction in the circulatory channels and alleviates swelling. Hence leaves ground in a paste is used; this paste is applied over lymphadenopathy. Leaf juice is applied on erysipelas.

Internal uses :

Digestive system : Being an appetizer, digestant and laxative, it is useful in anorexia, loss of appetite and gulma. Seed rubbed in butter-milk is useful in ascites.

Circulatory system : Raktagami, purifies blood, improves agni of rakta and alleviates oedema. It is therefore used in blood disorders like abscess caused by vata, kapha etc.

Respiratory system : Since it is snigdha and madhur, it acts as an expectorant. It is therefore useful in cough and hoarseness of voice. Raktagami, kaphanashak property is also helpful in cold and tuberculosis. Mixture of bharngi root juice and ginger juice is given in asthma to reduce the attacks of dyspnoea.

Reproductive system : In amenorrhoea, bharngi powder is used along with decoction of sesamum seeds (Vaghbatta Chi. 34/120).

Skin : Diaphoretic.

Temperature : Being ama digestant, hot (diaphoretic), it is used in fever. Cooked vegetable of bharngi leaves is given in malaria (Konkan).

Parts used : Root.

Dosage : 0.5 - 1.5 gm.

Formulations : Bharngiguda, Bharngyadi kwath, Bharngi sura.

Srotogamitva :

Dosha : Alleviates kapha, vata.

Dhatu : Rasa (menstruation), rakta (raktagulma), raktagami (rodhanashan).

Mala : Anthelmintic.

Organs : Respiratory - uterus (useful in fibroid, amenorrhoea).

References -

'भाङ्र्गी रूक्षा कटुस्तिक्ता रुच्योष्णा पाचनी लघु :दीपनी तुवरा गुल्मरक्तजिन्नाशयेद् ध्रवम् ।।
शोथकासकफश्वासपीनसज्वरमारुतान् ।' (भा.प्र.)
'भाङ्र्गी तु कटुतिक्तोष्णा कासश्वासविनाशिनी । शोफव्रणकृमिघ्नी च दाहज्वरनिवारिणी ।'

(86) BHRUNGARAJ

Eclipta alba Hask.

Kula : Bhrungaraj kula.

Family : Compositae.

Latin name : Eclipta = derived from ekleipo = to be deficient; alba = white.

Sanskrit names : Bhrungaraj (by which hair become humble bee coloured and beautiful),

For a person to be able to serve mankind, he has to be developed with good culture. This applies to dravyas too.

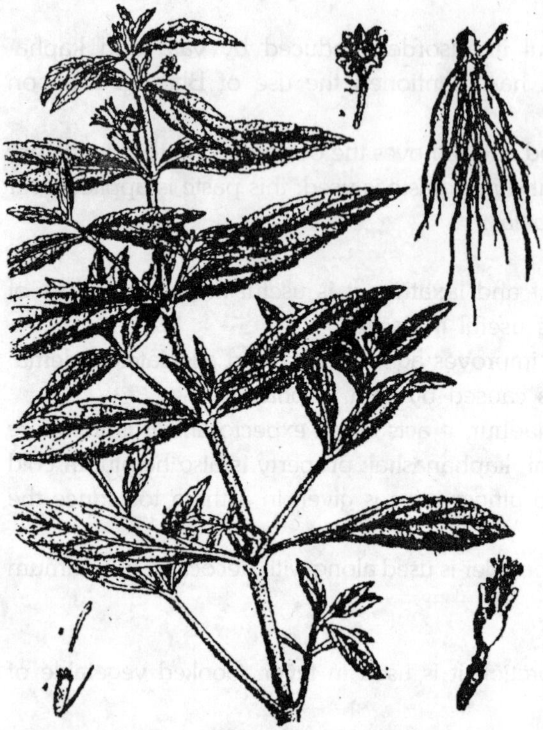

Markava (prevents greying of hair), Kesharanjana, Kesharaja, Ravipriya, Abhedakaraja, Keshali, Ravivallabha.

Botanical Description : A small herb having height 8-10 fingers. Trunk is blackish. Leaves - 3-5 cm in length, 1.5 - 2 cm. in breadth, having serrated margins. Flower stalk - elongated having white flower on its tip. Seed - black, elongated, like black cumin seed. A single fruit has many seeds. These herbs grow in rainy season and bear flowers and fruits in autumn. Maka should be used in autumn or after that.

Varieties : There are 3 varieties, mentioned in texts according to the colour of the flowers. 1) White 2) Yellow 3) Blue (white variety is described above). Yellow bhrungaraj is bigger than white one and leaves are also bigger. There is no certainty about the identity of blue bhrungaraj. But white bhrungaraj is used widely.

Habitat : All over India in moisture. Mainly grows in gutter water.

Chemical composition : It contains resin in large quantity and alkaloid known as ecliptin.

Properties :

Guna : ruksha, laghu; **Rasa** : katu, tikta; **Vipak** : katu; **Veerya:** ushna.

Karma :

Dosha : Kaphavatashaman. Kaphashaman by ruksha, laghu, katu, tikta and ushna and vatashaman by ushna property. It is useful in disorders induced by kapha and vata.

External uses : The herb alleviates swelling and pain, cleans and heals wounds, enhances complexion. But its main action is to promote hair growth and hair dye. Its paste reduces swelling and pain when applied over filariasis, glands, wounds and chronic ulcers. It helps in healing wounds and gives natural complexion to the skin. Drops of its juice are put in eyes and ear. It relieves conjunctivits if applied in eyes and earache, if applied in ear. The juice is applied over head to relieve headache. In migraine, bhrungaraj juice and goat's milk are used as nasal drops. Grey hair turns to black, if juice is applied over scalp.

Internal uses :

Central nervous system : Alleviates vata and acts as an analgesic. It is used in diseases like headache, vertigo etc. Bhrungaraj is effective in various vata disorders.

Eyes : It improves vision. It is used in night blindness and myopia.

Digestive system : Bhrungaraj is an excellent appetizer, digestant and liver stimulant. Its main action is on liver (and spleen). It improves the bilious flow. It is ama digestant, anthelmintic and

Properties (gunas) can be recognized by actvities (karmas) and dravyas are recognized by their gunas. A dravya, without gunas is unknowable. Therefore Ayurveda defines dravya as "Gunavatdravyam" - substance is as per the properties.

analgesic. It cures loss of appetite, indigestion, liver and spleen enlargements and ama disorders. A mixture of maka juice and castor oil is a good vermicide. It reduces mucous in the stool and foetid smell. Overall, maka can be described as a best medicine for digestive system.

Circulatory system : As it purifies blood, increases blood, reduces blood pressure and oedema, it is useful in blood disorders, anaemia, oedema and hypertension.

Respiratory system : Being an expectorant and raktagami, it is used in cough and asthma.

Urinary system : Kaphamedagami - It acts as a diuretic by alleviating kapha and meda. It reduces burning micturation. Mixture of roots and leaves + ajamoda is useful in all urinary disorders.

Reproductive system : Its seeds are ṣhukragami and spermatogenic. Hence it is used for virilisation.

Satmikaran : Maka promotes immunity and has rejuvenating action in anaemia and lipid disorders. But blue bhrungaraj should be used for rejuvenation.

Skin : It has diaphoretic action because it is rasa, rakta, mansagami. Useful in skin disorders, kilas urticaria, kshudrarogas. Also enhances complexion.

Temperature : Diaphoretic. Being ama digestant and being febrifuge, it is effective in many fevers like typhoid and malarial fever.

Parts used : Whole plant, seeds.

Dosage : Juice 6-12 ml; seeds : 0.5 to 1.5 gm.

Maka loses its potency by heating, hence fresh maka juice should be used.

Formulations : Bhrungaraj taila, Shadbindutaila, Bhrungarajadi churna, Bhrungarajghrit, Bhrungarajasava. Maka is an excellent rejuvenating drug. Its main action is to improve liver function. It improves all digestive and related functions, thus increasing weight and strength. If maka is taken everyday, it acts as an antiaging agent.

Maka is also hair rejuvenator.

Paste of maka + marva + henna applied over scars produced by burns prevents depigmentation of the skin and gives normal colour to the skin. Maka juice is used for bhavna in preparing many medicines (like Sutshekhar).

Srotogamitva :

Dosha : Alleviates kapha and vata.

Dhatu : Asthi (beneficial to teeth), rakta, meda (anaemia) and rejuvenator.

Mala : Hair (promotes healthy hair).

Organs : Eyes, head, intestines, liver, spleen.

References -

भृङ्गराजो भृङ्गरजो मार्कवो भृङ्ग एव च । अंगारकः केशराजो भृङ्गारः केशरञ्जनः ।।
भृङ्गारः कटुकस्तिक्तो रूक्षोष्णः कफवातनुत् । केश्यस्त्वच्यः कृमिश्वासकासशोथामपाण्डुनुत् ।।
दन्त्यो रसायनो बल्यः कुष्ठनेत्रशिरोऽर्तिनुत् ।' (भा.प्र.)
'ये मासमेकं स्वरसं पिबन्ति दिने दिने भृङ्गरजः समुत्थम् ।
क्षीराशिनस्ते बलवीर्ययुक्ताः समाः शतं जीवितमाप्नुवन्ति ।।' (वा.उ. ३९)
धात्रीतिलानभृङ्गरजोविमिश्रान् ये भक्षयेयुर्मनुजाः क्रमेण ।
ते कृष्णकेशा विमलेन्द्रियाश्च निर्व्याधयो वर्षशतं भवेयुः ।। (भै.र.)
'भृङ्गराजास्तु चक्षुष्यास्तिक्तोष्णाः केशरञ्जनाः । कफशोफविषघ्नाश्च तत्र नीलो रसायनः ।। (रा.नि.)

Rasa, veerya, vipak, guna, prabhav are all results of dynamic vibrations.

(87) MADANAPHALA
Randia dumetorum L.A.M.

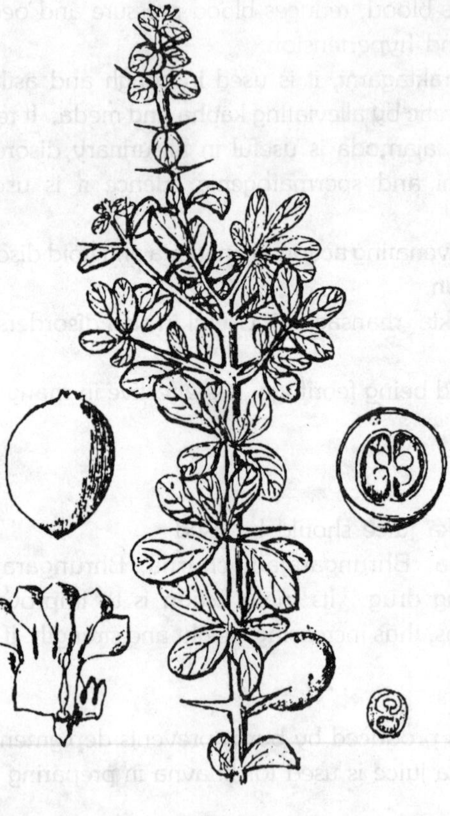

Gana : Vamaka, Phalini(C.); Urdhvabhagahara, Aragwadhadi, Mushkakadi (S.)
Kula : Manjishtha kula.
Family : Rubiaceae (Rubus = Red).
Latin name : Randia = In memory of Issac Rand, Botanist of Chelsea, London; dumetorum = of thorny bushes, of hedges - madanphala has many thorns.
English name : Emetic nut.
Sanskrit names : Madana (causing chhardana (causes emesis), Pindi (having round fruit), Shalyak (the tree has thorns), Vishapushpaka (flowers are poisonous), Ratha, Nut, Pinditaka, Harnya, Ghantakhya, Bastishodhana, Granthiphala, Golaphala, Vishamushkaka.
Botanical description : It is reticulated, thorny, medium sized tree. Leaves - like Achyranthes aspera, slightly round and long-sharp thorns are situated on either side of leaf axis. Flowers - yellowish white. Fruits - like naspati, fruits are round, yellow or dusky coloured. Fruit pulp - sweet and bitter. The pulp resembles walnut pulp. If this pulp is broken, 4 parts of seeds come out and they resemble inner portion of greater cardmum. These black seeds are called as 'madanphala pippali'. The tree bears flowers in summer and fruits in winter.
Habitat : Foothills of Himalaya, from Jammu to Sikkim, Sindh, Kuchabihar, Southern India and Maharashtra. In Maharashtra, there are many trees of emetic nut in places like Mahabaleshwar. In summer, the fallen ripe fruits spread a sweet smell resembling honey.
Chemical composition : Its fruit contains 33.3% saponin. Besides, it also contains valerenic acid, wax, resin. Seed contains a volatile oil.
Properties :
Guna : laghu, ruksha; **Rasa :** madhur, tikta, kashaya, katu; **Vipak :** katu; **Veerya :** ushna; **Prabhav :** vamak.
Karma :
Dosha : Kaphavatashodhaka and shamaka and pittanissaraka by ushna property. It eliminates kapha and pitta by emesis and pitta by purgation. It eliminates and alleviates vata. This action on vatadosha is carried out by using madanphala for asthapan and anuvasan.
External uses : Rind of emetic nut alleviates swelling and pain and cleans ulcers. The oil is used for

"Vrushyatva" is a strong dynamic vibration. The process of gensis of mankind, its growth, maintenance and decay depend on such vibrations.

massage in vata disorders. The paste is applied over painful and swollen joints in rheumatoid arthritis and abscess. Decoction is used for washing wounds. In abdominal pain, emetic nut rubbed in vinegar is applied over umbilicus.

Internal uses :

Nervous system : Rind of fruit alleviates vata. Generally decoction is used.

Digestive System : Madanaphala has been used so extensively for inducing emesis in shodhan chikitsa that its name has become syonymous with emesis. It is extremely suitable for emesis as it does not cause any complications. Fruit rind and seeds are used for emesis. Fruit is emetic and also purgative, cholagogue and anthelmintic. Rind is astringent.

To induce emesis, powder of whole fruit (approximately 3-4 masa) is soaked in 1/2 chhatak water overnight. This liquid is filtered through cloth and is given to the patient after adding honey and saindhav. Emesis starts in an hour if given on empty stomach. For instant emesis, dose of the seeds should be increased. It causes emesis in 15-20 min. If this fails to induce vomiting then warm water is given and the patient is encouraged to vomit. Repeated use of water with saindhav purifies stomach (amashaya) by eliminating kapha and pitta. This method is used in kapha dominant fever and amashayasth (developed in stomach) kapha disorders and also in constipation, gulma, helminthiasis. Emetic nut is used for emesis.

This type of emesis is useful in vomiting induced by kapha and pitta, acid-peptic disease. In dysentery, decoction of fruit rind is used to eliminate kapha and ama.

Circulatory system : Since it purifies blood and alleviates swelling, it is used in many blood disorders and oedema induced by kapha and pitta. Fruit ground in a paste is applied over abscess.

Respiratory system : Being an expectorant, it removes the obstruction of kapha and cures common cold, asthma and cough.

Reproductive system : Being an emmenagogue, it is useful in dysmenorrhoea and painful labour.

Skin : Fruit is diaphoretic and cures dermatoses. It can be used internally and externally in dermatoses.

Temperature : Since it is diaphoretic and dosha - purifier, it is used for instant relief in fever which occurs after meals and that which is induced by kapha.

Satmikaran : Madanphala is curative and antidode. It is used in obesity because it has a curating effect on the fats.

Parts used : Fruits, seed rind.

Dosage : Powder 1-3 gm. for emesis; decoction of fruit rind 15-30 tola.

Formulations : Madanadi lepa. There are many formulations of madanphala mentioned in Ayurvedic texts for emesis. Charaka alone has described 133 formulations in his Kalpa sthana. The term emesis reminds only a single drug i.e madanphala.

Dravyasiddhi : Before using madanphala for emesis it should be first purified as follows - on pushya, ashwini or mrigasheersha nakshatras in spring or summer, yellowish white fruits are collected. These fruits are wrapped in oil cakes, grass etc. The paste of cowdung is applied over it. This whole thing is kept under the heap of grains like yava, horsegram, moong and black gram for riping. After 8 days, when they become soft and sweet fragrant, they are removed and dried in shade. When totally dried, the inside pulp is removed and is mixed with ghee, curds, honey and paste of sesame seeds and dried. These are then stored and are used as per the need.

Ayurveda has imprinted deep in its heart and deeds that the treatment should cure but without any side effects.

Administration to produce emesis : Madanphala, preparation of which is described above and pippali powder, should be used for emesis. The patient should be given seven days of both internal and external oleation therapy as per the need. Minimum three days should be given. A day before emesis patient should be given anorexic drugs like meat soup, milk, curds, urad, sesame seed powder, khichri etc.

On second day in the morning, a diet of either milk with ghee or rice and ghee is given. Proper dose of madanphala-pippali powder soaked in any one of the decoctions of yashtimadhu, kanchanar, bitter bimbi, arka and apamarga should be given. It should be mixed very well, crushed and filtered. Then a small amount of saindhav, honey and warm water is added to the above mixture and given to the patient to drink. It should be given frequently in less quantity and wait for the emesis. Emesis should be continued till bile is seen in the vomitus. If emesis doesn't occur properly, the mixture of long pepper, amla, mustard, vacha and saindhav in warm water should be given.

Madanphala is the best emetic drug, but it is given with different anupan for different purposes. For vata disorders, it is given along with alcohol (souvirak), juice of sour fruits, sharbet, curds etc. For pitta disorders, with black dates, amla, honey, yashtimadhu, falsa, milk, sugarcane juice and for kapha disorders, with honey or cow's urine. There are very few drugs which alleviate dosha and mala without any adverse effect to body tissues. Madanphala tops the list of drugs which are most useful in carrying out the described action of detoxification by emesis or medicated enema.

Srotogamitva :

Dosha : Eliminates kapha and pitta, vata (carminative).

Dhatu : Rakta (cures abscess), rasagami.

Mala : Dececant (enema), detoxifies kapha mala.

Organ : Stomach.

References -

'राठको वृत्तपत्रोऽथ कंटकी पर्वतादिषु । विटपी मदनं तस्य फलं रेखाफलं स्मृतम् ।' (शि.)

'मदनो मधुरस्तिक्तो वीर्योष्णो लेखनो लघुः । वान्तिकृद्विद्रधिहरः प्रतिश्यायव्रणान्तकः ।।
रूक्षः कुष्ठकफानाहशोथगुल्मव्रणापहः ।' (भा.प्र.)

'मदनफलं वमनास्थापनानुवासनोपयोगिनाम् श्रेष्ठम् ।' (च.सू. २५)

'वमनद्रव्याणां मदनफलानि श्रेष्ठतमानि आचक्षतेऽनपायित्वात् ।' (च.क.१)

'मदनं सर्वगदाविरोधि च । मधुरं सकषायतिक्तकं तदरूक्षं सकटूष्णविज्जलम् ।
कफपित्तहृदाशुकारि चाप्यनपायं पवनानुलोमि च ।।' (च.क. ११)

'मदनः कटुतिक्तोऽथ कफवातव्रणावहः । श्लेष्मज्वरप्रतिश्यायगुल्मेषु विद्रधीषु च ।।
शोफस्यापि हरो बस्तौ वमने चेह शस्यते ।' (ध.नि.)

Ayurveda is a vast expanse of science but nearly everyone feels that he has understood it, and it is indeed Ayurveda's misfortune.

(88) MADHUYASHTI

Glycerrhiza glabra Linn.

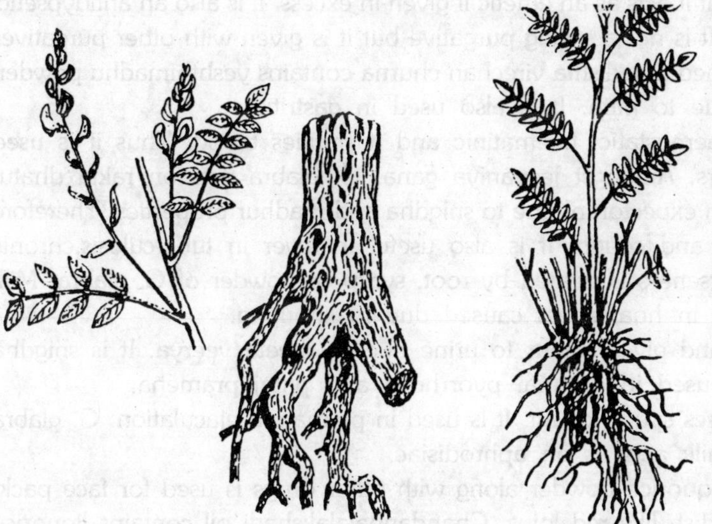

Gana : Kanthya, Jivaniya, Sandhaniya, Varnya, Kandughna, Mutravirajaniya, Shonitasthapan, Chardinigrahan, Snehopag, Vamanopag, Asthapanopag (C.) Kakolyadi, Sarivadi, Anjanadi (S.)

Kula : Shimbi kula.

Family : Leguminoceae (Legumen = pulse pod).

Latin name : Glycerrhiza (glykas = sweet), rhiza = root (the one whose root is sweet to taste); glabra = smooth and hairless.

English name : Liquorice.

Sanskrit names : Yasthimadhu, Madhuka, Yashti, Madhur, Atirasa, Saumya, Shoshapaha, Jalaja, Madhuparni.

Botanical Description : Perinneal shrub 1 to 1.5 mtrs. in height. Root - long, reddish yellow, root and bark give multiple branches. Leaves - compound leaflets. Flowers - pinkish. Pods - 3cm. long, flat. It contains 2-5 squared seeds. Flowers blossom in summer and seeds in rainy season.

Varieties : It has two varieties - sthalaja (terrestrial) and jalaja (aquatic). Jalaja is also called as madhulika or madhuparni and is rare. Sthalaja is of 3 types - 1) Egyptian 2) Arabic 3) Turkish. Their sweetness decreases successively.

Habitat : Egypt, Arab countries, Turkey, Iran, Afghanisthan, Asia minor, Mid Asia, South Europe and China. Nowadays it is cultivated in Punjab, Sindh and Peshawar. The roots of red gunja are sold as G. glabra in market.

Chemical composition : Root contains glycyrrhizin in the form of yellow powder. Its concentrate is available in the market and is called shirka in Marathi. Its black sticks are also available in market.

Properties :

Guna : guru, snigdha; **Rasa** : madhur; **Vipak** : madhur; **Veerya** : sheeta.

Karma :

Dosha : Vatashaman by guru, snigdha and madhur; pittashman by madhur rasa. Glabra is helpful in disorders induced by vata and pitta.

External use : It is a refrigerant, analgesic, antiinflammatory and helps hair growth. It is applied locally in poisoning and ulcerated wounds. Surgical wounds are healed with the local application

Vipak is not declared identical with rasa, but it is said to be a taste - comparable result because it does not directly come in contact with the tongue.

of yashtimadhu and ghee and pains are relieved (Su. 5).

Internal use :

Nervous system : It gives strength to nerves, thus it is useful in vatavyadhi and amavata.

Digestive system : Antiemetic, but it acts as an emetic if given in excess. It is also an antidypsetic, carminative, laxative and antacid. It is not a strong purgative but it is given with other purgatives to help purgation. Formulation named Swadishta virechan churna contains yeshthimadhu powder. It is useful in abdominal pain due to pitta. It is also used in gastritis.

Circulatory system : It is a haemostatic, haematinic and it purifies blood. Thus it is used in anaemia and bleeding disorders. Amongst jeevaniya gana, G. glabra acts on rakta dhatu.

Respiratory system : It acts as an expectorant due to snigdha and madhur properties. Therefore it is used in hoarseness of voice and cough. It is also useful in fever in tuberculosis,chronic fever, cough and chest pain. Hoarseness is treated by root, syrup or powder of G. glabra. Milk boiled with G. glabra is effective in hoarseness caused due to shouting.

Urinary system : It is diuretic and gives colour to urine due to sheeta veerya. It is snigdha and helps easy micturation thus used in dysuria, pyorrhoea and pittaj prameha.

Reproductive system : It increases sperm count. It is used in premature ejaculation. G. glabra powder with ghee, honey and milk acts as an aphrodisiac.

Skin : In summer and autumn, liquorice powder along with other drugs is used for face pack. It makes the skin smooth and reddish like red lotus. Chandanbalalakshadi oil contains liquorice because of which it is used to enhance complexion.

Temperature : Febrifuge, useful in chronic fever. Local application of it reduces the burning.

Satmikaran : Jivaniya (raktagami), sandhaniya (mansa), rasayan (sarvadhatugami), tonic. It is used in general debility. Yasthimadhu with increasing doses can be used as a rasayan.

Eye : It is beneficial to eyes. Decoction of yashtimadhu is used to wash eyes. It is used in conjunctivitis caused by vata-pitta.

Parts used : Root.

Anupan : Honey in cough and asthma, milk for aphrodisiac activity.

Dose : 1-2 gms. powder.

Formulations : Yashtyadi churna, Yashtyadipak, Yashtimadhvadi taila.

Srotogamitva :

Dosha : Pittaghna, vataghna.

Dhatu : Shukra, rakta (complexion enhancer), majja (beneficial to eyes), rasayani.

Mala : Promotes healthy hair, mutragami.

Organ : Eye.

References -

'यष्टिमधु तथा यष्टिमधुकं क्लीतकं तथा । अन्यत् क्लीतनकं तत्तु भवेत्तोयमधूलिका ।।
यष्टि हिमा गुरुः स्वाद्वी चक्षुष्या बलवर्णकृत् । सुस्निग्धा शुक्रला केश्या स्वर्या पित्तानिलास्रजित् ।।
व्रणशोथविषच्छर्दितृष्णाग्लानिक्षयापहा ।' (भा.प्र.)
'कर्ष मधुकचूर्णस्य घृतक्षौद्रसमन्वितम् । पयोनुपानं यो लिह्यान्नित्यवेगः स ना भवेत् ।।' (च.चि.२)
'मण्डूकपर्ण्याः स्वरसः प्रयोज्यः क्षीरेण यष्टीमधुकस्य चूर्णम् ।' (च.चि. १)

Is it possible that the after-tastes of some dravyas are caused by vipak? How do you respond to this idea?

(89) MARICHA
Piper nigrum Linn.

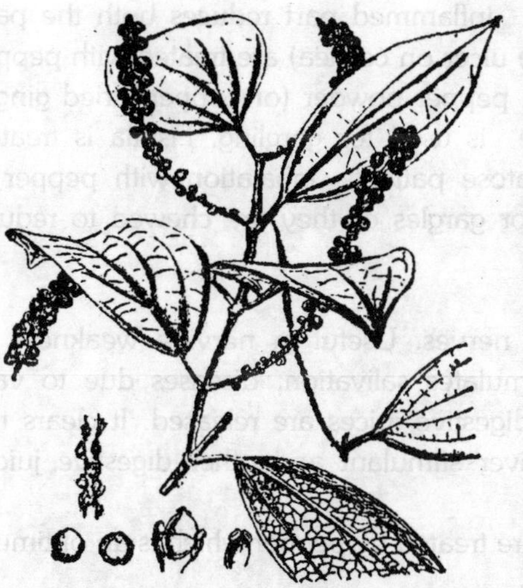

Gana :Deepaniya, Shulaprashamana, Krumighna, Shirovirechana (C.); Pippalyadi, Tryushan (S.)
Kula : Pippali kula.
Family : Piperaceae (Black pepper piper family).
Latin name : Piper = (Peperi - Gk.) or derived from Sanskrit word pippali), name of the plant used by Horace; nigra = black, slightly tinged with grey.
English name : Black pepper.
Sanskrit name : Maricha, Palita, Shyam (nigra), Kol, Yavaneshta (used in the Westen countries instead of chillies), Vrittaphala, Shakanga, Katuka, Krishna, Krimihara.
White Pepper : Sitamaricha, Shavala.
Botanical Description : It is a parasite which grows mostly on coconut and betel nut plants. The roots grow out of the nodes by which it creeps on the host. Leaves - resemble betel leaves, 12.7 cms. in length and 5-7 cms. broad, on the dorsal aspect they are five veined. Flowers small, unisexual and have airborne pollination. Fruit - round, grows in long clusters. When tender it is green in colour, turns red on ripening and black on drying.
The creeper is termed peppe vine (Mirwel). Flowering starts in summer and fruiting occurs in the monsoon. Just as there is a difference in action of fresh and dried pippali, similarly fresh and old black pepper differ in their actions and vipak. Vipak of black pepper is madhur.
Varieties : Some acharyas have defined a distinct category of white pepper. In the Keyadeva nighantu, there is a comment on dried pepper as a distinct variety. In the Raj nighantu, the seeds of drumsticks (Moringa oleifera) have been termed white pepper.
The fact is, if black pepper is soaked long enough in water and the pungent black skin is peeled off, the result is white pepper. This is the true white pepper. Then, with the removal of the skin the usual pungency and sharpness are also reduced. According to some experts, pepper is of two kinds based on where it grows 1) Oriental and 2) Western.
Habitat : Malaya, Singapore, Coochbihar, Assam, Kerala and Konkan.
Phytochemistry : The thin pungent skin of the fruit contains piperine, a volatile compound 5.9%, piperidine 5%, an aromatic oil 1-2% and 7 % fatty acids. The fruit pulp has a bitter resin called chavicin, starch, oil, gum, fats 1%, protein 7% and alkaloids 4%.
Properties :
Guna : laghu, tikshna; **Rasa** : katu; **Veerya** : ushna.
The green (fresh) fruit has madhur vipak but not ushna veerya.
Dosha : Ushna veerya = vatanashak; katu, ruksha and tikshna = kaphashaman and pitta vardhak.

Human body is made up of koshta, shakha and madhyam marg. At every level, gross and subtle digestion takes place. There is no place or time, when digestion does not occur.

External uses :
Its poultice is ushna, antiinflammatory and scraping agent. Therefore it used in newly formed boils, stye, abscess. It is also used in leucoderma, scabies etc. Pepper powder mixed with oil is also used locally. Application of pepper paste on an inflammed part reduces both the pain and inflammation. Night blindness, shukla (white opaque ulcer on cornea) are treated with pepper mixed with honey. In toothache, teeth are brushed with pepper powder (or pepper, dried ginger and long pepper powder) or decoction of this mixture is used for gargling. Fistula is treated with ksharasutra prepared with black pepper. In comatose patients, inhalation with pepper is given. In pharyngitis, black pepper decoction is used for gargles or they are chewed to reduce the inflammation.

Internal use:

Central nervous system : Stimulant and tonic for nerves. Useful in nervine weakness.

Digestive system : Being tikshna and ushna, it stimulates salivation, diseases due to vata and kapha are relieved, and appetite stimulating and digestive juices are released. It clears the deposits of kapha on the tongue and chest. It is a liver stimulant and other digestive juices are also released. It is a vermifuge.

Loss of appetite, indigestion, liver dysfunction and colic are treated by pepper which is an optimum remedy.

Circulatory system : It is a stimulant to circulatory system.The blockage in small capillaries is gradually removed on giving a very fine powder of black pepper in water. Useful in hepatitis, splenomegaly and chronic skin disorders.

Respiratory system : There is no better substance than pepper to reverse sluggishness of pranavaha srotas and reduce the mucous secretion.

Urinary system : Pepper corrects urinary disorders by reducing the viscosity of phlegm and its removal. It increases the flow of urine by stimulating the blood vessels in the kidneys.

Reproductive system : Its has a stimulating action on this system. It is useful in dysmmenorrhoea, amenorrhoea and impotency.

Skin : Stimulates the channels of sweat, causing perspiration and purifying the skin. Useful in reducing pruritus and skin diseases. Oil of pepper helps in reducing pruritus.

Temperature :

In intermittent fever : Pepper is used as a primary or adjunct therapy either daily or on alternate days or every two or three days. Specially white pepper is used in Vasanta Suvarna malati, to gradually increase the efficacy of tissue and reduce chronic cough. It is used in low fevers due to kapha.

Satmikaran : In a small dose, pepper stimulates the action of other drugs due to its strength. It opens up all the srotas, opening up even the narrow channels, with removal of even the deep rooted kapha dosha. Because of this effect, it has found place in trikatu, making it a well respected formulation in Ayurveda. Its supremacy of properties and actions makes it valuable.

Parts used : Fruit, leaf (for external use).

Dose: 0.25 to 0.5 gms.

Formulations: Marichadiguti, Marichadi taila, Marichadi ghrit, Marichadi churna, Shwasakuthar.

A dravya can affect a living body through its dynamic vibrations. It has no effect on a dead body.

Adulteration : Seeds of evening primerose are mixed.
Srotogamitva :
Dosha : Kaphavataghna, pitta vardhak.
Dhatu : Shukra.
Mala : Purisha (helminthiasis).
Organs : Respiratory (cough, asthma), (fresh pepper-beneficial to eyes), digestive system (dysentery).
References -

मरिचं कटुकं तीक्ष्णं दीपनं कफवातजित् । उष्णं पित्तकरं रूक्षं श्वासशूलकृमीन् हरेत् ।।
तदार्द्र मधुरं पाके नात्युष्णं कटुकं गुरु । किंचित्तीक्ष्णगुणं श्लेष्मप्रसेकि स्यादपित्तलम् ।।' (भा.प्र.)
'स्वादुपाक्यार्द्रमरिचं गुरु श्लेष्मप्रसेकि च । कटूष्णं लघु तच्छुष्कमवृष्यं कफवातजित् ।।
नात्युष्णं नातिशीतं च वीर्यतो मरिचं सितम् । गुणवन्मरिचेभ्यश्च चक्षुष्यं च विशेषतः ।। (सु.सू. ४६)
'नात्यर्थमुष्णं मरिचमवृष्यं लघु रोचनम् । छेदित्वाच्छोषणत्वाच्च दीपनं कफवातजित् ।।' (च.सू. २७)
'लिह्यान्मरिचचूर्णं वा सघृतक्षौद्रशर्करम् । सर्वकासहरं श्रेष्ठं लेह्यं कासार्दितो नरः ।।' (च.चि. २२)
'मनःशिलाले मारिचानि तैलमार्क पयः कुष्ठहरः प्रदेहः ।' (च.सू. ३)

(90) MISHREYA
Anethum sowa Roxb.

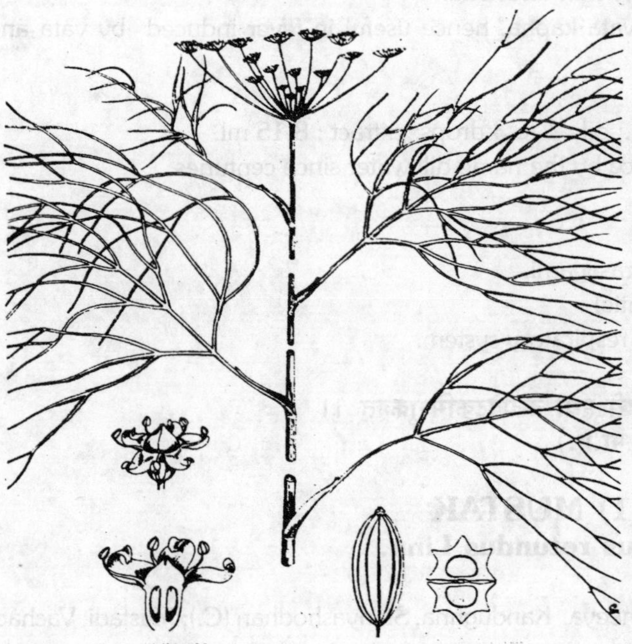

Kula : Shatapushpa kula.
Family : Umbellifereae - Producing an umbel of inflorescence - producing nearly equal branches from the same point, like the ribs of umbrella.
Latin name : Anethum = scented like anisi (dill), ano = upward, theo = I run = grows rapidly; sowa= derived from word 'sua'.
English name : Dill (Dill water available in the market is prepared from it). Sowa is used in preparing paediatric gripe water, gripe mixtures.
Snaskrit names : Mishreya, Shatavha, Shatapushpa, Mishi, Suvakpushpi, Madhavi, Karavi, Bahula, Suganda.
Botanical Description : A herb 30 cm. in height. Flowers - yellow. Fruit - small, blackish . Leaves - 5 to 6 cm. long, wing shaped and flowering, fruiting season is winter.

Habitat : All over India.
Chemical composition : Seed contains 3-4% volatile oil and also a stable oil.

The origin, development and destruction of the body is the result of all the dynamic vibrations and flow in srotasas.

Guna - laghu, ruksha, tikshna; **Rasa** : katu, tikta; **Vipak** : katu; **Veerya** : ushna.
Karma :
Dosha : Vatakaphanashak by ushna and tikshna properties. Useful in disorders induced by vata and kapha.
External uses : Analgesic, alleviates swelling, hence its oil is used for massage in pain in abdomen, flatulence, hemiplegia and rheumatic diseases. Oil is put in ear in earache. Decoction is used for fomentation on swelling and painful areas. Leaves ground in a paste are used for application on swelling. Leaves boiled in oil are good for poultice.
Internal uses :
Digestive system : It improves taste, it is an appetite stimulant and digestive. It is also laxative and vermicide. It is used in anorexia, emesis, loss of appetite, indigestion, flatulence, pain in abdomen and worms. Its extract is used widely in children's abdominal pain. Sowa is digestive.
Circulatory system : Cardiac stimulant, alleviates swelling, hence useful in cardiac debility and swelling.
Respiratory system : Being an expectorant, it is used in cough, dyspnoea and hiccoughs.
Urinary system : Being diuretic, it is useful in dysuria.
Reproductive system : Emmenagogue and galactagogue. It is used in conditions like ammenorrhoea and puerperal disorders. It improves lactation. Sowa has good action on vaginal pain. It is also shukranashini.
Skin : Being diaphoretic, it is used in many skin disorders.
Temperature : Febrifuge and alleviates vata kapha, hence useful in fever induced by vata and kapha.
Parts used : Seed, seed oil.
Dosage : Powder of seeds : 0.5 to 1 grm.; oil : 1 to 3 drops; extract : 8-15 ml.
Formulations : It is used widely in practice by the name dill water since centuries.
Srotogamitva :
Dosha : Alleviates vata, kapha
Dhatu : Shukra (reduces), galactagogue, rasagami.
Mala : Purisha (constipation), (anthelmintic)
Organs : Vagina (pain), digestive system, respiratory system.
References -
'मिश्रेयाः - विशेषाद् योनिशूलनुत् । अग्निमांद्यहरी ह्या बद्धविटकृमिशुक्रहृत् ।।
रूक्षोष्णा पाचनी कासकृमिश्लेष्मानिलान्हरेत् ।' (भा.प्र.)

(91) MUSTAK
Cyperus rotundus Linn.

Gana : Truptighna, Trushanigrahan, Lekhaneeya, Kandughna, Stanyashodhan (C.); Mustadi, Vachadi (S.)
Kula : Mustak kula.
Family : Cyperaceae.

Vipak causes microdigestion in shakhas and madhyam margas through dynamic vibrations. Its site of action is different from that of rasas.

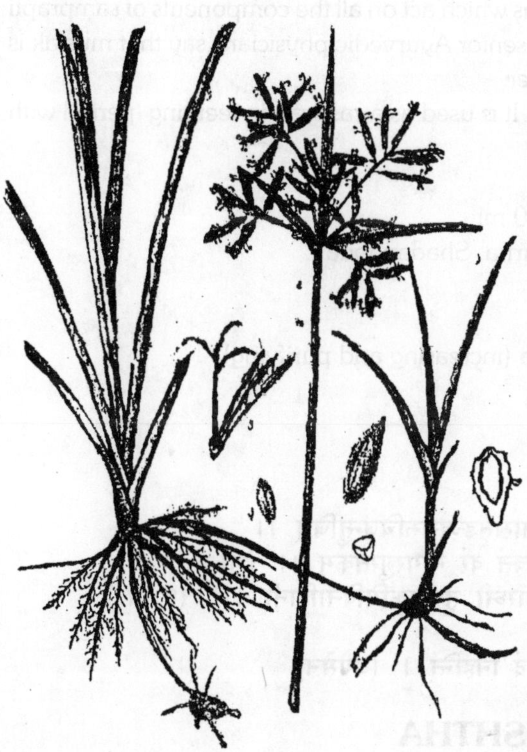

Latin name : Cyperus rotundus.

Sanskrit names : Jalad, Nagarmusta, Ghan, Shishira, Bhadra, Gudagranthi, Sugandhi, Hima, Balahak, Varid, Gundra.

Varieties : Bhadramustak, Nagarmustak, Kaivartmustak are the varieties which are described in nighantu. Out of them, nagarmustak is the best variety.

Botanical Description : It is a type of shrub belonging to grass variety varying in height from 0.3 to 1 metre. Leaves - long and thin similar to grass. Flowers - originate from the tip and are found in clusters. Fruits - are long. Roots - about 2 to 3 cms in thickness, blackish and aromatic.

Habitat : All over India in the vicinity of water.

Chemical composition : The roots contain fat, sugar, gum, starch, albumin, salt and aromatic oil.

Properties :

Guna : laghu, ruksha; **Rasa :** katu, tikta, kashay; **Veerya :** sheeta; **Vipak :** katu,

Karma :

Dosha : Kaphaghna by katu, tikta and kashaya and pittaghna by sheeta veerya.

External uses : Deodorant, corrosive when applied and rubbed on the skin and as a galactagogue when applied on the breast. In obese patients, powder is used for massage. Local application helps in pruritus and other skin disorders as well as in eye diseases.

Internal uses :

Nervous system : Brain and nervine tonic, hence its paste along with milk is given in brain impairment and convulsions.

Digestive system : Mustak is the best medicine for digestive system. Being bitter, it is appetizer, digestive, astringent, anthelmintic and antidipsetic. Hence it is used in anorexia, vomiting, indigestion, sprue and diarrhoea. Large dose is required for expelling worms. A mixture of mustak, karkatshringi and ativisha is good for infantile digestive disorders (balsanjivani churna).

Circulatory system : It is useful in blood disorders by enhancing raktagni and reducing kleda.

Respiratory system : It is found to be useful in respiratory disorders arising out of gastrointestinal pathology.

Urinary system : Diuretic, hence useful in dysuria, mainly when it is associated with digestive disorders.

Reproductive system : It is known to promote uterine muscle contractions and also breast milk purifier and promoter. Hence it is used in treating number of gynaecological and post-pailun conditions.

Skin : It is useful in number of skin disorders viz. pruritus, scabies and eczema etc.

Dietary and medicinal dravyas are conceptually and basically different but they are complementary to each other.

Temperature : Mustak is one of those very few dravyas which act on all the components of samprapti (pathogenesis) of fever. Even the Ayurvedic texts and senior Ayurvedic physicians say that mustak is the first drug which should be used in any type of fever.
Satmikaran : Useful as a general tonic and antidote. It is used as a rasayan in teething period with karkatshringi, ativisha and pippali.
Part used : Roots.
Dosage : Podwer - 1 to 3 gms.; decoction - 60 to 100 ml.
Formulations : Mustakadi kadha, Balasanjivani churna, Shadangodak.
Srotogamitva :
Dosha : Kaphaghna, pittaghna.
Dhatu : Rakta, rasa (fever), meda (digestive), stanya (increasing and purifying)
Mala : Purisha.
Organs : Digestive system.
(Best medicine for children = mustak)
References -
'मुस्तं हिमं कटु ग्राहि तिक्तं दीपनपाचनम् । कषायं कफपित्तास्रतृड्ज्वरारुचिजन्तुजित् ।।
अनुपदेशे यज्जातं मुस्तकं तत् प्रशस्यते । तत्रापि मुनिभिः प्रोक्तं वरं नागरमुस्तकम् ।।' (भा.प्र.)
मुस्ता तिक्तकषायातिशिशिरा श्लेष्मरक्तजित् । पित्तज्वरातिसारघ्नी तृष्णाकृमिविनाशिनी ।।'' (ध.नि.)
'मुस्ता संग्राहकदीपनीयपाचनीयानाम् ।' (च.सू. २५)
'क्वाथश्च मुस्तककृतः समधुः सुशीतः पीतः प्रवृद्धमतिसारगदं निहन्ति ।' (बंगसेन)

(92) MANJISHTHA
Rubia cordifolia Linn.

Gana : Varnya, Vishaghna, Jvarahar (C.); Priyangvadi, Pittasamshaman (S.)
Kula : Manjishtha kula.
Family : Rubiaceae (Rubia, ruber = red).
Latin name : Rubia = red (Its internal use gives red colour to breast milk and urine. Rub = indicating redness alluding to the dye obtained from fruit; cordifolia = cordia= heart, folia = leaves = heart shaped leaves.
English name : Indian Maddar.
Sanskrit names : Manjishtham, Harini, Rakta, Gauri, Rohini, Vijaya, Manjusha, Jvarahantri, Chadma, Ragangi, Rasayani, Tamramoola.
Botanical Description : It is a climber, whose branches spread for a long distance. Trunk - square shaped and reddish. Leaves - heart shaped, pointed, 6-12 cm. long, rough on upper surface and has superfluous hair on lower side. Stalk - its length double the length of leaves and has thorn like structures on it. Flower - small, yellowish white, with superfluous hair. Fruit - 1.5 cm long, round, fleshy, violet or black in colour. Root - reddish, long and thick.
Habitat : Western side of Himalayas, Neelgiri, Hilly areas, Manjishtha available in market is of 4 types : Nepali, Irani, Afghani and Hindustani. Amongst these, Afghani is of best quality and Hindustani of lower quality.

The first step in treatment is to change the diet suitably. This should be the frist thought.

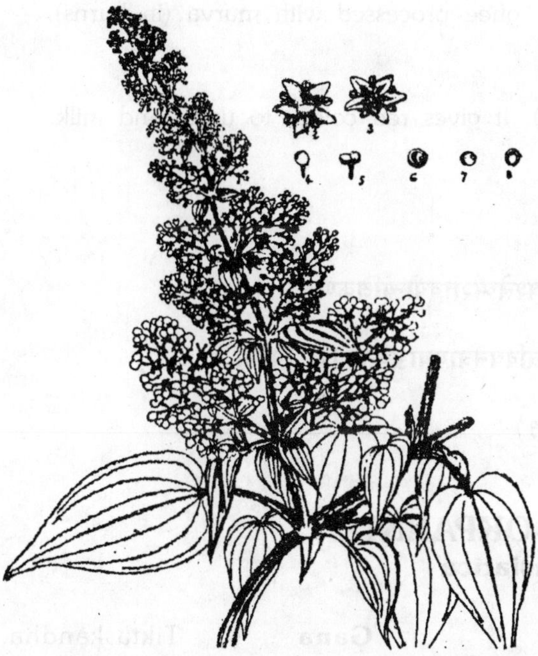

Chemical composition : Its root contains starch, sugar, gum, colouring matter, common salt. The red colour is due to perfurin. In addition, it has yellow gencoside, mangistin, garansin, algerin and zenthin. Oil is extracted from roots.

Properties :

Guna : guru ruksha; **Rasa** : kashay, tikta, madhur; **Vipak** : katu; **Veerya** : ushna

Karma :

Dosha : Kaphapittashamak, therefore useful in many kaphapittaj disorders.

External uses : It is antiinflammatory. It heals wounds and helps in skin disorders. Its lepa (paste) is applied on inflammation, ulcers and skin disorders.

Internal uses :

Nervous system : It gives relief to brain and nerves. Thus it is useful in nervous system disorders (But if given in excessive doses, it creates mania hallucinations.)

Digestive system : It is a good appetizer (deepan) and has good digestive capacity (pachan). It has astringent property that reduces motility and is anthelmintic. Therefore it is used in loss of appetite, amadosha, diarrhoea, dysentery associated with bleeding and different helminths.

Circulatory system : Being haemostatic, used in many blood disorders, raktapitta and skin disorders, ulcers, erysipelas etc.

Reproductive system : It stimulates uterus. It increases menstrual flow and it purifies breast milk. Therefore used in dysmenorrhoea, secondary amenorrhoea. It is used to purify uterus and breast milk after delivery. It also reduces fever.

Urinary system : It is antidiabetic, especially in manjishthameha, a type of pittaj prameha. In renal calculi, 1gm. manjishtha powder is given three times a day for 1 week. This removes the renal stone. If not, surgical opinion is advised.

Skin : It is used in skin diseases like leprosy, erysipelas, vitiligo and hypopigmentation. In these conditions manjishtha is given in honey.

Dhatugamitva : External as well as internal use of majishtha, arjuna bark, yashthimadhu and sugandhi vala is beneficial in fractures.

Temperature : It is used in fever, especially chronic pyrexia and fever after delivery.

Satmikaran : It has been proved beneficial in different skin disorders related with pigmentation, weakness, general debility and poisoning. Manjishtha improves voice.

Parts used : Root (used in opthalmic disorders and disorders of ear).

Dose : Decoction 60-120 ml.; powder - 1-3 gms (in excess causes hallucinations).

Formulations : Manjishthadi kadha, Manjishthadyark. Powder of manjishtha + chandan (in manjishthameha); manjishtha + raktachandan + ghee processed with murva (in burns).

Srotogamitva :

Dosha : Kaphaghna.

Dhatu : Rakta (skin disorders), meda (diabetes). It gives red colour to urine and milk.

Mala : Purisha (diarrhoea), mutra (diabetes).

Organ : Vagina, eye, ear, liver.

Prabhav : Antidote to poison.

References -

'मञ्जिष्ठा मधुरा तिक्ता कषाया स्वरवर्णकृत् । गुरुरुष्णा विषश्लेष्मशोथयोन्यक्षिकर्णरुक् ।
रक्तातिसारकुष्ठास्रवीसर्पव्रणमेहनुत् (भा.प्र.)
'मञ्जिष्ठामधुरा स्वादे कषायोष्णा गुरुस्तथा । कफोग्रव्रणमेहास्रविषनेत्रामयाञ्जयेत् ।।' (ध.नि.)
'मंजिष्ठा कुष्ठवैस्वर्यशोथघ्नी मूत्रकृच्छ्रजित् ।' (रा.व.)
'मंजिष्ठाचन्दनकषायं मञ्जिष्ठामेहिनं पाययेत् ।' (सु.चि. ११)

(93) MANDOOKPARNI

Centella asiatica

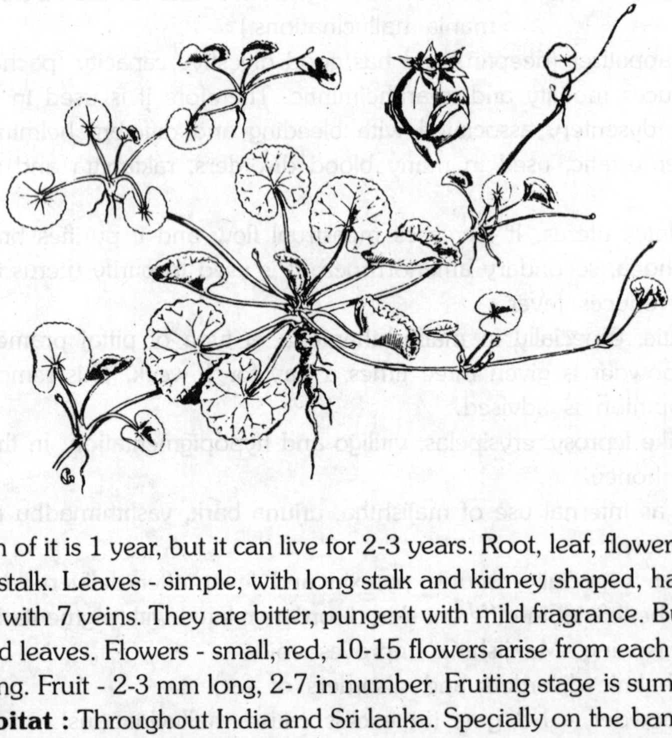

Gana : Tiktaskandha, Vayahsthapana (C) Tiktavarga (S.)

Family : Umbelliferae.

Latin name : Centella = many; asiatica = of Asia (Hydrocotyle asiatica).

English name : Indian pennywort.

Sanskrit names : Mandookparni (leaves look like frog), mandooki (like frog it is always near watery area), Ekuparni, Brahmamandooki.

Botanical description : A creeper growing in wet places. Life span of it is 1 year, but it can live for 2-3 years. Root, leaf, flowers and fruits arise from each node of the stalk. Leaves - simple, with long stalk and kidney shaped, having lenght and breadth 1.25 - 6.5 cm. with 7 veins. They are bitter, pungent with mild fragrance. But the taste and odour disappear in dried leaves. Flowers - small, red, 10-15 flowers arise from each flower stalk. The flowering stage is spring. Fruit - 2-3 mm long, 2-7 in number. Fruiting stage is summer. Root - thin and thread-like.

Habitat : Throughout India and Sri lanka. Specially on the banks of river, gutter, dams and mainly in rainy season. Also it is found in some foreign countries.There is one more variety known as

Body is made up of twenty gunas. Treatment consists of mobilising these gunas and this is done through dravyas.

Hydrocotyle rotundifolia (Roxb.) Rotundi = round, folia = leaves.
Chemical composition : It contains an alkaloid, hydrocortyline. Its fresh leaf contains asiaticoside, velerine, resin, fats, tanin, sugar, gum, salt, aluminium and alkaloids.
Porperties :
Guna : laghu, sara; **Rasa :** tikta; **Anurasa :** kashaya, madhura; **Vipak :** madhur; **Veerya :** sheeta; **Prabhav :** medhya and rasayana.
Karma :
Dosha : Tridoshashamak but mainly kaphapittashamak. It alleviates vata by madhur vipak, pitta by tikta, madhur, kashaya rasa, madhur vipak and sheeta veerya and kapha by tikta rasa and laghu guna. Useful in disorders induced by all three doshas.
External uses : Local application on the skin improves blood circulation. Leaves ground in a paste are used in dermatoses and many skin disorders. Powder or juice is applied over ulcers. Its paste is useful in acne.
Internal uses :
Nervous system : It is beneficial to intellect (medhya), that is, it enhances memory.
Hence it is used in weakness of brain, hysteria and epilepsy.
Digestive system : Its bitter taste improves appetite, hence it is used in loss of appetite. It acts as an astringent by astringent taste and cold property, hence useful in diarrhoea and sprue.
Circulatory system : Cardiac tonic and reduces oedema. It is used in oedema caused due to cardiac debility, lymphadenopathy and filariasis.
Respiratory system : It improves the voice by its expectorant action of bitterness. Also useful in cough and asthma.
Urinary system : Diuretic by sheeta veerya, hence it is used in dysuria. It should be given according to the stage of urinary disorders which are induced by pitta.
Skin : It improves blood circulation by vasodilating action. Therefore it is useful in many skin disorders. It has wound cleaning and healing property. Useful in dermatoses-specially granthik kushtha, chronic ulcers and tuberculous ulcers. It can be used in the secondary stage of syphilis when symptoms are present on the skin along with intradermal changes.
Temperature : Bitter taste is the best for fever and as mandookparni is bitter, it acts as an antipyretic. It digests ama (amapachana) and thus relieves fever.
Satmikaran : It is beneficial to physical strength and promotes longevity by its madhur vipak and sheeta veerya; mandookparni is a rejuvenating drug. Hence it improves the activities of each organ, gives strength and thus improves physical strength. Being vayahsthapan and balya, it is used in general debility.
Excretion : This drug is excreted through skin and kidneys, hence it stimulates both these organs.
Adverse effects : Its excess dose vitiates vata (sheetajanya vatavriddhi). It causes headache, giddiness and skin becomes erythematous with pruritus. In such conditions, either the dose should be reduced or the drug should be withdrawn totally.
Parts used : Whole plant.
Dosage : Juice 7-15 ml.; root powder : 360 - 900 mgm.; whole plant powder 3-5 gms. (Mandookparni should be dried in shade, otherwise oil in it gets evapourated. As it contains oil, its decoction should

While considering any treatment, one must not forget to add rejuvenating and energizing dravyas because medicines always have minute toxic effects.

not be done. It is used as a substitute for brahmi. It is used in children. It should be used fresh. Though mandookparni and brahmi resemble each other, they have different properties. They differ in class and properties.

	Brahmi	Mandookparni
Leaves -	slimy, many leaves on a single stalk.	rough, small, single leaf on single stalk.
Action :	on central nervous system.	on skin.

Srotogamitva :

Dosha : Alleviates pitta, sadhakpittasthapan.

Dhatu : Rakta, meda (urinary disorders), majja (beneficial to intellect), smrutiprada (memory enhancer) (rasayani).

Mala : Mutra (urinary disorders).

Organs : Indriyasthan, heart.

Mandookparni can be used as a rasayan in increasing dose.

References -

मण्डूकपर्णी.....प्रभृतीनि । रक्तपित्तहराण्याहुर्ह्य द्यानि सुलघूनि च कुष्ठमेहज्वरस्वासकासारुचिहराणि च।। कषाया तु हिता पित्ते स्वादुपाकरसा । हिमा । लघ्वी मण्डूकपर्णी तु........(सु. सू. ४६)

'ब्राह्मी हिमा सरा तिक्ता लघुः मेध्या च शीतला । कषाया मधुरा स्वादुपाकायुष्या रसायनी ।। स्वर्ण स्मृतिप्रदा कुण्ठपाण्डुमेहास्त्रकासजित् । विषशोथज्वरही तद्वन्मण्डूकपर्णिनी ।।' (भा.प्र)

'मण्डूकपर्ण्याः स्वरसः प्रयोज्यः ....। आयुःप्रदान्यामयनाशनानि बलाग्निवर्णस्वरवर्धानानि । मेध्यानि चैतानि रसायनानि ....। (च.चि. १)

'हतदोष एव प्रतिसंसृष्टभक्ः यथाक्रममागारं प्रविश्य णण्डूकपर्णीस्वरमादाय सहस्त्रसंपाताभिहतं कृत्वा यथाबलं पयसा पिबेत् । एवं दशरात्रमुपयुज्य मेधावीः वर्षशतायु वदति ।' (सु. चि. २८)

'रसो मण्डूकपर्ण्यास्तु प्रलेपात् पिटिकामयम् ।........ प्रणाशयेत् ।।' (शोढल)

(94) YAVANI

Trachispermum amami Linn. Sprague.

Gana : Sheetaprashaman (C.), Chaturbeeja (Bh.)

Kula : Shatapushpa kula.

Family : Umbelliferae = plants which bear umbels.

Latin name : Trachi = rough, sperma = seed.

English name : King's cumin.

Sanskrit names : Yawani, Deepyaka, Deepya, Vatari, Shoolhantri (the one who has a stomach ache, will ask for owa), Yawanika, Ugra, Teevragandha, Bhoomi, Agnigandha, Hridya, Agnivardha.

Botanical Description : A small shrub of height 3 to 4 ft. Leaves - appear like balantshep. Flowers - whitish and umbrella shaped. Seeds - small, yellowish, rust coloured. Flowering occurs in winter and seeds in summer.

Habitat : Found all over India as well as in Iran, Egypt, Afghanisthan.

Chemical composition : Aromatic oil is present in the seeds which solidifies on cooling and

At the inception of any scientific discipline, some axioms have to be taken for granted. Point and line in geometry are such axioms.

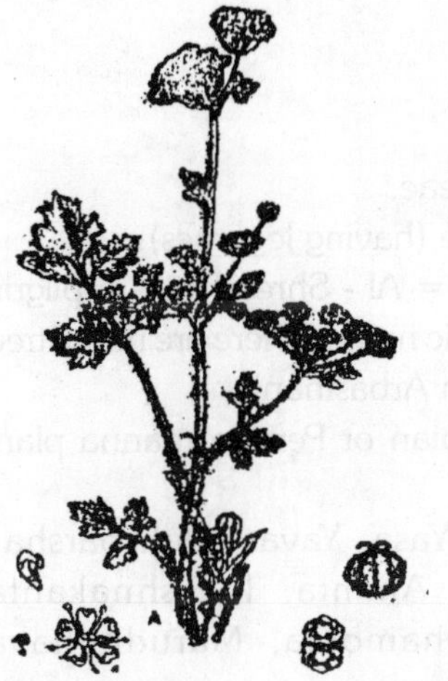

is called thymol cryst.

Properties :

Guna : laghu, ruksha, tikshna; **Rasa** : katu, tikta; **Vipak** : katu; **Veerya** : ushna.

Karma :

Dosha : Kaphavatanashak by tikshna and ushna, pittavardhak. Used in kaphavata diseases.

External uses : Being analgesic, antiinflammatory, laxative, antibacterial, complexion enhancer and antidote, its external application reduces oedema and pain, skin diseases, scorpion bite. It acts as an antibacterial and cleanses the wounds. In abdominal distention, its paste is applied on abdomen or poultice is used.

Internal use :

Digestive system : Being appetizer, deepan, pain killer, anthelmintic, it is used in anorexia, loss of appetite, indigestion, flatulence, abdominal pain, lump, spleenic enlargement and intestinal worms. Thymol cryst is used in hookworm and other infestations. It stops recurrence of worms.

Circulatory system : Being cardiac stimulant, it is used in cardiac debility.

Respiratory system : Kaphaghna and antiasthmatic, so used as powder or in bidi form. It acts as an expectorant, decreases suffocation, removes foul smell and is antibacterial.

Urinary system : Diuretic, useful in retention of urine.

Reproductive system : It is a uterine stimulant and hence used in dysmenorrhoea and in post partum conditions. It is an appetizer, carminative and reduces other symptoms. It is useful in puerperal disorders.

Skin : Being diaphoretic, it is used in skin disorders.

Fever : Used in fever with rigors.

Satmikaran : In doudenitis, also used in morphine addiction.

Parts used : Seeds, thymol cryst.

Doses : Powder 1-3 gms.; oil 15-30 drops; decoction: 15-30 ml., ark: 25-50 mgs.

Formulation : Yawanikadi kadha, Yavanikadi churna, Yavani shadhav, Yavanyarka. One who suffers from abdominal colic demands owa.

Srotogamitva :

Dosha : Pittavardhak, vatakaphakshayakarak.

Dhatu : Shukra, rakta (spleen).

Mala : Purisha (shodhan).

Organ : Dental diseases - alimentary system (appetizer).

References -

'यवानी पाचनी रुच्या तीक्ष्णोष्णा कटुका लघुः । दीपनी च तथा तिक्ता पित्तला शुक्रशूलहत् । वातश्लेष्मोदरानाहगुल्मप्लीहकृमिप्रणुत् ।।' (भा.प्र.)

'यवानी कटु तीक्ष्णोष्णा वातश्लेष्मद्विजामयान् । हन्ति गुल्मोदरं शूलं दीपयत्याशु चानलम् ।। (ध.नि.)

While practising Ayurveda, one has to traverse from gross to subtle, from the periphery to the centre and from manifest to the non-manifest.

(95) YAWASA
Alhaji mourorum

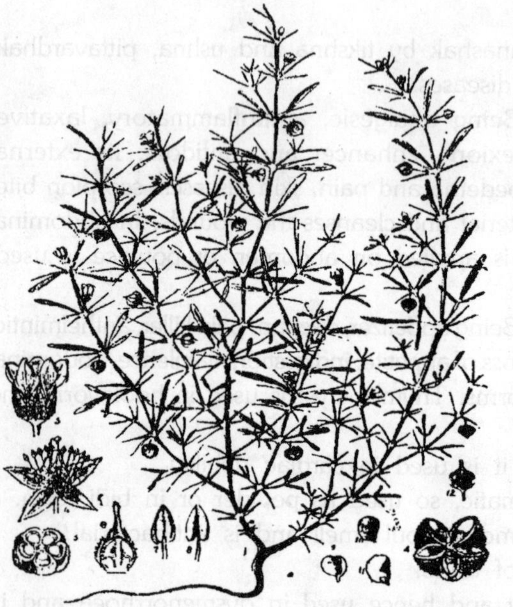

Kula : Shimbi kula.
Upakula : Papilionaceae.
Family : Leguminosae (having legumes).
Latin name : Alhaji = Al - Shree Haji - a pilgrim coming from Haj, Arabic name (There are many trees resembling dhamasa in Arbasthan).
English name : Arabian or Persian manna plant, camel thorn.
Sanskrit names : Yasa, Yavas, Duhsparsha (because of thorns), Ananta, Teekshnakanta, Samudranta, Deerghamoola, Marudhbhava, Gandhari, Dhanvayavas.
Botanical Description : A thorny plant of height 0.33 to 1 meter. It has many thin and long branches. Leaves - small, elongated, hairy, arise from the base of the thorn. Flowers - reddish, arise from the base of the thorn (same like leaves), flowering occurs in spring and fruiting in summer. The speciality of this plant is that it looks green even in summer. The gum derived from this plant is known as 'yasasharkara' (sugar of dhamasa). It is whitish red and crystalline.
Habitat : Western - north India (Marwad), Egypt, Syria, Messopotemia, Iraq, Persia, Arabia, Afghanisthan etc. Dates and dhamasa grow in sandy regions.
Chemical composition : It contains 'yasasharkara' (yasa sugar). If boiled with sour drugs, it gets converted into glucose. It also contains glucose.
Properties :
Guna : laghu, snigdha; **Rasa :** madhur, tikta, kashaya; **Vipak :** madhur; **Veerya :** sheeta.
Karma :
Dosha : Pittapradhan, kaphanubandhi, pittashamak by snigdha, madhur, sheeta and kaphashamak by tikta, kashaya properties. Chief property - pittashleshmaprashamana.
Enternal uses : It alleviates swelling and pain. It has haemostatic action hence it is used in piles specially bleeding piles. Piles are cleaned with the decoction and the paste of whole plant is applied over it. Leaf juice is used as nasal drops in headache. Oil boiled with dhamasa is used for massage in rheumatoid arthritis. Decoction is used for gargling in stomatitis and for cleaning wounds. It prevents pus formation.
Internal uses :
Nervous system : It has a tranquillising effect on the brain hence it is used in symptoms like syncope, vertigo and brain weakness.

In koshtha dietary-substrates start getting converted to various body constituents, the channels complete this function and Agni is responsible for the process.

Digestive system : It is an antiemetic, antidypsetic, mild-laxative and cholagogue. Therefore it is used in emesis, dyspepsia, constipation, jaundice and piles. Kapha and pitta work together in the lower part of the stomach. This is the field of action of dhamasa. It is used in healing ulcers of pylorus, duodenum etc.

Circulatory system : Being haemostatic and blood purifier, it is useful in haemorrhagic disorders and vatarakta. Hot infusion of dhamasa is given to prevent small pox.

Respiratory system : It is used in common cold, cough, asthma as it acts as an expectorant and reduces the irritation of respiratory organs. Besides this, whole plant is used for smoking. Decoction is used for gargling in throat manifestations.

Mansavaha srotas : Dhamasa is applied over neck stiffness.

Urinary system : It increases urination. Decoction is used in dysuria.

Reproductive system : Being spermatogenic, it is given in semen debility.

Skin : It can be used in various skin disorders by.

Temperature : Febrifuge and refrigerant by bitter and cold properties. Bitter taste is the best for fever. It can be used for cooling effect. It alleviates symptoms like vomiting, thirst and burning sensation etc. which are caused by vata and kapha in fever.

Satmikaran : It increases the physical strength and weight by unctuous and sweet properties.

Parts used : Whole plant and yasa sugar.

Dosage : Juice 8-16 ml.; decoction 48-100ml.; sugar - 2.5 gms.

Srotogamitva :

Dosha : Alleviates kapha, pitta (sweet and bitter - favourite food for pittaprakruti person).

Dhatu : Medaghna, raktagami.

Rasa : Fever, majja.

Mala : Purisha (laxative).

Organs : Respiratory, digestive systems.

References -

यासः स्वादुः सरस्तिक्तस्तुवरः शीतलो लघुः । कफमेदोमद भ्रान्तिपित्तासृक्कुष्ठकासजित् ।।
तृष्णाविसर्पवातास्त्रवमिज्वहरः स्मृतः ।' (भा.प्र.)
'यवासकः स्वादुतिक्तो ज्वरतृड्रक्तपित्तनुत्' । (ध.नि.)
'कषायमधुरा शीता सतिक्ता याशर्करा ।' (च. सू. २७)
'यवासशर्करा मधुरकषाया तिक्तानुरसा श्लेष्महरी सरा च ।' (से. सू. ४५)
'यवासाधूमपानेन कासो नश्यति तत्क्षणात् ।' (वैद्यामृत)

(96) RASONA
Allium sativum Linn.

Kula : Rasona kula.

Family : Liliaceae (From Lily family).

Latin name : Allium = garlic, sativum = cultivated.

English name : Garlic.

Sanskrit names : Rason (lacks only one rasa ie. lavana rasa), Lasuna, Arishta, Yavaneshta,

All stages in life from birth till death are due to the process of digestion-'Pak'. The process of 'Pak' never stops.

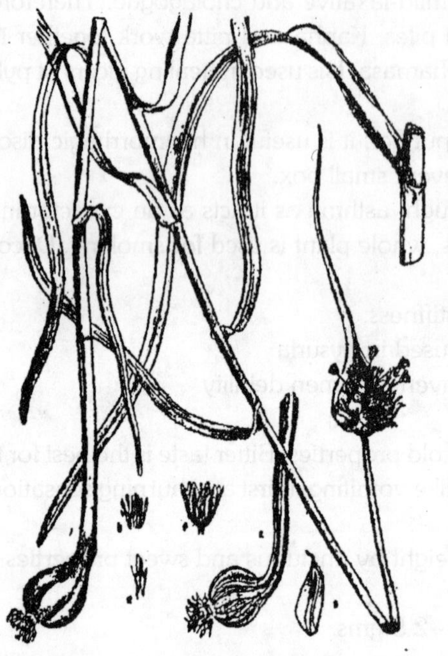

Mahaushadha, Bhutaghna, Ugragandha, Amlakant, Rasayanavara, Jugupsita.

Botanical Description : Garlic is a bulbous variety of plant. It is 30-60 cms. in height. Its stem is tender. Leaves - flat, thin and long. Infloresence - arises from the centre of the plant and bears flowers right at the top. Bulb - white, pinkish with 5 to 12 buds in it. Cold weather is the season for flowering and fruits.

Varieties : Two, 1) Rason and 2) Maharason. The bulb of Maharason is larger. Another (third) variety - garlic with single bud. This single bud variety is used extensively in medical pharmacopoea.

Habitat : All over India.

Chemical composition : Volatile oil, white liquid, albumin, sugar, jelly like substance. The volatile oil which is yellow in colour contains organic sulphur.

Properties :

Guna : snigdha, tikshna, pichchila, guru, sara; **Rasa** : Pancharasa. Mainly tikta and madhur. Different parts have different tastes viz., bulb - pungent, leaves-bitter, stem - astringent, stem tip-salty, seed - sweet; **Vipak** : katu; **Veerya** : ushna.

Karma :

Dosha : Kaphaghna by pungent and ushna; vatashamak by snigdha, pichchila, guru and ushna; raktapittavardhak by ushna and tikshna.

External uses : It is an antiinflammatory, pain killer and removes toxicity. In childhood cough, a necklace of garlic buds is worn. Garlic paste is used for swelling in rheumatoid arthritis, paralysis, sciatica, facial palsy and pain in the ribs. Juice is also used. Garlic juice is used in skin disorders like eczema. Swelling due to insect bites almost disappear on rubbing garlic juice or oil of garlic. A bud of garlic, inserted in the ear also relieves pain. If the uvula is elongated, juice of garlic brings it to normal.

Internal uses :

Nervous system : Used in paralysis, arthritis, sciatica and weak memory. Garlic juice is given internally in diminished vision.

Digestive system : In indigestion, low appetite, pain, constipation, worm infestation, piles - all diseases of vata and kapha, garlic is useful. Flatulence caused by food like rice can be avoided easily if cooked in garlic water.

Circulatory system : Oedema due to cardiac disorders is decreased by garlic.

Respiratory system : Being snigdha and tikshna, it decreases cough. Milk boiled with garlic reduces chronic cough, asthma, tuberculosis and hoarseness of voice. The volatile oil kills Mycobacterium tuberculi. Healing properties are therapeutic to inflammation patches in lungs.

Cough is demulcified by buds of garlic. In a persistent cough, a garland of garlic buds is put round the neck. In diseases of vata and kapha, garlic oil is rubbed on the chest.

Urinary system : It is useful in urinary disorders due to its tikta guna.

Reproductive system : Being pungent, pichchila and snigdha, it stimulates the production of semen. Thus it is of much use in paucity (weakness) of semen. Being a régulator of menstrual function it is used in dysmenorrhoea.

Satmikaran : Stimulant on all parts of the body. It alleviates psychological and mental troubles and is good rasayana (due to pichchila). In fractures of the bone, milk boiled with garlic is helpful.

Skin : As it contains organic sulphur, it is very effective in skin diseases, pruritus and eczema etc.

Temperature : Being antipyretic, diaphoretic and reducing ama, it is useful in fevers. In fever with rigours, garlic oil should be used for massage before the fever rises. It is used as a preventive medicine in enteric fever, diptheria etc.

Parts used : Bulb, oil.

Dose : Garlic bud paste - 1 to 6 gms; oil - 1 to 2 drops.

Formulations : Rasonvati, Rasonpinda, Rasonashtaka, Lasunadighrita, Rasona siddha taila.

Excretion : Garlic is excreted from skin, lung and kidneys. In the process, it enhances the action of all three organs. It is useful in hypertension.

Contraindication : Being tikshna and ushna, it is contraindicated in pregnancy and those with pitta prakruti because it aggravates pitta.

Antidote : Cold infusion of coriander seeds should be given repeatedly.

Srotogamitva :

Dosha : Pittavardhak + vataghna, kaphaghna.

Dhatu : Rakta (skin disorders), shukra (aphrodisiac), majja (brain tonic), asthi (repair of fracture), rasayana, mansameda (brimhana); raktapittavardhak.

Mala : Purisha (laxative, anthelmintic).

Organ : Respiratory system.

References -

'कृमिकुष्ठकिलासघ्नो वातघ्नो गुल्मनाशनः । स्निग्धश्चोष्णश्च वृष्यश्च लशुनः कटुको गुरुः ।।' (च. सू. २७)

'स्निग्धोष्णतीक्ष्णः कटुपिच्छिलश्च गुरुः सरः स्वादुरसश्च बल्यः ।
वृष्यश्च मेधास्वरवर्णचक्षुर्भग्नास्थिसन्धाकरो रसोनः ।।
हृद्रोगजीर्णज्वरकुक्षिशूलविबन्धगुल्मारुचिकासशोषान् ।
दुर्नामकुष्ठानल सादजन्तुसमीरणश्वासकफांश्च हन्ति ।।' (सु. सू. ४६)

रसोनोऽम्लरसोनः स्याद्गुरुष्णः कफवातनुत् ।
अरुचिकृमिहृद्रोगशोफघ्नश्च रसायनः ।।
रसोनोऽयो महाकन्दो गुञ्जनो दीर्घपत्रकः ।
पृथुपत्रः स्थूलकन्दो यवनेष्टो बले हितः (रा.नि.)
रसोनो बंहणो वृष्यः स्निग्धोष्णः पाचनः सरः ।
रसे पाके च कटुकस्तीक्ष्णो मधुरको मतः ।।
भग्नसंधानकृत कण्ठ्यो गुरुः पित्तास्रवृद्धिदः ।

The modern pharmacognosist must properly name and describe the form of the plants which are used in Ayurveda.

बलवर्णकरो मेधाहितो नेत्र्यो रसायनः ।।
'मद्यं मांसं तथाम्लं च हितं लशुनसेविनाम्
व्यायाममातपं रोषमतिनीरं पयोगुडम् ।।
रसोनमश्नन् पुरुषस्त्यजेदेतान्निरन्तरम् ।' (भा.प्र.)

(97) LATAKARANJ

Caesalpinia bondue Roxb.

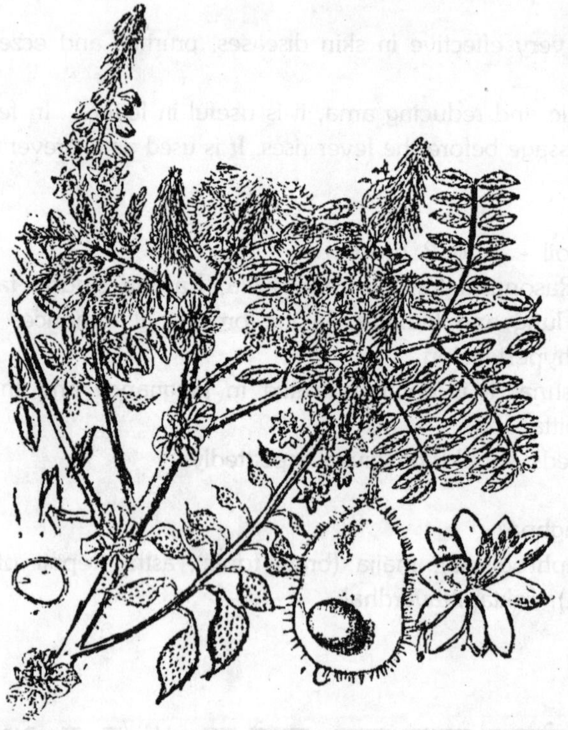

Gana : Adhobhaghara (S.)
Kula : Shimbi kula.
Family : Leguminosae.
Upakula : Caesalpin.
Latin name : Caesalpinia (from the name of the Botanist - Caesalpinus - Physician to Pope Clement VIII); bondue
English name : Fever plant.
Sanskrit names : Pooti karanj, Lata karanj, Ghrut karanj, Kantaki karanj, Kuberaksha, Prakeerya, Shakra, Veerasya, Najrabeejaka.
Botanical Description : A small shrub with a thorny stalk. Leaves - 3 cm. in length, wing shaped. Leaflets - twelve to sixteen in number. Flowers -yellow in colour. Fruit - 6 cm. in length, flat and thorny, 1 to 2 seeds. Shell is tough and bluish grey. Seed pulp is white in colour. Flowering - monsoon, fruiting in the winter.
Habitat : All over India, specially sea coast.
Chemical composition : The seeds contain a bitter principle 2% (it is called natin or bonducin), oil-25%, kshar - 3.57%, proteins - 20%, starch - 35.5%.

Properties :
Guna : laghu, ruksha, tikshna; **Rasa :** katu, tikta; **Vipak :** katu; **Veerya:** ushna.
Karma :
Dosha : Kaphavatashamak, used in kaphavata diseases. It is a cholagogue.
External uses : Local application of the leaves reduces inflammation and pain. Seed oil is applied in rheumatoid arthritis and osteoarthritis.
Internal uses :
Digestive system : As it is deepan, anuloman, liver stimulant, pitta rechan and vermicidal, it is used in loss of appetite, pain in abdomen, ascites, haemorrhoids, liver and splenomegaly and worms. Fried seed powder is used (dosage -0.75 to 1.5 gms) in pain due to antravriddhi. In indigestion, fried

pulp powder is given along with hot butter milk and asafoetida.
Circulatory system : Purifies blood, anti-infalmmatory and useful in blood diseases like syphilis.
Respiratory system : Juice of the tender leaves is used in cough and asthma as it reduces kapha and acts as antiasthmatic.
Reproductive system : Uterine stimulant, given after delivery, it involutes the uterus. Helps in fever, pain and inflammation .
Nervous system : The leaf oil is tonic for nerves. It is useful in convulsions.
Urinary system : Diuretic, so used in dysuria. In orchitis, tender leaves fried in castor oil are applied on testis.
Skin : As it is antidermatoses, it is used in dermatoses. Seed oil is applied on pimples.
Temperature : Antipyretic, especially if used regularly. Seeds containing tikta satva work as quinine. In malaria, seed powder + black pepper is given.
Satmikaran : As it is a pungent tonic, it is given in post pyrexial weakness. In jwara, bitter is the most important rasa.
Useful part : Seeds, roots, leaves.
Dosage : Seed pulp powder - 0.75 to 1.5 grms; root powder -1.25 to 2.5 gm.; leaf juice - 12 ml. to 24 ml.
Formulation : Shakravati.
Srotogamitva :
Dosha : Vatakaphaghna.
Dhatu : Rakta (acts on liver and spleen and secretes bile).
Mala : Purisha (sransan).
References -
'स्रंसनं कटुकं पाके लघु वातकफापहम् । शोथघ्नमुष्णवीर्यं च पत्रं पूतिकरञ्जम् ।।' (सु.सू. ४६)
'विरेचने प्रयोक्तव्यः पूतिकः ।' (च.सू. १)
'कुबेराक्षं यकृत्प्लीहवातघ्नं व्रणरोपणम् ।' (शो.)

(98) LAVANG

Syzygium aromaticum Merr perry.

Kula : Lavang kula.
Family : Myrtaceae (aromatic shrubs and trees of the tropics).
Latin name : Syzygium (conjuction caryophyllus); aromaticum = scented .
English name : Clove.
Sanskrit names : Lavang, Devkusum, Chandanpushpa, Shri, Varij (in marshyland), Shekhar, Tikshnapushpa, Divyagandha, Jalaji, Grahanihar.
Botanical Description : Tree full of green leaves, 10-13 mtrs. in height. Bark of trunk - yellowish white and tender. Branches appear from the bottom and are tender and directed downwards. Flowers - brown externally, four triangular petals (or sepals). Fruits - fleshy, 3 cms. long. Seed - single in each fruit. Flowering season is summer and fruiting in premonsoon. Flowering starts after nine years of plantation. Dried buds are sold in the market as clove.

All subtle and gross, visible and invisible processes in the universe lead to desirable or undesirable results in man.

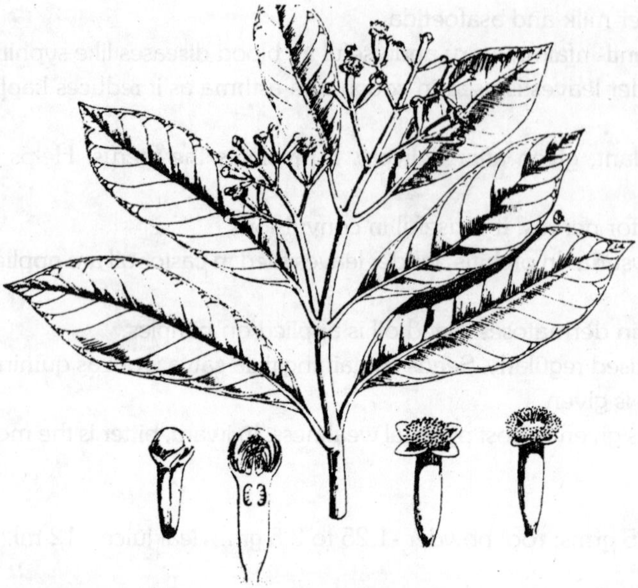

Habitat : Originally from Malaya - Sailibius island. At present it is being cultivated in Sumatra, Malakka, Zanjibar, Penang, Mauritius, Bornia, Brazil, Guyana, West Indies and Travancore in Southern India.

Chemical Composition : Gum and volatile oil 16-20%, resin 6%, euginine or cariophyllin, tanin, gum. Clove oil contains 85-92% eugenol.

Properties :

Guna : laghu, tikshna, snigdha; **Rasa** : katu, tikta; **Vipak** : katu; **Veerya** : sheeta.

Karma :

Dosha : Kaphaghna by tikta and katu, pittashamak by sheeta veerya. So useful in kaphapitta diseases.

External uses : It is stimulant, antimicrobial and tikshna, so it is applied locally in headache and sinusitis. Chewing of clove is useful in stomatitis and skin disorders. Clove oil is used for massage in rheumatoid arthritis, sciatica, backache and loss of libido (ordinary oil should be mixed with it). Oil swab is used in dental caries and toothache for reducing dental pain.

Internal uses :

Digestive system : Being pungent and bitter, it is an appetizer and digestive. Because of tikshna property, it stimulates salivary glands to increase salivary secretion. This relieves dryness of mouth, removes bad breath and cleans the oral cavity. Carminative and analgesic because of snigdha guna. Clove is a liver stimulant. It is useful in anorexia, loss of appetite, flatulence, abdominal colic, hyperacidity, nausea, thirst and liver disorders. In cholera, hot infusion prepared in 40:1 proportion is given to reduce vomiting, restlessness and thirst in a dose of 10-20 mls.

Circulatory system : Stimulates heart and circulation by tikshna property, increases blood pressure. Useful in blood disorders because of pungent and sheeta properties. It is used in cardiac debility, blood disorders and syphilis (Deokusumadi yoga is used in syphilis in South India.)

Respiratory system : Reduces cough, foul smell and breathlesness, stimulates respiratory mucosa causing expectoration. Cough, asthma and hiccups, cough of tuberculosis and bronchitis are treated effectively by clove.

Reproductive system : Aphrodisiac, galactagogue and purifies breast milk. In morning sickness (emesis) clove + honey is useful orally.

Urinary system : Diuretic, so useful in dysuria.

Skin : Clove is useful in many skin disorders by its stimulating action on skin.

Temperature : Useful in fever to reduce temperature. It is ama pachak and also relieves thirst and vomiting. Clove boiled in water is a good remedy for fever.

For acting on the molecules of the body, medicines too should be in molecular form - this can be understood by our comman sense.

Satmikaran : Katu, tikta, so used in tuberculosis and general debility, as a tonic.
Excretion : It is excreted through breath, bile, breast milk, sweat and urine.
Useful parts : Buds (clove).
Doses : 0.5 to 1.5 gm.; oil - 4 to 6 drops.
Formulations : Lavangadichurna, Lavangchatussam, Lavangadivati, Lavangodak.
Srotogamitva :
Dosha : Decreases kapha and pitta, vatanashak.
Dhatu : Rakta (bleeding disorders).
Mala : Purisha (malapachan).
Note : Effective in morning sickness.
References -
'लवंग देवकुसुमं श्रीसञ्ज्ञं श्रीप्रसूनकम् । लवंगं कटुतिक्तं च लघु नेत्रहितं हिमम् । दीपं पाचनं रुच्यं
कफपित्तास्रनाशनम् । तृष्णां छर्दि तथाध्मानं शूलमाशु विनाशयेत् ।।
कासं श्वासं च हिक्कां च क्षयं क्षपयति ध्रुवम् ।' (भा. प्र.)
'...लवंग च तिक्तं कटुकफापहम् । लघु तृषअणापहं वक्त्रक्लेददौर्गन्ध्यनाशनम् ।।' (सु. सू. ४६)
'धार्याण्यास्येन वैशद्यरुचिसौगन्ध्यमिच्छता ।...लवंगस्य फलानि च ।।' (च. सू. ५)
'पिपासायामनुत्क्लेशे लवंगस्याम्बु शस्यते ।' (च.द.)
'देवपुष्पोद्भवं तैलमग्निकृद्वातनाशनम् । दन्तवेष्टकफार्त्तिघ्नं गर्भिण्याः वमनापहम् ।।' (आ.स.)

(99) LODHRA
Symplocos racemosa Roxb.

Gana : Shonitasthapan, Sandhaniya, Purishasangrahaniya, Kashayaskandha (C.) Lodhradi, Nyagrodhadi.
Kula: Lodhra kula.
Family : Symplocaceae (stamens at the base) (sym = together) plants of symplocos.
Latin name : Symplocos = (GK) connection (stamens united at the base, having an inflorescence with a long undivided axis; racemosus = in form of a cluster of grapes (racemosus = a bundle of grapes)
Sanskrit names : Lodhra, Shabar, Galav, Lodhraka, Hema, Shabari, Tilwaktaru.
English name : Lodh bark tree.
Botanical Description : Medium high evergreen tree. Leaves are oblong, 9 to15 cms in length. Inflorescence - 6 to 11 cms. long with yellowish white flowers. Fruit is 2 cms in length and hard. Fruit rind is red.
Types : One type grows on the Himalayas at the height of 1 to 3 thousand meters. It is called as Symplocos crataigoides. This large tree is about 13 meter tall. Leaves are 6 to 9 cms long, 3 to 4 cms. broad, eggshaped and with corrugated borders. Inflorescence 3 to 15 cms long, fruit 1.5 to 2 cms long and round. The bark of this tree is of a smoky colour.
Habitat : Northern and Eastern India, Kerala, are specially rich in lodhra.
Chemical compositon : The bark contains loturine 0.06%, coloturine 0.02%, loturidine, clinovin and a dye. Ashes contain 18% sodabicarb. In spite of being astringent, lodhra does not contian

The food material gets converted into various constituents of the body by the action of agni. Life cannot be sustained without agni. तस्मिन नष्टे याति नाशमेत (ता.ति.)- If Agni is absent that leads to dissolution.

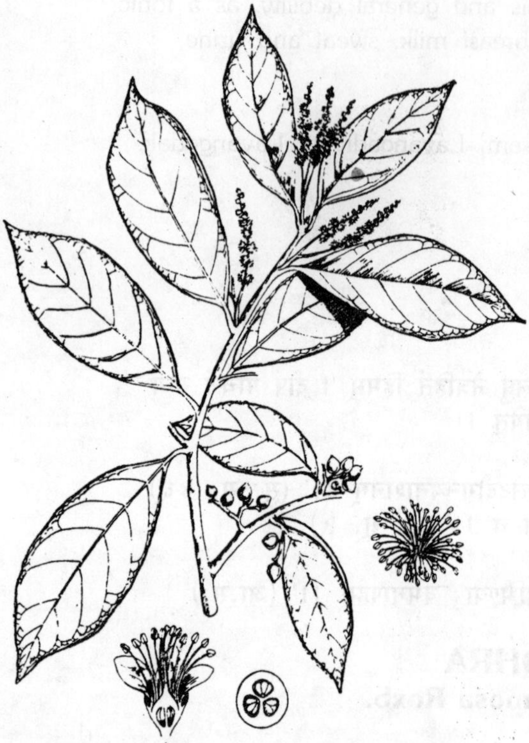

tannin.

Properties :

Guna : ruksha, laghu; **Rasa :** kashaya; **Vipak :** katu; **Veerya :** sheeta.

Karma :

Dosha : It is useful in removing kapha- pitta and diseases arising from these because of its kashaya sheeta guna.

System action and uses :

External uses : It removes oedema and is antileprosy, haemostatic and wound healing. Hence its paste is used in skin diseases, swelling, bleeding wounds and uclers. It reduces pain and oedema. Ear discharge is treated with the podwer of lodhra. Since it strengthens the gums, the powdered bark of lodhra is used in tooth powders.

Digestive system : It is astringent and hence is useful in diarrhoea, dysentery and tenesmus.

Circulatory system : Since it is a coagulant, it is used in bleeding disorders. It causes excellent vasoconstriction of capillaries thus stopping bleeding and reducing swelling.

Respiratory system : Lodhra reduces brochial secretion (mucoid discharge) and kapha, useful in kaphajkasa (and related diseases).

Reproductive system : Specially useful in inflammation of the uterus and reduces leucorrhea and menorrhagia. Decoction is used for uttarbasti or douche in diseases of the uterus.

Diseases of the eyes : Externally useful in conjunctivitis. The decoction is used for eye-washes. Poultice prepared from lodhra is used to foment the eyes. Its paste is applied around the eyes. For this, it may be used with yashtimadhu (jyeshthamadha), rasanjan and alum. This helps to set the paste and reduce the oedema.

Skin : Since it is kushthaghna, it is useful in skin diseases requiring purification of the skin.

Pyrexia : Antipyretic,hence useful in fevers originating from kaphapitta.

Pregnancy : When excessive foetal movements are felt in 7 th and 8 th month of pregnancy, lodhra powder should be given orally with honey.

Useful parts : Bark of the tree.

Dose : Powder - 1to 3 gms; decoction - 60 to 100 ml

Formulation : Lodharsava, Lodhradikadha. (This plant has become synonymous with the treatment of eye diseases and leucorrhoea).

Srotogamitva :

Dosha : Kaphapittaghna.

Dhatu : Rakta (raktapitta).

One should keep in mind that food and medicines are not nutrients to the body alone but they are also nutrients to the mind.

Mala : Purisha (grahi).
Avayava : Eyes (chakshu), uterus (constrictor).
References -
लोध्रोग्राही लघु:शीत:चक्षुष्य:कफपित्तनुत् ।
कषायो रक्तपित्तासृग्ज्वरातीसारशोथहृत् ।। (भा.प्र.)

(100) VACHA

Acorus calamus Linn.

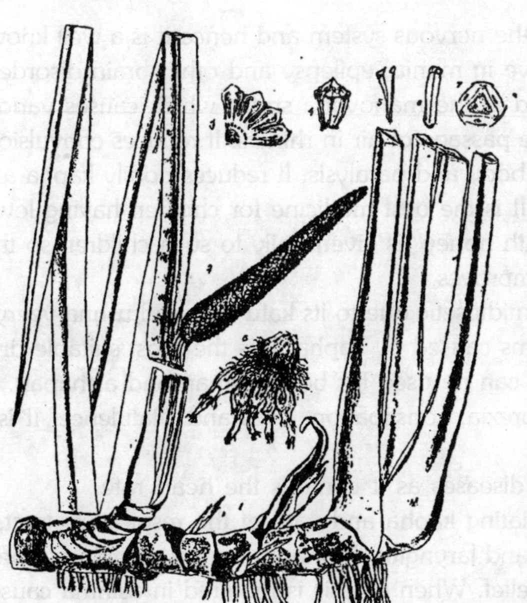

Gana : Virechan, Lekhaniya, Arshoghna, Triptighna, Asthapanopaga, Sheetaprashaman, Sangnyasthapan, Shirovirechan (C.); Pippalyadi, Vachadi, Mustadi, Vamana (S.)
Kula : Suran kula.
Family : Araceae - (Lat. arum) from Egyptian aron.
Latin name : Acorus, A = private, marked by the loss, kore = the pupil of the eye (for eye troubles); calamos = kalamos – (Gk.) a reed (various marshy or water plants, tall straight stem of one.)
English name : Sweet flag.
Sanskrit names : Vacha (increasing the vocabulory power), Ugragandha, Shadgrantha, (having 6 nodes), Golomi (like hair of cow), Shataparvika, Kshudrapatra (having tiny leaves), Lomasha, Bhadra, Rakshoghni.
Botanical Description : Evergreen rhizome having height of 150 cms. It spreads horizontally. Its width is like middle finger of hand. It has 6 hairy nodes which are fragrant and redish in colour. Leaves – shiny, green and elongated like the leaves of sugarcane. Flowers are yellowish white.
Varieties : In Bhavaprakash, 4 varieties are described - 1) Vacha 2) Parasikvacha (It is found in Iran and Kashmir). It is called as Balvacha. As it grows in Himalaya, it is called Haimavati. It is planted near Muslim grave, so it is called Majar Posh or Majar Munda. It has 3 types of flowers – 1) White, 2) Red and 3) Blue. In Charaka, it is included in lekhaniya gana and in mustadi gana in Sushruta (Lat. Iris versicolor).
3) Malay Vacha – It is also called as Mahabhari Vacha or Kulinjan.
4) Dweepantar Vacha - means Chopchini.
Habitat : Anup Pradesh, Assam, Manipur, Brahmadesh etc.
Chemical composition : Rhizome bark has 1.5 to 3.5% volatile oil which contains an asaryaldehyde. Besides, it contains acorine, eugenol, asarone, caffeine and little astringent matter.

If there are analogies in the degrees of rasa, then it will be reflected in vipak too and consequently it will lead to further results.

Properties :

Guna : laghu, tikshna, sara; **Rasa :** tikta, katu; **Vipak :** katu; **Veerya :** ushna; **Prabhav :** medhya.

Karma :

Dosha : Kapha and vatashamak by katu and ushna. Vatarodhanashak by alleviating kapha.

External uses : Being analgesic and antiinflammatory, its paste is useful in rheumatoid arthritis, osteoarthritis and hemiplegia. Its juice is used as ear drops for earache and tinnitus. The smoke is effective in painful piles. Pradhaman nasya of vacha is useful in heaviness of head, headache, lassitude, lethargy and excessive sleep. Vacha is also effective as an antiseptic on wounds. It is widely used as an antiseptic in animals for application on wounds.

Internal uses :

Nervous system : It is very useful in diseses of the nervous system and hence it is a well known medicine for brain since ages. It is highly effective in mania, epilepsy and other brain disorders. Vacha alleviates the excessive kapha accumulated in the manovaha srotas which causes various psychological disorders. It is helpful in clearing the passage of air in rhinitis. It reduces convulsions and pain. It is useful in spasmodic contraction of body and paralysis. It reduces bodily kapha and mental tamo dosha and restores consciousness. It is the best medicine for children having lower intellectual level. Vacha powder in small doses with honey is given daily to such children so that their body strength as well as intellectual level improves.

Digestive system : It acts as an appetizer and antidipsetic due to its katu rasa and ushna veerya. Vacha reduces abdominal colic by acting on worms caused by kapha. It is the most suitable drug for inducing emesis for removal of kapha. Vacha can be used for both, vaman and asthapan. Its emetic property is very useful in indigestion, anorexia, constipation, piles and flatulence. It is a digestive and clears the mouth.

Circulatory system : Vacha is used in heart diseases as it controls the heart rate.

Respiratory system : Since it is useful in alleviating kapha and vata of the respiratory tract, it is used extensively in cough, asthma, pharyngitis and laryngitis. In these diseases, keeping a piece of vacha in the mouth as a lozenge gives quick relief. When emesis is required in asthma caused by obstruction of kapha, 4 to 5 gms. of fresh vacha powder + 10 gms. of rock salt is given along with warm water. The patient is asked to drink 1 ltr. of warm water over it. This causes removal of kapha through emesis and the dyspnoea is reduced.

Urinary system : Vacha is useful in dysuria caused by kapha. It is also useful as a lithotrypsic.

Reproductive system : It is an oxytocic. A mixture of saffron, long pepper and vacha is used in painful labour. Vacha is also used in dysmenorrhoea. The most important action of vacha is to clear the obstruction caused by kapha. Vacha + saffron + long pepper should be used as a galactagogue in post partum conditions.

Skin : Since vacha is a diaphoretic, medogami and tvachagami, it is used internally as well as externally in many skin diseases. A formulation called vachadi siddha taila is very useful in chronic skin diseases due to its stimulant action on the skin.

Satmikaran : Since it has a curating action, it reduces obesity by alleviating kapha dosha and meda dhatu. Regular use of vacha in small doses acts as a rasayan on kapha and meda. It has been successfully used since ages on disorders of speech.

Ayurveda does not believe in absence of a dravya. It believes in instantaneous change of dravya. Both these are complementary to each other.

Temperature : Since it is a diaphoretic, it is useful in fever caused by obstruction of sweat. It is also useful in alleviating symptoms like drowsiness and delirium associated with high fever. Vacha alone is an extremely useful medicine for teething problems in children.
Parts used : Root (tuber).
Dose : Powder - 0.25 to 0.5 gms; for emesis - 1 to 2 gms powder. (Vacha loses its potency within a very short time after powdering. Hence it should be powdered only when required or alternatively, its tuber should be rubbed against a hard surface and the paste thus obtained should be used.)
Formulations : Saraswat churna, Medhya rasayan.
Srotogamitva :
Dosha : Vataghna, kaphaghna.
Dhatu : Majja (brain tonic).
Mala : Purisha (anthelmintic), mutra.
Manovaha srotas : Epilepsy, mania.
Organs : Stomach, mouth, heart.
References -
'वामनी कटुतिक्तोष्णा वातश्लेष्मरुजापहा । कण्ठ्या मेध्या च कृमिहृद्विबन्धाध्मानशूलनुत् ।। (ध. नि.)
'वचोग्रगन्धा षड्ग्रन्था गोलोमी शतपर्विका । क्षुद्रपत्री च मंगल्या जटिलोग्रा च लोमशा ।।'
वचोग्रगन्धा कटुका तिक्तोष्णा वान्तिवह्निकृत् । विबन्धाधअमानशूलघ्नी शकृन्मूत्रविशोधनी ।।
'अपस्मारकफोन्मादभूतजं त्वानिलान् हरेत् ।' (भा. प्र.)
'सौवर्ण सुकृतं चूर्णं कुष्ठं मधु धृतं वचा ।..... कुमाराणां वपुर्मेधाबलबुद्धिविवर्धनाः ।।' (सु. शा. १०)
गुडूच्यपामार्गविडङ्गशखिनीवचाभयाकुष्ठशतावरीसमाः ।
घृतेन लीढाः प्रकरोति मानवं त्रिभिर्दिनैः श्लोकसहस्त्रधारिणम् ।।' (भै.र.)
'यः खादेत् क्षीरभक्ताशी माक्षिकेण वचारजः । अपस्मारं महाघोरं सुचिरोत्थं जयेद्ध्रुवम् ।। (चक्र.)
'दिवारात्रिं वचाग्रन्थिं मुखं संधारयेत् भिषक् । तेन सौख्यं भवेत्तस्य मुखरोगाद्विमुच्यते ।।' (हा.)

(101) VATSANABH

Aconitum ferox Wall.

Kula : Vatsanabh kula.
Family : Ranunculacae (Rana = frog - Rana tigrina) Many species develop in marshy places.
Latin name : Aconitum = aconite – monk's hood; ferox = terrible, ferocious, very poisonous.
English name : Monk's hood, Aconite.
Sanskrit names : Vatsanabh (like the umbilicus of a calf), Visha (as it is a poison), Amrut (acts as elixir if used judiciously), Ugra, Mahaushadha, Garal, Maran, Nag, Stokaka.
Botanical Description : A shrub 30 to 60 cm. high. Leaves – like the leaves of water melon, short, and stalk with hairy structure. Flower stalk – straight. External flower is blue and resembling the flower of pea. Fruit – thorny like hurhur (tilwan). Seeds – black and winged. Root – is 9 cm. in length and 1.5cm. to 3 cm. in breadth. Externally it is brown in colour but inside it is white, oily and shiny. In some texts, it is described as the plant which has leaves like nirgudi. Shape is like umbilicus of a calf. No plant grows near this plant.
The plant is called bachanag. Some texts describe the rhizome of vatsanabh as resembling the udder

Ayurveda tells us that the effect of external substrates on the body and mind is by the representative agencies of the universe in the body.

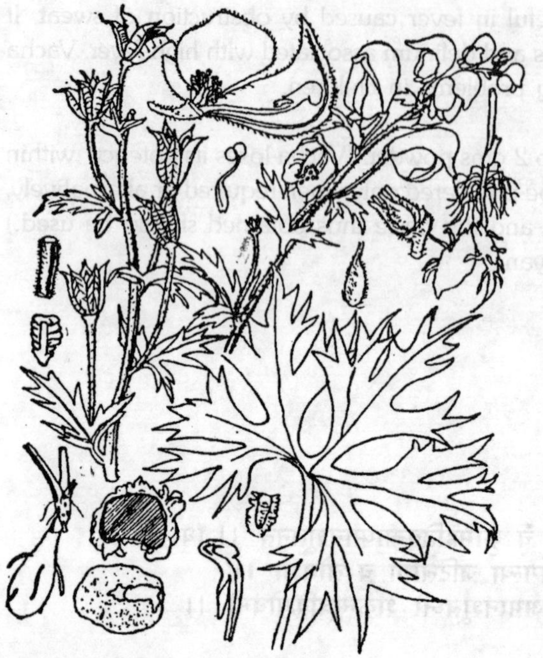

of cow, not more than 5 fingers in length. In India 24 types of vatsanabh are available. Bachanag is pungent to taste.

Habitat : In Himalayas from Sikkim to Garwhal at a height of 3000 to 5000 meters.

Chemical compostion : Aconitine (a toxin), picroeconine, benzoil, econine and homonepelin.

Types : Artificial bachanag is widely available in the market but real bachanag is of 2 types – white and black. Pure vatsanabh is actually white in colour but it becomes black after conditioning. This conditioning is required to protect it from insects. Vatsanabh, though poisonous, gets quickly infested with insects like ativisha.

Properties :

Guna : ruksha, tikshna, laghu, vyavayi and vikashi (these are the properties of visha).

Rasa : madhur; **Vipak :** madhur; **Veerya :** ushna.

Karma :

Dosha : Especially kaphavatashamak, ruksha, teekshna, laghu, kaphaghna. By madhur rasa pittashamak, by ushna veerya – vatashamak, vata kapha srotogami.

External uses : Application reduces pain and inflammation. It is applied after rubbing it with oil. On massaging, it stimulates the tip of sensory nerve fibres after which it produces tingling and numbness. It is absorbed faster through mucous membranes.

Internal uses :

Nervous system : It has no special effect on the brain. As it is vyavayi and vikasi and stimulates the tip of the nerve fibres, it acts as a depressant. It acts on motor nervous system also as a vasoconstrictor and above all on the vagus and respiratory system.

Digestive system : When it comes in contact with tongue it produces a tingling sensation initally then numbness, nausea and excessive salivation. In therapeutic doses it acts as an appetizer, deepan, pachan and reduces pain, parasthesia of stomach. It reduces gastric secretions and reduces kapha. It is a hepatostimulant.

Circulatory system : Impure vatsanabh has a depressant effect on the heart whereas purified vatsanabh acts as a cardiostimulant by its vyavayi and vikasi properties. This cardiostimulant property is enhanced if it is purified in cow's milk. Vatsanabh is used to alleviate oedema of any type.

Respiratory system : Kaphaghna. In small dose, it stimulates the respiratory system. It is useful in the pleuritis and pneumonitis.

Urinary system : Diuretic and reduces urinary calculi.

The constituents of the universe are transformed into human body. For health, we have to replete the body with these. That is our work.

Reproductive system : It is shukra stambhak and is useful in amenorrhoea.
Satmikaran : In very small dose, it is balya and nutritious (madhur rasa and madhur vipak).
Skin : Kushthaghna, diaphoretic.
Temperature : In jwara, it is the best medicine.
Excretion : It is chiefly excreted through the urine, saliva, bile and sweat.
Useful part : Rhizome.
Dose : 1.5 mg. (to be always given in lower doses). Must be used in winter and spring.
Formulations : Mrutyunjay Rasa, Hinguleshwar Rasa, Anand Bhairav Rasa, Panchavaktra, Laxmi Narayan, Tribhuvan kirti etc.
(Tribhuvan kirti has proved effective due to bachanag within it).
As it is a visha dravya, it should be used carefully. Initially it is stimulant and then depressant. Toxins act on marmas. Bachanag acts on heart. It acts on kaphavaha stotas.
Purification : Small pieces of bachanag are kept in cow's urine for 3 to 4 days. Then they are cleaned with fresh water and boiled in cow's milk for 3 hours. By this process, it gets purified. Only purified bachanag must be used and in little quantity only. To reduce toxicity of toxins, large quantity of cow ghee must be taken.
Srotogamitva :
Dösha : Kapha, vatavaha srotogami.
Dhatu : Raktagami, yakrutgami (it acts on liver), spleen, meda, rasayan.
Mala : Urine, sweat, saliva.

As bachanag is a cardiac depressant, arjuna bark is used after adminisration of bachanag, which is useful for heart. Ativisha also belongs to the same family as bachanag but it is an antitoxin.
References -
'विषं प्राणहरं प्रोक्तं व्यवायि च विकाशि च । आग्नेयं वातकफह्योगवाहि मदावहम् ।।
तदेव युक्तियुक्तं तु प्राणदायि रसायनम् । योगवाहि त्रिदोषघ्नं बृंहणं वीर्यवर्धनम् ।।' (भा.प्र.)
'वत्सनाभोऽतिमधुरः सोष्णो वातकफापहः सोष्णो वातकफापहः । कण्ठरुक्संनिपातघ्नः पित्तसंशोधनोऽपि च ।।' (रा.नि.)
'विषं रसायनं बल्यं वातश्लेष्मविकारनुत् । व्यवायि शीतनुद्दाहि कुष्ठशोथविनाशनम् ।।
अग्निमान्द्यश्वासकासप्लीहोदरज्वरापहम् कण्ठरुक्सन्निपातघ्नं मधुमेहहरं तथा ।।
प्रलेपाच्छ्वयथुं पीडामपचीं च विनाशयेत् ।'
विषं युञ्जीत नित्यं हि रसायनगुणैषिणः । घृतोपस्कृतदेहस्य विशुद्धस्य हिताशिनः ।।
सात्त्विकस्योते भानौ योज्यं शीतवसन्तयोः । ग्रीष्मे चात्ययिके व्याधौ न वर्षासु न दुर्दिने ।।
न क्रोधिनि न पित्तार्त्ते न क्लीबे राजवेश्मनि । क्षुत्तृष्णआभ्रमघर्माध्वव्याध्यन्तरनिपीडिते ।।
गर्भिण्यां बालवृद्धेषु न रूक्षेषु न मर्मसु । अभ्यस्तेऽपि विषे यत्नाद्वर्जनीयान् विवर्जयेत् ।।
कट्वम्ललवणं तैलं दिवास्वप्नानलातपान् । ब्रह्मचर्यं वरारोहे विषकाले समाचरेत् ।।
गव्ये क्षीरघृते पेये शाल्यन्नं गोधुमं तथा । शीतलं च पिबेत्तोयं मधुराणि च सेवयेत् ।।' (र. र. स. २९ अ)
बचनागाचे अतियोगावर :
'अतिमात्रं यदा भुक्तं तदाज्यं टंकणं पिबेत् । लिह्याद्वा मधुसर्पिभ्यां सम्पिष्टामर्जुनत्वचम् ।। (र.का.)

Whichever functional elements are in the human body also exist in the universe and vice versa.

(102) VARUN

Crataeva nurvala Roxb.

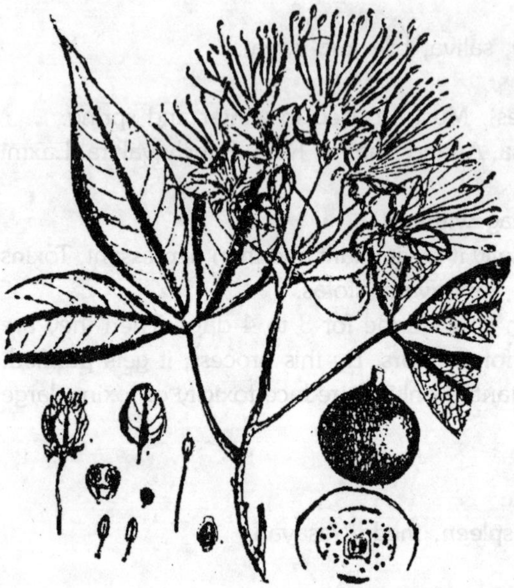

Gana : Varunadi, Vatashmarinashak, Kaphashmarinashak (S).
Kula : Varun kula.
Family : Capparidacae. (caper = kaparas) Gk. name of the family.
Latin name : Crataeva = Crativas – Gk. botanist who lived in the time of Crates; nurvala = (Nir – Malayalam) = water-water wood Apple (bilva) or religiosa = used for religious purpose.
English name : Three leaved caper.
Sanskrit names : Varun, Padap, Triparna, Bhramarpriya, Bilvapatra, Vruttaphala, Tiktashak, Setuvruksha, Ashmarighna.
Botanical Description : This tree is of 8 to 10 meter height. Bark – greyish in colour, bitter in taste, vertical striations. Leaves – approximately 18 cm. in length, like bilva patra, three leaves together. Among them, one leaf is oval in shape and having sharp tip, it gives strong smell after rubbing. Flowers – 6 to 9 cm. in length and are blue, white and fragrant. Fruits – like lemon. Pulp is yellowish and seeds are small. Fruit, when ripe, becomes red. The tree flowers in spring. Even the fresh bark can be powdered.
Habitat : All over India especially Madhya Pradesh, grown in the vicinity of temples in Bengal, Assam, Malabar.
Properties:
Guna : laghu, ruksha; **Rasa** : tikta, madhur, kashay; **Vipak** : katu; **Veerya** : ushna; **Prabhav** : bhedhan (ashmarighna).
Karma :
Dosha : Kaphavatashamak, therefore used in kapha vata diseases, vitiates pitta.
External uses : Bark powder applied on the skin, acts like application of mustard. So it is used in inflammation, abscess and lymphadenopathy.
Internal uses :
Digestive system : Deepan, anuloman, excretes pitta, bhedan, krumighna. Therefore used in distension, agnimandya, pain, liver diseases and worms.
Circulatory system : The decoction of the bark is used for purification of blood, gout, internal abscess and lymphadenopathy. In gandamala (cervical lymphadenopathy), varun + shunthi + bark of kanchanar is given.
Urinary system : It destroys urinary calculi, dysuria and pain in bladder. Its bark or decoction of the roots is used in these disorders. Its main action is on urinary calculi.In urinary calculi it is

The atomic elements of the universe are represented in the human body and these bring about good and bad effects in the body.

given along with apamarg, gokshur, yavakshar, punarnava and jyeshthamadh.
Temperature : Since it is a febrifuge, decoction of leaves is used in fever. Its application is done on the forehead to reduce giddiness in fever.
Satmikaran : It is bitter tonic. Juice of leaves is used as nutritious.
Parts used : Root, bark, leaves.
Dose : Decoction 60 to 100 ml.; juice – 12 to 24 ml.
Formulations : Varunadi quath, Varunadi Ghrit, Varunadi Tailam.
Srotogamitva :
Dosha : Pittavaha srotas (vitiates pitta), reduces kapha vata.
Dhatu : Rakta, meda (lymphadenopathy) to reduce fat, bone (abscess).
Mala : Urine (destroys urinary calculi); stool – (vermicidal).
Organs : Liver, kidney.
The smoke of dried leaves helps in deviated nasal septum (Sawant).
References -
'वरुण: पादप: तिक्त: त्रिपर्णो भ्रमरप्रिय: । बिल्वपत्रो वृत्तफलो बर्हपुष्प: कषायक: ।।' (शि.)
'वरुण: पित्तलो भेदी श्लेष्मकृच्छ्राश्ममारुतान् । निहन्ति गुल्मवातास्रकृमींश्चोष्णओऽग्निदीपन: ।।
कषायो मधुरस्तिक्त: कटुको रूक्षको लघु: ।' (भा. प्र.)
'वरुण: शीतवातघ्न: तिक्तों विद्रधिजन्तुजित् । तथा च कटुरुष्णश्च रक्तदोषहर: पर: ।।' (ध.नि.)
माक्षिकाढ्य: सकृत्पीत: क्वाथो वरुणमूलज: । गण्डमालां हरत्याशु चिरकालानुबन्धिनीम ।। (वृन्द)
'मूलं वरुणकस्य च। जलेन क्वथितं पीतमपक्वं विद्रधिं जयेत् ।।' (वृन्द)

(103) VASA

Adhatoda vasica Nees.

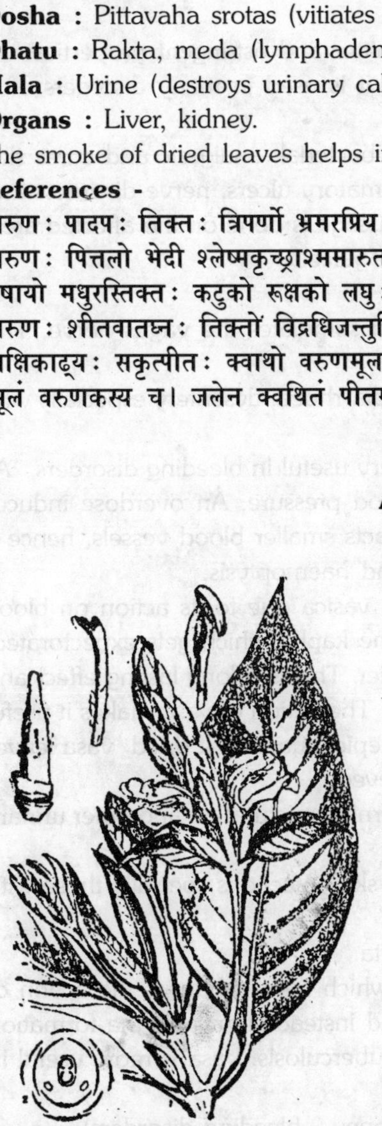

Kula : Vasa kula.
Family : Acanthacae (Gk. Akanthos = spine. Many species have thorns).
Latin name : Adhatoda. (It is the Malabari name of vasa); vasica = scented (fragrant), from the Sanskrit name 'vasak' meaning aromatic.
English name : Malabar Nut.
Sanskrit names : Vasak, Vasika, Vajidanta (white flowers resembling horse's teeth), Sinhasya, Bhishakmata, Vrusha, Sheetkarni, Panchamukhee, Maturka.
Botanical Description : The shrub is 1.5 to 3 mtrs in height. Leaves – 9 to 24 cm. in length. Flowers – white in colour, growing in a pattern resembling open jaws of a lion. The ovary has four seeds.
Varieties : A. vasica has 2 varieties - (1) white (2) black. The black variety is called asitparni. Its leaves are brown and flowers are red in colour. The branches have red nodes. Though this

shrub grows little high, it is less bitter. It is however used more widely.

Habitat : All over India, Brahmadesh, Singapore (white). Black adulsa grows mostly in the Himalayas at a height of 1.5 thousand meters.

Chemical composition : It contains an aromatic volatile oil, fats, vasicin, adhatodic acid, glycosides, resin, salt and a dye. A yellow xanthine exudes from the leaves. The root bark has more vasicin than the leaves.

Properties :

Guna : laghu, ruksha; **Rasa** : bitter, kashay; **Vipak** : katu; Veerya : sheeta.

Karma :

Dosha : Kaphashamak and vatavardhak by laghu, ruksha, bitter and astringent properties. Pittashamak by sheeta, bitter and astringent properties. Thus, it is used in many disorders of kapha and pitta.

External uses : The paste of leaves is antiinflammatory, antibacterial, analgesic and cures skin diseases. Local application of paste is useful in arthritis, inflammatory ulcers, nerve disorders and skin diseases. In disorders like amnesia and convulsions, oil massage is done on the affected area. To kill bacteria in ulcers, the affected area is washed with leaf juice.

Internal uses :

Nervous system : The use of vasa causes vaso dilation and stimulates the vagus nerve. This increases the heart rate and lowers blood pressure.

Digestive system : Being astringent and sheeta, it is useful in diarrhoea, dysentery especially with bleeding disorders.

Circulatory system : It acts on rakta dhatu. Therefore it is very useful in bleeding disorders. As it is a vasodilator, it increases the heart rate and reduces blood pressure. An overdose induces hypotension. It is also haemostatic and blood purifier. It contracts smaller blood vessels, hence it is useful in bleeding disorders, bleeding piles, menorrhagia and haemoptysis.

Respiratory system : This is the main area of action of A. vasica due to its action on blood flow and vagus nerve action, mainly on lungs. Vasa liquifies the kapha which gets expectorated. It causes bronchodilation and therefore breathing becomes easier. This is a long lasting effect and thus vasa is used in asthma, breathlessness and throat infection. The action of vasa makes it useful in chest congestion and tuberculosis. It has an effect similar to epicaquanine. If dried vasa leaves mixed with dhattura leaves are smoked, breathlessness is relieved.

Urinary system : It is a diuretic. Flowers are used in dysuria, burning micturation and other urinary disorders.

Skin : It is a diaphoretic and kushthaghna and thus useful in skin infections specially those with discharge and bleeding.

Temperature : Used in fevers induced by pitta and kaphapitta.

Satmikaran : Due to its tikta rasa, its stimulates rasa dhatu which then enhances the action of all dhatus. It stops the formation of kapha from rasa dhatu and instead stimulates the formation of successive dhatus like rakta, mansa etc. Thus it is useful in tuberculosis. Vasa is more useful in haemoptysis than bleeding per rectum.

Parts used : Root, root bark, leaves, flowers (leaf juice + honey - bleeding disorders).

Both hot and cold properties control each other. It is not possible for a single power to exist. Every force/power in the universe is relative and dependent on each other.

Dose : Leaf juice - 10 to 20 ml; flowers – 0.6 to 1.2 gms; root powder 250 to 625 mg.; root decoction - 40 to 80 ml.
Formulations : Vasavaleha, Vasakasav, Vasarishta, Vasapanak, Vasachandanadi taila, Vasaghritam, Vasaputapak, Gulkand of flowers.
The leaves of vasa are insecticidal. Water to which vasa leaves are added does not get spoilt. Fruits wrapped in vasa leaves do not rot. If manure containing vasa leaves is put in the fields then the grain from that crop does not get affected by pests. If vasa leaves are kept in woolen clothes then those clothes are protected from insects. Thus, vasa is pesticidal in addition to its antiasthmatic action. Application of leaves from the red flowering variety, mixed with coconut milk and heated, is used in breast abscess and mastitis.
Srotogamitva :
Dosha : Vitiates vata, kaphapittashamak.
Dhatu : Blood (raktapitta, kushtha), meda (meha), rasa (jwar, mansa, kshayanashak).
Mala : Pittasarak.
Organs : Pranvaha srotas, respiratory system, stomach (jwar, vomiting – asthma).
References -
'वासको वातकृत् स्वर्यः कफपित्तास्रनाशनः । तिक्तस्तुवरको हृद्यो लघुः शीतस्तृडर्त्तिहृत् ।।
श्वासकासज्वरच्छर्दिमेहकुष्ठक्षयापहः ।' (भा. प्र.)
'वृषपुष्पं... कफपित्तहरं तिक्तं शीतं कटु विपच्यते ।' (च. सू. २७)
'वृषागस्तयोः पुष्पाणि तिक्तानि कटु विपाकानि क्षयकासापहानि च ।' (सु. सू. ४६)
'वासायां विद्यमानायामाशायां जीवितस्य च । रक्तपित्ती क्षयी कासी किमर्थमवसीदति ।।?

(104) VIDANG
Embelia ribes Burm. F.

Gana : Krumighna, Truptighna, Shirovirechan (C.); Surasadi, Pippalyadi (S.), Trimada (Bhava Prakash).
Kula : Vidanga kula.
Family : Myrsinacae – somewhat similar looking gland dotted leaves (the Greek name by Dioscorides).
Latin name : Embelia = (amlika), the name 'embe' is derived from the Sinhali word for sour; ribes = rubarb's Arabic name.
Sanskrit names : Vidang, Chitratandul (on fruit there are white spots), Jantunashan, Vatari, Jantughnee, Jantughna, Krishnatandul.
Botanical Description : Big tree. Leaves -oval, pointed. Flowers - grow in cluster, when unripe – green and astringent in taste, when ripe - reddish coloured and sour (Ambat tingali). Fruit - contains greyish coloured seed and pulp. On external surface, there are small white spots. Commercially available vidang is adulterated with many similar looking substances.
Habitat : All over India in mountaineous areas. Always, one year old vidang must be used.
Chemical composition : Acid – 2.5%, volatile oil, stable oil, colouring agent, tannin, resin, cristebin, kshar.
Guna : katu; **Vipak** : katu; **Veerya** : ushna.

At the beginning of a particular science, one has to assume certain axioms, eg. line and dots in Geometry.

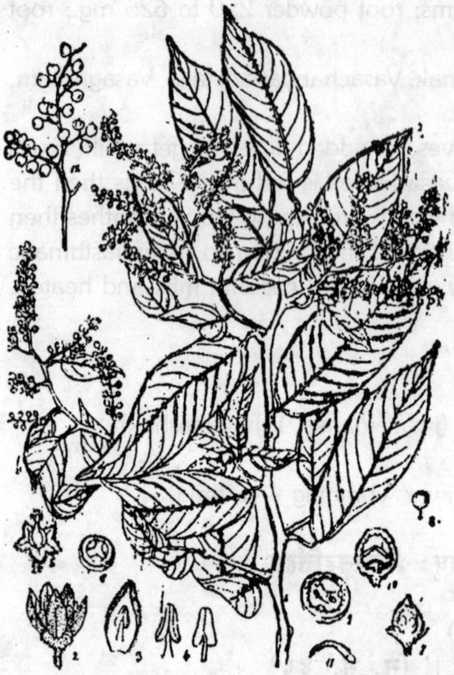

Karma :

Dosha : As it has ushna veerya, it is vatakaphanashak.

External uses : Bacteriocidal, kushthaghna and shirovirechan. Hence it is useful in dental caries, toothache etc. Decoction is used for gargles in dental diseases. External application is done in skin diseases. A fine powder of vidang is used for nasal administration (pradhaman nasya) in chronic rhinitis, jaundice and other diseases of the head.

Internal uses :

Nervous system : It is a nervine tonic. Vidang boiled in milk along with garlic is used in diseases of the brain and nervous system.

Digestive system : Deepan, pachan, anuloman but especially vermicidal. Vidang, along with warm water or buttermilk, is used in indigestion, vomiting, abdominal colic, flatulence, constipation and piles. In round worm, tape worm or thread worm infestation, 10 gms. of vidang powder is given on an empty stomach and then a purgative is given. This kills the worms which are expelled in the stools. After this, vidang churna is given in small quantity as a maintenance dose. Along with this, indrayava, seeds of palash and bark of neem are also useful. Continuous intake of vidang does not allow worms to survive in the intestines. It is used in all types of worms.

Circulatory system : It is useful in diseases due to blood impurities and in diseases caused by vitiation of meda. It purifies blood by optimizing its agni and is very useful in disorders of rasa dhatu and oedema.

Urinary system : It acts on the urinary system, diuretic, increases excretion of acid in the urine, useful in dysuria. Vidang causes red colouration of the urine.

Skin : It is useful for complexion and is kushthaghna. It is used in many skin diseases. Since there is an involvement of krumi in all types of kushtha, formulations of vidang are very useful in it. Local application of vidang is also useful in many skin diseases like scabies.

Satmikaran : Vidang is the greatest rasayan dravya. It gradually reduces the rigidity of the body, improves circulation, agni, appetite and texture of the skin. Vidang + iron formulations can be used as very good rasayan in children as well as in patients having anaemia.

Temperature : In jwara (fever) – to decrease the fever - vidang is given from time to time. Due to this, vomiting, dyspepsia decreases and by perspiration fever decreases. Vidang is a useful medicine in fever. In chronic cough and in rajyakshma (tuberculosis), milk boiled with vidang is useful.

Respiratory system : In rhinitis and in migraine, its fine powder is used for pradhaman nasya.

Useful part : Fruit (1 year old).

Dose : 1 to 2 gm. (for worms – 10 gm.)

Rasa is the life base of dravya. Once one is convinced with this whole truth, we can identify its physical gunas, veerya and vipak etc.

Formulations : Vidangadi churna, Vidangarishtam, Vidangadi loha, Vidang taila. (an application of vidang + ghee is used on trees affected with termites. The part affected with termite should be first scraped off and then vidang + ghee should be applied. Milk + water should be then applied on it.)

Vidang Tandula = Vidang in which the outer husk of the seed has been removed and which cannot germinate. Vidang beej = seeds = unaffected by insects which have the power to germinate. Germinating property is lost in vidang tandul.

Srotogamitva :

Dosha : Kaphaghna, vata and constipation.

Dhatu : Rakta (kushtha), meda (prameha), rakta (reduces shirorog), rasayan.

Mala : Purisha (laxative, tape worm), mutra.

Organs : Intestine, anus.

References -

'विडंगं कटुतीक्ष्णोष्णं रूक्ष वह्निकरं लघु । शूलाध्मानोदरश्लेष्मकृमिवातविबन्धनुत् ।।' (भा. प्र)

'विडंग.... तैलानि कटूनि कटुविपाकानिसराण्यनिलकफकृमिकुष्ठप्रमेहशिरोरोगापहराणि च (सु. सू. ४५)

'विडंगं कृमिघ्नानाम् श्रेष्ठम् (च. सू. २५)

'विडंगा कटुरुष्णा च लघु: वातकफार्तिनुत् । अग्निमांद्यारुचिभ्रान्तिकृमिदोषविनाशिनी ।।' (रा. नि.)

'विडंगतंडुलचूर्णमाहत्य यष्टिमधुयुक्तं यथाबलं शीततोययोगेनोपयुञ्जीत शीततोयं चानुपिबेत् ।.. एते खलु अर्शांसि क्षपयन्ति, कृमिनुपघ्नन्ति, ग्रहणधारणशक्ति जनयन्ति मासे मासे प्रयोगे वर्षशतमायुषोऽभिवृद्धिर्भवति । (सु. चि. २७)

(105) SHATAPUSHPA

Foeniculum vulgare Gaertn.

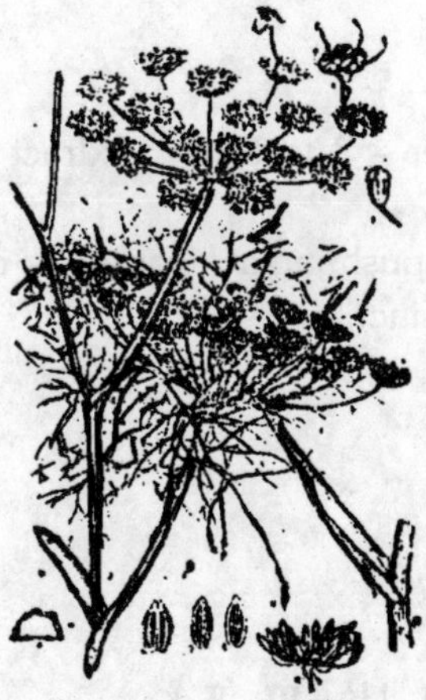

Gana : Asthapan (S.)

Kula : Shatapushpa kula.

Family : Umbelliferae (having nearly equal branches (ray like) from a point like the ribs of umbrella).

Latin name : Foeniculum = funnel. (Lat – foenum = hay, resemblence in odour); vulgare = common, ordinary.

English name : Fennel.

Sanskrit names : Shatahva, Shatapushpa (many flowers are situated in umbrella shape), Suvakpushpi, Sanghatpatrika, Vajrapushpa, Vanapushpa, Sugandha, Sookshmapatrika, Arvakpushpa, Madhurasa, Kshetra, Atilambi.

Botanical Description : An annual small herb and leaves – 5 to 10 cm. in length, winged. Flowers – yellowish white in colour. Fruits – oval in shape – green and having longitudinal striations.

Varieties : Basically its original variety is found in Egypt. Now it is also grown in Iran and Punjab. It is called anisoon, badiyaan or ainis. Latin name is Pimpinella anisam. In allopathy its oil (oleum anisi) is used. It has one wild variety as well. There is another

Every edible substance in its absorbed form, has to circulate along with the rasadhatu in the body and it has got to be excreted, too.

variety in which the seeds are small like jeerak with more frangrance.

Habitat : Everywhere in India.

Chemical composition : Its seeds contain a 3 to 5% volatile fragrant oil. It contains a compound called anithole which is now-a-days prepared artificially also.

Properties :

Guna : laghu, snigdha, tikshna; **Rasa** : madhur, katu, tikta; **Vipak** : madhur; **Veerya** : ushna.

Karma :

Dosha : Obviously, it is used in kapha vataj diseases.

Internal uses:

Nervous system : Brain tonic and useful for eyes. It is useful in weakness of brain and eye sight.

Digestive system : Reduces dyspepsia, vomiting, deepan, pachan, anuloman. Basically, it is purgative in nature. It is also used in distension, pain in abdomen, dysentery and piles. In dysentery, it acts as amapachak and anulomak of vata and it removes amadosha out of the body. Because of this, it reduces spasms. Fried fennel and ginger powder should be taken in spasmodic pain to reduce the spasm along with other medications. Root is used as purgative. In abdominal distension, all fragrant medicines (dravyas) are used. Dark, dried fennel is one of them. Milk boiled with fennel is an extremely useful remedy for abdominal colic in children.

Circulatory system : Useful for the heart. As it is rakta prasadan, it is useful in heart diseases and also in blood disorders.

Respiratory system : Kaphaghna and kapha expectorant. So used in kaphaj kasa and asthma.

Urinary system : Diuretic, useful in dysuria, urine retention, reduces burning micturation.

Reproductive system : Induces menstruation and increases breast milk secretion. Useful in dysmenorrhoea, menstrual obstruction and mastitis.

Skin : In kushtha, it induces sweating, removes blood impurities and acts as kushthaghna. It is applied locally on boils which occur due to heat in summer.

Temperature : Febrifuge and reduces burning.

Parts used : Seeds, seed oil, root, extract of seeds.

Dose : Seed powder – 3 to 6 gm.; oil – 5 to10 drops.; root powder – 3 to 6 gm.; extract – 24 to 48 ml.

Formulations : Shatapushpadi churna, Shatapushpadi ghrit, Shatapushparka (Fennel is eaten after meals for cleaning the mouth. It is considered as anti-aphrodisiac).

Srotogamitva :

Dosha : Vitiates pitta, kapha vata shamak.

Dhatu : Majja (medhya), shukra; rasa (jwar, increases breast milk).

Mala : Purisha (anuloman), urine (diuretic).

Organs : Eyes, stomach.

References -

'शतपुष्पा लघुतीक्ष्णा पित्तकृद्दीपनी कटुः । उष्णा ज्वरानिलश्लेष्मव्रणशूलाक्षिरोगहृत् ।।' (भा. प्र.)

शतपुष्पा कटुस्तिक्ता तीक्ष्णोष्णा दीपनी लघुः । पित्तला कफवातघ्नी मेध्या स्निग्धाज्वरापहा ।। निहन्ति शूलदाहाक्षिरोगतृष्णावमित्रणआन् । वन्या शताह्वा वृष्या च क्षतक्षीण हिता हिमा ।। अक्षिरुक्वातपित्तास्रक्षयघ्नी स्वादुतिक्तता ।' (कै.नि.)

An equillibrium is maintained in body's minute constituents and cells by prana and apana. Prana means intake and apana means output.

(106) SHATAVARI

Asparagus racemosus Willd.

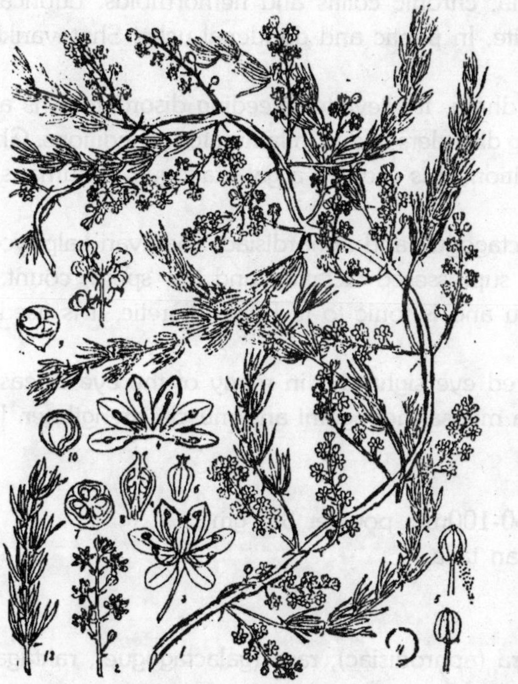

Gana : Balya, Vayasthapan, Madhurskandha (C.); Vidarigandhadi, Kantakpanchamoola, Pitta shaman (S.)

Kula : Rason kula.

Family : Liliaceae (Lat – Lilium = lily – Li = white).

Latin name : Asparagus = derivated from – A = intensive, sparasso = in allusion to strong prickles; racemosus = having an inflorescence with a long undivided axis (Raceme = inflorescence).

English name : Wild Asparagus.

Sanskrit names : Shatavari, Shatapadi (having over hundred rootlets), Vrushya, Deepya, Dweepshatru, Adharkanthika, Supatra, Bahumula, Shatahriya, Narayani, Laghuparnika, Shataveerya.

Botanical Description : It is a creeper. It has thorns on its stalk and it grows upward. Its branches are triangular, oily, and have striations on it. Leaves are very small, and like leafy vegetable shepu (in Marathi). Thorns – are 0.62 to 1.25 cm. in length and some what curved. Leaves – stalk 1.25 to 2.5 cm. in length and there are 2 to 6 together in bunch. Flower stalk- many branches with sub-branches, abundant flowers which are white, pink and fragrant. Fruit - like pods, 1-2 seeds. There are many thick oblong rootlets near the main root. These are used as medicine.

Varieties : There is another larger variety of this creeper called mahashatavari, sahasramooli or sahasra veerya (Aspargus armentosa - armed with thorns). The roots of this variety are longer and more spread out. Another thornless variety is found in the Himalayas at the height of 8-9 thousand meters and is known as Asparagus filicimis (thread like).

Habitat : All over India but found plentyfully especially in Northern India.

Chemicial composition : In fresh tuber, water soluble ingredient is 52.5%, fibre 33. 3% and water 9%. Water soluble ingredient contains sugar 7% and some mucilagenous principle.

Properties :

Guna : guru, snighdha; **Rasa :** madhur, tikta; **Vipak :** madhur; **Veerya :** sheeta.

Karma :

Dosha : Vatapittashamak so useful in many diseases.

External uses : Because of its shamak and balya actions, leaves boiled in oil are used for massage in head (brain) disease, vata disorders and weakness. Leaves are used in measles and smallpox.

Avasthapak is a natural consequence which cannot be avoided by each food material. Once considered and consumed, the freedom of dietary intake is over.

Internal uses : Shatavari is a brain tonic and pain reliever, gives energy to brain and nerves. It is used in epilepsy and syncope and vata disorders.

Digestive system : Enhances digestion, laxative, astringent. Because of its bitter rasa it is stomachic. Useful in loss of appetite, colic, gulma, chronic colitis and hemorrhoids. Lubricates internal skin and makes it soft. It increases appetite. In peptic and duodenal ucler, Shatavarikalp is used.

Circulatory system : Shatavari acts on rakta dhatu. It alleviates bleeding disorders. It is also cardiotonic. It is useful in cardiac disorders, bleeding disorders and in inflammatory conditions. Ghee boiled with shatavari can be useful in these condition. It is used as a galactagogue in humans as well as in animals.

Reproductive system : It is a foetal tonic, galactagogue and aphordisiac. Shatavari kalp works as rasayan in threatened abortion, menorrhagia, supressesed lactation and low sperm count.

Excretory system : It also acts on meda dhatu and is tonic to it. Being diuretic, it is used in dysuria. It gives strength to urinary bladder.

Eyes : It is an eye tonic, hence useful in impaired eye sight and in many of the eye diseases.

Satmikaran : Useful in general debility and as a mansa-medogami and muscle strengthner. It is also used in tuberculosis.

Parts used : Tuber.

Dosage : Juice of tuber 12-14ml.; decoction 60-100ml.; powder 3-6 gm.

Formulations : Siddhaghrita, Phalghrita, Narayan taila.

Srotogamitva :

Dosha : Vataghna, pittaghna, kaphaghna.

Dhatu : Rejuvenator, majja (brain tonic), shukra (aphrodisiac), rasa (galactagogue), raktagami (bleeding disorders.)

Mala : Purisha (astringent, antidiarrhoeal).

Organs : Eyes, stomach, liver, gall bladder, heart.

References -

'शतावरी गुरुः शीता तिक्ता स्वाद्वी रसायनी ।
मेघाग्निपुष्टि स्निग्धा नेत्र्या गुल्मातिसारजित् ।।
शुक्रस्तन्यकरी बल्या वातपित्तास्रशोथजित् ।
महाशतावरी मेध्या हृद्या वृष्या रसायनी ।।
शीतवीर्या निहन्त्यर्शोग्रहणीनयनामयान् ।
तदंकुरस्त्रिदोषघ्नो लघुरर्शःक्षयापहा' ।।' (भा.प्र.)
'वातपित्तहरी वृष्या स्वादुतिक्ता शतावरी । महती चैव हृद्या च मेध्याग्निबलवर्धिनी ।।
ग्रहण्यर्शोविकारघ्नी वृष्या शीता रसायनी । कफपित्तहरास्तिक्तातस्या एवांकुराः स्मृताः ।।' (सु. सू. ४६)
'शतावरी हिमा तिक्ता रसे स्वादुः क्षयास्र जित् । वातपित्तहरी वृष्या रसायनवरा स्मृता ।। (ध.नि.)
'भुक्त्वा वरीं क्षीरयुतां विलासी भुंक्ते शतं सुन्दरी! सुन्दरीणाम् ।' (वै. जी.) (अतिवृष्य)

Vipak being very important in the treatment of diseases of shakha, it has an independent place in our thoughts for therapy.

(107) SHARAPUNKHA

Tephrosia purpurea Linn.

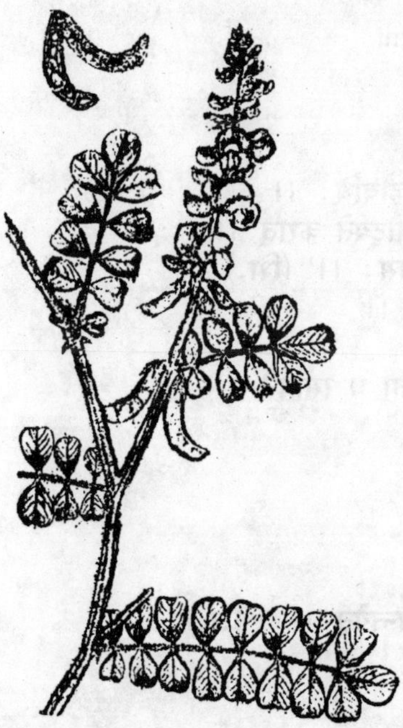

Kula : Shimbi kula.

Upakula : Aparajita kula (Papillionacae).

Family : Leguminosae.

Latin name : Tephrosia (Tephros = Ash grey) (Cinerious) colour of the leaves; purpurea = flowers purple.

English name : Purple tephrosia.

Sanskrit names : Sharapunkha, Sarpamukhi (cut off leaf angles look like open mouth of snake), Indupushpika, Kalsha, Pleehashatru, Neelavrukshakruti (leaves are like the leaves of Neeli).

Botanical Description : An annual herb, has many branches 5 to 7 cm. high. Leaves compound, 7 to 12 cm. in length, 13-21in number, with rounded tips. Flowers – red stalk, 5 to 7 cm. in length, legume – 2.5 to 5 cm. in length and curved. It contains 6 to 10 seeds. The plant flowers in the rainy season and fruits in winter.

Varieties : 2 types - (1) Red and (2) White (the above description is of red one). White sharapunkha is small and spreads on the ground and has hairy branches. Flowers are white. Its Latin name is Tephrosia villosa (rough haired.) It is a rasayani.

Habitat : All over India, but more in mountaineous areas.

Guna : laghu; **Rasa** : tikta, kashay; **Vipak** : katu; **Veerya** : ushna; **Prabhav** : bhedan.

Karma :

Dosha : Kaphavatashamak.

External uses : Reduces inflammation, kushthaghna, antidotal, bactericidal, wound healing and haemostatic. Useful in toothache.

Internal uses :

Digestive system : Rochan, deepan, anuloman, pitta sarak (optimises bile secretions) and krumighna. Root decoction is used in flatulence.

Circulatory system : Raktapittashamak, heamostatic (action on spleen, white sharapunkha is antiinflammatory).

Respiratory system : Expectorant.

Urinary system : Diuretic.

Reproductive system : Uterine stimulant, shukrastambhak.

Skin : Kushthaghna.

Temperature : Antipyretic – used in chronic fever.

Satmikaran : Antitoxic, white sharapunkha is rasayan.

Dosha : Useful in kapha vataj diseases.

It should be considered that there can be a single dravya which can bring about an increase or decrease in each one of the dosha-dhatu-malas.

Parts used : Root, panchang, kshar, seed.
Dose : Powder 3 to 6 gms.; juice - 12 to 24 ml.; kshar – 1 to 2 gms.
Srotogamitva:
Dosha : Vata (gulmaghna).
Dhatu : Blood (spleen, liver), rasa, rasayan, raktavahasrotogami.
Mala : Purish (vermicidal).
Prabhav : Antitoxic.
References -
'नीलिकाकृतिपत्रा च प्रसिद्धा भूमिमंडले । शिंबीफला रक्तपुष्पा नीलवर्णा महौषधिः ।।
शरपुंखेति विख्याता श्वेतपुष्पा क्वचिद् भवेत् । तस्याः पत्रं यदाकृष्य गृह्यते त्रोट्यते करात् ।।
तत्पत्रं जायते साक्षादूर्ध्व सच्छरपुङ्खवत् । इयमास्ते परीक्षास्याः औषधेः दिव्यतेजसः ।।' (शि.)
'शरपुङ्खा प्लीहशत्रुर्नीलवृक्षाकृतिश्च सा । शरपुंखा यकृत्प्लीहगुल्मव्रणविषापहः ।।
तिक्तः कषायाः कासास्रश्वासज्वरहरो लघुः।' (भा.प्र.)
'शरपुंखाः कटूष्णाश्च कृमिवातरुजापहाः । श्वेता त्वाशुगुणाढ्या स्यात् प्रशस्ता च रसायने ।।
कण्टपुंखा कटुष्णा च कृमिशूलविनाशिनी ।' (रा. नि)
'शरपुंखायाः कल्कः तक्रेण निषेवितो यथाग्निबलम् ।
यदि न जयति प्लीहानं शैलोऽपि तदा जले प्लवते ।।' (शो.)
'या विशालविटपा शरपुंखा मूलमात्मदशनैः मुहुरस्यः ।
चर्वितं निगिरितं विनिहन्ति प्लीहवृद्धिमकठोरभुजश्च ।।' (रा.मा.)
'मूलं च शरपुंखायाः पेषयेत्तडुलाम्बुना । पीत्वा च माषमात्रं तु अतिरक्तं प्रशान्तयेत् ।।' (भै.र.)

(108) SHAL
Shorea robusta Gaerth.

Gana : Vedanasthapan, Kashayaskandh, Asavyonivriksha (C.), Salsaradi, Lodhradi (S.)
Kula : Shal kula.
Family: Dipterocarpeae (Dipto = double, carpi = fruit).
Latin name : Shorea = name in honour of Sir Shore; robusta = strong (Latin – Robustus (Robur = strength), robust in appearance)
English name : Sal tree.
Sanskrit names : Shal (glorious), Ral, Sarjarasa, Kanakalodbhav, Shalsar, Rava, Maharoop, Dhoopan, Sarja, Dhoonak, Sarvarasa,
Botanical Description : This tree is tall and grows straight, leaving very little shadow. When young, the bark is tender; on ageing it becomes thick and rough. Trunk is strong and has much wood inside. Leaves - alternate, simple, 14 to 25 cm long and 10 to 12 cms. broad. Leaf stalk is 2.5 cm. in length. Flowers - white, yellow, tender, are hairy and grow in bunches. Fruits- 2.5 cm. in length, white and soft but on ripening become grey in colour. Flowering season is in March and fruiting in May- June. Its gum is called as ral. Shalniryas, sarjarasa, yakshadhoop are its synonyms. Its properties are like those of gandhabiroja. White shal is considered to be better than the red variety.
Habitat : Terai region in the Himalayas, in U.P. from Kangra to Assam, Panchamadhi, Coromandal.

Almost 80% of satva (essence) is obtained from Tinospora cordifolia plant, in the month of May. This must be thought of other plants too.

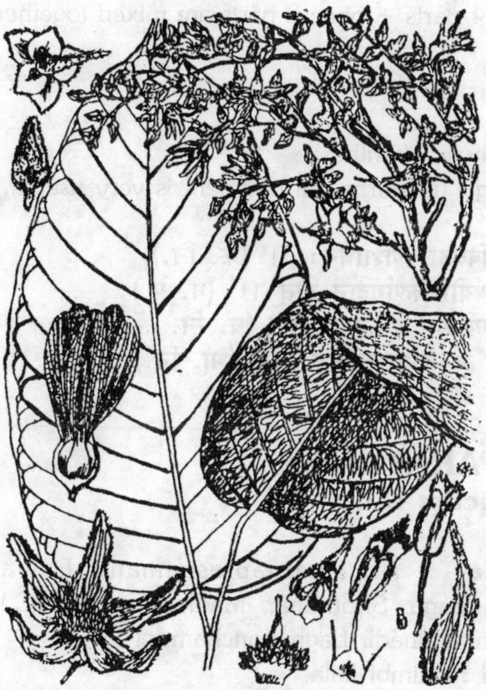

Chemical composition : Bark is astringent. After boiling in water, it looks like catechu.

Guna : laghu, ruksha; **Rasa :** Sal – astringent, bitter, pungent. Ral – astringent, sweet; **Vipak :** pungent; **Veerya :** bark – sheeta, ral – ushna veerya; **Prabhav :** skin – kaphapittashamak, ral – tridoshahara.

Karma :

Dosha : By prabhav it is tridoshaghna but being astringent, katu and bitter, it is kaphanashak. Ral is tridoshanashak and is useful in diseases caused by tridoshas.

External uses : Stimulant, analgesic, bactericidal. The ointment of ral cleanses wounds and heals them. It is useful in burns, dadru, vipadika etc. Dhoop (smoke of ral) is bactericidal in wounds and is useful in painful swelling. (Ral is used in Vipadika ointment, – Vagbhatta Chikitsa 19/77).

Internal uses :

Nervous system : Vataghna therefore analgesic. Used in ear diseases and used for eyes. Its bark decoction is given in any pain in the body. It is especially useful in contusions or in wounds. Application of the anjan of ral increases eyesight. In otorrhoea, the ear is washed by its bark decoction.

Digestive system : It acts as an astringent because of its kashaya rasa but ral is deepan and pachan. As it is pachan and astringent, it is useful in diarrhoea, raktaj pravahika and bleeding piles.

Circulatory system : Haemostatic hence used in bleeding and in haemolytic anaemia.

Respiratory system : Bark is kaphaghna. Ral is expectorant and it removes bad smell of kapha in cough and asthma. It acts as an antibacterial in the respiratory system.

Urinary system : Bark – antidiuretic and hence used in diabetes. Ral is useful in urinary tract infections and therefore used in pyuria.

Reproductive system : Reduces inflammation of the uterus.It is an aphrodisiac and is useful in menorrhagia and leucorrhoea. The decoction of the bark or ral is used in these diseases. For aphrodisiac action, 1.5 gm. ral powder in ½ sher milk is given.

Skin : Kushthaghna and antidiaphoretic agent. So used in kushtha and in excessive sweating.

Satmikaran : Since it is astringent, it is used for facilitating reunion of fractures. By ruksha guna it reduces meda. By these properties, it is useful in fractures, wounds and obesity.

Useful parts : Bark and niryas (ral) .

Doses : Bark decoction – 60 to 100 ml.; ral powder- 1 to 3 gm.

Formations : Sarjarasadi lepa, Vipadika lepa, Atasiadi lepa.

Since ral is ushna veerya, excess intake may cause increase in pitta dosha. In such cases, unctuous dravyas like milk + ghee should be given.

Out of twenty gunas, indriyas perceive only certain gunas or exactly opposite gunas.

Ral ointment : Ral 4 parts + wax 4 parts + teel oil 4 parts + ghee 3 parts are mixed together and slightly heated.

Srotogamitva :

Dosha : Kapha (kshapan).

Dhatu : Rakta, mansa, asthi (rejoins the fractures), shukra (virilizer).

Mala : Purisha (astringent), sweda (reduces sweating). (In burns, ral ointment is very useful).

References -

'शालः कषायो ग्राह्यसृग्ददग्धरुक्कफजिद्विमः। कर्णरोगहरो रूक्षो विषहा व्रणशोधनः ।।' (कै. नि.)

अश्वकर्णः कषायः स्यात् व्रणस्वेदकफक्रिमीन् । बध्नविद्रधिबाधिर्ययोनिकर्णगदान् हरेत् ।।' (ध. प्र.)

'कुष्ठकण्डूकृमिश्लेष्मवातपित्तरुजो जयेत् । सर्जयुग्मं कषायं स्याद्वर्ण्य रुक्षं कफापहम् ।।' (ध. नि.

'राल:स्वादुः कषायश्च स्तम्भनो व्रणरोपणः । विपादीभूतहन्ता च भग्नसंधानकृन्मतः ।।' (भा. नि.)

(109) SHALIPARNI

Desmodium gangeticum D.C.

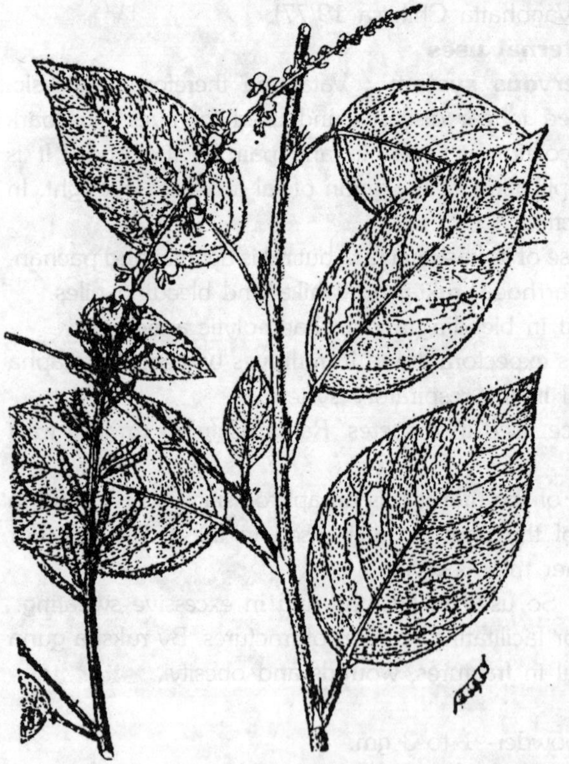

Gana : Angamardaprashaman, Balya, Snehopaga, Shothahar, Madhurskandha (C.); Vidarigandhadi, Laghupanchamool (S.).

Kula : Shimbi kula.

Upakula : Papilionaceae.

Family : Leguminoseae (Legumin = pod).

Latin name : Desmodium = (Gk. – Desmodion – little bond). Jointed pods and connected stamens.; gangeticum = pertaining to the Ganges.

Sanskrit names : Sudala, Chhalparni, Vidarigandha, Shothaghni, Shaliparni, Mahaklijanaka, Peetanee, Atiruha, Deerghanghree, Dhruvaparnee, Atiguha.

Botanical Description : A small herb 7 to 15 cm. high. Its stalk has slight edges. Leaves– like shala plant, length 0.75 to 1.25 mt. and breadth 1.5 to 5 cm., inferior surface of leaves hairy. Flowers – blue or pink, small, inflorescence is 15 to 30 cm. in length. Legume – tender, flat and curved, divided into 6 to 8 parts. The inflorescence stiks to clothes. Generally 6 to 8 legumes are together. In rainy season flowers appear and legumes in autumn. Commercially it is sold as shaliparni, in many varieties. One variety has 3 leaves and is called triparni.

Habitat : In the Himalayan foothills, all over India in the plains.

The sequence of the curriculum of studying medicine is as follows : health, then the health disturbances-diseases and the relevant dravyagunakarmas to reverse the disease.

Chemical composition : Its root has one yellow resin, oil and kshar. Its ash is 6%.
Guna : guru, snigdha; **Rasa** : madhur, tikta; **Vipak** : madhur; **Veerya** : ushna.
Karma :
Dosha : Tridoshashamak; due to snigdha and ushna properties, it is vatashamak, it is pitta shamak due to madhur rasa and since it is bitter and ushna veerya, it acts as kaphashamak. It is used in various tridoshaj diseases.
Internal uses :
Nervous system : As it is a nervine tonic, it is used in various vata disorders, especially in vata disorders of the heart. In palpitation, shalparni boiled in milk, is given to the patient.
Digestive system : Deepan, pachan, snehan, anuloman, astringent and deworming agent. Due to all these properties it is used in loss of appetite, koshthagata vata, haemorrhoids, diarrhoea and vomiting. It is also used as antihelminthiasis. Its root is used in vomiting.
Circulatory system : Useful for heart, antiinflammatory and raktasthapan. Due to these properties it is used in heart diseases, palpitations, blood disorders and cardiomegaly.
Respiratory system : Expectorant – so used in cough, urahakshata and rajayakshma (tuberculosis). Its decoction is given in haemoptysis.
Reproductive system : It is an aphrodisiac. It improves semen quality. Milk boiled with the roots of shalparni is useful for foetal nourishment.
Urinary system : As it is a diuretic, it is used in dysuria but it gives strength to the urinary system. It is used in diabetes.
Temperature : Antipyretic, especially in vishamjwara.
Satmikaran : It is included in balya, brihan and angamardaprashaman ganas. Besides, due to its all favourable properties, it is used as rasayana in weakness, kshaya – malnutrition and bodyache.
Parts used : Panchang especially root (it is not used – this is the reality).
Dose : Decoction 60 to 100 ml.
Formulations : Shalparnyadi kwath, Dashamloolarishtam.
Srotogamitva :
Dosha : Vata, tridoshanashak.
Dhatu : Rasa (bodyache), rasayanee, mansa, meda, shukra (virilizer).
Mala : Purisha, worms.
Organs : Heart, stomach (diseases originating in stomach, like vomitting).
Prabhav : Antitoxic, antiinflammatory.
References -
'शालपर्णी स्थिरा सौम्या त्रिपर्णी पीवरी गुहा । विदारिगन्धा दीर्घांघ्रिर्दीर्घपत्रांशुमत्यपि ।।
शालपर्णी गुरुश्छर्दिज्वरश्वासातिसारजित् । शोषदोषत्रयहरी बृंहण्युक्ता रसायनी ।।'
तिक्ता विषहरी स्वादुः क्षतकासकृमिप्रणुत्' (भा.प्र.)
'शालपर्णी रसे तिक्ता गुरुष्णा वातदोषजित् । विषमज्वरमेहार्शः शोथसंतापनाशिनी ।।
'विदारिगन्धा वृष्यसर्वदोषहराणाम् ।' (च. सू. अ. २५)

The following terms used during sacred-fast have become totally Indian - e.g. tea of China (chai), sago of java (sabudana), potatoes of Spain (butata) and dates of Arabastan (khajur).

(110) SHALMALI

Bombax malabaricum Schott and Endl.

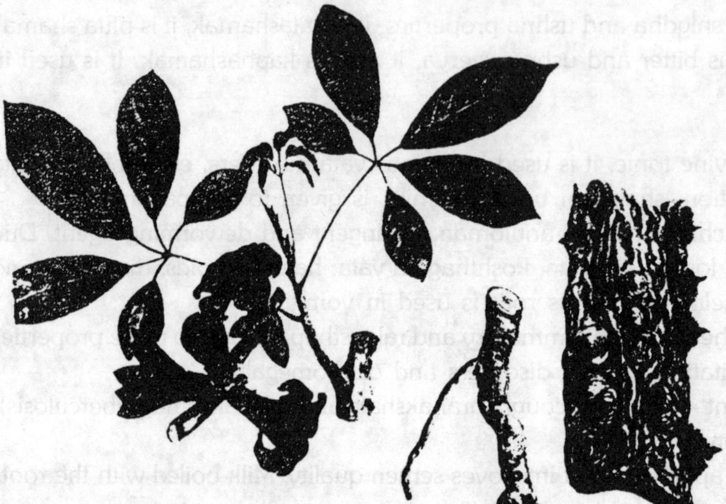

Gana : Purishavirajaneeyam, Kashayaskandha, Shonitasthapan, Vedanasthapan, (C.); Priyangvadi (S.)

Kula : Karpas kula.

Family : Malvaceae. (Latin name for mallow, Malakos = softening by emollient qualities.)

Latin name : Salmalia = (from Sanskrit name); malabarica = of Malabar.

English name: Silk cotton tree.

Sanskrit names : Shalmali, Poorani, Mocha, Raktapushpa, Sthirayu, (long life 6000 years), Toolini (from its fruit soft cotton comes out), Chirajeevi, Raktotpala, Rochana, Kumkuma.

Botanical Description : Big, tall tree having stout thorns. Leaves – like fingers of hand, about 10 to 15 cm. in length. Flowers – red, big petals. Fruits – 13 to 15 cm. in length, like banana, has 5 ovaries, within it is cotton and many black seeds. The seeds contain oil. Flowering season is the end of winter and fruiting occurs in summer. Its bark is cracked by termites and then latex oozes out. This is called as mocharas. It is honey-coloured.

Adulteration : In mocharas – gum of drumstick is added. But drumstick gum is heavy. Root of 1 to 2 years old tree of savaree is used as savar musali (semul musali).

Types : Another tree of semal which has fewer thorns and white flowers is called as koota shalmali (Eriodendron anfractuosom) = Twisted (Erio = wooly, Dendron = Tree). It is rare as compared to the red one.

Habitat : All over India, Sri lanka, Myanmar, Sumatra etc. Koota shalmali is seen more in South India.

Chemical composition : Seeds contain stable oil. Mocharas has tannic acid and gallic acid.

Properties :

Guna : laghu, snigdha, viscous; **Rasa** : sweet; **Vipak** : madhur; **Veerya** : sheeta.

Karma :

Dosha : Due to its snigdha, madhur properties, it acts as vatashaman and due to sheeta veerya, it is pittashaman. Mocharas is astringent and hence kapha pitta shaman. Its root, flowers and fruits are used in vata pitta disorders; mocharas is used in kapha pitta disorders.

A material which bring about rochan, deepan, sangraha and utsarjan, in that order, is mankind friendly.

External uses :
Bark – antiinflammatory, reduces burning sensation; flowers – haemostatic, mocharas – astringent and used in wound healing; thorns - lekhan and improves complexion.
In external bleeding – local application of flower juice or powder is done on the wound. Mocharas is used in oral ulcers and in tooth powders. A paste of the thorns prepared in milk is used for local application on the face in discolouration and hyperpigmentation. It is used in pichcha basti.
Internal uses :
Digestive system : Mocharas is astringent in property. So it is used in malena, diarrhoea, pravahika, raktaj pravahika, grahani, bleeding piles and other bleeding disorders.
Circulatory system : Flowers and mocharas are used as haemostatic.
Respiratory system : As raw fruit is astringent, it tones up the muscles of the throat and hence is used in cough.
Srotogamitva :
Dosha : Vitiates kapha, pittavatanashak.
Mocharas : Kapha pittaghna.
Dhatu : Vitiates blood, reduces meda, shukra (virilizer), rasayani.
Mala : Purisha (reduces motility), (virajaneeya), (malena); mutra - (raw fruit) calculi.
Organs : Liver, spleen.
Mocharas : Vata shaman.
Dhatu : Rakta.
Mala : Purishagrahi (reduces motility).
References -
'असारः शाल्मलीकूटो द्विधा स्थूलाणुकंटकः । पंचषट्वरपर्णो सुवाहो रक्ताब्जपुष्पकः ।।
फलं सतूलं चैतस्य रसो मोचरसाभिधः । षष्टिवर्षसहस्राणि बने जीवति शाल्मलिः ।।'(शि.)
'शाल्मली शीतला स्वाद्वी रसे पाके रसायनी । श्लेष्मला पित्तवातास्रहारिणी रक्तपित्तजित् ।।
मोचास्रावो हिमो ग्राही स्निग्धो वृष्यः कषायकः । प्रवाहिकातिसारामकफपित्तास्रदाहुत् ।।
कूटशाल्मलिकास्तिक्तः कटुकः कफवातनुत् । भेद्युष्णः प्लीहजठरयकृद्गुल्मविषापहः ।।
भूतानाहविबन्धास्रमेदः शूलकफापहः ।' (भा. प्र.)
'शाल्मलिः पिच्छिलो वृष्यो बल्यो मधुरशीतलः ।
कषाश्च लघुः स्निग्धः शुक्रश्लेष्मविवर्धनः ।।' (रा.नि.)
'शाल्मलीपुष्पशाकं तु घृतसैन्धवसाधितम् । प्रदरं नाशयत्येव दुःसाध्यं च न संशयः ।। (भा.प्र.)

(111) SHIGRU
Moringa oleifera Lam.

Gana : Swedopaga, Krumighna, Shirovirechanopaga (seeds), Katukaskandha (bark), Haritak Varga (C.), Varunadi, Shirovirechan (S.)
Kula : Shobhanjan kula.
Family : Moringaceae. In Malayalam, it is known as Muringi.
Latin name : Moringa = (because of above reason); oleifera = oil bearing.
English name : Drumstick plant or Horse.Radish Tree (because its legumes are like the sticks of

When a fire breaks out, one think about a fire-engine to extinguish it. Likewise the mention of amashaya, pittashaya and vatashaya should be associated with vaman, virochan and basti.

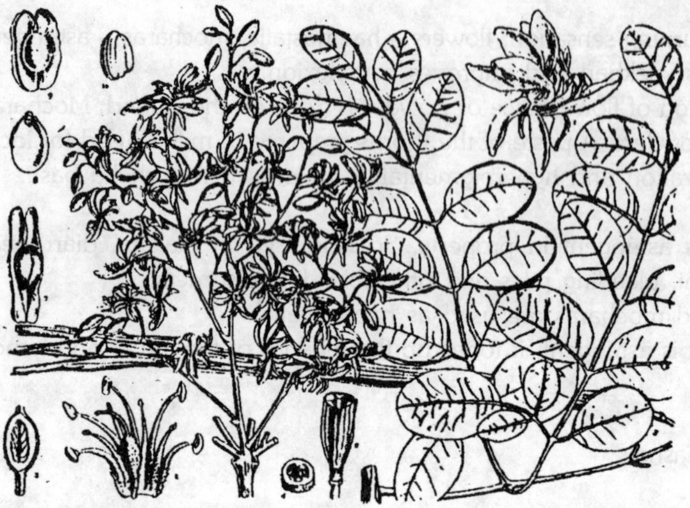

drum).

Sanskrit names : Shobhanjan (having fascinating appearance), Shigru (has sharp property), Teekshnagandha (bark is strong smelling), Mochak (relieves from diseases), Haritshak, Komalpatrak, Bahumoola, Danshamoola, Shigruka, Laghupatra, Moolakparni.

Botanical Description : Tree 7 to 8 mtr. high, with soft bark and wood. Leaves – compound, 14 to 24 cm. in length. Leaflets 6 to 9 in number, 1.25 to 1.5 cm. in length and slightly turned to inferior surface. Flowers - blue in clusters. Fruits – legume 15 to 25 cm.long, have 6 striations longitudinally, green - grey in colour. Seeds – have 3 striations and are winged and bitter in taste. Flowers – come in Feb. and legumes in March and April. These are used as vegetables. It tastes good in Dal, Kadhi, with Besan (gram flour). It contains vitamins – A, B, E, K. Fresh bark has strong odour.

Types : Depending on the types of flowers, it is classified into many types. But Bhavprakash has mentioned 2 types. (1) white and (2) reddish white. The white one is bitter in taste and reddish white is sweet in taste. Reddish white is called as madhu shigru while the white one is called as katu shigru. Katu is available everywhere, while madhu shigru is rare. But it is seen in Bengal (in Malda district), Rajputana and Sindh. Latin name of madhu shigru is Moringa coneanensis Nimmo. In Raja nighantu one more type is described as blue, which is very rare. Now-a-days sweet and bitter shigru are found. The legume of sweet shigru is sweet and that of bitter is bitter to taste. The bark of bitter variety has longitudinal striations. In sweet type, the bark is rough.

Habitat : In India and Myanmar.

Chemical composition : In bark, there is kshar tatva like sphatika, two types of resins, inorganic acid, slimy agent, 8% kshar. In root, there is a bad smelling volatile oil; seeds contain stable, clean, colourless oil 36.6%.

Properties :

Guna : laghu, ruksha, tikshna, sara; **Rasa :** katu; **Vipak :** katu; **Veerya :** ushna.

Karma :

Dosha : As it is laghu, ruksha, tikshna, katu (pungent), it is kaphashamak. By ushna veerya it is vatashaman. Useful in kapha vata disorders.

External uses : A paste of bark and leaves produces burning sensation, is antiinflammatory and acts on abscesses. It is applied topically on inflammation and abscess. Seed powder is the best shirovirechan nasya. Seed powder is administered nasally in headache and heaviness of the head produced by kapha. Seed oil is analgesic and antiinflammatory and hence used in rheumatoid

Why a clove tree (Syzygium aromaticum) flowers after 9 years? An answer to this question is in the following question - why a human female mentruates after 12 years?

arthritis and painful diseases for massage.

Internal uses :

Nervous system : As it is tikshna and ushna, it is a nerve stimulant.The non crystalline part of the bark is very strong and it acts through afferent nerves on the body. Because of this, it causes hypertension, increases heart rate and contracts the blood vessels. It lowers the function of muscles in respiratory as well as digestive system. Dilatation of pupil occurs similar to the action of adrenalin and ephedrin. Tender plant root is useful in epilepsy.

Digestive system : As it is pungent and tikshna, it improves appetite, is digestive, vidahi, grahi (reduces motility), analgesic, antibacterial and deworming agent. Madhu shigru is viscous and sweet and so it is purgative. In unassimilated internal abscess, madhu shigru is used in lunch, drink and in external application also. It is useful in loss of appetite, tastelessness, pain in abdomen, ascites, gulma and worms.

Circulatory system : Due to ushna guna it acts as a stimulant to heart, creates hypertension and is antiinflammatory. It is used in weakness of heart and inflammation.

Respiratory system : Kaphaghna. Useful in kaphaj kasa. Seed powder is useful for shodhan nasya.

Urinary system : As it is ushna, tikshna, it stimulates the kidneys and increases the quantity of urine. It is useful in dysuria and in increased acidity in urine. In calculi its decoction is useful. It is not used in hydronephorsis, as it irritates the kidneys and increases inflammation.

Reproductive system : It stimulates menstruation and as it is ushna and antiinflammatory, it is useful in dysmenorrhoea and obstructed menstruation.

Satmikaran : It controls medoroga and reduces effects of poison. It reduces shukra therefore one should not use it in conditions involving reduced shukra. It acts on shukra but reduces it.

Skin : Tikshna and ushna, induces sweating. Therefore its hot infusion is used in skin diseases. If there are maggots in the wound – fresh bark paste is applied and bandaged on the wound. Due to its smell, all maggots come out. (Turpentine and resin act similarly).

Temperature : Since it is a diaphoretic, its hot infusion is used in fever associated with rigors caused by obstruction of sweat. The legumes of shigru are used as diet in post - pyrexial conditions.

Eyes : The seeds are used for topical application in the eyes. It is useful in eye disorders produced by kapha.

Useful parts : Bark, legume, seed, oil, leaves.

Dose : Bark juice – 1to 2 spoon; bark decoction – 40 to 60 ml.; leaf juice – 2 to 4 spoon; seed powder – 1 gm.

Formulations : Shobhanjanadi powder for external application with water.

Excess intake : As it is ushna, tikshna, it produces raktapitta and burning sensation if taken in excess dose. It is contraindicated in pitta prakriti and raktapitta.

To counteract the effects of excessive intake of shigru, it should always be taken along with milk + ghee or alternatively, milk + ghee should be taken after it is administered. Cow's milk and ghee are more useful for this purpose.

(According to some experts, it is superior to penicillin in preventing inflammation and suppuration in traumatic wounds without any side effects as in penicillin).

__The most suitable vibration in the body may act on mind and work wonders.__

Srotogamitva :
Dosha : Kapha vataghna, vitiates pitta.
Dhatu : Meda (apachi), rakta (spleen), acts on blood, seeds are virilizer, bones – abscess.
Mala : Urine (calculi – root decoction), stool – purgative.
Organs : Heart, kidneys and the body elements where abscess occur.
Prabhav : Antitoxic.
References -
'शोभाञ्जनः शिग्रुतीक्ष्णगन्धकाक्षीवमोचकाः । तद्बीजं श्वेतमरिचं मधुशिग्रुस्तु लोहितः ।।
शिग्रुः सरः कटुः पाके तीक्ष्णोष्णो मधुरो लघुः । दीपनः रोचनो रूक्षः क्षारस्तिक्तो विदाहकृत् ।
संग्राह्यशुक्रलो हृद्यः पित्तरक्तप्रकोपणः । चक्षुष्यः कफवातघ्नो विद्रधिश्वयथुक्रिमीन् ।।
मेदोपचीविषप्लीहगुल्मगण्डव्रणान हरेत् । श्वेतः प्रोक्तगुणो ज्ञेयो विशेषाद्दीपनः सरः ।।
प्लीहानं विद्रधीं हन्ति व्रणघ्नः पित्तरक्तकृत् । शिग्रुवल्कलपत्राणां स्वरसः परमार्तिहत् ।।
चक्षुष्यं शिग्रुजं बीजं तीक्ष्णोष्णं विषनाशनम् । अवृष्यं कफवातघ्नं तन्नस्येन शिरोऽर्तिहृत् ।।' (भा. प्र.)
'शिग्रुतैलानि तीक्ष्णानि लघून्युष्णवीर्याणि कटूनि कटुविपाकानि सराण्यनिलकफकृमिकुष्ठप्रमेहशिरोरोगापहराणि चेति ।' (सू. सु. ४५)
'शिग्रुस्तिक्तःकटुश्चोष्णः कफशोफसमीरजित् । कृम्यामविषमेदघ्नो विद्रधिप्लीहगुल्मनुत् ।। (ध.नि.)
'सोंठ, सुहागा, सेंधा, गाँधी । सहिजन के रस में बरिया बाँधी ।।
सत्तर शूल औ अस्सी बाई । कहे धनन्तर छन मे जाई ।। (लोकोक्ति)
क्वाथश्चशिग्रुमूलोत्थः कटूष्णोऽश्मरिपातनः । वा. चि.
पानभोजनलेपेषु मधुशिग्रुः प्रयोजित ।' वा. चि.
दत्ता वापो यथादोषं अपक्वंहन्ति विद्रधीम् ।। वा. चि.

(112) SHIREESH
Albizzia lebbek Benth.

Gana : Vishaghna, Vedanasthapan, Shirovirechan, Kashayaskandha, (C.) Salsaradi (S.).
Kula : Shimbi kula.
Upakula : Mimosideae - resembling the sensitive plant mimosa (Gk). (Leaves sensitive and fold up on being touched).
Family : Leguminoseae.
Latin name : Albizzia = (Allbeetzy - Italian naturalist), (Pink shireesh or Nemu tree); lebbek = South African name of a similar plant.
Sanskrit names : Shireesh, Sitapushpa, Bhandik, Mrudupushpak, Uddanak, Shuktaru, Lomapushpak, Kapeetan, Shyamal, Shukapriya, Bhandil, Vipra, Plavavangak, Shukrapushpa.
Botanical Description : This tree is big and tall and has a height of 17 to 20 mtrs. These trees are planted on both the sides of the road. Leaves - compound, unctuous and hairy. Leaflet- wide, and there are 4 to 8 pairs. Flowers - white, frangrant and tender. Legume - 15 to 30 cm. long, 1.5 to 3 cm. wide, flat, tough and contains 6 to 10 seeds, which rattle when dried. Seeds - are brownish in colour, flat and circular. In winter leaves shed. Flowering season is monsoon and fruits come in spring (legume).
Types : Two types are seen - 1) white and 2) black (bark). Out of these, white is rare, its bark and stalk are white. Black shireesh is found abundantly and its bark is black.

As in human body the consideration of dosha is important, in plants also the consideration of guna is equally important.

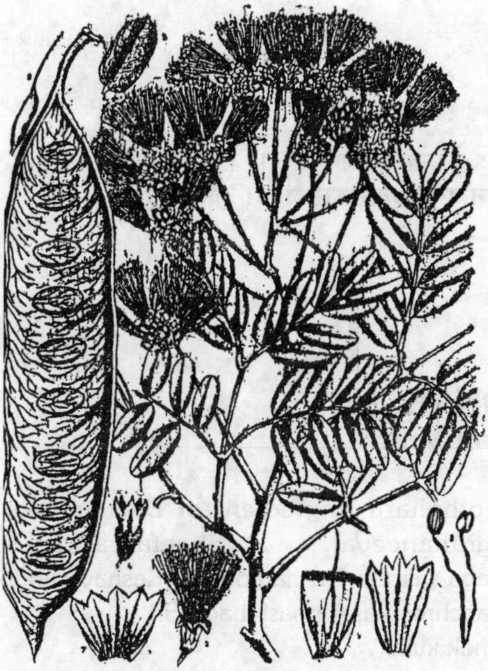

Habitat : Everywhere in India .
Chemical compostion : The bark contains sapponine.
Properties :
Guna : laghu, ruksha, tikshna; **Rasa :** kashaya, bitter, sweet; **Vipak :** katu; **Veerya :** mild ushna.
Karma :
Dosha : Tridoshashamak. It reduces vata by its ushna veerya and kapha pitta by kashaya and tikta rasa. Its overall action is to reduce all the three doshas. Very few dravyas have such action.
External uses : Anti-inflammatory, analgesic, antitoxic, beneficial to complexion, and beneficial to eyes. So used in inflammation, lymphadenopathy etc. Seed paste is applied in kushtha - dermatosis and in wounds, bark paste is applied. In toothache and looseness of tooth - gargling with bark decoction is done. In eye diseases, especially in night blindness, leaf juice or decoction is dropped in the eyes. Rubbed seeds are also used in eyes for application. It is also applied externally in various types of poisoning.
Internal uses :
Digestive system : Astringent, but in high doses vomiting occurs. Bark powder gives strength to the gums.
Circulatory system : Purifies blood, anti-inflammatory, useful in blood diseases, herpes, inflammation, lymphadenopathy. In all these diseases, bark decoction or seed powder is given.
Respiratory system : Shirovirechan (nasya) and kaphaghna. Therefore used in rhinitis, cough etc. In chronic kaphaja jwar seed powder is used for pradhaman nasya (nasal administration). In asthma, flower juice is given with honey and Piper longum (pippali) powder. The fragrance of flowers reduces the headache in migraine.
Reproductive system : It is virilizing. In poor semen quality, seed powder with milk is given for virilization. Flowers are used for delaying ejaculation. In puberty, delayed menstruation is treated with flower boiled in milk.
Skin : In dermatoses, seed powder is used.
Satmikaran : Antitoxic. In organic and inorganic poisoning, bark decoction or seed powder are used.
Parts Used : Bark, seeds, leaves, flowers.
Dose : Bark powder 3 to 6 gm.; seed powder - 1 to 2 gm.; leaf juice -12 to 24 ml.
Formulations : Mahashireesh Agad, Shireesharishta.
Srotogamitva :
Dosha : Tridosha (shaman).
Dhatu : Rasa (skin), rakta (herpes).

Even laboratory animals are not like human beings; no two human beings are alike. The same rule applies to plants too.

Mala : Reduces impurities in wounds.
Prabhav : Antitoxic.
Srotas : Respiratory system (asthma, cough).
References -
'शिरीषो मधुरोऽनुष्णस्तिक्तश्च तुवरो लघुः । दोषशोषविसर्पघ्नः कासव्रणविषापहः ।।' (भा. प्र.)
'तिक्तोष्णो विषहा वर्ण्यस्त्रिदोषशमनो लघुः । शिरीषकुष्ठकण्डूघ्नत्वग्दोषश्वासकासहा ।। (कै.नि.)
शिरीषो विषघ्नानाम् श्रेष्ठः । (च. सू. २५)
प्रभाव 'रसे शिरीषपुष्पस्य सप्ताहं मरिचं सितम् ।
भावितं सर्पदष्टानां नस्यपानाञ्जने हितम् ।। (च. चि. २५)

(113) SHYONAK

Oroxylum indicum Vent.

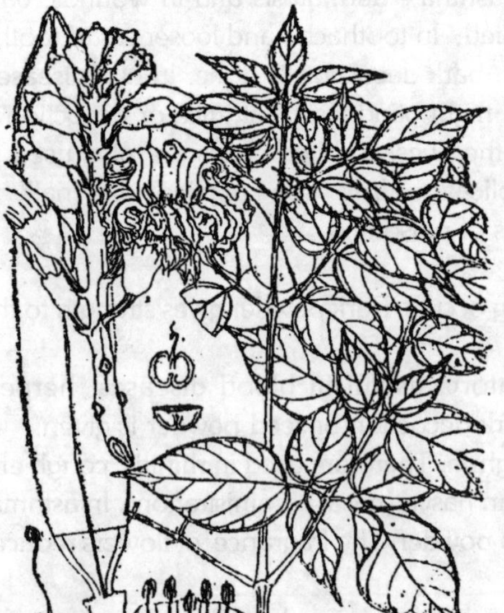

Gana : Shothahara (ingredient of Dashamoola), Purishasangrahaneeya, Sheetaprashaman, Anuvasanopaga (all the Dashamoolas), Kashayskandha (C.), Brihatpanchmoola, Ambashthadi (S.)
Kula : Shyonak kula.
Family : Bigoniaceae = (After the name of Dr. Begon, French patron of Botany).
Latin name : Oroxylum - Oros = mountain; xylon = weed - mountain weed.; indicum = of India.
English name : Indian trumpet flower.
Sanskrit names : Shyonak, Shukanasa, Ruksha, Katwanga, Katanbhar, Mayurjangha, Aralu, Priyajeeva, Kutannata.
Yellow shyonak - Pruthu shimbi, Bhalluk, Deerghavruntak, Peetavruksha, Mandookparna.
Botanical Description : A big tree 10 to 12 m. high. Leaves - compound, 0.5 to 1 mtr. in length and are bird shaped. There is a leaf at the end. Leaflet - 15 cm in length, 9 to 12 cm. broad, having a serrated margin and pointed at the tips. Flowers - stalk is 24 to 30 cms long, bigul shaped, with brinjal coloured flowers at the end of leaflet. Petals - are fleshy and have a bad smell. Legumes - 0.33 to 1 mtr. in length, winged and of breadth 4 to 6 cm. They contain cotton inside, for wind propagation of seeds. Flowers - in rainy season, fruiting in winter. Its wood is soft.
Types : There is another type too - a big tree with leaves like those of neem tree, with a bad smell.
Habitat : Everywhere In India and in Sri lanka.
Chemical composition : Its root bark contains oroxylin. Besides this, one bitter principle, pectin, fats, wax, chlorophyl, astringent principle, citric acid.

Dravya and its rasa, guna, vipak, prabhav, formulation and dose are to be individualized for the human being who is to be treated.

Properties :
Guna : laghu, ruksha; **Rasa :** bitter, astringent; **Vipak :** katu; **Veerya :** sheeta.
Karma :
Dosha : It is tridoshashamak. By its rasa and guna, it reduces kapha, by it sheeta veerya it is pitta shamak and as it reduces amadosha or pitta-kapha, it helps in 'Avrutta vata.' The avruttatwa of kapha and pitta on the vata is reduced by it. It is the speciality of shyonak. It is an extraordinary ingredient of brihatpanchamoola. It is anti-inflammatory and antipyretic.
External uses : As it is antiinflammatory, wound healing, analgesic,it is used in rheumatoid arthritis, osteoarthritis etc. In inflammation and painful diseases, tub bath is taken by its decoction. Its bark juice is used on wounds. Its root bark is boiled in sesame oil and is useful in otorrhoea.
Internal uses :
Nervous system : Useful in vata disorders and rheumatoid arthritis. Shyonak is the best medicine for such disorders.
Digestive system : Due to its bitter taste, it is deepan, pachan, appetizer and vermicidal. Its astringent bark juice is useful in diarrhoea and dysentery as astringent.
Circulatory system : It reduces amadosha in the blood circulation and helps in reducing inflammation. It is the best medicine in rheumatoid arthritis. (Aushadhee Sangraha - Dr. Desai).
Respiratory system : It is useful in kaphaj kasa (cough) and asthma (shwas).
Urinary system : In urinary system, it digests the ama and increases the quantity of urine. It reduces cystitis. It digests ama in the body and excretes dosha out of the body by urine.
Skin : Beneficial in amavata, vatavyadhi etc. as it is a diphoretic. But the disadvantage of it is that, it creates constipation.To counter act this, castor oil must be given along with it.
Temperature : In all types of fever, especially in sannipatic jwar for digestion of ama. By digestion of ama, swedwaha srotas open and diphoresis takes place If doshas are excreted through sweat and urine, fever decreases.
Satmikaran : Weakness due to amadosha gets reduced, increases appetite, digests the food, stomach is cleared, gradually strength increases.
Useful part : Root bark.
Dosage : 10 to 20 ratti; juice - 12 to 20 ml.
Formulations : Shyonak putpak, Brihatpanchamooladi decoction (decoction of bark is not done).
Srotogamitva :
Dosha : Tridoshanashak (sannipat jwara).
Dhatu : Meda (reduces meda), it digests ama in the dhatu.
Mala : Purisha (reduces motility), grahi, root bark is diphoretic.
Organs : Bladder, joints, respiratory system, middle channels.
Respiratory system : Cough, acts on middle channel.
References -
'श्योनाकः शोषणश्च स्यान्नटक्टवंगटुण्टुकः । मण्डूकपर्णपत्रोर्णशुकनासकुटंनटाः ।।
दीर्घवृन्तोऽरलुश्चापि पृथुशिम्बः कटम्भरः । श्योनाको दीपनः पाके कटुकस्तुवरो हिमः ।। ग्राही
तिक्तोऽनिलश्लेष्मपित्तकासामनाशनः ।' (भा. प्र.)

If Tinospora cordifolia is plucked during the month of May, nearly 80% of the essence (satva) can be obtained.

'टिण्टुकः शिशिरस्तिक्तो बस्तिरोगहरः परः । पित्तश्लेष्मामवातातीसारकासारुचुर्जयेत् ।। (ध.नि.)
स्योनाकयुगलं तिक्तं शीतलं च त्रिदोषजित् । पित्तश्लेष्मातिसारघ्नं सन्निपातज्वरापराहम् ।।' (ए. नि.)'

(114) SHANKHAPUSHPI

Convolvulus pluricaulis Chois.

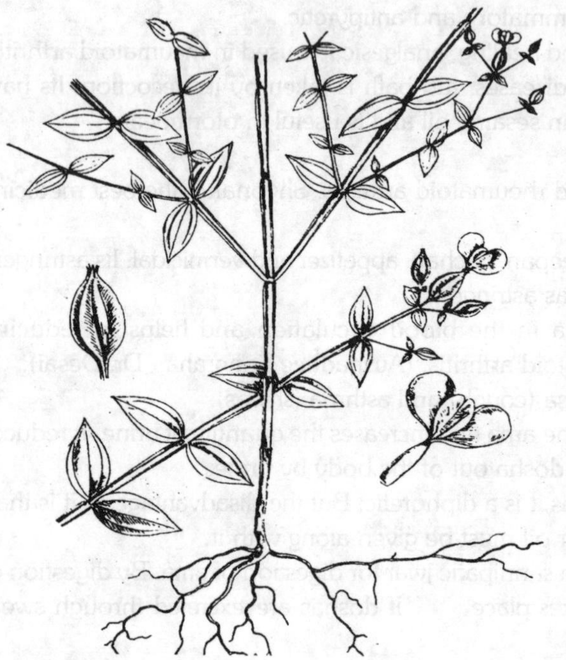

Kula : Trivrita kula.
Family : Convolvulaceae (twiner).
Latin name : Convolvulus (Convolvo = to twine) twinning.; pluri = many, caulis = stem (having many stems).
Sanskrit names : Shankhapushpi (bears flowers like shell), Kshirpushpi (milk-white flowers), Kusum (seeing the flower is auspicious), Supushpa, Medhya, Malavinashini, Shoolaghna, Smrutihita, Varnavilasini.
Botanical Description : This creeper is convula, perennial and with many branches. Stem - slightly quadrangular. Leaves thin, long, with three veins, without stalk and ciliated. Flowers - shell shaped, white. Fruits - small at the top or near the branches. Root - like rope or finger's thickness, 15-30 cm long, whitish or greenish.
Varieties : Three - white, reddish and bluish. But only the white one is used in medicine. Nighantus refer to red variety as sarpakashi and neelpushpi as vishnukranta (ie. Evolvulus alsiniodes).
Habitat : All over India - specially in rocky and open land.
Chemical composition : Cotains sedatives and tranquilisers.
Properties :
Guna : snigdha, pichchil, guru, sara; **Rasa** : kashaya, katu, tikta; **Vipak** : madhur; **Veerya** : sheeta; **Prabhav** : medhya (specific).
(Madhur vipaki though rasa is kashaya, katu and tikta).
Karma :
Dosha : Tridoshahar, but specially vatapittashamak. Snigdha, pichchil, guru gunas and madhur vipak makes it vatashamak, sheeta veerya - pittashamak and katu, tikta, kashaya - kaphashamak.
External uses : Kushthaghna and hair tonic. It is used in the form of paste in skin diseases and siddha oil for hair growth.
Internal uses :
Nervous system : It is a brain tonic, shamak, sedative and therefore it is used in epilepsy, insomnia and giddiness. In schizophrenia, it reduces the severity of attacks by its prabhav (shamak). Fresh

Honey, the best medicine for kapha, wouldn't be there if there were no flowers and the honey-bees.

juice 2-4 tolas overcomes schizophrenia by clearing the bowel.

Digestive system : Katu and tikta rasa improves appetite and digestion and pichchil and madhur vipak helps to improve peristalsis. This action of shankhapushpi is best for loss of appetite, flatulence and other vata conditions of bowel. Its peristaltic action helps to eliminate intestinal toxins and constipation.

Circulatory system : Cardiotonic, haemostatic. Useful in heart diseases, haemoptysis, haemetemesis and hypertension.

Respiratory system : It is an optimum expectorant by virtue of katu, tikta and snigdha property. Therefore it is used in cough caused by vatapitta and hoarseness of voice.

Urinary system : It is diuretic due to sheeta veerya, therefore useful in dysuria and urinary tract infections.

Reproductive system : It is a good aphrodisiac, implantative due to snigdha, pichchil and madhur vipak. In defecitve sperm conditions, uterine debility, abortions and cervical incompetence, shankhapushpi is considered as a good medicine.

Skin : Many skin diseases are cured because of its pittashamak and blood purifying actions. It is also used in syphilis.

Temperature : Sheeta veerya reduces burning sensation and fever accompanied by burning sensation.

Satmikaran : It improves somatic and psychological functioning by purification of malas and dhatus. Rasayan and balya properties make shankhapushpi a multifaceted useful plant. Syrup of shankhapushpi is used in summer to overcome burning micturation.

Parts used : Panchang (whole plant).

Dose : Decoction 20 to 30 ml.; powder 3 to 6 gms.; cold infusion 12 to 50 ml.

Formulations : Shankhapushpi syrup, Amrutadi rasayan. (It is always better to use its juice or sherbat. The identity of shankhapushpi has still not been ascertained.)

Srotogamitva :

Dosha : Vatashaman.

Dhatu : Majja (brain tonic, insomnia).

Mala : Purisha (laxative).

Organ : Brain.

Manovaha srotas : Epilepsy, schizophrenia.

References -

'शंखपुष्पी हिमा तिक्ता मेधाकृत् स्वरकारिणी । ग्रहभूतादिदोषघ्नी वशीकरणसिद्धिदा ।।' (रा.नि.)
शंखपुष्पी सरा स्वर्या कटुस्तिक्ता रसायनी । अनुष्णा वर्णमेधाग्निबलायुः कान्तिदा हरेत् ।।
'कल्कः प्रयोज्यः खलु शंखपुष्प्याः.... । मेध्याविशेषेण च शंखपुष्पी ।।' (च. चि. १)
तत्सेव्यं शंखपुष्पी च यच्च सेव्यं रसायनम् ।' (च. चि. १५)
'शंखपुष्पिकास्वरसा । उन्मादहतो दृष्टाः पृथगेते कुष्टमधुमिश्राः ।।' (चक्र.)
'क्षीरान्नभुक् पिबेत् यत्नात् विष्णुकान्तां सशर्कराम् ।
ऊर्ध्वरक्तार्दितः सम्यक् गव्येन पयसा सह ।।' (शोढल)

The resin (niryas) in the organism of the plant acts mainly as a combining and communication medium as in the human body blood does the same.

(115) SAPTAPARNA

Alstonia scholaris R.Br.

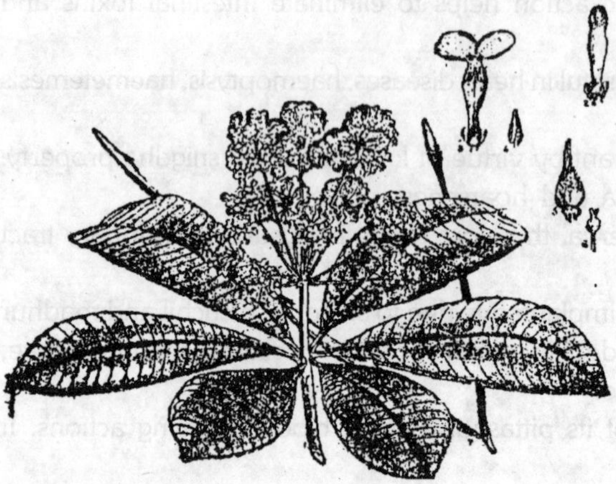

Gana : Tikta and Kashayaskandha, Kushthaghna, Udardaprashman, Shirovirechak (C.); Aragvadhadi, Lakshadi, Adhobhagahara (S.)

Kula : Kutaj kula.

Family : Apocynaceae (Dog's bane = poison).

Latin name : Alstonia = after the name of Dr. Alston, Prof. of Botany at Edinburgh; scholaris = pertaining to a school (Latin) - planks of the tree are used for making blackboards for use in schools.

Sanskrit names : Saptaparna (with 7 leaves), Vishaltvak (thick bark), Sharad (flowers bloom during autumn), Suparnak, Sahachhad, Yugmaparna, Munichhad, Bahuparna, Shalmalipatrak, Madagandha, Gandhiparna.

Botanical Description: This is an evergreen tree measuring 13 to 17 mtrs. in height. Bark - is thick, porous and white in colour. On cutting the bark, a milky white latex oozes out. Leaves - there are 7 leaves in each whorl, 10 to 15 cm. long, 3 to 4 cm. broad. The leaves are dark green in colour towards the apex and whitish towards the nodes. On plucking the leaves, milky white latex oozes out from the nodes. Flowers - the flowering season is autumn. Flowers are greeinsh white in colour, appear in bunches and have a strong odour. Fruits - the fruits are of legume type, measuring 30 cm. in length, flat and crooked. Seeds - are small and white in colour. Soft cotton envelopes both the sides of the seed. On ripening, the fruit bursts and the seeds are dispersed around by being carried with the wind. The tree flowers in autumn and fruits in winter.

Habitat : In the Himalayas, it grows at a height of one thousand mtrs. It is mainly found in Bengal, South India and West coast of India.

Chemical Composition : The bark contains ditamine and also akitannin, akikauchin, akisarin, akitin and akiratin.

Properties:

Guna : laghu, snigdha; **Rasa :** tikta, kashaya; **Vipak :** katu; **Veerya :** ushna.

Karma :

Dosha: Tridoshaghna, especially kaphavatashamak. It is mainly used for the treatment of diseases which arise due to tridosha and kaphavata.

External uses : It is useful in skin diseases and in wounds. The paste of the bark is applied in putrified wounds; tender leaves are first boiled, made into a paste and then applied on the wound.

While deciding the synonyms of the plants, the ancient Rishis have considered 3 doshas and 3 malas, 4 dishas (directions), 6 rasas, 7 colours and 7 dhatus.

Internal uses:

Digestive system : It stimulates the stomach, acts as an appetizer and also improves peristalsis. It is astringent and anthelmintic while the latex acts as a laxative and that is why it is used in ascites.

Decoction or the powder of bark is used for loss of appetite, abdominal pain, abdominal lump and dysentery. Bark and leaves increase appetite. Twigs of the tree are used for brushing teeth as it bacteriocidal. Saptaparna is also useful in thread worms and round worms.

Circulatory system : It acts as a blood purifier and cardiotonic. It is useful in splenomegaly, blood disorders and heart diseases.

Respiratory system : It is helpful in dyspnoea. The powder of flowers is used in headache for nasal administration.

Reproductive system : It improves appetite and is given to women after delivery. Saptaparna decreases fever, increases lactation and provides strength to women after delivery. A mixture of bark of saptaparna + vacha + ginger + is given to women from the first day of delivery to protect her from fever.

Skin : It is useful in skin diseases. Juice of the leaves is helpful in skin diseases and urticaria. Mixture of decoction + chopchini is used in skin diseases.

Temperature : It is antipyretic and is especially useful in malarial fever. Its effect is the same as that of quinine on fever, but has no side effects like those of quinine. It is also helpful in reducing the temperature in fever.

The paste of bark is applied over inflammed joints in chronic arthritis.

Satmikaran :

It acts as a tonic and reduces weakness; it is mainly used for weakness which arises after fever. Bark and leaves increase lactation.

Parts used : Bark, latex, flowers, leaves and extract.

Dose : Leaf juice - 10 to 20 ml.; decoction - 60 to 100 ml.; bark powder - 0.75 to 1.5 gms.; milk - 5 gms.

Formulations : Saptachhadadi kadha, Saptachhadadi taila, Saptaparna satvadi vati.

Srotogamitva :

Dosha: Tridosha (shamak).

Dhatu : Rakta (skin diseases), rasa (fever, lactation).

Mala : Purisha (laxative, worms).

Organ : Heart.

Stomach : Appetizer.

References -

'सप्तपर्णः शाल्मलीसदृशपत्रो गजमदगन्धपुष्पः शरदि विकसनशीलः उच्चैर्वृक्षः ।' (डल्हण)

'सप्तपर्णो गुच्छपुष्पो बहुत्वक् शाल्मलीच्छद्ः ।' (शि.)

'त्रिदोषशमनो हृद्यः सुरभिर्दीपनः सरः । शूलगुल्मकृमीन् हन्ति कुष्ठं शाल्मलिपत्रकः ।' (ध.नि.)

'सप्तपर्णो व्रणश्लेष्मवातकुष्ठास्रजन्तुजित् । दीपनः श्वासगुल्मघ्नः स्निग्धोष्णस्तुवरः सरः ।।' (भा.प्र.)

Would not the plants be cursing the " gentle men", who bring about their extinction by totally uprooting them, with a simlar fate?

(116) SARPAGANDHA

Rauwolfia serpentina Benth Ez Kurzaa.

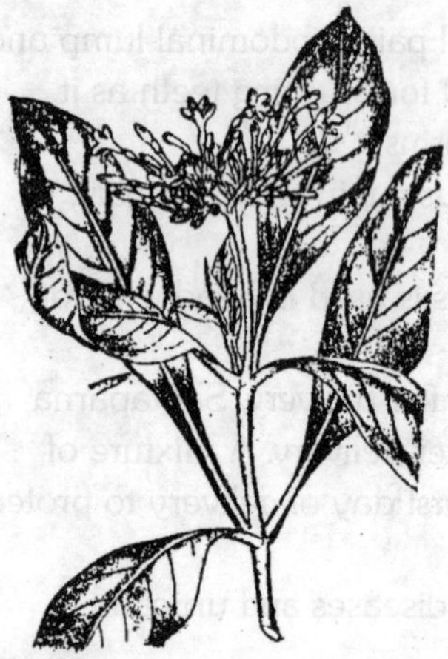

Gana : Aparajita (S.)

Kula : Kutaja kula.

Family : Apocynaceae (poisonous to dogs).

Latin name : Rauwolfia = Leonard Rauwolf - name of a physician at Augsberg, (Bavaria); serpentina = pertaining to serpents.

Sanskrit names : Sarpagandha (smell of serpents), Sarpakshi, Dhawalavitapa (pale bark), Nakuli, Sarpaangi.

Botanical Description : A shrub, 15 cm to 1 mtr. high. Trunk - bark is white with thin hair on it and 10 to 22 cms. long and 4 to 6 cms. broad. Leaves - light green on the lower aspect and dark green on the upper aspect, soft to touch. Flowers - white, pink or bluish white, around 3 cms. in size. One branch has many flowers in a bunch. Fruits - pea-sized, red or blue and 2 cms. in size. Flowering occurs in summer whereas fruiting occurs in winter. Roots - finger sized, thick. On breaking, it is circular with centripetal lines. Roots are haphazard and 48 cms. long.

Habitat : All over India, mostly in Bihar, Bengal, Konkan and Uttar Pradesh. Also found in Burma, Sri lanka, Java and Andamans.

Chemical composition : It contains salt, resin, white juice, gum, potassium carbonate, phosphate, calcium, caustic and manganese. In addition to these, there are about twenty five elements usually observed.

Properties :

Guna : ruksha; **Rasa :** tikta; **Vipak :** katu; **Veerya :** ushna; **Prabhav :** sedative, effective in mania and convulsions.

Karma :

Dosha : It is ushna, kaphavatashamak. Pittashamak by tikta rasa.

External uses : Juice of leaves can be applied to the eyes as a remedy for corneal opacity.

Internal uses :

Nervous systems : Being analgesic, sedative, vatashamak, it is used in insomnia and irritative conditions of the nervous systems. As it is used in mental disturbance, it is known as 'pagalpan ki jadi or pagalki buti'.

Digestive system : Because of ushna veerya and tikta guna, it acts as an appetizer, digestive, cholagogue, anthelmintic. Hence it is used in loss of appetite, helminthiasis etc. For pain in abdomen, 1 part of sarpagandha roots +2 parts of bark of kutaja +3 parts of roots of castor mixed with milk is given.

Circulatory system : Its salt reduces the heart rate and dilates the blood vessels with lowering of blood pessure. Because of this special property of reducing the blood pressure, it is a universally known medicine. Along with reducing blood pressure it causes drowsiness, reduces giddiness and mental tension. There is no other side effect. It is very effective on mental symptoms arising from hypertension. This is the reason why it is popular in the market as 'pagalki dava'.

Reproductive system : It reduces libido and increases menstrual bleeding. So it is used for priapism and excessive libido. It reduces pain of dysmenorrhoea. It is also used to increase uterine contraction during labour.

Temperature : Because of its tikta rasa it is amapachak as well as antipyretic, especially effective in fever caused by vata pitta, contageous fever and insomnia.

Satmikaran : It is antidote to snake bite.

Parts used : Roots (It is more useful when it is given with fragrant substance).

Dose : For hypertension 0.5 to 0.75 gms. of root powder, for insomnia 1 to 2 gms. and for mental condition 1.5 to 3 gms. are used. Reserpine alkaloid isolated from the plant is far more potent than panchang.

Formulations : Sarpagandhadi churna, Sarpagandha yoga, Sarpagandha vati (Maheshwari vati).

Precautions : It should be used only on established disease with mental disturbance. It should be used with caution in patients who are mentally as well as physically weak. The result of the medicine is expected within a week but within 3 to 6 weeks results are definitely seen. After stopping the medication its effect is washed out in 1 to 3 weeks. The blood pressure fluctuates according to change of body conditions, which does not happen with this medicine. It causes diarrhoea and bad dreams if given in a larger dose. Sarpagandha sometimes causes blocking of nose, weight gain, reduced libido and increased intestinal motility.

Contraindications : Bronchial asthma, duodenal ucler, hyperacidity, renal pain and mental instability.

Adulteration : Supply is much less than demand, so there are chances of adulteration.

Srotogamitva :

Dosha : Kaphavataghna.

Dhatu : Majja (sedative), rakta.

Mala : Purisha (laxative).

Organs : Heart, brain (manas - manovahastrotas - major effect).

Prabhav : Vishaghna - useful on snake bite, snakes which are commonly found in Konkan.

Orally : 10 to 20 gms. of root powder dissolved in cold water is given which is also locally applied on the affected area.

References -

'कुक्कुटी सर्पगन्धा च तथा काणविषाणिके । नैपाली हरितालञ्ञ रक्षोघ्ना ये च कीर्तिता ।। (सु. उ. ६०)
'वर्षासु छत्राकारा' (डल्हण)
ईषन्नीलारुणसुमदला पुष्पिता ग्रीष्मकाले । वर्षाकाले फलपरिचितिं नीलरक्तां दधाति ।।
मूलं यस्या हरिणधवलं स्थूलमन्त:स्थचक्रम् । चन्द्राख्या सा धवलविटपा सर्पगन्धा प्रसिद्धा ।।
सर्पगन्धाऽतितिक्तोष्णा रूक्षा कटुविपाकिनी । दीपनी पाचनी रुया शूलप्रशमनी सरा ।।
कफवातहरा निद्राप्रदा हृदवसादिनी । कामावसादिनी चैव हन्ति शूलज्वरकृमीन् ।।
अनिद्रां भूतमुन्मादमपस्मारं भ्रमं तथा । अग्निमान्ध्यं विषं रक्त-वाताधिक्यं व्यपोहति ।।' (स्व.)

Eclipta alba is a plant which, while growing in polluted and decaying soil, improves the environment. One wonders as to why not this plant also correct ecological damage in the human body?

(117) SARIVA

Hemidesums indicus R. Br.

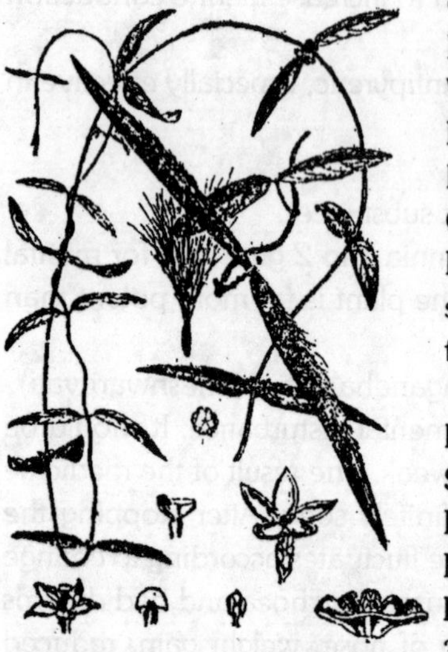

Gana : Stanyashodhan, Purishasangrahaneeya, Jwarahara, Dahaprashaman, Madhuraskandha (C.); Sarivadi, Vidarigandhadi, Vallipanchamool (S.)

Kula : Ark kula.

Family : Asclepiadaceae (milk weed), named after Askleplos - God of medicine.

Latin name : Hemi desmos - Half bond, so named in allusion to the subconnate filaments at their base - joint pods and connected stamens; indicus = of India

English name : Indian sarsaparila.

Sanskrit Names : White variety - Sariva, Sharda, Gopa, Dhavalsariva, Shariva, Nagjivha, Dhavala. Black variety - Krishnamula, Krishna, Chandansariva, Bhadra.

Botancial Description : It is a thin twisted creeper of length 1.5 - 3 mtrs. Leaves - compound and are of various sizes having length 3-12 cms. and breadth 1- 4 cms. Ventral surface of leaf is white with white veins on the dorsal surface with pointed ends. Flowers - arise from the nodes in bunches and are blue-green. Fruits - horn shaped at both ends, 12-15 cms. in size. Soft cotton comes out of the fruit. Root and stem are red externally and white internally. Fresh roots have camphor-like fragrance. Roots are deep and tapering.

Varieties : White and black. Black sariva is grey with purple veins. Two different plants are being used commercially as black sariva viz. 1) Cryptolepis buchanana Roem Schnlt. - its leaves are long, big, purple and when the leaves are broken, a sticky latex oozes out so this creeper is called jambupatrasariva. The other variety, Ichnocarpus frutescenes R.Br., belongs to the kutaja kula. Its leaves are small, close together and oblong. Fruits do not have any fragrance. Sariva which is without fragrance should not be used.

Habitat : All over India, mainly Bengal, Bihar, Maharashtra, Kerala and Sri lanka.

Chemical composition : It contains a substsance called coumarine, volatile oil, yeast and saponin.

Properties :

Guna : guru, snigdha; **Rasa :** madhur, tikta; **Vipak :** madhur; **Veerya :** sheeta.

Karma :

Dosha : Tridoshashamak. Vatashaman by madhur and snigdha, pittashamak by sheeta veerya and kaphashamak by tikta rasa.

External uses : Antiinflammatory, soothing, so used in burning sensation and inflammation. Juice is used in conjunctivitis.

Internal uses :

Digestive system : Being appetizer, digestive and laxative, it is used in the treatment of loss of appetite, diarrhoea, dysentery and mainly in malena.

Plants too suffer from infection, fluid loss, drying, infertility etc. Vrikshayurveda has considered all this.

Circulatory system : It is a blood purifier and antiinflammatory. Sariva is the best medicine for blood disorders, gout, soft chancre, secondary stage of syphilis, chornic rheumatoid arthritis, filariasis and cervical lymphadenitis.

Respiratory system : Being kaphaghna it is used in cough and asthma.

Reproductive system : Purifies breast milk, helps in conception. Decoction of sariva roots taken in pregnancy improves the complexion of the new born. It is useful in menorrhagia, leucorrhoea and abortion. It improves mobility of sperm. It cures lactating disorders.

Urinary system : It is a diuretic, increases urination by 2 to 4 times without affecting the kidneys. So used in dysuria and pittaj prameha.

Skin : Used in skin diseases, erysipelas, impetigo etc. and is used in blood and skin related disorders.

Temperature : Antipyretic and refrigerant (used in pittaj jwar and burning sensation). Hot infusion is given in raktagatjwar.

Satmikaran : Sariva is the best rejuvenator for skin. Useful in weakness, anaemia and tuberculosis. It also acts as an antidote.

Parts used : Bark of the root.

Dosage : Hot infusion -50 to 100 ml.; paste - 3 to 6 gms.

Mostly, decoction is not recommended since it contains volatile oils which may evapourate. It should be used in the from of sheeta, powder and hot infusion.

Formulations : Sarivadi phant, Sarivadi vati, Sarivadyavaleha, Sarivadyasav.

Phant should be started before pregnancy, since it prevents abortions and miscarriages caused by syphilis and it should be continued during pregnancy to improve the complexion of the new born. (Aushdhi sangraha, Dr. W.G. Desai). It acts better with guduchi.

Srotogamitva :

Dosha : Tridoshaghni.

Dhatu : Shukra (aphrodisiac), rakta (skin disorders), rasa (fever), meda (meha), rasayani - rasa, purifies lactation.

Mala : Purisha (diarrhoea), mutra (diuretic), sweda (diaphoretic).

Organ : Uterus (menorrhagia), fair complexion of new born baby.

References -

सारिवा दाडिमीपत्रा श्वेतरेखांकितच्छादा। दुग्धगर्भा शिंबिफला तूलिनी कृष्णवल्लरी।। (शि.)
सारिवा जम्बूपत्रा दुग्धगर्भा वल्ली स्वनामप्रसिध्दा कृष्णसारिवा.. चन्दनगंधा । (डल्हण.)
सारिवायुगलं स्वादु स्निग्ध शुक्रकरं गुरु । अग्निमांद्यारुचिश्वासकासामिवषनाशनम् ।।
दोषत्रप्रदरज्वरातीसारनाशनम् । (भा. प्र.)
सारिवे द्वे तु मधुरे पित्तवातास्त्रनाशने । कण्डूकुष्ठज्वरहरे मेहदुर्गनेधनाशने ।। (ध. नि.)
अनन्ता संग्राहकरक्तिपत्तप्रशमनानां श्रेष्ठ । (च. सू. २५)

Just like the human beings, the plants too must have the rules of vishamashan (abnormal intake), e.g. Ananshan, Adhyashana, Samushan (A thought !)

(118) HARIDRA
Curcuma longa Linn.

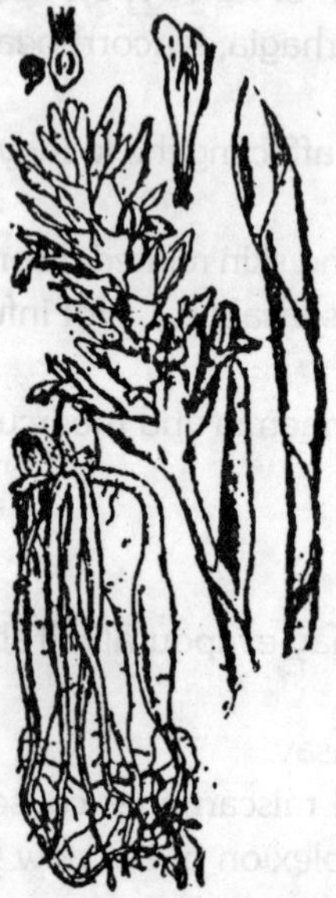

Gana : Kushthaghna, Tiktaskandha, Kandughna, Vishaghna, Shirovirechan (C.); Haridradi, Mustadi , Shleshmasanshaman (S.)
Kula : Haridra kula.
Family : Scitaminae (used with food stuff and condiments (zingiberae).
Latin name : Curcuma = Arabic name kurkum; longa = long.
English name : Turmeric.
Sanskrit names : Haridra (the one which improves skin complexion), Harita, Jayanti, Kanchani (which gives colour of gold), Nisha, Krumighna (which kills worms), Yoshitpriya.
Botanical Descripition : Annual shrub, rhizome grows underground. Leaves are 30-40 cms. in length and they smell like ginger. The petiole is long and broad like leaves and it smells like mango. The stalk of the flower is 12-16 cms. long and yellow flower grows at the tip. Fruit- oval with deep yellow pulp. The flowering of the plant occurs in the beginning of rainy season.
Habitat : All over India. In Maharashtra, Sangli is an important marketing centre. When stored in basement, it is well preserved for longer period.
Chemical composition : 1% volatile oil, resin, curcumin is responsible for its colour. Turmeric oil has a peculiar odour and taste.
Porperties :
Guna : ruksha, laghu; **Rasa :** tikta, katu; **Vipak :** katu; **Veerya :** ushna.
Karma :
Dosha : It is kaphavatanashak, pittasarak by ushna veerya, pittashamak by tikta rasa. Commonly used for disorders caused by tridoshas.
External uses : Local application of turmeric is antiinflammatory, analgesic and complexion enhancer. It cures skin disorders, has wound cleaning and healing properties. Turmeric smoke relieves hiccups, lowers respiration and also relieves pain caused due to scorpion bite. It is very strong in nature. Its paste acts as an antidote. Those who develope cough and other respiratory disorders by drinking milk can be treated by turmeric.
Internal uses :
Nervous system : Analgesic by ushna veerya. In cases of injury, a mixture of turmeric and jaggery administered orally reduces pain and promotes circulation.
Digestive system : Turmeric is better in taste, appetizer, laxative, cholagogue and anthelmintic. Because of these properties it is used for treating loss of appetite, hepatitis, constipation, ascites and worms. There is a wrong belief that turmeric causes jaundice or it is harmful in jaundice.
Circulatory system : Turmeric stimulates blood formation, circulation and it is also haemostatic.

The energy for work, in a human being, varies in different stages of life like childhood, youth and old age. It is possible that plants too may have similar changes (An idea!)

Turmeric is useful in treating anaemia, bleeding disorders and other blood diseases.

Respiratory system : Because of its tikta and tikshna properties, turmeric is useful as an expectorant. Kapha (mucous) developed due to drinking milk and other ailments due to kapha can be treated with turmeric. Inhalation of turmeric smoke reduces kapha.

Urinary system : Turmeric is a good antidiuretic but this action is carried out by digestion of ama, kapha and meda. Turmeric should be used in the form of decoction or powder in prameha. Bhasma of tin triturated with turmeric is an effective remedy for prameha.

Reproductive system : Haridrakhanda pak is administered in postpartum period because of its purifying effect on uterus and breast milk. Turmeric is also useful in shukrameha.

Skin : Turmeric is used in several skin diseases. It improves skin complexion. Itching and skin eruptions due to sheetapitta can be treated with turmeric. It is also useful in pruritus and urticaria.

Temperature : Because of its pittashamak and amapachak properties, turmeric is useful in high fever.

Satmikaran : Turmeric reduces and helps in treating weakness.

Parts used : Rhizome.

Dosage : 10-15 ml or powder 1-3 gm.

Formulations : Haridrakhanda.

Haridra is auspicious and leads the list in rituals of marriage etc. Kumkum is prepared from turmeric. Application of turmeric on the body before marriage is considered auspicious.

Srotogamitva :

Dosha : Kaphaghna, pittaghna.

Dhatu : Rasarakta (varnya), meda (urinary disorders), raktameda (anaemia), rakta (skin disorders).

Mala : Vermicidal.

Organs : Uterus, bladder.

Special property : Antidote.

References -

'हरिद्रा काञ्चनी पीता निशाख्या वरवर्णिनी । कृमिघ्ना हलदी योषित्प्रिया हट्टविलासिनी ।।
हरिद्रा कटुका तिक्ता रूक्षोष्णा कफपित्तनुत् । वर्ण्या त्वग्दोषमेहास्त्रशोषपाण्डुव्रणापहा ।।' (भा.प्र.)
'हरिद्रा तु रसे तिक्ता रूक्षोष्णा विषकुष्ठनुत् । मेहकण्डूव्रणान् हन्ति देहवर्णविधायिनी ।।
विशोधनी कृमिहरा पीनसारुचिनाशिनी ।' (ध.नि.)

(119) HARITAKI
Terminalia chebula Retz.

Gana : Triphala, Amalakyadi, Parushak, Trivrutt, Prajasthapana, Jwaraghna, Kushthanghna, Kasaghna, Arshoghna.

Kula : Haritaki kula.

Family : Combrataceae (after butterfly).

Latin name : Terminalia = proceeding from the extremity at the end; chebula = distorted from

If Ayurvedic Vaidyas were to be progressive, sophisticated, forword looking, updated, then they must learn to change with the evolving world.

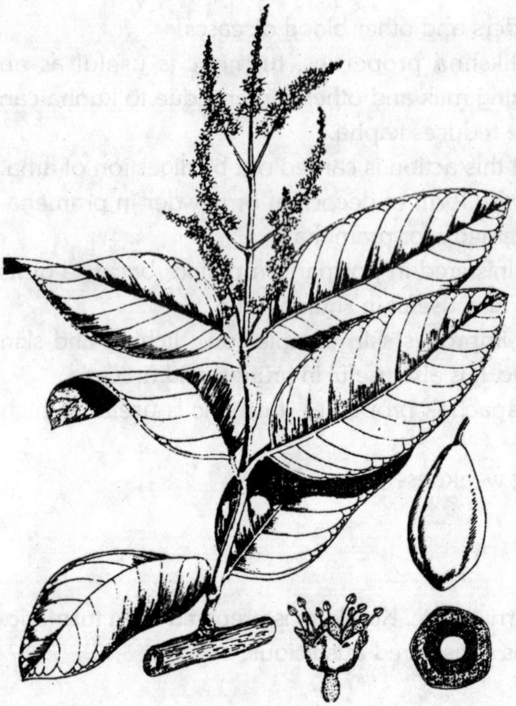

of the word kabul.

English name : Myrobalans; Chebulic myrobalan.

Sanskrit names : Haritaki, Haimamati, Shiva, Pathya, Rohini, Kayashta, Shreyasi, Chedanika, Pachani.

Botanical Descripition : A big tree, 25 to 30 mtrs in height. Its wood is hard and bulky. Leaves are 10-30 cm in length and are pointed. The vasculature of the leaves has 6 to 8 pairs of veins. The inferior aspect of the leaves show two small nodules near its attachment with the stalk. The flowers have short stalks, white or yellow in colour and have a strong smell. Fruits are 3 to 6 cms in length. Initially these are green but on ripening, they become yellowish brown. Each fruit contains one seed. Seeds are oval and hard. On breaking the shell of the seed, an oval shaped pulp is obtained.

Varieties : Depending on the fruits, haritaki is classified into seven types. Of these types, a type called vijaya is considered to be the best.

1) Vijaya - in Vindhya - oval in shape.
2) Rohini - found everywhere, round in shape.
3) Pootana - Sindh - small and less bulky.
4) Amruta - Champaranya - bulky .
5) Abhaya - Champadesha - fruit has five lines on it (eye diseases).
6) Jeevanti - Saurashtra - yellow in colour.
7) Chetaki - found in the Himalayas - having three lines on it.

In practice, however, three types of haritaki are found viz. 1) Bala haritaki 2) Chambhari (rangari) haritaki and 3) Survari haritaki. When the fruit of haritaki falls off from the tree, the seed gets hard, it is called bala haritaki. Sometimes, the fruits are plucked and dried while the seeds have not hardened; this is also called bala haritaki. Chambhari haritaki is an immature fruit of haritaki, whereas a fully mature fruit of haritaki is called survari haritaki. A fruit of haritaki which doesn't float in water, which is fresh, smooth, bulky, round in shape and weighs at least 26 grams is considered ideal for medicinal use.

Fruit - Initially is round in shape and is smooth but on drying 5 striae develope on it.

Habitat : Haritaki is found almost everywhere in India. This tree grows at places up to a height of about 2000 mtrs. from the sea level.

Guna : laghu, ruksha; **Rasa :** five rasas (lavana rasa is absent but kashaya rasa is predominant); **Vipak :** madhur; **Veerya :** ushna; **Prabhav :** tridoshahar.

Karma :

Dosha : By virtue of its madhur, tikta and kashaya rasa, it is pittaghna, by its katu, tikta and kashaya rasa, it is kaphaghna and by its amla and madhur rasa, it is vataghna. Haritaki is particularly vatashamak. It is helpful in many tridoshajanya diseases, particularly useful as a rasayan in vatavyadhi. Haritaki, which lacks lavana rasa, when given in combination with lavana rasa, acts as kaphaghni. It acts as pittaghni in combination with sugar and vataghni when given with ghee or gur (jaggery). Roasted haritaki can be used in tridoshaj diseases.

External uses : Local application of haritaki is antiinflammatory. In conjunctivitis, it can be used for application on the eyelids. A decoction of haritaki is used for washing wounds and also used for gargling in diseases of the mouth and throat.

Internal uses :

Nervous system : Useful in weakness of the nerves and brain as well as in vata disorders and diminished vision.

Digestive system : Useful in loss of appetite, pain in the abdomen, constipation, gulma, ascites, haemorrhoids, hepatomegaly, splenomegaly and parasites. It relieves constipation in chronic abodminal diseases and also helps in digestion of "ama". The bark of haritaki, if eaten after chewing it properly in the mouth, improves digestion. Powdered haritaki reduces constipation. A fine powder of haritaki is used as a tooth powder. It strengthens the gums.

Circulatory system : Since haritaki is raktagami (exhibiting much action on rakta dhatu), it is used in weakness of the heart, vatarakta and other disorders of the blood.

Respiratory system : Rhinitis (due to constipation), cough, hoarseness of voice, hiccups and dyspnoea are relieved by haritaki as it reduces congestion.

Reproductive system : Useful in shukrameha, leucorrhoea and acts as a uterine tonic.

Urinary system : Useful in dysuria, retention of urine, calculus (Haritakyasthi siddha dugdha) and kaphaj prameha.

Skin : Useful in erysipelas and other skin disorders, haritaki prevents accumulation of pus in skin diseases and acts as a rasayana. Haritaki + oil is extremely helpful in healing of wounds (especially in burns).

Temperature : Useful in typhoid fever and also chronic fever.

Restorative effect : Haritaki acts as a rejuvenator (by clearing the body of various malas). But for producing its rasayan effects, it needs various supportive dravyas in different seasons. Varsha (monsoon) - saindhav, sharad - sugar, hemant (winter) - sunthi, shishir - pippali, vasant (spring) - honey and greeshma (summer) - gur (jaggery).

Purgation induced by haritaki is relieved on its own. Bala haritaki is useful in haemorrhoids. It helps in clearing the bowels.

Part used : Fruit (various preparations of the ripe fruit).

Dose : 3 to 6 gms for shodhan (purgation); 1 gm for use as rasayana. Bala haritaki is given in a dose of 1 to 3 gms (Bala haritaki is not used as a rasayan since it is immature as far as its rasas are concerned.)

Formulations : Abhayadi modak, Abahayarishta, Pathyadivati, Pathyadikadha, Vyaghriharitaki leha, Agastiharitaki leha, Gandharvaharitaki churna.

Eventhough haritaki has excellent medicinal uses yet, considering its ruksha properties, it should not be used in patients who are low, malnourished, debilitated, who have lost considerable amount of

Just like in the human beings, in plants too - various stages of digestion - viz. Prapak, Vipak and Sthoola sookshma paka may be present.

blood (through blood letting), and pregnant women.
Vijaya - in all diseases; rohini - used in healing of wounds; pootana - for local application; amruta - for shodhana (removal of vitiated doshas form the body); abhaya - in diseases of the eyes; jeevanti - useful in all diseases.
The fruit of haritaki contains five rasas :
1) madhur (sweet) - the fruit pulp.
2) amla (sour) - the bulky portion of the fruit.
3) tikta (bitter) - seed.
4) katu - the covering of the fruit.
5) kashaya (astringent) - the hard portion of the seed.
Thus haritaki is pancharasatmak. Haritaki is a medicinal herb yet the Ayurvedic texts emphasize the use of haritaki as a medicine which has to be taken regularly. Regularizing all the normal functions of the body is also an important function of haritaki. Survari haritaki, chambhari (or rangari) haritaki and bala haritaki are the types of haritaki used in practice.
Srotogamitva :
Dosha : Haritaki is tridoshanashak by virtue of its prabhav, yet it is more effective on vata kapha.
Dhatu : Rasa, majja (brain tonic), rakta, mansa, rasayani, meda, asthi, shukra (through prolonged use, it increases the reproductive power).
Mala : Purisha (mild laxative), mutra (calculus) (dysuria).
References -
१.'विजया रोहिणी चैव पूतना चामृताभया ।
जीवन्ती चेतकी चेति पथ्यायाः सप्त जातयः ।।' (भा.प्र.)
२.'विन्ध्याद्रौ विजया हिमाचलभवा स्याच्चेतकी पूतना
सिन्धौ स्यादथ रोहिणी तु विजया जाता प्रतिस्थानके ।।
चम्पायाममृताभया च जनिता देशे सुराष्ट्राह्वये।
जीवन्ती च हरीतकी निगदिताः सप्त प्रभेदाः बुधैः ।।' (रा.नि.)
१.नवा स्निग्धा घना वृत्ता गुर्वी क्षिप्ता च याम्भसि । निमज्जेत् सा सुप्रशस्ता कथितातिगुणप्रदा ।।
नवादिगुणयुक्तत्वं तथैवात्र द्विकर्षता । हरीतक्याः फले यत्र द्वय तच्छ्रेष्ठमुच्यते ।।' (भा. प्र.)
२.पथ्याया मज्जनि स्वादुः स्नायावम्लो व्यवस्थितः
वृन्ते तिक्तस्त्वचि कटुरस्थिस्थस्तुवरो रसः ।। (भा. प्र.)
३.स्वादुतिक्तकषायत्वात् पित्तहृत् कफहृत्तु सा । कटुतिक्तकषायत्वादम्लत्वाद् वातहृच्छिवा ।। (भा. प्र.)
आयुर्वेदीय ग्रंथांतून त्रिफला स्वरूपात हिरडा पदोपदी वापरलला आढळून येतो आणि ते सकारण आहे. एवढे बहुकल्प, बहुगुणसंपन्न व योग्य औषध अन्य नाही. म्हणून हिरड्याचे स्थान सर्वश्रेष्ठ आहे.
'वासादलो द्रुमोऽद्रिस्थः फलं तस्य हरीतकी ।' (शि.)
'व्रणमुष्णं सरं मेध्यं दोषघ्नं शोथकुष्ठनुत् । कषायं दीपं चाम्लं चक्षुष्यं चाभयाफलम् ।।'(सु. सू. ४६)
'हरीतकी पञ्चरसाऽलवणा तुवरा परम् । रूक्षोष्णा दीपनी मेध्या स्वादुपाका रसायनी ।।
चक्षुष्या लघुरायुष्या बृंहणी चानुलोमनी । श्वासकासप्रमेहार्शः कुष्ठशोथोदरकृमीन् ।।
वैसर्प्यग्रहणीरोगविबन्धविषज्वरान् । गुल्माध्मानव्रणच्छर्दिहिक्काकण्ठहृदामयान् ।।
कामलां शूलमानाहं प्लीहानं च यकृद्वदम् । अश्मरीं मूत्रकृच्छ्रं च मूत्राघातं च नाशयेत् ।। (भा. प्र.)
'उन्मीलिनी बुद्धिबलेन्द्रियाणां निर्मूलिनी पित्तकफानिलानाम् ।
विस्रंसिनी मूत्रशकृन्मलानां हरीतकी स्यात् सह भोजनेन ।।' (भा. प्र.)

God wanted initially to create only plants but somewhere he made a mistake and moving animals too were created.

‘अन्नपानकृतान् दोषान् वातपित्तकफोद्भवान् ।
हरीतकी हरत्याशु भुक्तस्योपरि योजिता ।।’ (भा. प्र.)
‘हरीतकी पंचरसा च रेचनी कोष्ठामयघ्नी लवणेन वर्जिता ।
रसायनी नेत्ररुजापहारिणी त्वगामयघ्नी किल योगवाहिनी ।।’ (रा.नि.)
‘हरीतकी पथ्यानाम् श्रेण्ठा ।’ (च. सू. २५)
‘हरीतकीं पञ्चरसामुष्णामलवणां शिवाम् । दोषानुलोमनीं लघ्वीं विद्याद्दीपनपाचनीम् ।।
आयुष्यां पौष्टिकीं धन्यां वयसः स्थापनीं पराम् । सर्वदोषप्रशमनीं बुद्धिन्द्रियबलप्रदाम् ।।
कुष्ठं गुल्ममुदावर्त्तं शोषं पाण्ड्वामयं मदम् । अर्शांसि ग्रहणीदोषं पुराणं विषमज्वरम् ।।
हृद्रोगं सशिरोरोगमतिसारमरोचकम् । कासं प्रमेहमानाहं प्लीहानमुदरं नवम् ।।
कफप्रसेकं वैस्वर्य वैवर्ण्यं कामलां कृमीन् । श्वयथुं तमकं छर्दि क्लैब्यमंगावसादनम् ।।
स्रोतोविवन्धान् विविधान् प्रलेपं हृदयोरसोः । स्मृतिबुद्धिप्रमोहं च जयेच्छीघ्रं हरीतकी ।।’ (च. चि. १ -२९ ते ३४)
‘प्रमथ्या लेखनी लघ्वी मेध्या चक्षुर्हिता सदा । मेहकुष्ठव्रणच्छर्दिशोफवातास्रकृच्छ्रजित् ।।
वातानुलोमनी हृद्या सेन्द्रियानां प्रसादनी संतर्पणकृतान् रोगान् प्रायो हन्ति हरीतकी ।।’ (ध.नि.)

(120) HINGU
Ferula foetida Linn.

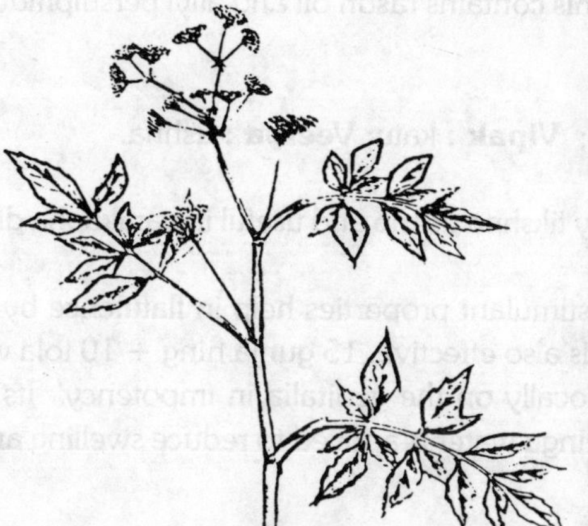

Gana : Sangnyasthapan, Deepaniya, Katukaskandha (C.) Pippalyadi, Ushakadi (S.)

Kula : Mandukparni kula.

Family : Umbellifereae, Umbel = bearing flowers with stalks nearly equal in length, spring from common centre.

Latin name : Ferula = Giant funnel (Pliny named this plant); foetida = foul smell.

English name : Asafoetida.

Sanskrit name : Hingu, Sahastravedhi (thousand actions), Jatuk (Jatu = gum), Balhik.

Botanical Description : A small perinneal shrub, 2 - 3 meter high. Leaves delicate, ciliated with 2-4 wings, stalk bears a single leaf with broken margin at the tip. Fruit 1 cm x 1cm; the latex is called hing.

Varieties : Two (1) white and (2) black. White variety oozes a latex which is scented, like diamond and crystal clear. This is called hirahing and is used in medicine. Black variety is foul smelling. Many varieties are available in the market, which are attributed to habitat, tree and mode of preservation. Chorabi, hita and talao hing are of good quality.

Collection is done by two methods :

(1) In summer the bark of a tree is scraped by a sharp knife just above the roots. Latex from this is

Doshanashak plants act on the particular dosha and its srotas but Vyadhinashak plants will act on the routes of all the constituents of Sumprapti (pathogenesis).

collected after 1-2 days. Latex can be collected from the same site after first collection. This process is repeated several times. Once the latex is exhausted, further latex is not obtained from the same plant. This latex is preserved carefully.
2) In the second method the trunk is cut horizontally and the latex is collected after accumulation. The same process is repeated till all latex from the tree gets exhausted. Hingu is useful in deciding the purity of kasturi.
Impure hingu : Wheat and gravel are mixed with it to increase the weight so it contains less hing. If dissolved in water, it settles at the bottom. Does not burn completely on fire. Also differs in smell and taste. It should not be used in medicine.
Pure hingu : When dropped in water, it slowly dissolves with a white edge and water turns milky white without a residue at the bottom. It should burn completely in fire.
It should be white in colour with sharp smell.
Process of purification : There are two methods of purification viz. (1) abharjit (2) bharjit.
1. In the first process, 1 part of hingu is dissolved in 8 parts of water and then dried on low flame in ghee layered iron pot.
2. In the second process, hing is roasted in cow-ghee till it becomes dry and rough.
Habitat : Iran, Turkey, Afghanistan, Punjab and Peshawar.
Chemical composition : 6 to 17 % volatile oil. This contains rason oil and allyl persulphide which emits a special smell. 65% resin, wax etc.
Properties :
Guna : laghu, snigdha, tikshna, sara; **Rasa :** katu; **Vipak :** katu; **Veerya :** ushna.
Karma :
Dosha : Ushna, kaphavatashamak, pittavardhak by tikshna ushna and useful in vatakapha diseases. But harmful in pitta.
External uses : Analgesic, vata alleviating and stimulant properties help in flatulence by topical application. Castor oil + hing douche (matrabasti) is also effective. 15 gunja hing + 10 tola water in douche is given in helminthiasis. Hing is applied locally on the genitalia in impotency. Its topical application is useful in cough and breathlessness. Hingu water is applied to reduce swelling and pain of guinea worm.
Internal uses :
Nervous system : It is stimulant, analgesic, sangnyasthapak and anticonvulsant by its ushna veerya. It is useful in paralysis, facial palsy, torticollis, sciatica and epilepsy.
Digestive system : Stimulates appetite, digestive and improves taste because of pungent and ushna property. Snigdha and tikshna guna helps to improve peristalsis, relieves colicy pain and intestinal worms. It is useful in loss of appetite, flatulence, tumour, pain, constipation and intestinal parasites. Roasted hingu should be used for treating digestive disorders. It is given at the beginning of meal in hypogastric pain and at the middle of the meal in epigastric (saman vayu) conditions. Thin paste of hing is applied on abdomen in flatulence in infants and middle aged patients.
Circulatory system : Cardiac stimulant, in vataj cardiac disorders, pericardial effusion, cardiac pain - karpurhingu vati is very useful in such conditions.
Respiratory system : Being tikshna, antibacterial and kaphavatahar, it is useful in asthma, cough,

pneumonia, chronic cough, whooping cough; karpurhinguvati or raw hingu is used in respiratory conditions.

Urinary system : In kaphavataj dysuria, it acts as diuretic. Hingu is excreted through urine, therefore useful in vataj dysuria and urinary bladder pain.

Reproductive system : It is an aphrodisiac by its ushna and tikshna property. Therfore it is useful in impotency. Helps ovulation. It helps to clean the uterus in postpartum conditions.

Satmikaran : It is a bitter tonic and increases strength. In general debility it increases appetite, and reduces weakness by this property.

Skin : It vitiates blood. It is a stimulant to the skin since it contains sulphur. It is used in itching. Hingu is excreted through skin.

Temperature : Febrifuge, sheetaprashaman, preventive in typhoid and useful in malarial fever.

Excretion : Through bronchi, skin and kidney.

Parts used : Latex.

Dose : 0.25 to 0.5 gm.

Formulations : Hingwashtak churna, Hingwadivati, Hingkarpurvati, Rajapravartinivati.

Note : Hingu roasted in ghee is used in gastroinstestinal conditions because unprocessed hingu causes irritation and inflammation. But the same hingu is effective in lung disorders by tikshna guna.

Contraindications : Liver and brain disorders and persons having pitta prakruti.

Antidote : Pomegranate, apple and sandal wood. Property of thousand actions makes hingu an important ingredient of panchapal. Its best action is seen in srotodushti caused by vatakapha derangement. It improves appetite, taste and digestion of food.

Srotogamitva :

Dosha : Vatakaphaghna, pittavardhak.

Dhatu : Rasa (menstruation), rakta, majja (fainting, epilepsy).

Mala : Anthelmintic.

Organ : Heart, eye, bronchi, skin, and urinary tract.

(Hingu is very useful in guinea worm infestation. 1 tola hingu is inserted in one coconut, wrapped with cotton and processed by putpak. Contents are consumed in a day followed by bath and dinner of curd and rice before sleep. All guinea worms die at first exposure; pain and inflammatory swelling also disappears.)

References -

सहस्रवेधि जतुकं बाह्लीकं हिंगु रामठम् । हिंगूष्णं पाचनं रुच्यं तीक्ष्णं वातबलासहृत् ।।
शूलगुल्मोदरानाहकृमिघ्नं पित्तवर्धनम् । 'स्त्रीपुष्पजननं बल्यं मूर्च्छापस्मारहृत् परम् ।।' भा.प्र.
'हिंगुनिर्यासश्छेदनीयदीपनीयानुलोमिकवातकफप्रशमनानाम् श्रेष्ठः ।' च. सू. २५
'हृद्यं हिंगु कटूष्णं चकृमिवातकफापहम् । विबन्धानाहशूलघ्नं चक्षुष्यं गुल्मनाशनम् ।।' रा.नि.

As a spoken language changes every 12 miles, what is the matter if the flora too have a minor change over a similar distance?

PART III

MEDICINAL PLANTS (CONTD.)

(1) ASHWAKARNA
Diptocarpus alatus Roxb.

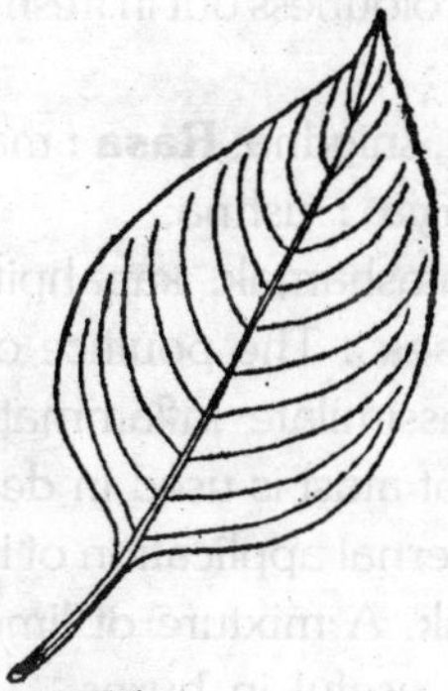

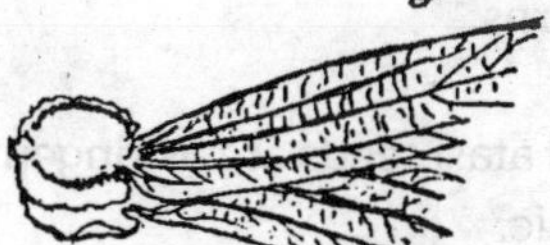

Kula : Shala kula.
Family : Dipterocarpiaceae – Di = 2, ptero = wing, having two wings to the fruit (carpus = fruit).
Latin name : Dipterocarpus = as given above, alatus = having wings.
Sanskrit names : Jarandrum, Ashwakarna, Deerghaparna, Kaushik, Tarkshya, Deerghavriksha.
Properties :
Guna : laghu, snigdha; **Rasa** : katu, tikta; **Dosha** : pittaghna, kaphaghna.
External uses : It reduces inflammation. Its external application helps in wound healing and early reunion of fractures.
Internal uses : It acts as a haemostatic. For obtaining its haemostatic action, its bark powder + ral is given in juice of vasa with honey. It is used in fever. It is used in diseases of pitta and kapha and also in disorders of rakta dhatu.
Srotogamitva :
Dosha : Kapha and pittanashak.
Dhatu : Meda (meha); rakta (dermatoses).
Mala : Mutra (reduces urinary discharges).
References -
अश्वकर्ण: कटुस्तिक्तो स्निग्ध: पित्तास्रनाशन: ।
ज्वरविस्फोटकण्डूघ्न: शिरोर्तिर्नाशनो 'नृपे' ।
मेहकुष्ठव्रणकफहर: प्रोक्तो 'गणे' तथा ।।

(2) ATASI
Linum usitaissimum Linn.

Kula : Atasi kula.
Family : Linaceae.
Latin name : Linum Gk. - Linon = flax (for weaving, oil for painting); usitaitissimum = common customary.
Sanskrit names : Atasi, Pichchila, Devi, Medagandha, Madotkata, Uma, Kshuma, Hemavati, Rudraneela, Masruna, Suvalkala.
Botanical Description : This is a herb attaining height of 1 to 1.25 metre. Leaves –long, narrow. Flowers – blue. Fruits – circular in shape with shallow seeds. Depending on the colour of seeds it is subdivided into 4 types, (1) white (2) yellow (3) red and (4) black.
Habitat : In India – Bengal, Bihar and Uttar Pradesh, Russia, Britain, Holand.

In padarthvignyan shastra, the basic figure of five is minimal whereas in Ayurveda it is three.

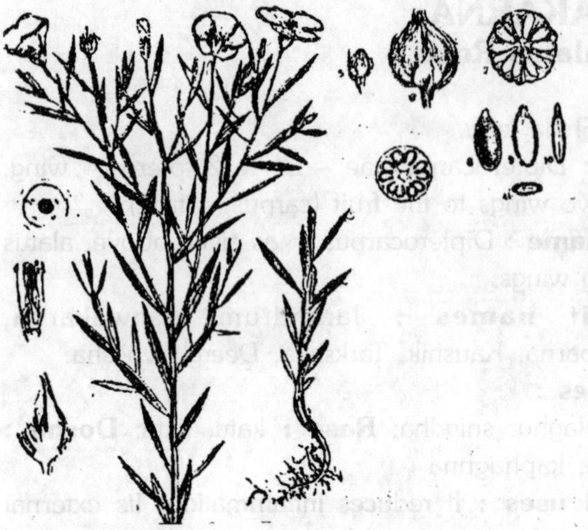

Chemical composition : Seeds have 37 to 44% oil. White seeds have more oil. Fresh oil is more viscous and colourless but in fresh air it gets solidified.

Properties :

Guna : guru, snigdha; **Rasa :** madhur, tikta; **Vipak :** katu, **Veerya :** ushna;

Dosha : vatashamak, kapahpittavardhak.

External uses : The poultice of the flour of atasi is used to assimilate inflammation. This external application of atasi is used in deeper inflammation also. The external application of its oil i.e. abhyanga is vatanashak. A mixture of lime water and oil of atasi is very useful in burns.

Internal uses :

Digestive system : Fried atasi seeds are astringent and reduce intestinal motility. Oil is a purgative. Flowers are cardiotonic.

Respiratory system : The decoction of the seeds of atasi is useful in cough, pleuritis, pneumonia and whooping cough in children. It works as an expectorant.

Urinary system : Hot infusion is useful in cystitis and pyuria. Seeds are not virilizing.

Srotogamitva:

Dosha : Vataghna, pittavardhak, kaphavardhak.

Dhatu : Rakta (asthma, cough etc, diseases of the lungs), shukra (seeds – avirilizing).

Organs : Eyes – oil not useful for eyes, intestines.

References -

'अतसी मधुरा तिक्ता स्निग्धा पाके कटुर्गुरुः । उष्णा दृक्शुक्रवातघ्नी कफपित्तप्रकोपिणी ।।' (भा.प्र.)

'अतसी तैलमाग्नेयं स्निग्धोष्णं कफपित्तकृत् । कटुपाकमचक्षुष्यं बल्यं वातहरं गुरु ।।

मलकृद्रसतः स्वादु ग्राहि त्वग्दोषहृत् घनम् । बस्तौ पाने तथाभ्यंगे नस्ये कर्णस्य पूरणे ।।

अनुपानविधौ चापि प्रयोज्यं वातशान्तये ।' (भा. प्र.)

(3) ARALU

Oroxylum indicum Vent.

Kula : Shyonak kula.

Family : Begnoniaceae (Michel Begon, French patron of Botany 1638 to 1710).

Latin name : Oroxylum = mountain wood (Oro = mountain, xylum = wood); indicum = of India.

Sanskrit names : Shyonak, Pruthushimbi, Shukanasa, Kutannat, Katwang, Mandukparna, Patrorna, Deerghavrunta, Aralu.

Yellow Shyonak : Bhallak, Deerghavrunta, Peetavruksha, Tentook, Bhootasara, Munidruma, Neesaar, Kunat, Virechan.

Botanical Description : It is a big tree of 10 to 12 metres height. Leaves are also big. Legume

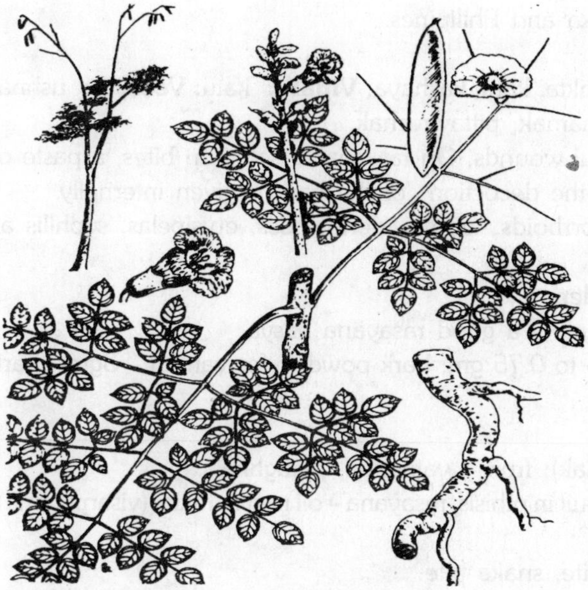

is very long and wide like a sword. Therefore its name is pruthushimbi. Leaf and flower stalks are also long (deerghavrunta). Flowers – red or purple. Petals of flowers have a bad smell and are fleshy. Seeds – shallow with wings, 0.75 cm. long and 1 cm. broad. It has some cotton also.

Habitat : All over India and Sri lanka.

Properties :

Guna : laghu, ruksha; **Rasa** : tikta, kashaya; **Vipak** : katu; **Veerya** : sheeta; **Dosha** : tridoshaghna. Shyonak is very useful on ama.

External uses : Root bark is useful in amavata, its kashaya i.e. decoction is used for external application as well as for internal use. Dashamoola contains shyonak.

Internal uses :

Digestive system : The juice of the root bark is useful in loss of appetite, anorexia, worms, loose motions, amoebiasis, inflammation etc. It is also used in disorders caused by ama.

Respiratory system : Useful in cough, asthma.

Urinary system : Cystitis. As it is a diaphoretic, it is used in disorders caused by obstruction of sweat.

Srotogamitva : Tridoshaghna (prabhav).

Dhatu : Meda, ama.

Mala : Sweda, mutra.

Organs : Joints (middle channel - madhyam margagami), bladder, digestive system (loss of appetite, dysentery, amoebiasis).

(4) ANKOT

Alangium lamarki Thw.

Kula : Ankol kula.

Family : Alangiacae (by Tamil name).

Latin name : Alangium (Azhincil from Tamil name); lamarki = from Lamark, French Naturalist.

Sanskrit names : Ankol, Deerghakeel, Rechi, Dhera, Ankod, Angulipatra, Drudhamoolak, Subhrapatra, Tamraphala, Kantaki, Mallika, Peetatamraphala, Gunaddhya, Kolak, Lambakarna, Rochan.

Botanical Description : This tree is of 3 to 8 meters height. Bark is 1.5cm. wide. Branches are white in colour. Leaves are thorny of 7 to 15 cm. length. Leaves and leaflets are odorous. In front of a leaf, there is one leaflet. Flowers bloom in clusters. Fruits are like those of leechi.

Madhur rasa is not heavy by itself. However, dravya belonging to madhur rasa is difficult to digest. It is desirable to bear this in mind.

Habitat : Konkan, China, Malaysia, Sri lanka and Philipines.

Properties :

Guna : laghu, snigdha, tikshna, sara; **Rasa :** tikta, katu, kashaya; **Vipak :** katu; **Veerya :** ushna; **Prabhav :** vishaghna; **Dosha :** kapahvatashamak, pittavirechak.

External uses : Its oil is applied on painful wounds. On rat, snake, scorpion bites, a paste of bark powder is applied. In these conditions, the decoction of the bark is given internally.

Internal uses : It is used in ascites, haemorrhoids, worms, dermatoses, erysipelas, syphilis as shodhan.

Fruits are used in pthisis and bleeding disorders.

Root bark and seeds are also used. Ankot's oil is a good rasayana nasya.

Dosage : As a diaphoretic and diuretic - 0.5 to 0.75 gm. bark powder; for vaman – 3gms. bark powder.

Srotogamitva :

Dosha : Kaphaghna, vataghna, pitta (virechak); fruit – vataghna, pittaghna.

Dhatu : Rakta (raktapittashamak); rasayana – fruit in pthisis, rasayana – oil nasya; rakta (visarpaghna).

Mala : Mutra, sweda.

Organs: Kidney, prabhav - vishaghna, rat bite, snake bite.

References -

'अंकौलोऽङ्गुलिपत्रः स्यात् पादपो दृढमूलकः । शुभ्रपुष्पो ताम्रफलः कंटकी वनवासी च ।।' (शि.द.)
'अंकोलः स्निग्धतीक्षोष्णः कटुको वातनाशनः । कुकुराखुविषं हन्ति ग्रहजन्तुविषापहः ।।
भूतहृद्विषहृत्वैव कणठशूलस्य शोधनः ।' (ध. नि.)
'अंकोटो दीर्घकीलः स्यादंकोलश्च निकोचकः । अंकोटकः कटुस्तीक्ष्णः स्निग्धोष्णस्तुवरो लघुः ।।
रेचनः कॉमिशूलामशोफग्रहविषापहा । विसर्पकफपित्तास्त्रमूषिकाहि विषापहा ।।
तत्फलं शीतलं स्वादु श्लेष्मघ्नं बृंहणं गुरु । बल्यं विरेचनं वातपित्तदाहक्षयास्त्रजित् ।।' (भा. प्र)
'अंकोलः कटुकः स्निग्धो विषलूतादिदोषनुत् । कफानिलहरः सूतशुद्धिकृत् रेचनीयकः ।। (रा. नि.)
अंकोलमूलकल्को वा बस्तमूत्रेण कल्कितः । पानालेपनयोः युक्तः सर्वाखुविषनाशनः ।। (अ. हृ.)
'नस्यं चांकोलतैलेन कुर्यान्मृत्युजरापहम् । निष्कार्धनिष्कं वर्षैकं जीवेद्वर्षशतत्रयम् ।। (र. र.)

(5) AGASTYAM
Sesbenia grandiflora.

Kula : Shimbi kula.

Family : Papilionaceae (like butterfly).

Latin name : Sesbenia = name of a botanist; grandiflora (grandi = big, flora = flower).

Sanskrit names : Agastee, Shighrapushpa, Agastya, Munidrum, Vranari, Deerghaphalak, Vakrapushpa, Surapriya, Vangasen, Madhuryati.

Habitat : In India - Bengal, Southern India, Gangetic plains.

Botanical Description : Early growing tree 8 to 10 mtrs high. Branches are wide spread. Leaves – have 41 to 61 leaflets. Flowers - white, boat shaped, long, flower in August. Legume – 30 cm. in length, oval in shape, having 4 angles. In India flowers and legumes are used as vegetables and for making pickles. There are 4 types, 1) white 2) yellow 3) bule and 4) red.

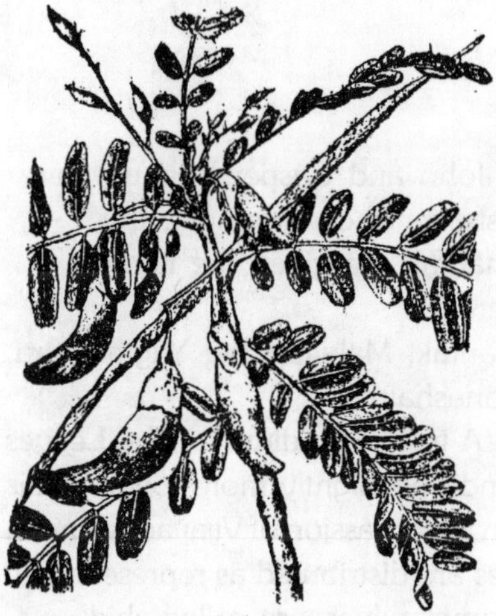

The white variety is most effective in night blindness and chronic rhinitis. Agasti is very useful in Vitamin A deficiency diseases.

Properties :

Guna : laghu, ruksha; **Rasa :** tikta; **Vipak** : madhur; **Veerya** : sheeta; **Dosha :** kaphapittashamak.

External uses : Bark and leaves are useful in inflammation and wounds.

Internal uses : Juice of leaves is useful in virechan nasya. Flowers are useful in opthalmic disorders. Agastee is a brain tonic and antitoxic.

Digestive system : Vegetable of flowers and leaves is useful in constipation. The juice of the bark is used in chronic intestinal disorders with honey. Juice of flowers is used in purification of silver. It is also used in loose motions.

Respiratory system : Pleuritis, cough, cold.

In kapha jwar, chaturthik jwar, sannipatik jwara, nasal administration of leaf juice is done.

Reproductive system : Useful in leucorrhoea.

Dosage : Leaf juice – 12 to 24 ml.; decoction - 48 to 100 ml.

Srotogamitva :

Dosha : Kaphaghna, pittaghna, vatavardhak.

Dhatu : Majja (medhya), asthi - majja (chaturthik jwar).

Mala : Purisha (leaves; flowers vegetables – reduces constipation).

Organs : Uterus – leucorrhoea, respiratory system.

References -

'सिद्धोऽगस्ति: पंक्तिपत्रो मृदुशिंबी महारुह: । अगस्त्यस्योदयं यावत् सपुष्प इव दृश्यते ।।' (शि.)
'अगस्त्य: पित्तकफजिच्चातुर्थिकहरो हिम: । रूक्षो वातकरस्तिक्त: प्रतिश्यायनिवारण: ।।'
तत्पुष्पं पीनसश्लेष्मपित्तनक्तान्ध्यनाशनम् ।' (भा. प्र.)
'अगस्त्यपत्रं कटुकं सतिक्तं गुरु कृमिघ्नं विशदं कफघ्नम् ।
'मुनिशिंबी सरा प्रोक्ता बुद्धिदारुचिदा लघु: । पाककाले तु मधुरा तिक्ता चैव स्मृतिप्रदा ।।
त्रिदोषशूलकफहृत् पांडुरोगविषापनुत् । शोषगुल्महरा प्रोक्ता सा पक्वा रूक्षपित्तला ।।' (नि.र.)
'वृषागस्त्यो: पुष्पाणि तिक्तानि कटुविपाकानि क्षयकासहराणि च।'
अगस्त्यं नातिशीतोष्णं नक्तान्धानां प्रशस्यते ।' (सु. सू. ४६.)
'अगस्तिपत्रं मरिचं मूत्रेण परिवेषितम् । नस्ये शस्तमपस्मारं हन्ति शीघ्रं नरस्य तु ।।' (हारीत चि. १९.)
'अगस्तिपुष्पचूर्णएन माहिषं जनयेद्धधि । तदुत्थनवनीतेन देहजं स्फुटनं जयेत् ।।' (भा. प्र.)
'चातुर्थिकहरं नस्यं मुनिद्रुमदलाम्बुना ।' (वै.जी.)
'नागरशोभाञ्जनयो: क्वाथ: शूलं विनाशयेत् त्रिदिनात् ।
मुनितरुवल्कक्वाथस्तद्वत् पटुरामठप्रतीवाप: ।। (वै. म.)

A dravya is either food or medicine, it undergoes a continuous change during digestion. One should think about it.

(6) ASHMANTAK
Bauhinia racemosa Roxb.

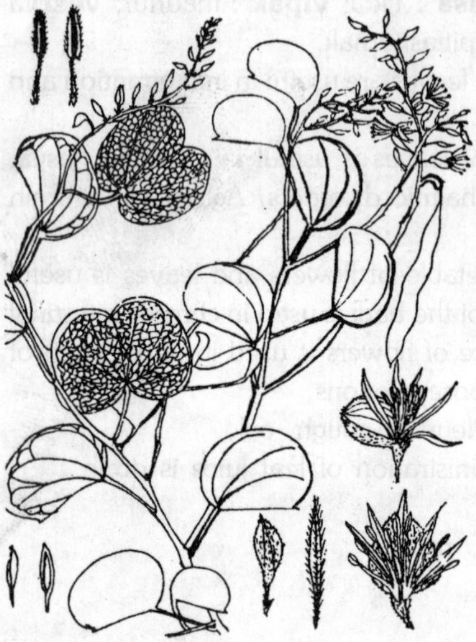

Family : Leguminoseae.
Latin name : Bauhinia (John and Casper Bahaun were two brothers; both botanists, in whose memory, the compound leaves of ashmantak are given the name); recemosa = flowers clustered.
Sanskrit names : Ashmantak, Malukapatra, Yugmapatra, Amlapatrak, Kushali, Papanashak
Botanical Description : A tree of medium height. Leaves – like kanchanar, compound and slightly more tough. Bidis are made from its leaves. On the occassion of Vijayadashmi(an Indian festival), these leaves are distributed as representative of gold. This tree has legumes which are called shid.
Properties :
Guna : kashay, ruksha; **Prabhav :** vishaghna.
Digestive system : Leaf juice mixed with powdered pepper is used in diarrhoea. Juice of leaves and onion juice are also used. Immature flowers are also given. A decoction of the bark is used in diarrhoea. In fever, when there is headache, external application of small leaves is done. In pyuria, juice of small leaves + milk is given. In ascites, root bark of kutaj is given in the leaf juice of karavellak and bhrungaraj.
Hepatitits : Decoction of root bark is useful.
Stomatitis : Decoction of root bark is used for gargling.
Srotogamitva :
Dosha : Kaphaghna, pittaghna.
Dhatu : Rakta (haemostatic), (hepatitis).
Mala : Purisha (sangrahi i.e. reduces the motility); mutra (increases quantity, pyuria).
Ashmantak – It prevents the formation of urinary stone and if formed, it acts as a lithotrypsic and throws it out through increased urine formation.

(7) AMLIKA
Tamarindus indica Linn.

Kula : Shimbi kula.
Family : Leguminoseae.
Latin name : Tamarindus = the distorted form of the Arabic name tamar – e – hind meaning 'ripe date of India'; indica = Indian.
Sanskrit names : Chincha, Chukrika, Chukra, Amlica, Shakchukrika, Amli, Sutattidi, Amla, Tittidika, Sukta, Suktika.

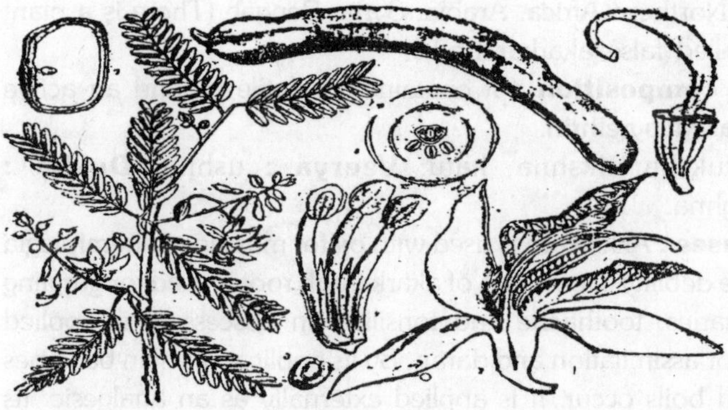

Botanical Description : It is a fast growing tall tree and is known by these names – chincha, tintini, imali, ambali, chinch, tamarind. Leaves – compound, leaflet – 20 to 40, round in shape. Flowers – in bunches, yellow in colour and boatshaped. Legume – 7 to 12 cm. long Seeds – are called as chinchoke in Marathi.

Habitat : All over India.

Chemical composition : Tartaric, citric, malic, acetic, potassium tartarate, etc. In the seed there is 63% carbohydrates.

Properties :

Guna : guru, ruksha; **Rasa :** amla; **Veerya :** ushna; **Dosha :** when ripe kaphapittanashak and vatanashak. Its sherbet is an effective pittashamak.

Uses : Tamarind and its seeds are applied externally on inflammation. Fruit is very good in taste and is used in anorexia, polydipsia, indigestion and liver disorders. In heart diseases, sherbet is given. Kshar is used in retention of urine and abdominal pain. (Shankhavati). Pulp and sherbet reduce the complication in fever. In cholera, tablets of fruits of tamarind and Semecarpus anacardium + salt are very useful.

Srotogamitva :

Dosha : Ripe fruit – pitta nashak.

Dhatu : Liver.

Mala : Mutra (retention of urine).

Organs : Heart.

(8) AKARKARABH

Anacyclus pyrethrom

Family : Compositeae.

Latin name : Anacyclus (Ana = like, kyklos = circle); pyrethrom (pyr = fire - due to pungent roots ?)

Sanskrit names : Akalla, Akorkaro, Akkirkaram, Akarkaram (Pellitory).

Botanical Description : On the stalk of the akarkarabh, at some distance there are nodes and hairy structures. Bark – brown in colour, bitter in taste. Root – 7 to 10 cm. in length. It is interesting to note that its root protects its potency till 7 years. Leaves – small, like the leaves of kapittha. Flowers – round in shape, flowering occurs in summer. Petals – white, pink, yellowish on the upper side. Fruits – shallow, oval in shape. The plant does not appear to be of Indian origin because it is not mentioned in Charaka samhita. But Bhavaprakash has described this plant just as he has mentioned tobacco plant which is not of Indian origin. Akarkarabh must have come from Arabastan.

Eventhough the gunas of a mango fruit change continuously during the process of ripening yet, its name remains constant.

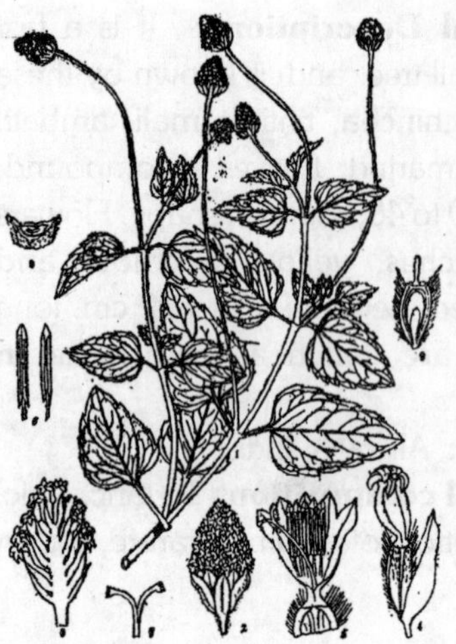

Habitat : Northern Africa, Arabia, Syria, Bengal. (There is a plant which is called false akarkarabh.)

Chemical composition : It contains a volatile oil and an active principle called pyrethrin.

Guna : ruksha, tikshna, katu; **Veerya :** ushna; **Dosha :** kaphavataghna.

External uses : Akkalkara is used with oil for massage in hemiplegia and nervine debility. Decoction of akarkarabh root is used for gargling in dental caries, toothache and tonsilitis. In abscess, it is applied externally for assimilation and daran. By its application, skin becomes reddish and boils occur. It is applied externally as an analgesic. Its nasya is given in chronic rhinitis and cold. It is used in various aphrodisiac oils prepared in unani medicine.

Internal uses : It is used internally in various types of vata disorders. A small dose of akarkarabh acts as an appetite stimulant in indigestion and pittakshaya. It increases heart rate. It is used in sexually transmitted diseases and inflammation. Useful in cough and hoarseness of voice. It is also used in children like Achorus calamus. It is useful in diabetes. It is also helpful in impotency caused by weakness of nerves. It is used as rasayana in kaphaj diseases.

If the root powder is given in a dose of more than 0.5 to 0.75 gm., it results in nausea, bleeding, increase in heart rate, unconsciousness etc. In such conditions, milk and other pittashamak dravyas should be used as antidotes.

Srotogamitva :

Dosha : Kaphaghna, vataghna, pittavardhak.

Dhatu : Majja (weakness), shukra (virilization).

Mala : Mutra (prameha).

Organs : Heart, lungs.

References -

'आकारकरभश्चैव कल्लकोऽथ ह्यकल्लकः । अकल्लकोष्णो वीर्येण बलकृत् कटुको मतः । प्रतिश्यायं च शोथं च वातं चैव विनाशयेत्' (भा. प्र.)

(9) ARANYA JEERAK

Centrotherum anthelminticum Wild Kurtze.

Kula : Bhringaraj kula.

Family : Campositae.

Latin name : Centrotherum = many spiked; anthelminticum = anthelmintic property.

English name : Purple Fleabane.

Sanskrit names : Bruhatpali, Sookshmapatra, Aranyajeer, Kana, Vanajeerak, Karajeeree.

Botanical Description : It is an annual herb which is 1 to 2 mtrs. high. Leaves – 7 to 16 cms. in length with pointed tip and serrated margins. Flowers – purple in colour. Seeds – blackish brown, oval shaped with 10 striations on them and has pungent odour. Flowering occurs in rainy season and seeds start growing in spring.

Habitat : All over India.

Chemical composition : Seeds contains 18% fixed oil.

Properties :

Guna : laghu, teekshna; **Rasa** : tikta; **Veerya** : ushna; **Dosha** : kapahavatanashak.

External uses : Local application reduces inflammation and pain, hence it is used in various skin disorders, lice and leucoderma (4 parts of kadu jeerak + 1 part of hartal + cow's urine is applied locally).

Internal uses : It is a good appetizer. It draws out the mucoid discharge by inducing vomiting. Respiratory disorders and worms in children are treated by a formulation called 'pleehodarari' which contains aranyajeerak. It purifies blood, acts as a diuretic and febrifuge. It is also useful in pueperal disorders. Mixture of aranyjeerak - 1gm. + black sesame - 1gm. in hot water is helpful in skin disorders. In chronic fever and animal induced toxins also, it is useful.

Dosage : Seed - 1 gm to 3 gms.

Somaraji is the name of bakuchi and also the synonym of kadujeerak.

Srotogamitva :

Dosh : Kapahghna.

Dhatu : Rasa – raktagata kapha (liver and spleen), rasa (galactagogue).

Mala : Purish shodhan, anthelmintic.

Organs : Spleen and liver.

(10) ADDHAH PUSHPI
Trichodesma indicum R. Br.

Kula : Shleshmantak kula.

Family : Boraginaceae.

Latin name : Trichodesma -thrix = a hair; indicum = Indian.

Sanskrit names : Addhah pushpi.

Botanical Description : It is a herb 0.5 to 0.50 feet. high and grows in rainy season. Branches - reddish green bending downwards and thorny. Leaves – 2 to 5 cms. in length and 2 to 3 cms. in breadth. Stalks of leaves are small. Flowers – whitish blue and hanging inversely, hence the name addhah pushpi. Fruit – white and ripe one is purple.

Habitat : All overs in India.

Properties :

Guna : laghu, snigdha; **Rasa** : katu, tikta; **Veerya** : ushna; **Dosha** : kaphavatanashak.

External uses : Reduces inflammation and pain by external application. Local application of the paste of whole plant is effective in osteoarthritis, inflammation and conjunctivitis. Its ash is used for cleaning the wounds and also useful in scabies.

Internal uses : Being an appetizer and digestive it is useful in agnimandya. It is also used in amoebic dysentery, blood disorders, dysuria, dysmenorrhoea and foetal anomalies

Permutations and combinations of rasas and anurasas are infinite. An intellegent person should use these judiciously, with proper methods.

Dosag : Root paste – 5 to 10 gms., juice of whole plant – 12 to 20 ml.
Srotogamitva :
Dosha : Kapha, vataghna.
Dhatu : Rakta, rasa (dysmenorrhoea), mansa (antiinflammatori), meda.
Mala : Mutra (dysuria).

(11) AMARVALLI

Cuscuta reflexa Benth Hook.

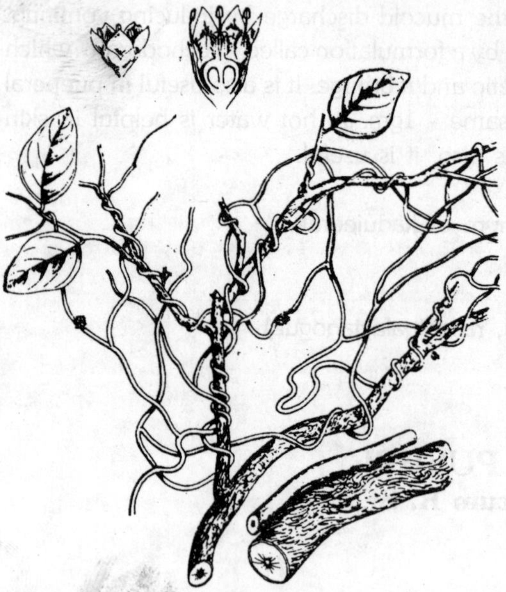

Kula : Trivrut kula.
Family : Convolvulaceae.
English name : Dodder.
Sanskrit names : Khavalli, Aakashvalli, Dusparsha, Vyomvallika, Swarnalata, Nirmuli, Aakashvel.
Botanical Description : It is a leafless delicate, yellow coloured creeper which is entangled like a web and grows on the trees of plumps and babbul. The root is not seen but it is inserted in the stalk of the tree and nourishes itself from it. Flowers – fragrant, white and appear in bunches. Fruits – pea shaped. Seeds – black in colour. Flowering season is spring while fruits occurs in summer.
If the seed is planted in the soil it grows easily, but when it grows on the tree it makes its own root in the stalk of the tree and the previous root dries up. This is its natural behaviour.
Habitat : All over India
Chemical composition : It contains quersetic and kuskutin.
Properties :
Guna : laghu, ruksha, picchila; **Rasa** : tikta, kashaya; **Veerya** : sheeta; **Dosha** : kapahpittanashak.
External uses : Useful in inflammation, pain, hair disorders and conjunctivitis.
Internal uses : It is an appetizer, digestive, liver stimulant, anthelmentic and reduces intestinal motility. Useful in cardiac and blood disorders. Seeds act as a cholagogue and also useful in dysuria, skin disorders, fever and general debility.
Dosage : Juice – 12 to 24 ml.; seed powder – 1 to 3 gm.
Srotogamitva :
Dosha : Kapha-pittaghna.
Dhatu : Rakta (liver stimulant), rasayani; shukra (potent aphrodisiac); mansa, meda, nutritious.
Mala : Hair, purisha (anthelmintic); mutra (diuretic); sweda (diaphoretic).
Organ : Heart

References -
'आकाशवल्ली तु बुधैः कथितामरवल्लरी । खवल्ली ग्राहिणी तिक्ता पिच्छिलाक्ष्यामयापहा ।।
तुवराग्निकरी हृद्या पित्तश्लेष्मामनाशिनी ।' (भा. प्र.)
'वृष्यवल्ली बलकरी परं वृष्या रसायनी । मूत्रकृत् स्वेदजननी पुष्टिदा कार्श्यवारिणी ।।
औपदंशिकरोगाँश्च हरेत् ।' (वै. श.)

(12) ASHVAGOLAM

Plantago ovata Forsk.

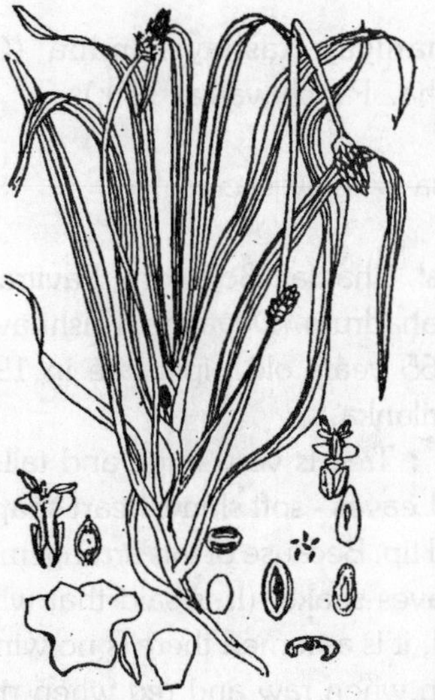

Kula : Isabgol kula.
Family : Plantaginaceae.
Latin name : Plantago = having a flat level surface; ovata = egg-shaped as solid as in outlined.
English name : Isabgol seeds.
Sanskrit name : Ashvakarnabeej (ashva=horse, karna = ears).
Botanical Description : Bark of seasonal shrub shows hard and thick cilia Leaves - long, slender with three prominent veins. Flowers bigonoas gynoecium, each gonad containing single seed. The seeds are light pink and resemble a boat or the ear of a horse. The moment they are immersed in water a gelatinous mucilage is formed.
Varieties : 1. white 2. red and 3. black (black should not be used for medicinal purpose).
Habitat : Iran, Punjab, Sindh. Grows in Karnataka and Bengal.
Chemical composition : It contains oil, albumin and abundant sticky mucilage. An excellent mucilagenous gel is formed, when 1 part of seed is mixed with 20 parts of water.
Properties :
Guna : snigdha, guru, pichchila; **Rasa** : madhur; **Veerya** : sheeta; **Dosha** : vatpittashamak and kaphavardhak.
External uses : Antiinflammatory, useful in headaches, oedema and boils.
Internal uses : Unctous, mild laxative, anthelmintic, antidote, cures ulcers. Roasted seeds are constipative due to loss of mucilagenous property. Seeds fried with ghee are useful in diarrhoea and dysentery. Also useful in dry cough, uremia, gonorrhoea and fever (pittajwar). Seeds are useful in chronic dysentery while powder in acute dysentery.
Dosage : 5-10 gms. Large dose causes loss of appetite which can be prevented if given with asav and arista.
Strotogamitva :
Dosha : Vatapittaghna, kaphavardhak.
Dhatu : Raktamansa (protects ulcers).
Mala : Purisha.

All individuals can be classified into various subsets for obtaining knowledge. Such a classification is the beginning of knowledge.

Organ : Digestive system, respiratory system.

References -

ईषद्गोलमश्वकर्णबीजं च स्निग्धजीरकम् । ईषद्गोलं गुरु स्वादु स्निग्धं शीतं च पिच्छिलम् ।।
स्नेहनं मूत्रजननं श्लेष्मनिःसरणं परम् । दाहतृष्णाहरं बल्यं ज्वरघ्नं चाथ शस्यते ।
प्रवाहिकातिसारामदाहतृष्णाज्वरादिषु । वातपित्तामये कासे दौर्बल्ये मूत्रकृच्छ्रजे ।। (स्व.)

(13) ASHVATTHA

Ficus religiosa Linn.

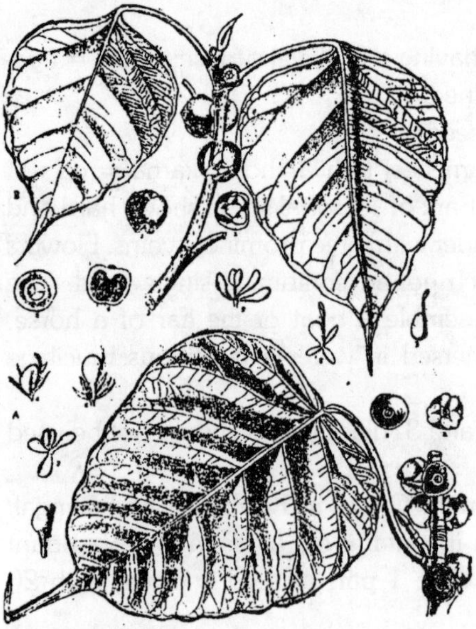

Gana : Mutrasangrahaniya, Kashayskandha (C.); Nyagrodhadi, Kshirivriksha, Panchavalkal (Bh.)

Kula : Vat kula.

Latin name : Religiosa = holy sacred.

Family : Urticaceae.

Sanskrit names : Pippal, Chaldal, Bodhidru, Pavitraka, Yadnik, Shreevriksha, Mahadrum, Devatma, Krishnavas. The author has seen 2265 years old pipal tree in 1961 at Anuradhapuram in Srilanka.

Botanical Description : Tree is very huge and tall. In old trees the bark cracks. Leaves - soft shiny, heart shaped with 5-7 veins and pointed tip. Because of this arrangement with a slight wind the leaves shake. (It is said that when the leaves of pipal are still, it is assumed there is no wind). Fruits - small round green when raw and red when ripe. Fruits appear in summer and ripe in monsoon. Old pipal tree produces a sealing wax which is known as krimij. A very small quantity of secretions falls on the ground from pipal tree. Hindus and especially Buddhists consider pipal tree as a very sacred tree.

Habitat : All over India and Sri lanka.

Chemical composition : Bark contains tannin, rubber and wax.

Properties :

Guna : guru, ruksha; **Rasa :** kashaya; **Vipak :** katu; **Veerya :** sheeta; **Dosha :** kaphapittashamak.

External uses : Complexion enhancer - paste of aerial roots is applied locally. The powder of bark is sprinkled on the wounds. Its latex is useful in reducing pain and swelling and also acts as haemostatic.

Internal uses : Being astringent bark is used in vomiting, diarrhoea, dysentery. Ripe fruits of pipal are used in stomachache and constipation. In diabetes fruits and bark are used . Decoction of the bark + honey and fruits are useful in gout, blood disorders and bleeding disorders. Powdered dry fruits are given for conception. Fruits, roots, bark and aerial roots processed in milk+ sugar + honey is prescribed as an aphrodiasiac. (Infertile couples are advised to worship pipal tree). Bark,

fruits and leaves are used for medicinal purpose.
Dosage : Juice - 12 to 24 ml.; decoction - 60 to 100 ml.; powder - 1 to 3 gms.
Srotogamitva :
Dosha : Kaphapittashamak.
Dhatu : Rakta (haemostatic, compexion enhancer); shukra (aphrodisiac), meda (diabetes).
Mala : Purisha and mutra (astringent).
References -
पिप्लो दुर्जरः शीतः पित्तश्लेष्मव्रणास्रजित् । गुरुस्तुवरको रूक्षो वर्ण्यो योनिविशोधनः ।।' (भा. प्र.)
'पिप्पलः सुमधुरस्तु कषायः शीतलश्च कफपित्तविनाशी ।
रक्तदाहशमनः स हि सद्यो योनिदोषहरणः किल पक्वः ।।' (रा.नि.)
'बोधिद्रुमकषायन्तु पिबेत्तं मधुना सह । वातरक्तं जयत्याशु त्रिदोषमपि दारुणम् ।।' (च.चि. २९)
'अश्वत्थफलमूलत्वक् शुङ्गसिद्धं पयो नरः । पीत्वा सशर्कराक्षौद्रं कुलिङ्ग इव हृष्यति ।। (सु. चि. ११)

(14) AKSHOTAK
Juglans regia Linn.

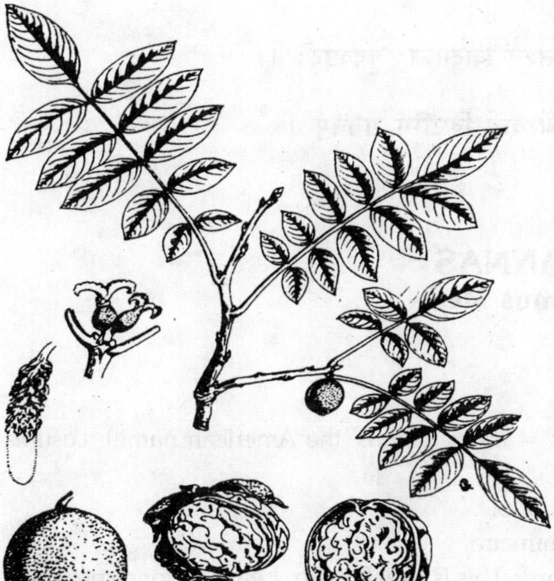

Kula : Akshot kula.
Family : Juglandaceae (juglans = walnut tree).
Latin name : Juglans = walnut tree; regia = royal.
English names : Walnut.
Sanskrit names : Akshot, Parvateeya, Kandaral, Bruhatchhada, Swadumajja, Vrittaphala, Madanahva, Shailbhava, Rekhaphala.
Botanical Description : It is a fragrant medium tree. External part of new branches are velvet like. Bark – 1.5 to 5 cms. wide, grey having, longitudinal gaps. Inner part of the stalk is grey having black spots. Leaves – compound, 15 to 30 cms. in length. Leaflets – 5 to 11 or 7 to 9 in pairs. 7 to 20 cms. in length and 5 to 10 cms. in breadth. Flowers – homosexual and 5 to 11 cms. in length. Fruits – circular with greenish striations on them and enclosed by tough covering. (To break a walnut there is a special nutcracker). It looks like a madanphala (Randia dumentorum). It has a single seed with two layers. This part resembles the brain in structure. It is edible. Flowering season is spring and fruiting season in autumn.
Habitat : In Himalaya about 1000 to 4000 mtrs. height. In Kashmeer it grows plentifully.
Chemical composition : It contains oxalic acid and barium, while pulp has 40 to 45% stable oil, acid and resin.

In the study of Dravyagunavignyan, guna is the most important. Absence of guna implies dosha.

Properties :

Guna : guru, snigdha; **Rasa :** madhur; **Vipak :** madhur; **Virya :** ushna; **Dosha :** vatashamak, kapha pitta vardhak.

External uses : Local application gives a good complexion, cures skin disorders, reduces inflammation and pain and hence is used in vata disorders. Bark has haemostatic property and its powder is used as a toothpowder which makes the gums strong. It is sold in Amritsar Swarna Mandir.

Internal uses : Nervine tonic, therefore used in paralysis, brain impairements, malnutrition. Being appetizer, unctous and mild laxative it is used in ascites and constipation. Fried walnut is given in dry cough.Pulp is useful in tuberculosis, general debility and as an aphrodisiac.

Dose : Oil - 12 to 24 ml.

Srotogamitva :

Dosha : Vataghna, kapha-pittavardhak.

Dhatu : Majja (tonic, paralysis, dystrophy and gout); mansa; meda (brinhan); shukra (aphrodisiac).

Mala : Purisha (snehan, laxative).

References -

'अक्षोट: शाखी सुमहद्दन्तिपत्रोऽथ तत्फलम् ।
पलमात्रं च गालाभं मध्ये प्रोन्नतरेखकम् ।।' (शि.)
'अखोट: पार्वतीयश्च फलस्नेहो गुडाशय: । कीरेष्ट: कर्परालश्च स्वादुमज्ज: पृथक्छद: ।।
रेखाफलो वृत्तफलो मदनाभफलश्च स: ।।' (नि.र.)
'अखोटकं गुणे स्निग्धं मधुरं रसपाकयो: । गुरूष्णबृंहणं वृष्यं बल्यं विष्टम्भि रोचनम् ।।
हृद्यं क्षयास्त्रपवनदाहघ्नं कफपित्तलम् ।' (नि.र.)
'अक्षोटकोऽपि वातामसदृश: कफपित्तकृत् ।' (भा. प्र.)

(15) ANANNAS

Ananas cosmus Mess.

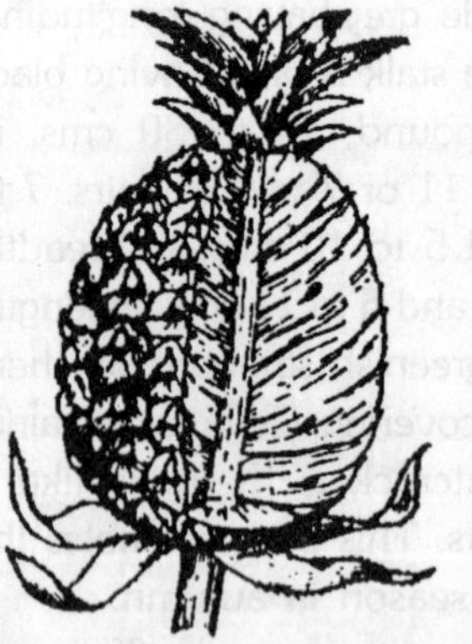

Kula : Ananas kula.

Family : Bromiliaceae.

Latin name : Ananas = (from 'Nanas' the American name); cosums = hairy.

English name : Pine apple.

Sanskrit name : Bahunetra.

Botanical Description : This is a leafy herb. Leaves – long spiky with serrated margins. Flowers – on those margins. Fruits – big like jackfruits. When unripe greenish and becomes yellow when ripes and has good smell. Its external surface is rough and dotted with dark spots which appear like many eyes. Seeds – small, oval and yellow. At the end of summer and during monsoon flowers and fruits occur.

Habitat : It is originally from Brazil. In 1513, it was brought in Europe. In 1564, portuguise have brought it into India. Now-a-days it is grown all over India.

Chemical composition : Its contains bromelin. It has a component which solidifies milk. Besides these there are many other components.

Properties :
Guna : guru, sniigdha; **Rasa :** madhur (ripe fruit); amla (unripe fruit); **Vipak :** madhur; **Veerya :** sheeta; **Dosha :** vata pitta shamak.
Internal uses : It is an appetizer and mild laxative. It is useful in jaundice. Sap of leaves is purgative as well as anthelmintic. Juice or murabba of ripe fruits is useful in heart diseases and also in bleeding disorders. Juice of unripe fruit is a uterine stimulant and emmenagogue If a woman in labour is given 1.25 sher juice of ripe fruit, she delivers spontaneously. Therefore it should not be given to pregnant woman. Juice of unripe fruit induces 3 months abortion in 12 hours. It is useful in renal calculi, dysuria and fevers.
Dosage : Fruit sap – 30 to 60 ml.; leaf sap – 12 to 24 ml.
Srotogamitva :
Dosha : Vataghna, pittaghna,
Dhatu : Rakta (jaundice, bleeding disorders and heart diseases); rasa (juice of unripe fruit - emmenagogue).
Mala : Mutra (dysuria); purisha (leaf sap - purgative).
Organ : Pine apple juice - abortefacient.

(16) AAVARTANI

Helicteres streptocarpus/isora

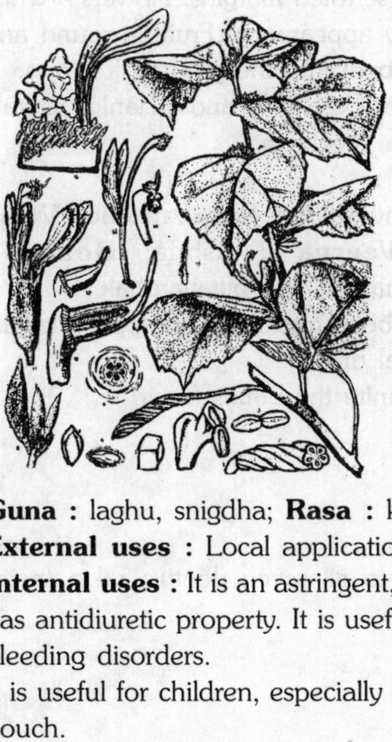

Kula : Pishach karpas.
Family : Sterculiaceae.
Latin name : Helicteres - heli-sunloving, teres = round twisted; strepto carpus - strepto = twisted, carpus = fruit; isora - iso = equal.
Sanskrit name : Avartani.
Botanical Description : It is a herb belonging to pishach karpas kula with height of 2 to 4 mtrs. Fruits - black, 2.5 to 6 cms. in length and twisted, therefore it is called as avartaphala. Leaves – like that of parushak. with 5 to 7 veins on them. Flowers – curved, red and found in various shapes.
Habitat : Madhya Pradesh, Western India and Sri lanka.
Properties :
Guna : laghu, snigdha; **Rasa :** kashaya; **Veerya :** sheeta; **Dosha :** tridoshaghna.
External uses : Local application has haemostatic and wound healing properties.
Internal uses : It is an astringent, analgesic (fruit oil) and anthelmintic. Decoction of the root bark has antidiuretic property. It is useful in diarrhoea, dysentery, abdominal pain, worms and internal bleeding disorders.
It is useful for children, especially in intestinal disorders and is the main content of grandmother's pouch.

The flowers of Bahava (Cassia fistula) are incomparable. Hence the tree is called 'Rajavruksha' (The king amongst trees).

Srotogamitva :
Dosha : Tridoshaghna.
Dhatu : Rakta (haemostatic - external as well as internal bleeding).
Mala : Purish and mutra (astringent).
Organs : Intestine, urinary system and circulatory system.

(17) ASTHISANHARAK

Vicisus quandriangularis

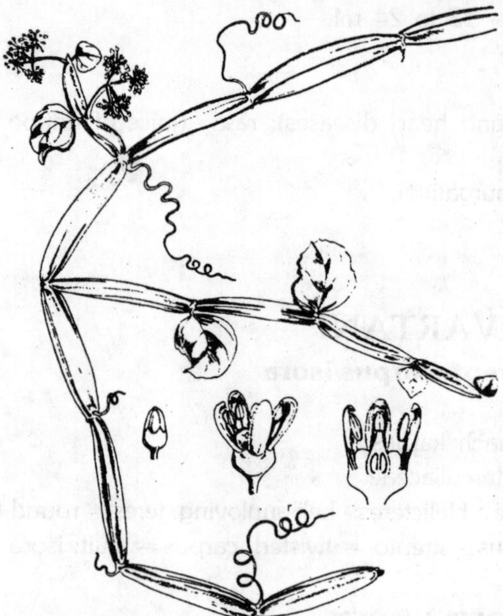

Kula : Draksha kula.
Family : Vitaceae = plant of vitis vine, tribe.
Latin name : Vicisus – intruns; quadriangularis - quadri = four, the stalk has 4 edges.
Sanskrit names : Asthishrunkhala, Vajravati, Vajrang, Kroshtughantika, Granthiman, Vajravallari, Vajri, Asthisandhanini.
Botanical Description : It is a creeper having green and quandrangular stalk which have nodes in between. Therefore it looks like a chain. Leaves – small, divided into 3 to 5 parts and have serrated margins. Flowers – white with a hairy appearance. Fruits – round and red. If it is bent into the ground, it grows.
Habitat : In South India and Sri lanka, its stalk is used as a vegetable.
Properties :
Guna : laghu, ruksha; **Rasa** : madhur; **Vipak** : amla; **Veerya** : ushna; **Dosha** : kaphavatashamak and pittavardhak.
External uses : It has haemostatic and joining properties. In bone fractures, it is applied locally or its oil is applied. In nasal bleeding, its juice is used as nasal drops.
Internal uses : In bone fractures its juice is given orally to unite the bones faster.
Parts used : Stalk and leaves.
Dosage : Juice – 12 to 24 ml.
Srotogamitva :
Dosha : Vatashleshmaghna; pittavardhak.
Dhatu : Asthi (joins bones); shukra (aphrodisiac); nutritious to all seven dhatus; rakta (nasal bleeding).
Mala : Purisha (laxative and anthelmintic).
Organs : Eyes (eye diseases).

References -

'अस्थिसंहारकः प्रोक्तो वातश्लेष्महरोऽस्थियुक् । उष्णः सरः कृमिघ्नश्च दुर्नामघ्नोऽक्षिरोगहृत् ।
रूक्षः स्वादुर्लधुर्वृष्यः पाचनः पित्तलः स्मृतः । भिषग्वरैर्यथा नाम फलं चापि प्रकीर्तितम् ।।'
'काण्ड त्वग्विरहितमस्थिशृंखलायाः माषआर्द्रद्विदलमकञ्चुकं तदर्धम् ।
संपिष्टं तदनु ततस्तिलस्य तैले संपक्वं वटकमतीव वातहारि ।।' (भा. प्र.)
'वज्रवल्ली सरा रूक्षा कृमिदुर्नामनाशिनी । दीपन्युष्णा विपाकेऽम्ला स्वाद्वी वृष्या बलप्रदा ।।
अस्थिसंधानजननी वातश्लेष्महरा लघुः ।' (कै. नि.०
'अर्शसां तु विशेषेण हिता चैवाग्निदीपनी । चतुर्धारा काण्डवल्ली भूतोपद्रवकुष्ठहा ।।' (नि.र.)
'संघृतेनास्थिसंहारम् ....। संधियुक्तेऽस्थिभग्ने च पिबेत् क्षीरेण मानवः ।।' (च.द.)

(18) ARISHTAK

Sapindus trifoliatus Linn.

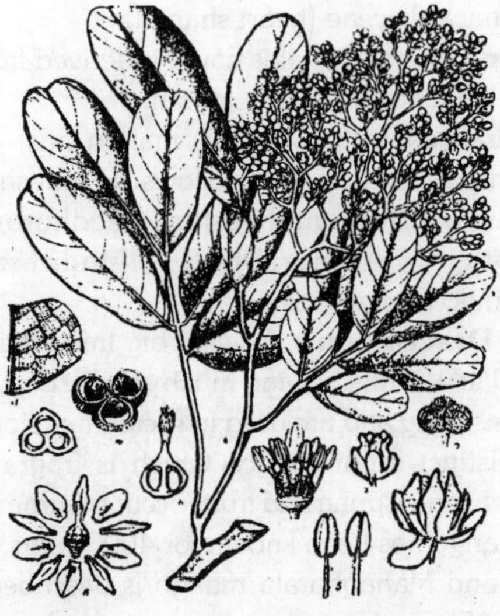

Kula : Arishtak kula.

Family : Sapindaceae (a group from which soap is derived).

Latin name : Sapindus = which yields soap; trifoliatus = having three leaves.

Sanskrit names : Rithakaranj, Gucchapushpak, Mangalya, Kumbhabeejak, Prakeerya, Phenil, Garbhapati, Raktabeeja, Rakshabeeja.

Botanical Description : This tree is 8 to 10 mtrs. high and has many branches with leaves and leaflets. Flowers are white. Fruits are round, trifoliated and occur in spring. It has two varieties.

Habitat : All over India.

Chemical composition : It contains 11.5 % saponin, 10% glucose. Seed contains 30% oil.

Properties :

Guna : laghu, snigdha, tikshna; **Rasa :** katu, tikta; **Vipak :** katu; **Veerya :** ushna; **Prabhav :** vamak (emetic); **Dosha :** tridoshaghna.

External use : Antiinflammatory.

Internal uses : It purifies vitiated kapha and pitta by emetic and purgative actions whereas alleviates vata by snigdha and ushna properties. Seed is intoxicant, while fruit rind has oxytropic action. In migraine, its water or powder is used as a nasya. In morphine poisoning, it is given orally to induce emesis.

Parts used : Fruit.

Dosage : For emesis - 3 to 6 gms., for purgation - 4 to 8 gms.; for medicinal purpose - 0.5 to 1 gm.

Srotogamitva :

Dosha : Tridoshaghna, kaphapittashodhan.

Dhatu : Rasa (induces emesis); rakta (cures dermatoses); meda(lekhan).

Dravyas which are beneficial to the body and the toxic dravyas, both are products of panchamahabhootas and they will act as to their properties.

Mala : Kaphashodhan (mala of rasa dhatu).
Organs : Uterus (induces abortion), oxytropic (in the form of nasya in migraine).
References -
'अरिष्टको गुच्छफलः सर्वतिक्तश्च मंजरी ।' (शि.)
'अरिष्टकस्तु मंगल्यः कृष्णवर्णोऽर्थसाधनः । रक्तबीजः पीतफेनः फेनिलो गर्भपातनः।।
अरिष्टकस्त्रिदोषघ्नो ग्रहजिद् गर्भपातनः।' (भा. प्र.)
'रीठाकरंजस्तिक्तोष्णः कटुः स्निग्धश्च वातजित् । कफघ्नः कुष्ठकण्डूवर्तिविषविस्फोटनाशनः ।। (रा. नि.)
'अरिष्टः कटुकः पाके तीक्ष्णोष्णो लेखनोऽगुरुः । दोषत्रयहरो गर्भपातनो ग्रहशान्तिकृत् ।।
तज्जलं वामकं पानान्स्याच्छीर्षरूजापहम् । अर्धशीर्षव्यथां हन्ति, वमनाद्विषनाशनः ।।' (नि.सं.)

(19) AMRA

Mangifera indica Linn.

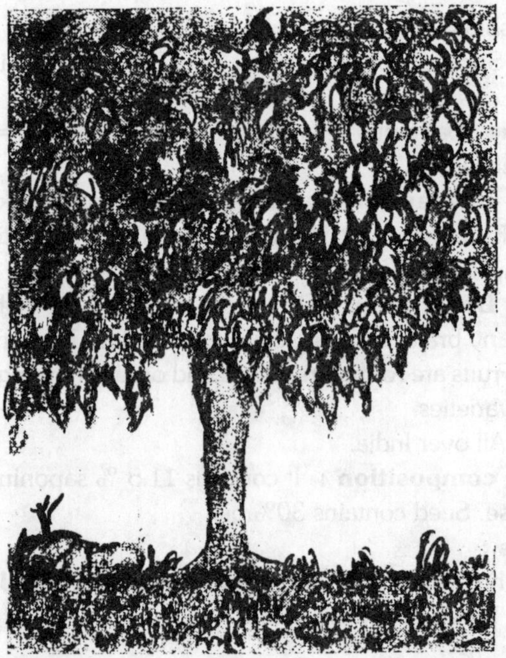

Kula : Amra kula.
Family : Anacardiaceae (heart shaped).
Latin name : Mangifera - this name is derived from malayalam language; indica = Indian.
Sanskrit names : In Sanskrit, mango has 63 names. Some of them are as follows : Kamashar, Madhavdruma, Bhrungubheeshta, Seedhurasa, Vasantdoota, Atisaurabha, Madirasav, Kokilabandhuk, Shukapriya.
Botanical Description : A very big tree having height of 10 to 12 mtrs. giving much shade. Leaves -13 to 16 cms. long and are used in sacred functions. It has a distinct inflorescence which is fragrant. Flowering season is spring and fruits occur in summer. (In India, mango has been known for 4000 years. In Ramayana and Mahabharata mango is described.) In the years 1556 to 1605, there was a garden having 1,00,000 Langada Mango trees in Bihar. This garden was named as 'Lakh Baug'. There are approximately 1000 varieties of mango fruit. Some of them are - Banganpalli, Cherukurasam, Suvarnarekha, Neelam, Jahangeer, Phajarie, Khas, Ulkhas, Jardalu, Himsagar, Shahpasand, Rogani, Rajapuree, Vansharaj, Alfanzo, Pareira, Fernandin, Totapuree, Mundappa, Dashehari, Langada, Zafaran, Rumanee etc. As the tree ages, the number of fruits it bears also increase. There is the largest mango tree in Burelgaon at Ambala district. Its stem has diameter of 9.75 mtrs. and its branches spread about 2258 square mtr. area. And every year this tree bears about 170 quintal fruits.
Chemical combination : Fruit contains 61.5% cellulose and vit. C.
Properties:
Guna : guru, snigdha, laghu, ruksha; **Rasa :** kashaya, madhur, amla; **Veerya :** sheeta.

Mango has different properties according to its stages. Bark, leaves, flowers and seeds are kapha pittashamak, haemostatic and wound healing. Ripe mango is vatapittashamak. Raw fruit is tridoshakarak.

Raw mango - appetizer, improves digestion and vitiates rakta pitta. 'Panha'(sherbet) reduces burning.

Leaves - antiemetic. In pyuria leaf juice is useful.

Flowers - astringent, antidiarrhoeal.

Bark - astringent heals the wounds and reduces inflammation of uterus.

Seed - anthelmintic reduces inflammation of uterus, antidiuretic, constipative and useful in menorrhagia and leucorrhoea.

Ripe mango - unctous, laxative, cardiotonic, haemostatic, aphrodisiac, gives strength and improves complexion.

Srotogamitva :

Dosha : Raw fruit - tridosh prakopak , ripe fruit - vata pitta shamak.

Dhatu : Bark, leaves, flowers and seed - raktagami (haemostatic); mansagami (wound healing). Raw fruit- rakta pitta prakopak; seed - rakta (stops menorrhagia); ripe fruit - raktagami (haemostatic), shukra - aphrodisiac, mansa meda (brumhan), rakta (improves complexion), rejuvenation.

Mala : Mutragami (leaf juice - pyruia), seed (antidiuretic, purisha (antidiarrhoeal, seed-anthelmintic).

Organs : Intestine, uterus.

References -

आम्रपुष्पमतीसारकफपित्तप्रमेहनुत् । असृग्दरहरं शीतं रुचिकृद् ग्राहि वातलम् ।
आम्र बालं कषायाम्लं रुच्यं मारुतपित्तकृत् । तरुणं तु तदत्यम्लं रूक्षं दोषत्रयास्रकृत् ।।''
पक्कं तु मधुरं वृष्यं स्निग्धं बलसुखप्रदम् । गुरु वातहरं हृद्यं वर्ण्यं शीतमपित्तलम् ।।
कषायानुरसं वह्निश्लेष्मशुक्रविवर्धनम् ।'
मन्दानलत्वं विषमज्वरं च रक्तामयं बद्धगुदोदरं च ।
आम्रातियोगो नयनामयं च करोति तस्मादति तानि नाद्यात् ।।'
(या श्लोकात सांगितलेले विकार आंब्याचा अतियोग झाल्याने होणारे आहेत.)
शुण्ठ्यंससोऽनुपानं स्यादाम्राणामतिभक्षणे । जीरकं वा प्रयोक्तव्यं सह सौवर्चलेन च ।। (हा त्यावरील उपाय आहे.) (भा. प्र.)
'आम्रबीजं कषायं स्याच्छर्द्यतीसारनाशनम् । ईषदम्लं मधुरं तथा हृदयदाहनुत् ।।'
आम्रस्य पल्लवो रुच्य: कफपित्तविनाशन: (भा. प्र.)
रक्तपित्तकरं बालमापूर्ण पित्तवर्धनम् । पक्वमाम्रं जयेद्वायुं शुक्रमांसबलप्रदम् ।। (च. सू.)
पित्तानिलकरं बालं पित्तलं बद्धकेशरम् । हृद्यं वर्णकरं रुच्यं रक्तमांसबलप्रदम् ।।
कषायानुरसं स्वादु वातघ्नं बृंहणं गुरु । पित्ताविरोधि संपक्वमाम्रं शुक्रविवर्धनम् ।। (सु: सू. ४६)
'त्वङ्मूलपल्लवं ग्राहि कषायं कफपित्तजित् ।' (ध. नि.)
'आम्रत्वचा कषाया च मूलं सौगन्धि तादृशम् । रुच्यं संग्राहि शिशिरं पुष्पं रोचनदीपनम् ।।' (रा. नि.)

Rasa-veerya-vipak-guna and prabhav are latent or unmanifest in a dravya. These act only when the dravya comes in contact with the body.

(20) AVARTAKI

Cassia auriculata Linn.

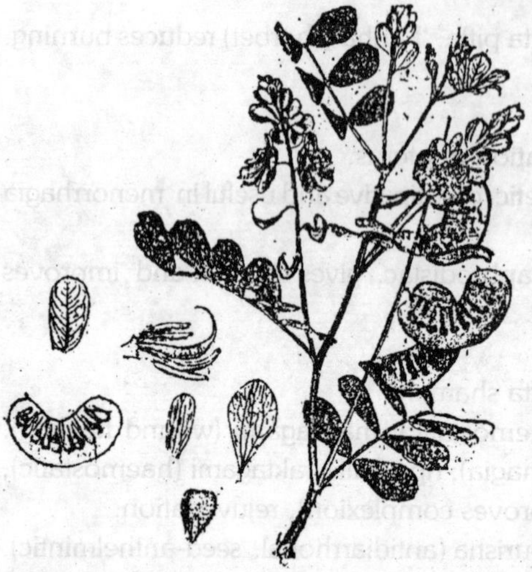

Kula : Shimbi kula.

Family : Leguminoseae.

Latin name : Cassia- from the name 'Kasian' (Gk); auriculata = small eared.

Sanskrit names : Vibhandi, Manodnya, Mahada, Charmaranga, Vamavarta, Mahajalini, Peetapushpa, Taravar, Aaval.

Botanical Description : A tree of height 1 to 3 mtrs. with yellow flowers. Legume contains 10 to 20 seeds. This tree is useful for dyeing leather.

Habitat : Maharashtra, Gujarat, Rajasthan, South India, Sri lanka.

Chemical composition : Bark contains 25% tanin.

Properties :

Guna : laghu, ruksha ; **Rasa :** tikta, kashaya; **Veerya :** sheeta; **Dosha :** kapha-pittashamak; **Karma :** astringent, krumighna, antidiuretic, (flowers) shukrastambhan, decreases uterine secretions (panchang). Besides that reduces dermatoses.

External uses : It is useful in wounds and conjunctivitis.

Internal uses: Astringent, anthelmintic, antidiuretic

It is useful in diarrhoea, dysentery, worms, bleeding disorders, diabetes (flowers or seeds), vaginal discharges and skin disorders.

Dosage : Bark decoction - 60 to 100ml., juice of flowers - 12 to 24 ml., seeds powder - 2 to 4 gms.

Srotogamitva :

Dosha : Kaphaghna, pittaghna.

Dhatu : Shukra (stambhan - flowers), rakta - (cures dermatoses and haemostatic).

Mala : Purisha (diarrhoea, dysentery and worms) (cures diarrhoea with bleeding per rectum); mutra - pramehaghna (seeds and flowers).

Organs : Uterus (cures menorrhagia), eyes (conjunctivitis - external use).

References -

आवर्तकी कषायातिस्तंभनी तिक्तशीतला । रक्तपित्तातिसारघ्नी कृमिकुष्ठविनाशिनी । नेत्ररोगे प्रमेहेच तत्पुषं तु प्रयुज्यते ।।

(21) AAYAPANAM

Eupatorium triplinerve Vent.

Kula: Bhringaraj kula.

Family: Compositeae.

Latin name: Eupatorium = Mithridates Eupator, King of Pontus (Dead sea) who discovered one of the species to provide an antidote for poison; triplinerve= having three nerves.

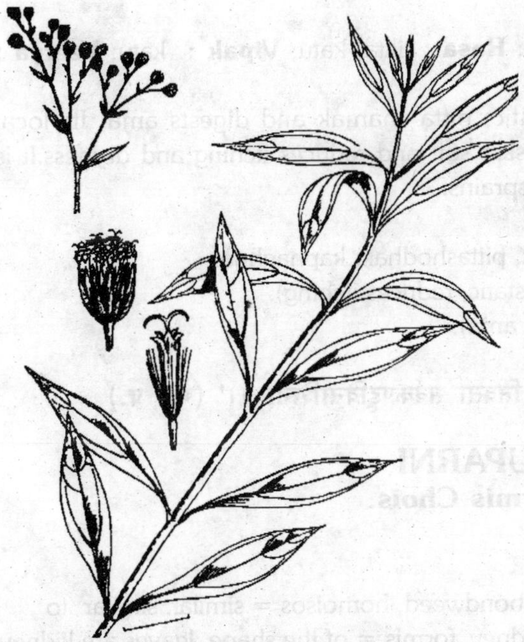

Botanical Description : A shrub 60 cm to 1.25mtr. high. Branches - reddish, hairy and straight. Leaves - opposite, 5 to 7 cms. in length, 2 cms. wide, tender with sharp tip, red having 3 venations. It is fragrant when crushed. Flowers - violet

Habitat : Basically Brazilian plant and also grows plentifully in Bengal.

Chemical composition : Volatile oil,aayapanin and many astringent components.

Properties :

Guna : laghu, ruksha; **Rasa :** tikta, kashaya;

Veerya :ushna; **Dosha :** kapha pittaghna.

External uses : It acts on raktadhatu and alleviates pitta, therefore it acts as a haemostatic and is useful in cleaning and healing wounds and as an antidote for poisons.

Internal uses : Cardiac stimulant. It is also useful in bleeding disorders, haematuria, diarrhoea with bleeding per rectum, skin disorders and urinary disorders caused due to vitiated pitta in which different shades of urine are seen. It plays an important role in menorrhagia. In fever with rigors, decoction of leaves is used.

In America, aayapan is a wellknown medicine for fever.

Parts used : The whole plant.

Dose : Juice - 3 to 6 ml; hot infusion - 30 to 100ml; powder - 2 to 4 gms.

Srotogamitva:

Dosha : Kaphaghna, pittaghna.

Dhatu : Raktagami - pittashaman (useful in bleeding disorders, haematuria etc. mainly menorrhagia).

Mala : Different shades of urine - Prameha

Organ : Uterus.

(22) AAMRAGANDHI HARIDRA

Curcuma amada Roxb.

Kula : Haridra kula.

Family : Scitaminaceae.

Latin name : Curcuma= Arabic name of turmeric; amada.

English name : Mangoginger.

Sanskrit names : Aamaharidra, Aamragandha, Kapoorharidra, Sugandha.

Botanical Description : A herb which looks like turmeric . Leaves - 0.6 to 1 mtr. long.Rhizome round, stout and resembles ginger. Flowering occurs in autumn.

Habitat : Bengal, West India (pickles and chutnies are made).

Plants impart more physical and mental strength through direct use and seeing respectively. One must contemplate one's mind on it.

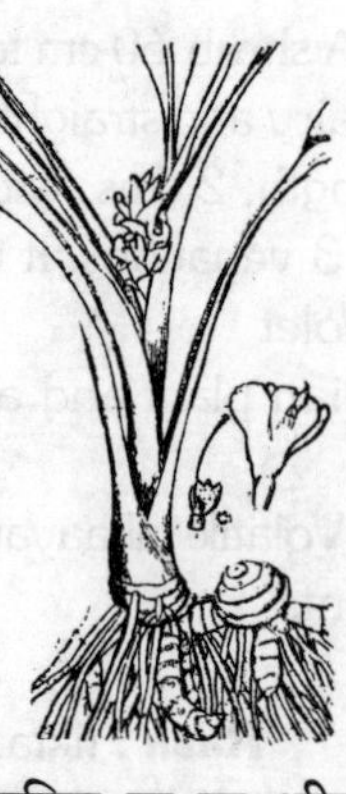

Properties :

Guna : ruksha, laghu; **Rasa :** tikta, katu; **Vipak :** katu; **Veerya :** sheeta.

Uses : It is haemostatic, pitta shamak and digests ama. Its local application makes the skin soft and reduces itching and dryness.It is also applied locally on sprains.

Srotogamitva :

Dosha : Vatavardhak, pittashodhak, kaphaghna.

Dhatu : Rakta (haemostatic, reduces itching).

Mala : Purisha (digests ama).

References -

'आम्रगन्धिहरिद्रा या सा शीता वातला मता । पित्तहन्मधुरा तिक्ता सर्वकण्डूविनाशिनी ।।' (भा. प्र.)

(23) AAKHUPARNI

Ipomoea reniformis Chois.

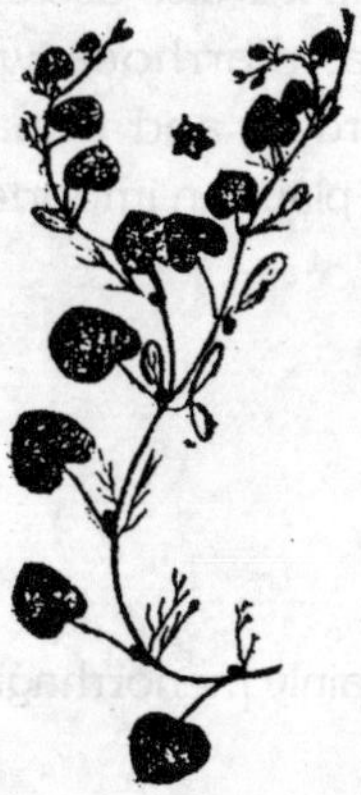

Family : Convolvulaceae.

Latin name : Ipomoea - Ips = bondweed, homoisos = similar, similar to bondweed; reniformis - ren = kidney, formis = of the shape, leaves are kidney shaped.

Sanskrit names : Aakhukarni is the appropriate name. Aakhu = rat, leaves resembles the ears of rat, hence the name aakhukarni. Shubhashreni, Krushika, Dravanti, Undirkarnika, Chitra, Sukarni, Nyagroodhi, Bhoomiradashrava, Mooshik karnika.

Botanical Description : A creeper grows especially in black ground. Leaves have curved edges. The plant grows everywhere.

Properties : Shodhan, diuretic, rejuvenative, anthelmintic, laxative and cures skin disorders.

Uses : Roti made up of rice with juice of aakhuparni is given along with oil of vidang and salt for deworming.(Charak and Sushrut). Juice is used orally in skin disorders.

Dose : Hot infusion is prepared using 0.6 to 1.2 gms. of crude powder which is used for deworming.

Srotogamitva :

Dosha : Vataghna, kaphaghna.

Dhatu : Rasayan, rakta (cures skin diseases).

Mala : Worms, mutragami.

References -

आखुपर्णी कटुस्तिक्ता कषाया शीतला लघुः । विपाके कटुका । मूत्रकफामयकृमिप्रणुत् ।।

(24) AMLAVETAS
Garcinia pedunculata

Kula : Nagakeshar kula.
Family : Guttifereae (gutta = drop; ferae = yielding).
Latin name : Garcinia = after the name of Dr. Garcia; pedunculata (pedinculate) - peduncle - stalk of flowers, fruits or cluster, especially main stalk bearing solitary flower or subordinate stalk, having a peduncle or flower stalk.
Sanskrit names : Vedhu, Rasamla. Veeravetas, Vetasamla, Amlasar, Bhedan, Raktasar, Shankhadravi, Mansadravi. (Chukra is considered as a representative of amlavetas).
Botanical Description : It is 20 mtrs. high tree. Leaves are 15 to 30 cms. in length. Androecium is bigger than gynaecium. Fruits - small yellow fruits like musk melon with 8 to 10 seeds.Fruit pulp - sour.
Properties :
Guna : laghu, ruksha, teekshna; **Rasa :** extremely sour; **Vipak :** amla; **Veerya :** ushna; **Dosha :** kaphavatashamak and pittavardhak.
Uses: It promotes all the digestive properties. It is used in cardiac debility and pain, cough, asthma, hiccups, sinusitis, dysuria and calculi.
Commercially branches of revandachini are sold as amlavetas. Charak has mentioned amlavetas in phalavarg, so it should be considered as fruit.
Srotogamitva :
Dosha : Pittavardhak, kaphaghna, vataghna.
Dhatu : Rakta (spleen).
Mala : Hair, purisha (purgative).
Organ : Heart, respiratory system , urinary system (calculi, dysuria).
It is used as a digestive with goat meat.
(Iron gets dissolved when needles and hooks are penetrated in amlavetas fruit.)
References -
'अम्लवेतसमत्यम्लं भेदनं लघु दीपनम् । हृद्रोगशूलगुल्मघ्नं पित्तलं लोमहर्षणम् ।।
रूक्षं विण्मूत्रदोषघ्नं प्लीहोदावर्त्तनाशनम् । हिक्कानाहारुचिश्वासकासाजीर्णवमिप्रणुत् ।।
कफवातामयध्वंसि छागमांसद्रवत्वकृत । चणकाम्लगुणं ज्ञेयं लोहसूचीद्रवत्वकृत् ।।' (भा.प्र.)
'अम्लवेतसो भेदनीयदीपनीयानुलोमिकवातश्लेष्महराणाम् ।' (च. सू. २५)

(25) IRIMED
Acacia catechu

Kula : Shimbi kula.
Upakula : Mimososeae (babbul).
Family : Leguminoseae.
Latin name : Acacia = Akazo Gk = I sharpen, many of the species have sharp spines; catechu = betal nut.

A man can harbour both love and anger simultaneously. Similarly a plant also harbours opposite properties like guru, laghu, snigdha etc. at the same time.

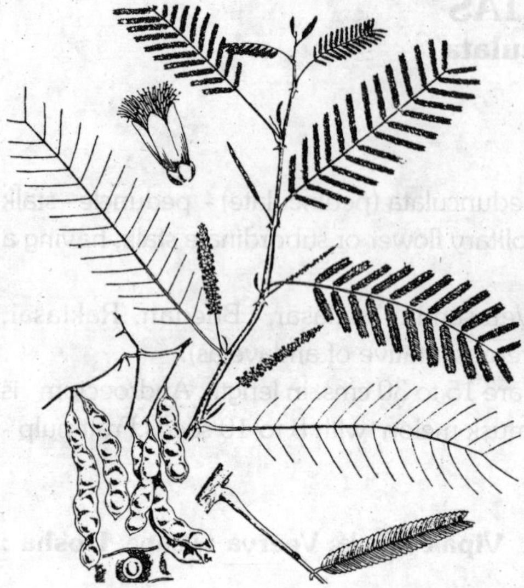

Sanskrit names : Khadir, Balapatra, Khadyapatri, Vakrakanta, Yadnyang, Dantadhavan, Gayatree, Kushthari, Medhya.

White Khadir - Shwetasar, Karmuk, Kubja Kantak, Somasaar, Somavalka.
Red Khadir - Raktasar, Tamrakanta, Bahushalya, Kushthatodan.

Varieties : It belongs to shimbi kula and kashayaskandha. Kushthaghna is prabhav of this varga. It has 5 varieties - shweta, raktakapish, rakta, krushna and vit. The fifth variety is called as arimed or irimed because it smells like stools or fats. All these varieties belong to acacia class.

Botanical Description : It is a tree of medium height. Stem - rough and thorny. Leaves - resemble the leaves of babool and are 7 to 10 cms. in length. Leaflet - 30 to 50 in pairs. Flowers - yellow, small having 3 petals. Legumes - 5 to 10 cms. in length, flat, shining and contain 5 to 8 round seeds.

Habitat : In Himalaya at the height of 2000 mtrs. and usually grows in dry weather.

Chemical composition : It contains 35% catechu and 57% astringent principle.

Properties :

Guna : laghu, ruksha; **Rasa:** tikta, kashaya; **Veerya:** sheeta; **Prabhav :** kushthaghna; **Dosha:** kapha-pittashamak.

Uses : Astringent, cures skin disorders, improves the taste, anthelmintic, haemostatic,blood purifier, antiinflammatory, antidiuretic, shukraghna, reduces laxity of uterus. Therefore it is used in bleeding disorders, dental diseases, hoarseness of voice, vitiligo, dermatoses, diarrhoea, worms, anaemia, cough, urinary disorders,menorrhagia and splenomegaly.

Srotogamitva :

Dosha : Kaphaghna, pittaghna and vatavardhak.

Dhatu : Rakta (prabhav - kushthaghna, haemostatic, blood purifier, antiinflammatory and reduces splenomegaly).

Mala : Mutra (antidiuretic and urinary disorders), purisha.

Organ : Uterus (reduces laxity, menorrhagia).

Prabhav : Kushthaghna.

(26) IKSHWAKU
Lagenaria siceraria Standle.

Kula : Koshataki kula.

Gana : Vaman, Phalinee, Urdhwabhagahar.

Family : Cucurbitaceae (Lat. cucurbita = a gourd - ornamental and edible gourds (big fruit) etc.

Latin name : Lagenaria = bottle like; siceraria = intoxicating.

English name : Bitter gourd.
Sanskrit names : Ikshwaku (Lord Ram's family), Pindaphala, Dantabeeja, Katutumbi, Tiktaalabu.
Botanical Description : Long creeper. Leaves - having diameter of 15 cms. and pentagonal. Flowers - homosexual, yellow, flower stalk -15 cms.
Varieties : 2 - sweet and bitter.
Habitat : All over India.
Chemical composition : It contains 90.36% water, ether extract, alkaloids, saponin. Seeds contains stable oil.
Properties :
Guna : Kapha-pittashodhan, shirovirechak, useful in kapha pittaj disorders.
Uses : Its juice is used as a nasya in jaundice and headache due to kapha dosha. Its oil is useful for shodhan therapy in inflammation, lymphadenitis, wound and dermatoses, cough, asthma, vomiting, fever, syncope, blood disorders.
Dose : Juice 3 to 6 ml.
Srotogamitva :
Dosha : Pittaghna, kaphaghna.
Dhatu : Rasa, rakta (cough, asthma).
Mala : Aamashayagata kapha.
Organ : Stomach.

(27) ISHWARI

Aristolochia indica Linn.

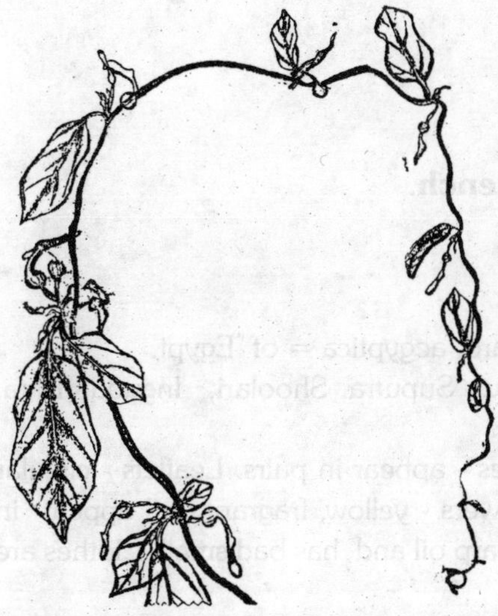

Kula : Ishwari kula.
Family : Aristolochiaceae.
Latin name : Aristolochia - aristos = best; lochia = parturation, it is supposed to have medicinal quality for easing birth; indica = Indian.
English name : Indian Birthvart.
Sanskrit names : Ishwari, Rudrajata, Sugandhika, Patravalli, Dhana, Rudralata, Sugandhapatra, Sauputra, Netrapushkar, Nakuli.
Botanical Description : It is a creeper having a long lifespan. Stem - small and hollow. Branches - tender. Leaves - 5 to 10 cms. in length and 2.5 cms. wide, pointed but wider at the end. Each leaf has 3 to 5 venations. Flowers - greenish white, 2.5 to 7 cms. in length. Fruits -round but becomes umbrella shaped when ruptures. Seeds - triangular and have wings. Roots- have frangrance like camphor. Flowers and fruits occur in rainy season.
Habitat : Nepal, South India, Bengal.

Vata vruddhi is the expression by those affected constituents of the body the properties of vata. Contrary to this vata kshaya.

Chemical composition : Roots contain volatile oil and dyeing agent.
Properties :
Guna : laghu, ruksha, tikshna; **Rasa :** katu, tikta, kashaya; **Veerya :** ushna; **Dosha :** tridoshahara, especially kaphavata nashak.
External uses : Its paste is used locally in snake bite, wound and painful inflammation.
Internal uses : It acts as a stimulant in vata disorders, depression and psychosomatic disorders. It is a good appetizer, laxative, analgesic, astringent and anthelmintic. Hence it is used in various internal disorders. It is also useful in cholera, teething disorders in children, cardiac debility and blood diseases. In children, leaf juice is used in cough and cold (by emetic action).It is useful in dysmenorrhoea, amenorrhoea. Pippalimool + ishwari is given in postnatal period.
It is used for shodhan in dysuria, skin diseases, typhoid, fever caused due to all the three doshas and puerperal fever.
Leaf juice or powdered roots are given in different poisons of snake, scorpion, spider and rat.
Dose : Root powder - 0.75 to 1.5 gm.; leafjuice - 4 to 12 ml.
Srotogamitva :
Dosha : Tridoshahara (especially kaphavata nashak).
Dhatu : Majja (Vata disorders, depression and psychosomatic disorders), blood diseases.
Mala : Purisha (astringent, anthelmintic and useful in cholera).
Organs : Internal channel, uterus.
Special action : Antidote to various poisons.
References -
'नाकुली तुवरा तिक्ता कटुकोष्णा नियच्छति । भोगिलूतावॉश्चिकाखुविषज्वरकृमित्रणान् ।।' (भा. प्र.)
'नाकुली कटुका तिक्ता तथोष्णा कृमिरोगहृत् । वृश्चिकोन्दुरुसर्पादिविषं नाशयति क्षणात् ।।
तुवरा च त्रिदोषघ्नी कन्देऽप्येते गुणा स्मृताः' । (ग.नि.)

(28) INGUDI
Balanites aegyptica Plench.

Kula : Ingudi kula.
Family : Simarubaceae.
Latin name : Balanites - balanus = nut, fruit rind is very hard; aegyptica = of Egypt.
Sanskrit names : Hingupatra, Vishakanta, Anilantak, Gaur, Suputra, Shoolari, Inguda, Tikta, Pootikantak, Angarvriksha.
Botanical Description : A plant 3 to 6 mtrs. high. Leaves - appear in pairs. Leaflets - circular ventrally. At the base of each leaf, there is a hard thorn. Flowers - yellow, fragrant and appear in bunches. Fruits - ovalshaped. Seeds - pentagonal, contains sharp oil and has bad smell. Clothes are washed with these fruits. It is used as a soap.
Habitat : Rajasthan, Gujarat etc.
Chemical composition : Its bark contains saponine.

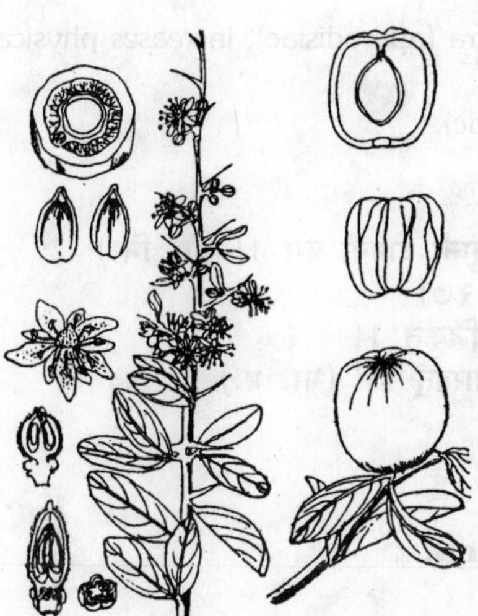

Properties :

Guna : laghu, snigdha; **Rasa :** tikta, katu; **Vipak :** katu; **Veerya :** ushna; **Prabhav :** krimighna; **Dosha :** vata-kaphanashak.

Uses : Oil has antimicrobial activity, it promotes hair growth, helps in healing of wounds and burn injuries. Bark is a strong purgative. Ingudi is an appetizer, anthelmintic, blood purifier and is useful in cough, asthma (fruitpulp),dysuria and leucoderma etc.

Srotogamitva:

Dosha : Vata-kaphaghna.

Dhatu : Mansa (wound healing), rakta (purifier), rakta meda (vitiligo), rasayani, shukra (reduces strength and antifertility).

Mala : Beneficial to hair (oil), purisha (bark - purgative) anthelmintic, useful in dysuria (increases formation of urine).

Organ : Eyes (diminishes vision).

References -

'इङ्गुदः कुष्ठभूतादिग्रहव्रणविषक्रिमान् । हन्त्युषअणः श्वित्रशूलघ्नस्तिक्तकः कटुपाकवान् ।।' (भा. प्र.)
'इङ्गुदी मदगन्धा स्यात् कटूष्णा फेनिला लघुः । रसायनी हन्ति जन्तुवातामयकफव्रणान् ।।' (रा. नि.)
'कांमिघ्नमिंगुदीतैलमीषत्तिक्तं तथा लघु । कुष्ठामयकृमिहरं दृष्टिशुक्रबलापहम् ।।' (सु. सू. ४५)

(29) UPAKUNCHIKA

Nigella sativa Linn.

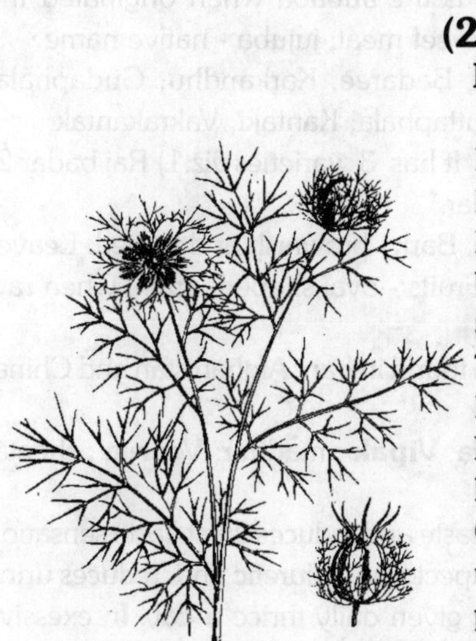

Kula : Vatsanabh kula.

Family : Ranunculaceae (grows in the marshy land.)

Latin name : Nigella = fennel flower - love in mist, devil in bush; sativa = cultivated.

Sanskrit names : Upakunchika, Deepya, Kalee, Manodnya, Taruna, Jeerna, Sushavi, Pruthveeka, Kalika, Bashpika.

Botanical Description : A shrub imported from South Europe. Now-a-days all over India.

Properties :

Guna : laghu, ruksha, tikshna; **Rasa :** katu, tikta; **Veerya :** ushna; **Vipak:** katu; **Dosha :** kaphavatashamak and pittavardhak.

Uses : Oxytrophic and galactogogue.It is used for external application in alopecia. It is used as a nasya in jaundice and headache.It is also used in round worms.

Dose : 1 to 3 gms.

Srotogamitva :

Dosha : Vataghna, kaphagna and pittavardhak.

Ayurveda is incomplete without the concept of avrutta. But in recent times, this concept has been lost.

Dhatu : It digests ama in all dhatus, majja (brain tonic), shukra (aphrodisiac), increases physical strength, rasa (breast milk).
Mala : Purisha (astringent, foul smell scavenger and anthelmintic).
Organs : Uterus (purification), eyes (beneficial to eyes).
References -
'पृथ्वीका कटुतीक्ष्णोष्णा वातगुल्मामदोषनुत् । श्लेष्माध्मानहराजीर्णआ जन्तुघ्नी दीपनी परा ।। (रा. नि.)
'.... कुञ्चिका..... । रोचनं दीपनं वातकफदौर्गन्ध्यनाशनम् ।।' (च. सू. २७)
'जीरकत्रितयं रूक्षं कटूष्णं दीपनं लघु । संग्राहि पित्तल मेध्यं गर्भाशयविशुद्धिकृत् ।।
ज्वरघ्नं पाचनं वृष्यं बल्यं रूच्यं कफापहम् । चक्षुष्यं पवनाध्मानगुल्मच्छर्धतिसारहृत् ।।' (भा. प्र.)

(30) UNNAV
Zizyphus jujuba Mill & Lamk.

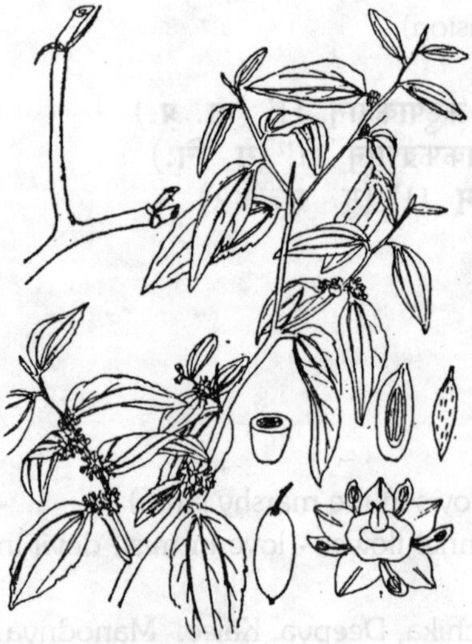

Gana : Hridya, Hikkanigrahana, Shramahara, Swedopaga, Aragvadhadi, Vatasamshaman.
Kula : Badar kula.
Family : Rhamnaceae (Rhamnus = ancient Gk name, The Drug cascura is obtained from the bark of one specy).
Latin name : Zizyphus = from the Egyptian name of one Sp. Z. jububa with dark red fruit is the Jubaba when originated the victorian word Jujbe for a sweet meat; jujuba - native name.
Sanskrit names : Badar, Badaree, Karkandhu, Gudaphala, Baleshta, Drudhabeeja, Vruttaphala, Kantaki, Vakrakantak.
Botanical Description : It has 3 varieties viz.1) Raj badar 2) Badar and 3) Kshudra badar.
A medium high thorny tree. Bark - brownish and torned. Leaves - 2.5 to 7.5cms. in length. Fruits - oval shaped, green when raw and yellow when ripes.
Habitat : All over India also found in Iran, Afghanistan and China.
Properties :
Guna : guru, snigdha, pichchila; **Rasa :** amla, madhur, kashaya; **Vipak :** madhur; **Veerya :** sheeta;
Dosha : vata-pittashamak.
Uses : Refrigerant, cleanes and heals the wounds, improves the taste and reduces thirst. Taste sensation vanishes for some time when leaves are chewed. It acts as an expectorant, diuretic and reduces urine sugar. In ikshumeha, powdered leaves in a dose of 3 gms are given daily thrice a day. In exessive thirst, sharbat of ripe fruit is given.
Srotogamitva :
Dosha : Vata-pitta-kaphanissarak.
Dhatu : Shukra (aphrodisiac), rasa - rakta (foam reduces burning sensation in fever), snayu (hoarseness of voice), meda (ikshumeha).

Mala : Purisha (strong purgative).
Organ : Uterus (cures menorrhagia).
References -

'सौवीरं बदरं शीतं भेदनं गुरु शुक्रलम् । बृंहणं पित्तदाहास्रक्षयतृष्णानिवारणम् ।।
कोलं तु बदरं साम्लं रुच्यमुष्णं च वातहृत् । कफपित्तकरं चापि गुरु सारकमुच्यते'।।
अम्लं स्यात् क्षुद्रबदरं कषायं मधुरं मनाक् । स्निग्धं गुरु च तिक्तं च वातपित्तापहं स्मृतम् ।।
शुष्कं भेद्यग्निकृत् सर्वं लघु तृष्णआक्लमास्रजित् ।' (भा. प्र.)
'बदरं मधुरं स्निग्धं भेदनं वातपित्तजित् । तच्छुष्कं कफवातघ्नं पित्तेन च विरुध्यते' (च. सू. २७)
'कर्कन्धुकोलबदरमामं पित्तकफावहम् । पक्वं पित्तानिलहरं स्निग्धं सुमधुरं सरम् ।।
पुरातनं तृट्शमनम् श्रमघ्नं दीपनं लघु ।' (सु. सू. ३९)
'राजबदरः सुमधुरः शिशिरो दाहार्तिपित्तहरः । वृष्यश्च वीर्यवृद्धिं कुरुते शोषश्रमं हरते ।।' (रा. नि.)
'तस्य मज्जा तु तुवरो मधुरो वीर्यवर्धनः । श्वासकासतृषादाहच्छ्र्दिमारुतपित्तजित् ।।' (रा.नि)
बदरीपत्रकल्कं वा घृतभृष्टं ससैन्धवम् । स्वरभेदे च कासे च लेहमेतत् प्रयोजयेत् ।।' (च. चि. २२)
'सममधुगुडभागं श्लक्ष्णकर्कन्धुचूर्णम् । प्रदरशमनमुक्तं योषितां खाद्यमानम् ।।' (शो.)
'बदरीपल्लवोत्थश्च तथैवारिष्टकोद्भवः । फेनिलायाश्च यः फेनः तैदाहे लेपनं शुभम् ।।' (च. चि. १२)
तैलोन्मिश्रैः बदरकपत्रैः संमूर्च्छितैः समुपनद्धः । मुशलेन पीडितोऽनुयातिप्लीहा पयोभुजोनाशम् ।। (वा. चि.)

(31) UTANGANAM
Blepharis edulis Pers.

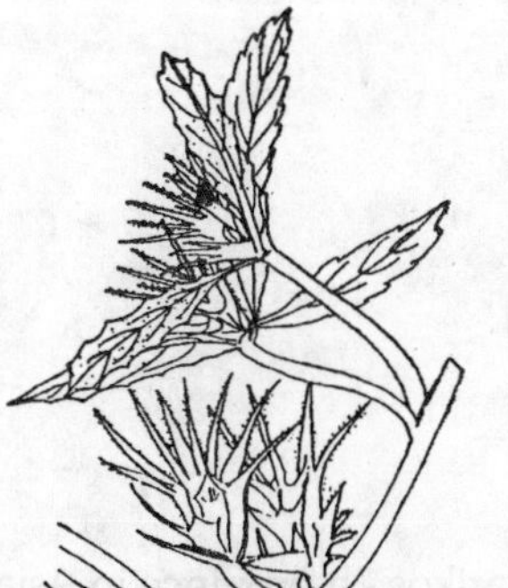

Kula : Vasa kula.
Family : Acanthaceae.
Latin name : Blepharis - blepharon = eyelid; edulis = eatable.
Sanskrit names : Utangan, Utangjan, Utingan.
Botanical Description: A shrub having fruits small, peach coloured, unctuous, shiny with 2 seeds. Seeds - heart shaped, flat, hairy and swells when soaked in water. This solution becomes slimy.
Habitat : Iraq, Iran, Afghanistan, Sindha and Punjab.
Chemical composition : Seeds contain mucilagenous substance.
Properties :
Guna: guru, snigdha, pichchila; **Rasa** : madhur, tikta; **Veerya** : ushna;
Dosha: tridoshahara.
Uses : It promotes spermatogenesis. It is an aphrodisiac and diuretic.

Srotogamitva :
Dosha : Tridoshahara.
Dhatu : Shukra.
Mala : Mutra (diuretic).

Treatment is education to the body (not punishment). Toxins punish the body.

(32) USHABA
Smilax zeylanica Linn.

Kula : Rasona kula.
Family : Liliacae (Lilium = Lily)
Latin name : Smilax = Sarsaparila plant Gk, smile = rasping or scrapping - the prickly stems. A graping chisel; zeylanica = of ceylon or ornata.
Sanskrit names : Kalika, Kalashak, Kalik, Vipindruma, Krushnavarna, Shraddhashaka.
Botanical Description : It is wild thorny creeper. Leaves - oval, 15 to 30 cms. in length and width with 7 to 9 venations. Flowers and fruits appear in bunches. Each fruit contains 1 to 3 seeds. Roots - reddish and those also appear in bunches and have plenty of secondary roots. The plant Ushaba magarbee is also known as Salasa. But this plant basically grows in South and central America.
Habitat : In wet mountainary area.
Chemical composition : Fats, glucose, glucosides, dyeing agent, saponin, gum and starch.
Properties :
Guna : laghu, ruksha; **Rasa :** tikta; **Vipak :** katu; **Veerya :** ushna; **Dosha :** tridoshashamak.
Uses : It is mainly used as a blood purifier in blood diseases and veneral diseases like syphilis etc.
Dose : Root powder - 3 to 6 gms; decoction - 5 to 10 ml.
Formulation : Majoon ushaba.
Srotogamitva :
Dosha : Tridoshashamak.
Dhatu : Rakta (as a blood purifier in various blood disorders).
Mala : Mutra (purifier).

(33) ERANDAKARKATI
Carica papaya Linn.

Kula : Erandakarkati kula.
Family : Passifloraceae - Lat. passio = suffering and flos = a flower.
Latin name : Carica = erroneously thought to have come from carica - karikos - a province in Asia minor; papaya = popai, Papaw.
Sanskrit names : Erandakarkati (as it is originated from Brazil, it has fewer sanskrit names), Talapatri, Chhatrapatra, Saptangulpatra, Ashakhavriksha, Dugdha, Pachani, Mansapachani.
Botanical Description : A tree 7 to 8 mtrs. high. Branches - absent. Stalk - straight and rough. Leaves - resemble the leaves of castor and have 7 angles. Stalk of leaf is 1 mtr. in length and hollow. Flowers - homosexual. Fruits - oval, when raw are green and yellow when ripe. Raw fruit oozes latex on cutting. Seeds - numerous and blackish grey.
Habitat : Not basically Indian but mainly from South America and Brazil. The Portugese brought it to India. Papeeta is its Portuguese name, however now it grows all over India.
Chemical composition : The main component papain solidifies and digests milk. It is mostly found in fruit, but also found in the other parts. Besides, there are many other components in the

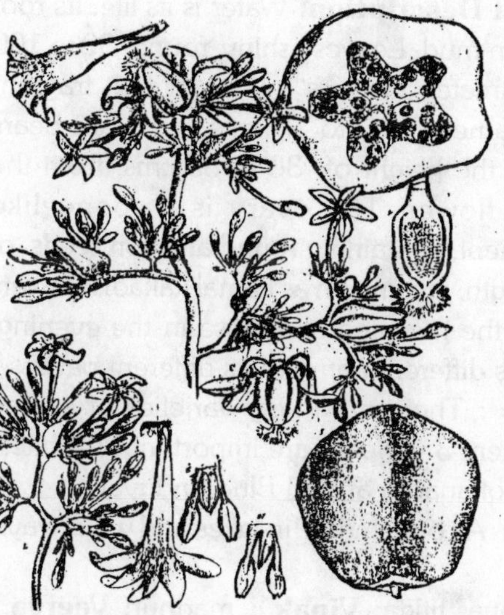

fruit.

Latex from fully grown raw fruit is collected, dried and powdered for medicinal use.

Properties :

Raw papaya - **Guna :** laghu, ruksha, tikshna; **Rasa :** katu, tikta; **Vipak :** katu; **Veerya :** ushna; **Dosha :** pittashamak (ripe papaya), vata kaphashamak (raw papaya).

Uses : Latex - lekhan, it is used locally in throat disorders, glossitis, skin diseases and glandular enlargements. Scorpian bite is treated by local application of latex. In vata disorders, leaves are tied over affected area. Oil derived from seeds is useful in paralysis and facial palsy. In filaria, paste of the leaves is applied. Papaya has good digestive property. One part of latex can easily digest 250 times flesh (meat). 3 gunja i.e. 375 mgs. of dried latex digests 1/2 lit. milk easily. It is also effective as a deworming agent. Carpene present in the leaves reduces heart rate and relaxation period is increased. Being an expectorant, it is used in cough and asthma. Hot infusion is used in dysuria and fever. Latex and seeds are used in amenorrhoea and dysmenorrhoea. Raw papaya causes abortions.

To avoid the after effects of colitis, papaya is the best medicine.

Dose : Hot infusion - 4 to 8 gms, latex - 6 to 12 ml, digestive principle -1 to 5 gunja (125 - 625 mgs), powdered seeds - 4 to 8 gunja.

Srotogamitva :

Dosha : Raw papaya - vata kaphashamak, ripe fruit - pittaghna.

Dhatu : Rasa (amenorrhoea, dysmenorrhoea - latex and seeds are useful).

Mala : Mutra (dysuria - hot infusion of leaves), purisha (worms - latex is useful).

Organs : Heart (carpene present in the leaves reduces heart rate), papaya is the best medicine for - after effects of colitis.

(Special note - If a pregnant woman eats raw papya, then there is possibility of abortion)

(1 part of latex digests 250 times meat easily. On scorpion bite latex is applied locally).

(34) KAMALAM
Nelumbo nucifera

Kula : Kamal kula.

Family : Nymphaceae (bears seven coloured lotuses).

Gana : Utpaladi gana, Mutravirajaneeya.

Latin name : Nelumbo = Indian name. This was previously known as nelumbium - neeram = water, biyam = bean; nucifera - nunci = nut, fera = bearing. Kamal seed is a tough shelled seed.

Sanskrit names : Pathoj, Kamal, Padma, Nalin, Ambhoj, Salilaja, Aravinda, Mahotpala, Rajeev, Sarasija. (Besides these, there are hundred of names according to the varieties).

All sufferings initially disturb the mind. And when everything is well, it is felt by the mind. Ayurveda does not classify diseases solely as mental or somatic.

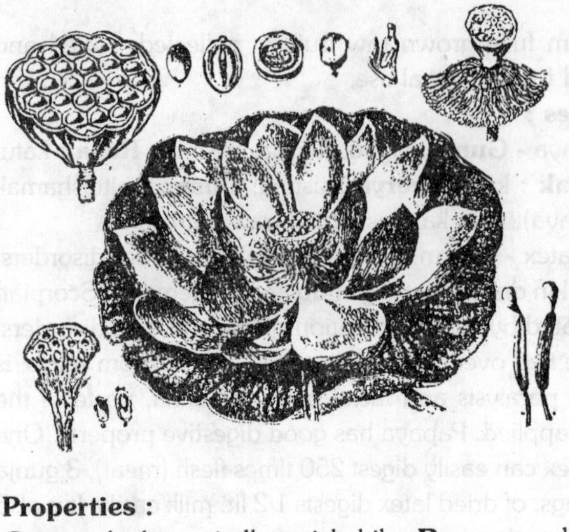

Botanical Description: Water is its life. Its root is dipped in mud. Leaves - shiny, round, 30 to 100 cm. in diameter. Flowers - white or red, fragrant having diameter 10 to 15 cms.The plant bears flowers at the height of 30 to 35 cms. from the stalk of flower. The ovary is a spongelike compartment, containing round and soft seeds of 4 cms. length, are known as kamal kakadi. Flowers bloom in the morning and close in the evening. Kamal has different name to its different parts.

Varieties : There are many varieties of kamal. Among them 3 varieties are important,1) White, 2) Red (Kokanada) and 3) Blue (Induvar).

Habitat : All over India, in lakes and waterways.

Properties :

Guna : laghu, snigdha, pichchila; **Rasa :** madhur, kashaya, titkta; **Vipak :** madhur; **Veerya :** sheeta; **Dosha:** kapha-pittashaman.

Uses: It is a refrigerant. Being a brain tonic, it enhances the intellectual power and it promotes sleep. It acts as an astringent in vomiting, thirst and diarrhoea associated with bleeding per rectum. Its special function is to protect the heart from excessive heat. As it alleviates pitta dosha, it is useful in various bleeding disorders. It is useful in foetal growth. It plays an extraordinary role in urinary disorders caused due to pitta, high grade fever, toxicity especially in paediatric diseases, in which children become weak.

Srotogamitva :

Dosha : Kaphaghna, pittaghna; (seeds - tridoshahara).

Dhatu : Rakta (erysipelas, complexion enhancer), rasa, shukra (seeds - aphrodisiac).

Mala : Purisha (seeds - astringent, constipative).

Organ : Uterus (seeds - stabilizes the foetus).

Prabhav : Antidote to poisons.

References :

'कमलं शीतलं वर्ण्यं मधुरं कफपित्तजित् । तृष्णादाहास्रविस्फोटविषवीसर्पनाशनम् ।।' (भा. प्र.)

'उत्पलकुमुदपद्मकिंजल्कः सांग्रहिकरक्तपित्तप्रशमनानाम् ।' (च. सू. २५)

उत्पलानि कषायानि रक्तपित्तहराणि च ।' (च. सू. २७)

सतिक्तं मधुरं शीतं पद्मं पित्तकफापहम् ।' (सु. सू. ४६)

'पद्मबीजं हिमं स्वादु कषायं तिक्तकं गुरु । विष्टम्भि वृष्यं रूक्षं च गर्भसंस्थापकं परम् ।।
कफवातहरं बल्यं ग्राहि पित्तास्रदाहनुत् ।' (भा. प्र.)

(35) KAREER

Capparis decidua

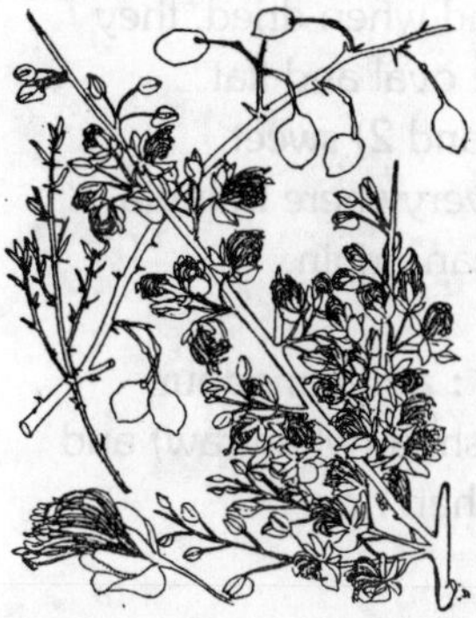

Family : Capparidaceae.

Latin name : Capparis = derived from the Arabic name 'kabar'; decidua = decido = to fall down, to cut off, finally falling. This tree looks like as if all the leaves are plucked off.

Sanskrit names : Nishpatrak, Kaveer, Karir, Tikshnakantak, Mruduphala, Tikshnasaarak, Suphala, Ushtrapriya, Apatra.

Botanical Description : A thorny shrub 2 to 3 mtrs. high with very few small leaves, hence it is called as 'Apatra'. Flowers - pink with much of honey. Pickles are made from its berries.

Habitat: It grows in Marvad, Punjab, Kutch and sandy areas.

Chemical composition : Buds contain capric acid.

Properties :

Guna : laghu, ruksha; **Rasa :** tikta, katu; **Vipak :** katu; **Veerya :** ushna; **Dosha :** vata-kaphanashak.

Uses : Analgesic and cleans wounds. Toothache is relieved by chewing its sprouts. It is very useful in haemorrhoids and worms.

Srotogamitva :

	Kareer	**Flowers of Kareer**
Dosha :	Kaphaghna, vataghna.	Vataghna.
Dhatu :	Digestion of amadosha.	
Mala :	Diaphoretic, purisha (purgative - haemorrhoids), diuretic.	

Fruits of kareer : Kaphaghna, vataghna.

References -

करीरः कटुकस्तिक्तः स्वेद्युष्णो भेदनः स्मृतः । दुर्नामकफवातामगरशोथव्रणप्रणुत् ।।' (भा. प्र.)
'करीरः कटुकस्तिक्तो लघूष्णो भेदनो जयेत् । दुर्नामकफवातामगरशोफकृमिव्रणान् ।।' (कै. नि.)
'करीरकुसुमानि कटुविपाकानि वातहराणि सृष्टमूत्रपुरीषाणि च ।
करीरफलानी च स्वादुतिक्तकटूष्णानि कफवातहराणि च ।' (सु. सू. ४६)
'लवणं ह्यर्कपत्राणि करीरतरुजान्यपि । मद्येरम्लैश्च युक्तानि युक्त्या क्षारं दहेत् पुटे ।।
सुखोदकेन मद्यैर्वा रसैरम्लैश्च पाययेत् । पीतः क्षारो ह्ययं हन्याद् वाताशांस्यिचिरेण तु ।।' (ग. नि.)

(36) KARMARANGA

Averrhoa carambola

Kula : Changeri kula.

Family : Geraniaceae (geranos = crane) The beaklike stigma.

Latin name : Averrhoa = in the memory of an Arabic physician in Spain; carambola = from its Indian name karmarak.

Sanskrit names : Karmarak, Karmar, Dharaphala, Peetaphala , Mugdarphala, Mugdarak, Karmarang, Nagaphala.

Ayurveda gives more importance to the stages of the diseases than the name of the disease. The stages of the dosh-dhatu-malas are more important than the names of the diseases.

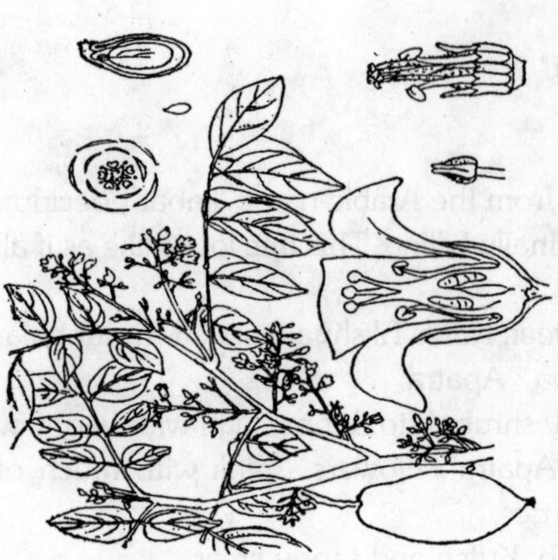

Botanical Description : This is a tree having a height of 7 to 10 mtrs. It has many branches and oval leaves. Flowers are reddish white in colour. Fruits contain 4 to 5 seeds. (When raw, they are green and when dried, they become yellow coloured). Seeds are oval and flat.

Types : There are 2 types, 1) sour and 2) sweet.

Habitat : Eventhough it is found everywhere in India, some scientists consider it of American origin.

Properties :

Fruit - Guna: laghu, ruksha; **Rasa :** amla, madhur, kashaya; **Vipak :** amla; **Veerya :** ushna (when raw) and madhur vipaki and sheeta veerya when ripe.

Karmaranga

Raw fruit	Ripe fruit
1) Sour	Sweet
2) Amla vipaki	Madhur vipaki
3) Ushna veerya	Sheeta Veerya
4) Kaphavata shaman	Pittashaman
5) Useful in Kaphavataj diseases	Pittaj diseases

Ripe fruit : is useful in dyspepsia, tastelessness, loss of appetite, bleeding piles, colitis, bleeding disorders, fever, burning sensation and weakness.

	Raw	Ripe
Srotogamitva:		
Dosha:	Kaphavataghna	pittaghna
Dhatu :	Mansa, meda, rakta, rasa	
Mala :	Purisha (astringent)	
Organ :	Intestine	

References -

'कर्मरगं हिमं ग्राहि स्वाद्वम्लं कफवातहृत् ।।' (भा. प्र.)

'कर्मारकोऽम्ल उष्णश्च वातहृत् पित्तकारकः । पक्वस्तु मधुराम्लः स्यात् बलपुष्टिरुचिप्रदः ।।' (रा. नि.)

(37) KATU TUMBI

Lagenaria sisereriya Stadle.

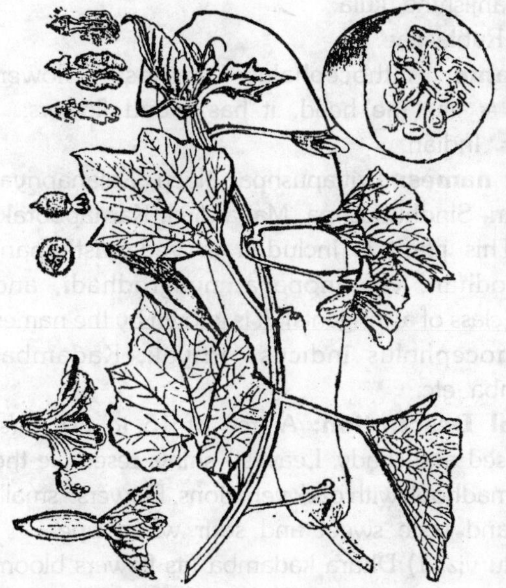

Kula : Koshataki kula.

Family : Cucurbitaceae.

Latin name : Lagenaria = bottle like.

English name : Bitter Gourd.

Varga : It is included in vamanvarga, Phalineevarga and urdhvabhagahar.

Sanskrit names : Ishwaku, Katutumbi, Titlauki, Kadvi, Tumbadi.

Botanical Description : A creeper spreads over a long. Leaves - 18 cm in diameter, tender and pentagonal. Flowers - yellow, homosexual with 18 cms. long flower stalk. Fruit - resembles sweet gourd.

Habitat : All over India.

Chemical composition : Fresh fruit has 90% water content. Seeds contain a stable oil.

Properties :

Guna: laghu, ruksha, tikshna; **Rasa** : tikta, katu; **Vipak** : katu; **Veerya** : sheeta; **Dosha** : kapha - pitta shodhan and shaman.

External uses : Nasya, antimicrobial, antiinflammatory, cleans wounds and cures dermatoses. Its juice is used as a nasya in jaundice and headache due to kapha dosha. Gargling of its juice is helpful in dental caries. Its oil is used externally in inflammation, glandular enlargements, lymphadenopathy, wounds and dermatoses.

Internal uses : Its fruit, seeds and leaves induce vomiting as well as purgation. It is used as a shodhak in cough, asthma, toxicity, vomiting, fever, unconciousness. It is a good expectorant. Roots are more effective in inflammation and blood diseases.

Dose : Leafjuice - 6 to 12 ml; seed powder - 1 to 3 gms.

Srotogamitva :

Dosha : Kaphashodhan, pittashodhan.

Dhatu : Rasa (cleans the wounds, cures dermatoses), rakta(jaundice - nasya) (cough).

Organ : Chest, stomach and intestine.

References -

'कटुतुम्बी हिमाऽहृद्या पित्तकासविषापहा । तिक्ता कटुर्विपाके च वातपित्तज्वरान्तकॉत् ।।' (भा. प्र.)
'कटुतुम्बी कटुस्तीक्ष्णा वान्तिकृच्छ्रासवातजित् । कासघ्नी शोधनी शोफव्रणशूलविषापहा ।।' (रा. नि.)
'कासश्वासविषच्छर्दिज्वरार्त्ते कफकर्शिते । प्रताम्यति नरे चैव वमनार्थ तदिष्यते ।।' (च. क. ३)
'तुम्बी... स्नेहास्तिक्तकषाया अधोभागदोषहराः कृमिकफकुष्ठानिलहरा दुष्टव्रणशोधनाश्च ।' (सु. सू. ४५)

(38) KADAMBA

Anthocephalus indicus A. Rich.

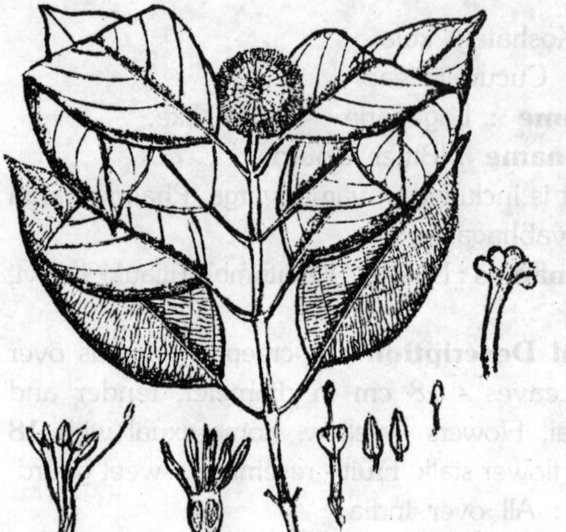

Kula: Manjishtha kula.

Family: Rubiaceae.

Latin name: Anthocephalus - anthos = flower, cephalus = like the head, it has round flowers; indicus = Indian.

Sanskrit names: Vrittapushpa, Neep, Lalanapriya, Kadambari, Sindhupushpa, Madadhya, Karnapoorak.

Varga: This plant is included in vedanasthapan, shukrashodhan, vamanopaga, nyagrodhadi, and rodhradi (class of astringents). It is known by the names viz. Anthocephalus indicus Priyak, Kadamba, Rajkadamba etc.

Botanical Description: A tree of 15 to 20 mtrs. high, densed and shady. Leaves - shiny, resemble the leaves of madhook with dark venations. Flowers - small, yellowish orrange. Fruits - like small balls, hard and taste sweet and sour when ripe.

Varieties: 3 varieties are mentioned in Raja Nighantu viz. 1) Dhara kadamba (its flowers bloom in monsoon), 2) Dhooli kadamba (its flowers bloom in spring) and 3) Bhoomi kadamba (having small flowers).

Habitat: Bengal, Uttar Pradesh and Madhya Pradesh. It is also described in the epics of Lord Krishna.

Properties:

Guna: laghu, ruksha; **Rasa:** katu, kashaya, tikta; **Veerya:** sheeta; **Prabhav:** vishaghna; **Dosha:** tridoshahara.

External uses: Warm leaves are tied on wounds to reduce inflammation. In conjunctivitis, the paste of bark is applied to eyelids. Wounds are washed and cleaned by the decoction of its leaves.

Internal ues: Decoction of leaves and gum are analgesic. In diarrhoea, bleeding per rectum and colitis, decoction of the bark is used. Juice or powder of bark + jeerak + sugar, is effective in vomiting.

Exessive thirst in fever is reduced by fruit juice.

It is used in bleeding disorders, oedema and cough. Decoction of roots is useful in calculi, and dysuria. In spermatorrhoea and vaginal disorders, decoction of bark is used. Menorrhagia is treated by leaf juice or decoction. Fruit juice promotes breast milk. In various skin diseases, bark paste is applied locally. Its bark is the best medicine to reduce burning sensation in fever. It is also useful in general debility and toxicity.

Parts used: Bark, leaves and fruits.

Dose: Bark powder - 0.5 to 1 gm; fruit juice - 12 to 24 ml; leaf juice - 12 to 24 ml.

References -

'सुगन्धिपुष्पः स्वाद्वम्लपक्वसस्यो महोन्नतः । मधूकपत्रसदृशपत्रो राजकदम्बकः ।।' (शि. द.)
'कदम्बस्तिक्तकटुकः कषायो वातनाशनः । शीतलः कफपित्तार्तिनाशनः शुक्रवर्धनः ।
त्रिकदम्बाः कटुर्वर्ण्या विषशोफहरा हिमाः । कषायास्तिक्तपित्तघ्ना वीर्यवृद्धिकराः पराः ।।' (रा. नि.)
'कदम्बस्तु कषायःस्याद्रसे शीतो गुणेऽपि च । व्रणसंरोहणश्चापि कासदाहविषापहः ।।' (ध. नि.)
'कदम्बो मधुरःशीतःकषायो लवणो गुरुः । सरोविष्टम्भकृद्रूक्षः कफस्तन्यानिलप्रदः ।.' (भा. प्र.)
'शीतवीर्यं तत्प्रवालं कषायं दीपनं लघु । रक्तपित्तातिसारघ्नमरोचकविनाशनम् ।।' (नि. र.)
'तत्फलं मधुरं शीतं गुरु पित्तास्रवातजित् ।' (कै. नि.)

(39) KAKUNDAR
Blumea lacero D. C.

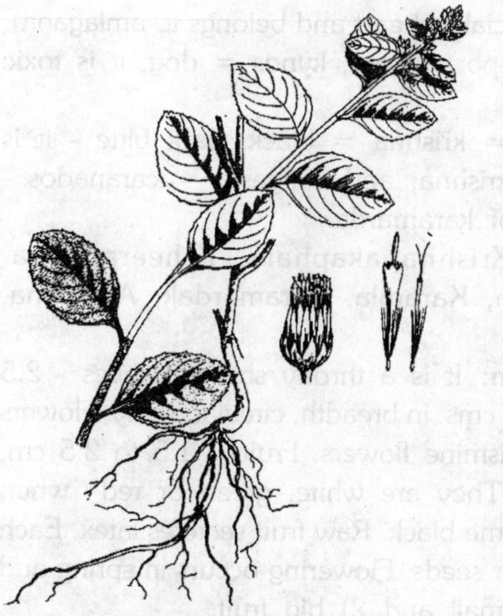

Kula: Bhringaraj kula.
Family: Compasiteae.
Latin name: Blumea = flowers; lacero = torn, irregularly cleft.
Sanskrit names: Kukurunda, Tamrachooda, Sookshmapatra, Mriducchada, Kukudru, Kukurbandha, Kukurunda.
Botanical Description: A shrub of 30 to 60 cms. high. Leaves - stout like kasani, hairy with strong smell. Flowers - tiny, yellowish, hairy and heterosexual. Seeds - small, black. Upper part of the plant is red in colour. These plants grow in rainy season and dry up in summer (which is used as a medicine). Flowering and fruiting occur in winter.
There are many varieties of this plant.
Habitat: In watery but at the height of 700 mtrs. but grows all over India.
Chemical composition: It contains volatile oil and comphor which is known as Nagee or patri camphor and has properties similar to bhimseni camphor.
Properties:
Guna: laghu, ruksha, tikshna; **Rasa:** tikta, kashaya; **Veerya:** ushna; **Dosha:** kaphapitta shamak.
Uses: Leaf juice or powder is used as a nasya in rhinitis, headache. Warm leaves are tied on inflammation. Conjunctivitis is treated by local application of leaf juice. The leaf juice kills maggots and is also used in wounds. Being appetizer, laxative, liver stimulant and anthelmintic properties, it is used in ascites, worms, liver disorders, haemorrhoids. In haemorrhoids, mixture of leaf paste and black pepper is given.
As it acts on rakta dhatu, it is used in blood disorders, bleeding disorders and oedema. It is useful in rhinitis, cough, asthma, fever and menorrhagia.
Especially in rabies, 6 gms. of root powder is given along with the water. (It acts by its emetic action).

Agni holds a unique place in treatment. Without agni neither health nor treatment exists.

Srotogamitva:
Dosha: Kaphaghna, pittaghna.
Dhatu: Rakta - liverstimulant - hepatitis.
Mala: Leaf juice kills maggots.
Prabhav: Emetic (in rabies).
References -
'कुकुन्दरस्ताम्रचूड : सूक्ष्मपत्रो मृदुच्छद : ।'
'कुकुन्दर :कटुस्तिक्तो ज्वररक्तकफापह : । तन्मूलमार्द्रं निक्षिप्तं वदने मुखशोषहृत् ।।' (भा. प्र.)

(40) KARAMARDA
Carissa congesta Linn.

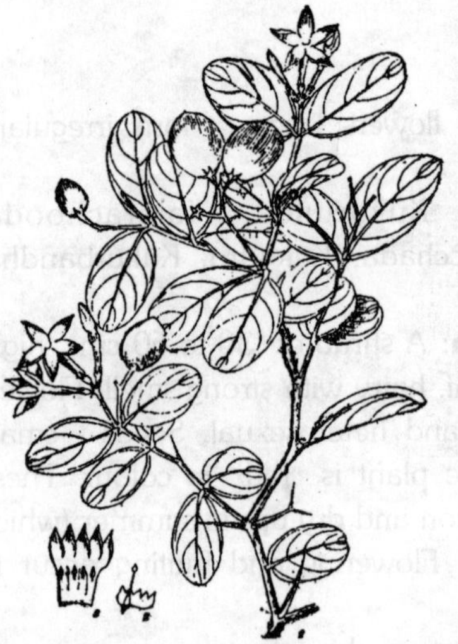

Kula: Kutaj kula (beneficial to heart and belongs to amlagana).
Family: Apocynacae (apo = from, kynos = dog; it is toxic to dogs).
Latin name: Carissa = krishna = black, dark blue - it is the modified word of krishna; and congesta = caranados - is the modified word of karamarda.
Sanskrit names: Krishnapakaphala, Ksheeraphena, Saamlapushpa, Sushen, Karamla, Karamardak, Aavighna, Panimarda, Dindima.
Botanical Description: It is a throny shrub. Leaves - 2.5 to 7.5 cms. in length, 3.5 cms. in breadth, circular, shiny. Flowers - white and resemble jasmine flowers. Fruits - 1.5 to 2.5 cm, either oval or circular. They are white, green or red when raw and when ripe become black. Raw fruit secretes latex. Each fruit contains 4 triangular seeds. Flowering occurs in spring and fruits occur in summer. Fruits are of 2 varieties - 1) Small and 2) big fruit.
Habitat: Punjab, Bengal, Brahmadesh and mostly grows in sandy, dry mountainous area.
Chemical Composition: It contains salycilic acid.
Properties: Even though it is guru, snigdha, there is difference between the properties of raw fruit and ripe fruit.
Raw fruit - **Rasa:** amla; **Vipak:** amla; **Veerya:** ushna; **Dosha:** vatashamak, kapha pitta vardhak.
Ripe fruit - **Guna:** singdha; **Rasa:** madhur; **Vipak:** madhur; **Veerya:** sheeta; **Dosha:** Vatapittashamak.
Root - **Rasa:** tikta; **Vipak:** katu; **Veerya:** ushna; **Dosha:** kaphavatashamak.
Uses: Raw fruit - It improves the taste, appetizer, astringent and useful in excessive thirst, anorexia and diarrhoea.
Ripe fruit - alleviates pitta dosha, useful in bleeding disorders and skin diseases.
Root - useful in cough, asthma, skin diseases, typhoid and persistent fever. Decoction of leaves is given in typhoid.
Dose : Juice - 12 to 40 ml; decoction - 60 to 100 ml.

Srotogamitva:
Raw fruit - **Dosha:** vataghna, kapha pittavardhak. Ripe fruit - vata-pittaghna.
References -
'करमर्दः सुषेणः स्यात् कृष्णपाकफलस्तथा । तस्माल्लघुफला या तु सा ज्ञेया करमर्दिका ।।
करमर्दद्वयं त्वाममम्लं गुरु तृषाहरम् । उष्णं रुचिकरं प्रोक्तं रक्तपित्तकफप्रदम् ।।
तत्पक्वं मधुर रुच्यं लघु पित्तसमीरजित् ।' (भा. प्र.)
'लवङार्द्रकसंयुक्तं सुपिष्टं वआरिणा युतम् । कारमर्द करैर्मर्दं सप्तभागसितान्वितम् ।।
वातहृद्रुचिदं बल्यं हृद्यमम्लतरं स्मृतम् । रक्तपित्तकरं चोक्तम् कण्ठ्यं करमर्दकम् ।।' (क्षे.कु.)

(41) KATAK

Strychnos potatorum Linn.

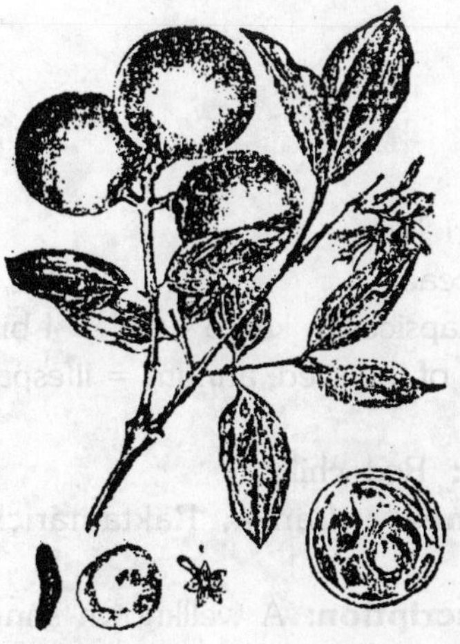

Gana: Parushakadi.
Kula: Karaskar - Kuchala kula.
Family: Loganiaceae.
Latin name: Strychnos = Gk. name for solanum and allied = poisonous; potatorum = pertaining to drink.
English name: Clearing nut.
Sanskrit names: Chakshushya, Nirmali, Ambuprasad, Kata, Tiktaphala, Ruchya, Chhedaneeya, Lekhanatmak, Dridhaphala, Kattha, Ruchishna, Shodhan.
Botanical Description: A tree 10 to 20 mtrs. high. (higher than Strychnos nuxvomica). Flowers - yellow. Fruits - black. Seeds - like the seeds of Strychnos nuxvomica, but small, double convexed, white and hard.
Habitat: South India, Bengal and Brahmadesh.
Chemical Composition: Seeds contain bruesin.
Properties:
Guna: laghu, vishad; **Rasa:** madhur; **Veerya:** sheeta; **Dosha:** kapha-vatashamak.
Uses : To purify water. When its seeds are rubbed in water and added to impure water, all the impurities in the water settle at the bottom and water is purified. Sushrutacharya has mentioned kataka as a best drug to purify the water.
External uses: It is rubbed in honey and applied in the eyes as a anjan in corneal ulcer and chronic conjunctivitis. Powdered seeds along with the honey are applied on the abscess.
Internal uses : Its seeds are appetizer, astringent and also improve the taste. Large dose causes emesis. It is useful in anorexia, diarrhoea and swellings.
It is a diuretic and is used in dysuria, pyuria, ikshumeha. Roots are used in dermatoses.
Dose: Seeds - 1 to 2 gms., for emesis - 6 gms.
Srotogamitva:
Dosha: Kapha-vataghna (fruit - vatavardhak).
Dhatu: Rakta, meda (urinary disorders, anaemia, jaundice, dermatoses).

Depending upon the causes there are various stages and consequently the symptoms of diseases. Hence there must be a difference in treatment, too.

Mala: Purisha (astringent), mutra (diuretic).
Prabhav: Beneficial to eyes.
References -
‘कतं कतफलं कात्थं श्लक्ष्णं वारिप्रसादनम् । तोयप्रसादनफल चक्षुष्यं लेखनात्मकम् ।।
कतकं तुवरं तिक्तं विशदं शीतल लघु । विकाशि मधुरं छेदि चक्षुष्यं कफवातनुत् ।।
तृष्णां दाहं विषं गुल्मं हन्ति तोयमलापहम् ।’ (कै. नि.)
‘तस्यैव च फलं पक्वं वातकृन्मेहनाशनम् । सुपिच्छिलं छर्दिकरं श्लेष्मपित्तप्रसेककृत् ।।
शोफपाण्डुप्रतिश्यायकामलागरनाशनम् । कतकस्य च मूलं तु सर्वकुष्ठप्रणआशनम् ।।’ (कै. नि.)
‘कतकं शीतलं प्राहुस्तृष्णाविषविनाशनम् । नेत्रोत्थरोगविध्वंसिविधिनाऽञ्जनयोगतः ।।
कतकस्य फलं तिक्तं चक्षुष्य शीतलं मृदु । वारिप्रसादनं कृच्छ्रशर्करामश्मरीं जयेत् ।।’ (ध. नि.)
‘पयःप्रसादी कतकः कतकं तत्फलं च तत् । कतकस्य फलं नेत्र्यंजलनिर्मलताकरम् ।।
वातश्लेष्महरं शीतं मधुरं तुवरं मधु ।’ (भा. प्र.)

(42) KATUVEERA

Capsicum annum Linn.

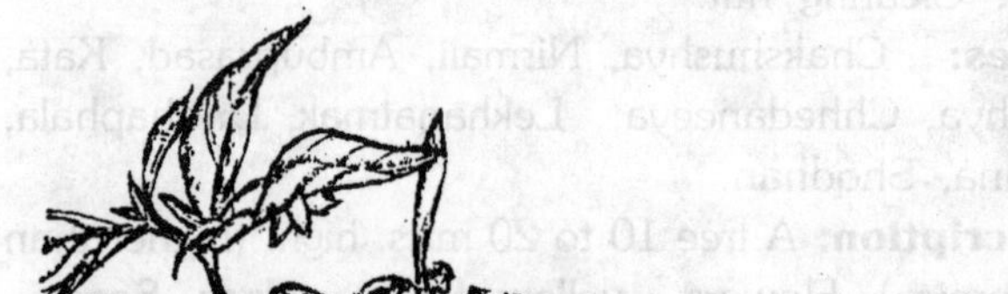

Kula: Kantakari kula.
Family: Solanceae.
Latin name: Capsicum - kapto - Gk. = I bite = the pungency of the seed; annum = lifespan of 1 year.
English name: Red chilly.
Sanskrit names : Lanka, Raktamarich, Katuveera.
Botanical Description: A wellknown shrub having lifespan of 1 year or many years. Leaves - oval with narrow tip. Fruits - green when raw and red when ripe. (Green colour is a indication of peacefullness, sacred while red colour indicates anger, irritant to nerves, exactly opposite to green colour. Some fruits are yellow also. Seeds - numerous like brinjal.
Habitat: All over India, it is cultivated.
Chemical composition: Pungency is due to capsikine - a volatile alkaloid.
Properties:
Guna: laghu, ruksha, tikshna; **Rasa:** katu; **Vipak :** katu; **Veerya:** ushna; **Dosha:** kapha-vata shamak and pittavardhak.

External uses: Lekhan, vitiates blood, antipruritic, analgesic, antiinflammatory. It reduces low backache and sciatic pain by external application. In throat disorders, gargling is done by its hot infusion. It is also used in dog bite.

Internal uses: 1 to 2 gms. of chilly powder along with honey is useful in rheumatoid arthritis, delirium and alcoholism. It creates excess salivation. It is an appetizer, digestive and laxative but causes burning sensation. Green chilly acts as a cardiac stimulant and also aphrodisiac. If given in small dose acts as a diuretic in retention of urine. In cholera, asafoetida + comphor + red chilly powder improves digestion as well as patient does not develope weakeness. It is also useful in fever and obesity. Burning sensation is relieved by milk and ghee.

Srotogamitva:

Dosha: Kaphaghna, pittavardhak.

Dhatu: Rakta (vitiates), cardiac stimulant (green chilly), shukra (aphrodisiac), meda (fat metabolism).

Mala: Mutra (diuretic if given in small dose).

Organ: Digestive system (asafoetida + camphor + red chilly - digestive).

References -

'कटुवीरोज्ज्वला तीक्ष्णा तीर्रशक्त्यजडे तथा । कटुवीराग्निजननी बलासग्नी च दाहिनी ।।
हन्त्यजीर्ण विसूचीं च व्रणं क्लिन्नं सुदारुणम् । तन्द्रां मोहं प्रलापं च स्वरभेदमरोचकम् ।।
नरं लुप्तधरं क्षीणं सन्निपातनिपीडितम् । नष्टेन्द्रियगणं तीक्ष्णा मृत्योराकृष्य जीवयेत् ।।' (आत्रेयसंहिता)

(43) KANKOLAM

Piper cubeba Linn.

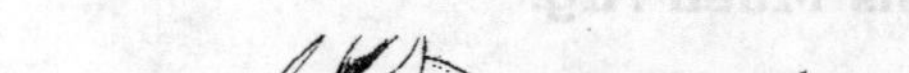

Kula: Pippali kula.

Family: Piperaceae.

Latin name: Piper = Gk. pipto, Latin - piper, peper, suggested derivation from Gk - pepto = to digest; cubeba = Kabab = local name.

Sanskrit names: Gandhamarich, Kritaphala, Kulak, Katukphala, Dweep, Mareech, Triputa, Kola, Chakrabeeja, Koshaphala, Katuphala.

Botanical Description: A creeper with leaves 12 to 14 cms. long, oval and tapering towards the tip. Flowers - small, homosexual and appear in bunches. Fruits - circular, look like black pepper and appear in bunches. They have very strong odour or pungent. It feels cool to taste. It bears flowers and fruits in autumn.

Habitat: Indonesia, Malaysia, Karnataka and Mahabaleshwar.

Chemical composition: It contains an essential oil 10 to 15%, cubabin, cubebic acid, fats, wax, starch, gum etc.

The principal goal of Ayurveda is to protect and promote health. Other considerations come later. But in reality, the concept is reversed.

Properties:
Guna: laghu, ruksha, tikshna; **Rasa:** katu, tikta; **Veerya:** ushna; **Dosha:** kaphavatashamak.
External uses: Vitiates blood, stimulant, antiinflammatory, deodorant and has wound healing property. It is applied locally on inflammed sites. In oral , dental and throat disorders, kankol is kept in the mouth. It is also used in toothpowders. In impotency, it applied on penis. Its powder is used as a nasya in heaviness of head. Local application of its powder acts as a deodorant.
Internal uses: It improves the taste and is good appetizer, digestive and laxative, so used in various internal diseases.
In cough and asthma, it acts as an expectorant. It is a good cardiac tonic.It is used in dysmenorrhoea, amenorrhoea, loss of libido, impotency and dysuria.
Dose: Fruit powder - 1 to 3 gms, oil - 5 to 20 drops.
Srotogamitva:
Dosha: Kaphaghna, vataghna.
Dhatu: Rakta (antiinflamatory), mansa (wound healing), shukra (external application on the penis).
Mala: Sweda (deodorant), mutra (dysuria).
References -
कङ्कोलं कटु तीक्ष्णोष्णं वक्त्रजाड्यहरं परम् । दीपनं पाचनं रुच्यं कफवातनिकृन्तनम् ।।' (रा. नि.)
कङ्कोलकं.... कटुतिक्तं कफापहम् । लघु तृष्णापहं वृष्यं वक्तदौर्गन्ध्यनाशनम् ।।' (सु. सू. ४६)

(44) KAMPILLAKA
Mallotus philippinensis Muell Arg.

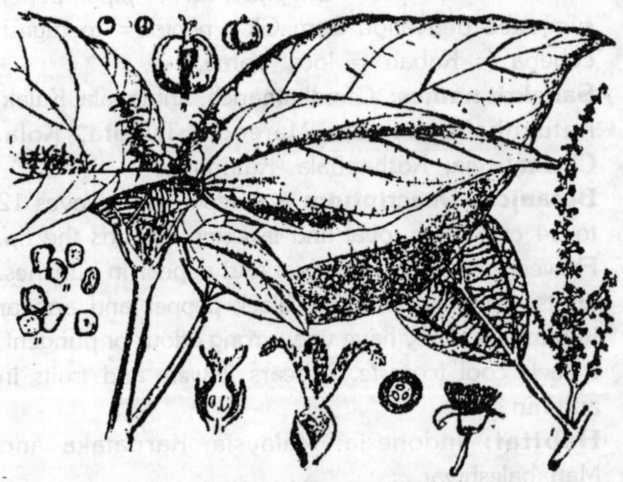

Gana: Virechan (C.); Adhobhagahara, Shyamadi (S.)
Kula: Eranda kula.
Family: Euphorbiaceae = in the memory of the scientist Euphorbus.
Latin name: Mallotus = like the shape of Melon; philippinensis = in island Phillipines (Rottlera tinctoria - to dye silk).
Sanskrit names: Kampillaka, Raktang, Rechee, Rechanak, Ranjan, Lohitanga, Karkash, Raktachoornak, Kapilo, Kamala dye.
English name: Monkey face tree (mouth becomes red like monkey when its fruit is held in the mouth).
Botanical Description: Evergreen tree 8 to 10 mtrs. high. Leaves - like udumbar and has 2 nodes at the base of the leaf stalk. Ventrally it has 3 red veins. Flower stalk is red. Fruit

- small, having 3 compartments and appear in bunches. On the ripe fruit there is red powder which falls off when fruits are rubbed. It is called as kapila. Seeds - circular and smooth. Flowering occurs in autumn and fruits in spring. (Observation : Pure kapila powder doesn't get dissolved in water. It floates on the upper surface of water. It is inflammable like alcohol. It dissolves in ether and alkaloids. When kapila powder is smeared on paper with a wet finger, it turns the paper yellow. It is soft to touch, light and odourless. It is adulterated by brick powder.)

Habitat: India, Sri lanka, Brahmadsh, Malaysia, Singapore, China, Africa and Australia.

Chemical composition: It contains 80% reddish yellow resin and also many other components.

Properties:

Guna: laghu, ruksha, tikshna; **Rasa** : katu; **Veerya:** ushna;**Dosha:** kaphavatashamak and pittavardhak.

External uses : Useful in dermatoses, cleans and heals the wound. It should be mixed with oil and honey and then applied to ulcerated and pyogenic wounds.

Internal uses : It is used in flatulence, ascites, constipation, worms. It kills and expells the worms. There is tradition of using mild laxative along with it. It is very strong for the persons with mrudu koshtha. Kapila + swadishta virechan choorna is a good remedy for worms. It is useful in blood diseases, calculi, impotency and dermatoses.

Dose : Powder on the fruit - 2 to 3 mgs; for children - 1 to 2 mgs. (Kapila developes nausea) (Kapila powder is used to dye silk).

Srotogamitva :

Dosha: Kaphaghna , vataghna, pittakarak.

Dhatu : Rasa (dusted on pyogenic wounds), rakta (blood disorders and dermatoses), shukra (impotency).

Mala: Mutra (calculi).

References -

इष्टिकाचूर्णसंकाशः चन्द्रिकाढ्योऽल्परेचनः । सौराष्ट्रदेशे वृक्षस्य फलरेणुः कपिल्लकः ।।' (शि.)
काम्पिल्लः कफपित्तास्रकृमिगुल्मोदरव्रणआन् । हन्ति रेची कटूष्णश्च मेहानाहविषाश्मनुत् ।।' (भा. प्र.)
कम्पिल्लको विरेची स्यात् कटूष्णो व्रणनाशनः । गुल्मोदरविबन्धाध्मश्लेष्मकृमिविनाशनः ।। (ध. नि.)

(45) KANKUSHTHA

Garcinia morella Desr.

Kula: Nagakesar kula.

Family: Guttifereae.

Latin name: Garcinia = after the name of Dr. Garcia; morella = bitter kind of cherry. Indian gamboge (Vaidya Bapalal Vaidya).

Sanskrit names: Kankushtha, Kalakushtha, Virang, Shodha, Kalapalak, Kakakushtha, Rechan, Kolavaluka, Rochan, Jalavaluka.

Botanical Description: Medium sized tree.

Properties:

Rasa: tikta, katu; **Vipaka:** katu; **Veerya:** ushna; **Dosha:** kaphavataghna.

We must understand the technical language and definitions of Ayurveda. One must not have wrong concepts about vata etc.

Indications: Haermorrhoids, tumour, wounds, pain, inflammation, flatulence and worms.
Uses: It is a strong purgative and hence used in ascitis, worms, hypertension. Also useful in amenorrhoea. It is a good complexion enhancer.
Parts used: Gum.
Dose: 30 to 60 mgs.(along with volatile drugs), toxic dose - 1 drm, higher dose leads to severe emesis, purgation, pain and finally the death.
Srotogamitva:
Dosha: Kaphavataghna.
Dhatu: Rakta (useful in hypertension), rasa (amenorrhoea).
Mala: Purisha (strong purgative).

(46) KATPHALA
Myrica nagi Thumb.

Gana: Sandhaneeya , Shukrashoddhan, Vendanasthapan (C.); Lodhradi, Surasadi (S.).
Kula: Katphala kula.
Family: Myricaceae.
Latin name: Myrica = name of Venus; nagi = Chinese or Japanese name of this plant.
English name: Box myrtle (Myristica malabarica).
Sanskrit names: Ramapatri, Katphala, Somavalka, Kumudika, Bhadravati, Krishnagarbha, Ugragandha, Ranjank, Laghu kashmari.
Botanical Description: Evergreen medium high tree, very dense leaved and fragrant. Bark - red, hard having diameter 10 cms. and has small oval spots inside. Wood heart - grey and hard. Leaves - 10 to 12 cms. in length and fragrant. Flower stalk - small, soft and hairy. Flowers - red, unisexual - female and male flowers on different trees. Fruits - 1.5 to 1.75 cm. in length, when ripe red, sour and sweet. It bears flowers during winter and fruits in summer.
Habitat: Punjab, Garwhal, Kumaon, Khasi hills and Sylhet.
Chemical Composition: It contains an astringent principle, glucose and salts.
Properties:
Guna: tikshna; **Rasa:** katu, tikta, kashaya; **Vipak:** katu; **Veerya:** ushna; **Dosha:** vatakapha shamak and pittavardhak.
External uses: Bark powder is used as a nasya for rhinitis, unconsciousness and headache. Bark powder - is applied on wounds and for removing maggots. It is also used to warm body parts on excessive sweating. In vata disorders, powder mixed with oil is used for massage. Decoction is used for gargling in oral diseases and toothache. A vaginal suppository made up of the powder contracts the uterus and reduces dysmenorrhoea.
Internal uses: It is a nervine tonic and useful in vata disorders like facial paralysis. It is also used in anorexia, cardiac debility, haemoptysis, oedema, cough, asthma, rhinitis, urinary disorders, skin diseases and fever.
Note - It is harmful to liver and spleen.

Srotogamitva :
Dosha: Vataghna , kaphaghna, pittavardhak.
Dhatu: Majja (cures unconsciousness by nasya), shukra (shodhan), rakta (haemoptysis, cough), meda (urinary disorders and mumps), rakta (acts on liver and spleen but harmful).
Mala: Sweda (excessive sweating - applied on body).
Organ: Uterus (vaginal supository - uterine contractions). Nasya - shiroshuddhi occurs faster.
References -
'कट्फलः सोमवल्कस्च कैटर्यः कुम्भिकापि च । श्रीपर्णिका कुमुदिका भद्रा भद्रवतीति च ।।
कट्फलस्तुवरस्तिक्तः कटुर्वातकफज्वरान् । हन्ति श्वासप्रमेहार्शः कासकण्ड्वामथारुची: ।।' (रा. नि.)
'कटफलं मधुयुक्तं वा मुच्यते जठरामयात् ।' (च. चि. १०)
'प्रियंगुकाकट्फलशंखगैरिकाः पृथक् पृथक् चन्दनतुल्यभागिकाः ।
सशर्करास्तण्डुलधावनाप्लुताः रक्तं सपित्तं शमयन्ति योगाः ।।' (च. चि. ४)
'ध्रेयं कट्फलचूर्णं वा ।' (सु. उ. २६)
'कट्फलचूर्णान्तर्गलघर्षो गलगण्डमपहरति ।' (च. द.)

(47) KARPOOR

Cinnamomum camphora Nees and Eberm.

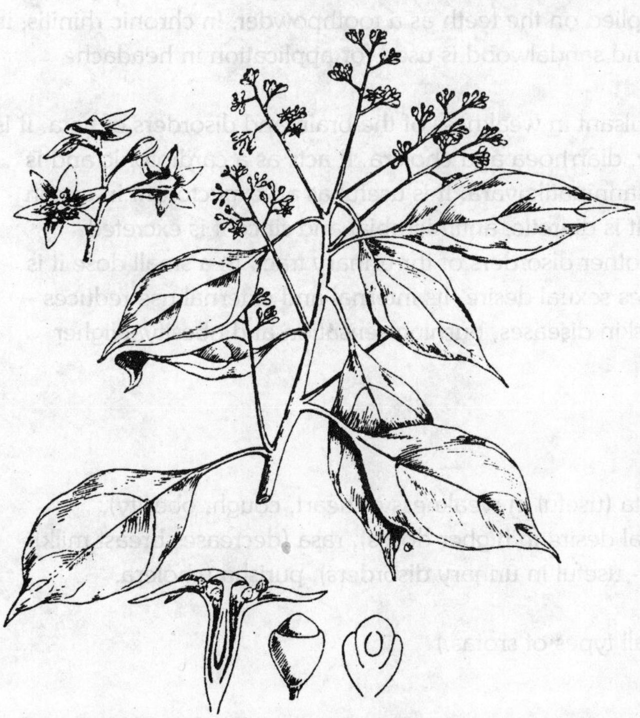

Kula: Karpoor kula.
Family : Lauraceae.
Latin name : Cinnamomum = from its Arabic name kinamon; camphora = cognate of karpoor.
Sanskrit names : Ghanasar, Chandra, Hima, Karpoor, Sheeta, Sheetakara, Shashank, Shambhav, Sheetanshu, Himavaluka, Shila, Himkara, Gaur, Tushar. All the names of moon are given to karpoor.
Bheemsenee Kapoor: Bheemsenee, Potas, Panshoo, Sheetakar, Shankaravas, Pinja, Abdasara, Jootika, Patrika. There is another type of karpoor called 'cheen karpoor'.
Botanical Description : This is an evergreen tree growing upto a height of 10 to 13 mtrs. Bark - though rough externally, is smooth internally. Leaves - alternate, yellowish green, resembling tejpatra. Flowers - greenish yellow inflorescence. Fruits - pea-shaped and are in bunches. The tree has camphor-like fragrance. Flowering occurs in spring and fruiting in summer. One tree yeilds upto 4 to 5 kgs. of camphor.

Eight types of surgical procedures have their origin in kayachikitsa (internal medicine). This statement is 101% true.

Varieties: Depending on its habitat, karpoor is of three types -
1) Bheemsenee - Bornio, Sumatra.
2) Japanese (Chinese kapoor) - China, Japan.
3) Indian - Dehradoon, Neelgiree, Calcutta etc. The trees are small having a strong fragrance like Ocimum sanctum.
Depending on its method of preparation, it is of 2 types - Pakavidhi and Apakva (superior).
Depending on its colour, it is of three types -
1) Riyahi (Apakva, bheemsenee).
2) Kaisoori - Formosa, camphor, apakva, white in colour.
3) Kaphoormoti - like sand. It is prepared by pak vidhi.

Properties :

Guna: laghu, tikshna; **Rasa :** tikta, katu, madhur; **Vipak :** katu; **Veerya:** sheeta; **Dosha:** tridoshanashak.

External uses : Karpoor is widely used in external applications. It is used in ointments for wounds.

It is mixed with oil and is applied in rheumatoid arthritis. Its powder is applied on eczema. A mixture of camphor and peppermint is used as an analgesic. In opthalmic disorders, it is applied on the eyes and in dental diseases, it is applied on the teeth as a toothpowder. In chronic rhinitis, it is used as a nasya. A mixture of karpoor and sandalwood is used for application in headache caused by fever.

Internal uses : It is used as an anticonvulsant in weakness of the brain and disorders of vata. It is useful in oral diseases, anorexia, flalulence, diarrhoea and cholera. It acts as a cardiotonic and is especially useful as a cardio-protective in sannipatik jvara. It is useful as an expectorant in cough and asthma. It is also used in dermatosis. It is diuretic, antimicrobial and since it is excreted through the urine, it is used in pyuria and other disorders of thr urinary tract. In a small dose it is aphrodisiac while in higher doses, it reduces sexual desire. Its internal and external use reduces breast milk secretion. Karpoor is useful in skin diseases, burning sensation and obesity. Higher doses may cause toxicity.

Dose : 125 to 375 mg.

Srotogamitva :

Dosha: Tridoshanashak.

Dhatu : Majja (anticonvulsant, tonic), rakta (useful in weakness of heart, cough, obesity), aphrodisiac (in a small dose, reduces sexual desire in higher doses), rasa (decreases breast milk).

Mala: Mutra (it is excreted through urine - useful in urinary disorders), purisha (cholera, diarrhoea).

(Karpoor is useful in clearing blockage of all types of srotas.)

(48) KADALI

Musa paradisiaca

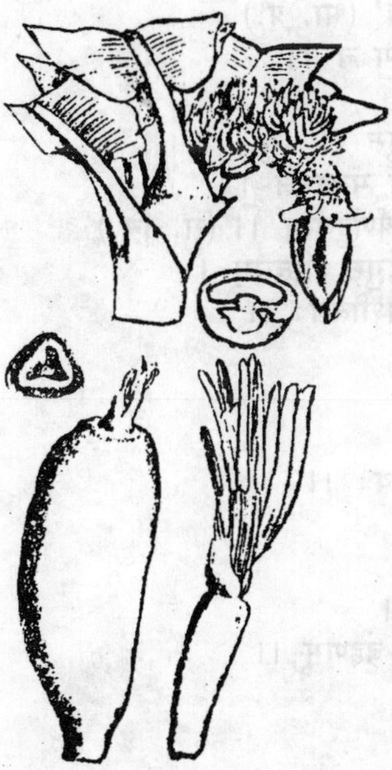

Kula: Haridra kula.

Family: Scitaminaceae.

Latin name: Musa = muza - from the Egyptian name; paradisiaca = of paradise.

Sanskrit names: Kadali, Sukumar , Rambha, Swaduphala, Deerghapatra, Kashthirasa , Amrit, Balak priya, Urustambha, Tantu vigraha.

English name: Banana, plantain.

Botanical Descriptuion: It is 1 to 4 mtrs. high. Stalk of this plant is made up of layer of leaves Leaves - long and wide. Flowers - 1.25 to 2 mtrs. long and appear in inflorescence and grow through leaves. Fruits - appear in bunches having different lengths. Wild variety of banana has black big seeds. (These seds are used in small pox as a preventive measure as well as for treatment). **Varieties:** There are many varities of banana.

Habitat: India, surrounding islands.

Chemical composition: Ripe fruit contains 22% sugar, starch, albuminoid, vitamins C, B and A. In short it is a nutritious fruit.

Properties:

Guna: snigdha; **Rasa:** madhur, kashaya; **Veerya :** sheeta; **Dosha:** vatapittashamak, kaphavardhak.

External uses: Fruit pulp, leaves and flowers are applied on burnt injuries. In dysuria, paste of the rhizome is applied on the lower abdomen. Mixture of turmeric and bananakshar is applied on sidhma kushta. Its kshar acts as a lekhan dravya.

Internal uses: Being shamak and brain tonic, juice of stalk is used in hysteria and epilepsy. Raw as well as ripe banana are used in diarrhoea and dysentery. In excessive thirst, sharbat of ripe fruits is given. In cholera, its juice is given to reduce thirst.

Flowers and ripe fruits are used in bleeding disorders. Ripe fruit acts as an expectorant if given in dry cough. Juice is used in dysuria while fruit in urinary disorders. In seminal debility, vaginal discharges and burning sensation, ripe banana is useful. Juice of stalk is an antidote to morphine and arsenic toxicity.

Dose: Juice - 3 to 6 tsf; kadalikshar - 4 to 8 gunja (0.5 - 1 gm.); sharbat - 1.5 to 20 ml.

Srotogamitva:

Dosha: Fruit - Vatapittaghna, kaphavardhak.

Dhatu: Majja, rakta (pitta -flowers and ripe fruits are given), shukra (reduces debility), mansa meda (brimhan).

Mala: Purisha (in cholera, juice of stalk is used), dysuria (stalk juice), manovahasrotas(hysteria and epilepsy - stalk juice - shamak and brain tonic).

Antidote: Juice of stalk is given in morphine and arsenic toxicity.

Eclipta alba, Kolista, Aconitum ferox, Aconitus heterophyllum, Centella asciatica, Piper longum etc. are the plants found near water. That is their nature.

References -

'मोचाफलं स्वादू शीतं विष्टम्भि कफनुदू गुरु । स्निग्धं पित्तास्रतृ डदातृक्षतक्षयसमीरजित ।।
पक्वं स्वादू हिमं पाके स्वादू चृष्यं च बृंहणम् । क्षुत्तृष्णानेत्रगदहन्मेहघ्नं रुचिमांसकृत् ।।' (भा. प्र.)
कदल्याः कुसुमं स्निग्धं मधुरं तुवरं गुरु । वातपित्तहरं शीतं रक्तपित्तक्षयप्रणुत् ।।' (भा. प्र.)
'सम्पक्वं पनसं मोचं राजादनफलानि च । स्वादूनि सकषायाणि स्निग्धशीतगुरुणि च ।।
कषायविशदत्वाच्च सौगन्ध्याच्च रुचिप्रदम् ।' (च)
'मौचं स्वादुरसं प्रोक्तं कषायं नातिशीतलम । रक्तपित्तहर वृष्यं रुच्यं श्लेष्मकरं गुरु ।।' (सु.)
'रम्भापक्वफलं कषायमधुरं बल्यं च शीतं तथा पित्तघ्नास्रविमर्दनं गुरुतरं पथ्यं च मन्दानले ।
सद्यः शुक्रविवृद्धिदं क्लमहरं तृष्णापहं कान्तिदम् दीप्ताग्नीसुखदं कफामयकरं संतर्पणंदुर्जरम् ।। (रा. नि.)
'मोचागुर्वी हिमा स्निग्धा स्वाद्वी पित्तास्रनाशिनी । भ्रमघ्नी योनिगदनुत् तत्काण्डंगुरु शीतलम् ।
बल्यः कदल्याः कन्दः स्यात् कफपित्तहरो गुरुः । वातलो रक्तशमनः कषायो रुक्षशीतलः ।।
कर्णशूलं रजोदोषं सोमरोगं नियच्छति ।'
'रम्भातोयं शीतलं ग्राहि तृष्णाकृच्छ्रन् मेहान् कर्णरोगातिसारान् ।
अस्थिस्रावं स्फोटकान् रक्तपित्तं दाहं हग्यादसत्रयोनिविशेषान् ।।'
'कदलीकुसुमं तिक्तं कषायं ग्राहि दीपनम् । उष्णवीर्यं बलासघ्नं तादृशास्तत्सटादयः ।।'
तृट्रक्तपित्ताक्षिगदप्रमेहान् फलं कदल्यास्तरुणं निहन्ति ।
संग्राहकं तिक्तकपायरूक्षं रक्तातिसारं शमयेत् ज्वरं च ।।
ईपत्कपायमधुरं मध्यमं कदलीफलम् । गुर्वग्निसादकृत्वक्तु कटुतिक्तरसा लघुः ।।
मोचं पक्वं स्वादु पाके सकषायं हिमं गुरु । मांसलं श्लेष्मलं रुच्यं वृष्यं विष्टम्भि बृंहणम् ।।
स्निग्धं क्षतक्षयक्षुतृड्वातपित्तास्रदाहजित । (कै. नि.)

(49) KASHERUK

Scirpus grosus Linn.

Kula: Mustak kula.
Family: Cyperaceae (from kyperus - old Gk. name).
Latin name: Scirpus = club rush or bull rush; grosus = large.
English name: Water chestnut.
Sanskrit names: Gunthakanda, Kaseru, Kshudramusta, Kaseruka, Sugandhi, Sukanda, Gandha kandak (pigs like the rhizomes very much), Sukareshta.
Botanical Description: Annual plant grows in marshy area. Stalk - 15 to 180 cms. long, digitate and triangular. Leaves - long and wide. Inflorenscence - 90 cms. in length. Fruits - small, grey or black. Rhizome - appear like nutmeg, oval, black and hairy while internally white. It is sweet to taste and fragrant. Flowers occur in rainy season followed by fruits. This is the description of small kaseru. There is one more variety called raj kaseru (raj = big). The rhizome of the raj kaseru is big and it is used for medicinal purpose. Its latin name is Scirpus tuberose.
Habitat: Equatorial areas in India and China.
Chemical composition: Its rhizome contains 63% starch, 7% proteins, 7% gum and ash.
Properties:
Guna: guru, ruksha; **Rasa:** madhur, kashaya; **Vipak:** madhur; **Veerya:** sheeta; **Dosha:** pittashamak, vatakaphavardhak.

External uses: In eye diseases, paste of kaseru and yashtimadhu is applied. It is also applied on burns, boils and inflammations.
Internal uses: It is used in thirst, vomiting and diarrhoea. In cholera, its rhizome rubbed with rose water is given which helps in reducing the symptoms. It is a cardiotonic. In jaundice, flowers are used. It is also used in seminal debility, urinary disorders, fever, burning sensation and general debility. It is a galactagogue also.
Dose: Rhizome - 1.5 to 2 gms.
References -
'कशेरु द्विविधं तत्तु महद्राजकशेरुकम् । मुस्ताकृति लघु स्याद्यत्तच्चिचोढमिति स्मृतम् ।'
कशेरुकद्वयं शीतं मधुरं तुवरं गुरु । पित्तशोणितदाहघ्नं नयनामयनाशनम् ।।
ग्राहि शुक्रानिलश्लेष्मारुचिस्तन्यकरं स्मृतम् ।' (भा. प्र.)
'गुरु विष्टम्भिशीतौ च शृंगाटककशेरुकौ ।' (सु. सू. ४६)
'कशेरुकं हिमं रूक्षं मधुरं तुवरं गुरु । संग्राहि शक्रल स्तन्यकफमारुतवर्धनम् ।।
पित्तशोणितदाहघ्नं नयनामयनाशनम् । वृष्यं मेहं तृषां हन्याद्विष्टम्भि कृमिकारि च ।।
कशेरुकस्य पुष्पं तु पित्तघ्नं कामलापहम् ।' (कै. नि.)
'तत्र पूर्वोक्तैः कारणैः पतिष्यति गर्भे... पयसा पाययेत् कशेरुशृंगाटकशालू ककल्कं वा ।' (सु. शा. १०)

(50) KANDEER

Ranunculus sceleratus Linn.

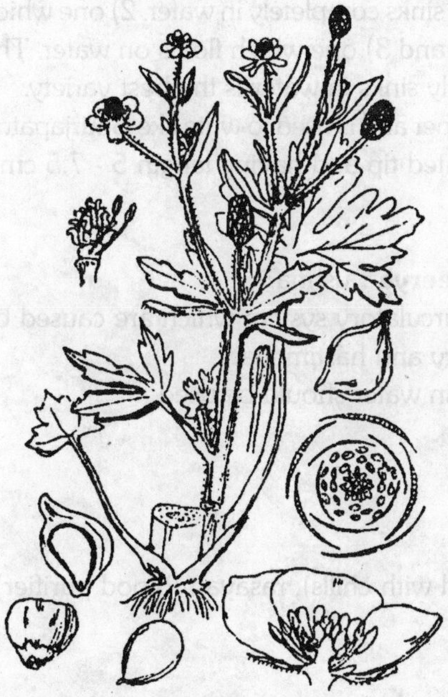

Kula: Vatsanabh kula.
Family: Ranunculaceae.
Latin name: Ranunculus = water celery, rana = frog, inhibiting in marshy places; sceleratus = acrid, biting, bitter.
Sanskrit names: Kandeer, Kandakatuka, Nasasanvedan, Agrakanda, Toyavalli, Karavalli, Ugrakanda, Katilla, Nasalivedan.
Botanical Description: A shrub growing in marshy area.
Properties:
Guna: ruksha, tikshna; **Rasa:** katu, tikta; **Veerya:** ushna;
Dosha: kaphavatashamak and developes blisters. It is very tikshna and toxic, so it should be used carefully.
External use: In lymphadenitis and buboes of plague, it is applied locally. It is also applied on penis in loss of libido.
Srotogamitva :
Dosha: Vataghna, kaphaghna, pittavardhak.
Dhatu: Rasa, rakta, meda (tumour) (buboes of plague), shukra (loss of libido - paste is applied), rakta (spleen).
Mala: Cleans the nasal cavity.
Organ: Stomach (mandagni), intestines (laxative).
Prabhava: Antidote to poison but itself is toxic.

The mere name 'Dashamoolarishta' itself will not generate any action. The formulation requires the specific ten roots mentioned as dashamoola to be active. This holds true for other formulations also.

References -

काण्डीरः कटुतिक्तोष्णः सरो दुष्टव्रणार्त्तिजित्। लूतागुल्मोदरप्लाहशूलमन्दाग्निनाशनः ।। (ध. नि.)

(51) KASHTHAGARU

Aquilaria agallocha

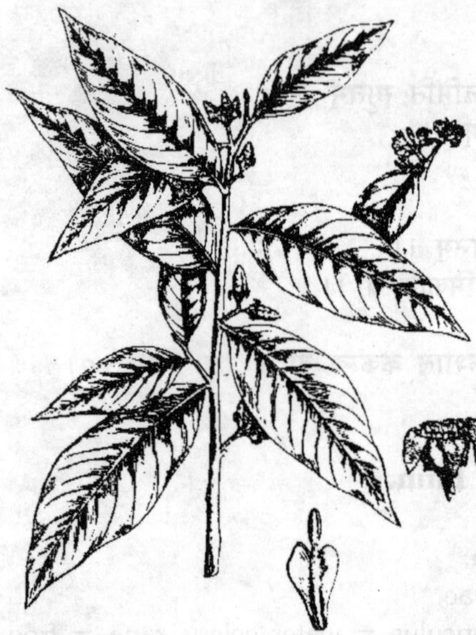

Gana : Sheetaprashamana, Shwasahara, Shirovirechana, Tiktaskandha (C.); Eladi, Salasaradi, Shleshmasamshamana (S.).

Kula : Aguru kula.

Family : Thymelaceae.

Latin name : Aquilaria agallocha = similar to agaru.

English name : Eaglewood.

Sanskrit names : Peetak, Varnaprasadana, Anaryaka, Krumijagdha, Kashthak, Laghuchandan, Agnikashtha, Narendra, Vanadruma. Kashthagaru is one of the varieties of agaru. There are 4 varieties of agaru - 1) Krushnagaru, 2) Kashthagaru (yellow), 3) Dahagaru and 4) Mangalyagaru. Mangalyagaru is the best among them.

There are another 3 varieties depending upon the sinking test viz.1) one which sinks completely in water, 2) one which partly sinks in water and 3) one which floats on water. The one which completely sinks in water is the best variety.

Botanical Description : Tall evergreen tree. Bark - thin like paper and is used to write like Bhurjapatra. Wood - fragrant. Leaves - similar to leather but thin with pointed tip and having length 5 - 7.5 cms. Flowers - white, appear in a cluster.

Properties :

Guna : laghu, ruksha, tikshna; **Rasa :** tikta; **Vipak :** katu; **Veerya :** ushna.

Uses : It is useful in disorders of digestive, respiratory, and circulatory system which are caused by vata and kapha. It is an aphrodisiac. It is used in bladder laxity and hastimeha.

Parts used : Stem extract and oil. Krushnagaru which sinks in water should be used.

Dose : Powder - 0.5 to 1.75 gm, oil - 1 to 6 drops.

Formulation : Agurvadi oil for massage.

Srotogamitva :

Dosha : Vatakaphaghna and pittavardhak.

Dhatu : Shukra (aphrodisiac), rasa (useful in fever associated with chills), rasayan (blood purifier).

Mala : Beneficial to urinary bladder.

Organ : Digestive system.

(52) KARPAS
Gossypium herbaceum

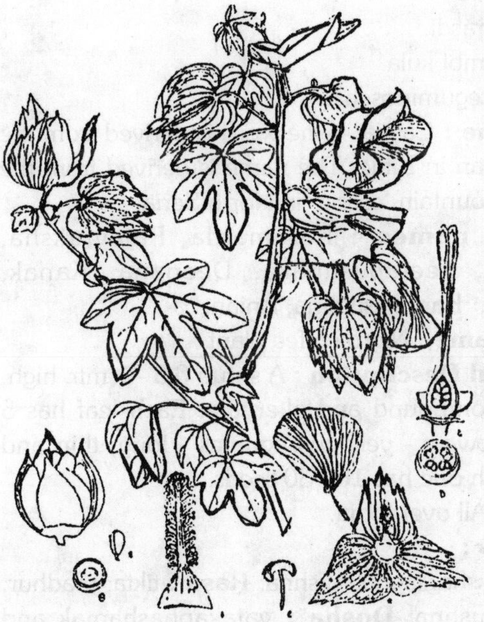

Kula : Karpas kula.
Family : Malvaceae.
Latin name : Gossypium = originated from Arabic name Goz = soft substance - one of its varieties. Some of them are G. barbadense and G. herbaceum etc. Former is a good variety; herbaceum = means grassy, herba = grass, barbadensis = from the island of Barbados in West Indies.
Sanskrit names : Karpas, Nagnajit, Tundi, Sarni, Chavya, Pathya, Somavalli, Vamani, Vishaghni, Stanyadabeeja.
Botanical Description : A tree known to every one belongs to its own kula i.e. Karpasa kula. It has other varieties like Aranyakarpasi, Devakapashi etc. They all are 3 - 4 mtrs. high. Leaves - resemble castor or papaya laeves with 3 - 5 ends. Flowers - yellow, (flowers of devakarpas are red) come in winter. Fruit - contains cotton and black seeds.
Habitat : All over India but mainly in Bengal, Gujarat, Maharashtra and Tamilnadu.
Chemical composition : Seeds contain 10 to 29 % oil.
Properties :
Guna : laghu, singdha; **Rasa :** madhur,kashaya; **Vipak :** madhur; **Veerya :** slight ushna; **Dosha :** vatashamak but kaphapittavardhak.
Uses : External appliction has analgesic and wound healing property. Seedpulp is beneficial to nervous system . Flowers are stimulant and pleasant to mind. Seedpulp is a good laxative. Leaf juice is viscous and flowers, being liver stimulant are used in jaundice. They are also used in psychosomatic disorders. Decoction or powder of roots is given in amenorrhoea and dysmenorrhoea. It is used in postpartum period to contract uterus, to avoid puerperal disorders and as a haemostatic. Excess dose may cause abortion. Cotton is used as a galactogogue and aphrodisiac.
Srotogamitva :
Dosha : Vataghna, kaphavardhak (seed).
Dhatu : Rakta (vardhak), (galactogogue - seed), rasagami, shukra (seed).
Mala : Mutra (diuretic).
Organs : Ears (tinnitus, purulent or other discharges).
References -
'काप्रासको लघुः कोष्णओ मधुरो वातनाशनः । तत्पलाशं समीरघ्नं रक्तकृन्मूत्रवर्धनम् ।।
तत्कर्णपिडकानादपूयस्त्रावविनाशनम् । तद्बीस्तन्यदं वृष्यंस्निग्धं कफकरं गुरु ।।' (भा. प्र.)
कार्पासिका किंचिदुष्णआ कषाया मधुरा लघुः ।' (कै. नि.)

A disease may have many features but the treatment should be targetted to the root cause. For a tree, the roots require to be nurtured with water and manure.

(53) KASAMARDA
Cassia occidentalis

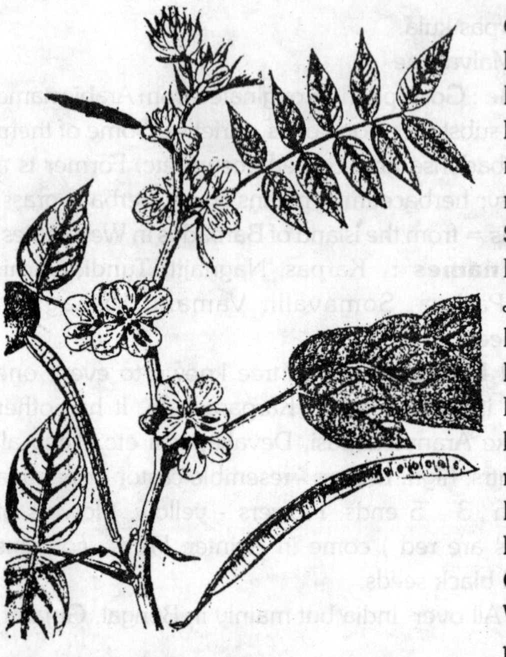

Gana : Surasdi.
Kula : Shimbi kula.
Family : Leguminoseae.
Latin name : Cassia = the word is derived from the name kashan in Bible. The name is derived from the name of mountain 'cassia' in North Seria.
Sanskrit names : Kasamarda, Rajavruksha, Kasaghna, Peetapushpaka, Deepana, Kanak, Jaranakala, Kartakasaghna, Anjan.
English name : Nigro coffee plant.
Bdotanical Description : A shrub 0.5 - 1 mtr. high. Leaves - compound and alternate. Each leaf has 5 leaflets. Flowers - yellow. Legumes - long, thin and round. Each one has 10 - 30 seeds.
Habitat : All over India.
Properties :
Guna : ruksha, laghu, tikshna; **Rasa :** tikta, madhur; **Veerya :** ushna; **Dosha :** vatakaphashamak and pittasarak.

Uses : It is used in dermatoses and poisons. Useful as an analgesic in vata disorders. Being carminative and cholagogue, it is used in ascites, loss of appetite and constipation . Effective in cough and asthma. Leaf juice + honey is used in whooping cough. Also useful in dysuria, ikshumeha, swelling, dermatoses and filaria.

Dose : Leaf juice - 6 to 12ml; seeds - 1to 2 gms; decoction of roots - 48 to 96 ml.

Srotogamitva :
Dosha : Kaphavataghna, pittashodhan.
Dhatu : Meda (filaria, ikshumeha), rakta (dermatoses).
Mala : Purisha (constipative), mutra (cures dysuria).
Organ : Respiratory system.
Note - Root powder is put in ear in scorpion sting.

References -
'कासमर्द: सुतिक्त: स्यान्मधुर: कफवातजित् । विशेषत: पित्तहर: पाचन: कण्ठशोधन: ।।' (ध. नि.)
'कासमर्दकपत्राणां यूष...... हिक्काश्वासनिवारण: ।' (च. चि. १७)
कासमर्दकबीजानि मूलकान्नं तथैव च । गन्धपाषाणमिश्राणि सिध्मानां परमौषधम् ।।' (च. द.)
'जम्बीरस्वरसे पिष्टंकासमर्दाङ्घ्रिलेपनम् ।
विचर्चिकानां सर्वेषां परमौषधमुच्यते ।।' (वैद्यमनोरमा)
'कासमर्दशिफाकल्कं गव्येनाज्येन य: पिबेत् ।
श्लीपदं वातजं तस्य नाशमायाति सत्त्वरम् ।।' (वङ्गसेन)

'यः कासमर्दमूलं वदने प्रक्षिप्य कर्णे फुत्कारम्
मनुजो दधाति शीघ्रं जयति विषं वृश्चिकानां सः ।।' (च. द.)

(54) KARAVELLA

Momordica charantia

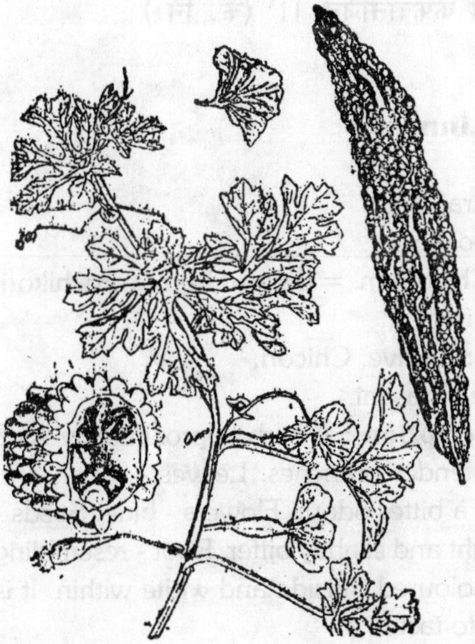

Gana : Tikta skandha (C.)
Kula : Koshataki kula.
Latin name : Momordica - original Latin name mordeo = one bite, appears jagged as if bitten; charantia.
English name : Momordica, bitter gourd.
Sanskrit names : Angarvelli, Sushavi, Pacharu, Kantaphala, Peetapushpa, Sukumari, Aphala, Akhili, Rajavalli.
Botanical Description : Annual creeper. Leaves - round, hairy with irregular margins. Flowers - yellow, homosexual. Fruits - 2.5 to 7 cms. long, green with tapering ends and triangular spikes on the surface. Seeds - 1.3 cm. in size, flat. Fruits are used as vegetable.
Varieties : There are two varieties - 1) large - karavellak and 2) small - karavelli.
Habitat : All over India.
Chemical composition : It contains a bitter principle and fresh fruit contains 88.45 % fluid.

Properties :
Guna: laghu, ruksha; **Rasa :** tikta; **Veerya :** ushna; **Dosha :** tridoshashamak.
External uses : It has analgesic, wound cleaning and healing properties. It is useful in burning sensation, dermatoses and piles. It is beneficial to the eyes. Leaf juice is applied on eyes in night blindness.
Internal uses : Being an appetizer, digestive, cholagogue, purgative and anthelmintic, it is used in anorexia, loss of appetite, ama dosha, liver disorders, piles and helminthiasis. It is a blood purifier, antiinflammatory, diuretic, emmenagogue and galactogogue. It alleviates kapha, hence it is useful in blood disorders, inflammation, asthma, cough, dysmenorrhoea, amenorrhoea, disorders of lactation, calculi,urinary disorders, dermatoses. fever, obesity and poisoning. Experience has shown that it is an excellent remedy for high sugar levels in blood and urine.
Dose : Juice of whole plant and fruit - 10 to 30 ml.; for inducing emesis - 100 ml.
In case of overdose, rice mixed with ghee is given.
Srotogamitva :
Dosha : Tridoshashamak.
Dhatu : Rasa (galactogogue, dysmenorrhoea, amenorrhoea), mansa (wound healing), rakta, meda (anaemia), rakta (dermatoses, liver disorders, high blood sugar, bleeding disorders).

If we imbibe regularly all rasas in our diet, then there will not be any necessity of treatment. This is the seminal key to remain healthy.

Mala : Mutra (calculi, urinary disorders), purisha (helminthiasis).
Organ : Intestine.
References -
‘कारवेल्ली पीतपुष्पा मंडपी चीरितच्छदा ।’ (शि.)
‘कारवेल्लं सकटुकं कटुपाकमवातलम् । दीपनं भेदनं तिक्तमवृष्यमाहिमं लघु ।।
त्वरोचकपित्तास्रकफपाण्डुव्रणक्रिमीन् । श्वासकासप्रमेहाश्मकोठकुष्ठज्वरानपि ।
कारवेल्लीफलं वन्यं ज्वरार्शःकृमिनाशनम् । कासघ्नं दीपनं हृद्यं सतिक्तं कफवातजित् ।।’ (कै. नि.)

(55) KASANI
Chicorium intybus Linn.

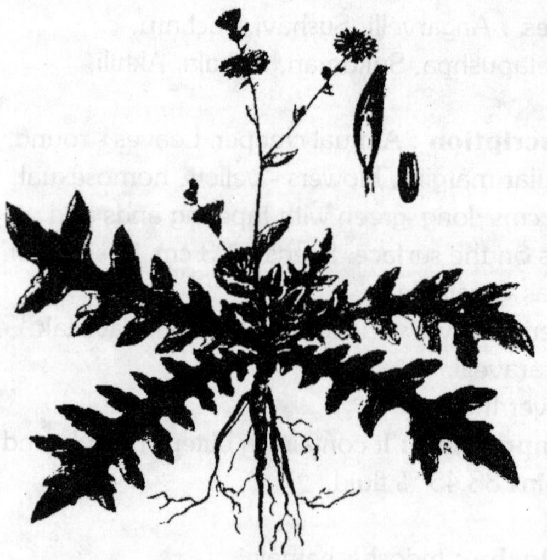

Kula : Bhrungaraj kula.
Family : Compositeae.
Latin name : Chicorium = derived from wordchikori; intybus = word indive.
English name : Endive, Chicori.
Sanskrit name : Kasani.
Botanical Description : A herb approximately 1 - 2 mtrs. high with tender branches. Leaves - rough and rectangular with a bitter odour. Flowers - blue. Seeds - white or grey, light and slightly bitter. Root - resembling cow's tail. Ash coloured outside and white within. It is slimy and bitter to taste.
It has 2 varieties wild and urban, which is cultivated in vegetable pots.
Habitat : It grows at the height of 2000 mtrs. in Himalaya. Also in south and west India, Kashmir, Punjab, Iran and Europe.
The different parts have different chemical properties.
Guna : laghu, ruksha; **Rasa :** tikta; **Veerya :** sheeta (roots - ushna), hence useful in disorders induced by kapha and pitta.
Uses : Leaves ground into paste are applied on swelling induced by pitta dosha. Because of its calming action on the brain, sherbat made of seeds is used in insomnia. Being an appetizer,liver stimulant and cholagogue, it used in diseases which are caused due to impaired agni, liver disorders and obstructive jaundice. Root and seed are used in blood disorders and dysuria. Root is mainly used in dysmenorrhoea and other menstrual disorders. Also useful in fever, pitta, disorders, burninig sensation and general debility.
Srotogamitva :
Dosha : Kaphaghna, pittasarak.
Dhatu : Majja (calming action, useful in insomnia), rasa (menstrual disorders), rakta (liver stimulant, useful in blood disorders).
Mala : Mutra (useful in dysuria).

(56) KAKAMACHI
Solanum nigrum Linn.

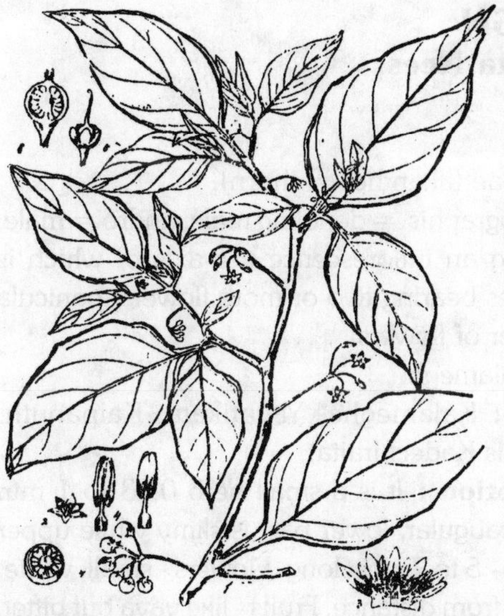

Kula : Kantakari kula.
Family : Solonaceae.
Latin name : Solanum = comforting, having sedative qualites; nigrum = niger - black.
English name : Garden night shade.
Sanskrit names : Kakamachi, Dhwankshamachi, Vayasavha, Vayasi, Sarvatikta, Bahuphala, Katphala, Rasayani, Kakamata, Gucchaphala, Swadupaka.
Botanical Description : This is a shrub with irregular branches and grows upto a height of 30 cm. to 1mt. Leaves - 5 cm. to 7 cm. in length and 2.5 cm to 3.75 cm in breadth. Flowers - small and white. Fruits - small, spiral, smooth, green when unripe but turn blue on ripening, in bunches. The plant flowers in rainy season an fruits in spring.
Habitat : Found all over India.
Chemical composition : Solenin is present in fruits.

Properties :
Guna : laghu, snigdha; **Vipak:** katu; **Veerya:** anushna; **Doshaghnata:** tridoshaghna.
Uses : It is used extensively in inflammation, osteoarthritis, wounds, orchitis, liver enlargement and ascites. Its decoction is used for gargling in stomatitis, throat infeciton and tonsilitis. Warm decoction is used locally in earache. Its juice is used for nasal administration in nasopharyngial diseases and in eye disorders. Being a digestive, it is used in loss of appetite, common cold, liver diseases, piles, ascites, dysentery, splenomegaly, heart disease and oedema (used as a vegetable). The powder of the fruit is used in hoarseness of voice, cough and asthma. It can also be useful in renal disorders, gonorrhoea, dysuria, skin disorders and chronic fever.
Parts used : Whole plant.
Dose : Juice of the whole plant - 10 to 20 ml.; powder of the fruits - 1 to 3 gm.
Percaution : Large dose causes vomiting, diarrhoea, thirst, abdominal colic, headache, delirium, seizures, coma and sometimes even death.
Antidote : The treatment should be done similar to dhatura poisoning.
Srotogamitva :
Dosha : Tridoshaghna.
Dhatu : Shukra (brimhan), rasayana (nourishes all the seven dhatus), rasa (fever), meda (antidiabetic), rakta (dermatoses).
Mala : Purisha (purgative).
References -
'काकमाची त्रिदोषघ्नी स्निग्धोष्णा स्वरशुक्रदा । तिक्ता रसायनी शोथकुष्ठार्शोज्वरमेहजित् ।।'
'कटुर्नेत्रहिता हिक्काछर्दिहृद्रोगनाशिनी ।' (भा. प्र.)

There has to be no opportunistic and unwholesome compromises in science scriptures. In reality, this is rampant.

'त्रिदोषशमनी वृष्या काकमाची रसायनी । नात्युष्णशीतवीर्याच भेदनी कुष्ठनाशिनी ।.' (च. सू. २७)
'ईषत्तिक्तं त्रिदोषघ्नं शाकं कटु सतीनजम् । नात्युष्णशीतंकुष्ठघ्नं काकमाच्यास्तु तद्विधम् ।।' (सु. स. ४६)

(57) KALAMEGH

Andrographis paniculata Nees.

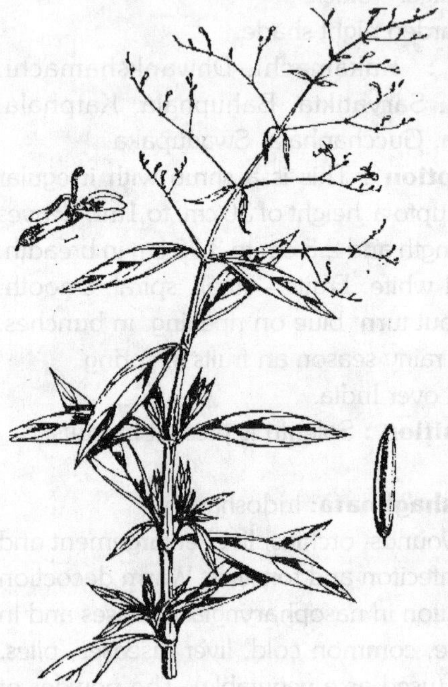

Kula : Vasa kula.

Family : Acanthaceae (akanthos = thorn).

Latin name : Andrographis = denoting male, andro = male; paniculata = having an inflorescence the axis of which is divided into branches bearing two or more flowers; panicula = tuft, a loose cluster of flowers.

English name : Kalamegh.

Sanskrit names : Kalamegha, Yavatikata, Kalpanath, Palekiraita (another is Kadechiraita).

Botanical Description : It is a small herb 0.03 to 1 mtr. high. Stem - quandraugular, lower part is slimy while upper part is hairy. Leaves - 5 to 7 cms. long. Flowers - small, white, look like mosquitoes from distance. Fruits - like yava but bitter. Seeds - numerous quandrangular. Whole plant is very much bitter. The plant bears flowers and fruits from autumn to winter.

Habitat : All over India but mainly in Bengal and Assam.

Chemical composition : The whole plant contains kalameghin and chlorophyll in large quantities.

Guna : laghu, ruksha, tikshna; **Rasa** : tikta; **Vipak** : katu; **Veerya** : ushna; **Dosha** : kaphapittahara. **Uses** : Being an appetizer, liver stimulant, laxative and vermifuge, it is used in loss of appetite, liver and spleen enlargement, constipation, jaundice and worms.

In fever with rigors, mixture of black pepper and kalamegh is useful. It is also effective in chronic fever and general debility.

Dose : Powder of whole plant - 0.5 to 1.25 gm, juice - 2 to 4 ml, decoction - 20 to 40 ml.

Srotogamitva :

Dosha : Kaphaghna and pittahara.

Dhatu : Rakta (liver stmulant, cholagogue, liver and spleen enlargement, blood metabolism).

Mala : Purisha (laxative - constipation and worms).

Organs : Internal organs.

References -

शंखिनी तिक्तला चैव यवतिक्ताऽक्षिपीडकः । ते गुल्मगरहृद्रोगकुष्ठशोफोदरादिषु ।।
विकासितीक्ष्णत्वाद् योज्ये श्लेष्माधिकेषु तु ।
'नातिशुष्कं फलं ग्राह्यं शंखिन्याः निस्तुषीकृतम् ।।' (?)

(58) KEETAMARI

Aristolochia bracteata Retz.

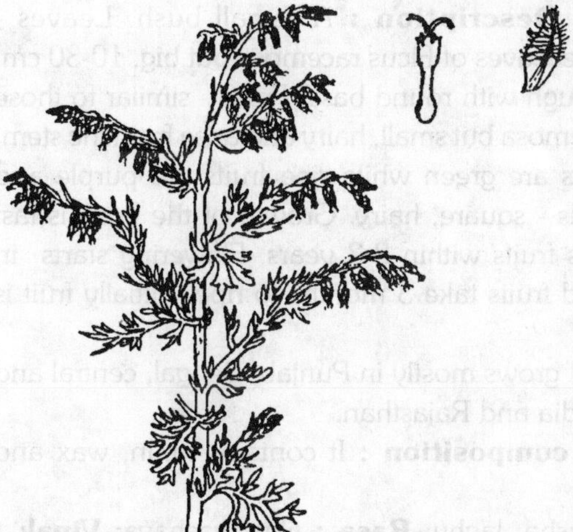

Kula : Ishwari kula.

Family : Aristolocihaceae.

Latin name : Aristolochia = aristos = best, lochia = parturation. Its supposed medicinal properties for easing birth; bracteata - bracted = small leaf or scale below calyx provided with bracts (modified laeves on the peduncle).

English name : Worthwort.

Sanskrit names : Dhoomrapatra, Keetamari, Keedamari, Paniri.

Botanical Description : A perennial creeper 30 cm. to 1 mtr. high. Leaves - broad having length and breadth 2.5 - 7 cms. Flowers - purlpe, appear in clusters. Frutis - 2.5 cm. long. Seed - triangular. It bears flowers and fruits after monsoon.

Habitat : Confluence of Ganga and Yamuna, western and southern India, Bihar, Sindh and Bundel khanda.

Chemical composition : It contains irritatant oils and potassium chloride.

Guna : laghu, ruksha, tikshna; **Rasa :** tikta (the whole plant is bitter); **Veerya :** ushna; **Dosha :** kaphavatashamak

External uses : Insecticide (Keetamari) and heals chronic ulcers. Juice is applied.

Internal uses : It is an appetizer, laxative and anthelmintic. It is useful in oedema, cough and by its stimulating action on uterus, it is effective in dysmenorrhea and amenorrhoea. Being a diaphoretic, it is used in fever, specially in periodical fever as a preventive therapy.

It is used as a tonic in diseases like anaemia in which body tissues are laxed.

Dose : Whole plant 3 gms.

Srotogamitva :

Dosha : Kaphavataghna.

Dhatu : Rasa (dysmenorrhea), rakta, meda (anaemia -tonic).

Mala : Purisha, sweda (useful in fever).

(Cures dysmonorrhoea and amenorrhoea by stimulating uterus).

(59) KAKODUMBAR

Ficus hispida Linn.

Kula : Vata kula.

Family : Urticaceae (urticae = nettle).

Latin name : Ficus = from fag, hebrew name of fig; hispida = having bristles.

Ayurveda considers a well-nourished balanced muscular body to be better than an obese body (sthaulya). This statement is made after an immense thought.

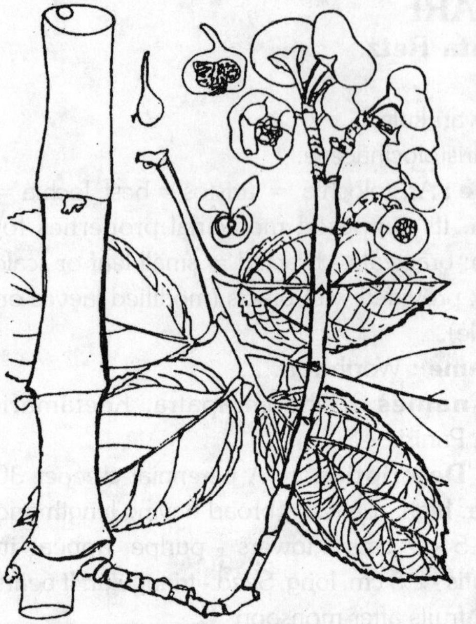

Sanskrit names : Malayu, Kathina, Kushtaghni, Falguni, Falini, Hemadugdhika, Kharapatrika (rough leaves), Garbhasanrakshak, Stanyapradayini.

Botanical Description : A small bush. Leaves - resemble the leaves of Ficus racemosa but big, 10-30 cm. long and rough with round base. Fruits - similar to those of Ficus recemosa but small, hairy and arise from the stem. Unripe fruits are green while ripe fruits are purple and sweet. Seeds - square, hairy. Growth of the bush is fast and it bears fruits within 2-3 years. Flowering starts in summer and fruits take 3 months to ripe. Initially fruit is very hard.

Habitat : It grows mostly in Punjab, Bengal, central and southern India and Rajasthan.

Chemical composition : It contains tanin, wax and saponin.

Guna : ruksha, laghu; **Rasa :** tikta, kashaya; **Vipak :** katu; **Veerya :** sheeta; **Dosha :** kaphapittashamak.

External uses : The paste of rootbark or latex is applied on dermatoses and vitiligo. Latex developes blisters on the skin and acts as a curative agent. Powder and decoction are used in ulcers. Ripe fruit ground in a paste is applied on lymphadenitis.

Internal uses : Decoction or powder of fruits is used in constipation, ascites, piles and jaundice. Ripe fruit is used as a haemostatic agent. It is used as a tonic, aphrodisiac and galactogogue. Root and fruit are useful in dermatoses. The plant has chief action on vitiligo. In Rabies, rootbark 1 tola + datura seeds 1tola is given with ricewater.

Dose : Bark powder - 2 to 5 gms. (for detoxification), as a tonic 1 to 2 gms; fruit - 1/2 to 1.

Srotogamitva :

Dosha : Kaphaghna and pittaghna.

Dhatu : Rakta , meda (external use on dermatoses and vitiligo), meda (paste of fruits - lymphadenitis), rasa (ripe fruit - galactogogue), shukra (ripe fruit - aphrodisiac), rakta (jaundice, anaemia and bleeding piles) haemostatic (ripe fruit).

Mala : Purisha (purgative).

Note : Effective medicine for vitiligo and useful in rabies.

References -

'काकोदुम्बरिका फल्गुर्मलयूर्जघनेफला । मलयूः स्तम्भकृत्तिक्ता शीतला तुवरा जयेत् ।।
कफपित्तव्रणश्वित्रकुष्ठपाण्डूवर्शकामलाः ।' (भा. प्र.)

'फल्गुस्तु तुवरा तिक्ता शीतला स्तम्भनी जयेत् । कफपित्तव्रणश्वित्रकुष्ठपाण्डूवस्त्रकामलाः ।।
फलं तु शीतलं स्वादु कषायं गुरु तर्पणम् । शुक्रलं मधुरं पाके स्निग्धं विषट्म्भि बृंहणम् ।।
ग्राहि वातकफपित्तक्षतदाहविषास्त्रजित् ।' (कै. नि.)

'भद्रासंज्ञोदुम्बरीमूलतुल्यं दत्वा मूलं क्षोदयित्वा मलय्वाः ।
सिद्धं तोयं पीतमुष्णे सुखोष्णं स्फोटाञ्श्विस्त्रे पुण्डरीके च कुर्यात् ।।

द्वैपंदग्धं चर्म मातंगजं वा भिन्ने स्फोटे तैलयुक्तं प्रलेपः ।' (सु. चि. ९) ।
'काकोदुम्बरमूलन्तु धुस्तूरफलकान्वितम् । पिबेत्तण्डुलतोयेन सारमेयविषापहम् ।।' (वंगसेन)

(60) KUMUD
Nymphaea stellata Linn.

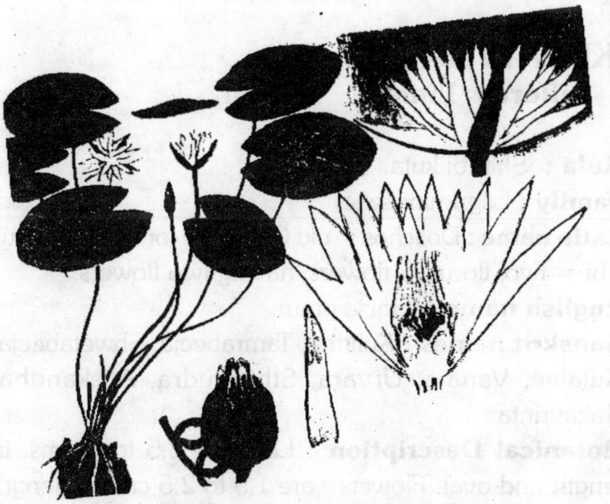

Gana : Mutravirajaneeya.
Kula : Kamal kula.
Family : Nymphaceae.
Latin name: Nymphaea - nymphs = half divine in mythology. These water lillies are in seven colours - white, yellow, pink, rose, purple, red and blue; stellata = star like or radiating like the points of a star glittering.
Sanskrit names : All names of white lotus can be used for kumud (part - II, plant no. 34), Kalhar.
Botanical Description : It grows in water. The speciality of this plant is that its flowers bloom on moonrise and close up in the morning. A tubular stalk is present upto the water level. Hence leaves and flowers both float on water. Seeds - small, round. Unripe seeds are red and ripe seeds are black. Though it has many varieties like white, red, blue and etc., white variety is used for medicinal purposes.
Habitat : It grows in lakes in India.
Properties : Similar to lotus. **Rasa** : madhur, tikta, kashaya; **Veerya** : sheeta; **Dosha** : pittashamak.
Uses : Useful in fever, bleeding disorders, excessive thirst and burning sensation. This plant boiled in a milk or its paste mixed with milk is used to prevent abortion. It is used in fever so that the vital organs like heart can tolerate the body heat.
Srotogamitva :
Dosha : Pittashamak.
Dhatu : Rakta (bleeding disorders, burning sensation), shukra , artava.
Mala : Diuretic.
Organ : Uterus (chief action is to prevent abortion), heart (for tolerating body heat in fever).
References -
'श्वेतं कुवलयं प्रोक्तं कुमुदं कैरवं तथा । कुमुदं पिच्छिलं स्निग्धं मधुरं ह्लादि शीतलम् ।।' (भा. प्र.)
'पतिष्यति गर्भे.... क्षीरमुत्पलादिसिद्धं पाययेत् । .... पयसा पाययेत् उत्पलादिकल्कं वा ।' (सु.शा. १०/५७)

It is no wonder that the body made up of prithvi and jala prefers madhur rasa which is also made up of prithvi and jala. Yet it should be consumed in moderation.

(61) KUNDARU
Coccinia indica WLA.

Gana : Moolanee (C.); Urdhvabhagahara (S.).
Kula : Koshataki.
Family: Cucurbitaceae.
It is described as Bimbi - plant no.162 in the same part.

(62) KULATTHA
Dolichos biflorus Linn.

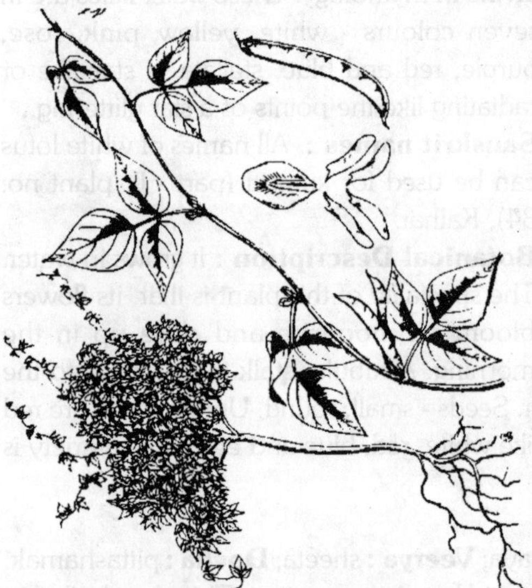

Kula : Shimbi kula.
Family : Leguminoseae.
Latin name : Dolichos = old Gk. name for bean; biflorus - bi = two, florus = flowers, having two flowers.
English name : Horse gram.
Sanskrit names : Kulittha, Tamrabeeja, Shwetabeeja, Kulalee, Vanaja, Urvara, Sthirmudra, Aliskandha, Kakavrinta.
Botanical Description : Leaves 2.5 to 5 cms. in length and oval. Flowers - are 1.5 to 2.5 cms. in length and yellow. Legumes - 2.5 to 5 cms. long, slightly curved and contain 5 to 6 flat seeds which are called as kulitha. Chakrapani, commentator of Charak samhita has described 4 varieties viz. white, red, black and chitra. There are another 2 varieties, urban and wild.
Habitat : All over India, at the height of 1000 mtrs.
Properties :
Guna : laghu, ruksha, tikshna; **Rasa :** kashaya; **Vipak :** amla; **Veerya :** ushna; **Prabhav :** bhedan;
Dosha : kaphavatashamak, acts on blood, vitiates blood causing bleeding disorders.
External use : Powder of kulattha if applied to whole body reduces excessive perspiration.
Internal uses : Being carminative, purgative, anthelmintic, uterine stimulant, diuretic, antipyretic, lekhan, shukranashan and causes burning sensation, it is used in inflammation (by diaphortic action), eye disorders (by local application), flatulence, liver and spleen enlargements, tumours, pains, haemorrhoids, worms, chronic rhinitis, cough, asthma, hiccups, dysmenorrhoea and calculi. In all above disorders, soup of kulattha is useful. It acts on rakta dhatu, causes acidity, bleeding disorders and impotency, helps in fat metabolism. Buttermilk added to kulattha soup forms tasty curry.
Parts used : seeds.
Dose : Powder - 2 to 4 gms.
Srotogamitva :
Dosha : Kaphaghna, vataghna, pittavardhak (developes bleeding disorders).

Dhatu : Rakta (developes bleeding disorders, reduces hepatosplenomegaly), shukra (causes impotency), rasa (dysmenorrhoea), meda (metabolism).
Mala : Sweda (in excesssive sweating its powder is applied to whole body), urine (diuretic, lithotripsic), purisha (purgative).
Organs : Respiratory and circulatory systems.
References -
कुलत्थः कटुकः पाके कषायः पित्तरक्तकृत् । लघुर्विदाही वीर्योष्णः श्वासकासकफनिलान् ।।
हन्ति हिक्काश्मरीशुक्रदाहानाहान् सपीनसान् । स्वेदसंग्राहको मेदोज्वरकृमिहरः सरः ।। (भा. प्र.)
कुलत्थिका कटुस्तिक्ता स्यादर्श:शूलनाशिनी । विबन्धाध्मानशमनी चक्षुष्या व्रणरोपणी ।।' (रा. नि.)
'उष्णाः कषायाः पाकेऽम्लाः कफशुक्रानिलापहाः ।
कुलत्थाः ग्राहिणः कासहिक्काश्वासार्शसां हिताः ।।' (च.)
'कषायस्वादुरूक्षोष्णाः कुलत्था रक्तपित्तलाः । पीनसश्वासकासार्शोहिध्मानाहकफानिलान् ।।'
कनन्ति शुक्राश्मरींशुक्रंदृष्टिंशोथंतथोदरम् । ग्राहिणओलघवस्तीक्ष्णाः विपाकेऽम्लाः विदाहिनः ।।

(63) KUMKUM
Crocus sativus Linn.

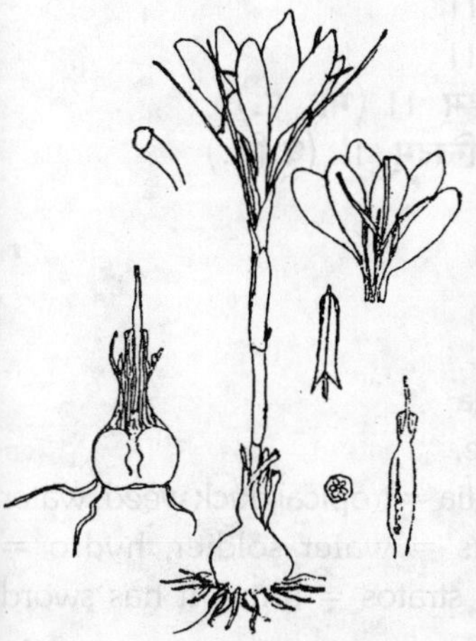

Gana : Shonitasthapan, Eladi.
Kula : Keshar kula.
Family : Iridaceae.
Latin name : Crocus = name adopted from Theophratus; sativus = cultivated.
English name : Saffron (it is obtained from anthers of two spp).
Sanskrit names : Ghusrun, Rakta, Kashmir, Balhik, Kesar, Kashmiraj, Kumkum, Agneeshekhar, Asrugvar, Shatha, Shonit, Pitaka, Rudhir.
Botanical Description : It is a shrub. Leaves are seen towards the base of the stem and are compactly arranged. Flowers - either 2 to 3 flowers are in a bunch or one solitary flower is found besides each leaf. Flowers are voilet in colour. On every flower, there are 3 yellow coloured stamens. Seeds - the ovary is trilobed and in each lobe many round seeds are found. The stalk of gynaecium is made up of three fibres and each fibre has a red coloured stigma. This is known as kesar. Each flower yeilds three fibres of kesar and twenty flowers yeild 120 mg. kesar. The plant flowers in autumn.
Habitat : It is basically an Asian plant but now it is grown in Spain, Iran and Kashmir.
Chemical compostition : It contains a dye, volatile oil 8 to 13.4 %, crocin and picrococin. (Kashmiri kesar is brown, thin, smells like lotus and has a colour similar to that of the rising sun. It is considered to be the best. Balhikaj kesar is thin, whitish and smells like kevada. It is of moderate quality. Parasdeshaj kesar is thick, whitish and smells like honey. It is of inferior quality.)
Properties :
Guna: snigdha, laghu; **Rasa:** katu, tikta; **Vipak:** katu; **Veerya:** ushna; **Dosha :** tridoshahara.
External uses : It improves complexion and hence is used for application on hyperpigmented

The intensity of sweetness of a substance experienced by one person may not be the same as experienced by another since no two persons are identical.

lesions of the skin. It is also used for application in headache. Its paste is applied on wounds. For weak eye sight, a mixture of rosewater and kesar is put in the eyes. Its paste is also used in hepatitis. It is useful in nervous debility, migraine, rheumatoid arthritis, pain caused by vata, loss of appetite, liver disorders, heart diseases and blood disorders.
Kesar is used in dysuria. It is also useful in impotency, dysmenorrhoea, amenorrhoea and painful labour. It is very useful in small pox. It has also been used as a rejuvenator since ancient times. (According to Shri Priyavrat Sharma, this plant survives for many years. But my opinion is that it is a very small shrub living for about 1-2 years. I have seen it grown in Kashmir. It hardly achieves a height of 10 to 15 cms. from the ground.)

Srotogamita :

Dosha : Tridosha and kaphavataghna.

Dahtu : Rakta (improves complexion, useful in hyperpigmented spots, liver, blood and heart diseases and small pox), majja (debility), shukra (impotency), rasa (dysmenorrhoea, amenorrhoea).

Mala : Mutra (useful in dysuria).

References -

कुङ्कुमं घुसृणं रक्तं काश्मीरं पीतकं वरम् । संकोचं पिशुनं धीरं बाह्लीकं शोणिताभिधम् ।।
काश्मीरदेशजे क्षेत्रे कुङ्कुमं यद्भवेद्धि तद् । सूक्ष्मकेसरमारक्तं पद्मगन्धि तदुत्तमम् ।।
बाह्लिकदेशसंजातं कुङ्कुमं पाण्डुरं मतम् । केतकीगन्धयुक्तं तन्मध्यमं सूक्ष्मकेसरम् ।।
कुङ्कुमं पारसीकं यन्मधुगन्धि तदीरितम् । ईषत्पाण्डुरवर्णं तत् ह्यधमं स्थूलकेसरम् ।।
कुङ्कुमं कटुकं स्निग्धं शिरोरुग्व्रणजन्तुजित् । तिक्तं वमिहरं वर्ण्यं व्यङ्गदोषत्रयापहम् ।। (भा. प्र.)
'कुङ्कुमं कटुकं तिक्तमुष्णं श्लेष्मसमीरजित् । व्रणदृष्टिशिरोरोगविषहृत् कायकान्तिदम् ।' (ध.नि.)

(64) KUMBHIKA

Pistia stratiotus Linn.

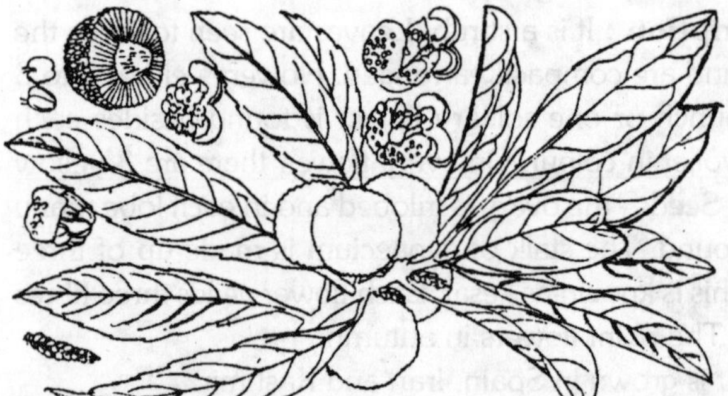

Kula : Suran kula.

Family : Araceae.

Latin name : Pistia = tropical duck weed, water lettuce; stratiotus = water soldier, hydro = charitacae, Gk.- stratos = army. It has sword like leaves.

English name : Tropical Duck weed.

Sanskrit names : Variparni, Varimooli, Jalakumbhi.

Botanical Description : It is a stalkless plant and grows in the pool or lakes. Leaves - 2.6 cm. to 10cms. long, fleshy and round. Flowers - homosexual, its frill like ovary contains many ovoid seeds. Flowering season is summer followed by fruits.

Habitat : India, Asia, Africa, America.

Chemical composition : It contains sodium, potassium, magnesium, calcium carbonate, iron salylic acid.

Properties :

Guna : laghu, ruksha ; **Rasa :** tikta, madhur; **Veerya :** sheeta; **Dosha :** tridoshashamak.

External uses : It is used to remove bedbugs and lice. Leaves ground into paste and applied on fesh wounds, act as a hemostatic and also reduces burning sensations. Bhasma is applied on pruritus and ringworm infection.

Internal uses : Being carminative, laxative and hemostatic, it is used in constipation and dysentery associated with bleeding per rectum. In bleeding disorders, its bhasma is given along with cow's urine. It is used in cough and asthma as an expectorant. It is also used in dysuria, fever, burning sensation and general debility.

Dose : Juice of whole plant - 12 to 24 ml.

Srotogamitva :

Dosha : Tridoshashamak.

Dhatu : Rakta (as a hemostatic in fresh wounds, bleeding disorders and dysentery with bleeding per rectum), meda (mumps).

Mala : Purisha (mild laxative).

References -

'वारिपर्णी हिमा तिक्ता लघ्वी स्वाद्वी सरा कटुः । दोषत्रयहरी रूक्षा शोणितज्वरशोषकृत् ।। (भा. प्र.)
जलकुंभीकजं भस्म पक्वं गोमूत्रगालित् । पिबेत् कोद्रवतक्राशी गलगंडोपशान्तये ।।' (वृंद)

(65) KASH

Saccharum spontaneum Linn.

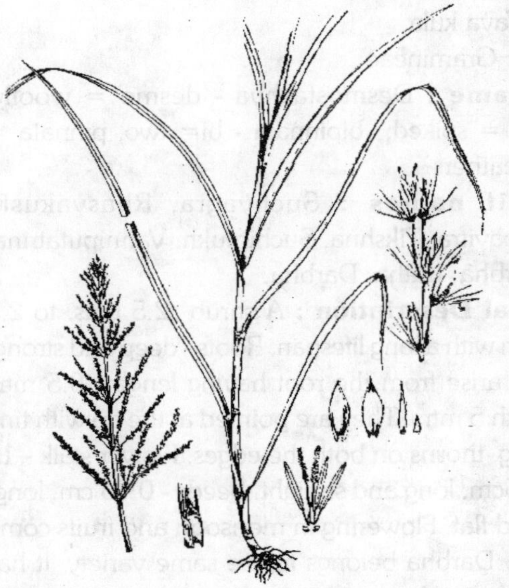

Gana : Mootra virechaneeya, Stanyajanan (C.); Trinapanchamool (S.).

Kula : Yava kula.

Family : Gramineae.

Latin name : Saccharum = from arabic name souker - sugar; sopntaneum = growing wild, sponta = of one's own accord - no need of cultivation.

English name : Thatch grass.

Sanskrit names : Kandekshu, Shwetachamar, Ishika, Ikshur, Sharad, Sitpushpak, Nadeya, Darbhapatra, Lekhani.

Botanical Description : A shrub growing in moist and shallow area is 12.5 to 15 cms. high. Stalk - strong. Leaves - thin and with folded margins. Stalk of flower - 2.5 to 5 cms. long and having white coloured flowers in bunches. Flowers occur in autumn and fruits in winter. Boru reed which is used for writing belongs to the same family and its latin name is Saccharum fuscum.

Habitat : India (at about 1600 mtrs. of height), Sri lanka, South Europe and Australia.

Since the tongue is predominant in aap mahabhoota, it perceives rasa which is also predominant in the same mahabhoota. The same rule applies to all the other senses.

Properties :
Guna : laghu, singdha; **Rasa :** madhur, tikta; **Vipak :** madhur; **Veerya :** sheeta; **Dosha :** vatapitta shamak.
Uses : It acts on rakta dhatu vitiated by vata and pitta. It is useful in bleeding disorders, in digestion due to pitta, diarrhoea with bleeding per rectum, bleeding piles, menorrhagia, burning sensation and pthisis. Because of its diuretic and lithotripsic properties, it is used in dysuria and calculi. It is also used as a galactogogue.
Dose : Decoction of roots - 2 to 4 ounces.
Formulations : Trinapanchmool kwath, Kushavleha, Kushadya ghrit.
Srotogamitva :
Dosha : Vataghna, pittaghna.
Dhatu : Rakta (bleeding disorders, diarrhoea with bleeding per rectum, haemorrhoids, menorrhagia), rasa (galactogogue), reduces fats.
Mala : Diuretic (dissolves calculi).
References -
'कास :स्यान्मधुरस्तिक्त : स्वादुपाको हिम : सर : । मूत्रकृच्छ्राश्मदाहास्रक्षतपित्ताक्षिरोगजित् ।। (भा. प्र.)
'कासेक्षुर्मधुरस्तिक्त : स्वादुपाको हिमो जयेत् । मूत्रकृच्छ्राश्मरीदाहरक्तपित्तज्ञतज्ञयान् ।।' (कै. नि.)

(66) KUSHA
Desmostachya bipinnata Staff.

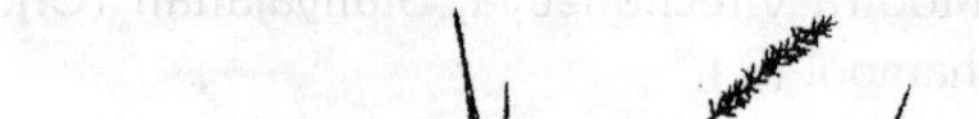

Gana : Mutravirechaneeya, Stanyajanan, Madhurskandha (C.); Trinapanchamool (S.).
Kula : Yava kula.
Family : Gramineae.
Latin name : Desmostachya - desmo = woolly, stachyus = spiked; bipinnata - bi= two, pinnata = having feathers.
Sanskrit names : Suchyagra, Rhasvakush, Brahmapavitra, Tikshna, Suchimukh, Vahniputatrina, Mridudarbha, Kutha, Darbha.
Botanical Description : A shrub 2.5 cms. to 2.5 mtrs. high with a long lifespan. Roots - deep and strong. Leaves - arise from the root having length 0.5 mtrs and width 5 mtrs. They are pointed at the tip with tiny and string thorns on both the edges. Flower stalk - 15 cm. to 45cm. long and straight. Seeds - 0.75 cm. long, ovoid and flat. Flowering in monsoon and fruits come in winter. Darbha belongs to the same variety. It has long and rough leaves.
Habitat : All over India.

Properties :

Guna : laghu, singdha; **Rasa** : madhur, kashaya; **Vipak** : madhur; **Veerya** : sheeta; **Dosha** : tridoshaghna but pittakaphaghna.

Internal uses : As it is haemostatic, it is used in diarrhoea and dysentery with bleeding per rectum, menorrhagia and other bleeding disorders. It is a galactogogue. It has diuretic and lithotripsic properties, hence it is used in dysuria and calculi. Its decoction is helpful in skin disorders.

Part used : Root.

Dose : Decoction - 50 to 100 ml.

Formulations : Trinapanchamool kwath, Kushavaleha, Kushadya ghrit.

Srotogamitva :

Dosha : Tridoshaghna.

Dhatu : Rasa (galactogogue), rakta (haemostatic - bleeding disorders).

Mala : Mutra (diuretic, dissolves calculi), purisha (diarrhoea, dysentery with bleeding per rectum).

Organ : Uterus (menorrhagia).

References -

'दर्भद्वयं त्रिदोषघ्नं मधुरं तुवरं हिंमम् । मूत्रकृच्छ्राश्मरीतृष्णाबस्तिरुक्प्रदरास्त्रजित् ।।' (भा. प्र.)

'दर्भः स्निग्धो हिमः स्वादुःकषायः कफपित्तहा । विसर्पदाहकृच्छ्राश्मतृष्णाबस्तिविकारनुत् ।।' (कै. नि.)

'कुशमूलं समुद् धृत्यपेषयेत्तण्डुलाम्बुना । एतत् पीत्त्वात्र्यहान्नारी प्रदरात् परिमुच्यते ।।' (वृन्द)

(67) KEMBUK

Brassica olerecca

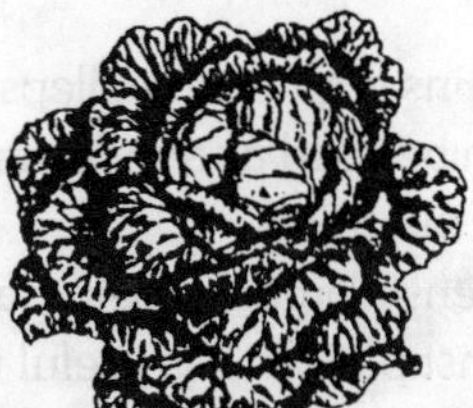

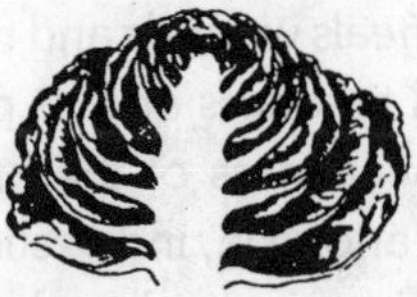

Family : Crucifereae (four petals cross shaped).

Latin name : Brassica = cabbage; olerecca = eatable garden herb.

English name : Cabbage.

Sanskrit names : Kembuka, Kemuk, Kembu, Supatra, Swalpavitap, Swadukanda.

Properties :

Guna : laghu; **Rasa** : tikta; **Vipak:** katu; **Veerya** : sheeta; **Dosha** : kaphapittatmak.

Uses : Appetizer, digestive, cardiotonic, febrifuge. It is useful in dermatoses, cough, urinary disorders and bleeding disorders. Charak has indicated it in retention of urine.

Srotogamitva :

Dosha : Vatavardhak, kaphapittakshapanak.

Dhatu : Rasagami.

Compared to a 'vaidya's' therapy, Ayurvedic treatment is more effective. What does that mean? Need we say that?

(68) KETAKI

Pandanus tectorius Soland Ex Parkino

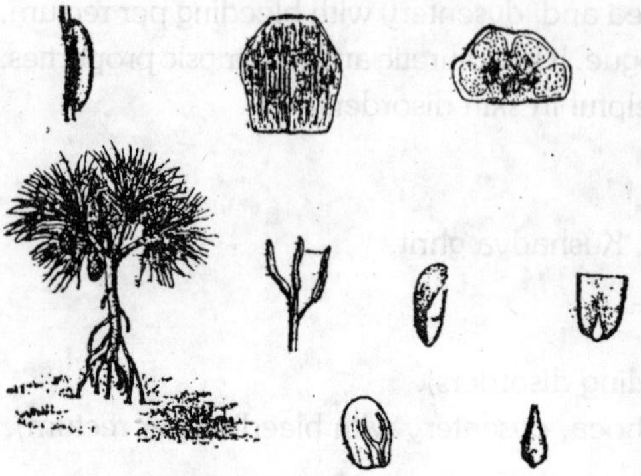

Family : Pandanaceae (screw pine).
Latin name : Pandanus = from a river in Italy, screw pine; tectorius = of roof,covered.
English name : Screw pine.
Sanskrit names : Tikshnapushpa, Vikala, Dhoolipushpika., Medhya, Shivdvishta, Nrupapriya, Deerghapatra, Sthirgandha. Suavarna ketaki is one of the varieties of ketaki which is also known as Hemaketaki, Kanak, Kamakhagadalu, etc.
Botanical Descriptuion : This plant is similar to the plant of date but is only 7 to 6 hands high. Its stalk is crooked with branches. There are many acrial roots vatavriksha and they penetrate into the ground. Mid part of the stalk is tender. Leaves - 4 to 6 mtrs. long and bent, shiny green having marginal spikes. Male flower is white with fragrance, arising from the mid part of the stalk. Flowers are homosexual. Female flower is yellow and smaller than male flower and is more fragrant. It is called as suřvarna ketaki. Fruit - like orange but hard. Flowering occurs in rainy season and fruiting in autumn.
Varieties : Two - 1) Male green flowers = Ketak; 2) Female yellow flowers = Suvarna ketaki.
Chemical composition : It contains an essential oil.
Properties :
Guna : laghu, singdha; **Rasa :** madhur, tikta, katu; **Vipak :** katu; **Veerya :** anushna; **Dosha :** tridoshashamak but especially kaphapittashamak. Its katurasa and vipak are not so strong. If it had been of ushna veerya, the functions would have been stronger.
External uses : Its oil is applied topically on painful back. Nasya of pollengrains is given in epilepsy. Oildrops are used in otalgia. Pollengrain powder heals wounds and reduces can be used as deodorant. Fragrance of ketaki reduces mental and physical tiredness and is pleasing to the mind.
Internal uses : It is used as a brain tonic in weakness of the brain and sense organs. Being an appetizer, digestive and carminative, it is used in anorexia, indigestion and constipation. It is useful in palpitations and blood diseases. Roots are used in urinary disorders. Its oil is used to treat infertility and to prevent abortion. Flower is an aphrodisiac. It is used in measles, small pox and other skin diseases to lessen the rash.
Useful parts : Flowers and roots.
Dose : Ketaki arka (extract) - 4 to 6 drops, ketakdrink (sharbat) - 1 to 2 ounces.
Srotogamitva :
Dosha : Tridoshashamak, mainly kaphaghna and pittaghna.
Dhatu : Majja (prashamak, tonic), rakta (blood diseases - measles, small pox), meda (roots in urinary disorders), shukra (flower -aphrodisiac).
Mala : Sweda (deodorant).
Organ : Uterus (used in infertility), manovaha srotas (pollengrains for nasya).

References -

'केतकः सूचिकापुष्पो जम्बुकः क्रकचच्छदः । सुवर्णकेतकी त्वन्या लघुपुष्पा सुगन्धिनी ।।'
केतकः कटुकः स्वादुर्लघुस्तिक्तः कफापहः । उष्णस्तिक्तरसो ज्ञेयः चक्षुष्या हेमकेतकी ।। (भा. प्र.)
'पुष्पाणां प्रवरं हेमकेतकीपुष्पमुच्यते ईषदुष्णं सुगन्धं च सुतिक्तं दृष्टिदायकम् ।।' (कै. नि.)
'केतकी कटुका पाके लघुतिक्ता कफापहा ।।' (ध. नि.)
'केतकीकुसुमं वर्ण्यं केशदौर्गन्ध्यनाशनम् । हेमाभं मदनोन्मादवर्धनं सौख्यकारि च ।।
तस्य स्तनोऽतिशिशिरः कटुः पित्तकफापहः । रसायनकरो बल्यो देहदार्ढ्यकरः परः' ।। (रा. नि.)

(69) KOSHAMRA

Schleichera trijuga Willd.

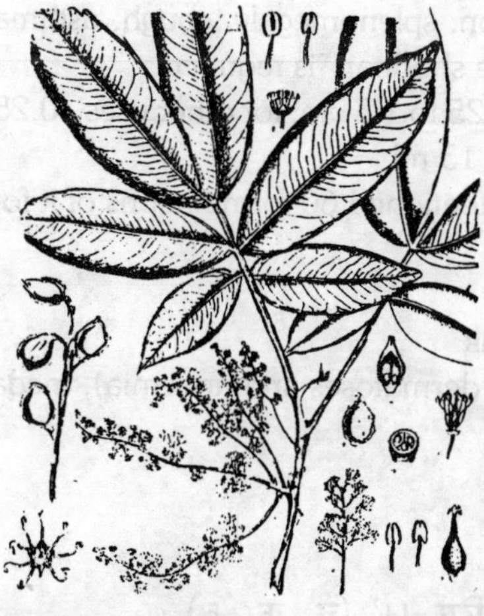

Family : Sapindaceae.
Latin name : Schleichera = from August Schleichera; Trijuga = with three pairs of leaflets.
English name : Ceylon oak.
Sankrit names : Ghanaskandha, Vanamra, Kshudramra, Raktamra, Lakshavriksha, Suraktak, Jatudrima, Krumitaru.
Botranical Description : It is a beautiful tree with fruit of the size of Myristica fragrance having 1 to 3 seeds. It is sour to taste. Wood - hard and strong (It is used to make oil). Bark and seeds are used in medicine. In Bengal, seeds are called as paka. Oil which is known as makasar oil promotes hairgrowth and reduces dandruff. It is also used in scabies, bodyache and headche. Bark rubbed in water is applied on scabies, abscess and lower backache.

Srotogamitva :
Dosha : Vataghna.
Dhatu : Rakta (by external application).
Mala : hair (oil promotes hair growth).

(70) KOSHATAKI

Luffa acutangulata Roxb.

Gana : Vaman, Phalinee, Ubhaybhagahara, Urdhvabhagahara (S.).
Kula : Koshataki kula.
Family : Cucurbitaceae.
Latin name : Luffa = Malayalam name; acutangulata = sharp edged, acute pointed angles, striations of sweet gourd.
English name : Ribbed gourd.
Sanskrit names : Koshataki, Kritachhidra, Sutika, Mridanga phalini, Koshavati, Karkoti, Tiktaghotali, Jyotsna, Katudalinee, Devadali.
Botanical Description : A creeper with fruit 7.5 to 12.5 cms. long. There are 10 straitions on its

If preventive modalities are used in proper time then the number of operations will be reduced. (Then what will the surgeons do?)

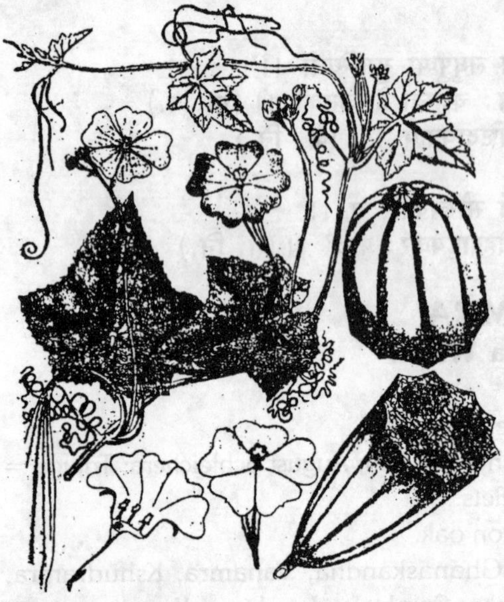

upper surface. Fruit pulp is white and has no specific odour. Seeds are greyish with black spots.

Varieties : There are 2 varieties, 1) Sweet (for vegetables) and 2) Bitter (for medicine).

Habitat : Bitter variety grows in jungles, especially in Bengal and South India.

Properties :

Guna : laghu, ruksha, tikshna; **Rasa :** tikta, katu; **Vipak** : katu; **Veerya :** ushna; **Prabhav :** Ubhayatobhagahara.

Uses : It is used for shodhan in kapha-pitta disorders (emesis and purgation). It is used in ascites, tumour, blood disorders, inflammation, splenomegaly, cough, asthma and dermatoses where shodhan is required.

Dose : For emesis - 1.25 to 1.5 gm, for other uses - 0.25 to 0.5 gm, juice - 8 to 15 ml.

Charakacharya had mentioned 60 formulations of it for shodhan.

Srotogamitva :

Dosha : Kaphaghna (shodhan), pittaghna (shodhan), vatavardhak.

Dhatu : Rasa (fever), rakta (inflammation, splenomegaly, cough, dermatoses and anaemia), meda (urinary disorders).

Mala : Purisha (purgation).

Organs : Stomach and chest.

References -

'अत्यर्थं कटुतीक्ष्णोष्णं गाढेष्विष्टं गदेषु च । कुष्ठपाण्ड्वामयप्लीहशोथगुल्मगरादिषु ।।' (च. क. ६)
'राजकोशातकी शीता मधुरा कफवातकृत् । पित्तघ्नी दीपनी श्वासज्वरकासकृमिप्रणुत् ।।' (भा. प्र.)
'कोशातकी... प्रभृतीनि । रक्तपित्तहराण्यहुर्हृद्यानि सुलघूनि च ।।
कुष्ठमेहज्वरश्वासकासारुचिहराणि च ।।' (सु. सू. ४६)
'कृतवेधन... तैलानि तीक्ष्णानि लघून्यण्णवीर्याणि कटूनि कटुविपाकानि
सराण्यनिलकफकृमिकुष्ठप्रमेहशिरोरोगापहहाणि च ।' (सु. सू. ४५)

(71) KOKILAKSHA

Astercantha longifolia Nees.

Kula : Vasa kula.

Gana : Shukrashodhan (C.)

Family : Acanthaceae (having spikes).

Latin name : Asteracantha = asterius = star-like, cantharus = tankard (a large drinking vessel); longifolia - longi = long, folia = leaves (having long leaves).

Sanskrit names : Kokilaksha (the plant which has flowers like the eyes of cuckoo), Ikshur, Shringali, Shrinkhala, Ranak, Shrigalghanti, Vajrasthishrinkhala, Vajrakantak, Kshurak, Vajra, Shrinkhalika.

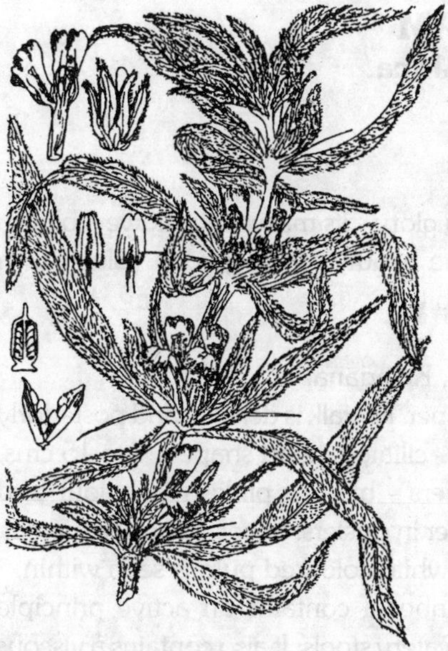

Botanical Description : It is a thorny plant with a height of about 1 to 1.5 mtrs. Its stalk has joints similar to those seen on sugarcane. The stalk is quandrangular and without branches. At each joint on the stalk, there are 5 to 6 leaves and sharp, yellow thorns. Above the leaves, there are brinjal coloured flowers growing on all sides. Each ovary has 4 to 8 seeds. If these are soaked in water, then the water becomes viscous. Flowering and fruiting occurs in winter. At some places, another variety having white flowers is seen.

Habitat : Always grows in marshy lands in Konkan, Bengal and Bihar.

Chemical composition : Seeds contain 31 % viscous principle, 21 to 23 % yellowish, sweet stable oil.

Properties:

Rasa : madhur, tikta; **Veerya :** sheeta ; **Doshaghnata:** vatapittashamak and vitiates kapha.

Seeds: are used in weakness of the nerves, vata disorders, rheumatiod arthritis, desentery, seminal weakness, impotency, dysuria, calculi and cystitis.

Leaves: are used in jaundice, hepatomegaly and gout as a vegetable.

Root: dysuria, calculi, cystitis, inflammation, bleeding disorders, gout and anaemia.

Dose: Juice of panchang - 24 to 50 ml.; decoction - 60 to 100 ml.; seeds - 1 to 3 gms.; kshar - 2 to 5 ratti.

Its seeds are used in tonic preparations.

Srotogamitva :

Dosha : Decreases vata and pitta, increases shuddha kapha.

Dhatu : Majja (balya), increases shukra, rakta (bleeding disorders , vatarakta, jaundice, hepatomegaly, ascites), mansa, meda (anabolic).

Mala : Mutra (dysuria, dissolves gallstones), purisha (dysentery).

Organ : Bladder.

References -

'कण्टकी दीर्घपत्रश्च पत्वलेषु प्ररोहति:' (शि.)

'क्षुरक: शीतलो वृष्य: स्वाद्वम्ल: पिच्छिलस्तथा ।

तिक्तो वातामशोथाश्मतृष्णादृष्ट्यनिलास्त्रजित् ।।' (भा. प्र.)

'कोकिलाक्षस्तु मधुर: शीत: पित्ताश्मरिप्रणुत् । वृष्य: कफहरो बल्यो रुच्य: संतर्पण: पर: ।।' (रा. नि..)

'स्वयंगुप्तक्षुरकयो: फलचूर्णं सशर्करम् । धारोष्णेन नर: पीत्वा पयसा न क्षयं व्रजेंत् ।।' (सु. चि. २६)

'कोकिलाक्षकनिर्यूह: पीतस्तच्छाकभोजिना । कृपाभ्यास इव क्रोधं वातरक्तं नियच्छति ।।' (वा. चि. २२)

'शोथनुत् कोकिलाक्षस्य भस्ममूत्रेण वाम्भसा ।' (च. द.)

The power of all actions resides in seed-form in the body. Treatment provides either internal or external stimulus to these and once that is achieved, a disease gets cured.

(72) KRISHNABEEJAM

Ipomoea hederacea Linn-Joca.

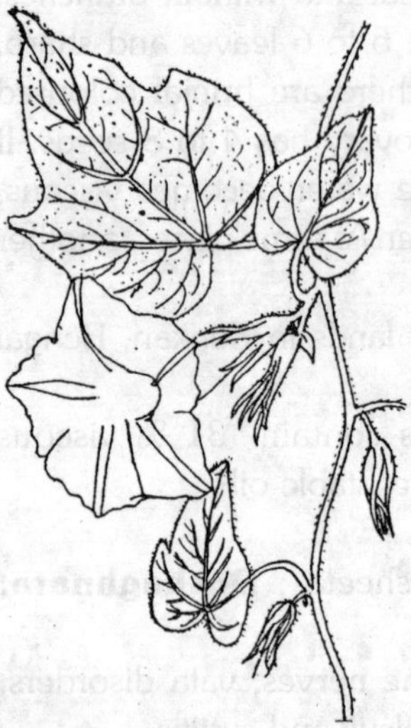

Kula : Trivrutta kula.
Family : Convolvulaceae.
Latin Name : Ipomoea = morning glory - its marvellous flowers bloom in the morning and these add to the beauty of the garden (Blue dawn flower); hederacea = ivy like in habit.
English Name : Forbitis seeds.
Sanskrit Names : Krishnabeejam, Kaladana.
Botanical Description : It is a creeper. Its stalk is delicate and posteriorly it has strong, curled tendrils. Leaves - ciliated, heart shaped, 7 to 15 cms. long and are mostly trilobed. Flowers - blue or pinkish in colour and commonly 1 to 5 flowers grow together in clusters. Seeds - black, triangular. On removing the rind of the seeds, white coloured pulp is seen within.
Chemical composition : Krishnabeeja contains an active principle called forbistine (8 %) which causes watery stools. It also contains a viscous oil (14.4 %).

Properties:
Guna: laghu, ruksha, tikshna; **Rasa** : katu, madhur; **Veerya** : ushna; **Dosha** : vatakaphahara, pittashodhak.
External uses: It is acts as a scraping agent by external application. Its external application is done in kaphaj skin disorders for lekhan. By its tikshna property, it acts as lekhan.
Internal uses:
Since it removes the doshas from the body, it is used in diseases like ascites and oedema which require continuous removal of doshas. For the same reasons it is also used in fever, constipation, headache, flatulence and helminthiasis. Worms are killed and expelled out by krishnabeeja. It is used in a dose of 1 to 3 gms. in gout, rheumatoid arthritis, oedema, dysuria, amenorrhoea and dysmenorrhoea. The seeds are dried, roasted, powdered and then used for medicinal purposes. To avoid abdominal spasm, it is given along with gulkanda, haritaki, fennel etc.
Srotogamitva :
Dosha : Vataghna, kaphaghna, pittashodhan.
Dhatu : Rakta (gout), rasa (rajodosha).
Mala : Dysuria, purisha (shodhaneeya, anthelmintic).
References -
'रेचनं श्यामबीजं स्याच्छ्रोथोदरविनाशनम् । ज्वरे पुरीषसंगे च दारुणे शिरसो गदे ।।
उदावर्त्ते तथानाहे बुधैरेतत् प्रयुज्यते ।' (आ. वि.)

(73) KHATMI

Althaea officinalis

Kula : Karpas kula.

Family : Malavaceae.

Latin name : Althaea = altheo = to cure, remedial qualities of some spp.; officinalis = of the shop, available in the market.

Since the plant is found in Iran, it doesnot have a Sanskrit name, but can be named as Vartulapushpa.

Botanical Description : It is a herb having a height of 1 to 1.25 mtrs. and it has big, hairy leaves. The leaves are circular with serrated edges. Flowers - are of many colours. Seeds - are flat and circular. In summer, the plant oozes out a reddish-yellow gum. This plant can be used for medicinal purposes if two years old.

Habitat : Iran and Kashmir.

Properties:

Guna : singdha, pichchil, guru; **Rasa :** madhur; **Vipak :** madhur; **Dosha:** tridoshashamak but especially vatapittashamak. It is a kaphasarak.

Uses : External application of the seeds and leaves is done in inflammed wounds, breast abscess, pleuritis and pneumonitis. In inflammation of the throat, decoction of the roots is used for gargling. In diarrhoea caused by pitta, decoction of the roots is given by rectal administration in the form of a special enema called pichcha basti. Its decoction is also useful in colitis, dysentery, rhinitis and cough caused by vatapitta.

Srotogamitva :

Dosh : Vata, pitta (tridoshanashak), kaphanissarak.

Dhatu : Rakta, mansa, meda (reduces obstruction), rasa.

Mala : Purisha (dysentery - pichcha basti).

Organ: Pleura, intestines, respiratory system.

(74) KHARJOOR

Phoenix sylvestris Roxb.

Gana: Shramahara, Virechanopaga, Madhurskandha, Kashayskandha, Phalasava (C.)

Kula: Narikel kula.

Family: Palmae.

Latin name: Phoenix = Gk. name of the tree; sylvestris = sylvisticus = of the wood lands.

Sanskrit names: Kharjoor, Kharaskandha, Dushpradharsha, Durarooha, Nihshreni, Kashaya, Yavaneshta, Haripriya.

English name: Date.

Botanical Description: It is a tree growing to a height of 10 to 13 mtrs. Its trunk is straight, greyish and the stalk of the leaves is attached to the trunk. Leaves - 15 to 17.5 cm. long. Leaflets - 15 to 30 cm. long and 2.5 cm. wide, pointed at the tips and arranged opposite to each other. There is one

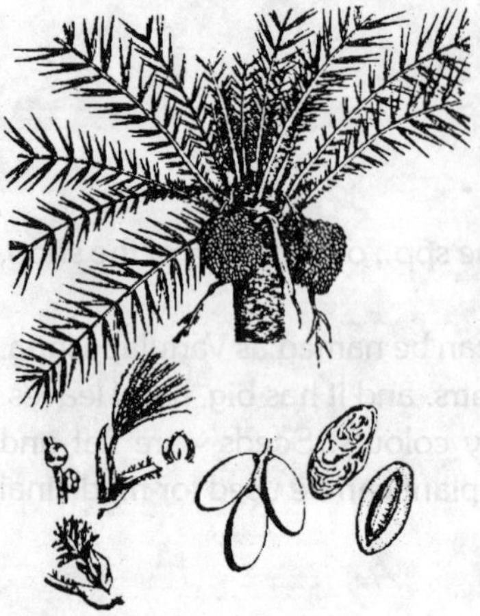

leaflet at the tip of each leaf. Each leaf has at its base a thorn which is 10 cm. long. Only the female khajoor plant bears fruits. Fruits - 2.5 to 3 cm. long, round and yellowish in colour. On ripening, they become red in colour. The fruit contains an oblong seed. Flowers - bloom in summer and later on fruiting occurs. Juice obtained from its trunk is called khajuri. When the juice ferments after some time, it becomes an alcoholic beverage. Jaggary is prepared from its juice.
Types: 1) Khajoor 2) Pindakharjoor (fruit is big, fleshy, Gostan khajoor). Besides, other varieties like Rajakharjoori, Madhukharjoori, Bhookharjoori, Sulemani khajoor etc. are also described in the nighantus.
Habitat: All over India. Pindakharjoor is basically from North Africa, Egypt, Syria and Arabasthan. But now a days, it is also cultivated in Punjab and Sindh.
Chemical composition: Pindakharjoor contains iron, mucilagenous substance and calcium.
Properties:
Guna: snigdha, guru; **Rasa:** madhur; **Veerya:** sheeta; **Vipak:** madhur; **Dosha :** vatapittashamak.
External uses: Roots are analgesic. In toothache, decoction of the roots is used for gargling or root powder is applied on the tooth.
Internal uses: It alleviates vata and acts as a nervine tonic and a tranquiliser. It is useful in fainting, giddiness, intoxication, lower backache and sciatica. It reduces polydipsia, vomiting, diarrhoea, weakness of the heart, cough, asthma, hiccups, seminal weakness and dysuria. In fever, its sherbat is given. Its sherbat is also useful in various debilitating diseases like tuberculosis and fever. Kharjuri is useful in tuberculosis.
Dose: Fruits - 5 to 7; juice - 50 to 100 ml.
References -
'खर्जुरीत्रितयं शीतं मधुरं रसपाकयोः । स्निग्धं रुचिकरं हृद्यं क्षतक्षयहररं गुरु ।।
तर्पणं रक्तपित्तघ्नं पुष्टिविष्टम्भशुक्रदम् । कोष्ठमारुतहृद् बल्यं वांतिवातकफापहम् ।।
ज्वरातिसारक्षुतृष्णाकासश्वासनिवारकम् । मदमूर्च्छामरुत्पित्तमद्योद्भूतमदान्तकृत् ।। (भा. प्र.)
खर्जूरीतरुतोयं तु मदपित्तकरं भवेत् । वातश्लेष्महरं रुच्यं दीपनं बलशुक्रकृत ।।' (भा. प्र.)
'मधुरं बृंहणं वृष्यं खर्जूरं गुरु । रसे पाके च मधुरं खार्जूरं रक्तपित्तनुत् ।। (सु. सू. ४६)
दाहघ्नी मधुरास्रपित्तशमनी तृष्णार्तिदोषापहा,
शीता श्वासकफश्रमोदयहरा सन्तर्पणी पुष्टिदा ।
वह्नेर्मान्द्यकरी गुरुर्विषहरा हृद्या च दत्ते बलं,
स्निग्धा वीर्यविवर्धनी च कथिता पिण्डाख्यखर्जुरिका ।।' (रा. नि.)

(75) KHOOBAKALA
Sisymbrium irio

Kula: Rajika kula.
Family: Cruciferae (cruci = cross; ferae = having cross shaped four petals).
Latin name: Sisymbrium = tansy mustard; irio.

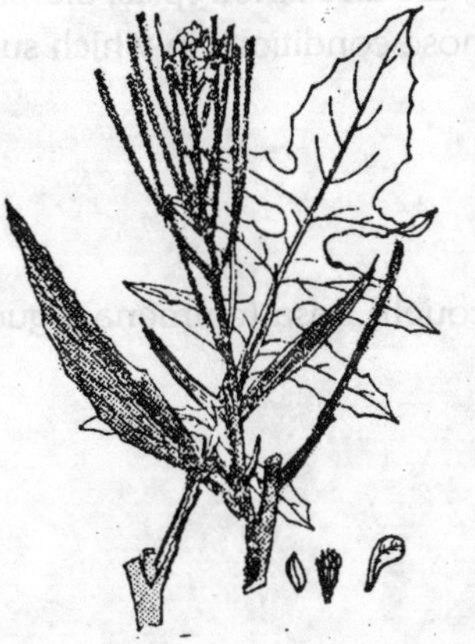

English name: Hedge-mustard.
Botanical Description: It is a shrub of Rajika kula and is similar to the shrub of mustard. It also grows as a weed in the fields of wheat and methika. Seeds - are reddish yellow and are smaller than poppy seeds.
Properties:
Guna: snigdha, guru, pichchil; **Rasa:** madhur, tikta; **Vipak:** madhur; **Veerya:** ushna; **Dosha :** vatapittashamak and kaphanissarak.
Uses: It reduces vomiting and polydipsia. External application is useful in conjunctivitis and in breast abscess. In measels, the leaves of khoobakala are spread over the patient's bed and the patient is made to lie on them. This facilitates early recovery. It is useful in reducing the thirst and vomiting in cholera.
Srotogamitva:
Dosha: Vataghna, pittaghna, kaphanissarak.
Dhatu: Rasa, rakta.
Mala: Purisha (reduces the toxicity in cholera).
Organs: Eyes, breasts.

(76) GARJARAM
Daucas carota Linn.

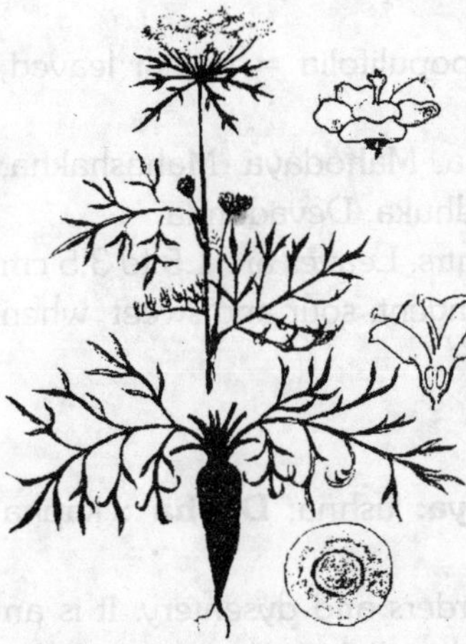

Kula: Shatapushpa kula.
Family: Umbellifereae.
Latin name: Daucas = Latin name; carota = old generic name.
English name: Carrot.
Sanskrit names: Garjar, Pindamool, Peetak, Swadumool, Supeet, Naranga, Pingalmool, Peetakanda.
Botanical Description: It is a shrub of about 1 mtr. height. Leaves - 5 to 8 cm long and have cilia on them. Flowers - white in colour. Fruits - small, white in colour and resemble the fruits of fennel. Roots - red in colour and tapering towards the end like cow's tail. It is an eatable.
Habitat: All over India.
Chemical composition: The root contains carotene, glucose, starch, pectin, malic acid, lignine, salt, albumin, terpine and a high quantity of iron. The seeds contain a yellow coloured and strong odoured oil.
Guna: laghu, tikshna, snigdha; **Rasa:** madhur, tikta; **Veerya:** ushna; **Dosha :** tridoshashamak
Uses: The seeds are applied on inflammation. Its powder is applied on fresh wounds. A preparation (pak) made from its roots is useful in weakness of the brain and nerves. Garjaram is appetizer, unctuous, carminative and astringent. Because of these properties, it is used in anorexia, flatulence, chronic dysentery, haemorrhoids, ascitis and other diseases caused by disorders of digestion. A sweet

In any dravya even though rasa and vipak are exactly opposite, they will not eliminate each other. This is natural and innate to the dravya.

dish (halwa) prepared from it is given in heart diseases and blood disorders. Since it is an expectorant, it is useful in cough and asthma. Seeds are aphrodisiac in property. They are also lithotrypsic, diuretic, emmenagogue and oxytocic in nature. Hence garjaram is used in all those conditions in which such actions are required.

Dose: Root juice - 20 to 40 ml.; seed powder - 3 to 6 gm.;

Srotogamitva:

Dosha: Tridoshashamak.

Dhatu: Majja (weakness), rakta (bleeding disorders, blood diseases, cough), rasa (emmenagogue), shukra (seeds - aphrodisiac).

Mala: Purisha (constipative), mutra (lithotrypsic, diuretic).

Organs: Uterus (oxytocic, induces abortion - seeds).

References -

'गुञ्जनो मूलकैस्तुल्यो रक्तकन्दो रसालु च ।' (शि.)
'नारंगवर्णकश्चैव स्वादुमूलश्च स स्मृतः ।' (रा. नि.)
'गाजरं मधुरं तीक्ष्णं तिक्तोष्णं दीपनं लघु । संग्राहि रक्तपित्तार्शोग्रहणीकफवातजित् ।।' (भा. प्र.)
बीजं चोष्णं मतं चास्य वृष्यं वै गर्भपातकृत् ।' (रा. नि.)
'ग्राही गृंजनकस्तीचक्ष्णो वातश्लेष्मार्शसां हितः ।' (च.)

(77) GANGERUKI
Grewia populifolia

Kula: Parushaka kula.

Family: Tiliaceae (Lime like tree).

Latin name: Grewia = Patron of Botany - Mr. Nahemiah Grew; populifolia = poplar leaved, perpetually trembling leaves.

Sanskrit names: Mahabala, Nagabala, Kharagandha, Chatuhphala, Mahodaya, Mahashakha, Mahapatra, Mahaphala, Vishwadeva, Arishta, Kharva, Rhaswa, Gavedhuka, Devadanda.

Botanical Description: It is a herb with a height of about 1.5 to 3 mtrs. Leaves are 1.5 to 3.5 cm long. Flowers are white in colour and slightly frangrant. Fruits are astringent, sour and sweet when ripe.

Habitat : Western India.

Properties:

Guna: laghu, ruksha; **Rasa:** kashaya, madhur; **Vipak:** katu; **Veerya:** ushna; **Dosha :** kapha pittashamak.

Uses: It is useful in cleansing and healing of wounds, bleeding disorders and dysentery. It is an astringent and is a haemostatic. It is applied on fresh wounds. Few people call this plant as nagabala.

Srotogamitva:

Dosha: Pittaghna, kaphaghna.

Dhatu: Rakta (bleeding disorders), mansa (healing).

Mala: Purisha (in dysentery associated with bleeding as an astringent).

The juice of its root is applied on wounds inflicted by sharp weapons immediately after the injury. This acts as an analgesic and facilitates quick healing.

References -
'गांगेरुकं... । मधुरं सकषायं च शीतं पित्तकफापहम् ।।' (च. सू. २७)
'सकषायं हिमं स्वादु धान्वनं कफवातजित् । तद्वद् गांगेरुकं विद्यात् ।।' (सु. सू. ४६)
'खड्गादिच्छिन्नगात्रस्य तत्कालं पूरितो व्रणः । गांगेरुकीमूलरसैर्जायते गतवेदनः ।।' (शा.)

(78) GIRIPARPAT
Podophyllum hexandrum

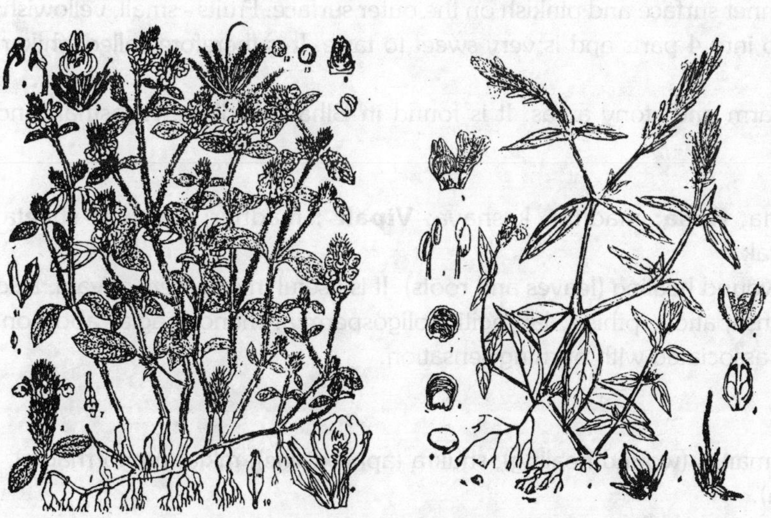

Kula: Daruharidra kula.
Family: Berberideae (plants of the Berberis Tribe).
Latin name: Podophyllum = podo = foot, duck's foot leaved; hexandrum = hexa = six, andrus = anthered.
Botanical Description : It is a small shrub with a height of about 15 to 30 cm. having a stalk which grows straight. Leaves are like the leaves of papaya. Flowers are white in colour with a pinkish tinge. Fruits - are 2.5 to 30 cm. long, red in colour and resemble the fruits of cucumber. Fruit has many seeds and is edible.
Habitat: It grows in the Himalayas, Kashmir, Kangra, Kulu, Chamba, Simla and Sikkim above 2033 mtrs. This shrub always grows in shade.
Properties:
Guna: laghu, ruksha, tikshna; **Rasa:** tikta, katu; **Vipak:** katu; **Veerya:** ushna; **Dosha :** kaphapittahara, it is especially pittashodhak.
Uses : It acts as an irritant and a scraping agent on external application. It acts specifically on the liver. Since it is a cholagogue, it is used in many diseases like jaundice which involve vitiation of pitta. If given in excess, it causes irritation of the intestines. This irritation can be counteracted by snigdha, madhur and sheeta dravyas.
Srotogamitva:
Dosha: Pitta (shodhan), kaphaghna.
Dhatu: Rakta (cholagogue).
Mala: Purisha (bhedan).
Organs: Liver, intestine.

The purgative property of astringent haritaki (Terminalia chebula) remains intact even during transition and digestion. This happens because agni can differentiate. That is why agni is most important to life.

(79) GUDASHARKARA
Grewia hirsuta

Kula: Phalasa kula.
Family: Tiliaceae (Lime tree).
Latin name: Grewia = after Mr. N. Grew - patron of Botany; hirsuta = having long distinct hair.
Botanical Description: It is a herb having a height of about 1.5 to 2 mtrs. Leaves - tapering at both the ends, serrated, with tiny hair on them and 2 to 3 flowers arising from the base of each leaf. Flowers - are yellowish on the inner surface and pinkish on the outer surface. Fruits - small, yellowish; on ripening, the fruit breaks up into 4 parts and is very sweet to taste. It is therefore called 'shikari meva'.
Habitat : It grows in hilly, warm and stony areas. It is found in Bihar, Vindhya, Rajasthan and Konkan.
Properties :
Guna: guru, pichchil, snigdha; **Rasa:** madhur, kashaya; **Vipak :** madhur; **Veerya:** sheeta; **Doshaghnata:** Vatapittashamak.
Uses: It is a haemostatic and wound healing (leaves and roots). It is useful in disorders of vata, acid peptic diseases, flatulence, constipation, pthisis, laryngitis, oligospermia, menorrhagia, abortion, dysuria, pyuria and in malaria associated with burning sensation.
Srotogamitva:
Dosha: Vataghna, pittaghna.
Dhatu: Rakta (haemostatic), mansa (wound healing), shukra (aphrodisiac), rakta (menorrhagia).
Mala: Mutra (useful in dysuria).
Organ: Uterus (useful in preventing abortion).

(80) GUNJA
Abrus precatorius

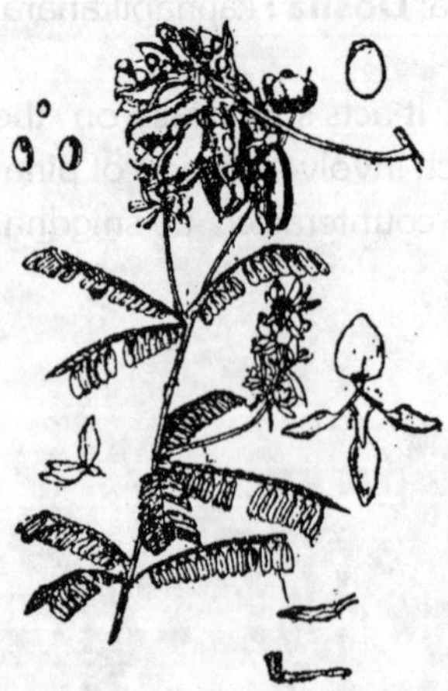

Kula: Shimbi kula.
Upakula: Aparajita - Papilionaceae.
Family: Leguminoseae.
Latin name: Abrus = delicate leaves; precatorius = of prayers = seeds of this plant are used for making rosaries.
English name: Indian licorrice root.
Sanskrit names: Gunja, Choodamani, Raktaphalika, Kakanantika, Kakadani, Kakachinchi, Krushnaraktika.
Botanical Description: A creeper with many branches. Leaves resemble tamarind leaves having 20-40 leaflets. Flowers are pink, bluish and appear in cluster. Legumes are 1.5 - 3.5 cm. long containing red, white and black coloured seeds. Red coloured seeds have black spot on their tips. Root and leaves are sweet like that of G. glabra.

It is of 3 varieties - white (seeds of which are used in medicine), red and black (roots and leaves of all these 3 varieties are used in medicines).

Habitat : This creeper grows in India, Sri lanka and Sayam.

Properties: Seed - **Guna :** laghu, ruksha, tikshna; **Rasa:** tikta, kashaya; **Vipak:** katu; **Veerya:** ushna

Root: madhur and snigdha.

Seeds alleviate kapha and vata; leaves and roots alleviate all the three doshas.

Seeds ground in a paste are applied over skin disorders, dermatoses, chronic ulcers and alopecia. Paste of the leaves is applied over inflammations and wounds. Oil boiled with the leaves is used for massage in vata disorders. Nasya of powdered seeds is given in headache.

Milk boiled with the leaves is given in hoarseness of voice, impotency, dysuria and general debility. Powdered seeds in excess dose causes toxic symptoms like cardiac arrest etc. Juice of tandulja + sugar is an antidote to these symptoms. Seeds are purified by boiling them in kanji or cow's milk for three hours.

Dose: Seed powder - 0.5 to 1.5 ratti; root powder - 0.25 to 0.5 gms.

Dosha: Kaphavata (seed), tridoshanashak (leaves and roots).

Dhatu: Muscles (hoarseness of voice - milk boiled with the leaves); shukra (milk boiled with the leaves - aphrodisiac).

Mala: Mutra (dysuria - milk boiled with leaves), keshya - enhances hair growth.

References -

''गुञ्जावल्ली तु मधुरा चिंचापत्री सुशिम्बिका । बीजं कृषारूणं श्वेतं जायते सर्वभूमिषु ।।' (शि.)
'गुञ्जाद्वयं तु केश्यं स्यात् वातपित्तज्वरापहम् । नेत्रामयहरं वृष्यं बल्यं कण्डूव्रणापहम् ।।
मुखशोषभ्रमश्वासतृष्णामदविनाशिनी । कृमीन्द्रलुप्तकुष्ठानि रक्तबद्ध बलापि च ।।' (भा. प्र.)
'गुञ्जा सोष्णा रसे तिक्ता कषाया कफपित्तहा । चक्षुष्या शुक्रला केश्या त्वच्या रुच्या बलप्रदा ।।
इन्द्रलुप्तहरा तीव्रा सविषा मदमोहकृत् । हन्ति रक्षोग्रहविषं कण्डूकुष्ठविषक्रिमीन् ।।' (कै. नि.)
'मूलं तु मधुरं तिक्तं मुखशोषहरं परम् । मुखपाकहरं पत्रं, सर्वं श्वेताभवं शुभम् ।।' (नि. स.)
'गुंजाद्वयं च शीतोष्णं बीजं वान्तिकरं, शिफा । शूलघ्नी विषकृत् पत्रं वश्ये श्वेता प्रशस्यते ।।' (ध. नि.)

(81) GORAKSHA

Adansonia digitata

Kula: Karpasi Kula.

Family: Malvaceae.

Latin name: Adansonia = after an eminent French scientist and traveller; digitata = finger shaped.

Sanskrit name: Gorakshakarkati.

Botanical Description: It is a huge tree. Base of the stem is bigger than any other tree. It bears bottel or cucumber shaped fruits which are surrounded by a hard shell and have greenish yellow cilia.

Properties: Kernel of the fruit - cardiotonic, sheeta and laxative. Leaves - astringent. Bark -sheeta, appetizer, astringent and causes lowering of heart rate. Because of their resin content, the leaves are used for local application in inflammations.

Ayurveda doesnot accept abhav padarth. All actions are carried out by bhav padarth. What can poor abhav achieve?

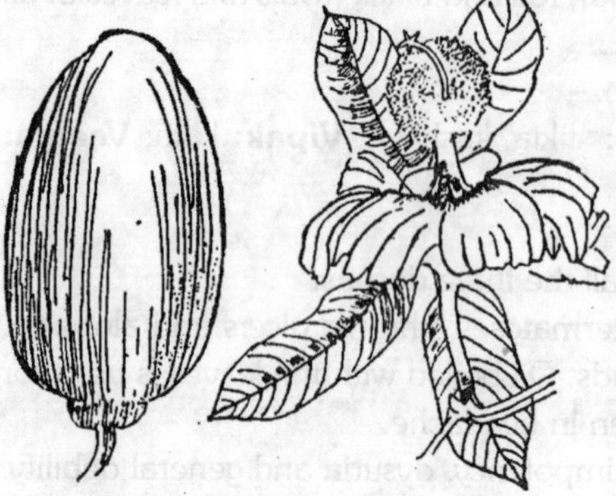

Uses: Fever - kernel of the fruit in a dose of 1 to 2 gms. is given in typhoid fever. Juice of the kernel reduces the temperature. Thirst - juice of the kernel along with sugar reduces thirst.

Fever - Decoction of the bark is used to reduce the pulse rate.

Pthisis - Juice of the kernel alleviates night sweats.

Respiratory tract - A mixture of pulp of the fruit 1.5 gms + dry fig totally cures asthma. Juice of the kernel is given in dysentery, diarrhoea and acid-peptic disorders.

Parts used: Fruits, leaves and bark.

Srotogamitva:

Dosha: Pittaghna.

Dhatu: Rakta (alleviates pitta in the blood), rasa (fever).

Mala: Purisha (antidiarrhoeal).

Organs: Respiratory system, heart (reduces the pulse rate).

(82) GOJIVHA

Onosma bracteatum Wall.

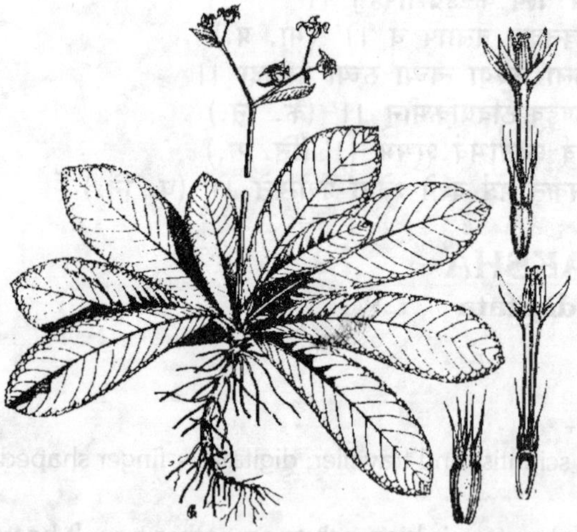

Kula: Shleshmantaka kula.

Family: Boraginaceae.

Latin name: Onosma = onos = ass, Rutton root (it was said to be pleasing to animals); bracteatum = bracted = small leaf or scale below calyx.

Sanskrit names: Gojivha, Kharapatra, Darvipatra, Vrushajivha, Gajaban, Gavajbana.

Botanical Description: A small herb spreading on the ground. Leaves - big, fleshy, rough like cow's tongue and have small, round spots on them. Flowers - blue, appear in clusters and become red on drying. Leaves and flowers, when soaked in water, form a sticky substance.

Habitat: In the Himalayas at a height of 3 - 4 thousand meters and also in Kashmir, Kumaon, Iran, Afghanistan.

Chemical composition: Leavs contain 27% calcium, potassium, sodium and iron.

Properties:

Guna: lahgu, snigdha, madhur, tikta; **Vipak:** madhur; **Veerya:** sheeta. It alleviates vata and pitta.

Uses: Its local application has cooling and wound-healing properties. Bhasma of leaves is applied over stomatitis and wounds. Being beneficial to majja dhatu, it is useful in hysteria and mental

debility. Being carminative and mild laxative, it is used in jaundice, udavarta and constipation. It is also used in cardiac impairment, rheumatoid arthritis and chancres. Its expectorant activity is seen in cold, cough, asthma, pleuritis and throat irritation. It is used along with Glycerrhiza glabra and Viola odorata. Being a diuretic, it is useful in dysuria and pyuria. It reduces the pyrexial complications and weakness.
Parts used: Leaves and fruits are used.
Dose: Leaves 4 to 6 gms.; flowers - 3 to 6 gms.
Srotogamitva:
Dosha: Vata pitta kapha nissaraka.
Dhatu: Majja (tonic), rakta (jaundice, chancre), all dhatus (rejuvenator by digestion of ama).
Mala: Purisha (mild laxative), mutra (diuretic).

(83) CHAKRAMARDA

Cassia tora Linn.

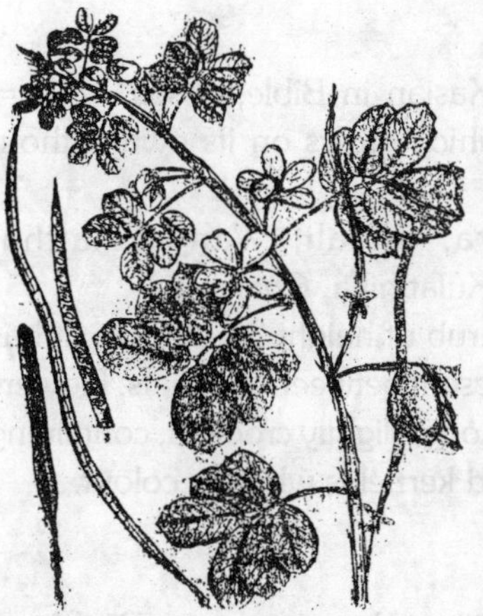

Kula: Shimbi kula.
Family: Leguminoseae.
Latin name: Casia = cognate of Kasian in the Bible; tora = Singhalese name of the plant.
English name: Ringworm plant.
Sanskrit names: Edagaja, Prapunnada, Dadrughna, Vimarda, Shakunashana, Chakri, Chakragaja, Drudabeeja, Meshavha, Vyavartaka, Punnata, Khurjughna, Gajakya, Mesha.
Botanial Description: A herb of having a height of approximately 0.5 - 1 mtr. It has a bad odour. Leaves - compound and get closed in the evening. Flowers - yellow. Legumes - 10 -15 cm long, quandrangular. Each legume contains 20 -30 seeds. Flowering occurs in rainy season and fruiting in winter.
Habitat : It grows throughout India.

Properties:
Seed: laghu, ruksha, katu, ushna; **Leaves:** madhur and sheeta veerya.
It alleviates kapha and vata and its local application is antipruritic and has antidotal activities.
Seeds ground in a paste with sour drugs (curds, lemon) is useful in disorders such as scabies and ringworm. Useful in raktagata kapha-vata disorders. Being carminative, vermifuge and liver stimulant, it is effective in vata-kaphaj disorders, dermatoses, worms, piles, gulma, cough and asthma. Also useful in toxic and lipid disorders. A drink made from its seeds tastes like coffee. It purifies the blood and cures many skin disorders.
Dose: Seeds 1 to 3 gms.; leaf juice 3 to 6 ml.
The main activity of the plant is against ringworm infestation. Seeds ground in a paste with latex of Euphorbia nerifolia and cow's urine are applied over keloids.

If the minute representatives of the universe in the body itself become depleted, then external medicines however strong, will not have any effect.

Srotogamitva:

Dosha: Vatakaphaghna.

Dhatu: Meda (reduces fats), rakta (cures ringworms, infections, complexion enhancer, liver stimulant).

Mala: Purisha (worms).

Organs: Respiratory system, digestive system, circulatory system.

References -

चक्रमर्दः कटूष्णः स्यात्मेदोवातकफापहः । दद्रुकण्डूहर:कान्तिसौकुमार्यकरो मतः ।।' (ध.नि.)

'चक्रमर्दः प्रपुन्नाडो दद्रुघ्नो मेषलोचनः । पद्माटः स्यादेडगजः चक्री पुन्नाट इत्यपि ।।'

'चक्रमर्दो लघुः स्वादू रूक्षः पित्तानिलापहः । हृद्यो हिमः कफश्वासकुष्ठदद्रुकृमीन् हरेत् ।।

हत्युष्णंतत्फलंकुष्ठकण्डुदद्रुविषानिलान् । गुल्मकासकृमिश्वासनाशनं कटुकंस्मृतम् ।। (भा. प्र.)

(84) CHAKSHUSHYA

Cassia absus Linn.

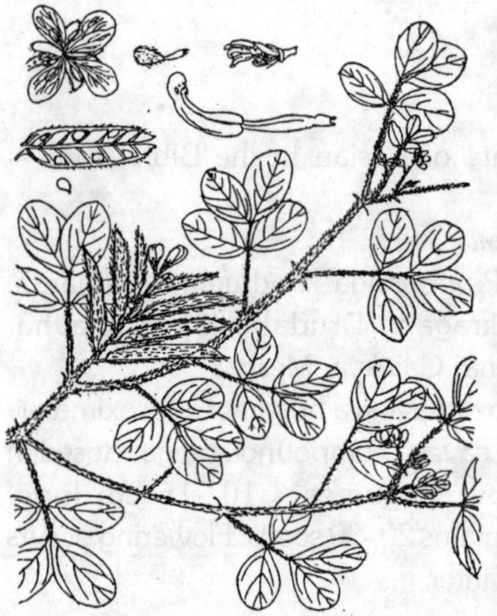

Kula: Shimbi kula.

Upakula: Caesalpinaideae.

Family: Leguminoseae.

Latin name: Cassia = from Kasian in Bible; absus - (ab = away; sus = sow) = a plant which grows on its own without sowing - wild.

Sanskrit names: Chakra, Kulali, Vanyakulattha, Aranyakulatthika, Lochanhita, Kulatthika, Chakrak.

Botanical Description: A shrub of height 30 - 60 cm. It has leaves and leaflets. A gland is present between 2 leaflets. Flowers - reddish, legume is 2.5 - 3.7 cm long, slightly crooked, containing 5 shiny, dusky black seeds. Seed kernel is white in colour.

Habitat: Throughout India.

Properties:

Guna: ruksha; **Rasa :** kashaya, tikta; **Veerya:** sheeta; **Prabhav:** chakshushya, **Dosha :** kapha-pittashaman.

It is an antiinflammatory, beneficial to the eyes, astringent, haemostatic, diuretic and antidote in nature. It has action on meda dhatu. It has anti-obesity properties.

Uses: Its paste is applied over eye-lashes. Its fine powder is applied in eye disorders like conjunctivitis. Paste is applied over wounds, mainly ulcers of genital organs. It is useful in colitis, dysentery, lower intestinal haemorrhagic disorders, diarrhoea, dysuria and calculi. The seeds of C. absus are roasted with any flour and then they are seperated from the flour used for roasting. The outer cover is removed and the inner core is made to a fine powder for its use in eyes.

Srotogamitva:

Dosha: Kaphaghna, pittaghna.

Dhatu: Rakta (anti-inflammatory - haemorrhagic disorders), rakta, mansa (mainly useful in ulcers of genital organs).

Mala: Purisha (colitis, dysentery, diarrhoea), mutra (dysuria, calculi).
Organs: Because of its chakshushya prabhav, its powder is applied in many eye disorders.
References -
चक्षुष्या दृक्प्रसादा च सैव प्रोक्ता कुलत्थिका । कुलाली लोचनहिता कुम्भकारी मलापहा ।।
हिमा प्रोक्ता कषाया च विषं स्थावरजंगमम् । छिनत्ति योजिता सम्यक नेत्रस्रावाननेकशः ।।
सा च विस्फोटकण्डूवर्त्तिव्रणदोषनिबर्हणी । (ध. नि.)
'कुलत्थिका तु चक्षुष्या कषाया कटुका हिमा ।
विषविस्फोटकण्डूर्तिव्रणदोषनिबर्हिणौ ।।' (रा. नि.)

(85) CHANCHU
Corchorus acutangulus

Kula: Parushaka kula.
Family: Tiliaceae.
Latin name: Corchorus = jute; acutangulus = acute = sharp, angulus = having angles.
Sanskrit names: Chincha, Chanchoo, Chanchuki, Deerghapatra, Satiktata.
Botanical Description: This shrub grows in rainy season and has a life span of one year and then dries off. Stalk is 2.5 - 5 cm. long. Leaves are 5 - 7.5 cm. long and 1.25 - 3.5 cm. broad, with serrated margins. Flowers - yellow. Fruit looks like a horn having 6 striations on it. It contains slimy seed. Leaves are edible.
Habitat: It is of many varieties and it grows throughout India.
Properties:
Guna: guru, snigdha, pichchil; **Rasa :** madhur, kashaya; **Vipak:** madhur; **Veerya:** sheeta (but seeds are katu and ushna veerya).
It is tridoshashamak by prabhav.
External use: Local application has antispetic and wound healing properties.
Internal uses: It is unctuous, mild laxative and astringent. It is antihaemorrhagic, aphrodisiac and diuretic.
Srotogamitva:
Dosha: Pittaghna, tridoshaghna (by prabhav).
Dhatu: Rakta (alleviates pitta), shukra (aphrodisiac), mansa (wound healing), tonic for all dhatus (pichchil, guru, snigdha).
Mala: Mutra (diuretic), purisha (astringent).
Organs: Genital organs, intestine (astringent).
Prabhav: Rat poison (seeds are useful), brain tonic.
References -
चञ्चुः शीता सरा रुच्या स्वाद्वो दोषत्रयापहा ।
धातुपुष्टिकरी बल्या मेध्या पिच्छिलिका स्मृता ।। (भा. प्र.)
'चंचुस्तु मधुरा तीक्ष्णा कषाया मलशोषणी ।
गुल्मोदरविबंधार्शोग्रहणीरोगनाशिनी ।।' (रा. नि.)
'लघुः पाके च जन्तुघ्नः पिच्छिलो व्रणिनां हितः ।

Just as some diseases are never dwidoshaj, similarly certain combinations of two mahabhootas do not exist. Prabhav is responsible for this.

कषायमधुरो ग्राही चुचुस्तेषां त्रिदोषहा ।।' (सु. सू. ४६)
'चंचुबीजं कटूष्णं चंचु गुल्मशूलोदरार्त्तिजित् ।
विषत्वग्दोषकंडूघ्नमाखोर्दुष्टविषापहम् ।।' (नि. र.)

(86) CHANDRASHUR
Lepidium sativum

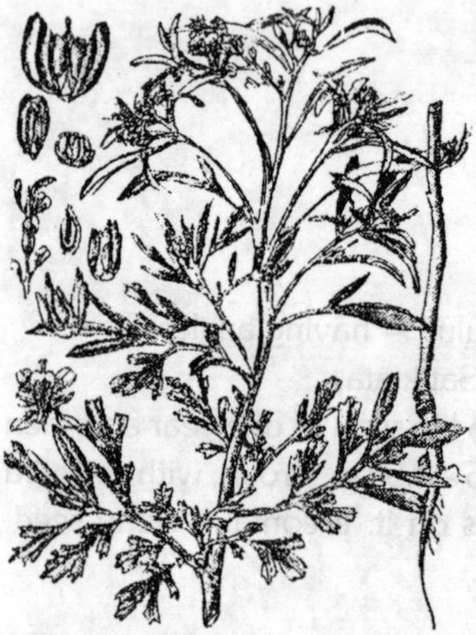

Kula: Rajika kula.
Gana: Chaturbeeja (Bhavaprakash).
Family: Cruciferae (having cross shaped four petals).
Latin name: Lepidium = resembling cress or pepper wort; sativam = cultivated.
Sanskrit names: Chandrashur, Chandrika, Charmahantri, Pashumehanakarika, Nandinee, Karavee, Bhadra, Vasapushpa, Suvasara.
Botanical Description: The shrub is 2.5 to 5 cm. high. Leaves – resemble those of coriander. Seed – is red and boatshaped. When sowed, it grows in 2-3 days.
Habitat: India and Tibet.
Properties:
Guna: laghu, snigdha, pichchil; **Rasa:** katu, tikta; **Vipak:** katu; **Veerya:** ushna; **Dosha:** vata-kaphashamak.
External uses: It alleviates pain and inflammation of joints by local application.
Internal uses: It is an appetizer, carminative, diuretic and blood purifier. It is also useful as an aphrodisiac, emmenagogue and galactagogue. Its rejuvenating property is helpful in post partum period. It is also useful in gout.
Srotogamitva:
Dosha: Vataghna, kaphaghna.
Dhatu: Rakta, mansa, meda, rasa (menstruation and breast milk), shukra (aphrodisiac).
Mala: Purisha.
Organ: Uterus.
References -
'चन्द्रशूरं हितं हिक्कावातश्लेष्मातिसारिणाम् । असृग्वातगदद्वेषि बलपुष्टिविवर्धनम् ।।' (भा. प्र.)
'वरकृष्णो वातशूलगुल्मघ्नः स्तन्यपुष्टिकृत् । बल्यो वाजीकरः पानाल्लेपाच्छोणितशूलनुत् ।।' (शो.)

(87) CHAMPAK
Michelia champak

Kula: Champak kula.
Family: Magnoliaceae.
Latin name: Michelia = after an Italian botanist; champak = from the Indian name.
Sanskrit names: Swarnapushpa, Champeya, Sheetalacchada, Brungamohi, Sheetal, Bhramaratithi,

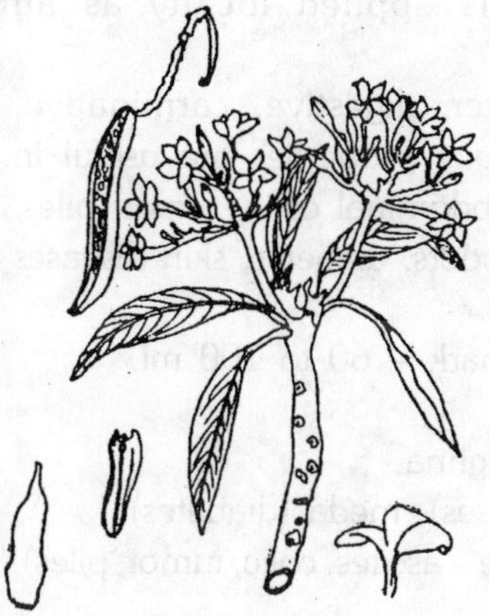

Sthirgandha, Hemapushpa, Peetpushpa.
Botanical Description: This is an evergreen tree. Flowers – dark yellow and have a slightly stingent smell.
Habitat: All over India
Varieties: Two - 1) Peeta champak 2) White champak.
Properties:
Guna: laghu, ruksha, tikshna; **Rasa:** katu, kashaya, madhur; **Vipak:** katu; **Veerya:** sheeta;
Dosha: kaphapittashamak.
Uses: Local application of flowers is done in headache and burning. Internally, it is soothing, hemostatic and antipyretic. The bark is used as a preventive in malarial fever. Flowers are used in dysuria and pyuria.
Srotogamitva:
Dosha: Kaphaghna, pittaghna, vataghna.
Dhatu: Rakta (bleeding disorders), gout.
Mala: Mutra (dysuria), anthelmintic.
Organ: Head.
Special character: Katu vipak but sheeta veerya.
References -
'चम्पक:कटुकस्तिक्त: कषायो मधुरो हिम: । विषक्रिमिहर: कृच्छ्रकफवातास्रपित्तजित् ।।' (भा. प्र.)
'चम्पक: कटुकस्तिक्त: शिशिरो दाहनाशन: । कण्डूकुष्टव्रणहर: कफपित्तविनाशन: ।।' (रा. नि.)
'चम्पकं कटुकं तिक्तं कषायं मधुरं हिमम् । निहन्ति कफपित्तास्रमूत्रकृच्छ्रविषक्रिमीन् ।।' (कै. नि.)

(88) CHIRIBILVA
Holoptelea integrifolia Planch.

Kula: Vata kula.
Gana: Lekhaneeya, Bhedaneeya, (C.); Shleshmasanshaman (S.)
Family: Urticaceae.
Latin name: Holoptelea = holo = all, ptelia = winged fruit; integrifolia = having leaves with unbroken smooth edges.
Sanskrit names: Prakeerya, Chirbilva, Putikaranj, Putik, Kalimarak, Puti, Karanjik, Chilbill, Navili.
Botanical Description: Medium sized tree with white coloured branches. Leaves – 2.5 to 20 cms. long and 5 to 10 cms. broad, egg shaped, pointed with transparent spots. Dried leaves exhibit small elevations on the ventral surface. Flowers – small, green and in clusters. Fruits – winged with bent tips. Flowering season is summer followed by fruiting. Leaves and trunk have an offensive odour.
Habitat: All over India, in small hilly areas.
Properties:
Guna: laghu, ruksha; **Rasa:** tikta, kashaya; **Vipak:** katu; **Veerya:** ushna; **Dosha:** kaphapitta shamak

In this world no two substances are totally identical to each other then how can two persons be?

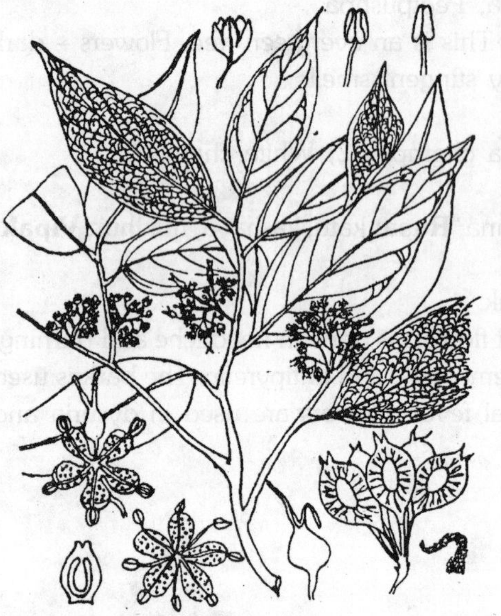

External use: Bark is applied locally as an antiinflammatory.

Internal uses: Appetizer, digestive, carminative, anthelmintic and cholagogue properties are useful in loss of appetite, ascites, abdominal colic, tumor, piles. Also useful in blood disroders, diabetes, skin diseases and obesity.

Dose: Decoction of the bark – 60 to 100 ml.

Srotogamitva:

Dosha: Kaphaghna, pittaghna.

Dhatu: Rakta (skin diseases), meda (diabetes).

Mala: Purisha (cholagogue – ascites, colic, tumor, piles).

References -

करंजी स्तंभनी तिक्ता तुवरा कटुपाकिनी ।
वीर्योष्णा वमिपित्तार्श: कृमिकुष्ठप्रमेहजित् ।। (भा. प्र.)

(89) CHUKRAM

Rumex vesicarius Linn.

Kula: Chukra kula.

Family: Polygonaceae (Poly = many, gona = angle).

Latin name: Rumex = Latin name – Duck, sorrel; vesicarius = bladdered.

English name: Country sorrel.

Sanskrit names: Chukram, Chukrika, Patramla, Rochani, Shatvedhani.

Botanical Description: An annual herb growing 15 - 30 cm. high. Leaves – egg-shaped, 2.5 to 7.5 cm in length, showing 3 - 5 veins. Fruits – small, white or brownish containing very small seeds. It is used commonly as a vegetable. Another variety found in the Himalayas is known as chulmora (Rumex hastet).

Habitat: In the hilly areas of India.

Chemical composition: Fresh leaves contain 92% water. Dried leaves contain 57.86% carbohydrates.

Properties:

Guna: laghu, ruksha; **Rasa:** amla, madhur; **Vipak:** amla; **Veerya:** ushna; **Dosha:** vatashamak, kaphapittavardhak. **Seed:** pittashamak (slimmy and sheeta).

External uses: Useful as an analgesic, anti-inflammatory and antitoxic (scorpion bite). Leaf juice is used for gargles in toothache.

Internal uses: Leaves are appetizer, digestive, purgative and liver stimulant but seeds are snehan and constipative. Therefore leaves are used for loss of taste, thirst, nausea, loss of appetite, jaundice,

tumour, colic and piles whereas seeds are used in dysentery along with isabgol. Seeds are also very useful in dysuria and burning micturition. Juice of the leaves is used in palpitation. (Chukra is said to cause dhatukshaya).
Dose: Juice of whole plant – 10 to 20 ml.; seed powder – 3 to 5 gms.
Srotogamitva:
Dosha: Vataghna, kaphapittavardhak (seed – pittashamak).
Dhatu: (Leaves) Rakta (jaundice, liver stimulant).
Mala: Mutra (dysuria), purisha (bhedan).
Organ: Heart (palpitations).

(90) CHORAK
Anjelica glouca Edgw.

Gana: Eladi gana, Sugandhi gana.
Family: Umbelliferae.
Latin name: Anjelica = angelic virtues in medicine; glouca = blue, grey, green.
Sanskrit names: Shankit, Dushpatra, Kshemak, Ripu, Ganahas, Kopanak, Phalchorak, Nishachar, Dhanhara.
Botanical Description: The shrub grows 10 cm. to 18 cm. high.
Habitat: Kashmir, Nepal.
According to Dalhan, this plant resembles granthiparni but according to others it is sthaunak – chor ova.
Properties: It is fragrant, appetizer, digestive, stimulant and laxative. Therefore, it is useful in indigestion, constipation and debility.
Uses: Epilepsy, hiccups, dyspnoea, rhinitis etc.
Parts used: Root.
Srotogamitva:
Dosha: Vataghna, kaphaghna.
Dhatu: Rakta.
Mala: Purisha (laxative).
Organ: Digestive system, respiratory system and nervous system.
References -
रोचको मधुरस्तिक्त: कटु: पाके कटुर्लघु: ।
तीक्ष्णो हृद्यो हिमो हन्ति कुष्ठकण्डुकफानिलान् ।।

(91) CHAUHAR
Artimisia maritima Linn.

Kula : Bhringaraj kula.
Family : Compositeae.
Latin name : Artimisia = one of the names of Diana; maritima = of the seaside.

For detection of taste the tongue is continuously wetted by saliva. This flow never stops. Even if it stops for a moment, what can happen?

English name : Wormseed.
Sanskrit names : Chauhar, Chaurapurva, Parsikyavani, Jantunashan, Chorahva.
Botanical Description : This herb belongs to bhringaraj kula. It is known as keetmariyavani, kirmali ajavayan, kirmali ajama, wormseed etc.
Habitat : This plant grows at the height of 2-3 thousand mtrs. in the Himalayas, Kumaon, Kashmir, Afghanisthan, Persia, Tiber etc.
Chemical composition : It contains a camphor-like fragrant volatile oil. Flower contains 1.75% santonin. It turns yellow on exposure to sunrays or on preservation.
Properties:
Guna : laghu, ruksha, tikshna; **Rasa :** tikta, katu; **Veerya :** ushna; **Prabhav :** anthelmintic.
External uses : Analgesic, anti-inflammatory, wound healing and hair tonic. Therefore oil is used for massaging in inflammatory conditions or oil packs in wound healing. Its ash mixed in oil is applied on scalp for baldness.
Internal uses : It is especially known for anticonvulsant property. It is therefore used in tetanus and convulsive disorders to overcome convulsions. Excess dose results in uneasiness and delirium.
Alimentary system : It acts as an appetizer, carminative, hepatic stimulant and powerful anthelmintic. It is especially useful in round worms (Ascaris lumbricoidus) and thread worms. A full dose is given on empty stomach at bed time followed by a purgative in the morning. Dead worms are expelled. In chronic infestation, the same dose is repeated after a week.
Urinary system : It acts as a diuretic, acidic urine turns greenish yellow while alkaline shows violet colour.
Reproductive system : It is used as an emmenagogue and spermatogenic. It is also useful in fever with rigors and dyslipidemia.
Dose : Panchang 2 to 3 gms.; santonin - 60 to 180 mg.
Santonin toxicity causes headache, vomiting, diarrhoea, fainting, lock jaw, coldness of skin, slowing of the heart and pulse rate, dark yellow urine, tremors and some times skin rash. Santonin and chauhar could be sometimes fatal.
Srotogamitva :
Dosha : Vataghna, kaphaghna, pittavardhak.
Dhatu : Majja, rakta (liver), shukra (aphrodisiac), rasa, meda.
Mala : Purisha (anthelmintic), mutra (diuretic).
Organ : Intestine.

(92) CHHATRAK
Psolliota campestris

Kula : Chhatrak kula.
Family : Agaricaceae.
Latin name : Psolliota = plants mostly roughened; compestris = of the fields, of the plains or Agaricus albus.
English name : Mushroom , Touchwood.

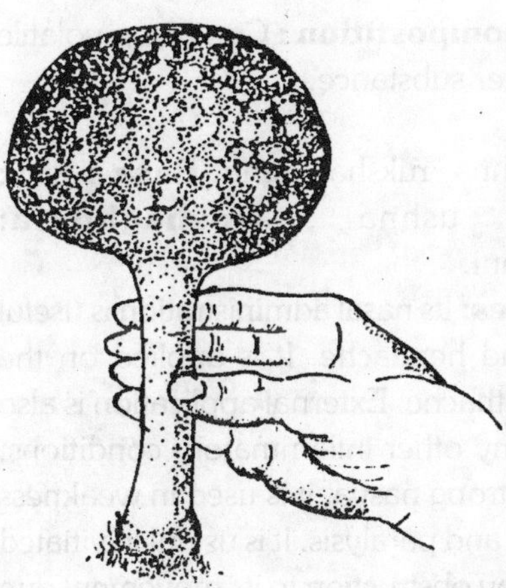

Sanskrit names : Sansvedajashak, Bhumichhatra, Shileendhrak.
Botanical Description : The herb resembles an umbrella. Non poisonous variety is used as a vegetable. It is known as dog's umbrella.
There are 200 consumable varieties. They are nutritious and spermatogenic.
Varieties : There are many varieties which are broadly classified into two - 1) Non poisonous and 2) Poisonous.
The non poisonous variety is not black in colour, is very fragile, breaks easily and has an unclear ring below the umbrella. The poisonous variety is foul smelling, has many colours and also has a big ring below the umbrella.
Habitat : Hilly areas of Punjab; Kashmir etc. It is cultivated like vegetables in USA, Germany, France and East Asia.
Properties:
Guna : guru, singdha; **Rasa :** madhur; **Vipak :** madhur; **Veerya:** sheeta; **Dosha:** vata pittashamak and kaphavardhak.
Uses : Used as an aphrodisiac in seminal debility and rejuvenating in pthisis, emaciation and rhinitis (along with milk).
Dose : Panchang - 3 to 6 gms.
Srotogmitva :
Dosha : Vatapittaghna, kaphavardhak.
Dhatu : Shukra, mansa, meda (rejuvenating).
References -
'सर्पच्छत्रकवर्ज्यांस्तु बहव्योऽन्याश्छत्रजातयः ।
शीताः पीनसर्कत्र्यश्च मधुरा गुर्व्य एव च ।।' (च. सू. २७)

(93) CHHIKKIKA
Centipeda minima

Kula : Bhringaraj kula.
Gana : Shirovirechaneeya (C.) Mustadi (S.)
Family : Compositeae.
Latin name : Centipeda = cent = 100, peda = foot; minima = small.
English name : Sneeze wart.
Sanskrit names : Chhikkika, Tikshna, Ghrandukhahda, Chhikkani, Kashvakrut, Nakachhikkani, Mecheta.
Botanical Description : Annual shrub of 10 - 15 cm. height. Stalk shows branches and subbranches with bristly hairs. Branches - spreading on the ground. Leaves - oval, 1 to 2.5 cm. long with soft bristly hairs. Flowers - small, stalkless, yellow, in a cluster. Fruits - with small hairs; the shrub grows at the end of the winter.

Rasa (as Dhatu) suggests ceaseless motion for 24 hours. It never stops. If it stops it is not Rasa.

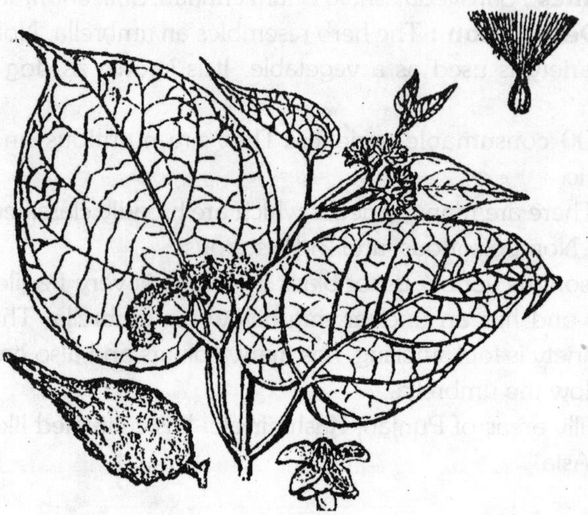

Chemical compostition : Contains a volatile oil and a bitter substance.

Properties:

Guna : tikshna, ruksha, laghu; **Rasa :** katu; **Veerya :** ushna ; **Doshaghnata:** kaphavataghni.

External uses: Its nasal administration is useful in rhinitis and headache. It is applied on the cheeks in toothache. External application is also useful in many other inflammatory conditions. Since it is a strong nasya, it is used in weakness of the nerves and paralysis. It is useful in vitiated vata caused by obstruction to its movement due to kapha.

Internal uses : Since it is a stomachic, appetizer and anthelminic, it is useful in anorexia, reduced appetite and intestinal worms. Also useful in blood disorders, hepatosplenomegaly, skin diseases, impotence due to obesity.

Parts used : Seeds.

Dose: 1 to 3 gms.

Srotogamitva :

Dosha : Vataghna , kaphaghna.

Dhatu : Rakta (hepatosplenmegaly).

Mala : Purisha (anthelmintic).

Organ : Nose.

References -

'छिक्कनी क्षवकृत्तीक्ष्णा छिक्किका घ्राणदु:खदा । छिक्कनी कटुका रुच्या तीक्ष्णोष्णा वह्निपित्तकृत् । वातरक्तहरी कुष्ठकृमिवातकफापहा ।।' (भा. प्र.)

'छिक्किका छिक्कपत्रा च नासासंवेदनस्तथा । क्षवक: क्षुरकस्तीक्ष्ण: क्रूर उद्वेजनस्तथा ।
क्षुधातिजननो राजक्षवको क्षुद्बिबोधन: । क्षवक: कटुक: पाके रसे रुच्यग्निपित्तकृत् ।।
तीक्ष्णोष्ण: कफवातास्रदृक्कुष्ठकृमिजिल्लघु: ।।' (कै. नि.)

(94) JAYANTI

Sesbania egyptica

Kula : Shimbi kula.

Family : Leguminoseae.

Latin name : Sesbania = of Sesban; egyptica = of Egypt.

Sanskrit names : Harita, Jaya, Vijaya, Sukshmamoola, Vikranta, Aparajita, Sheetala, Vatala, Galgandahari.

Botanical Description : This plant belongs to shimbi kula. The tree grows to a height of 2-3 mtrs.

Leaves resemble the leaves of Tamarindus indica. One leaf has 20-24 leaflets which have a bitter taste. The legume contains 20 to 25 small seeds.

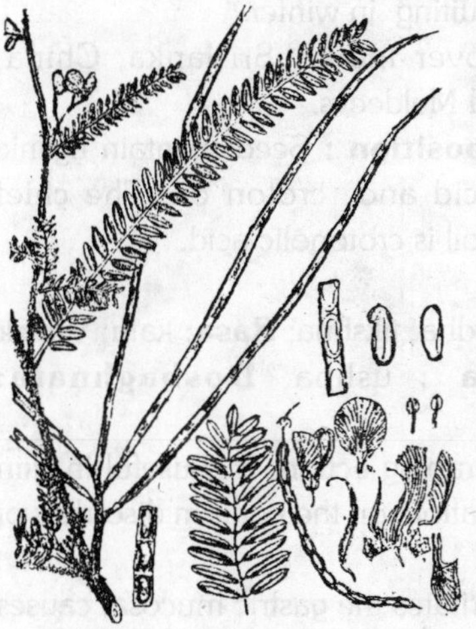

Habitat : Originally from Africa, but now available in south India, Sri lanka and Sayam.

Properties:

Guna : laghu ruksha; **Rasa:** katu, tikta; **Vipak :** katu; **Veerya :** ushna; **Prabhav :** antidotal, antipyretic; **Dosha :** kaphapittashamak, tridoshaghna.

External uses : Its application is useful as an analgesic and for wound cleansing. Also useful in hairfall and greying of hair. (It is said that it reduces scorpion poisioning by holding the fresh root in hand.)

Internal uses: Seeds are used in loss of appetite and diarrhoea. A vegetable recipe prepared from its leaves is useful in chronic rhinitis. In leucoderma, root is used along with milk. Flowers mixed with jaggery and rice given for three days after menstruation acts as a contraceptive. But the seeds are emmenagogue. To prevent small pox, 20 - 25 seeds are crushed and given with cow's ghee.

Parts used: Root, bark, leaves and flowers.

Dose: Powder - 2 to 6 gms.; juice - 10 to 20 gms.; decoction - 50 to 100 gms. The juice of the leaves is used in the purification processes of many metals.

Srotogamitva:

Dosha: Pittakaphaghna, tridoshahara.

Dhatu: Rakta, meda (leucoderma), rasa (menstruation).

Mala: Mutra (dysuria).

Organ: Uterus (contraceptive).

References -

'बलामोटा सूक्ष्ममूला जयन्ती विजया जया । हरिता चैव विज्ञेया सूक्ष्मपत्त्रापराजिता ।।
बलामोटा कटुस्तिक्ता लघुः पित्तकफापहा । मूत्रकृच्छ्रं विषं हन्ति विवादे कुरुतेजयम् ।।' (कै. नि.)
'श्वेतजयंतीमूलं पीतं पिष्टञ्च पयसैव । शिवत्रं निहन्ति नियतं रविवारे वैद्यनाथाज्ञा ।।' (भै. र.)

(95) JAYAPAL
Croton tiglium

Kula : Eranda kula.

Family : Euphorbiaceae.

Latin name : Croton = kroton - a tick; tiglium = a small beam.

English name : Kroton.

Sanskrit names : Dantibeeja, Rechak, Sarak, Tittiriphal, Maladravi, Beejarechani, Kumbhibeeja, Shodhani, Ghantabeeja.

Botanical Description : This is an evergreen small tree. Leaves - 5 to 10 cm. long, slimmy, oblong,

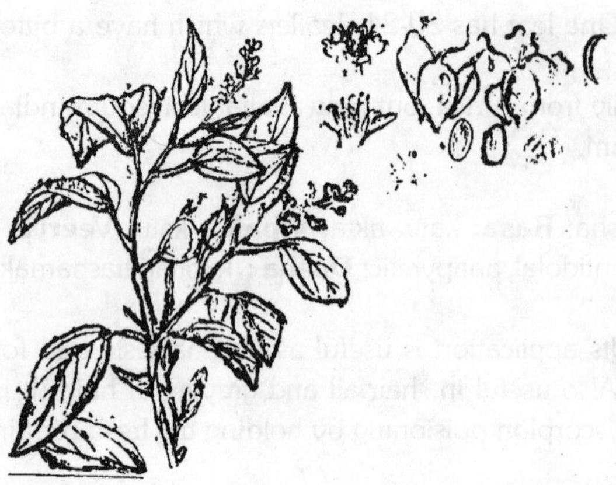

with 3 - 5 venis. Flowers - unisexual, greenish yellow, in clusters. Fruits - 2 -5 cm. long, oval but triangular. Seeds - brown in colour. Flowering occurs in summer and fruiting in winter.

Habitat : All over India , Sri lanka, China, Lakshadeepa and Maldeevs.

Chemical composition : Seeds contain tiglinic acid, crotonic acid and croton oil. The chief ingredient of the oil is crotonolic acid.

Properties:

Guna: guru, singdha, tikshna; **Rasa:** katu; **Vipak** : katu; **Veerya** : ushna; **Doshaghnata:** kaphavatahara.

External uses: It is an irritant on local application and has a scraping action. It is useful in skin diseases and hairfall (seeds are used). It is also used for local application on the penis in disorders of erection.

Internal uses : It is an appetizer, purgative and anthelmintic. It irritates the gastric mucosa, causes griping pain, inflammation of the intestinal mucosa and results in diarrhoea. Therefore it is used to reduce the water content of the blood in many conditions. It is also used in reduced appetite, chornic constipation, intestinal worms, ascites, intracranial haemorrhage and anasarca. Seeds triturated in lemon juice are used as eye drops in snake poisoning.

Dose: Seeds - 30 to 60 mg.; oil - 0.5 to 1 drop.

Antidote for toxicity : Drugs of madhur rasa and sheeta veerya like milk, cow's ghee, butter milk, lemon juice etc.

Purification of seeds : The rind of the seeds is removed and then boiled in cow's milk for 1-2 hours. The seeds are then washed with hot water and triturated with lemon juice. Lastly, they are dried in sunshine and preserved for use.

References -

'जयपालो दन्तिबीजं विख्यातं तिन्तिडीफलम् । जयपालो गुरुस्तीक्ष्णो रेची पित्तकफापहा ।।' (भा. प्र.)

'जेपालः कटुरुष्णश्च कृमिहारी विरेचनः । दीपनः कफवातघ्नो जलोदरविनाशनः ।।' (रा. नि.)

'जयपालभवां मज्जां भावयेन्निम्बुकद्रवैः । एकविंशतिवेलं तु ततो वर्त्ति प्रकल्पयेत् ।।'

'मनुष्यलालया घृष्ट्वा ततो नेत्रे तयाऽञ्जयेत् । सर्पदष्टविषं जित्वा संजीवयति मानवम् ।।' (शा.)

'नागदन्ती कटुस्तिक्ता रूक्षा वातकफापहा । मेधाकृद् विषदोषघ्नी पाचनी शुभदायिनी ।।
गुल्मशूलोदरव्याधिकण्ठदोषनिकृन्तनी ।' (रा. नि.)

(96) JATI
Jasminum grandiflorum

Kula : Parijatak kula.

Gana : Kushthaghna.

Family : Oleaceae.

Latin name: Jasminum = from the original Arabic name - yasmin; grandiflorum = large flowers.

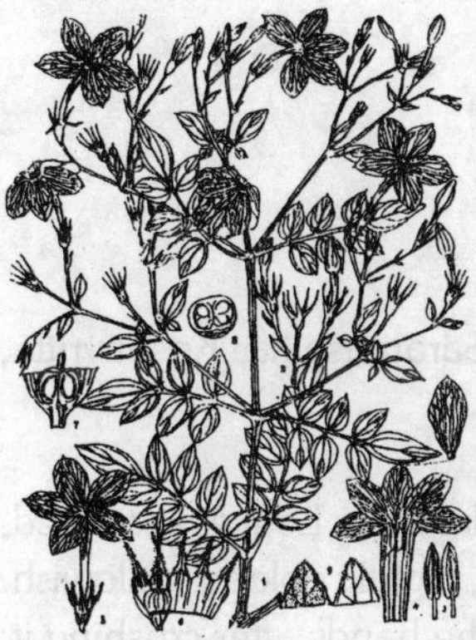

English name : Spainsh Jasmine.
Sanskrit names : Jatik, Manognya, Sumana, Rajputri, Priyamvada, Malati, Hrudyagandha, Chetika, Telbhavini.
Botanical Description : This is a slender creeper, bearing hard and angular branches. Leaves - compound with three paired foliates ending with a single leaf at the tip. Flowers - white, fragrant, with five petals. Flowering occurs in rainy season.
Varities : Two 1) white and 2) yellow (swarna).
Habitat : Found all over India.
Chemical composition : Salicylic acid and jasminine alkaloid.
Properties:
Guna : laghu, singdha, mridu; **Rasa:** tikta, kashaya; **Vipak :** katu ; **Veerya** : ushna; **Dosha** : tridoshaghni.
External uses : The leaves are chewed for oral hygiene. It relieves stomatitis and strengthens teeth and gums. Flowers are aphrodisiac. Leaves and roots are used for cleaning and healing wounds. Decoction is used as gargles for stomatitis. Local application of root or oil is useful in paralysis, bell's palsy etc. Roots are applied on the penis in loss of libido. Also useful in itching and skin diseases.
Ear conditions - leaves are boiled in oil which is then used as ear drops.
Eye conditions : leaves and flowers are tied on the eyes or their juice is used as eye drops.
In urinary disorders, the flowers or leaves are applied locally on the hypogastric region for relieving cystitis and retention of urine.
Internal uses: Blood diseases, dysuria, amenorrhoea, impotence, skin diseases and poisoning.
Parts used: Leaves, root, flowers.
Dose : Decoction 50 to 100 ml.; powder - 1 to 3gms.
Formulations: Jatyadi taila, ghee or varti (thread).
Srotogamitva :
Dosha : Tridoshaghni.
Dhatu : Shukra (aphrodisiac), rakta (bleeding disorders), rasa (menstrual disorders).
Mala : Mutra.
References -
'जातिर्जाती च सुमना मालती राजपुत्रिका । चेतिका हृद्यगंधा च सा पीता स्वर्णजातिका ।।
जातीयुगं तिक्तमुष्णं तुवरं लघु दोषजित् । शिरोऽक्षिमुखदन्तार्तिविषकुष्ठव्रणास्त्रजित् ।।' (भा. प्र.)
'मालती तुवरातिक्ताकटूष्णादोषनाशिनी । शिरोक्षिमुखदन्तार्त्तिविषकुष्ठव्रणास्त्रजित् ।।' (कै. नि.)
'मुखपाके सिरावेधः शिरः कायविरेचनम् । कार्यञ्च बहुधा नित्यंजातीपत्रस्य चर्वणम् ।। (भा. प्र.)
'जातीपत्ररसैस्तैलं विपक्वं पूतिकर्णजित् ।' (च. द.)

The etymological interpretation of the names of the plant is both enlightening and entertaining. But how many individuals are expert in it?

(97) JEEMUT
Luffa echinata Roxb.

Kula : Koshataki kula.
Family : Cucurbitaceae.
Latin name : Luffa = Malayan name; echinata = sea urchin like.
Sanskrit names : Jeemutaka, Kantaphala, Ghora, Karkati, Deodali, Saramushika, Koshavritta, Akhuvishaha, Romashpatrika.
Varieties : 1) White 2) red and 3) yellow.
Botanical Description : This is a slender creeper with thin and pentangular stalk. Leaves - serrated, round shaped, 2.5 to 5 cm. long. Flowers - small, white. Fruits - spiny, netted, slightly oblong, yellowish. Seeds - small, panchang is very bitter to taste. Even repeated washing of the hands after crushing it, does not remove the bitterness.
Habitat : North-west India, East Bengal.
Properties:
Guna : laghu, ruksha, tikshna; **Rasa :** katu, tikta; **Vipak :** katu; **Veerya :** ushna; **Dosha:** tridoshahara, kaphapittahara.
External uses : Juice is applied on wounds. A rectal suppository made from its fruits is used in piles. Juice in the form of nasya (nasal drops) is used in jaundice, epilepsy and sinusitis. Intense rhinorrhoea is observed after nasal administration of the juice.
Internal uses : Large dose is emetic whereas a small dose is appetizer, liver stimulant and cholagogue. Therefore it is useful in loss of appetite, hepatosplenomegaly, jaundice and piles. It is also useful in blood disorders, oedema, cough, asthma, hiccups, dysuria, dysmenorrhoea, obstructed labour and skin diseases.
Srotogamitva :
Dosha : Tridoshahara, specially kaphahara, pittasarak.
Dhatu : Rakta (jaundice, liver spleen enlargement), majja (epilepsy), rasa (dysmenorrhoea, fever).
Mala : Mutra (dysuria), pruisha.
Organ : Head, uterus, obstructed labour, stomach (emetic).
References -
'जीमूतकं त्रिदोषघ्नं यथास्वौषधकल्पितम् । प्रयोक्तव्यं ज्वरश्वासहिक्काद्येष्वामयेषु च ।।' (च. क. २)
'देवदाली तु तिक्तोष्णा कटुः पाण्डुकफापहा । दुर्नामश्वासकासघ्नी कामलाशोथनाशिनी ।।' (रा. नि.)
'देवदाली रसे पाके तिक्ता तीक्ष्णा विषापहा । वामनी हन्ति गुदजकफशोफामकामलाः ।।
ज्वरकासारुचिश्वासहिध्मापाण्डुक्षयकृमीन् ।' (के.)

(98) JEEVANTI
Leptadenia reticulata

Kula : Arka kula.
Gana : Jeevaneeya, Madhur, Kakolyadi.
Family : Asclepiadaceae.

Latin name : Leptadenia = lepto = slender, thin, small, fine; reticulata = finely netted; reticulum = a small net.
Sanskrit names : Jeevanti, Payaswini, Bhadra, Mangalya, Yashskari, Shrungati, Kanjika, Shashibeeja, Pingala.
Botanical Description : This slender creeper grows in rainy season. Leaves are heart shaped, white and fleshy. Flowers are bluish, yellowish-green. Legumes are like horns, 5 - 10 cm. in length. Raw legumes are used as vegetables and are superior in vegetables.
Types : Jeevanti is of two types -1) white latex - jeevanti; and 2) yellow latex - swarna jeevanti.
Habitat : Plenty in west and south India.
Properties :
Guna: laghu, singdha, madhur; **Rasa :** madhur; **Veerya :** sheeta. With these properties, jeevanti is useful in all the three doshas. It is especially vatapittanashak.
External uses: It is used for application as an ointment in allergy due to pitta.
Internal uses: Jeevanti soothes the digestive system and is used in constipation and colitis. It is a cardiotonic and cures bleeding disorders. It is also used in bronchitis as an expectorant. It is an aphrodisiac and improves seminal quality through its specific action on the reproductive organs. It is also used in spermatorrhoea. Since it is a diuretic, it is used in dysuria, burning micturition and pyuria. Useful in fever, burning, pthisis and also in defective eyesight.
Dose: Root powder : 1 to 3 gms.; decoction - 50 to 100 ml.
Formulations: Jeevantyadi ghrit, Jeevantyadi taila.
Srotogamitva :
Dosha : All three doshas specially vata-pittanashak.
Dhatu : Rakta (pittashamak), shukra (aphrodisiac).
Mala : Mutra (diuretic), purisha (constipative).
Organ : Eyes (improves eyesight).
References -
'जीवन्ती शीतला स्वादु:स्निग्धा दोषत्रयापहा । रसायनी बलकरी चक्षुष्या ग्राहिणी लघुः ।।' (भा. प्र.)
'जीवन्ती मधुरा शीता रक्तपित्तानिलापहा । क्षयदाहज्वरान् हन्ति कफवीर्यविवर्धनी ।।' (रा. नि.)
'जीवन्ती मधुरा शीता सुस्निग्धा ग्राहिणी लघुः ।
चक्षुष्या सर्वदोषघ्नी बल्या वृष्या रसायनी ।।' (कै. नि.)
'चक्षुष्या सर्वदोषघ्नी जीवन्ती मधुरा हिमा । शाकानां प्रवरा' (ध. नि.)
'चक्षुष्या सर्वदोषघ्नी जीवन्ती समुदाहता ।' (सु. सू. ४६)
'जीवन्तीशाकं शाकानाम् श्रेष्ठा ।' (च. सू. २५)

(99) JUPHA
Hyssopus officinalis Linn.

Kula : Tulasi kula. (Jupha is a Persian and Arabic name.)
Family : Labiateae.
Latin name : Hyssopus = a plant of Dioscoridus; hyssop = culinary herb (culina = kitchen); officinalis = available in market.

Ayurveda gives importance to focusing thought on the patient and not on the disease. It considers "patient" and not the disease. (Treat the patient and not the disease.)

Botanical Description : This scented shrub spreads on the land. Each knob of branches bears a yellow flower.
Habitat : Iran, Sayam, Punjab, Kashmir.
Chemical composition : Tannin, resin, fat, starch, slimy substance and a greenish yellow oil 25% to 50%.
Properties :
Guna: laghu, ruksha, tikshna; **Rasa :** tikta, katu; **Vipak :** katu; **Veerya :** ushna ; **Dosha:** kaphavatashamak, pittasarak.
External uses : Lekhan and anti-inflammatory.
Internal uses : Since it is carminative, hepatostimulant, cholagogue and anthelmintic, it is useful in constipation, ascites, hepatosplenomegaly and intestinal worms.
Respiratory system : Being an expectorant it is used in rhinitis, cough, asthma and pneumonitis.
Srotogamitva :
Dosha : Kaphaghna, vataghna, pittasarak.
Dhatu : Rakta (hepatosplenomegaly).
Mala : Purisha (cholagogue, laxative, anthelmintic).
Organ : Respiratory system (expectorant, pneumonitis etc.)

(100) ZANDU

Tagetus erecta Linn.

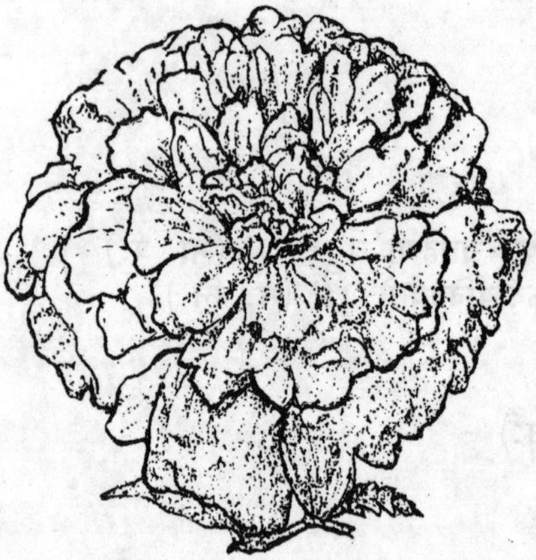

Kula : Bhringaraj kula.
Family : Compositeae.
Latin name : Tagetus = marigold, tages = an Etruscan God; erecta = straight.
Sanskrit names : Zandu, Salpushpa, Zenduk.
Botanical Description : This is a small plant. Its stalk and branches are angular and bear bristle hairs. Leaves - regularly placed, foliated and with hairs. Flowers - dark yellow. Seeds - black and oblong. Flowering - in October (around Dassera). Many varieties are found.
Habitat : Though imported from Mexico, it is found all over India.
Properties :
Guna : laghu, ruksha; **Rasa:** tikta, kashaya; **Veerya :** sheeta; **Dosha :** kaphapittashamak. It has a specific activity on the rakta dhatu.
External uses : Its hemostatic and antiinflammatory properties are helpful in injury and ulcers. Leaves and flowers are used for local application.
Internal uses : Since it is a blood purifier and hemostatic it is useful in blood disorders, bleeding diathesis, bleeding piles and menorrhagia. Flowers fried in ghee are given orally.
Parts used : Flowers or leaf juice.

Dose : Juice 10 to 20 gms.
Srotogamitva :
Dosha : Kaphapittaghna.
Dhatu : Rakta (hemostatic), in bleeding diathesis - specially in reducing kaphapitta from the blood.
References -
झण्डुः कटुकषाया स्यात् ज्वरभूतग्रहापहा ।। (रा. नि.)

(101) TAMALPATRA
Cinnamomum tamal Iners.

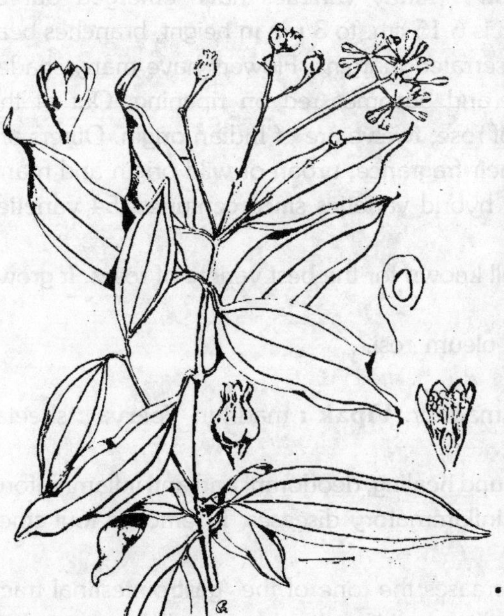

Kula : Karpur kula.
Family : Lauraceae.
Latin name : Cinnamomum = (Cinamon); tamal = from the name tamal.
English name : Leaf of cinamon tree.
Sanskrit names : Tamalpatra, Patra, Palash, Chhandan, Ram, Tapasaj, Gopan, Anshuk, Tejpatram.
Botanical Description : This is a strong and medium high tree. Branches - round, evergreen, bears leaves throughout the year and fragrant. Bark - thin, tough, rough with folds. Bark is called tejapatra or patraj.
Habitat : At the foot hills of Himalayas.
Properties: Ushna, laghu,appetizer, diaphoretic, diuretic, vataghna and stimulant. **Dosha** : kaphaghna.
Uses :
Alimentary system : Indigestion , loss of appetite, colic and diarrhoea.
Reproductive system : It is used in uterine inertia. It also helps fertilization and overcomes habitual abortion. It is useful in postpartum amenorrhoea. Bark decoction is used in gonorrhoea.
Srotogamitva :
Dosha : Vatakaphaghna.
Dhatu : Rasa (emmenagogue).
Mala : Sweda (diaphoretic), mutra (diuretic), purisha.
Organ : Uterus (inertia).

Keeping the fundamental of Ayurveda intact, there is a lot of scope for development of this science. But this demands a forward-looking intelligence.

(102) TARUNI
Rosa centifolia

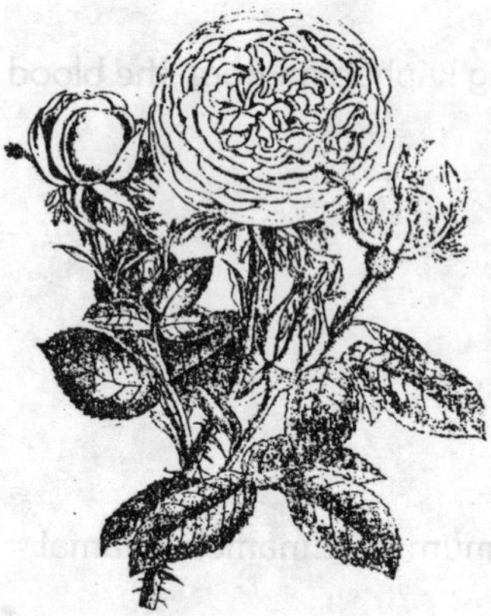

Kula : Taruni kula.
Family : Rosaceae.
Latin name : Rosa = Latin name, a root word for colour in many languages; centifolia = hundred petals.
English name : Rose.
Sanskrit name : Shatapatri, Karnika, Charukeshara, Ramtarani, Bhrungeshta, Saha, Gandhaddhya, Bhrungavallabha.
Botanical Description : Many varieties have emerged out of hybridization. The shrub is 6.15 cm. to 3 mt. in height, branches bear thorns. Leaves - have serrated margins. Flowers have many shades of colours. Fruit - oval and becomes red on ripening. Out of the innumerable varieties of rose, twelve are of Indian origin. Others are of foreign origin. They are classified on the basis of their fragrance, urban or wild origin and many other factors. Due to innumerable attempts to create hybrid varieties since centuries, 54 varieties of roses are available at present.
Habitat : In India, Kashmir, Garhwal, Santhal are well known for the best variety of roses. It grows at a height of 1000 mtrs. from sea level.
Chemical composition : It contains an oil called oleum rosi.
Properties:
Guna : laghu, singdha; **Rasa** : tikta, katu, kashaya, madhur; **Vipak** : madhur; **Veerya** : sheeta; **Prabhav** : heart tonic; **Dosha** : tridoshaghna.
External uses : It improves complexion and acts as wound healing, deodorant and anti inflammatory. It is therefore useful in disorders of complexion and inflammatory diseases. It removes foul smell of sweat.
Internal uses : It acts as a brain tonic as well as increases the tone of the gastrointestinal tract. It is a hepatoprotective and is useful in all digestive disorders like diarrhoea and dysentery. It is useful in diseases of the heart, bleeding disorders and other blood diseases. It is useful in fever and burning sensation. Rose buds increase the bulk of solid excreta. It is also useful in impotency.
Dose : Powder - 1 to 3 gms.; gulkanda 10 to 20 gms.; arka 20 to 40 gms.
Srotogamitva :
Dosha : Tridoshaghna.
Dhatu : Shukra, majja, rakta, raktamansa.
Mala : Sweda (deodorant), purisha.
References -
शतपत्री तरुण्युक्ता कर्णिका चारुकेशरा । महाकुमारी गन्धाढ्या लाक्षा वृष्यातिमंजुला ।।
शतपत्री हिमा हृद्या ग्राहिणी शुक्रला लघुः । दोषत्रयास्त्रजिद्वर्ण्या कट्वी तिक्ता च पाचनी ।।' (भा. प्र.)

(103) TAGAR

Valerian wallichi Dc.

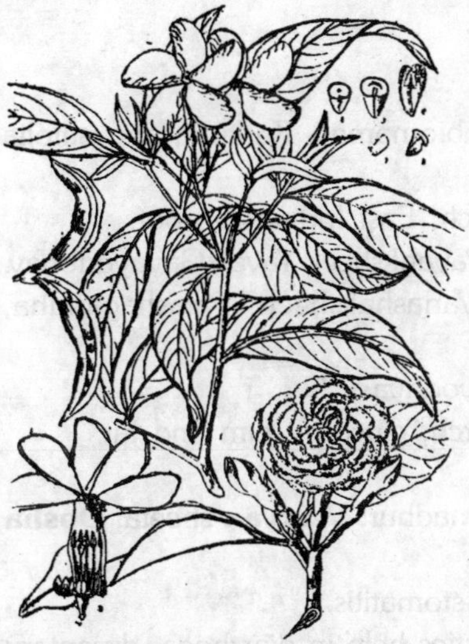

Kula : Jatamansi kula.

Gana : Sheetapradhaman, Tiktaskandha, Eladi gana.

Family : Valerianaceae.

Latin name : Valerian = (ward, spike) Lat. to be strong (Valerius, who drove away the Roman kings, first used it.); wallichi = after Dr. Wallich.

Sanskrit names : Vakra, Kutil, Vinamra, Kunchit, Shatha, Nihusha, Dandahasta, Pinditagarak, Parthiv.

English name : Indian valerian.

Botanical Description : This is a long living tree. Trunk - small. Leaves - broad, with tender hair, stalk - 5 to 7 cm. long with hair. Flowers - white or pink, flowering occurs in July. Fruiting - in September, October. Fruits also have hair on them. Root - 1.25 to 2.5 cm. long, fragile, bent and have a strong odour.

Varieties : In Nighantu, two varieties are described - 1) Tagar and 2) Pindatagar. The latter variety is less fragrant and slightly round.

Habitat : France, Italy, Africa, Sayam, U. A. E., Persia, India (Kashmir to Bhutan) at the height of 1.5 to 3 thousand mtrs.

Chemical composition : Root contains volatile oil, yellow and bitter substances and a sweet chemical.

Properties:

Guna: laghu, snigdha, sara; **Rasa :** tikta, katu; **Veerya :** ushna; **Dosha :** tridoshahara.

External uses : It is used for local application in wound healing, fractures and rheumatoid arthritis. Decoction helps in wound healing and also as an analgesic.

Internal uses : It is mainly useful in Bell's palsy, hemiplegia, epilepsy, osteoarthritis, rheumatoid arthritis and gout. It reduces pain, convulsions and nourishes the central nervous system. Since it is an appetizer, digestive, antispasmodic, laxative and hepatostimulant, it is useful in loss of appetite, colic, flatulance, hepatomegaly , jaundice, ascites, splenomegaly etc. It is cardiostimulant, but in large doses it causes hypotension. It is also useful in cough, asthma, retention of urine, impotency and dysmenorrhoea.

Also useful in debility, poisoning, skin disorders, blood disorders and chronic fever.

Dose : Root powder - 1 to 3 gms.

Overdose causes fainting, hiccups and vomiting. Antidote - dried black grapes.

References -

'तगरं स्यात् कषायोष्णं स्निग्धं दोषत्रयप्रणुत् । दृक् शीर्षविषदोषघ्नं भूतापस्मारनाशनम् ।।' (ध. नि.)
'तगरं कटुकं तिक्तं कटुपाकरसं लघु । स्निग्धोष्ण तुवरं भृतमदापस्मारनाशनम् ।।
विषचक्षुः शिरोरोगरक्तदोषामयापहम् ।' (कै. नि.)
'कालानुसार्यं तगरं कुटिलं नहुषं नतम् । अपरं पिण्डतगरं दण्डहस्तं च बर्हिणम् ।।
तगरद्वयमुष्णं स्यात् स्वादु स्निग्धं लघु स्मृतम् । विषापस्मारशूलाक्षिरोगदोषत्रयापहम् ।।' (भा. प्र.)

Ayurveda more than on substances, is based on their antecedant philosophy. Ayurveda is in the tradition of tatwas. It is not dependent on only dravyas.

(104) TAVAKSHEERAM

Curcuma angustifolia Roxb.

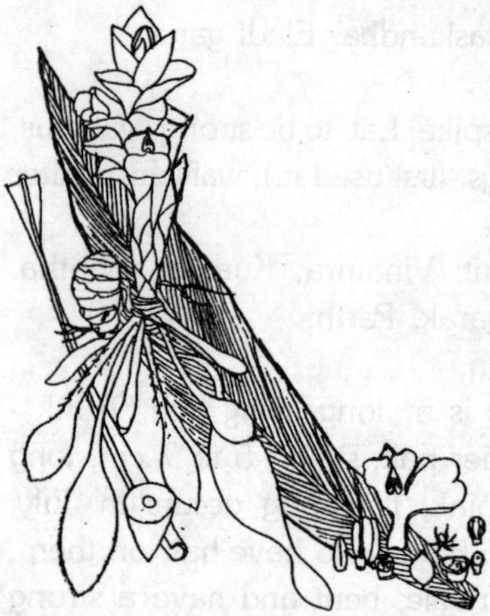

Kula : Haridra kula.

Family : Scitaminaceae.

Latin name : Curcuma = Arabic name - Kurkum; angustifolia = having narrow leaves.

English name : Curcuma starch, East Indian Araroot.

Sanskrit names : Tavaksheer, Payahksheer, Yavaj, Gavayodbhav, Vanshya, Godhumsambhuta, Vanashaksheeri, Palashagandha, Parthivi.

Habitat : Himalayas, Bihar, Ayodhya.

Chemical composition : Starch, glucose, gum and fat.

Properties :

Guna : laghu, singdha; **Rasa** : madhur; **Veerya** : sheeta; **Dosha** : vatapittashamak.

External uses : It is used for local application with honey in stomatitis.

Internal uses : Its unctuous, carminative and astringent properties help in diarrhoea, dysentery and flatulance. It is also a cardiotonic, aphrodisiac and diuretic.

Dose: Tuber powder - 10 to 20 gms. with porridge is useful in reducing intestinal inflammation.

Srotogamitva :

Dosha : Vataghna, pittaghna.

Dhatu : Rakta (bleeding disorders), shukra (aphrodisiac).

Mala : Mutra (diuretic) , purisha (constipative).

(105) TAMRAPARNA

Saraca indica Linn.

Kula : Shimbi kula.

Gana : Kashay, Vedanasthapan (C.); Lodhradi (S.)

Family : Leguminoseae.

Latin name : Saraca = after Dr. Sarasin - French physician, indica = of India.

English name : Ashoka tree.

Sanskrit names : Ashok, Hemapushpa, Vanjul, Tamrapallav, Kankeli,Pindapushpa, Gandhapushpa, Nat, Ashogham.

Botanical Description : The tree is 8 to 10 mtrs.high and leaves resemble mango leaves. Tender leaves are red and soft. Flowers - grow in clusters, intially yellowish brown but then turn to red and are scented. Legumes - 7 to 25 cms. long, 4 to 5 cm. broad, flat and containing 4 to 8 oblong, flat seeds. Flowering occurs in spring and fruiting in autumn.

Habitat : Bengal , south India, Burma.

Chemical composition : Bark contains metoxylene and a small amount of iron.

Properties:

Guna : laghu, ruksha; **Rasa** : kashaya, tikta; **Vipak:** katu; **Veerya** : sheeta; **Doshaghnata** : kaphapittaghna.

External uses : Local application is done in pain and poisoning.

Internal uses : Its astringent property is useful in diarrhoea, dysentery, intestinal worms, thirst etc.

Circulatory system : (Flowers and trunk) Menorrhagia, dysmenorrhoea, bleeding diathesis, oedema and burning due to inflammation. Also useful in dysuria and urinary calculi. It is specially useful in uterine inertia, pain, menorrhagia and leucorrhoea.

Dose : Milk boiled with its bark is given. Bark decoction - 10 to 20 gms.; seed powder - 1 to 3 gms.; flower powder - 1 to 3 gms.

Formulations : Ashokarishta.

Two varieties : True and false. False variety is decorative and not of medicinal use.

Srotogamitva :

Dosha : Kaphapittaghna.

Dhatu : Raktagami (bleeding disorders, menorrhagia, burning sensation).

Mala : Mutra (dysuria), purisha (antidiarrhoeal).

Organ : Uterus (menorrhagia, leucorrhoea).

(106) TAALMULI
Asparagus adscendens Roxb.

Kula : Rason kula.

Family : Liliaceae.

Latin name : Asparagus = Gk. asperaso = to rip, the sharp spines on some spp.; adscendens = ascending.

Sanskrit names : Musali, Suvaha, Godhapadi, Hemapushpi, Deerghakandika, Hiranyapushpi, Khalini, Vrushyakanda, Mahavrusha.

Botanical Description : This herb belonging to the shatavari kula is a small plant growing without support and with spikes. Stalk - big, thick and large, does not require support unlike Asparagus racemosus. The stalk is long, large, round, tall and oily. Branches are hollow, greyish, bent downwards but of the ascending type. The entire plant is spread with long, thick and straight spikes which are 1.25 to 1.75 cms. long. The stalks which resemble the leaves are 1.25 to 5 cms in length, round and 6 to 20 in bunches. Root - white, oblong and in bunches, called safed musali.

Varieties : Two 1) white which is described above and 2) black is called talmuli belonging to Amarilidaceae family and known as Curculigo ochioides. This herb is small, leaves 3 to 4 of 15 - 45 cm. length. Flowers - yellow, seeds black and shining.

Habitat : Western Himalayas, Punjab, Gujarat, Maharashtra, Madhya pradesh, Rajasthan.

Chemical composition : It contains starch 43.5 %, resin, astringent and viscous substances.

Properties:

Guna : guru, snigdha; **Rasa** : madhur, tikta ; **Vipak** : madhur; **Veerya** : ushna; **Dosha** :

Vyadhi-pratyaneek-dravyas (dravyas targetted to act on the disease) act on all doshas, dhatus, malas and other constituents of body and that is how their action is completed.

tridoshahara, vatapittashamak.

Internal uses :

Reproductive system : Aphrodisiac, helps in spermatogenesis.

Urinary system : It is a diuretic. It is predominantly used for its rejuvenating, anabolic and tonic properties. It is used in piles, spermatorrhoea and pyuria.

Dose : Tuber powder - 3 to 6 gms.

Formulations: Musali pak, Musalyadiyoga.

Srotogamitva :

Dosha : Tridoshahara, specially vatapittaghna.

Dhatu : Shukra (aphrodisiac), mansa, meda (brimhan), rasayana.

Mala : Mutra (diuretic).

Organ : Colon (piles).

References -

'मुशली मधुरा वृष्या वीर्योष्णआ बृंहणी गुरू । तिक्ता रसायनी हन्ति गुदजान्यनिलस्तथा ।।' (भा. प्र.)

(107) TAAL

Borassus flabellifera Linn.

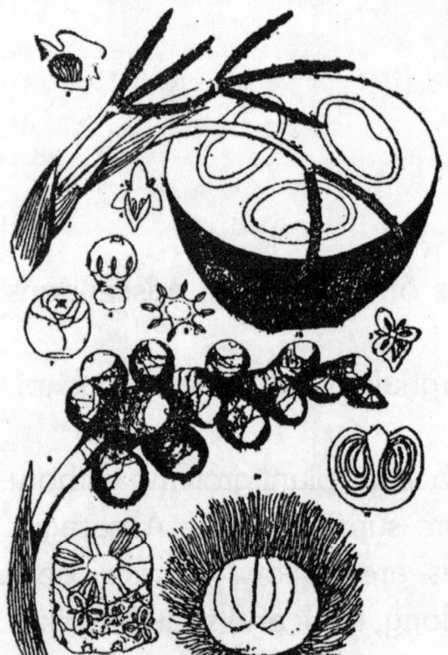

Kula : Narikel kula.

Gana : Madhur, Kashayskandha, Patrasav (C.); Salsaradi, Shirovirechan , Madhurskandha(S.)

Family : Palmae.

Latin name : Borassus = juice which flows from wounded spathe of this plam (spathe = large bract); flabellifera = yielding fan leaves.

Sanskrit names : Patri, Deerghaskandha, Dhvajadruma, Trunraj, Madhurasa, Deerghapadap, Chirayu, Taruraj, Gajabhaksha.

Botanical Description : This tree grows 20 to 21 mtrs. high, without branches. Leaves - 3 to 5 mtrs. long, fan shaped, veins elevated and extended upto the tip of the leaf. Leaf stalk is covered with black pointed spikes on both the sides. Flowers - unisexual. The male plant bears only flowers while the female plant bears fruits. Flower stalk resembles the legume of Cassia fistula and is round and long. Each stalk holds 15 to 20 fruits in a bunch. Fruits - round hard, violet in colour, but turn to a yellowish shade on ripening. The kernel of the fruit is fibrous. The inside of the fruit contains 2/3 part of sweet water. Flowering occurs in spring and fruiting in summer. Juice which flows from the wounded spathe is called tadi.

Properties:

Guna : guru, snigdha; **Rasa :** madhur; **Vipak :** madhur; **Veerya :** sheeta; **Dosha :** vatapittashaman.

External uses: Leaf juice is hemostatic, refrigerant and antiinflammatory. It is therefore used for wound healing. Pulp of the fruit is used in skin diseases.

Internal uses : Leaf juice acts as a brain tonic, antipyretic and refrigerant. It is therefore useful in typhoid fever as a supportive therapy for controlling delirium and supporting cardiac strength. Also useful in bleeding disorders, syphilis and blood diseases.

Raw fruit pulp - useful in constipation , fresh juice - useful in loss of appetite, thirst, debility and anuria. Flower kshar - in splenomegaly and tumor (kshar + jaggary in combination). Ripe fruit - cardiac debility, for spermatogenesis and skin disorders. Sugar obtained from its juice - in debility. Root juice - whooping cough. Flower stalk (decoction) - dysmenorrhoea, amenorrhoea.

Dose : Juice - 10 to 20 ml.; tadi - 50 to 100 ml.; salt 1 to 2 gms.

Srotogamitva :

Dosha : Vataghna , pittaghna.

Dhatu : Majjabalya, rakta, shukra, rasa.

Mala : Purisha, mutra.

Organ : Heart.

References -

'तालस्तु लेख्यपत्रः स्यात्तृणराजो महोन्नतः । पक्वं तालफलं पित्तरक्तष्लेष्मविवर्धनम् ।।
दुर्जरं बहुमूत्रं च तन्द्राभिष्यनदशुक्रदम् । तालमज्जा तु तरुणः किंचिन्मदकरो लघुः ।।
श्लेष्मलो वातपित्तघ्नः सस्नेहो मधुरः सरः । तालजं तरुणं तोयमतीव मदकृन्मतम् ।
अम्लीभूतं तदा तु स्यात् पित्तकृद्वातदोषहृत् ।' (भा. प्र.)
'तालशस्यानि सिद्धानि....। बृंहणस्निग्धशीतानि बल्यानि मधुराणि च ।।' (च. सू. २७)
'फलं स्वादुरसं तेषां तालजं गुरुपित्तजित् । तद्बीजं स्वादुपाकं च मूत्रलं वातपित्तजित् ।।
स्वादुपाकरसान्याहुः रक्तपित्तहरांस्तथा । शुक्रलाननिलघ्नांश्च कफवृद्धिकरानपि ।।' (सु. सू. ४६)
'फलं स्वादुरसं पाके तालजं गुरु पित्तजित् । तद्बीजं स्वादु पाके तु मूलं स्याद्रक्तापर्तताजत् ।। (ध. नि.)
'तालपुष्पभवः क्षारः सगुण्डः प्लीहनाशनः ।' (च. द.)
'उन्मादे समधुः पेयः शुद्धो वा तालशाखजः । रसः..... (च. द.)

(108) TILPARNI
Gynandropsis gynandra

Kula : Varun kula.

Family : Capparidaceae (plants of caper shrub).

Latin name : Gynandropsis - combining both sexes when the stamens are attached to the pistils (as in orchids); gynandra - pentaphylla = five leaved.

Sanskrit names : Ajagandha, Kharpushpa, Ugragandha, Brahmakarma, Pashugandha, Kabari, Suvarchala, Shabarigandha, Tungi.

Botanical Description : This plant is an annual shrub. It smells like goat skin and so called ajagandha or ugragandha (some call it suvarchala or adityabhakta). Leaves - 3 to 7 in number. Flowers - small, white or yellow.

Habitat : Tropical region - India.

Properties:

Guna : ruksha, laghu, tikshna; **Rasa :** katu, **Vipak :** katu; **Veerya :** ushna; **Dosha :** vatakaphanashak

Uses : It is an anticonvulsant, analgesic, anthelmintic, diaphoretic, antipyogenic and stimulant. Leaf juice is used in earache. Decoction of the seeds is used in chronic wound as an antiseptic. External

The plants, trees and forests envolved earlier on the earth than human beings. Nature planned it like that.

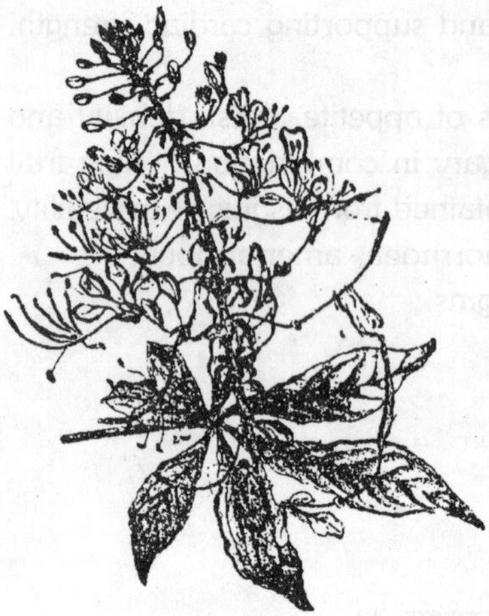

application in elephantiasis results in vesicle formation through which the fluid oozes out thereby reducing the oedema. Seed powder is given in round worms along with sugar followed by castor oil. Overdose causes acidity.

Srotogamitva :

Dosha : Vataghna, kaphaghna, pittavardhak.

Dhatu : Shukra , rasa, meda.

Mala : Purisha, sweda.

Organ : Heart, ear, intestine.

References -

'अजगन्धा कटूष्णा स्याद्वातगुल्मोदरापहा ।
कर्णव्रणार्त्तिशूलघ्नी कृमिघ्नी च ज्वरापहा' ।। (रा. नि.)
'अजगन्धा कटुः पाके रसे रूक्षाग्निदीपनी ।
हृद्या रूच्या लघुस्तीक्ष्णआ दृक्शुक्रकफवातहा ।' (के. नि.)

(109) TINTIDIK

Tamarindus indica

Kula : Shimbi kula.

Upkula : Ceasalpiniaceae.

Family : Leguminosae.

Latin name : Tamarindus = from the Arabic name Tamar-I-Hind; indica = Indian.

English name : Tamarind tree.

Sanskrit Names : Chincha, Chukrika, Chukra, Samlika, Shakchukrika, Amli, Sutittidi, Amla, Tittidika, Sukta, Suktika, Chinchika, Dantashatha, Yamadutika.

Botanical Description : The tree is 15 to 16 mtrs. high. Leaves - compound with many leaflets. Flowers - in bunches, yellow, boat-shaped. Legumes - 7.5 to 15 cms. long. Seeds are called chinchoka.

Habitat : All over India and Burma.

Chemical composition : Fruit pulp contains various acids. Seed contains 63.22 % starch.

Properties:

Guna : guru, ruksha; **Rasa** : amla; **Vipak:** amla; **Veerya** : ushna; **Dosha : Ripe -** tridoshanashak; **Raw -** raktapittakarak Syrup of ripe fruit is pittaghna.

Uses: Local application of leaves and seeds reduces inflammation. Flower pulp is used in conjunctivitis. Ripe fruit - anorexia, thirst, loss of appetite and liver disorders. Fruit - kernel used in abdominal colic, tumor (ingredient of shankha vati). Syrup is used in heart diseases and vomiting associated with fever.

Useful parts : Fruit, seed, leaves, flower.

Srotogamitva :

Dosha : Unripe - vataghna, pittakaphavardhak. Ripe - pittakaphavataghna.

Dhatu : Rakta (reduces burning sensation).

Mala : Unripe - constipative. Ripe - laxative.
References -
'अम्लिकाम्ला गुरुर्वातहरी पित्तकफास्रकृत् । पक्वा तु दीपनी रूक्षा सरोष्णा कफवातनुत् ।।' (भा. प्र.)
'चिञ्चात्यम्ला भवेदामा पक्वा तु मधुराम्लिका । वातघ्नी पित्तदाहास्रकफदोषप्रकोपनी ।।
अम्लिकायाः फलं त्वाममत्यम्लं लघु पित्तकृत् । पक्वंतु मधुराम्लंस्यादृभेदि विष्टम्भवातजित् ।।
पक्वचिंचाफलरसो मधुराम्लो रुचिप्रदः । शोफपाककरो लेपाद् व्रणदोषविनाशनः ।।
चिञ्चापत्रं च शोफघ्नं रक्तदोषव्यथापहम् । तस्य शुष्कत्वचाक्षारः शूलमन्दाग्निनाशन. ।।' (रा. नि.)
'अम्लिकायाः फलं पक्वं तस्मादल्पान्तरं गुणैः ।' (च.)

(110) TINISH
Ougeinia dalbergioides

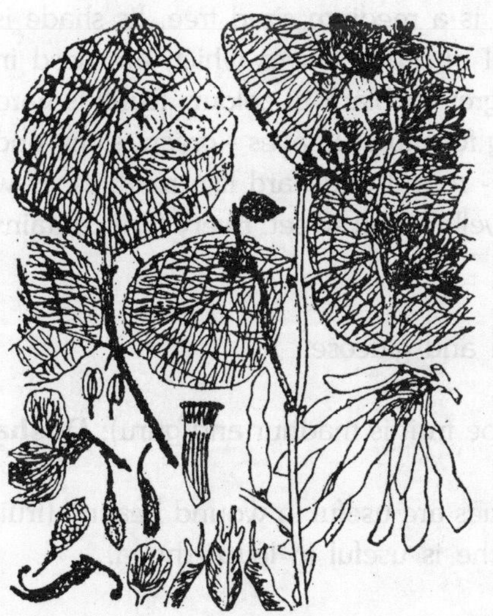

Kula : Shimbi kula.
Gana : Salsaradi.
Family : Leguminosae.
Latin name : Ougeinia = the palace of Ujjain was constructed from the timber of this tree; dalbergioides = after Nicholas Dalberg, a Sweedish Botanist who lived for 110 years (from 1720 to 1830 A. D.)
Sanskrit names : Tinish, Syandan, Rathadru (wood is used to prepare chariots).
Botanical Description : This tree grows up to a height of 7 to 15 mtrs. Bark is whitish, reddish or blackish in colour. On piercing the trunk, a red and granular gum oozes out. The leaves and leaflets resemble those of palash. The last leaf is very big. Flowers are reddish, pink and in bunches. Legumes resemble ground nut containing 2-3 seeds.
Habitat : Ample in the Himalayas.

Properties:
Guna : laghu, ruksha; **Rasa** : kashaya; **Veerya** : sheeta; **Dosha** : kaphapittashamak
Bark and gum are astringent, hemostatic, antidiuretic, antidermatoses and rejuvenating. Therefore they are useful in oedema, leucoderma and other skin diseases. Internally, it is used in diarrhoea, dysentery, blood disorders, diabetes, skin diseases, debility etc.
Dose : Decoction - 10 to 100 ml.; gum - 0.5 to 1 gm.
Srotogamitva :
Dosha : Kaphaghna, pittaghna.
Dhatu : Meda, rakta, raktameda.
Mala : Purisha (diarrhoea, dysentery), mutra (antidiabetic).
References -
तिनिशः श्लेष्मपित्तास्रमेदः कुष्ठप्रमेहजित् ।
तुवरः शिवस्रदाहघ्नो व्रणपांडुकृमिप्रणुत् ।। (भा. प्र.)

Henceforth it is necessary to recognize a plant by only one Sanskrit name. It is the need of the day.

(111) TINDUK

Diospyros tomentosa Roxb.

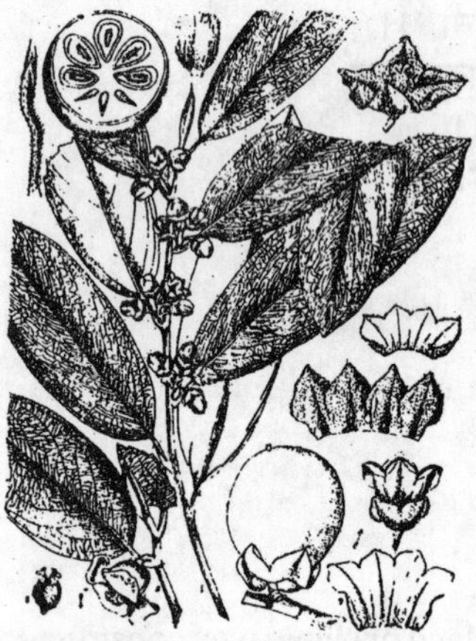

Kula : Tinduk kula.

Gana : Udardaprashaman, Nyagrodhadi.

Family : Ebenaceae (of the ebony wood).

Latin name : Diospyros = fruit of the god; tomentosa = densely covered with short, soft tangled hair.

English name : Gaub tree or Embroypteris.

Sanskrit Names : Tinduk, Neelsar, Atimuktak, Sphurjak, Tushta, Syandan, Raman, Rava, Asitkarak, Gabha, Tendu. (Leaves are used for preparing bidi.)

Botanical Description : This is a medium sized tree. Its shade is thick since the branches are full of green leaves which are used in preparing bidi. Trunk - bark is grey or black in colour. Trunk is hard and black and is used in making furniture. Leaves - green, slimy and long, arranged in two rows. Flowers - white, fragrant. Fruits - round and hard like marbles. Raw fruits are green and astringent to taste while the ripe ones are yellow and sweet. Every fruit contains 6 to 8 kidney-shaped seeds.

Habitat : All over India, Madhya pradesh, Maharashtra.

Chemical compostion : Raw fruit contains tannin, pectin and glucose.

Properties:

Guna : laghu, ruksha; **Rasa** : kashaya; **Veerya** : sheeta; (ripe fruit is madhur and guru); **Dosha** : kapahpittashamak.

External uses : Its hemostatic and antiinflammatary properties are useful in wound healing (fruit or bark powder). Gargling helps in stomatitis, uvulitis. Douche is useful in leucorrhoea.

Internal uses:

Fruit or bark decoction is used in diarrhoea and dysentery. In bleeding disorders and other diseases of the blood, ripe fruit syrup or bark decoction is used. Chewing of tablets prepared from the bark acts as antitussive. Also useful in diabetes, spermatorrhoea, premature ejaculation, menorrhagia, leucorrhoea, hiccups, skin disorders, typhoid fever and poisoning.

Parts used : Bark, raw fruit, ripe fruit, seeds, oil of seeds.

Dose : Decoction 40 to 80 ml.; powder of seeds - 1 to 3 gms.; oil - 10 to 20 gms.

Srotogamitva :

Dosha : Kaphaghna, pittaghna, (raw fruit - vataghna).

Dhatu : Rakta, rasa, shukra.

Mala : Purisha (dysentery, diarrhoea), Mutra (diabetes).

References -

'तिन्दुकः स्फूर्जकः कालस्कन्धश्चासितकारकः ।
स्यादामं तिन्दुकं ग्राहि वातलं शीतलं लघु ।।
पक्वं पित्तप्रमेहास्रश्लेष्मघ्नं मधुरं गुरु ।' (भा. प्र.)

(112) TILAM

Sesamum indicum Linn.

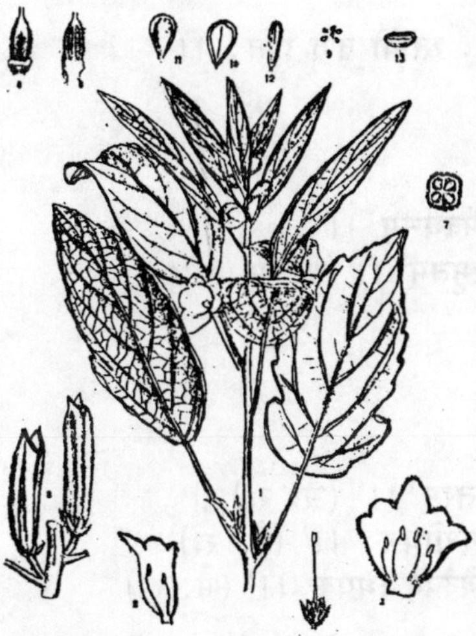

Kula : Tila kula.
Family : Pedalianeae (of the pedalium tribe).
Latin name : Sesamum = from English name; indicum = Indian.
English name : Sesamum.
Sanskrit names : Tila, Homadhanya, Pavitra, Pitrutarpan, Papaghna, Pootadhanya, Jartil, Vanodbhav.
Botanical Description : Annual herb of 1 mt. height. Stalk bears soft, tender hair. Leaves - 7-12 cm. long. Flowers - tender, ciliated, bluish, whitish, brown or yellowish. Seeds - small, white, brownish or black. Depending on the colour of the seeds, it is of three varieties. White seeds yield more oil whereas the black variety is considered to be the best for medicinal use.
Habitat : All over India.
Chemical composition : It contains oil 50 - 60 % and proteins 22 %.

Properties:

Guna: guru, singdha; **Rasa** : madhur; **Uprasa** : kashaya, tikta; **Vipak** : madhur; **Dosha** : vatashamak, kaphapittaprakopak, tridoshaghna (after processing).

Uses : Sesamum is an excellent snehan and analgesic and is very useful for wound healing, dental health, skin and hair. It is very useful in dry skin and bodyache by acting as vatashaman. Its snigdha guna increases the oleation by overcoming dryness (Ch. sutra). In paralysis, oil is used for massaging and also internally. Local application of oil pack in the anal region reduces the pain of piles. Oil massage is used in fractures and wounds. Decoction of the roots and leaves is used for washing the hair which is helpful in hair growth and making them black and soft.

Tila is a brain tonic and is aphrodisiac. It is useful in dysmenorrhoea, diabetes and gum and teeth problems (seeds are given for chewing). It increases meda-mansa (weight). In bleeding piles, it is given along with butter. Also used in pyuria.

Among all the available oils, tila oil is considered to be the best for nourishing all the seven dhatus of the body. Therefore, it is useful as both food as well as medicine.

Srotogamitva :

Dosha : Vataghna, kaphapittavardhak.
Dhatu : Mansa, shukra, meda, majja, asthi, rakta, rasayana.
Mala : Keshya, purisha (increasing the bulk), mutra (antidiuretic).

References -

'स्निग्धोष्णो मधुरस्तिक्त: कषाय: कटुकस्तिल: ।
त्वच्य: केश्यश्च बल्यश्च वातघ्न: कफपित्तकृत् ।। (च. सू. २७)
'ईषत् कषायो मधुर: सतिक्त : सांग्राहिक: पित्तकरस्तथोष्ण: ।
तिलो विपाके मधुरो बलिष्ठ: स्निग्धो व्रणालेपन एव पथ्य: ।।

In Botany, many families are named after scientists, professors and Gods etc. Similarly names are derived from the morphology of the plant.

दन्त्योऽग्निमेधाजननोऽल्पमूत्रस्त्वच्योऽथ केश्योऽनिलहा गुरुश्च ।
तिलेषु सर्वेष्वसितः प्रधानो मध्यः सितो हीनतरास्तथाऽन्ये ।।' (सु. सू. ४६)
'तिलः कृष्णः सितो रक्तः स वन्योऽल्पतिलः स्मृतः ।
तिलो रसे कटुस्तिक्तो मधुरस्तुवरो गुरुः ।।
विपाके चापि मधुरः स्निग्धोष्णः कफपित्तकृत् । बल्यः केश्यो हिमस्पर्शस्त्वच्यः स्तन्यो व्रणे हितः ।।
दन्त्योऽल्पमूत्रकृद्ग्राही वातघ्नोऽग्निमतिप्रदः ।
कृष्णः श्रेष्ठतमस्तेषु शुक्रलो मध्यमः सितः ।।
अन्ये हीनतराः प्रोक्तास्तज्ज्ञैः रक्तादयस्तिलाः ।।' (भा. प्र.)
'कषायानुरसं स्वादु सूक्ष्ममुष्णं व्यवायि च । पित्तलं बद्धविण्मूत्रं न च श्लेष्माभिवर्धनम् ।।
वातघ्नेषूत्तमं बल्यं त्वच्यं मेधाग्निवर्धनम् । तैलं संयोगसंस्कारात् सर्वरोगापहं स्मृतम् ।। (च. सू. २७
'नवनीततिलाभ्यासात् केशरनवनीतशर्कराभ्यासात् ।
दधिसरमथिताभ्यासादर्शांस्यपयान्ति रक्तानि ।।' (च. चि. १४)
'तिलकुसुमलवणगोजलकटुतैलं लौहभाजने कृत्वा ।
शोषितमर्कमयूखैः पादस्फुदनं निहन्ति लेपेन ।।' (भै. र.)
'तिलैश्च गुटिकां कृत्वा लेपयेज्जठरोपरि । गुडिका शमयस्येषा शूलं चैवातिदूस्तरम् ।।' (भै. र.)
'तिलकल्कः सलवणः द्वे हरिद्रे त्रिवृद्घृतम् । मधुकं निम्बपत्रं च लेपःस्याद् व्रणशोधनः ।।' (भै. र.)
'तिलैरणअडातसीबीजसर्षपैः परिलिप्य च । श्लेष्मगुल्मपयः पात्रैः सुखोष्णैः स्वेदयेद् भिषक् ।।' (भै. र.)

(113) TOOD
Morus alba

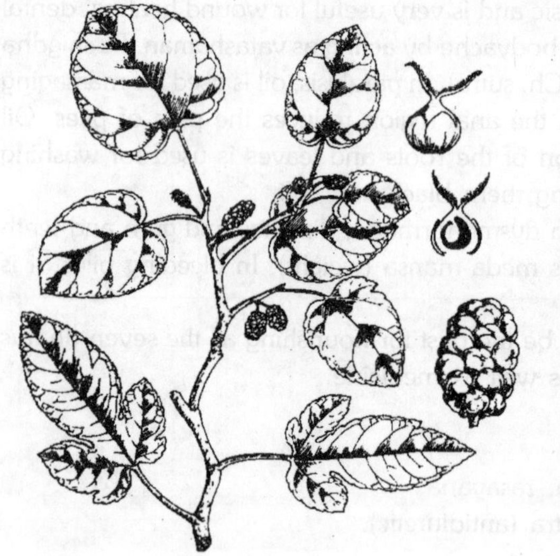

Kula : Vata kula.
Family : Uritcaceae (like a nettle) (nettle = sting).
Latin name : Morus = Latin name of black mulberrry; alba = white.
Sanskrit names : Toota, Sthool, Brahmadaru, Madhupippali.
Botanical Description : This is a tree of medium height. Trunk - browinsh or yellowish grey in colour. Leaves - 5 - 10 cm. long, oval and margin denticulated with three veins at the base. Stalk - 2.5 to 5 cm. long. Flowers - unisexual, small, white. Fruits - like Piper longum, oblong but large. Flowering occurs in winter and fruiting in summer. The leaves are useful as silk worms' food.
Varities : Two 1) white fruits - large and sweet and 2) brown black fruits - slightly sour-sweet.
Habitat : All over India.
Chemical composition : Fruit contains sugar, pectin, citrate, mallate etc.
Properties:
Guna : guru, singdha; **Rasa** : madhur; **Vipak** : madhur; **Veerya** : sheeta (raw fruit - amla vipaki and ushna veerya); **Dosha** : vatapittaghna.

External uses : Leaves are used for wound healing, especially for bed sores. Decoction of leaves is useful as gargles in stomatitis and pharyngitis.
Internal uses: Ripe fruit is appetizer and carminative. Bark is purgative and anthelmintic. Fruits and bark are used in loss of appetite, flatulence, constipation and intestinal worms. It is very useful in tape worm. Syrup of ripe fruits is useful in heart diseases, bleeding disorders, burning sensation and debility.
Dose : Bark decoction - 50 to 100 ml.; fruit juice - 20 to 50 ml.
Srotogamitva :
Dosha : (Ripe) vataghna, pittaghna; (Raw) pittavardhak.
Dhatu : Rakta (wound, bed sores), mansa (stomatitis).
Mala : Purisha (tape worm, bark - purgative).
References -
'तूदं पक्वं गुरु स्वादु हिमं पित्तानिलापहम् । तदेवामं गुरु सरमम्लाष्णं रक्तपित्तकृत्त ।।' (भा. प्र.)
'तूदस्य तु फलं स्वादु बलवर्णाग्निवृद्धिकृत् । तूदं तु मधुराम्लं स्याद् वातपित्तहरं सरम् ।।
दाहप्रशमनं वृष्यं कषायं कफनाशनम् ।' (ध. नि.)

(114) TAILPARNI

Eucalyptus citriodora Heok.

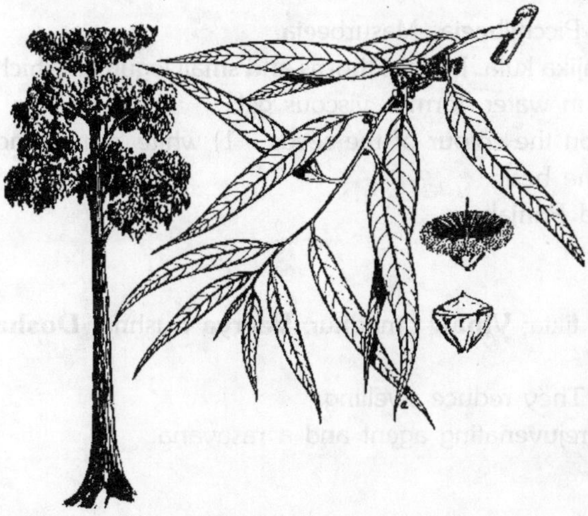

Kula : Lavang kula.
Family : Myrtaceae (Held sacred to Venus).
Latin name : Eucalyptus - eu = good, kalypto = conceal, the calyx which covers the flowers, falls off like a cap. All with white flowers; citriodora - citrus = lemon, odor = smell.
Sanskrit names : Sugandhapatra, Haritparni, Raktaniryas.
Botanical Description : The tree rapidly achieves a good height. The trunk is straight and long. Leaves - oblong and emit a pleasant odour on crushing. Its wood is used for railway tract sleepers.
Habitat : Australia (originally), now found in India, hills and mountains of Nilgiri, gardens etc.
Chemical composition : Oil contains eucalyptol 50 - 60%. Mites do not attack the tree.
Varities : About 600 species are found in Australia. (The author has himself seen many of these varieties in the National Botanical garden of Canberra.)
Properties:
Guna : laghu, singdha, tikshna; **Rasa :** katu, tikta, kashaya; **Vipak :** katu, **Veerya :** ushna;
Dosha : kaphavatashamak.
External uses : Old, preserved oil is useful in pyogenic infections. It is used to prepare ointments.

The study of the origin of the names of plants gives unusual joy to experts.

Mixture of eucalyptus oil and mustard oil is used in osteoarthritis. Inhalation of oil in hot water vapours is useful in various lung conditions. Its analgesic property is useful in headache, bodyache and neuropathy. Enema of oil and water is useful in thread worms.

Internal uses : In small doses, it is a cardiostimulant but in large dose causes cardiac arrest. Oil is useful in loss of appetite and flatulence. Enema of the oil is given in worms. Gum is used in diarrhoea, dysentery, bronchiectasis and lung infections. Oil is useful in cystitis and chronic pyuria. Decoction of dry leaves is useful in chronic fever and typhoid fever. It is a diaphoretic.

Doses : Leaf powder - 0.5 to 1 gm.; decoction - 20 to 50 gms.; gum - 0.25 to 0.5 gm.

Srotogamitva :

Dosha : Kaphaghna, vataghna.

Dhatu : Rasa, rakta (pulmonary infection).

Mala : Sweda, purisha (diarrhoea, dysentery), pulmonary congestion; mutra (pyogenic infection).

(115) TODARI
Lepidium iberis

Kula : Rajika kula.

Family: Crucifereae (cross shaped four petals).

Latin name : Lepidium = pleasant, charming; iberis = of Iberia.

English name : Papergrass.

Sanskrit names : Kantavruksha, Laghuphala, Picchilbeeja, Masurbeeja.

Botanical Description : The plant belongs to rajika kula. It bears thorns and small legumes which contain minute seeds. The seeds, when dipped in water, form a viscous gel.

Varities : There are three varieties depending on the colour of the seeds - 1) white 2) red and 3) yellow. The last variety is considered to be the best.

Habitat : Southern Europe to Siberia, Iran and Punjab.

Chemical composition : Seeds contain sulphur.

Properties:

Guna : guru, snigdha, pichchil; **Rasa :** madhur, tikta; **Vipak :** madhur; **Veerya :** ushna; **Dosha :** tridoshaghna.

External uses : Seeds are irritant to the skin. They reduce swelling.

Internal uses : It is useful as an aphrodisiac, rejuvenating agent and a rasayana.

Srotogamitva :

Dosha : Tridoshaghni.

Dhatu : Shukra, mansa, medogami.

Organ : Reproductive system.

(116) TRAPUSHA
Cucumis sativum

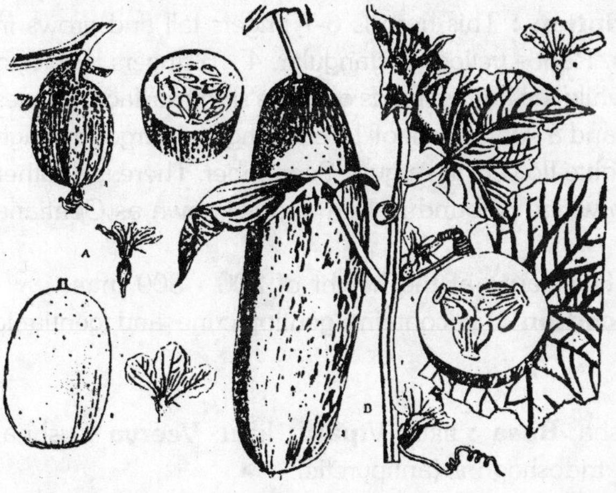

Kula : Koshataki kula.

Family : Cucurbitaceae (bearing round large fruits).

Latin name : Cucumis = cucumber; sativum = cultivated.

Sanskrit names : Trapusi, Peetapushpi, Kantalu, Trapuskarkati, Bahuphala, Koshaphala, Tundilphala, Muni.

Botanical Description : Creeper with leaf stalk, 5 - 7 cm. long, bearing pentangular broad leaves of 7 to 17 cm. diameter. Flowers - yellow, unisexual. Fruit - greenish-white or greenish yellow. Stalk bears spikes. Seeds - plenty, flat, oblong, tapering at both ends, shining and white.

Varities : 1) Small and 2) large.

Habitat : All over India, specially in temperate and sandy land.

Chemical composition : Seeds contain a stable oil, starch and sugar.

Properties:

Guna : laghu, ruksha; **Rasa:** madhur; **Veerya:** sheeta; **Dosha** : pittashamak, vatakaphavardhak. It reduces burning, thirst, promotes diuresis and strength. Seed oil is used in burning, insomnia and frontal headache.

Internal uses : Useful in thirst, jaundice, bleeding disorders, anuria and burning sensation. Cold drink prepared from the seeds is used in summer for soothing effect.

Srotogamitva :

Dosha : Pittaghna, vatakaphavardhak.

Dhatu : Rasa , rakta.

Mala : Mutra (seed).

References -

'स्वादुपित्तापहं शीतं रक्तपित्तहरं परम् ।
तद्बीज मूत्रलं शीतं रूक्षं पित्तास्रकृच्छ्रजित् ।। (मा. प्र.)

(117) TRAYAMANA
Gentiana kurroa

Kula : Bhunimba kula.

Gana : Tikta (C.) Lakshadi (S.)

Family : Gentianaceae (Ranunculaceae?)

Man is not the only one who treats his malady. Even animals and birds do it. There are many such examples in Ayurveda.

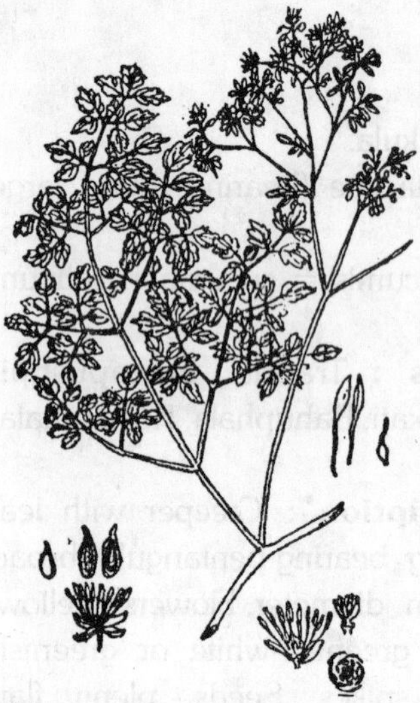

Latin name : Gentiana = leaves resemble gentiai; kurroa or Thalictrum foliotosum.

English name : Gold thread.

Sanskrit names : Balabhadra, Trayamana, Trayanti, Girisanuja.

Botanical Description : This herb is 6-7 fingers tall and grows in the cracks of rocks. Root - yellow, rectangular, 4 - 6 fingers long and peneterates deep while the herb spreads over the stony surface. Leaves - 3 to 4 in number and a flower stalk of 15 cm. length emerges through them to bear 3 - 4 blue flowers in August, September. There is another variety of this herb which is found in Iran and is known as Gentiana dahurica.

Habitat : In the Himalayas at the height of 200 - 300 mtrs.

Chemical composition : It contains gentiopicrine and gentianic acid.

Properties:

Guna: laghu, ruksha; **Rasa :** tikta; **Vipak :** katu; **Veerya :** ushna;

Dosha : kaphavatashamak and pittashodhak; tridoshaghni (antipyretic).

External uses : Used for application in wounds, skin disorders and alopecia.

Internal uses : It is an appetizer, digestive, cholagogue, carminative, laxative and anthelmintic. It is therefore useful in loss of appetite, liver disorders, piles, colic, tumor and ascites. It is also useful in blood disorders, dysmenorrhoea, disorders of breast-milk secretion, anuria and skin diseases. It is a well known antipyretic drug. It is useful in anaemia and post pyretic debility.

Parts used : Panchang and roots.

Dose : Syrup - 10 to 20 ml.; powder - 3 to 6 gms.

Srotogamitva :

Dosha : Kaphaghna , pittashodhini.

Dhatu : Rakta (liver disorders), rasa (dysmenorrhoea, antipyretic), raktamajja.

Mala : Hair tonic, purisha (purgative), mutra (anuria).

References -

'त्रायन्ती तुवरा तिक्ता सरापित्तकफापहा । ज्वरहृद्रोगगुल्मास्त्रभ्रमशूलविषप्रणुत् ।।' (भा. प्र.)

'त्रायमाणाशृतं वापि पयसा ज्वरितः पिबेत् ।' (च. चि. ३)

(118) DAMANAK

Artemisia vulgaris Linn.

Kula: Bhringaraj kula.

Family: Compositeae (Composite head of tiny flowers).

Latin name: Artemisia = one of the names of Diana (used for flavour); vulgaris = common, ordinary.

Sanskrit names: Danta, Muni, Pundarik, Brahmajata, Jatil, Pavitrak, Dandi, Vinit, Devshekhar, Tapasviputra.

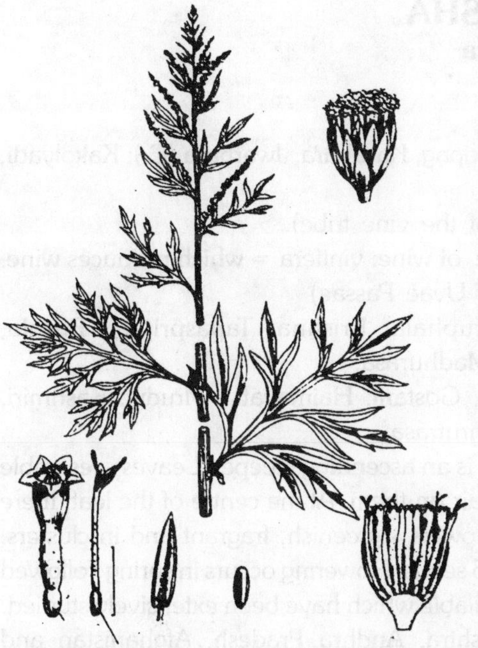

Botanical Description: This shrub grows 30 to 60 cms. tall. Leaves and branches are small. Flowers and leaves emit a stingent odour.

Chemical composition: It contains a camphor-like volatile oil and also yavakshar in large quantity.

Habitat : All over India.

Properties:

Guna: laghu, ruksha, tikshna; **Rasa:** tikta, kashaya; **Vipak :** katu; **Veerya :** ushna; **Dosha:** tridoshahara.

Uses: It is an analgesic and antiinflammatory. Because of its analgesic property and action on the nervous system, it is useful in vata disorders. Since it is an appetizer, digestive, carminative and cholagogue, it is useful in loss of appetite, constipation, flatulence and colic. It clears the bile through stools. Its kshar is used in ascites.

Cardiovascular system: It is a cardiostimulant and hence useful in cardiac oedema. It purifies blood.

Respiratory system: By its expectorant action, it is useful in cough, bronchitis, breathlessness and asthma.

Urinary system: It is a diuretic and therefore used in dysuria.

Reproductive system: It is an aphrodisiac and helps uterine contractions. Therefore it is used in amenorrhoea, dysmenorrhoea and impotency.

Temperature: In fever, it reduces bodyache, insomnia and sweating. It is more effective in anaemia if given with loha bhasma.

Parts used : Panchang, flowers and leaves.

Dose: Juice - 5 to 10 ml.; powder - 0.75 to 1 gm.

Srotogamitva:

Dosha: Tridoshahara.

Dhatu: Raktameda (anaemia), rasa (bodyache, amenorrhoea, dysmenorrhoea).

Mala: Mutra (diuretic), purisha (bile excretion through stool).

Organ: Heart, uterus, respiratory organs.

References -

'दमनस्तुवरस्तिक्तो हृद्यो वृष्यः सुगंधिकः । ग्रहणोविषकुष्ठास्रक्लेदकण्डूत्रिदोषजित् ।।' (भा. प्र.)

'दमनः स्याद्रसे तिक्तो विषघ्नो भूतदोषनुत् । त्रिदोषशमनो हृद्यः कण्डूकुष्ठापहः स्मृतः ।।' (ध. नि.)

Modern botanical science is a compilation since ancient times. Information on new plants is being added continuously to it. However, some of the information is also getting outdated.

(119) DRAKSHA

Vitis vinifera

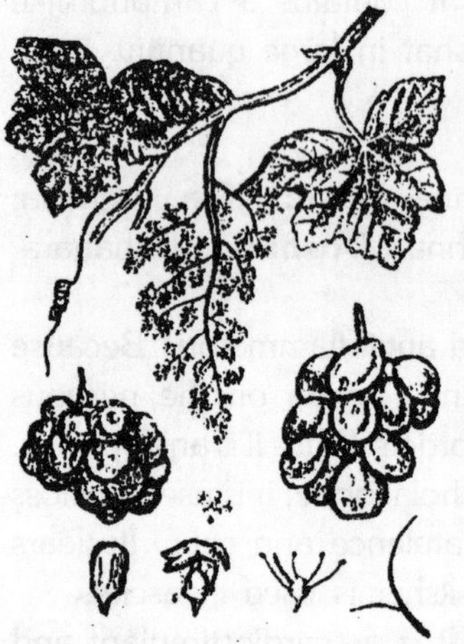

Kula: Draksha kula.
Gana: Snehopag, Virechanopag, Kasahara, Jwarhara (C.); Kakolyadi, Parushakadi (S.)
Family: Vitaceae (plants of the vine tribe).
Latin name : Vitis = name of wine; vinifera = which produces wine.
English name: Grape (or Uvae Passae)
Sanskrit names: Charuphala, Krishna, Tapaspriya, Rasala, Amrutphala, Phalottama, Madhurasa.
Black grape: Mrudvika, Gostani, Haimavati, Mrudvi, Kashmiri, Shataveerya, Madhuli, Amrutrasa.
Botanical Description: It is an ascending creeper. Leaves - resemble bitter gourd but have fine hair on them. At the centre of the leaf, there are 4 to 5 veins in pairs. Flowers - greenish, fragrant and in clusters. Fruits are oblong, having 4 -5 seeds. Flowering occurs in spring followed by fruiting in summer. Now-a-days many varieties are available which have been extensively studied.
Habitat: North-west India, Punjab, Kashmir, Maharashtra, Andhra Pradesh, Afghanistan and Baluchistan.
Chemical composition: Fruits contain water 72.8 to 77.2 %, sugar 15.69 to 18.6 % and other chemical substances.
Properties: Grape is described as the best fruit because of its extremely beneficial properties.
Guna: snigdha, guru, mridu; **Rasa:** madhur; **Vipak:** madhur; **Veerya:** sheeta.
Internal uses: Useful in thirst, bleeding disorders, burning, gout, pthisis, pleurisy, tuberculosis, cough, asthma, dysuria, burning micturition, wasting etc.
Srotogamitva :
Dosha: Vataghna, pittaghna, vatapittashamak.
Dhatu: Mansa, shukra, rakta, saptadhatu, rasa.
Mala: Purisha (laxative), mutra (purifier).
Organ: Heart, uterus.
References -

'तृष्णादाहज्वरश्वासरक्तपित्तक्षतक्षयान् । वातपित्तमुदावर्त्तं स्वरभेदं मदात्ययम् ।।
तिक्तास्तयामास्यशोषं कासं चाशु व्यपोहति । मृद्विका बृंहणी वृष्या मधुरा स्निग्धशीतला ।। (च. सू. २७)
'तेषां द्राक्षा सरा स्वर्या मधुरा स्निग्धशीतला । रक्तपित्तज्वरश्वासतृष्णादाहक्षयापहा ।।' (सु. सू. ४६)
'द्राक्षा पक्वा सरा शीता चक्षुष्या बृंहणी गुरुः । स्वादुपाकरसा स्वर्या तुवरा सृष्टमूत्रविट् ।।
कोष्ठमारुतहृद् वृष्या कफपुष्टिरुचिप्रदा । हन्ति तृष्णाज्वरश्वासकासवातास्रकामलाः ।
'कृच्छ्रास्रपित्तसम्मोहदाहशोषमदात्ययान् ।' (भा. प्र.)
'द्राक्षा तु मधुराऽम्ला च शीता पित्तार्त्तिदाहजित् ।
मूत्रदोषहरा रुच्या वृष्या सन्त्तर्पणी परा ।।' (रा. नि.)

(120) DUGDHAPHENI
Taraxacum officinale Weber.

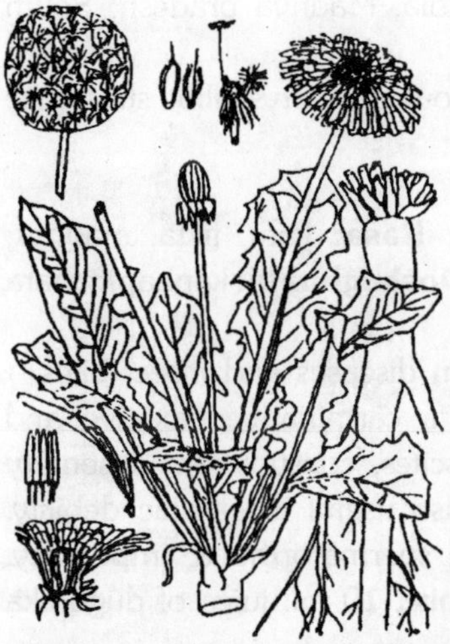

Kula: Bhringaraj kula.
Family: Compositeae (composite head of tiny flowers).
Latin name: Taraxacum = Dandelion - possibly a reference to medicinal qualities; officinale = available in market.
Sanskrit names: Dugdhapheni, Payaswini, Lutari, Dudhal, Dudhali.
Botanical Description: This is a shrub which survives for many years. Leaves - emerges from the base of the stem, just above the roots. Leaves are 7-10 cms. long and torn. Flowers - yellow, 7.25 to 10 cm long, appear at the end of flower stalk. Milky white latex oozes out from all the parts of the plant.
Habitat: Himalayas, Tibet, Nilgiri.
Chemical composition: White latex contains taranacin and taraxacerin. Root contains inulin 25% besides pectin and starch.
Properties:
Guna: laghu, ruksha, tikshna; **Rasa:** tikta; **Vipak:** katu; **Veerya:** ushna; **Dosha:** kaphapittahara.
External uses : Its application is very useful in chronic nonhealing ulcers.
Internal uses : Since it is an appetizer, hepatic stimulant, cholagogue, purgative and antimicrobial, it is useful in loss of appetite, jaundice, ascites etc.
Its rejuvenating, blood purifying and diuretic action is useful in oedema, skin diseases, inflammation and anuria. It is beneficial in chronic fever, general debility and poisoning.
Dose: Root powder - 0.75 to 1.25 gms.; decoction - 25 to 50 ml.
Srotogamitva :
Dosha: Kaphaghna, pittaghna.
Dhatu: Rasapachan, rakta (jaundice), rasayana.
Mala: Mutra (dysuria).

(121) DUGDHIKA
Euphorbia thymifolia

Kula: Erand kula.
Family: Euphorbiaceae (Name of the discoverer).
Latin name: Euphorbia = Spurge milk wort; Euphorbus = physician to the King of Mauretamia; thymifolia (Thymus = (Gk) thuo = perfume). (Leaves of this plant are similar to thymus).
Sanskrit names: Rajakshava, Dugdhanika, Dugdhika, Swadupushpika, Ksheerani, Ksheerika, Sheeta, Sheetambu, Madhuparnika.
Botanical Description: This is an annual creeper spreading on the land. Some times it grows vertically. Trunk - tender with plenty of branches, bristly hair and 10 - 25 cm. long. Leaves - small,

Madhur rasa produces certain vibrations on the tongue. If one can stimulate similar vibrations, perception of madhur rasa is possible.

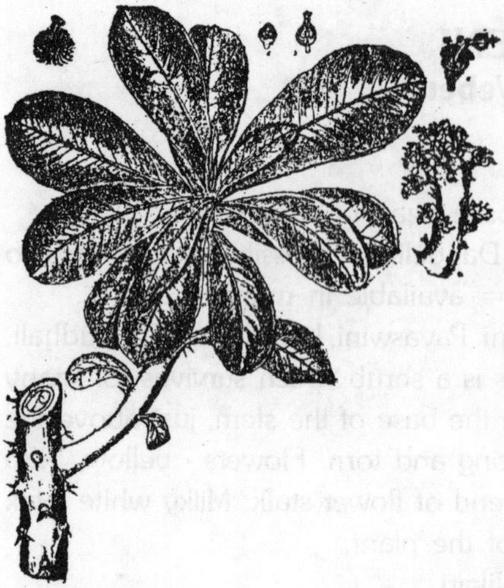

oblong. Fruits - small and smooth. Seeds - smooth and blue.
Varities: 1) Large 2) Medium and 3) Small. It is also classified as 1) white and 2) red. The red variety is small and is used in medicine.
Habitat: Tropical parts of India, Madhya pradesh, South India and Bengal.
Chemical composition: It contains a crystalline substance similar to quarcentine.
Properties:
Guna: guru, ruksha, tikshna; **Rasa:** katu, tikta, madhur; **Vipak:** katu; **Veerya:** ushna; **Doshaghnata:** kaphapittahara and vatavardhak.
External uses: Useful in skin diseases and insect bites.
Internal uses: Since it is a carminative, laxative and anthelmintic, it is useful in ascites, constipation, dysentery and worm infestation. It is also useful in cardiac debility, syphilis, gonorrhoea, chronic cough, breathlessness, anuria, pyuria, spermatorrhoea, impotency, skin disorders and ammenorrhoea. It is useful in eczema. In snake bite, 10 ml. juice of dugdhika + black pepper powder is given.
Dose: Juice - 5 to 10 ml.; decoction - 20 to 40 ml.
Srotogamitva:
Dosha: Kaphaghna, pittaghna, vatashamak.
Dhatu: Rakta, rasa, shukra.
Mala: Mutra, purisha.
References -
'दुग्धिकोष्णा गुरु रूक्षा वातला गर्भकारिणी । स्वादुक्षीरा कटुस्तिक्ता सृष्टमूत्रमलापहा ।।
स्वादुर्विष्टम्भिनी वृष्या कफकोष्ठकृमिप्रणुत् ।।' (भा. प्र.)

(122) DWIPANTAR VACHA
Smilax glabra Roxb.

Kula: Rason kula.
Family: Liliaceae (plant of the Lily tribe).
Latin name: Smilax = Sarasaparila plant. Gk. Smile = rasping, the prickly stems; glabra = smooth, not having hairs (or china).
English name: China root.
Sanskrit names: Dwipantarvacha, Chopchini, Topchini.
Botanical Description: It is an ascending and spreading type of creeper. Leaves - oval. Flowers - small, white. Roots - thick, heavy and brown coloured. This tuber is itself known and used as chopchini. Another plant, Smilex china, is also considered to be chopchini.
Habitat: The plant is originally from China and Japan but now also growing in Assam.
Chemical composition: Root contains fat, sugar, glucoside, pigments, saponine, gum and starch.

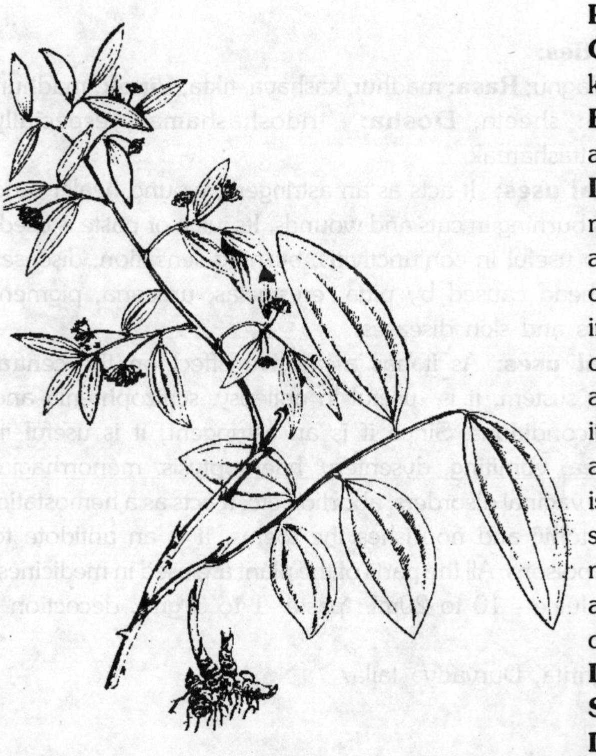

Properties:

Guna: laghu, ruksha; **Rasa:** tikta; **Vipak:** katu; **Veerya:** ushna; **Dosha:** tridoshanashak.

External uses: Its local application is helpful as an analgesic and anti-inflammatory.

Internal uses: As it is a vatashamak and nervine tonic, it helps in schizophrenia, epilepsy and other brain disorders. Its digestive, carminative and laxative properties are useful in loss of appetite, flatulance, abdominal colic, constipation and intestinal parasites. Since it is a blood purifier and has anti-microbial activity, it is very useful in secondary and tertiary syphilis and cervical adenitis. Milk boiled with chopchini is used in skin diseases, impotency and other seminal disorders. A special preparation (pak) made from its tuber is used in gonorrhoea and associated arthritic symptoms, fever and general debility.

Dose: Tuber powder - 3 to 6 gms.

Srotogamitva:

Dosha: Tridoshanashak.

Dhatu: Majja, shukra, meda, in all the stages of syphilis for rasadi dhatus.

Mala: Purisha (anthelmintic).

Organ : Manovahasrotas (schizophrenia, epilepsy).

(123) DURVADWAYAM

Cynodon dactylon Linn.

Kula: Yava kula.

Gana: Prajasthapan and Varnya (C.)

Family: Gramineae (This family contains 126 species).

Latin name: Cynodon = cyno = kyno = dog; dactylon = fingered.

English name: Conch grass.

Sanskrit names: Green - Shataveerya, Harit, Shambhavi, Shyama, Shanta, Anushnavallika.

White - Shwetadurva, Sitakhya, Chanda, Bhadra, Bhargavi, Gaura, Vighna.

Botanical Description: Durva is a creeper which spreads on the ground. Its stem bears numerous knots from which roots appear and help it in spreading. Leaves - 2.5 to 10 cm. long and narrow. Stalk of flowers is 2.5 to 5 cm. in length with green or violet colour. Seeds are very minute.

Varieties: There are three varieties (1) white (described above) - this is used in medicine (2) blue - this spreads over a large area and is also called as ananta, sahasraveerya, lata etc. and (3) ganda durva (gandiri) - this grows near the edges of small ponds.

For achieving the unity of India, the common sanskrit names of plants have played a major role.

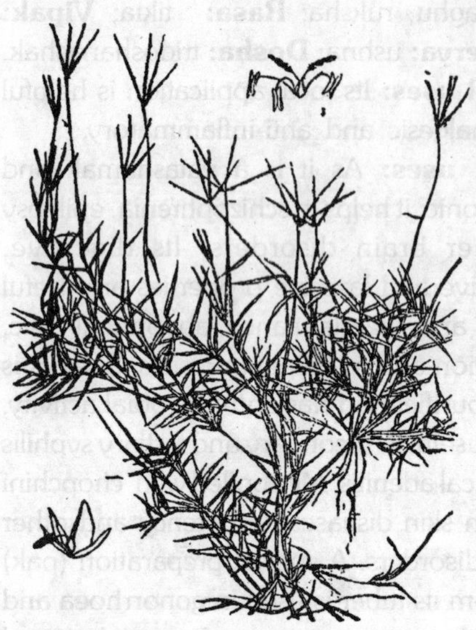

Properties:

Guna: laghu; **Rasa:** madhur, kashaya, tikta; **Vipak:** madhur; **Veerya:** sheeta; **Dosha:** tridoshashamak, especially kaphapittashamak.

External uses: It acts as an astringent, wound healer and reduces burning in cuts and wounds. Its juice or paste is used. It is also useful in conjunctivitis, burning sensation, diseases of the head caused by pitta, erysipelas, urticaria, pigment disorders and skin diseases.

Internal uses: As it has a positive effect on the central nervous system, it is useful in epilepsy, schizophrenia and painful conditions. Since it is an astringent, it is useful in diarrhoea, vomiting, dysentery, haemoptysis, menorrhagia, syphilis, vaginal disorders, abortion etc. It acts as a hemostatic, uterine tonic and nourishes the foetus. It is an antidote to various poisons. All the parts of the plant are used in medicines.

Dose: Juice - 10 to 20ml.; paste -1 to 3 gm.; decoction - 50 to 100 ml.

Formulations: Durvadi kwath, Durvadya ghrita, Durvadya taila.

Srotogamitva:

Dosha: Tridosha, kaphaghna, pittaghna.

Dhatu: Rakta (hemostatic, improves complexion, erysipelas, bleeding disorders), foetus (nutritive).

Mala: Purisha (constipative, dysentery).

Organ: Uterus (abortion, uterine bleeding).

Manovahasrotas : Schizophrenia, epilepsy.

Antidote to poisons (vishaghna).

References -

'दूर्वा शीता कषाया च रक्तपित्तकफापहा ।' (ध. नि.)

'दूर्वा: कषाया: मधुराश्च शीता: पित्ततृषारोचकवान्तिहन्त्र्य: ।
सदाहमूर्च्छाग्रहभूतशान्तिश्लेष्मश्रमध्वंसनतृप्तिदाश्च ।।' (रा. नि.)

'दूर्वा तु रक्तपित्तघ्नी कण्डूत्वग्दोषनाशिनी ।' (रा. व.)

'दूर्वा स्वाद्वी हिमा तिक्ता कषाया जीवनी जयेत् । कफपित्तास्त्रवीसर्पतृष्णादाहत्वगामयान् ।।' (कै. नि.)

'वृक्षादनी पयस्या च लता चोत्पलसारिवा । यथासंख्यं प्रयोक्तव्या: गर्भस्त्रावे पयोयुत: ।।' (सु. शा. १०)

(124) DHAV
Anoceissus latifolia Wall.

Kula : Haritaki kula.

Gana : Salsardi gana.

Family : Combretaceae.

Latin name : Anoceissus = ano = up; latifolia = broad leaved (or Conocarpus latifolia).

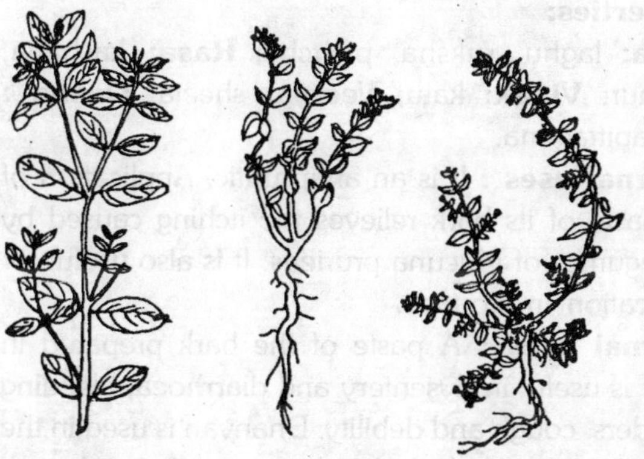

Sanskrit names : Dhava, Dathataru, Gaur, Madhurtwak, Shuklavriksha, Pandutaru, Dhaval, Spirodatha, Shakat.

Botanical Description : This is a huge tree growing up to a height of 28 mtrs. Its bark is greenish white. Leaves - 4 to 8cm. long and 2.5 to 5 cm. broad, smooth. Flowers - round and in bunches. Latex oozes out from the tree.

Habitat : Himalayas, Sri lanka.

Properties:

Guna: laghu, ruksha; **Rasa** : kashaya, madhur; **Vipak** : katu; **Veerya** : sheeta; **Dosha** : kaphapittashamak.

Uses: Its decoction is used for washing and healing of wounds. Since it is an astringent and hemostatic, it is useful in diarrhoea, dysentery, bleeding piles, bleeding diorders and other blood diseases. Its antidiuretic action helps in diabetes mellitus. It is used as a tonic and also in skin diseases. It acts as an antitoxic in scorpion and snake bite.

Dose : Decoction - 50 to 100 ml.; latex - 0.5 to 1 gm.

Srotogamitva :

Dosha : Kaphaghna, pittaghna.

Dhatu : Rakta, raktamansa, rasayana, raktameda.

Mala : Purisha, mutra (antidiuretic).

Organ : Digestive system.

Prabhav : Scorpion and snake poisoning.

References -

'धवो दढ़तरुः गौरः कषायो मधुरत्वचः । पाण्डुतरुः पीतफलो धवलश्च भरोद्वहः ।।' (शि.)

'धवः शीतः प्रमेहार्शः पांडुपित्तकफापहः । मधुरस्तुवरस्तस्य फलं तु मधुरं मनाक् ।।' (भा. प्र.)

(125) DHANVAN

Grewia tiliofolia

Kula : Parushak kula.

Family : Tiliaceae = lime tree (brasswood).

Latin name : Grewia = after Mr. Nahemiah Grew, Scientist; tiliofolia = lime tree like leaves or G. elasica.

Sanskrti names : Raktakusum, Dhanurvruksha, Mahabal, Rujapaha, Pichchilak, Swaduphala, Gotradrum, Dharman, Saravrikshak.

Botanical Description : The tree grows 13-16 mtrs. in height, bark is rough and white internally. Leaves - alternate, equidistant, round and with bristly hair. Flowers - yellow, small. Fruits - pea-shaped and black in colour.

Habitat : Western parts of India, Burma, Sri Lanka.

During the Charaka period, Ayurveda was not the only medical science which was practised. Physicians were prevalent who followed different systems of medicine.

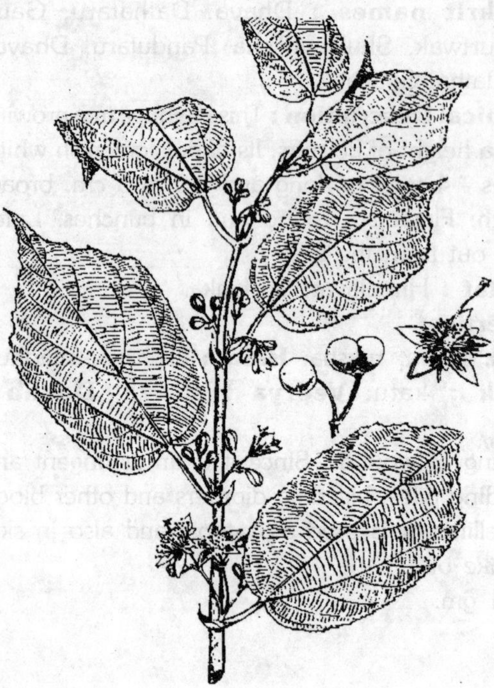

Properties:
Guna: laghu, ruksha, pichchil; **Rasa:** kashaya, madhur; **Vipak:** katu; **Veerya:** sheeta; **Dosha** : kaphapittaghna.
External uses : It is an antipruritic. Application of the paste of its bark relieves the itching caused by the legumes of Mucuna pruriens. It is also useful for application in wounds.
Internal uses : A paste of the bark prepared in water is useful in dysentery and diarrhoea, bleeding disorders, cough and debility. Dhanvan is used in the preparation of pichcha basti (a formulation administered rectally). It is used as an emetic in opium poisoning.
Srotogamitva :
Dosha : Kaphavataghna (pittaghana).
Dhatu : Rakta, asthi.
Mala : Purisha (pichcha basti in diarrhoea).
Organ : Intestines, circulatory system, respiratory system.
Antidote for itching caused by Mucuna pruriens and opium poisoning.
References -
'धन्वंगस्तु धनुर्वृक्षो गोत्रवृक्षः सुतेजनः । धन्वंगः कफपित्तास्रकासहृत्तुवरो लघुः ।।
बृंहणो बलकृद्रूक्षः सन्धिकृद् व्रणरोपणः ।' (भा. प्र.)
'.... धन्वनम् । मधुरं सकषायं च शीतपित्तकफापहम् ।' (च. सू. २७)
'फलं तस्य हिमं स्वादु कषायं कफवातजित् ।' (कै. नि.)
'सकषायं हिमं स्वादु धान्वनं कफवातजित् ।' (सु. सू. ४६)

(126) DHAMARGAV
Luffa cylindrica M. Roem Linn.

Kula : Koshataki kula.
Family : Cucurbitaceae.
Latin name : Luffa = Malayan name; cylindrica = round and oblong like a cylinder.
English name : Wash sponge.
Sanskrit names : Mahakoshataki, Mahajalini, Dhamargav, Koshaphala, Hastighosha, Mahaphala, Ghoshak, Hastiparni.
Botanical Description : Leaves are pentangular and dentate, 15 cms. in diameter. Flowers - yellow, unisexual. Fruits - oblong, 26 cm. x 45 cms. long with white streaks on them. Seeds - black and winged.

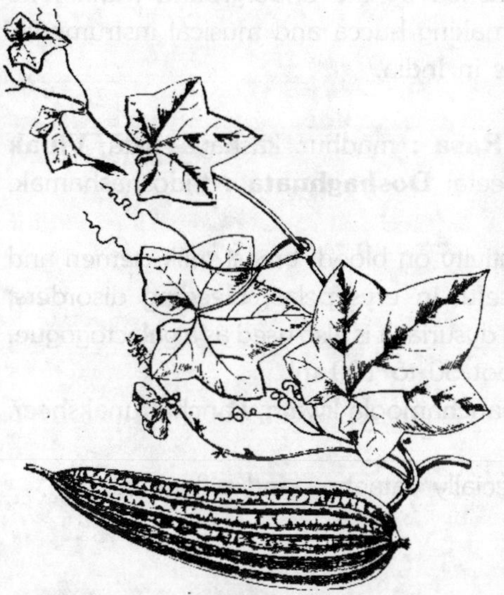

Varieties : There are two varieties - 1) bitter and 2) sweet. The former variety is used in medicine while the latter is used as a vegetable.

Habitat : All over India. Bitter variety grows in the forest. The bitter variety is described here.

Chemical composition : It contains colosynthine and luffein.

Properties:

Guna : laghu, ruksha, tikshna; **Rasa :** tikta, katu; **Vipak** : katu; **Veerya :** ushna; **Prabhav :** vamak (emetic); **Dosha** : kaphapittaghna by emesis.

Uses : The bitter variety is emetic and purgative. Therefore, it is useful in ascites, cough, asthma and hoarseness of voice (by expectoration of mucous). It is useful in blood disorders, oedema and acts as an antidote in poisons.

Parts used : Fruits, flowers, leaves.

Dose : Powder - 1 to 3 gms.; juice - 3 to 6 ml. (Charaka, in the Kalpa sthana, like many other plants, has mentioned 60 formulations of dhamargava.)

Srotogamitva :

Dosha : Kapha (purification), pitta (purification), vataghna.

Dhatu : Rakta (purification), rakta (bleeding disorders).

Mala : Purishashodhan (ascites).

Organ : Large intestine, stomach. It is used as an antidote to poisons.

References -

'कोशातकी सुतिक्तोष्णआ पक्वामाशयशोधनी ।' (ध. नि.)

'गरे गुल्मोदरे कासे वाते श्लेष्माशयस्थिते । कफे च कण्ठवक्त्रस्थे कफसञ्चयजषु च ।।
रोगेष्वेषु प्रयोज्यं स्यात् स्थिराश्च गुरवश्च ये ।' (च. क. ४)

'महाकोशातकी स्निग्धा रक्तपित्तानिलापहा ।' (भा. प्र.)

'अन्या स्वादुस्त्रिदोपघ्नी ज्वरस्यान्ते हिता स्मृता ।' (ध. नि.)

(127) NALA

Arundo donax Linn.

Kula : Yava kula.

Gana : Trunapanchamoola (S.)

Latin name : Arundo = a reed; donax = distaff cane, great reed.

English name : Reed.

Sanskrit names : Nada, Kushirandhra, Keechak, Vanshavar, Dhaman, Vibhishan, Chhidranta, Mrudupatra, Randhrapatra.

Botanical Description : The tree grows to a height of 3-6 mtrs. and resembles a cane tree. Stalk - small, thin, yellowish and hollow. Leaves - small, thin but like bamboo leaves. Flower stalk - ash

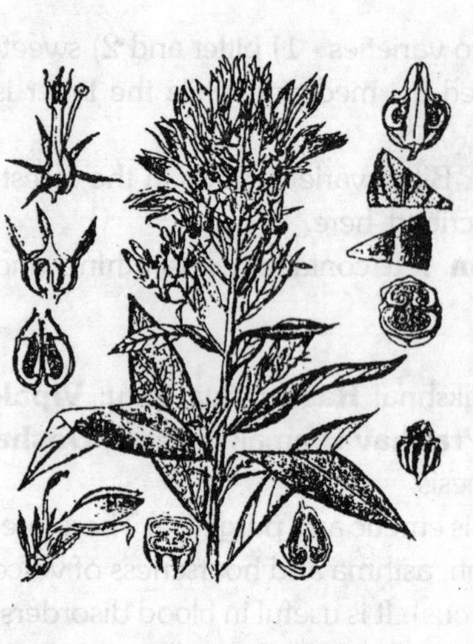

grey, fast growing, nourished by the underground trunk. The hollow stalk is used in making hucca and musical instruments.
Habitat : Marshy lands in India.
Properties:
Guna: laghu, singdha; **Rasa :** madhur, kashaya, tikta; **Vipak :** madhur; **Veerya :** sheeta; **Doshaghnata :** tridoshashamak, vatapittashamak.
Uses : It has specific activity on blood, breast milk, semen and urinary system. It is useful in erysepelas, bleeding disorders, oligospermia, cystitis and dysuria. It is also used as a galactogogue.
Dose : Decoction of root 50 to 100 ml.
Formulations : Trunapanchamoola kwath, Panchatrunaksheer.
Srotogamitva :
Dosha : Tridosha, especially vataghna and pittaghna.
Dhatu : Rasa, rakta, medogami, shukra.
Mala : Cystitis (diuretic, lithotripsic).
References -
'वंशपत्रो मृदुच्छदः । छिद्रांत्रो नर्तको रन्ध्री मृत्युपुष्पो विभीषणः ।।'
'नलस्तु मधुरस्तिक्तः कषायः कफरक्तजित् ।' (भा. प्र.)
'नलः शीतः कषायश्च पित्तमूत्रविनाशनः ।' (ध. नि.)
'देवनालोऽतिमधुरो वृष्य ईषत् कषायकः । नलः स्यादधिको वीर्ये शस्यते रसकर्मणि ।।' (रा. नि.)

(128) NADIHINGU
Gardenia gummifera Linn F.

Kula : Manjishtha kula.
Family : Rubiaceae.
Latin name : Gardenia = (cape jasmin) American Dr. Garden (Gardinia was the favourite button hole of Edwardians); gummifera = oozing latex.
English name : Dikamali Resin.
Sanskrit names : Nadihingu, Hingushivatika, Hingupatri, Jantuka, Ramathi, Vanshapatri, Pindahva, Suveerya, Hingunadika.
Botanical Description : The shrub is small, leaves resembling guava leaves but are slightly big and long. A yellow coloured latex oozes out from its branches on piercing the bark and from the angles of leaf stalks. It solidifies on exposure to air. Since it has an odour similar to asafoetida, it is called hingupatri. A small tablet of dikamali held in the mouth doesnot dissolve easily.
Habitat : Maharashtra, Madhya pradesh, South India, Burma etc. Generally grows in hilly areas.
Properties:
Guna: laghu, ruksha, tikshna; **Rasa:** katu, tikta; **Veerya:** ushna; **Dosha:** kaphavatashamak
External uses : It is antimicrobial, wound healing and analgesic. It is useful in toothache and teething problems of children (rubbing latex to the gums).

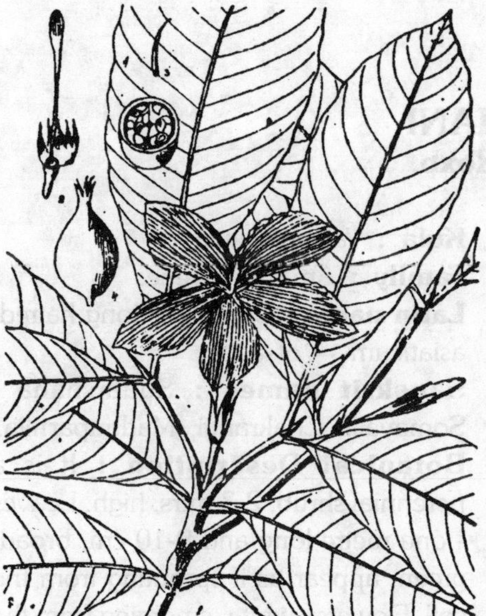

Internal uses : It is an appetizer, digestive, carminative and anthelmintic. Therefore it is useful in anorexia, loss of appetite, indigestion, constipation, flatulence, ascites, piles, intestinal parasites etc. It is one of the best medicines for the alimentary tract. It is useful in tape worms. Latex with lemon juice is useful in cardiac disorders and splenomegaly by expelling vata and enhancing peristalsis. It is also useful in chronic cough, breathlessness, hiccups and skin diseases. In malaria, it is used for reducing the fever, cold and rigors. It is a lipolytic and therefore used in lipid disorders.

Dose : Latex 250 to 500 mgm.

Srotogamitva :

Dosha : Kaphaghna, vataghna

Dhatu : Asthi, rakta, rasa, meda.

Mala : Purisha.

Organs : Intestines, heart, urinary bladder.

References -

'नाडीहिङ्गु कटूष्णं च कफवातार्त्तिशान्तिकृत् । विष्ठाविबन्धदोषघ्नमानाहामयहारि च ।।' (रा. नि.)

'हिङ्गपत्री भवेद्रुच्या तीक्ष्णोष्णा पाचनी कटुः । हृद्बस्तिरुग् विबन्धार्श:श्लेष्मगुल्मानिलापहा ।।' (भा. प्र.)

(129) NAGADANTI
Croton oblongifolia

Kula : Erand kula.

Family : Euphorbiaceae.

Latin name : Croton = kroton - a tick; oblongifolia = with oblong leaves.

Sanskrit names : Shwetaghanta, Madhupushpi, Vishodhini, Nagasphota, Nagachatra, Vichakshana, Sarpapushpa, Shuklapushpi, Swaduka.

Botanical Description : The tree grows abundantly in south Konkan and Bengal. Leaves - oblongifolines like mango. Bark - ash grey and slimy. Leaves - 15 to 30 cm. long, both sides are slimy. Flowers - faint green and in clusters. Root - twisted, flat, with a thick skin, externally rough, ash coloured, internally yellow with grey spots. The bark is pungent and smells like camphor.

Properties: It is pungent to taste and is very useful in all types of inflammation - internal as well as external. It is more effective in acute inflammation.

Guna : laghu; **Rasa :** katu; **Vipak :** katu ; **Veerya :** ushna; **Dosha :** pittashodhak, therefore it is very useful in hepatitis.

Uses : In Konkan, it is a well known remedy for snake bite. 10 to 20 gms. of nagadanti is given to the victim after every two hours.

Srotogamitva :

Dosha : Pittavirechak.

In plant kingdom, there are some trees that live upto 3000 years. Similarly there are sky-high trees which are 300 ft. in height.

Dhatu : Rasa, rakta.
Mala : Purisha (purgative).

(130) NAGADAMANI

Crinum asiaticum Roxb.

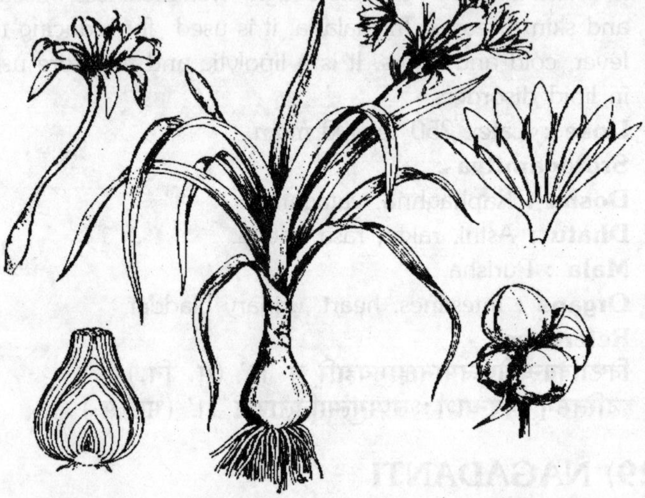

Kula : Valamuli kula.
Family : Amaryllidaceae.
Latin name : Crinum = long haired; asiaticum = of asia.
Sanskrit names : Sudarshana , Somavalli, Chakrangi, Madhuparnila.
Botanical Description : It is a perennial shrub, 2-3 mtrs. high. Leaves - one metre long and 9-10 cm. broad, green, appear as if sprouting from the soil. Flowers - white, emerging from the middle of the trunk. Flowering occurs from April to August. Fruit - slightly round.
Properties :
Guna : ruksha, tikshna; **Rasa** : madhur, tikta; **Vipak** : madhur; **Veerya** : ushna; **Dosha** : vatakaphanashak.
External uses : Juice of the leaves is used in otorrhoea and earache. Local fomentation as well as application of leaves is done in osteoarthritis. Local application of tuber in piles reduces the pain. It is insecticidal if leaves are hung in the house.
Internal uses : Used for removal of poison by emesis and diarrhoea, also used in oedema, skin diseases and especially in fever.
Parts used : Leaves and tuber.
Dose : Leaf juice - 0.5 gm.; tuber powder - 0.5 to 1 gm.
Srotogamitva :
Dosha : Vatakaphaghna.
Dhatu : Rakta.
Mala : Shodhan.
References -
स्वादूतिक्तोष्णा कफशोकास्त्रवाताजित् ।

(131) NARIKEL

Cocos nucifera Linn.

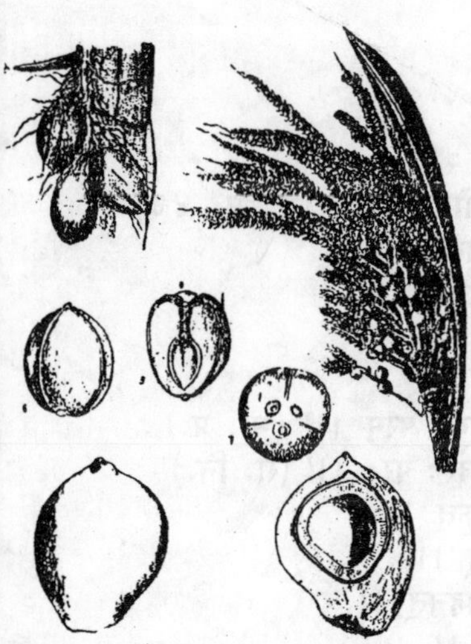

Kula : Narikel kula.

Family: Palmae (leaves resemble the palm of hand).

Latin name : Cocos = from the Portugese word coco = monkey.The nut resembles the head of a monkey; nucifera = (nuci = nut, fera = yielding).

English name : Coconut.

Sanskrit names : Naliker, Rasaphal, Sutung, Kurchasekhar, Neertaru, Mangalya, Dakshinatya, Duraruha, Jalakaranja.

Botanical Description : The tree is 13 to 20 mtrs. high with a trunk having diameter of 30 to 60 cms. The trunk is thick, blackish, showing circles on external surface.

Leaves - compound 4 to 5 mtrs. long. Leaflets -30 to 60 cms. long, green with pointed tips (vein is used for preparing broom). Stamen - small, yellow. Fruit - oval, large 15 - 25 cms. long, hard capsule and full of water. Flowering and fruiting occurs throughout the year.

Stages - 1) Young (only water inside the fruit), 2) Medium (water along with soft morrow) and 3) Mature (hard morrow with little water). Ultimately, only hard morrow remains without water.

Habitat : Sea shore (South India, Konkan, Bengal, Sri Lanka, Burma etc.)

Chemical composition : Elements useful to life are found at different stages of maturity. Matured fruit contains 60-70% oil with vitamins A and B.

Properties :

Guna : snigdha; **Rasa :** madhur; **Vipak :** madhur; **Veerya :** sheet; **Prabhav :** keshya;

Dosha : vatapittashamak.

External uses : Water from the fruit is applied in small pox to reduce the burning sensation. Oil is hair tonic. Kernel oil is best for skin diseases especially eczema. Oil is mixed with camphor. Powder of kernel mixed with dry ginger is used in oral infection.

Internal uses : Water is pittashamak, and is useful in indigestion, raktapitta, hiccups, dysuria, other urinary disorders, fever, excessive thirst and burning sensation.

Kshar - Strong purgative.

Oil - Antibacterial, useful in pthysis similar to cod liver oil.

Flowers - Astringent, useful in polyuria and bleeding per rectum.

Matured fruit - Aphrodisiac, emmenagouge and majjagami.

Fresh fruit - Anabolic.

Tender coconut - Useful in urinary disorders, hyperacidity, bleeding disorders, pain induced by pitta and as a carminative.

Parts used : Flower, fruit, root, kshar, oil, etc.

Dose : Fruit - 25 to 35gm.; oil -10 to 20 drops; kshar - 250 to 500 mgm. Sugar is used as antidote for indigestion caused by narikel.

One of the French revolutionaries, who was to be hanged, sent two flowers of Lilly, as remembrance to his daughter. He did this only 2 days before his execution.

Srotogamitva :
Dosha : Vataghna, pittaghna, kaphavardhak.
Dhatu : Rasa, rakta, shukra, mansa, meda, majja.
Mala : Mutra (diuretic), purisha (constipative - flower).
Prabhav : Keshya (oil).
References -

'नारिकेलफलानि च । बृंहणस्निग्धशीतानि बल्यानि मधुराणि च ।। (च. सू. २७)'
'नालिकेरं गुरु स्निग्धं पित्तघ्नं स्वादु शीतलम् । बलमांसप्रदं हृद्यं बृंहणं बस्तिशोधनम् ।।' (सु. सू. ४६)
'नारिकेलो दृढफलो लांगली कू र्चशीर्षकः । तुंगः स्कन्धफलश्चैव तृणराजः सदाफलः ।।
नारिकेलफलं शीतं दुर्जरं बस्तिशोधनम् । विष्टम्भि बृंहणं बल्यं वातपित्तास्रदाहनुत् ।।
विशेषतः कोमलनारिकेलं निहन्ति पित्तज्वरपित्तदोषान् ।
तदेव जीर्णं गुरुपित्तकारि विदाहि विष्टम्भि मतं भिषग्भिः ।।
तस्याम्भः शीतलं हृद्यं दीपनं शुक्रलं लघु । पिपासापित्ताजित् स्वादु बस्तिशुद्धिकरं परम् ।।' (भा. प्र.)
'नारिकेलो गुरुः स्निग्धः शीतः पित्तविनाशनः । अर्धपक्वस्तृषाशोषशमनो दुर्जरः परः ।।' (रा. नि.)
'नारिकेलं हिमं स्निग्धं स्वादुपाकरसं गुरु । तर्पणं प्रीणनं वृष्यं बृंहणं बलमांसकृत् ।।
विष्टम्भि दुर्जरं हृद्यं श्लेष्मलं बस्तिशोधनम् । दाहक्षतक्षयहरं वातपित्तास्रनाशनम् ।।'
तस्योदकं हिमं स्निग्धं मधुरं बस्तिशोधनम् । दीपनं शुक्रलं वृष्यं हृद्यं तृट्पित्तदाहनुत् ।।
नारिकेलोद्भवं तैलं बृंहणं बलवर्धनम् । केश्यं पित्तानिलहरं दन्त्यं मधुरमेव च ।।
'नारिकेलप्रसूनं तु रक्तपित्तप्रमेहनुत् । रक्तातिसारं हरति महालोहितनाशनम् ।।
शीतलं सोमरोगघ्नं विबन्ध कुरुते भृशम् ।' (कै. नि.)

(132) NIRVISHA
Delphinium denudatum

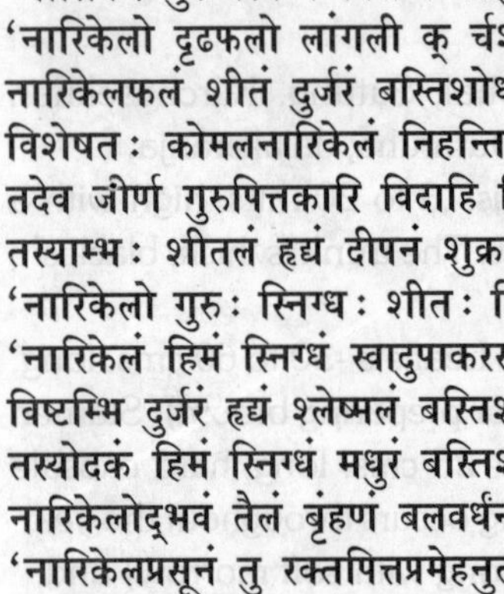

Kula : Bachanag kula.
Family : Ranunculaceae (marshy land).
Latin name : Delphinium = Dolphin - resemblance to the spur on the dolphin head; denudatum = nude, unclothed.
Sanskrit names : Nirvisha, Upavisha, Vishaha, Vishahantrika, Vivisha, Vishabhava, Avisha, Vishavairini.
Botanical Description : A very small herb. Five varieties are described in Unani medicine.
Habitat: Himalaya at the height of 3-4 thousand metres.
Properties :
Guna : laghu, ruksha; **Rasa :** tikta; **Veerya :** ushna; **Dosha :** tridoshashamak.
Uses : Local application of nirvisha is the best antidote in poisoning by snake, strychnine and digitalis.
Srotogamitva :
Dosha : Kaphaghna, vataghna.
Dhatu : Raktagami, mansavardhak.
Mala : Malashoshani.
Organ : Heart.

(133) NEELEE

Indigofera tinctoria Linn.

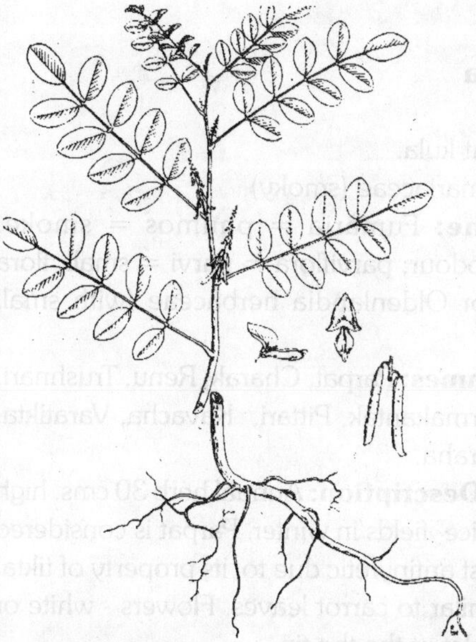

Kula : Shimbi kula (having legumes).

Family : Leguminoseae.

Latin name : Indigofera = Indigo = blue, fera = offering; tinctoria = of the dyer's.

English name : True indigo, Dyer's indigo (useful to dye maker).

Sanskrit names : Neela, Tutya, Radni, Kalika, Shyama, Shodhani, Gramya, Neelkeshi, Truni.

Botanical Description : A tree 2 to 2.5 mtrs. high with white trunk. Leaves - resemble Tephrosia purpurea. Flowers - blue or rose coloured. Legume - 1 to 2 fingers in length, bent at the tip containing 8-10 seeds.

Habitat : Bihar, Bengal, Orissa, Sindh, Madhya Pradesh, Maharashtra. Cultivation is reduced due to synthetic variety being available. Herb is kept under water to obtain 50% blue dye. It contains Indican.

Properties :

Guna : laghu, ruksha; **Taste :** tikta; **Vipak :** katu; **Veerya :** ushna; **Dosha :** kaphavatashamak.

External uses : Its lekhan property is useful for treating cataract and other eye conditions (seed powder).It is used as an analgesic in piles and rheumatoid arthritis. It is also useful in wound healing and skin diseases. Alcohol extract kills mites and lice. Leaves are used to dye and nourish hair.

Internal uses: It is useful in fainting,delirium, constipation, rheumatoid arthritis, hiccups, hepatosplenomegaly, worms, colic, gout, oedema, cough, breathlessness, calculus and anuria. In dog bite, 60 gms. of leaf juice with equal quantity of cow's milk is given to prevent hydrophobia. Root decoction is used in arsenic poisoning.

Dose : Panchang decoction - 60 to 100 ml.

Srotogamitva :

Dosha: Kaphavataghna.

Dhatu: Rakta, majja.

Mala: Purisha, keshya, mutra.

Organ: Intestine.

Prabhav: Antidote for rabies and arsenic poisoning.

References -

'नीली तु नालिनी तूली काला दोला च नीलिका । रञ्जनी श्रीफला तुत्था ग्रामिणा मधुपर्णिका ।।
क्लीतिका कालकेशीच नीलपुष्पा च सास्मृता । नीलिनी रेचनी तिक्ता केश्या मोहभ्रमापहा ।।
उष्णा हन्त्युदरप्लीहवातरक्तकफानिलान् । आमवातमुदावर्त्त मंदच विषमुब्दतम् ।।' (भा. प्र.)
'नीली तिक्ता रसे पाके सरोष्णा भ्रममोहकृत् । कफानिलहरा केश्या प्लीहोदरविषापहा ।।
वातरक्तमुदावर्त्तमामवातगदं हरेत् ।।' (कै. नि.)

Plants sense human feelings and emotions. Man too should also imbibe in him the language of plants.

'नीली तिक्ता रसे चोष्णा कटिवातकफापहा । केश्या विषोदरं हन्ति वातासृक्कृमिनाशिनी ।।' (ध. नि.)
'नीली तु कटुतिक्तोष्णा केश्या कासकफामनुत् । मरुद्विषोदरव्याधिगुल्मजन्तुज्वरापहा ।।' (रा. नि.)

(134) PARPAT
Fumaria parviflora

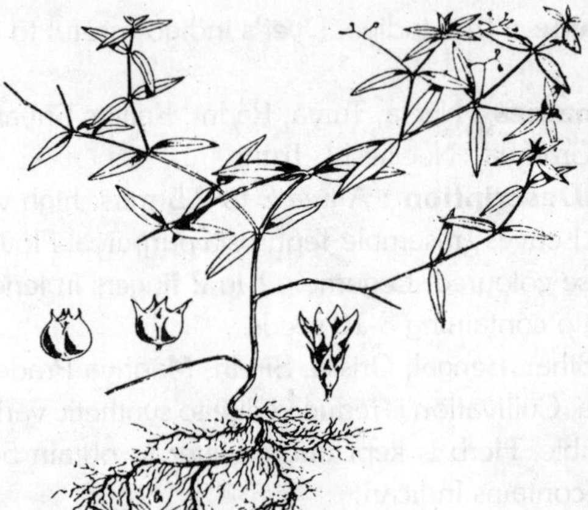

Kula: Parpat kula.
Family: Fumariaceae (smoky).
Latin name: Fumaria = phumos = smoke, unpleasant odour; parviflora = parvi = small, flora = flowers or Oldenlandia herbaceae (with small flowers).
Sanskrit names: Parpat, Charak, Renu, Trushnari, Kharak, Varmakantak, Pittari, Kavacha, Varatikta, Varak, Atisaraha.
Botanical Description: Annual herb 30 cms. high growing in rice fields in winter. Parpat is considered to be the best antipyretic due to its property of tikta. Leaves - similar to carrot leaves. Flowers - white or rosy red, violet at the the tip.

Habitat: On the bank of the Ganges and in the Himalayas.
Properties:
Guna: laghu; **Rasa:** tikta; **Vipak:** katu; **Veerya:** sheeta; **Dosha:** kaphapittanashak.
Uses : Useful in delirium, fainting,intoxication, excessive thirst, anorexia, loss of appetite, hepatomegaly, jaundice, bleeding disorders and gout. Fever, thirst and burning sensation are the symptoms for which parpat is the most useful remedy. It is useful in skin, liver and kidney diseases as it is excreted through these organs.
Srotogamitva:
Dosha: Pittaghna, kaphaghna and slightly vatavardhak.
Dhatu: Rakta (bleeding disorders), rasa (fever), rakta, majja (intoxication).
Mala: Purisha (constipative), sweda, mutra.
Organ: Skin, liver, kidney.
References -
'पर्पटो वरतिक्तश्च स्मृतः पर्पटकश्च सः । कथितः पांशुपर्यासयस्तथा कवचनामकः ।।
पर्पटो हन्ति पित्तास्रभ्रमतृष्णाकफज्वरान् । संग्राही शीतलस्तिक्तो दाहनुद्वातलो लघुः ।।' (भा. प्र.)
'पर्पटः शीतलस्तिक्तः पित्तश्लेष्मज्वरापहः । रक्तदाहरुचिग्लानिमदभ्रमविनाशनः ।।' (ध. नि.)
'पर्पटाः तिक्ताः पित्तकफापहाः ।' (सु. सू. ४६)
'शाकं पार्पटकं च यत् । कफपित्तहरं तिक्तं शीतं कटु विपच्यते ।।' (च. सू. २७)
'मुस्तपर्पटकोशीरचन्दनोदीच्यनागरैः शृतशीतं जलं देयं पिपासाज्वरशान्तये ।।' (च. चि. ३)

(135) PARUSHAK
Grewia asiatica Linn.

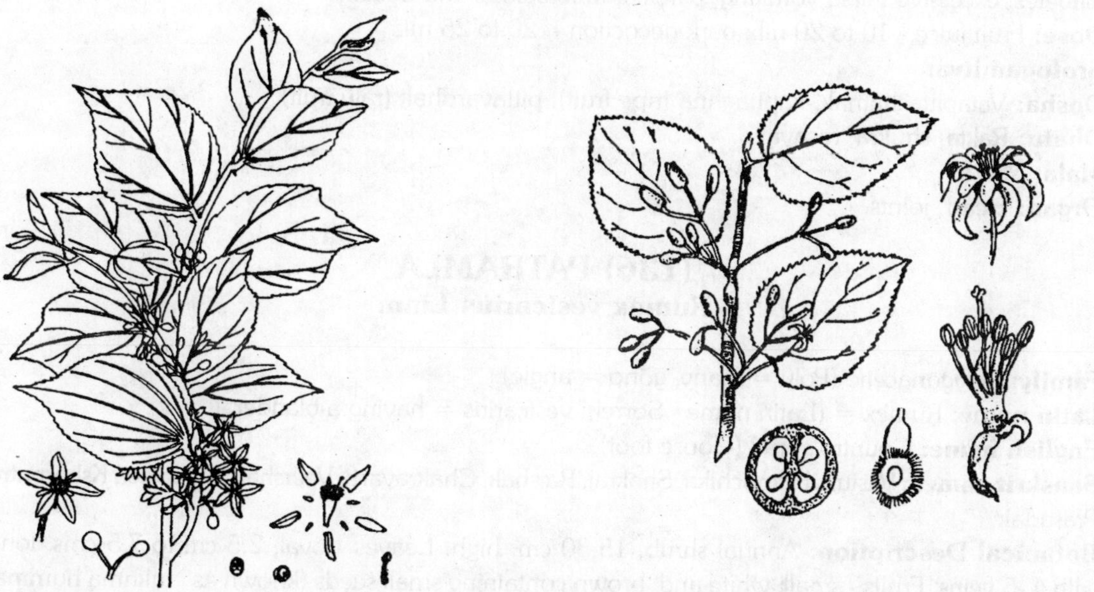

Kula: Parushak kula.
Family: Tiliaceae (resembling leaves of lemon).
Latin name: Grewia = after the name of a scientist, Grew Nehemiah; asiatica = of Asia.
Sanskrit names: Parushak, Neelparna, Giripilu, Alpagasthi, Atimandal, Roshan, Dhanvancchada, Parimandal. (Charaka includes this plant in Virechanopag, Shramahar, Jwarahar, Madhur varga and Asavyoni while Sushruta has described a separate parushakadi gana).
Botanical Description: A tree 8-9 mtrs. high,with grey bark. Leaves - borders are dentate. Flowers - small, yellow. Fruits - round, large, pea shaped, green when raw and pungent, brown when unripe. On ripening, they become violet and sweet.
Varieties: There are two varieties - 1) Amlavarga - Falasasharbati, raw is sour and ripe is sweet and juicy. 2) Madhurvarga - Falasashakari - raw is sweet-sour, ripe is sweet and less juicy.
Habitat: All over India.
Chemical composition: Fruit contains acid, sugar and a viscous substance.
Properties:
Guna: laghu, snigdha; **Rasa:** madhur, amla, kashaya; **Vipak:** madhur (ripe fruit), amla (raw fruit); **Veerya:** sheeta; **Dosha:** vatapittashamak, kaphavardhak, raw fruit - pittavardhak.
External uses: Paste of leaves and buds is applied on abscess. Paste of bark is used in osteoarthritis,while that of root is used for inducing abortion (applied on umbilicus, hypogastric region and external genitalia). Fruit infusion is used for gargle in oral conditions.
Internal uses: Used in anorexia, loss of appetite, diarrhoea, dysentery (raw fruit) whereas ripe fruit

When there was no language, the words flower and leaf were indicated by drawing their pictures.

is given in thirst and as an adjuvant to emetic drugs, also useful in heart diseases and bleeding disorders. Bark decoction is useful in rheumatoid arthritis, asthma, haematuria, burning micturation, diabetes, excessive thirst, vomiting, pyrexia, tuberculosis and debility.
Dose: Fruit juice - 10 to 20 ml.; bark decoction - 20 to 25 ml.
Srotogamitva:
Dosha: Vatapittashamak, kaphaghna (ripe fruit), pittavardhak (raw fruit).
Dhatu: Rakta, shukra, rasayana.
Mala: Mutra.
Organ: Heart, joints.

(136) PATRAMLA
Rumex vesicarius Linn.

Family: Polygonaceae (Poly = many, gono = angle).
Latin name: Rumex = (Latin name - Sorrel); vesicarius = having a bladder.
English name: Country sorrel (Goose foot).
Sanskrit names: Vastuk, Hilmochika, Shakraj, Rajshak, Chakravarti, Veershak, Shakveer, Ksharpatra, Prasadak.
Botanical Description: Annual shrub, 15-30 cm. high. Leaves - oval, 2.5 cm to 7.5 cms. long, with 4 -5 veins. Fruits - small, white and brown containing small seeds (known as `tukhma hummaj' in Unani science.) Leaves are consumed as vegetable.
Properties:
Guna:laghu, ruksha; **Rasa:** amla, madhur; **Vipak:** amla; **Veerya:** ushna; seeds are slimy and sheeta veerya; **Dosha:** vatashamak, kaphapittakar, seeds - pittashamak.
Uses : Leaves stimulate appetite and are digestive, hepatostimulant and laxative. Seeds are unctuous but constipative. It is used in anorexia, jaundice, colic and piles. In dysentery, it is used with isabgol. Also useful in palpitations.
Srotogamitva:
Dosha: Vataghna, kaphapittaghna, pittasarak.
Dhatu: Rakta.
Mala: Purisha (laxative), mutra.
Organ: Heart.
References -
'चुक्रिका स्यात्तु पत्राम्ला रोचनी शतवेधनी । चुक्रा त्वम्लतरा स्वाद्वी वातघ्नी कफपित्तकृत् ।।
रुच्या लघुतरा पाके वृन्ताकेनातिरोचनी ।' (भा. प्र.)
'चुक्रं स्यादम्लपत्रं तु लघूष्णं वातगुल्मनुत् । रुचिकृद्दीपनं पथ्यमीषत्पित्तकरं स्मृतम् ।।' (रा. नि.)

(137) PADMAKAM

Prunus cirasoidus Linn.

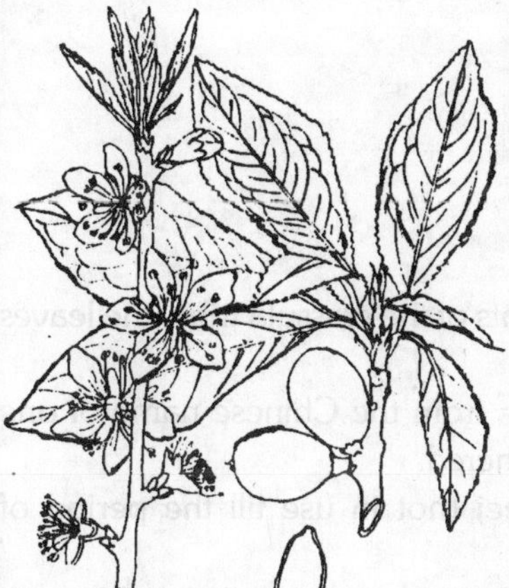

Kula: Taruni kula.

Family: Rosaceae.

Latin name: Prunus = frosted, snowy; cirasoidus or Prunus padum.

Sanskrit names: Padmakam, Preetak, Palay, Sheetal, Padmakashtha, Padmavriksha, Malaya, Hemapatra, Garbhasansthapan.

English name: Bird cherry.

Botanical Description: It is a large tree, very decorative after flowering. It is included in the Vedanasthapan, Varnya, Kashayskandh, Sarivadi and Chandanadi ganas, all of which contain pittashamak dravyas. Stalk is round, reddish with knobs and fragrant like lotus. Skin - brown. Flowers - whitish, brownish, appear through sepals. Fruits - round, astringent, sour, containing hard seed with slight flesh, useful for consumption. Fresh stalk should be used.

Habitat: Himalaya, Simla, Gadhwal, Sikkim, Nepal, Bhutan.

Chemical composition: Skin contains hydrocyanic acid.

Properties:

Guna: laghu, snigdha; **Rasa:** kashaya, tikta; **Vipak:** katu; **Veerya:** sheeta; **Prabhav:** tridoshahar;

Dosha: stalk - kaphapittashamak, bark - vatashamak.

Uses: External application of the paste is useful as refrigerant, anti-pruritic and complexion enhancer. When used internally, it acts as an appetite stimulant, digestive, astringent, analgesic, cardiotonic, diuretic (seeds), aphrodisiac, spermatogenic, febrifuge and antidermatosis. Due to these properties, it helps in the conditions of neurogenic pain, loss of appetite, laxity of stomach, vomiting, thirst, obesity, bleeding disorders, breathlessness, hiccups, abortion etc. It also acts as rejuvenating agent. Seed pulp is used in urinary calculi.

Dose: Bark - 0.5 to 2 gm.; infusion - 30 to 40 ml. Decoction should not be prepared and the bark should be used cautiously.

Srotogamitva:

Dosha: Tridoshahar prabhav, stalk - kaphapittaghna, bark - vataghna.

Dhatu: Rakta, shukra, meda, rasayan, rasa (febrifuge).

Mala: Mutra (calculus), seed (diuretic).

References -

'पद्मकः सूक्ष्मविछिन्नपत्रोऽद्रौ पादपोऽफलः । ईषत्पद्मसुगंधि स्यात् पद्मकं रक्तवल्कलम् ।।
पद्मकाष्ठं नवं ग्राह्यं रक्तपीतं च वर्णतः ।' (शि. द.)
'पद्मकं शिशिरं स्निग्धं कषायं रक्तपित्तनुत् । गर्भस्थैर्यकरं प्रोक्तं ज्वरच्छर्दिविषापहम् ।।
मोहदाहज्वरभ्रान्तिकुष्ठविस्फोटशान्तिकृत् ।' (ध. नि.)
'पद्मकं शीतलं तिक्तं रक्तपित्तविनाशनम् ।' (रा. नि.)

When alphabet was not evolved, flowers were used to convey messages.

'पद्मकं तुवरं तिक्तं शीतलं वातहल्लघु । विसर्पदाहविस्फोटकुष्ठश्लेष्मास्रपित्तनुत् ।।
गर्भसंस्थापनं वृष्यं वमिव्रणतृषाप्रणुत् ।' (भा. प्र.)
'उशीरकालीयकलोध्रपद्मक...। पृथक्पृथक्चन्दनतुल्यभागिकाः सशर्करास्तण्डुलधावनाप्लुताः ।।
रक्तं सपित्तं तमकं पिपासां दाहं च पीताः शमयन्ति सद्यः ।' (च. चि.)

(138) PARNABEEJ

Kalanchoe pinneta Pers.

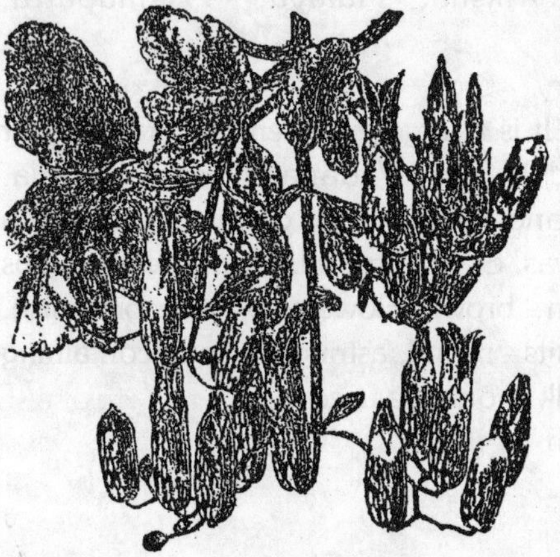

Kula: Parnabeej kula.
Family: Crassulaceae (plants of the crassula tribe, the leaves are fleshy and succulent).
Latin name: Kalanchoe = from the Chinese name of one the species; pinneta = feathered.
Sanskrit name: Parnabeej (not in use till the period of Vagbhatta).
Botanical Description: The height of the plant is 30 cm to 1 mtr. It is also known as panphuti, dhanvantari, etc. It contains three leaflets which are 10-20 cm. long and fleshy, oval, with serrated margins. Flowers - 2 inches long, red coloured. Legume - divided into four parts, contains plenty of seeds. Serrated margin bears reproductive capacity and can give rise to a new plant so it is called parnabeej. Large variety of parnabeej in Bengal is called himsagar.
Habitat: Tropical regions, Bengal.
Chemical composition: Leaves contain calcium sulphate, oxalate and tartaric acid.
Properties:
Guna: laghu, ruksha; **Rasa:** kashaya, amla; **Vipak:** madhur; **Veerya:** sheeta; **Dosha:** vatapittashamak.
Uses: Externally, it is used in bleeding wounds for hemostasis and healing. Internally, the juice of the leaves in a dose of 3 to 6 ml. is given in dysentery, bleeding piles and menorrhagia.
Srotogamitva:
Dosha: Vataghna, pittaghna.
Dhatu: Rakta, mansa.
Mala: Purisha (dysentery).

(139) PARNAYAVANI
Coleus amboinicus Benth.

Kula: Tulsi kula.
Family: Labiateae (lipped flowers).
Latin name: Colens = Gk, koleos = a sheath (refering to the way the base of the stamens are combined); amboinicus = ambo - pulpit = a raised platform.
English name: Country borage.
Sanskrit names: Parnayavani, Karpurvalli, Pashanbhedi.
Botanical Description: A perennial, hairy shrub, very frangrant and with bristly hair. Trunk is 30 cm. to 1mtr. high and delicate. Leaves - 6cm. long, dentate, thick with pungent smell. Flowers - small, violet, flowering at the end of winter and fruiting in summer.
Habitat: Originally from Malaysia. Now all over India.
Chemical composition: It contains a volatile oil and an essential principle called karvaerole.
Properties:
Guna: laghu, ruksha, tikshna; **Rasa:** katu, tikta; **Veerya:** ushna; **Dosha:** kaphavatashamak, anticonvulsive.
Uses: Internally, it is an optimum medicine for the alimentary system. It is used in anorexia., loss of appetite, indigestion, constipation, hepatosplenic disorders, abdominal colic, diarrhoea, duodenitis and intestinal worms. It is very effective in diarrhoea due to cholera; initially 15ml of the juice should be given followed by 8 ml. every two hours till diarrhoea stops. It is bacteriostatic but not bacteriocidal. Also useful in cardiac debility, cough, breathlessness, hiccups, dysuria and urinary calculi.
Dose: Leaf juice - 6 to 12 ml. (sedative in large dose).
Srotogamitva:
Dosha: Kaphaghna, vataghna.
Dhatu: Rasa, rakta.
Mala: Purisha (cholera), mutra (calculi).

(140) TALEES
Abies webbiana

Kula : Devdar kula.
Family : Conifereae (Latin - Conifer, cona = a scaly multiple fruit), pine family.
Latin name : Abies = a pine tree; webbiana = Mr. P. Barkar Webb, a naturalist).
English name : Himalayan silver fir.
Sanskrit names : Taleespatra, Shukodar, Arkavedha, Ghanacchada, Neelambar, Talipatra, Amalakipatra, Tulasipatra, Granthikapatra.
Botanical Description : A huge tree of 60 to 70 mtrs. high with diameter of 10 mtrs. Tender branches are small, grey and hairy. Leaves - 3 to 6 cms. long with bent tips and tips have two spines. Dorsally leaves are slimy while ventrally it has long medial line. Leaves arise like spring form the stem. Fruit - 16cm. long, oblong, violet or green. Seeds - winged and 2-3 cms. long. This plant is known by three different names, out of which thuner is a poisonous plant.

Anyone who destroys a plant which is a friend of mankind, is either a demon or a butcher.

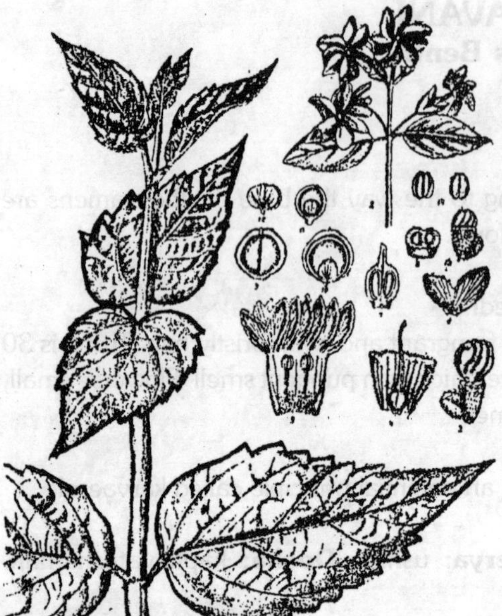

Habitat : In Bhutan, Afghanisthan and Baluchistan, at the height of 3 - 5 thousand mtrs.
Chemical composition : Leaves contain taxin and volatile oil.
Properties :
Guna : laghu,tikshna; **Rasa:** tikta; **Veerya:** ushna; **Vipak:** madhur; **Dosha:**kaphavatashamak.
External use : Analgesic.
Internal uses : Being an appetizer and carminative, it is used in anorexia, loss of appetite and flatulence. By tikta, katu, tikshna and ushna properties, it is useful in cough, asthma, hoarseness of voice and tuberculosis. Inflammation of urinary tract and dysuria are treated as it is a diuretic.
It is also used in fever due to vitiated vata and kapha, chest pain, general debility and pthisis.
Parts used : Leaves.
Dose: 1/2 to1 gm.
Formulations : Talisadichoorna, Talisadivati etc.

Strotogamitva :
Dosha : Vatakaphaghna.
Dhatu : Rasagami.
Mala : Urinary tract.
References -
तालीसपत्रं तिक्तोष्णं, मधुरं कफवातनुत् ।
कासहिक्काक्षयश्वासच्छर्दिदोषविनाशकृत् ।। (रा. नि.)

(141) PANAS
Artocarpus heterophyllus Lam.

Kula : Vata kula.
Family : Urticaceae (Lat. nettle) from urtice = toting property of the hairs of the plant.
Latin name : Artocarpus - artos = bread, carpos = fruit, bread fruit; heterophyllus - hetero = unequal, dissimlar leaved.
English name : Indian Jack tree.
Sanskrit names : Mahasarja, Phalin, Phalavrukshak, Kashtaphala, Aashay, Garbhakantak, Kantakiphal, Bruhatphal, Sthulkantaphala.
Botanical Description : A huge tree grows 15 - 20 mts. high. Leaves - thick with three veins. Flowers - unisexual. Fruit - 10-20 cms. long and 16-30 cm. broad having thorns all over the surface. It weighs about 5 to 20 kg. Pulp of unripe fruit is white while that of ripe is yellow. Seeds - 2.5 to 3 cm. long. slightly traingular and contains oil. It bears flowers in November and fruits in

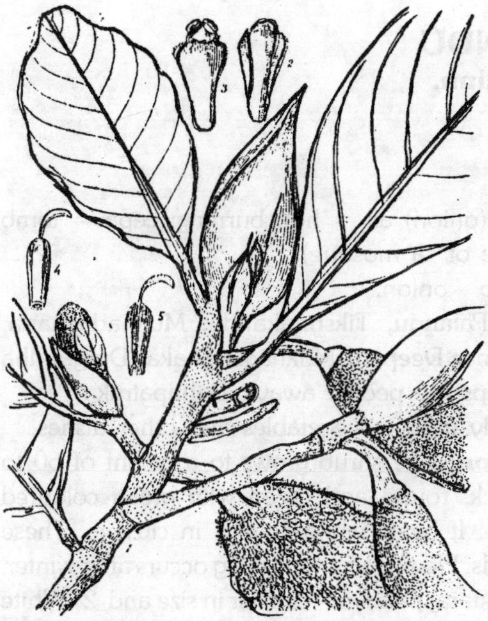

April and May. Furits also hang from the trunk. Fruits and seeds are edible. Seeds are roasted and eaten while fibrous part is cooked as vegetable.

Varieties : Two, 1) Kapa and 2) Barka.

Habitat : All over in India, specially in southern region.

Chemical composition : Ripe fruit contains 69.20% water. Seeds contain 41.95% starch and oil. Bark exudes a latex called phanasamba.

Properties :

Guna : guru, snigdha; **Rasa :** madhur, kashaya; **Vipak :** madhur; **Veerya :** sheeta; **Dosha :** vatapittashamak. (Raw fruit - kaphavatavardhak).

External use : Latex is used as antiinflammatory and wound healing agent. Phanasamba is effective in stomatitis.

Internal uses : Pulp is guru and constipative. Decoction of root is an astringent and is given in diarrhoea. Ripe fruit is spermatogenic, brimhan and used in bleeding disorders. Decoction of roots and leaves is useful in skin disorders while decoction of leaves is given as antidote to poisons.

Parts used : Roots and leaves.

Dose : Decoction of leaves and roots - 30 to 100 ml.

Srotogamitva :

Dosha : Vatapittaghana, kaphavardhak.

Dhatu : Ripe fruit - rakta (bleeding disorders), mansa (brimhan), shukra (aphrodisiac).

Mala : Purisha (constipative).

Because of its guru and constipative properties, it is contraindicated in disorders where shodhan is required.

References -

'पनसः कण्टकिफलः पनसोऽतिबृहत्फलः । पनसं शीतलं पक्वं स्निग्धं पित्तानिलापहम् ।।
तर्पणं बृंहणं स्वादु मांसलं श्लेष्म भृलंश । बल्यं शुक्रप्रदं हन्ति रक्तपित्तक्षतव्रणान् ।
आमं तदेव विष्टम्भि वातलं तुवरं गुरू । दाहकृन्मधूरं बल्यं कफमेदोविवर्धनम् ।।
पनसोभ्दूतबीजानि वृष्याणि मधुराणि च । गुरूणि बद्धविट्कानि सृष्टमूत्राणि संवदेत् ।।
मज्जा पनसजो बृष्यो वातपित्तकफापहः । विशेषात् पनसो वर्ज्यो गुल्मिभिर्मन्दवह्निभिः ।' (भा. प्र.)
'पनसं सकषायं तु स्निग्धं स्वादुरसं गुरु ।' (सु. सू. ४६)

As much as the desired effect of guna is increased by medicines so much, in equal proportion, the medicine will decrease the undesirable effects of the opposite guna.

(142) PALANDU

Allium cepa Linn.

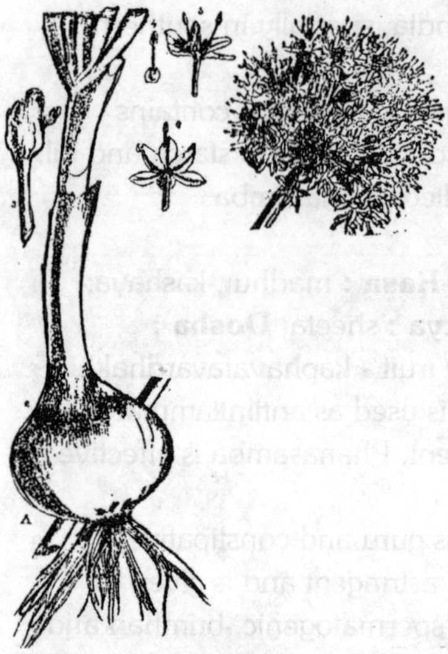

Kula: Rason kula.
Family: Liliaceae.
Latin name: Allium (onion) all = hot, burning; cepa = tomb (shaped like the dome of a mosque).
English name: Bulb - onion.
Sanskrit names: Palandu, Tikshnakanda, Mukhadushana, Shudrapriya, Krumighna, Deepan, Mukhagandhaka, Durgandha (one onion a day keeps the people away), Bahupatraka.
This plant is commonly used in vegetables and other dishes.
Botanical Description: The shrub grows to a height of 60 to 90 cms. Leaves - thick, round and green with green coloured flower stalk at the top. It bears white flowers in clusters. These produce triangular seeds. Flowering and fruiting occurs after winter.
Varieties: 1) Red - raktaraj palandu - smaller in size and 2) White - shwetakshir palandu - larger in size.
Habitat: All over India. Onions growing in Maharashtra are large in size.
Chemical composition: It contains an oil having pungent taste and offensive smell, sulphur, quercetin, sylapicrin, syllamarin, syllanine etc.
Guna: guru,snigdha; **Rasa:** madhur,katu; **Vipak:** madhur; **Veerya:** ushna. Onions decrease vata and increase pitta.
External use: Analgesic, antiinflammatory, tonic, enhances eyesight and reduces otalgia. Pain due to bronchitis is controlled with a warm poultice of grated onion. In skin infections, onion is applied externally as a poultice. In weak eyesight, onion juice mixed with honey is used as eye drops. In ear ache, warm onion juice is used as eardrops.
Internal uses: Onions reduce vata and cause an increase in raja and tama. It is therefore useful in arthritic pain, sciatica, hysteria and hydrophobia. It improves digestion and helps in constipation, piles and jaundice. Onions are also used in rectal prolapse. It is useful in cardiac debility, bleeding disorders, dry cough, dysuria, azoospermia, impotency, dysmenorrhoea, cholera, plague and skin diseases.
Dose: Juice - 10 to 30ml. Seed powder - 1 to 3 gms. Onions are not beneficial to those with pittaprakruti and brain weakness. The antidote in these cases is pomegranate juice.
Srotogamitva:
Dosha: Vataghna, kaphapittavardhak.
Dhatu: Majja; rakta (raktapitta, kamala); shukra (vrushya).
Mala: Purisha (cholera), mutra (dysuria).
Manovahasrotasa: Amedhya.

References -
‘पलाण्डुर्यवनेष्टश्च दुर्गन्धो मुखदूषकः । पलाण्डुस्तु गुणैर्ज्ञेयो रसोनसदृशो बुधैः ।।
स्वादुः पाके रसेऽनुष्णः कफकृन्नातिपित्तलः । हरते केवलं वातं बलवीर्यकरो गुरुः ।।’ (भा. प्र.)
श्लेष्मलो मारुतघ्नश्च पलाण्डुर्न च पित्तहृत् । आहारयोगी बल्यश्च गुरुर्वृष्योऽथ रोचनः ।। (च. सू. २७)
‘नात्युष्णवीर्योऽनिलहा कटुश्च तीक्ष्णो गुरुर्नातिकफावहश्च ।
बलावहः पित्तकरोऽथ किञ्चित् पलाण्डुरग्निं परिवर्धयेत्तु ।।
स्निग्धो रुचिष्यः स्थिरधातुकारी बल्योऽथ मेधाकफपुष्टिदश्च ।
‘बीजं पलाण्डोः वृष्यं स्यात् दंतकीटप्रमेहजित् ।’ (नि. र.)
‘रसखड्यूषयवागूसंयुक्तः केवलोऽथवा जयति ।
रक्तमतिवर्त्तमानं वातञ्च पलाण्डुरुपयुक्तः ।।’ (च. चि. ९)
‘लशुनानन्तरं वायोः पलाण्डुः परमौषधम् ।
यस्योपयोगेन शकाङ्गनांना लावण्यसारादिविनिर्मितानाम् ।
कपोलकान्त्या विजितः शशाङ्को रसातलं गच्छति निर्विषण्णः ।।
स्निग्धाङ्गत्वं गौरता कान्तिमत्ता वह्नेर्दीप्तिश्चर्मशुद्धिर्वृषत्वम् ।
सम्प्राप्यन्ते यन्त्रणोद्वेगयुक्तैर्यस्याभ्यासाद्दीर्घमायुः सुखं च ।।
लभते बलवर्णौजः स्वरसौमनस्यतेजांसि ।
क्षीणशकृत् बधिरोऽपि च रसोनवत्तद्रसं पीत्वा ।।’ (गदनिग्रह)

(143) PLAKSHA
Ficus lacor Buch - Ham.

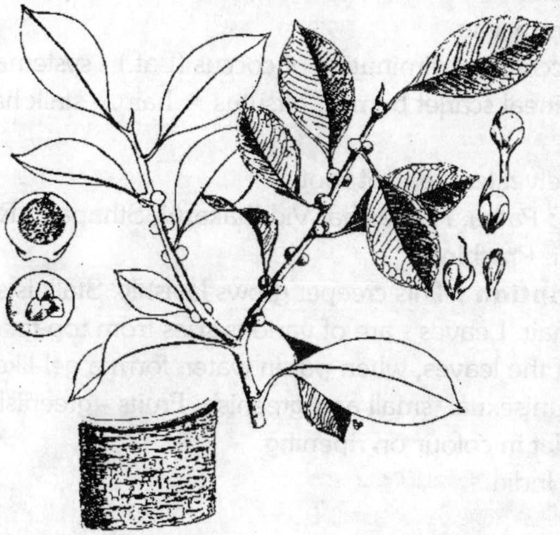

Kula : Vata kula.
Family : Urticaceae.
Gana : Mutrasangrahaneeya, Kashayskandha (C.); Nyagrodhadi (S.); Kshirivriksha, Panchavalkal (Bh.).
Latin name : Ficus = from an original Arabic word meaning fig; lacor = or thespasia populuca = divine.
English name: Wave leaved fig tree.
Sanskrit names : Plaksha, Jati, Parkati, Pakativruksha, Pakar.
Botanical Description : It is a huge tree with a greenish grey bark. Leaves - resemble the leaves of Ficus racemosus but are smaller. Leaves have 4 -10 pairs of veins. Leaf-stalk is sour. Fruits - whitish, round and small. Flowering occurs in summer and fruiting in monsoon.
Habitat: All over India.
Properties:
Guna: laghu, ruksha; **Rasa:** kashaya; **Vipak:** katu; **Veerya:** sheeta; **Dosha:** kaphapittashamak.
External use : It possesses hemostatic, antiinflammatory and wound healing properties. It is

The words guna and dosha are mutually related. Therefore as often as one thinks of gunas, one has to think of doshas too and vice-versa.

therefore useful for application in bleeding, inflammation, erysipelas and wounds in the form of ointment or powder. It is also used for gargles in stomatitis.

Internal use : Since it is a tranquiliser, it is used in conditions like delirium, fainting, giddiness etc. It is useful in diarrhoea and dysentery as an astringent. As it is a hemostat, it is useful in bleeding disorders. Its decoction is used for vaginal douche as well as orally in menorrhagia and leucorrhoea. A vaginal suppository made from its powder can also be used. In diabetes, it acts as antidiuretic. A widely used local ointment for burns contains plaksha.

Dose : Bark decotion - 50 to 100 ml.

Srotogamitva :

Dosha: Kaphaghna, pittaghna.

Dhatu : Rakta.

Mala: Purisha.

Organ: Vagina, brain (fainting, delirium).

References -

'प्लक्षः कषायः शिशिरो व्रणयोनिगापहः । दाहपित्तकफास्रघ्नं शोथहा रक्तपित्तहत् ।।
रक्तदोषहरो मूर्च्छाप्रलापभ्रमनाशनः ।' (भा. प्र.)

(144) PATAL GARUDI

Cocculus hirsutus

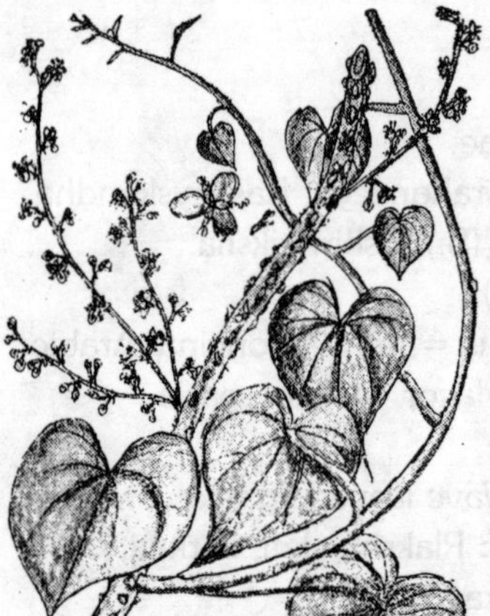

Kula : Guduchi kula.

Family : Menispermaceae.

Latin name : Cocculus = diminutive of coccus (Lat.) - systematic name for the cochineal scarlet berries; hirsutus = hairy - stalk has white hair.

English name: Velvet leaf, parrot root.

Sanskrit names : Patha, Ambastha, Viddhakarni, Sthapani, Rasa, Ekashthila, Papveli, Prachina.

Botanical Description : This creeper grows lavishly. Stalk is soft with white bristly hair. Leaves - are of various sizes from top to bottom. Powder of the leaves, when put in water, form a gel-like colloid. Flowers - unisexual, small and greenish. Fruits - greenish when raw and violet in colour on ripening.

Habitat: All over India.

Properties :

Guna: laghu, snigdha, pichchil; **Rasa :** katu; **Vipak:** katu; **Veerya:** ushna; **Prabhav:** antitoxin; **Dosha:** tridoshaghna.

External use: Application of the paste is used as an antitoxic and soothing agent.

Internal use: Since it is an appetizer, digestive and purgative, it is helpful in loss of appetite. It is useful in bleeding disorders. It is useful in many disorders of blood and also in bronchitis. Its juice is used as an aphrodisiac. Its juice mixed with sugar, is used in burning micturation, anuria and gonorrhoea. Root is locally applied in snake bite.

Srotogamitva:

Dosha: Kaphaghna, vataghna.

Dhatu: Shukra, rakta.

Mala : Mutra (reduces burning micturition).

Organs : Respiratory system.

It is useful as an antidote in snake bite.

References -

हिलहिण्टो महामूल: पातालगरुडाह्वय: ।
छिलिहण्ट: परं वृष्य: कफघ्न: पवनापह: ।। (भा. प्र.)

(145) PARIS

Thespesia populnea

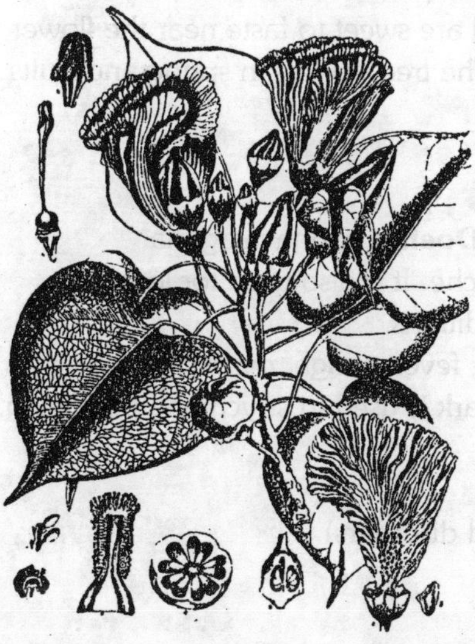

Kula : Karpas kula.

Family : Malvaceae.

Latin name : Thespesia = divine, frequently planted about temples and churches; populnea = (public) poplar like.

English name : Heart wood, Portia tree, Tulip tree.

Sanskrit names : Paris, Phalish, Kapichudha, Kapitan, Pushpashvattha. The colour of the flowers changes in the evening.

Botanical Description : The tree is known as paris, paras pimple, etc. It is a huge tree having leaves which resemble pipal leaves. It bears large, yellow flowers. Fruit contains thick yellow latex. Bark and ripe fruits are used in medicine. Branches are very strong and elastic and therefore they are used in making parallel bars.

External use : Ash of ripe fruits mixed in oil is applied in skin disorders like scabies, ringworm and eczema. Internally, decoction of bark is also given in the same disorders.

Srotogamitva :

Dosha: Kaphaghna.

Dhatu: Rasa, rakta.

Mala : Sweat glands.

The seven dhatus constitute the stable foundation of the body and only that treatment is the best which is not obstructive to these. On the other hand, it reinforces their strength.

(146) PARIBHADRA
Erithrina variegata

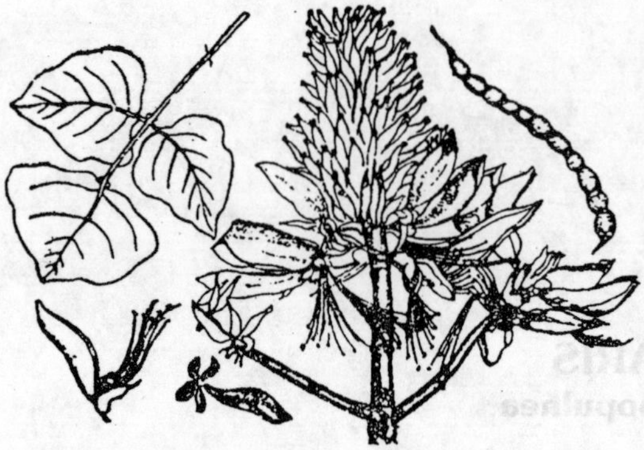

Kula : Shimbi kula.
Family : Leguminoseae.
Latin name : Erithrina = Erithros = red (Gk.) - colour of the flowers; variegata = variagated, diversify in colours - flowers marked with irregular patches of different colours.
English name : Indian coral tree.
Sanskrit names: Paribhadra, Phalabhadra, Raktakeshar, Kantaki, Parijatak, Kantakiparijatak. (Latex of the leaf is applied on corns.)
Botanical Description : This thorny tree is 3-8 mts. high. Leaves - three in number. Flowers - red in colour and are sweet to taste near the flower stalk. Legumes - contain 3 to 8 seeds which are 2.5 cms. long. The tree flowers in spring and fruits in summer.
Habitat : Found in gardens and jungles all over India.
Properties:
Guna: laghu, tikta; **Rasa:** katu; **Vipak:** katu; **Veerya:** ushna; **Dosha:** kaphavataghna.
External uses : Juice of the leaves is used as ear drops in earache. It is also used for local application in swelling, skin disorders, wounds and otorrhic conditions.
Internal uses : It is used in convulsions, insomnia, dermatoses, fever, cough, dysuria, dysmenorrhoea and lipid disorders. An alkaloid present in the bark is used in strychnine poisoning.
Srotogamitva :
Dosha: Kaphaghna, vataghna (flowers - pittaghna).
Dhatu: Rakta (dermatoses), rasa (dysmenorrhoea), meda (lipid disorders).
Mala: Mutra (dysuria).
Organs: Uterus, genital organs.
References -
पारिभद्रोऽनिलश्लेष्मसोफमेदःकृमिन्हरेत् । तत्पुष्पं पित्तरोगघ्नं कर्णव्याधिविनाशनम् ।। (कै. नि.)
पारिभद्रः कटूष्णः स्यात्कफवातनिकृन्तनः । अरोचकहरः पथ्यो दीपनश्चापि कीर्त्तितः ।। (रा. नि.)

(147) PASHANBHED
Bergenia ligulata Wall.

Kula : Pashanbhed kula.
Gana : Mutravirechaneeya, Veertaradi.
Family : Saxifragaceae - amarantanceae (Saxi = rock breaking).
Latin name : Bergenia = after the name of K.A. Von Bergen, German Botanist; ligulata = strap like or Colus aromaticus.

English name: Iris sp.
Sanskrit names: Pashanbhed, Ashmaghna, Shilabhed, Ashmabhedak, Upalbhadi, Nagbhid, Shiligarbhak, Pashan, Ashmabhedan.
Botanical Description : This small herb survives for many years and is found in hilly and rocky regions. Its stalk emerges from the cracks in the rocks. Root is 2.5 cm. thick and red in colour. Leaves - round, 7.5 to 12.5 cm. in diameter, fleshy, dentate, greenish on the upper surface and reddish on the lower surface. Flowers - whitish, brownish or bluish.
Habitat : Himalayas at the height of 2 thousand mtrs.
Chemical compostion : It contains tannic acid, gallic acid, starch, calcium oxalate etc.
Properties :
Guna: laghu, snigdha, tikshna; **Rasa:** kashaya, tikta, **Veerya:** sheeta; **Prabhav:** ashmarighna (lithotripsic); **Dosha :** tridoshashamak.
External uses : It is antiinflammotry, wound healing, hemostatic, cardiotonic, antipyretic and antitoxic. Its local application is useful in conjunctivitis. In teething problems, it is rubbed with honey on the gums.
Internal uses : It is used in diarrhoea, dysentery, tumours, piles, splenomegaly, heart diseases, bleeding disorders, cough, leucorrhoea, menorrhagia and dysmenorrhoea. But it is especially useful in urinary calculi and dysuria. It is also useful in turbidity of urine. It is an antidote to morphine.
Dose : Root 1 to 3 gms.
Srotogamitva:
Dosha: Tridoshaghna.
Dhatu: Rakta (bleeding disorders, splenomegaly, menorrhagia), raktamansa (wound healing), rasa (dysmenorrhoea), asthi (teething problems).
Mala : Mutra (urinary calculi).
Prabhav : Lithotripsic.
Organ : Urinary bladder, heart, uterus.
References -
अश्मभेदो हिमस्तिक्तः कषायो बस्तिशोधनः । भेदनो हन्ति दोषाशोंगुल्मकृच्छ्राश्महृद्रुजः ।।
योनिरोगान् प्रमेहांश्च प्लीहशूलव्रणानि च ।' (भा. प्र.)

(148) PARIJATAK

Nyctanthus arbortristis Linn.

Kula: Parijatak kula.
Family: Oleaceae. Olive tree tribe.
Latin name: Nyctanthus (Nyct = night; anthus = flowering (night flowering); arbortristis = (Arbor = tree, tristis = weeping, gloomy, flowers dropping like tears).
English name: Night jasmine.
Sanskrit names: Shefalika, Mandar, Rajpushpi, Parijatak, Prajakta, Harishringar, Pushpak, Nalkumkumak, Kharapatrak. (Red stalks of flowers are cut, dried in the sun and stored to be used

To start the treatment by employing vishaushadhi (poison-drugs), is a feature of intellectual bankruptcy. It is also an insult of the human body.

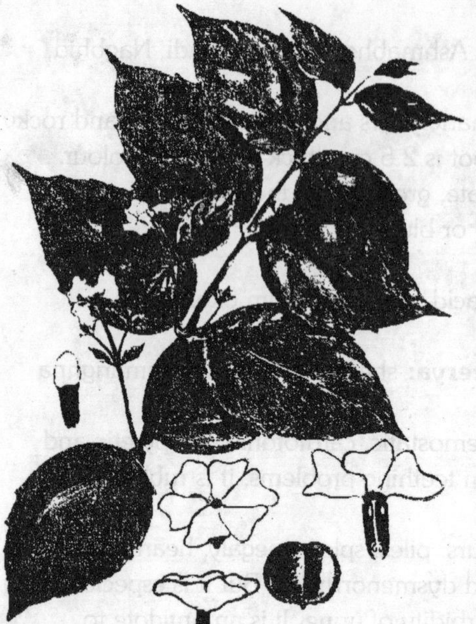

for dying clothes and as a colouring agent for sweets and other eatables. Poets in India have compared the lips of beautiful women to the flowers of this tree.)

Botanical Description: A tree of 3 - 10 mts height. Leaves - facing forwards, 10 to 12.5 cm long, 5 to 6.25 cm broad, rough. Upper surface is green and the lower surface is white. Petals are yellowish red and very attractive in appearance. Therefore it is compared to the lips of a young lady. Flowers - white, fragrant and delicate. Flowers bloom in the night and fall off in the morning on the ground below the tree. Ovary is flat, bilobular with two seeds. (Children play with these seeds and call them as coins).

Habitat: All over India. Flowers contain fragrant oil, flowering occurs in monsoon.

Properties :

Guna: laghu, ruksha; **Rasa** : tikta; **Veerya:** ushna; **Dosha:** kaphavatahar and pittashodhan. **Uses** : Seeds are used as antihelminthics and in alopecia. Rough leaves are used for scrapping the margins of wounds. Leaf juice is used in loss of appetite, piles, liver disorders, biliary disorders and intestinal worms. Powder prepared from leaves or bark is given in cough and asthma. Also useful in dysuria, chronic fever and snake poisoning. Decoction of leaves is very useful in fever with rigors.

Dose: Juice of leaves - 10 to 20 gms.; powder - 1 to 5 gunja.

Srotogamitva:

Dosha: Kaphaghna, vataghna, pittashodhak.

Dhatu: Rakta (liver - leaf juice).

Mala: Hair (seeds), mutra (dysuria - barkpowder), sweda (decoction of leaves).

Organ: Respiratory tract (cough - decoction of leaves).

References -

'शेफालिः कटुतिक्तोष्णा रूक्षा वातक्षयापहा । स्यादङ्गसंधिवातघ्नी गुदवातादिदोषनुत् ।।' (रा. नि.)

'प्राजक्तः पारिजातश्च हारिशृंगारपुष्पकः । नालकुंकुमको रागपुष्पी च खरपत्रकः ।।' (नि. सं.)

'रसः प्राजक्तपत्रस्य ज्वरघ्नो तिक्तकः स्मृतः । पर्णखण्डसमायुक्ता त्वचा कासविनाशिनी ।।

(149) PEELU

Salvadora persica

Kula : Peelu kula.

Family : Salvadoraceae. Kiknel oil plant ?

Gana : Virechan, Virechanopag, Shirovirechan, Jwarhara, Katu.

Latin name : Salvadora = Salvadore - Spanish Botanist; persica = peach - old generic and latin name.

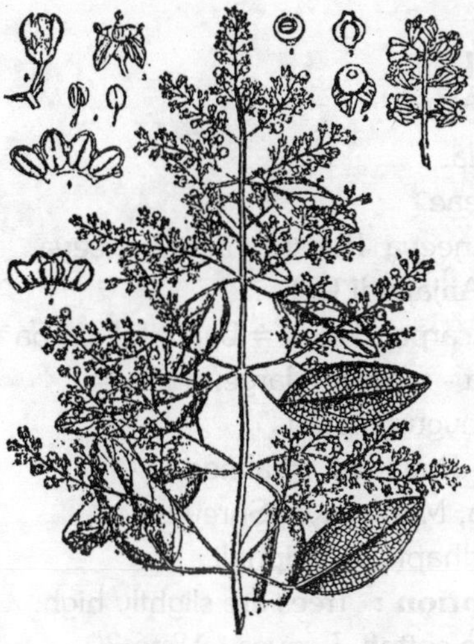

English name : Toothbrush tree.
Sanskrit names : Small variety - Peelu, Sheetasaha, Gudphala, Virekphal, Shakhi, Shyam, Karabhapirya. Large variety - Mahapeelu, Rajpeelu, Mahavriksha, Madhupeelu, Teekshnavriksha.
Botanical Description : The shrub grows from 0.3 to 1 mt. high. Trunk is uneven with numerous branches which are bent downwards and break easily. Leaves - facing upwards, fleshy, thick, oval, 2.5 to 5 cm. long and 2.5 cm. broad. Flowers - greenish, grow at the tip of the branches. Fruits - very small, fleshy, red on ripening and give a pungent odour on breaking. Fruit contains a single seed. Flowering is followed by fruiting in summer. Large variety is called brihat peelu (Salvadore oleoides).
Habitat : Iran , Afghanisthan, Punjab, Sindh, Baluchisthan, Rajasthan, Gujarat, South India and Sri lanka. Bark also gives a pungent smell.
Chemical composition : Bark of root contains resin, pigments, trimethylamine and chlorine. Fruit and seeds also contain different chemical substances.
Properties:
Guna : laghu, singdha, tikshna; **Rasa :** katu, tikta madhur; **Veerya :** ushna; **Dosha :** kaphavatashamak, pitta vardhadk; **Ripe fruit :** madhur vipaki and anushna, therefore tridoshahara.
External use : Seed oil being antiinflammatory and analgesic, is used in rheumatoid arthritis for massage. Root bark is irritant and causes rash, itching and burning by applying on the skin. Warm leaves are applied locally in piles, tumours and painful joints. Branches are used as tooth brush. Seed powder and bark of root is applied in snake bite.
Internal uses : Ripe fruit acts as a laxative, seeds as purgative and leaves as purifier. Flowers and fruits are inhaled to give relief in common cold and breathlessness by clearning respiratory passage. Fruit juice is used for nasal administration in worm infestation of the nasal cavity. Fruit is used in impotency and root bark in amenorrhoea.
Parts used : Fruit, seed, root, skin, leaves.
Dose : Fruit juice - 5 to 10 gms.; seed powder - 1 to 3 gms; leaf powder - 1 to 3 gms.; seed oil is called as kharvan taila.
Srotogamitva :
Dosha : Kaphaghna, vataghna, pittavardhak.
Dhatu : Shukra , rasa.
Mala : Purisha (ripe fruit - laxative), nasal worm infestation.
Organ : Respiratory tract.
References -
'तिक्तं पित्तकरं तेषां सरं कटु विपाकि च । तीक्ष्णोष्णं कटुकं पीलु सस्नेहं कफवातजित्‌ः । (सु. सू. ४६)
'पीलु... दोषघ्नं गरहारि च ।' (च. सू.२७)
'पीलु श्लेष्मसमीरघ्नं पित्तलं भेदि गुल्मनुत्‌ । स्वादु तिक्तं च यत्‌ पीलु तन्नात्युष्णं त्रिदोषहृत्‌ ।।' (भा. प्र.)

Before including from the thousands of plants some as medicinal plants "whether or not these are harmful to our body?" must be found out.

(150) PRIYANGU

Callicarpa macrophylla Vaul.

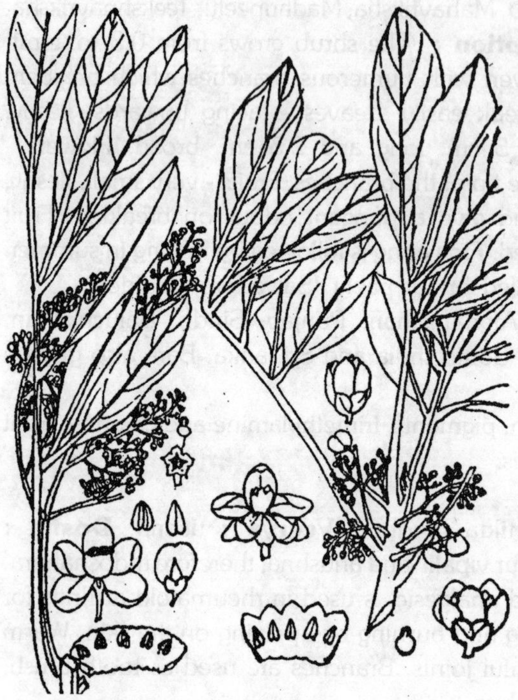

Kula : Nirgundi kula.
Family : Verbeneceae.
Gana : Mutravirajaneeya, Purishasangrahaneeya (C.); Priyangvadi, Anjanadi (S.).
Latin name : Callicarpa - kalos = beautiful, carpa = fruit; macrophylla - macro = large, philla = leaved (or Aglaria roygurghiana).
Sanskrit names : Priyangu, Phalinee, Parnabhedini, Peeta, Mangalaya, Shreyasi, Varnabhedini, Gandhaphali, Striphali.
Botanical Description : Trees are slightly high. Branches - hairy like cotton. Leaves - 18 to 30 cms.long, rectangular with sharp tips and serrated margins. Smooth from upper surface and hairy from ventral surface. Flowers - small, pink appear in inflorescence. Fruits - fleshy, white divided into four compartments each having a single seed. Ripe fruits look spongy.
Varieties : Two, 1) Priyangu and 2) Gandhapriyangu which is called as gavhala in marathi.
Habitat : Himalaya, Grass land, Baluchistan.
Properties :
Guna : guru, ruksha; **Rasa :** tikta, kashaya, madhur; **Vipak :** katu; **Veerya :** sheeta; **Dosha :** tridoshaghna.
External uses : Useful in burning sensation, headache, excessive perspiration, ulcers and rheumatoid arthritis.
Internal uses : Used in painful conditions. Also useful in loss of appetite, colic, tumors, dysentery, blood disorders, bleeding disorders, pittaprameha , skin disorders, general debility and poisons.
Dose : Gandhapriyangu powder - 200 to 500 mgs; Priyangu powder - 1 to 2 gms. and Priyangvadi taila.
Strotogamitva:
Dosha : Tridoshaghna.
Dhatu : Rakta (diarrhoea with bleeding per rectum, blood disorders, skin diseases and bleeding disorders).
Mala : Purisha, mutra (pittaprameha), excessive perspiration (external use).

References -
'प्रियंगुः शीतला तिक्ता तुवरानिलपित्तहृत् । रक्तातीसारदौर्गन्ध्यस्वेददाहज्वरापहा ।।
गुल्मतृड्विषमेहघ्नी तद्वद्गन्धप्रियंगुका ।' (भा. प्र.)
'प्रियंगुः शीतला तिक्ता मोहदाहविनाशिनी । ज्वरवान्तिहरा रक्तमुद्रिक्तं च प्रशामयेत् ।।' (ध. नि.)
'गन्धप्रियंगुः शोणितपित्तातियोगप्रशमनानाम् श्रेष्ठा ।' (च. सू. २५)
'पीतः प्रियंगुकाकल्कः । सक्षौद्रस्तण्डुलाम्बुना । रक्तस्रावं जयेच्छीघ्रं धन्वमांसरसाशिनः ।।' (च. चि. १०)

(151) PEETAMOOLA
Rueum emodi Wall.

Kula : Chukra kula.
Family : Polygonaceae (having many angles).
Latin name : Rueum; emodi = from the Himalayan mountains.
English name : Indian rubarb.
Sanskrit names : Amlaparni, peetamula, Revandachini.
Botanical Description : A tree 1.5 to 2 mtr. high. Bark - greenish grey. Trunk - thick, long with many thick branches bearing leaves. Leaves - resemble pippal leaves but smaller and their stalks are 30 - 40cms. long. Flowers - resemble flowers of Calotropis procera. Fruits - violet and 1.5 cm. long. Root - large, thick, browinsh yellow. It turns saliva yellow when chewed. Leaves and branches are sour to taste. It bears flowrs and fruits in monsoon.
Habitat : Many varieties are found in Himalaya where it grows at the height of 3-4 thousand mtrs. and also in Sikkim and China.
Chemical composition : Leaves contain Oxalic acid while root contain acids, resin, mucin, tannic acid, starch, pectine etc.
Properties:
Guna : laghu, ruksha, tikshna; **Rasa :** tikta, kashaya, katu; **Veerya :** ushna; **Dosha :** kaphapittahar.
External uses : Useful in skin diseases and inflammatory conditions.
Internal uses : In small dose of 120 to 350 mgs, it causes salivation, increases appetite, stimulates liver and acts as an astringent. Large dose (1 to 1.5 gm) increases intestinal secretions, peristalsis and causes purgation. It also developes gripping pain and stops diarrhoea abruptly due to its astringent property. It acts as an expectorant, diuretic and is useful in amenorrhoea and general debility. Also useful in children's diarrhoea.
It is excreted through breast milk, urine and stool.
Dose : Root 120 mgs. (as a tonic), 1 to 2 gms. (as a purgative).
Srotogamitva :
Dosha : Kaphapittahar.
Dhatu : Rasa (acts on breast milk and appetizer), rakta (liver stimulant).
Mala : Purisha (astringent), mutra (excreted through urine).

Shlokas on the plants describing their guna-karma, also indicate their dosh-dhatu-mala gamitva. This point of view should be understood.

(152) PUNNAG
Calophyllum inophyllum

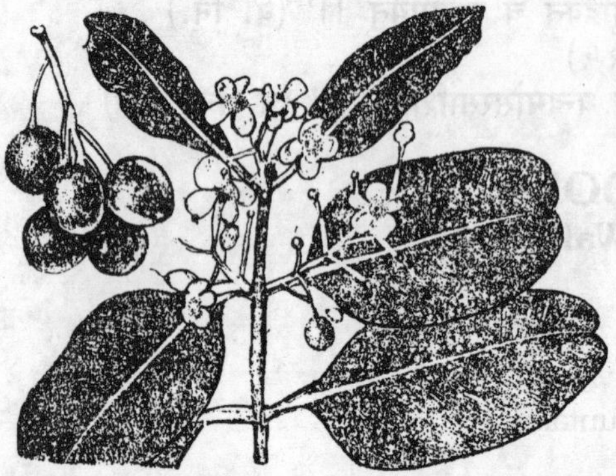

Kula : Nagkesar kula.
Family : Guttifereae. Yielding gum, resin or dye.
Latin name : Calophyllum - kalos = beautiful, phyllum = leaved; inophyllum - ino = fibrous, leaved.
English name : Alexandrian laurel (Pinne oil tree).
Sanskrit names : Punnag, Purusha, Rakta vriksha, Devavallabh, Surapanika, Sugandhipushpa, Surapati, Champak.
Botanical Description : A evergreen beautiful tree 7-8mtrs. high. Leaves - oval like that of banyan tree. Flowers - white and fragrant. Fruits - ripe fruits are round and yellow. They occur in rainy season. Seeds - contain oil.
Habitat : Coastal region of India and fruits are found floating on sea water.
Properties :
Guna : laghu, ruksha; **Rasa :** madhur, kashaya; **Vipak :** madhur; **Veerya :** sheeta; **Dosha :** kaphapittashamak.
External uses : Oil is lekhan, analgesic and alleviates vata. Latex has wound healing property.
Internal uses : It has astringent, diuretic and hemostatic properties. Decoction of bark is used in diarrhoea, dysentery, bleeding disorders. Seed oil is used in dysuria and pyuria.
Strotogamitva :
Dosha : Pittaghna, kaphaghna, vataghna (oil).
Dhatu : Rakta (hemostat), bark - bleeding disorders.
Mala : Purisha (astringent), mutra (diuretic), seed oil - dysuria, bark -diarrhoea and dysentery with bleeding per rectum.
Organs : Intestine, liver and urinary tract.
References -
पुन्नागो मधुरः शीतः सुगंधिः पित्तनाशकृत् (रा. नि.)

(153) PISHACH KARPAS
Abroma augusta

Kula : Pishach karpas kula.
Family : Sterculiaccae. Buddha's coconut.
Latin name : Abroma - A = not, broma = food. If eaten it has ill effects; augusta = majestic, exalted.
Engilsh name : Devil's cotton.
Botanical Description : A small tree 3 mtrs. high. Threads come from stem bark. Flowers - violet, hanging downwards and appear in bunches. Fruits - pentagonal with five compartments containing

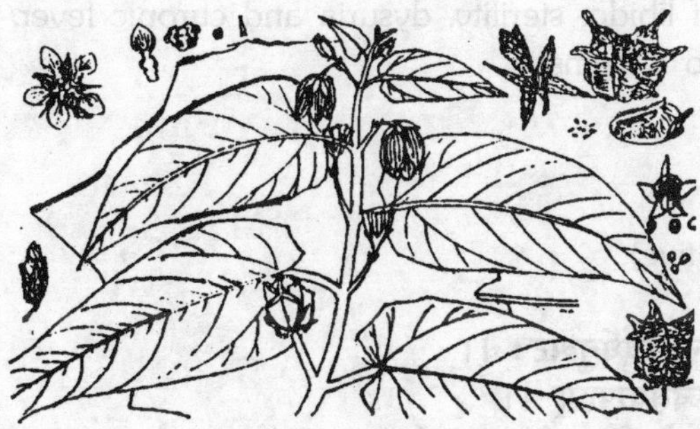

plenty of black seeds. It blossoms in the month of August and September.

Habitat : Bengal and Sikkim.

Properties :

Guna : laghu, ruksha (roots) and tikshna, snigdha (leaves); **Rasa** : katu, tikta; **Vipak** : katu; **Veerya** : ushna; **Dosha** : kaphavatashamak.

Uses : It mainly acts on the uterus as a tonic, stimulant and emmenagogue. It is useful in dysmenorrhoea and also regularises the menstrual flow. It is given three days prior and two days after the menstrual cycle. Also useful in pyuria.

Strotogamitva :

Dosha : Kaphaghna, vataghna.

Dhatu : Rasa (emmenagogue).

Mala : Mutra (gami - pyuria).

Organ : Uterus (tonic).

(154) PRIYAL

Buchanania latifolia

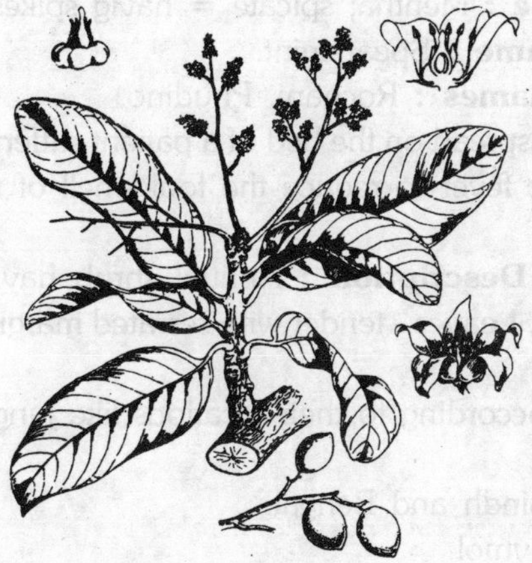

Gana : Udarda prashaman, Shramahar.

Kula : Amra kula.

Family : Anacardiaceae. Monkey nut like.

Latin name : Buchanania = Dr. Bhuchanan Hamilton; latifolia = broad leaved.

Sanskrit names : Priyal, Kharaskandh, Bahalvalkal, Snehabeej, Lalan, Tapaspriya, Charoli, Chiraunji, Karaka.

English name : Kaddappa almond.

Priyal is heavy to digest and generates ama dosha.

Botanical Description : A tree 16 mtrs. high. Bark - 3cm. thick and rough. Leaves - broad and long. Flowers - occur at the tip of branches, blue, white . Fruits - round, slightly flat, black, fleshy and mild sour to taste. Fruitpulp is small, white and oily.

Habitat : Grows in hilly region.

Chemical Composition : It contains 28% pulp and seeds contain 58% fixed oil.

Properties :

Guna : snigdha, guru; **Rasa** : madhur; **Vipak** : madhur; **Veerya** : sheeta; **Dosha** : vatapitta shamak.

External uses : Its powder is used for rubbing in skin disorders and pruritus. Oil is used in lymphadenitis and hair fall.

Generally, the malayanas which give rise to the disease are not even examined. Then the possibility of treating these, based on such findings, is indeed remote.

Internal uses : It is useful in cough (seeds), loss of libido, sterility, dysuria and chronic fever.
Dose : Bark decoction - 30 to 100 ml; priyal -12 to 24 gms.
Strotogamitva :
Dosha : Vataghna, pittaghna (fruitpulp).
Dhatu : Shukra (seeds), mansa - meda (brimhan).
Mala : Mutra (dysuria), purisha (fruitpulp - constipative).
References -
प्रियालस्तु खरस्कन्धश्चारो बहुलवल्कलः । राजादनस्तोपसेष्टः सन्नकद्रुर्धनुष्पटः ।।
चारः पित्तकफास्रघ्नस्तफलं मधुरं गुरु । स्निग्धं सरं मरुत्पित्तदाहज्वतृषापहम् ।।
प्रियालमज्जा मधुरो वृ,यः पित्तानिलापहः । हृद्योऽतिदुर्जरः स्निग्धो विष्टम्भी चामवर्धनः ।।' (भा. प्र.)
'वातपित्तहरं वृष्यं प्रियालं गुरु शीतलम् । प्रियालमज्जा मधुरो वृष्यः पित्तानिलापहः ।। (सु. सू. ४६)
'गुरुष्णस्निग्धमधुराः..... बलप्रदाः । वातघ्नाः बृंहणाः वृष्याः कफपित्ताभिवर्धनाः ।।
प्रियालमेषां सदृशं विद्यादौष्ण्यं विना गुणैः ।' (च. सू. २७)
'प्रियालतैलं मधुरंगुरुश्लेष्माभिवर्धनम् । हितमिच्छन्ति नात्यौष्ण्यात् संयोगे कफपित्तयोः ।। (च. सू. २७)

(155) PUTIHA
Mentha spicate

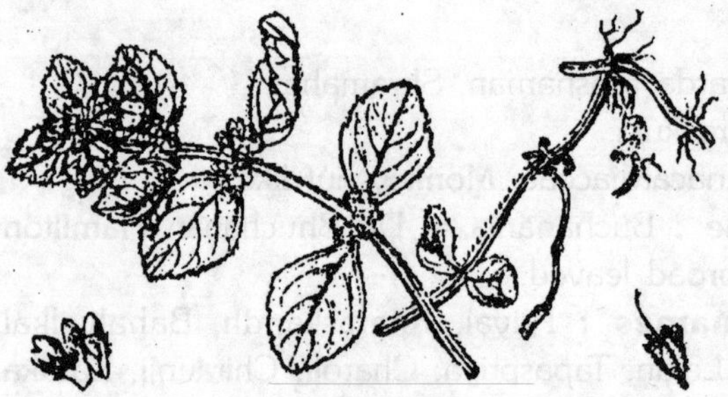

Kula : Tulasi kula.
Family : Labiateae, lipped flowers.
Latin name : Mentha; spicate = havig spikes.
English name : Spear mint.
Sanskrit names : Rochani, Phudino.
(Leaves are spread on the bed of a patient suffering from enteric fever to reduce the foul smell of the body).
Botanical Description : Annual shrub having strong smell. Leaves - tender with serrated margins. Flower stalk bears inflorescence all around .
Varities : It has many varieties. They are also classified according to their locations like jungle, mountains and narshy land.
Habitat : All over India, mainly in Himalaya, Kashmir, Sindh and Bengal.
Chemical composition : Leaves and flowers contain thymol.
Properties :
Guna : laghu, ruksha, tikshna; **Rasa :** katu; **Vipak :** katu; **Veerya :** ushna; **Dosha :** kaphavatashamak.
External uses : Analgesic, deodorant, antiseptic and wound healing. Its oil is also is used. Leafjuice mixed with water is used for gargles as a mouth freshner. Leaves are spread on the patient's bed suffering from fever.
Internal uses : Its paste is used as an appetizer, antiemetic, carminative and anthelmintic. Juice is used in cardiac debillty, cough, asthma, hiccups. It is also useful in dysuria, amenorrhoea, dysmenorrhoea, puerperal fever, skin diseases, common fever and poisoning.

Dose : Leaf juice - 10 to 20 ml; hot infusion - 20 to 40 ml; oil - 2 to 3 drops. Pudina extract is available in the market.

Strotogamitva :

Dosha : Kaphaghna, vataghna.

Dhatu : Mansa (wound healing), rasa (amenorrhoea, dysmenorrhoea, puerperal fever and typhoid).

Mala : Purish (anthelmintic).

Organs : Digestive system, respiratory system (deodorant).

References -

'पूतिहा कटुरुष्णश्च रोचनो दीपनो लघुः। हन्ति वातकफाध्मानशूलच्छर्दिकृमींस्तथा ।' (स्व)

'रोचनी वह्निजननी वक्त्रजाड्यनिषूदनी । कफवातहरी बल्या छर्दरोचकवारिणी ।।' (व. द.)

(156) PUTRANJEEVAK

Putranjiva roxburghii Roxb.

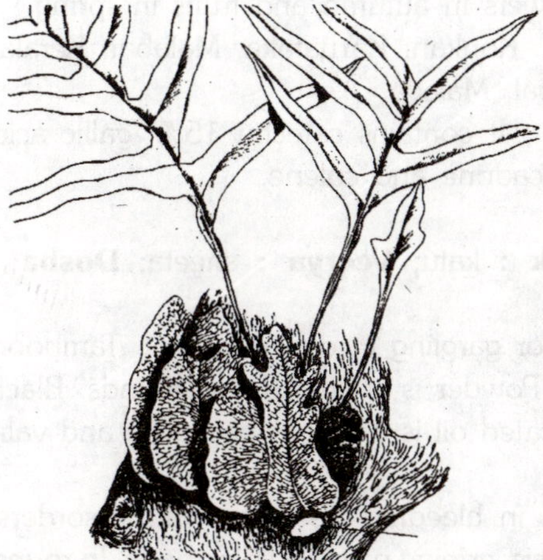

Kula : Eranda kula.

Family : Euphorbiaceae (scientist's name).

Latin name : Putranjiva = name of the plant, roxburghii = from Roxburgh - scientist's name.

Sanskrit names : Putranjeev, Pavitra, Garbhad, Sutajeevak, Kutajeeva, Apatyajeeva, Siddhid, Arthasadhak, Garbhakar.

Habitat : Tropical territory of India.

Botnical Description : A medium high tree.

Properties :

Guna : guru, ruksha; **Rasa** : madhur, lavan, katu; **Vipak** : katu; **Veerya** : sheeta; **Dosha** : vatakaphanashak.

External uses : Its paste is useful as an analgesic in headache, inflammation and abscess.

Internal uses : Aphrodisiac and bebeficial to foetus. Decoction of leaves and fruits is given in fever and common cold.

Parts used : Leaves, fruits, seeds.

Strotogamitva :

Dosha : Vatakaphaghna.

Dhatu : Shukra, artav (beneficial to foetus).

Mala : Purisha, mutra.

References -

पुत्रजीवो गुरुर्वृष्यो गभ्दिः श्लेष्मवातहृत् । सृष्टमूत्रमलो रूक्षो हिमः स्वादुः कटुः कटु ।।

पुत्रजीवो हिमो वृष्यः, श्लेष्मदो गर्भजीवदुः । चक्षुष्यं, पित्तशमनो, दाहस्तृष्णाहरो 'नृपे' ।।

श्लेष्मवातहरः प्रोक्तो वेद्यैर्मदनपालके । सृष्टमूत्र मलापघ्नो, भावे गुरु कटुः पटूः ।।

It is indeed difficult to understand the depth of the genius of the Sages and Munis who founded Ayurveda; the depth is awesome.

(157) PUGA

Areca catachu Linn.

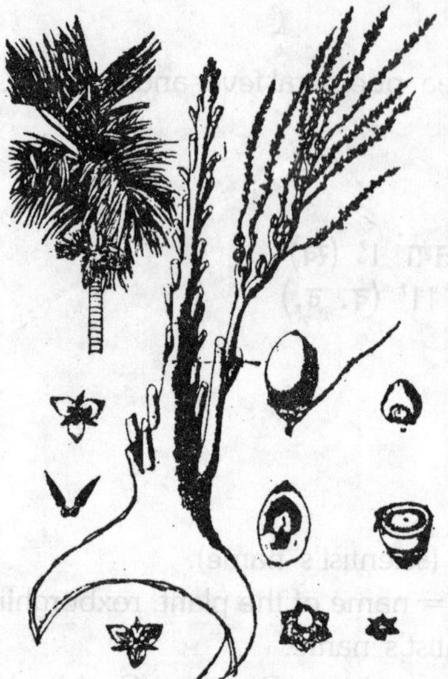

Kula : Narikel kula.

Family : Palmeae. Palm plants.

Latin name : Areca = old name from Malabar; catachu = derived from catechu, betle nut.

Sanskrit names : Kramuk, Puga, Pugavriksha, Deerghapadap, Vallataru, Drudhavalka, Chikkan, Guvak, Shupari.

Botanical Description : A tree 10-15 mtrs. high having no branches. Leaves - 1.5 to 2 mtrs. Leaflets - 30 to 50 cms. long, slender and hairy. Flower stalk - hard and branched. Fruits - appear in bunches, 3 - 6 cms, round, smooth and hard. Green when unripe and yellowish red when ripes. Catachu is obtained after removing the hard rind. It bears flowers in autumn and fruits in spring.

Habitat : Tropical region, Konkan, Karnataka, Malabar, Kerala, Tamil Nadu, Assam, Bengal, Malaya.

Chemical composition : It contains catechu 15%, gallic acid 14%, ericolin, ericane, ericadrine and colene.

Properties :

Guna : guru, ruksha; **Rasa** : kashaya, madhur; **Vipak** : katu; **Veerya** : sheeta; **Dosha** : kaphapittanasak, trioshashamak - roasted with sand.

External uses : Hemostatic and wound healing. Used for gargling in oral disorders. Tampoon dipped in its decoction is kept in vagina in leucorrhoea. Powder is sprinkled on wounds. Black powder of nut is used in tooth powder. Massage of medicated oil is useful in backache and vata diseases.

Internal uses : It reduces blood pressure and is useful in bleeding disorders, vata disorders, stomatitis and bad breath. Over dose results in hyperperistalsis, griping pain and diarrhoea. In round and flat worms, 3 gm. betle nut + 2 gm. lemon juice (or 250 ml. of milk) given after a fast of 12 to14 hours kills and expells the worms. Also useful in anorexia, loss of appetite, spermatorrhoea, leucorrhoea and polyuria.

Dose : Nut - 1to 3 gms. It is intoxicant because of its vikasi guna. In such condition water, milk and milk products should be used.

Strotogamitva :

Dosha : Kaphaghna, pittaghna (tridoshaghna if roasted with sand).

Dhatu : Rakta (hemostatic, wound healing - externally), shukra (spermatorrhoea), majja (intoxicant).

Mala : Purisha (anthelmintic), mutra (polyuria).

References -

'पूगं गुरु हिमं रूक्षं कषायं कफपित्तजित् । मोहनं दीपनं रुच्यमास्यवैरस्यनाशनम् ।।
आर्द्र तद् गुर्वभिष्यन्दि वह्निदृष्टिहरं स्मृतम् । स्विन्नं दोषत्रयच्छेदि दृढमध्यं ततुत्तमम् ।।' (भा. प्र.)
('गव्यकरीषघ्राणाज्जलपानाल्लवणभक्षणाद्वापि ।
शाम्यति पूगीफलमदश्चूर्णरजः शर्कराकवलात् ।।' (ग. नि.)

(158) BADARAM

Zizyphus sativus

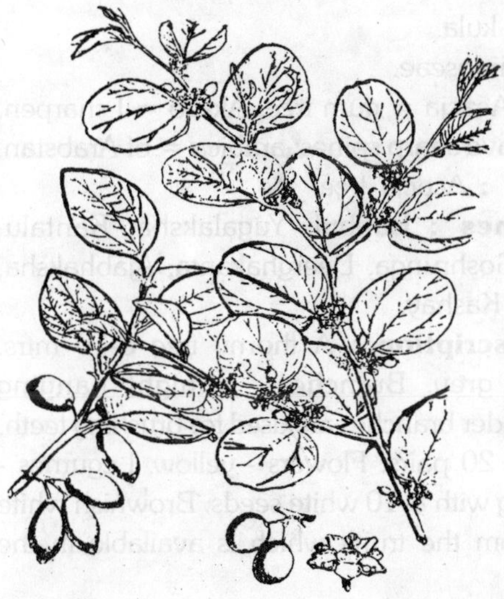

Gana : Hrudya, Hikkanigrahan, Udardaprashaman, Aragvadhadi, Vatashamanadi.

Kula : Badar kula.

Family : Rhamnaceae Buckthorn (Rhamnus family).

Latin name : 1) Zizypus = Egyptian name; sativus = cultivated.

2) Rajbadar - Zizypus jujuba.

3) Kshudra badar - Zizypus nummularia = monkey wort like, round and flat like a coin.

Varieties : There are three varieties viz. 1) Sauveer - large, sweet and grows in Marwar, 2) Kol - medium and 3) Karkandhu - wild variety.

Another five varieties - 1) Karkandu, 2) Badar, 3) Kol, 4) Sauveer and 5) Sitrachatee. Fruit size becomes bigger in ascending order.

English name : Jujube, Bherefruit tree, Indian plums.

Sanskrit names : Karkandhu, Badari, Kol, Phenil, Kuval, Sauveer, Ajapriya, Koli, Visham, Abhaykantak.

Botanical Description : There are three main varieties namely, 1) Rajbadar 2) Badar and 3) Kshudrabadar. It is a medium sized tree with spikes. Bark - grey and torn. Rajbadar variety is used in medicine.

Habitat : Kashmir, Iran, Afghanistan, China and all over India.

Properties :

Guna : guru, snigdha, picchil; **Rasa** : amla, madhur, kashaya; **Vipak** : madhur; **Veerya** : sheeta; **Dosha** : vatapittashamak.

External uses : Paste of the leaves has refrigerant, wound cleaning and healing properties. It is also used to treat abscess.

Strotogamitva :

Dosha : Vataghna, pittaghna.

Dhatu : Mansa (wound healing), rakta (splenomegaly).

Mala : Acts on intestines.

Organ : Spleen.

One should not compromise the basic principles of Ayurveda but in other matters, changes suitable to the times are inevitable.

(159) BABBUL

Acacia arabica Wild.

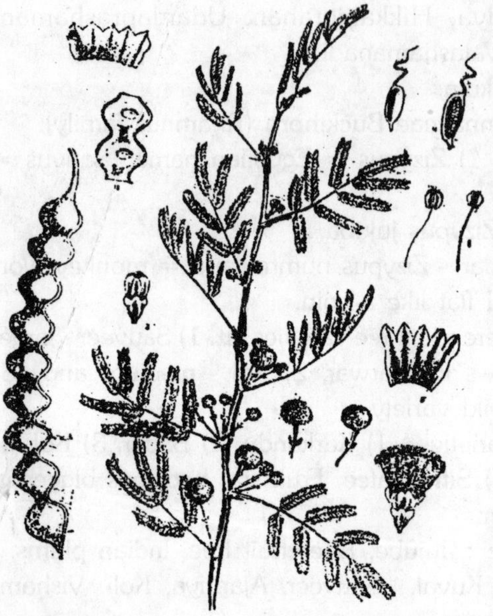

Kula : Shimbi kula.

amily : Leguminoseae.

Latin name : Acacia = gum tree, Akazo = I sharpen, many species have sharp spines; arabica = of Arabstan.

English name : Acacia tree.

Sanskrit names : Babbul, Yugalaksha, Kantalu, Tikshakantak, Goshrunga, Deerghakanta, Ajabhaksha, Sukshmapatra, Kashay.

Botanical Description : A thorny tree 8-10 mtrs. high. Trunk - grey. Branches - straight hanging downwards. Tender branches are used for brushing teeth. Leaflets - 10 to 20 pairs. Flowers - yellow. Legumes - 7 to 10cms. long with 8-10 white seeds. Brownish white gum exudes from the trunk which is available in the market.

Habitat : All over India.

Chemical composition : Bark and legumes contain an astringent principle.

Properties :

Guna : guru, ruksha; **Rasa** : kashaya; **Veerya** : sheeta; **Dosha** : kaphapittashamak.

Gum - Guna : guru; **Rasa** : madhur, kashaya; **Vipak** : madhur; **Veerya** : sheeta; **Dosha** : vatapittashamak.

External uses : Being a blood purifier, hemostatic, vasoconstricting and healing property , its powder is sprinkled on burnt injuries and bleeds. Decoction of bark is used for uttar basti (enema through vagina) in leucorrhoea. It is also used for tub bath in rectal prolapse and for gargles in oral disorders.

Internal uses : Useful in diarrhoea, dysentery, piles, helminthiasis, bleeding disorders, cough and urinary disorders. Gum is used in dysuria and loss of libido. In premature ejaculation, powder of raw legume + sugar is found useful.

Dose : Bark decoction - 30 to 80 ml; powder of legumes - 3 to 6 gms; paste -4 gms; and gum - 3 to 6 gms.

Formulations : Babbularishta, Lavangadi vati.

Strotogamitva :

Dosha : Kaphaghna, vatapittaghna (gum).

Dhatu : Rakta (purifier, hemostatic,wound healing, bleeding disorders), muscles (tub bath in rectal prolapse), shukra (aphrodisiac - gum), asthi (joining property).

Mala : Purisha (dysentery), mutra (urinary disorders).

References -
'बब्लूल:कफनुद्र ग्राही कुश्ठक्रिमिविषापह:।' (भा. प्र.)
'बब्लूलस्य तु निर्यासो ग्राही पित्तानिलापह: । रक्तातिसारपित्तास्रमेहप्रदरनाशन: ।।
भग्नसंधानक: शीत: शोणितस्रुतिवारण: ।' (आ.सं.)
'बब्लूलस्य फलं रूक्षं विशदं स्तम्भनं गुरु । कषायं मधुरं शीतं लेखन कफपित्तहत् ।।' (नि. र.)

(160) BAKULA

Mimusops elingi Linn.

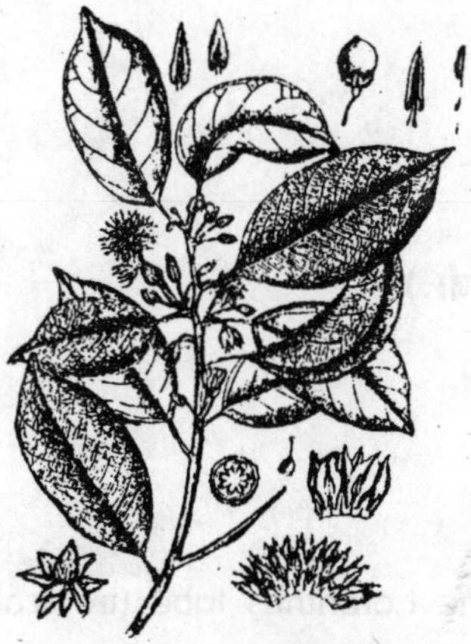

Kula : Madhuk kula.
Family : Sapotaceae (Plants of the sapota, vegetable egg tribe).
Gana : Dantadardhyakar.
Latin name : Mimusops = mimo = an ape, monkey flower; elingi = Malayan name.
English name : Mimusops.
Sanskrit names : Bakul, Sidhugandha, Madhupushpa, Sthirkusum, Shardik, Karak, Goodhapushpa, Madyamoda, Madhugandha.
Botanical Description : This evergreen tree is 15 mtrs. high and provides a thick shade. Bark is ash coloured an broken. Trunk is hard, heavy, brownish externally and red from inside. Leaves - 9 cm. long and 6 cm. broad, pointed with serpentile ends. Flowers - white in colour and give out a sweet fragrance even on drying. Flowers are preserved by making garlands out of them. Fruits - oblong, green when raw, astringent and sticky. Ripe fruits are yellow, sweet and easily breakable. Flowering season lasts for 6 months from April-May. Male plant bears flowers only whereas female plant bears flowers and fruits. The flowers, fruits and plants of brihat bakul are larger.
Habitat : All over India, especially in Konkan, Burma, Sri Lanka.
Chemical composition : Bark is astringent, flowers contain volatile oil. Seeds contain stable (non volatile) oil while the pulp of fruit contains sugar.
Properties :
Guna: guru; **Rasa:** katu, kashaya; **Veerya:** anushna; **Dosha:** kaphapittaghna.
External uses : Flowers act as nervine tonic and generate freshness of mind. Powder of the flowers is used for nasal administration in headache. Bark powder is used for strengthening gums and teeth and in pyorrhoea.
Internal uses : Decoction of the bark is astringent and is therefore used in diarrhoea, dysentery and intestinal worms. Alcoholic extract of flowers is useful in heart diseases as it acts specifically on the heart and blood. Flowers and bark have good hemostatic activity and are therefore used in menorrhagia, leucorrhoea, spermatorrhoea, cystitis, gonorrhoea etc. Ripe fruits are used as general tonic.
Dose: Decoction of the bark - 50 to 100ml.; powder of flowers - 1 to 2 gms.; fruits - used as a food item.

In a living human being mutually opposite twenty gunas interplay harmoneously, day and night; both the actions are occuring together.

Formulation: Bakuladya taila.
Strotogamitva :
Dosha : Kaphapittaghna.
Dhatu : Majja, rakta, shukra.
Mala : Purisha (astringent).
Organs : Urinary bladder, heart.
References -
'बकुलस्तुवरोऽनुष्णः कटुपाकरसो गुरुः । कफपित्तविषश्वित्रकृमिदन्तगदापहः ।।' (भा. प्र.)
'तत्फलं मधुरं स्निग्धं कषायं विशदं हिमम् । कफपित्तहरं हृद्यं दन्त्यं ग्राहि च वातलम् ।।' (कै. नि.)
'सुगन्धि विशदं हृद्यं बाकुलम्' (सु. सू. ४६)
'दन्तचाले तु गण्डूषो बकुलत्वक्कृतो हितः'
चलदन्तस्थिरकरं कुर्याद्बकुलचर्वणम् । (च. द.)
'दन्तास्तु बीजैबकुलद्रुमस्य स्थानच्युता अप्यचला भवन्ति ।' (शो.)
'सोऽयं सुगन्धिमुकुलो बकुलो विभाति वृक्षाग्रणीः प्रियतमे ! मदनैकबन्धुः ।
यस्य त्वचैव चिरचर्वितया नितान्तं दन्ता भवन्ति चपला अपि वज्रतुल्याः ।।' (वै.जी.)

(161) VANDAK
Dendrophthoe falcata

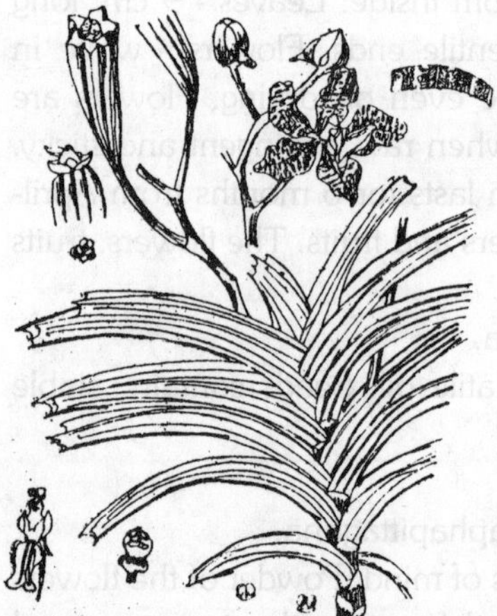

Kula : Vandak kula.
Family : Loranthaceae. Plants of the Loranthus tribe (tropical evergreen parasites).
Gana : Mutravirechaneeya (C.); Veertarvadi (S.)
Latin name : Dendrophthoe = dendros = tree; falcata = sickle like.
English name : Parasite or loranthus coriaceus.
Sanskrit names : Vrikshadani, Vandak, Vriksharuha, Shekhari, Kamrupa, Taruruha, Kamini, Padmarupini.
Women, having a tendency of abortion or having signs of abortion in the third month of pregnancy, should be given the powder of vrikshadani along with milk to strengthen the implantation. At this stage, the foetus is also a type of parasite which is nourished by this parasitic plant.
Botanical Description : This is a parasitic shrub growing on mango and Acacia arabica trees. Branches are small and greyish in colour. Leaves - 9 to 16 cm. long and 3 to 6 cm. broad, oval and thick. Flowers - brown, blue or white. Fruits - small, oblong, brownish, sweet, sticky and in bunches.
Properties :
Guna: laghu, ruksha; **Rasa:** kashaya, tikta, madhur; **Vipak:** katu; **Veerya:** sheeta; **Dosha:** tridoshashamak.
External use : It is used for local application in oedema and wounds.

Internal use : Since it is a nervine tonic and an anticonvulsant, it is useful in hysteria, epilepsy and tetanus. Being a constipative, it is useful in diarrhoea and amoebic dysentery. Leaves are useful in heart diseases, hypertension, blood disorders, bleeding diathesis, cough and breathlessness. As it is a diuretic, it is used in nephritis and urinary calculi.
Special note - Vandak growing on Ficus racemosa is useful for implantation of foetus in threatened abortion in the third month of pregnancy.
Parts used : Leaves, flowers.
Dose : Juice of the flowers and leaves - 5 to 10 ml.
Srotogamitva :
Dosha : Tridoshashamak.
Dhatu : Majja (anticonvulsant), rakta (bleeding disorders).
Mala : Mutra (urinary calculi).
Organ : Uterus (implantation), heart.
References -
बन्दाक: स्याद्धिम: तिक्त: कषायो मधुरो रसे । मांगल्य: कफवातास्त्ररक्षोव्रणविषापह: ।। (भा. प्र.)
वृक्षादनी हिमा तिक्ता कषाया मधुरा रसे । अश्मरीकफवातास्त्ररक्षोव्रणविषापहा ।।' (कै. नि.)
'वन्दाकमौदुम्बरमादरेण वन्ध्यांगना पुष्पविशुद्धिवारे ।
पूर्व विरिक्ता लभते कुमारं छागस्य दुग्धेन सह प्रपीय ।।' (वै. म.)

(162) BIMBI
Coccinia indica

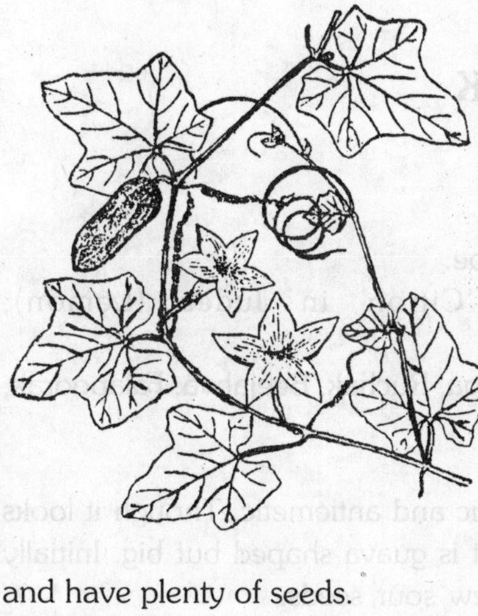

Kula : Koshataki kula.
Family : Cucurbitaceae (Gourd tribe).
Gana : Moolini (C.); Urdhvabhagahara (S.)
Latin name : Coccinia = cocci = berry, indica = indian.
English name : Large flowered bryonia.
Sanskrit names : Bimbi, Raktaphala, Tundi, Tundikeri, Bimbika, Oshtopamaphala, Peeluparni.
Botanical Description : It is a perennial ascending creeper also known as kundaru, telakucha, tindora etc. Its stalk is pentangular, leaves triangular or pentangular, dentate, slightly twisted, 4 to 6 cms. in length and 7-8 cms. broad. Flowers - unisexual, white, large and in bunches. Fruits - unctuous, fleshy, tapering at both ends, initially green and red when ripe. The fruits are marked with 10 white stripes and have plenty of seeds.
Varieties : Two - bitter and sweet. The bitter variety is found in the wild and all its parts are bitter to taste. The sweet variety is used as a vegetable.
Habitat : All over India, Bengal, Bihar.
Chemical composition : It contains resins, starch, sugar, gum and fats.

The son of man, whether he likes it or not is totally dependent - a robot of the programmed rules of universe.

Properties:
Guna: laghu, ruksha, tikshna ; **Rasa:** katu, kashaya; **Veerya:** ushna; **Prabhav:** vamak and rechak; **Dosha:** kaphapittashodhan.
Uses: Application of the leaves reduces inflammation. Juice of the leaves cleanses wounds. Raw fruit is chewed in stomatitis. Since it is an appetizer, emetic, laxative and hepatostimulant, it is used in anorexia, jaundice and other liver disorders. It reduces the diseases of blood caused by kaphapitta. It is useful in cough and asthma as it is an expectorant. Juice of the roots in a dose of 10 ml. or root powder 3 to 6 gms. is useful in pyuria and diabetes. It is also useful in skin diseases and fever.
Parts used : Panchang.
Dose: Juice - 10 to 12 ml.; powder - 3 to 6 gms.
In small doses, it acts as a rasayana due to its bitter taste.
Srotogamitva:
Dosha: Kapha (removal by emesis), pitta (removal by purgation).
Dhatu: Rasa (emetic), rakta (purgative, jaundice, liver, kaphapitta shodhan), mansa, meda (diabetes).
Mala: Mutra (pyuria, diabetes).
Organ: Stomach
References -
'तुण्डिका कफपित्तासृक्शोथपांडुज्वरापहा । श्वासकासापहं स्तन्यं फलं वातकफायहम् । (ध. नि.)
'तिक्तं प्रसूनं पित्तघ्नं तत्परं कामलापहम् ।' (कै. नि.)
'तिक्तबिम्बीफलं तिक्तं पित्तघ्नं वातकोपनम् । विषघ्नमतिरुच्यं स्यात् गुरु श्लेष्मकरं न च ।।
शोफास्त्रपाण्डून् जयति न मेध्यं छर्दिकृत् परम् ।।' (कै. नि.)

(163) BEEJAPOORAK
Citrus medica Linn.

Kula: Jambir kula.
Family: Aurantiaceae, Rutaceae = plants of the ruta, rue, tribe.
Latin name: Citrus = named after city called 'Citron' in Judea (Lemon); medica = for medicinal purpose.
Sanskrit names: Beejapur (full of seeds), Mahalunga, Matulunga, Ruchak, Beejahva, Falapoorak, Lunga, Amlakesar.
English name: Citron tree.
Botanical description: It is an excellent appetizer, cardiotonic and antiemetic. Though it looks like the tree of kagadi limbu, its leaves are big and broad. Fruit is guava shaped but big. Initially it is green, then it becomes yellow. Fruit has thick bark and few sour seeds.
Varieties : Sweet and sour.
Habitat: It grows in north, east and south India.
Chemical composition: It contains 76% citrin.

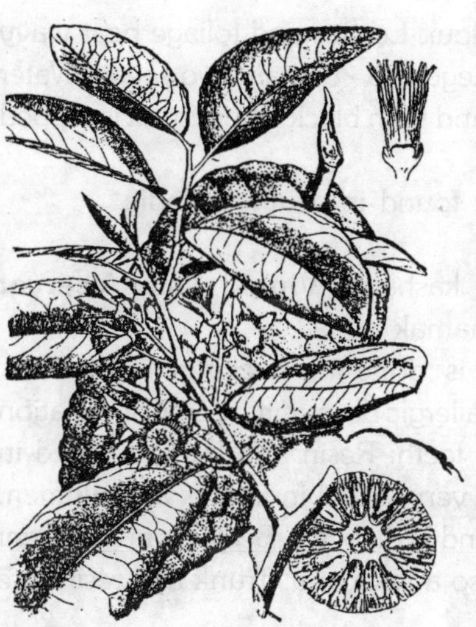

Properties:
Sour beejapooak - Guna: tikshna, **Rasa:** amla, **Vipak:** amla, **Veerya:** anushna, **Dosha:** kaphavatashamak. **Sweet beejapoorak - Guna:** snigdha, **Rasa:** madhur, **Vipak:** madhur, **Veerya:** sheeta, **Dosha:** vatapittashamak.
Uses : Warm leaves are applied over inflammed area to relieve pain and swelling. Seeds are useful externally for scorpion bite. Beejapoorak (mahalung) is extremely useful in alcohol intoxication. It is also useful in vomiting, liver disorders, pain, abdominal tumour, piles and dysentery. Fruits and seeds are used in amenorrhoea.
Srotogamitva:
Dhatu: Rakta, majja (brain tonic).
Mala: Kesar - purisha sangrahi (dysentery).
Organ: Heart, digestive system, brain, respiratory system.
Prabhav: Antidote (scorpion).
References -
'बीजपूरो मातुलुङ्गो रुचकः फलपूरकः । बीजपूरफलं स्वादु रसेऽम्लं दीपनं लघु ।।
रक्तपित्तहरं कण्ठजिह्वाहृदयशोधनम् । श्वासकासारुचिहरं हृद्यं तृष्णाहरं स्मृतम् ।।' (भा. प्र.)
'शूलेऽरूचौ विबन्धे च मन्देऽग्नौ मद्यविप्लवे । हिक्काश्वासे च कासे च वम्यां वर्चोगदेषु च ।।
वातश्लेष्मसमुत्थेषु सर्वेष्वेवोपदिश्यते ।' (च. सू. २७)
'लघ्वम्लं दीपनं हृद्यं मातुलुन्गमुदाहृतम् । त्वक्तिक्ता दुर्जरा तस्य वातक्रिमिकफापहा ।।
स्वादु शीतं गुरु स्निग्धं मांसं मारुतपित्तजित् । मेध्यं शूलानिलच्छर्दिकफारोचकनाशनम् ।।
दीपनं लघु संग्राहि गुल्मार्शोघ्नं तु केशरम् । शूलाजीर्णाविबन्धेषु मन्देऽग्नौ कफमारुते ।।
अरुचौ च विशेषेण रसस्तस्योपदिश्यते ।' (सु. सू. ४६)
'बालं पित्तमरुत्कफास्रकरणं मध्यं च तादृग्विधम् ।
पक्वं वर्णकरञ्च हृद्यमथ तत् पुष्णाति पुष्टिं बलम् ।।
शूलाजीर्णविबन्धमारुतकफश्वासार्त्तिमन्दाग्निजित् ।
कासारोचकशोकशान्तिदमिदं स्यान्मातुलुङ्गं सदा ।।' (रा. नि.)

(164) BEEJAK
Pterocarpus marsupium Linn.

Kula: Shimbi kula.
Family: Leguminosae.
Upkula: Aparajita (Pappilionaceae).
Latin name: Pterocarpus = ptero - with wings, carpus - fruit; marsupium = bears pouch in flowers; marsupium = purse (Animals like kangaroo which have a pouch are called marsupials).
English name: Kino tree.
Sanskrit names: Beejak, Vijaysar, Peeyasal.
Botanical Description: The tree grows to 10 - 15 mtrs. in height, smoky skin of the trunk bears

If the concepts of tadgamitva, praspanda and samanya-vishesha are abandoned, no dravyagunavignyan can exist.

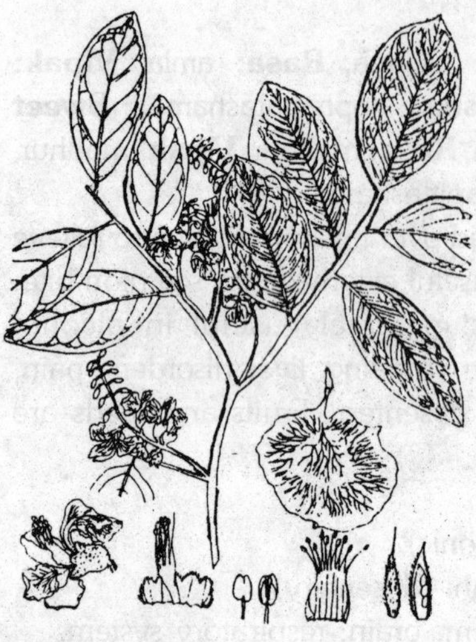

vertical slits. Gum is red in colour. Leaves and foliage bear wavy margin. Flowers - yellowish. Legumes - contain two seeds. Water turns yellow at the beginning and then black when trunk is dipped in it.

Habitat: It is predominantly found in southern India.

Properties:

Guna: laghu,ruksha; **Rasa:** kashaya; **Vipak:** katu; **Veerya:** sheeta; **Dosha:** kaphapittashamak

Uses: External application is done in swelling, erysepelas, leucoderma, dermatoses and allergic dermatitis. Local application of the resin strengthens loose teeth. Resin and bark are used in diarrhoea and dysentery. It is very useful in infants and women, raktagami vatapitta disorders and in diabetes. Beejak is an excellent remedy for fractures and is also a rasayana. Trunk and resin are used.

Dose: Decoction - 50 to 100 ml.; powder - 3 to 6 gms; gum - 250 to 500 mg.

Srotogamitva:

Dosha: Kapha, pitta.

Dhatu: Raktagami (oedema, erysepalas, leucoderma, dermatosis),medogami , rasayan, rakta (cohesive).

Mala: Purisha, mutra.

Organ: Intestines.

(165) BOLAM
Commiphora myrrh

Kula : Guggulu.

Family : Burseraceae.

Latin name : Commiphora myrrh.

Botanical Description : Tree resembles guggul tree. Latex is known as Hirabol. It is in the form of small balls which when mixed together forms to large ball. It is red, bitter and fragrant. It is available in 2-3 varieties.

Habitat : Originated in north east part of Africa and now found in U.A.E., Persia, Sayam, India etc. But Hirabol of Macca is of supreme quality.

Properties :

Guna : ruksha, laghu; **Rasa :** tikta, katu, kashaya; **Vipak :** katu; **Veerya :** ushna; **Dosha :** tridoshahar, vatakaphaghna.

External uses : Useful in rheumatoid arthritis, gout, sciatica and in oral diseases for gargling. Bolam rubbed in human milk is used as eyedrops in conjunctivitis and purulent discharges.

Internal uses : It is used in vata disorders, anaemia, gout, blood disorders, cough, asthma, dysuria, amenorrhoea and dysmenorrhoea.

Strotogamitva :
Dosha : Tridoshahar, but pittavirechak.
Dhatu : Rakta, manasa (oral diseases), raktameda (anaemia), rasa (amenorrhoea, dysmenorrhoea).
Mala : Mutra (dysuria).
Organ : Joints.

(166) BHAVYAM
Dillenia indica

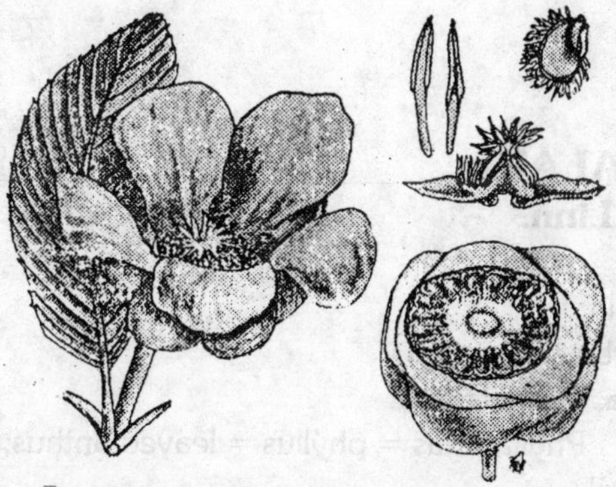

Kula : Bhavya kula.
Family: Dilleniaceae (plants of the tribe of the Sandpaper tree). (Dillania).
Latin name : Dillenia = after Johanon Akob Dillen - a scientist; indica = of India.
Sanskrit names : Bhava, Bhavya, Bhavishya, Bhavan, Vaktrashodhan, Pichchilbeeja, Romaphal.
Botinacl Description : The tree is of medium height. Its fruits are hard with bristles and contain seeds inside. Leaves are dentate.
Properties:
Guna : guru; **Rasa :** madhur, amla, kashaya; **Vipak :** amla; **Veerya :** sheeta; **Dosha:** vatashamak, kaphapittavardhak. It improves taste and oral hygiene.
Internal use : It is a cardiotonic, expectorant and antipyretic. Leaves are used in dysentery.
Srotogamitva :
Dosha : Pittaghna, shleshmavardhak.
Dhatu : Rakta, mansa, rasa.
Mala : Purisha (constipative).
Organ : Mouth, heart.
References -
'हृद्यं स्वादु कषायाम्लं भव्यमास्यविशेदनम् । पित्तश्लेष्मकर ग्राहि गुरु विष्टम्भिशीतलम् ।।' (सु. सू. ४६)
'मधुराम्लकषायं च विष्टम्भि गुरु शीतलम् । पित्तश्लेष्मकरं भव्यं ग्राहि वक्त्रविशोधनम् ।।' (च. सू. २७)

(167) BHANDEER
Clerodendron infortunatum

Kula : Nirgundi kula.
Family : Verbenaceae.
Latin name : Clerodendron = Kleros = chance, dendron = tree (uncertainty of medicinal qualities); infortunatum = with no luck - without medicinal property, unhappy, unlucky.
Botinical Description: This shrub grows to 3 mtrs. in height and emits a foul smell from all its parts. It is bitter to taste.

Forests (jungles) are the wealth of nation. These jungles enhance the bliss of human life (Mangal). Therefore the word 'mangal' should replace the word 'jungle'!

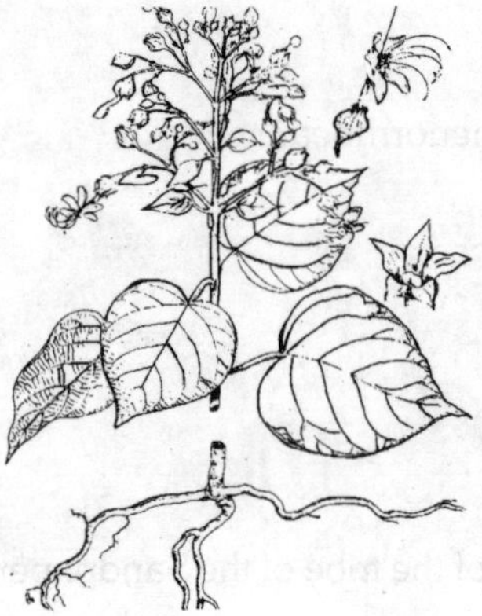

Properties and uses : It is bitter, overcomes tiredness and loss of appetite. It is a mild purgative, cholagogue and anthelmintic. In diarrhoea, its root powder is given along with butter milk. In dermatoses, it is used internally as well as externally.

Dose : Powder of leaves - for children - 250 mg. to 1 gm. mixed with honey and fragrant drugs; for adults - 2 to 6 gms.

Srotogamitva :

Dosha : Pittanissarak.

Dhatu: Meda, asthi, majja.

Mala : Purisha.

(168) BHUMYAMALAKI
Phyllanthus niruri Linn.

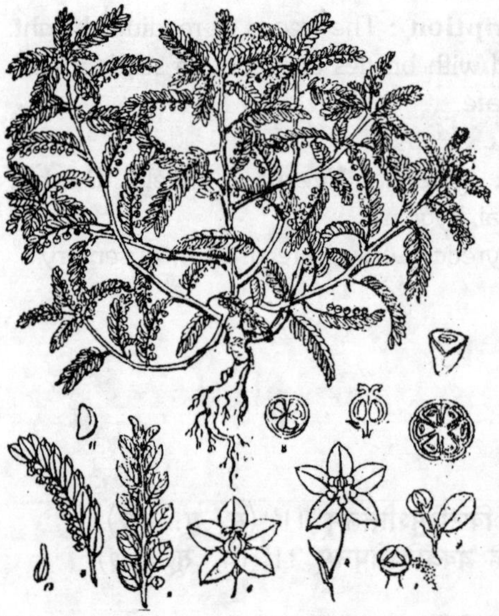

Kula: Erand kula.

Family: Euphorbiaceae.

Gana: Kasahara, Shwasahara.

Latin name: Phyllanthus = phyllus = leaved anthus; urinaria (or niruri).

Sanskrit names: Vrushya, Bhudhatri, Vishwaparni, Bindupatri, Bahuveerya, Tamalaki, Uttama, Bahuputra, Shiva. (Bhumyamalaki is very useful in urinary disorders caused by pitta. It restores the natural colour of the urine in paitik (diabetes) meha.)

Botanical Description: Perennial herb, 18 to 24 cm. in height. Leaves - small, bearing leaflets. Flowers - yellow. Fruits - grow on the under surface of the leaves, like Emblica officinalis, and are tripartate. Seeds - whitish, tender. The shrub grows in rainy season, flowering occurs in autumn followed by fruiting.

Varieties: - 1) white and 2) brown. The branches of the brown variety are brown in colour.

Habitat: All over India, Assam, Bihar, South India.

Chemical composition: Contains phyllenthin.

Properties:

Guna: laghu,ruksha; **Rasa:** tikta, kashaya, madhur; **Veerya:** sheeta; **Dosha:** kaphapittashamak.

External uses: Paste of the leaves is applied on wound, oedema and dermatitis. Paste prepared from leaves crushed with salt is used in fractures for external application. An application of bhumyamalaki roots + rice gruel + salt is useful in eye diseases. Nasya of the juice of roots mixed

with sugar is used for hiccups.
Internal uses: It is an appetizer, digestive, liver stimulant, laxative, carminative and alleviates thirst. It is therefore useful in diarrhoea and dysentery. It is useful in bleeding disorders since it is raktagami and kaphapittashamak. Seed + rice water is useful in menorrhagia, leucorrhoea, dysuria, diabetes, skin diseases, chronic malarial fever and hepatic splenomegaly.
Dose: Decoction of panchang - 10 to 20 ml.; powder - 3 to 6 gms.
Srotogamitva:
Dosha: Kaphapittaghna.
Dhatu: Asthi (in fractures), rasa (appetizer, digestive), rakta (stimulates liver), useful in menorrhagia, bleeding disorders, cough and asthma.
Mala: Purisha (constipative), urine (dysuria), pyuria.
References -
'भूधात्र् वातकृत्तिक्ता कषाया मधुरा हिमा । पिपासाकासपित्तास्त्रकफपाण्डुक्षतापहा ।।'
'तामलकी हिमा तिक्ता कषाया मधुरा लघुः । रोचनी पांडुपित्तास्त्रकफकुष्टविषापहा ।।
जयेच्छवासतृषादाहहिष्माकासक्षतक्षयान् ।' (कै. नि.)
'भूधात्रीतुकषायाम्लपित्तमेहविनाशिनी । शिशिरामूत्ररोगार्तिशमनीदाहनाशिनी ।।' (रा. नि.)
'भूम्यामलकीबीजं सु पीतं तण्डुलवारिणा । दिनद्वयत्रयेणैव स्त्रीरोगं नाशयेद् ध्रुवम् ।।'

(169) BHURJA
Betula utilis D.Don.

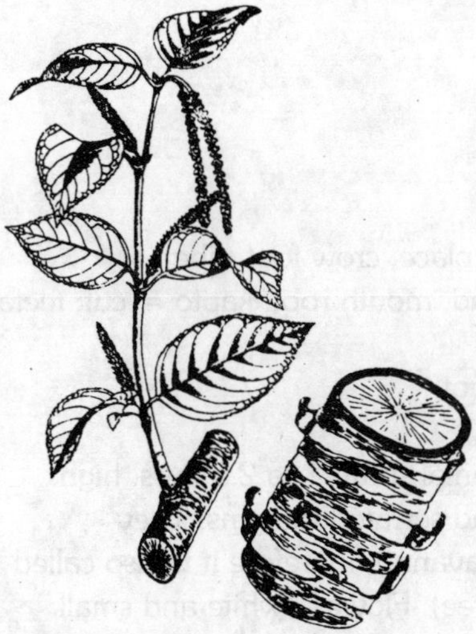

Kula : Bhurja kula.
Family : Betulaceae (Plants of the birch tribe) (Betula).
Latin name : Betula = Birch - Latin name; utilis = useful, serviceable.
English name: Jacquemon tree, Birch tree.
Sanskrit names: Valkadruma, Sucharma, Bhurjapatrak, Chitratvak, Bindupatra, Rakshapatra, Vichitrak, Bhutaghna, Mrudupatra. (The bark of this plant was used for writing before the discovery of paper).
Botanical Description : The tree is 15-20 mtrs. high. Bark - tender, shiny, brownish white and thin like paper having verticle stripes. Central part of the trunk is white with reddish spots. Leaves - 4 to 6 cm. long and 1.5 inch broad, with a long tip, spotted and dentate margin. Seeds - winged. Flowering occurs in summer and fruiting in autumn.
Habitat : Himalayas at the height of two thousand metres, Sikkim and Bhutan.
Chemical composition: Betulin and a volatile oil.
Properties:
Guna : laghu, snigdha; **Rasa :** kashaya; **Vipak :** katu; **Veerya :** ushna; **Prabhav :** antibacterial;

Every human being uses at last fifteen large trees during his lifetime. One should at least plant these many trees.

Dosha: tridoshashamak.
External uses : Since it is an insecticidal, its decoction is used for washing wounds which also helps in healing. In otalgia, the ear is first washed with the decoction of its bark and then medicated oil, prepared from its bark is put as ear drops. Its fumigation is done in grahabadha.
Internal use : It is useful in conditions like hysteria, epilepsy, tetanus, clonic and tonic contractions. It is also useful in diarrhoea and dysentery as it is a constipative. Since it is a hemostatic, it is used in bleeding disorders. Cough, lipid disorders and poisoning are other conditions in which it is found useful.
Dose : Bark powder - 1 to 3 masha (975 mgm. to 2.92 gm.); decoction - 5 to 10 tolas (50 to 100 gms.)
Srotogamitva :
Dosha : Tridoshashamak.
Dhatu : Rakta, meda, mansa.
Mala : Purisha.
Organ : Brain (fumigation is done in mania).
References -
भूर्जः कषायो जयति बलासं पित्तशोषितम् । मेदोभूतग्रहरक्षः कर्णरोगविषप्रणुत् ।।' (कै. नि.)
'भूजपत्रः स्मृतो भूर्जश्चर्मी बहुलवल्कलः । भूर्जी भूतग्रहश्लेष्मकर्णरुक् पित्तरक्तजित् ।।
कषायो राक्षसघ्नश्च मेदोविषहरः ।' (मा. नि.)
'भूर्जो वल्कद्रुमो भूर्जः सुचर्मा भूर्जपत्रकः । चित्रत्वग्विन्दुपत्रश्च रक्षापत्रो विचित्रकः ।।
भूतघ्नो मृदुपत्रश्च शैलेन्द्रस्थो द्विभूमितः । भूर्जः कटुकषायोष्णो भूतरक्षाकरः परः ।
त्रिदोषशमनः पथ्यो दुष्टकौटिल्यनाशनः ।।' (रा. नि.)

(170) MAMEERA
Coptis teeta

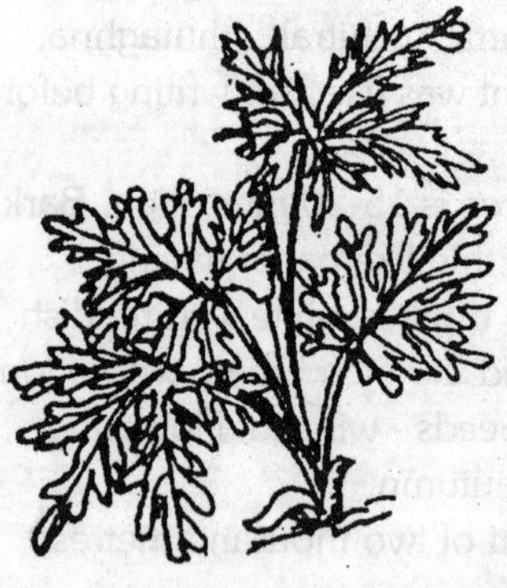

Kula : Vatsanabh kula.
Family : Ranunculaceae (marshy place, crow foot tribe).
Latin name : Coptis = gold thread, mouth root, kapto = cut; teeta = covered with short silky hair.
English name : Golden thread root.
Sanskrit name : Peetmula.
Botanical Description : A perrenial shrub 1 to 2.5 mtrs. high. Leaves - compound with round and serrated margins. They resemble an old quarter rupee (chavanni), therefore it is also called as 'Chavanni gaccha' (gaccha = tree). Flower - white and small. Root - black externally and yellow internally.
Properties :
Guna : ruksha; **Rasa :** tikta; **Veerya :** ushna; **Dosha :** kaphapittahar.
External uses : Its juice is used as eye drops in conjunctivitis along with other medicines. Also used in leucoderma.

Internal uses : Appetizer, digestive because of its bitterness. As it is hepatostimulant, it is useful in obstructive jaundice. Also useful in oedema, cough with expectoration, asthma, dysuria, pyruia, typhoid fever, dermatoses and leucoderma.
Parts used : Roots.
Dose : 1to 2 gms. 2 - 3gms. as a prophylactic drug in typhoid fever, as a toinc - 5 to10 ratti (0.5 to 1gm.)
Adulteration : Thalictrum foliolosum is mixed with mameera.
Srotogamitva :
Dosha : Kaphapittaghna.
Dhatu : Rakta (hepatostimulant), rasa (fever, dermatoses).
Mala : Mutra (diuretic, useful in pyuria).
Organs : Eye, liver, respiratory system, digestive system.
References -
ममीरा पीतमूला स्यात् हिमाचलसमुद्भवा । वृत्तदन्तुरपत्रा च सितपुष्पाऽतितिक्तिका ।।
पीतमूला कटुस्तिक्ता रूक्षोष्णा दीपनी सरा । चक्षुष्या पाचनी रूच्या कफपित्तहरा मता ।।
यकृदुत्तेजनी चैव विषमज्वरनाशिनी । नेत्रामये यकृद्रोगे कुष्टे शोथे कफामये ।।
कासे श्वासे तथा मूत्रकृच्छे मेहे च पूयजे । ज्वरौत्तरिकदौर्बल्ये ज्वरे चापि प्रशस्यते ।।' (स्व.)

(171) MAKHANNAM

Euryale ferox

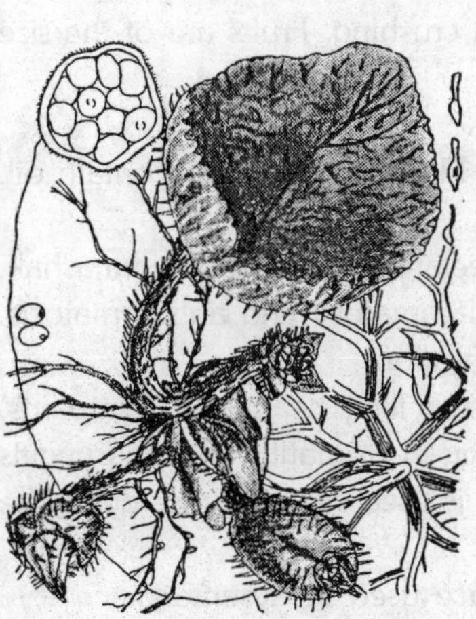

Kula : Kamal kula.
Family : Nymphoeacae.
Latin name : Euryale = Eurya - Gk. eurys = large flowers, broad anthes; ferox = fierce-bristled.
Sanskrit names : Makhanna, Padmabeejabh, Paneeyaphal (this plant grows in water).
Botanical Description : Leaves, fruits and stem bear thorns; leaves float on the surface of water and are round with a diameter of 0.6 to 1.5 mtrs. Flowers - 3 to 6 cm. long. Fruits - oval, containing 4 to 20 black coloured seeds. Roasted seeds are sold in the market.
Habitat : North Bihar and Northen India.
Properties:
Guna: guru, ruksha; **Rasa:** madhur, kashya, tikta; **Vipak :** madhur; **Veerya :** sheeta; **Dosha :** tridoshashamak, especially pittashamak.
Uses: Since it is an astringent, cardiotonic, hemopoetic and spermatogenic, it is useful in dysentery, haemetemesis, bronchitis, asthma, difficult labour, leucorrhoea, spermatorrhoea and in post partum period.
Srotogamitva :
Dosha : Kaphavataghna, especially pitta.

Whenever any organ or part of the body is mentioned, its constituents and respective srotas should be visualised.

Dhatu : Shukra (aphrodisiac), rakta (bleeding disorders), anabolic.
Mala : Purisha (constipative), antidiuretic (roasted seeds).
Organs: Uterus, respiratory system.
References -
'मखान्नं पद्मबीजस्य गुणैस्तुल्यं विनिर्दिशेत् ।' (भा. प्र.)
'विष्टम्भि वृष्यं रूक्षं च गर्भसंस्थापकं परम् । कफवातहरं बल्यं ग्राहि पित्तास्रदाहनुत् ।।' (भा. प्र.)

(172) MADAYANTIKA

Lawsonia inermis Linn.

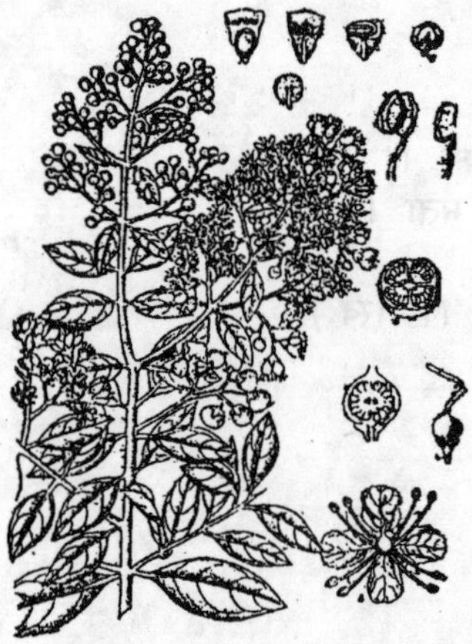

Kula: Madayantika kula.
Family: Lythraceae (plants of purple loose strife).
Latin name: Lawsonia = after Mr. M. A. Lowson, FRS, who assisted in preparation of flora of British India; inermis = smooth stemmed, without spines or alba = white.
English name: Henna, samphire.
Sanskrit names: Timir, Kokadanta, Dwivrunta , Nakharanjak.
This plant is commonly used for colouring palms, soles and hair especially on auspicious occassions like marriages for cosmetic purposes.
Botanical Description: It is a shrub with sweet smelling white flowers. Leaves give a red colour on crushing. Fruits are of the size of peas, with small seeds inside.
Habitat: Grows all over India.
Chemical composition: The leaves contain 12 to 15% of dye. Flowers and seeds contain oil.
Properties:
Guna: laghu, ruksha; **Rasa:** tikta, kashaya; **Vipak:** katu; **Veerya:** sheeta; **Dosha:** kaphapittanashak.
Uses: It is an anlgesic, reduces oedema, and is astringent, antiinflammatory and antidermatosis. It improves complexion and hair growth and reduces burning sensation.
External application of the paste is useful for burning of hands and feet, headache, jointpains, inflammation, ulcer and skin diseases. Decoction is used for gargling in stomatitis and pharyngitis (as an astringent). A combination of henna and Indigofera tinctoria is used externally for dying the hair black. Flowers are used as refrigerant and in insomnia.
Seeds - Extract of seeds stimulates the spleen and liver and hence used in dysentery.
The juice of the leaves is given orally in jaundice.
Flowers - Since the flowers are useful in heart conditions, its hot infusion is used in heart diseases.
Leaves - The juice or decoction of the leaves is used in diseases of the blood. The leaf juice is used in oedema.
Since it is a diuretic, leaf juice + sugar are used in dysuria and pyuria. It reduces burning in the urine and soothes the urinary tract. The decoction of the leaves is used in dermatoses and syphilis. Hot infusion of the flowers is given in fever.

Dose: Juice 5 to 10 ml. , powdered seeds - 1 to 3 gms.
Formulations: Madayantyadi churna.
Srotogamitva:
Dosha: Kaphaghna, pittaghna (burning sensation).
Dhatu: Rakta (deramatoses, burning sensation, bleeding disorders, jaundice, vertigo, urticaria, wounds), rasa (fever).
Mala: Purisha (diarrhoea), mutra (dysuria), kesha (hair dye).
Immature flowers: Cardiotonic (hot infusion).

(173) MADHUK

Madhuka indica Jf. Gmel.

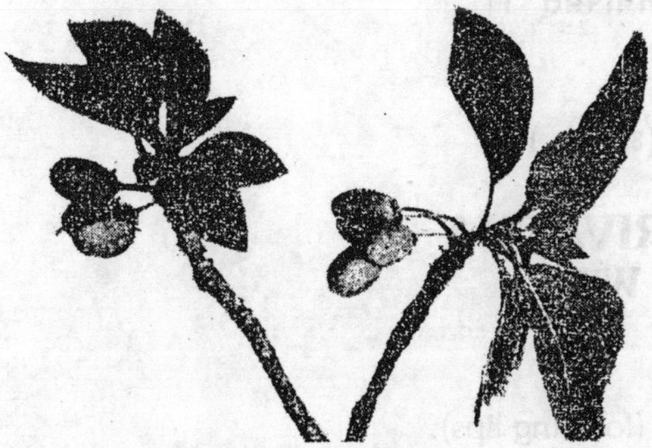

Kula : Madhuk kula.
Family : Sapotaceae (Plants of the Sapota, vegetable egg).
Latin name : Mudhuka = from the Sanskrit name - madhuk; indica = Indian or Bassia = after Fernando Bassi, Curator of the Botanical garden of Bologna, Italy; latifolia = broad leaves.
English name : Indian butter tree, Mahwa tree.
Sanskrit names : Madhuk, Teekshnasar, Vanaprastha, Madhusrav, Dholaphala, Swadupushpa, Madhushthil, Madhulak. (Amongst the many reasons behind tigers turning man eaters, one of the reasons is the practice of collecting the flowers of madhuk. Usually, tribal women go to the jungles in early morning to collect the flowers fallen during the previous day. One of them may fall prey to a tiger looking for a hunt. Once a tiger tastes human blood, he becomes a man eater.)
Botanical Description : It is an evergreen tree growing to a height of 10-16 mtrs. Bark - blackish or greyish in colour, torn, but the wood is brownish. Leaves - 8 to 15 cm. in length, oblong, oval, with 10 to 12 veins. Flowers - white, juicy and contain a sugar-like substance. Fruits - oblong, 1/2 inch long, initially green and then turning to yellow. Fruit contains 1-4 red coloured seeds. The tree flowers in summer and fruits in rainy season.
Chemical composition: The seeds contain 55% stable oil.
Variety: One of the varieties called jalamadhuk grows in marshy land. The sweet portion of the flowers gets quickly converted to alcohol. The flowers are used to make liquor.
Properties:
Guna: guru, snigdha; **Rasa:** madhur, kashaya; **Veerya:** sheeta (dry flowers are ushna); **Dosha:** vatapittashamak.
Uses : Massage done with the oil prepared from madhuk is analgesic. Flower juice is rubbed on the skin in dermatoses and is used as nasal drops in pittaj headache. Flower pulp is given along with milk in nerve disorders as a nervine tonic. Decoction of the flowers or madhukarishta is used

If one were to think of dosha, dhatu and mala, one should concurrently visualize srotas of the same.

in diarrhoea, dysentery and thirst and it is a carminative and astringent. Juice of fresh flowers is used in bleeding disorders. It is used in bronchitis and asthma as an expectorant and in hiccups. Flowers are aphrodisiac and galactogouge and hence used in seminal debility and reduced breast milk secretion. The pulp of the seeds is used to prepare vaginal suppository for inducing menstrual bleeding. Madhuk is also useful in dysuria, fever, burning and pthisis.

Parts used : Flowers, fruits, bark, seeds, oil and leaves (Oil is used in preparation of soap as well as for cooking purposes.)

References -

'मधूकपुष्पं मधुरं शीतलं गुरु बृंहणम् । बलशुक्रकरं प्रोक्तं वातपित्तविनाशनम् ।।'
कलं शीतं गुरु स्वादु शुक्लं तत् वातपित्तनुत् । अहृद्यं हन्ति तृष्णास्रदाहश्वासक्षतक्षयान् ।।' (मा.प्र.)
'रक्तपित्तहराण्याहुर्गुरूणि मधुराणि च । बृंहणीयमहृद्यं च मधूककुसुमं गुरु ।।
वातपित्तोपशमनं फलं तेनोपदिश्यते ।' (सु. सू. ४६)
'मधूकपुष्पस्वरसं श्रृतमर्धक्षयीतम् । क्षौद्रपादयुतं शीतं पूर्ववत् सन्निधापयेत् ।।
तं पिबन् ग्रहणीदोषान् जयेत सर्वान् हिताशन: ।' (च. चि. १९)
'सद्यश्च्युतं स्थूलमधूकपुष्पं संशोधितं केशरधूलिवर्जितम् ।
संपाचितं शुभ्रसिताघृताभ्यां सजीरकं जीवनदं हि जीविनाम् ।।' (क्षे. कु.)

(174) MAHABHARIVACHA

Alpinia galanga Willd.

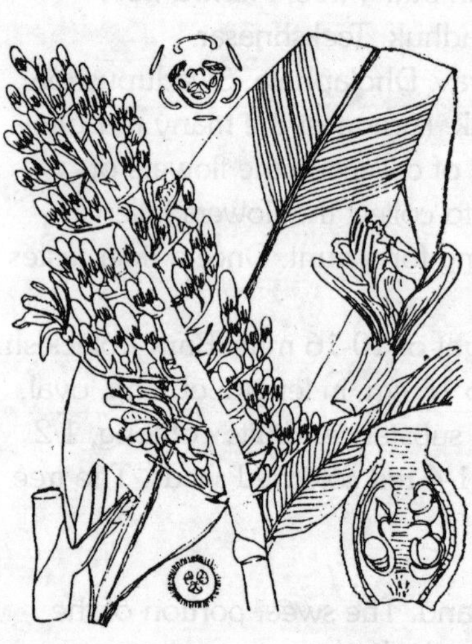

Kula : Haridra kula.

Family : Scitamineae (forming lips).

Latin name : Alpinia = Indian shell flower, Alpini = Italian botanist; galanga = galanthus = snow drops.

Sanskrit names : Kulaj, Gandhamoola, Kulanjan, Gandhabeeja, Ugragandha, Sugandha, Mahabhairavacha, Malayavacha.

English name : Greater galangal, Java galangal.

Botanical Description : A shrub 1.25 to 2 mtrs. high. Leaves are 30 to 60 cms. long, 12 to 18 cms broad, upper surface is smooth and the undersurface is hairy. Flowers - small, greenish white and bent. Fruit - round, like a lemon but red in colour (fuirt is called galanga cardamum). Seeds - light, flat, triangular and fragrant. Flowering occurs in summer. Root - resembles potato and its pieces are available in the market.

Habitat : Origin in Java, Sumatra, also found in Southern India and Bengal. One Chinese variety is also available in the market.

Chemical composition : Camphoride, galangin, alpinin. Fresh roots contain a volatile oil.

Properties:

Guna: laghu, tikshna, ruksha; **Rasa:** katu; **Veerya :** ushna; **Dosha:** kaphavatashamak, aggravates pitta.

External uses : Since it eliminates cold and acts as a stimulant, it is rubbed on the body in conditions in which the body becomes hypothermic due to excessive perspiration.
Internal uses : It is mainly useful in diseases caused by vata. Chewing mahabharivacha improves the taste. It is extremely useful in cardiac diseases caused by vata, hoarseness of voice, stammering, cough, breathlessness, polyuria and impotency. (It causes sexual stimulation if kept in the mouth.)
Dose : Powder of root - 1 to 2 gms.
Srotogamitva :
Dosha : Kaphaghna, vataghna, pittavardhak.
Dhatu: Mansa, meda, shukra.
Mala : Sweda, mutra (antidiuretic).
References -
'सुगन्धाप्सु प्रगन्धा च विशेषात्कफकासनु त् । सुस्वरत्वकरी रुच्या हृत्कण्ठमुखशोधनी ।।' (भा. प्र.)
'कुलञ्जोचो गन्धमूलश्च तीक्ष्णमूलः कुलञ्जनः । कुलञ्जः कटुतिक्तोष्णो दीपनो मुखदोषनुत् (रा. नि.)
'कुलिञ्जनं कटुतिक्तमुष्णं चाग्निप्रदीपनम् । रुच्यं स्वर्यं च हृद्यं च मुखकण्ठविशुद्धिकृत् ।।'
मुखदोषं कफं श्वासं कासं वातं ध्रुवंजयेत् । बृहत्कुष्ठगुणैर्ज्ञेयंन्यूनमस्मादिति स्मृतम् ।।'

(175) MAYURSHIKHA
Adiantum caudatum Linn.

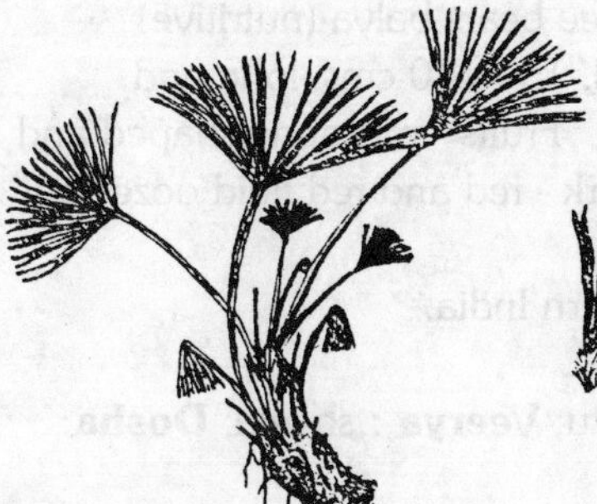

Kula: Hansapadi kula.
Family : Polypodiaceae (Polypody).
Latin name : Adiantum = adianthos (Gk.) = dry, unwetted (The way water is shed by the leaves and during a shower the leaves remain apparently unwetted); caudatum = cauda = tail, having a tail.
Sanskrit names : Mayurshikha, Madhuchchada.
Botanical Description: This is a leafy shrub belonging to the hanspadi kula. Leaves - 5 to 10 cms. long and in bunches, originating right from the roots. Leaflets - facing upwards, five in number, broader towards the tips and look like the feather of a peacock. Spores are found at the borders of the leaves from which the plant can reproduce. Different varieties are found.
Habitat : This plant generally grows in the rainy season on old stony or muddy walls and dries in the summer.
Properties:
Guna : laghu, ruksha; **Rasa:** tikta, kashya, madhur; **Vipak :** katu; **Veerya :** sheeta;
Doshaghnata : kaphapittashamak.
Uses : It acts as an astringent in alimentary system and a hemostatic in circulatory system. It is therefore useful in diarrhoea, dysentery, bleeding disorders, intestinal worms, skin diseases and as an antipyretic.

Even if Chandan (sandalwood) and Chitraka (Plumbago zeylanicum) are planted in the same soil, the trees will certainly carry out the transformations useful to their unique needs.

Dose : Panchang decoction - 7 to 15 ml.
Srotogamitva : -
Dosha : Kaphapittaghna.
Dhatu : Rakta (astringent, hemostatic), rasa (fever), meda (diabetes).
Mala : Stool (bacillary dysentery).
References -
मयूराहशिखा प्रोक्ता सहस्राहिमधुच्छदा । नीलकंठशिखा लघ्वी पित्तश्लेष्मातिसारजित् ।।' (भा. प्र.)
'मयूराह शिखा शीता कषाया कटुपाकिनी । लघ्वी पित्तकफौ रक्तमतीसारं विनाशयेत् ।। (कै. नि.)

(176) MANSAROHINI
Soymida febrifuga

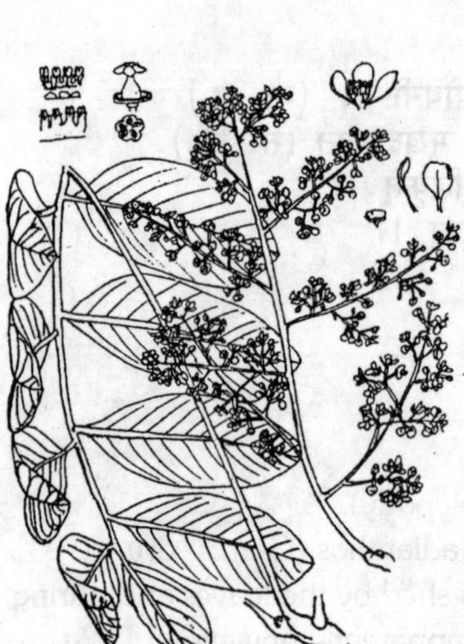

Kula : Nimba kula (bead tree tribe).
Family : Meliaceae.
Latin name : Soymida = semida - Telugu word - genetive of somi - from Swami = deity, used for sacred pillers in temples; febrifuga = to bring down temperature in human febrile conditions.
Sanskrit names : Mansarohini, Atiruha, Vritta, Praharvalli, Vikasha, Kasha, Mansarakta, Pishitrohini, Agniruha.
Botanical Description : The tree bears balya (nutritive) property. Leaves - feather shaped, 15 to 40 cms. long and compound. Leaflets - 3 to 6 pairs. Fruits - mrudung shaped and apple sized with seeds inside. Bark - red and red fluid oozes out on cutting.
Habitat: North -west and southern India.

Properties :
Guna : laghu, ruksha; **Rasa :** kashaya, katu, madhur; **Vipak :** katu; **Veerya :** sheeta; **Dosha:** kaphapittashamak.
External uses : Astringent and antiiflammatory. Decoction is used for gargling, in oral and dental disorders while as vaginal douche in leucorrhoea. Fruits are used as complexion enhancer.
Internal uses: It acts as an astringent in diarrhoea, dysentery and bleeding disorders. Its healing property is useful in bone fractures, muscular sprain and chest injury.
Dose : Powder - 1 to 3 gms; decoction - 20 to 40 ml. Higher dose causes vertigo, unconsciousness and syncope which should be treated with snigdha and sweet drugs.
Strotogamitva :
Dosh : Tridoshanashak, especially kaphapittaghna.
Dhatu : Shukra (aphrodisiac), mansa (wound healing property), rakta (complexion enhancer), asthi (joining property).
Mala : Purisha.
Organ: Circulatory system.

Manovaha strotas: Higher dose causes adverse effects.

References -

'स्यान्मांसरोहिणी वृष्या सरा दोषत्रयापहा । रसे पाके तु कटुका तुबरा शीतला च सा ।।' (भा. प्र.)

'सप्तरात्रं स्थितं क्षीरे छागले रोहिणीफलम् । तेनैव पिष्टं सुश्लक्ष्णं सवर्णकरणं हितम् ।' (सु. चि. १)

(177) MASHAPARNI

Phaseolus mungo

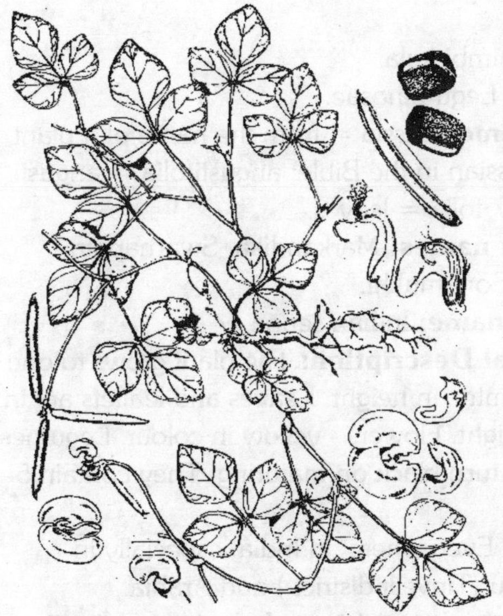

Gana : Jeevaneeya, Shukrajanan, Madhurskandha.

Kula : Shimbi kula.

Family : Leguminoseae (seed vessels with one cell and two valves).

Upakula : Aparajita - Pappilionaseae.

Latin name : Phaseolus = a little boat like; mungo.

Sanskrit names : Krishnavrinta, Kamboji, Hayapucchika, Mansamasha, Sinhamukhi, Swadumasha, Mahasaha, Ardramasha, Sinhavinna.

Botanical Description : A creeper is also known as Teramnus labialis. Leaves - 2 to 4 cms. long, compound and trifoliate. Leaflets - oval shaped. Flower stalk - bears violet flowers. Legume - 3 to 6 cms. long, slightly crooked containing 8 to 10 seeds.

Habitat : Mainly India.

Properties :

Guna : laghu, snigdha; **Rasa :** madhur, tikta; **Vipak :** madhur; **Veerya :** sheeta; **Dosha:** vata pittashamak, kaphavardhak.

Internal use : It is used in the treatment of Bell's palsy, hemiplegia, rheumatoid arthritis, bleeding disorders, abdominal colic, spermatorrhoea, burning sensation and pthisis. Charak has advised to feed the cow with leaves of mashaparni and to consume cow's milk as an aphrodiasic.

Parts used : Whole plant and roots. Usually mudgaparni and mashaparni are used in combination.

Strotogamitva :

Dosha : Vatapittaghna, kaphavardhak.

Dhatu : Rakta (bleeding disorders), shukra (spermatorrhoea and aphrodisiac), rasayan.

Mala : Purisha (astringent).

Organs : Joints, brain and intestines.

References -

माषपर्णसदृक् पर्णा रोमालुर्वनसम्भवा । मार्जारमोदनी माषपिण्ढी च वक्रमालका ।।

हयपुच्छसमाकारा मधुरा पर्वतोभ्द्वा ।' (शि.)

माषपर्णी हिमा तिक्ता स्निग्धा शुक्रबलासकृत् । मधुरा ग्राहिणी शोथवातपित्तज्वरास्रजि त् ।।' (भा. प्र)

'माषपर्णी रसे तिक्ता वृष्या दाहज्वरापहा । शुक्रवृद्धिकरी बल्या शीतला पुष्टिवर्धनी ।।' (रा. नि.)

Dosha-viparit treatment counteracts the dosha; vyadhi-viparit treatment acts through being doshadushyasthangami - a trasort and localization in the vitiated dosha and its locus.

'सहाद्वयं.... ज्ञेया विपाके मधुरा रसे च बलप्रदा: पित्तनिर्वहणाश्च । (सु. सू. ४६)
'माषपर्णाभृतां धेनुं गृष्टिं पुष्टां चतु:स्तनीम् । समानवर्णवत्सांच बुद्धिमान ।
रोहिणीं अथवा कृष्णां ऊर्ध्वश्रुंगी अदारुणां ।
इक्ष्वादामर्जुनादांवा सान्द्रक्षीरां च धारयेत् । केवलं तु पय: तस्या श्रृतं वा श्रृतमेव वा ।।
शर्करामधुसर्पिभि: युक्तं तद् वृष्यमुत्तमम् ।' (च. चि. ३/४)

(178) MARKANDIKA

Cassia angustifolia Vahl.

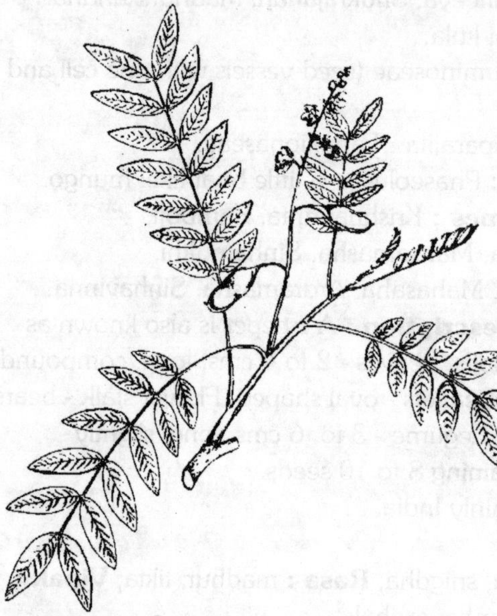

Kula: Shimbi kula.
Family: Leguminosae.
Latin name: Cassia = from the name of a plant called kassian in the Bible; angustifolia = angusti = narrow, folia = leaves.
Sanskrit names: Markandika, Swarnapatri, Sanaya, Sonamukhi.
English name: Indian senna.
Botanical Description: The plant grows to one and half mtrs. in height. Leaves and leaflets are in pairs of eight. Flowers - yellow in colour. Legumes flat and turn black on maturing. They contain 5-6 seeds.
Habitat: Everywhere in India, especially in Tamilnadu (Tinvelli district) and Arabia.
Chemical composition: It contains cathartic acid which is responsible for its purgative action.

Properties:
Guna: laghu, ruksha, tikshna; **Rasa:** katu, tikta; **Veerya:** ushna; **Vipak:** katu; **Dosha:** vatakaphashamak.
Uses: It is applied externally in skin diseases. It is an emetic, laxative, mild purgative, cholagogue, enhances peristalsis and secretion of the intestines. It causes griping pain in higher doses. It also acts as anthelmintic. It is useful in conditions like constipation, fever, ascites, rheumatoid arthritis, gout and in blood disorders.
Parts used: Leaves and fruits.
Dose: Powder - 1 to 3 gms. (mild purgative); 6 to 9 gms. (purgative to wash out colonic kapha pitta).
It is excreted through all the body secretions even in breast milk (causes diarrhoea in breast fed babies).
Srotogamitva:
Dosha: Kaphavatapittashodhani.
Dhatu: Rasa, rakta, liver.

Mala: Purisha (purgative, anthelmintic).
Organs: Digestive system, intestine.

(179) MAYAPHALAM
Quercus infectoria Oliv.

Kula: Mayaphal kula.
Family: Cupuliferae (Bowl - Basin).
Latin name: Quercus = Quer = fine, cuez = tree (Celtic); infectoria = of the dyers, stained.
English name: Gall, Magic nut.
Sanskrit names: Mayaphal, Mayiphala, Chidraphala (small holes on the fruit), Mayika , Mayi.
(The name mayaphal is a misnomer. Mayaphala is not actually a fruit but a coccoon of an insect made by using the juice of the tree. It is hollow from within.)
Botanical Description: This is a shrub with a greyish trunk. Leaves - long, oblong, with dentate margins. Flowers - unisexual. Fruits - small, round, yellowish with a single seed. An insect called Sinips galli tinctoria sucks the juice from its branches and makes a coccoon-like shelter for itself in which it lays its eggs. This is called mayaphal.
Varieties: There are four varieties - 1) Blue 2) Black 3) Green and 4) White.
The first three varieties are superior whereas the last variety is considered to be inferior.
Habitat: U.A.E., Asia minor, Syria, Persia.
Chemical composition: Mayaphal contains 50 to 70 % gallotannic acid and 3% tannic acid.
Properties:
Guna: laghu, ruksha; **Rasa:** kashaya; **Vipak:** katu; **Verya:** sheeta; **Dosha:** Kaphapittashamak.
External uses: It is used as a hair dye. Since it is an astringent and wound healing, it stops bleeding from wounds. It is used for gargling in pharyngitis and stomatitis. Its powder is used for application in rectal prolapse, piles and wounds. Application of its powder is done in excessive sweating.
Internal uses: It is a strong constipative (also causes vomiting in excess dose). It is useful in diarrhoea (colonic), dysentery, bleeding piles, bleeding diathesis, cough, polyuria, diabetes, pyuria and leucorrhoea. Its vaginal suppository is used in leucorrhoea. In case of poisonong by strychnine, dhattura, aconite, morphine or antimony, its decoction is given repeatedly in large doses after a proper stomach wash.
Dose: Powder - 1 to 2 gms.
Srotogamitva:
Dosha: Kaphapittaghna.
Dhatu: Rakta, mansa, meda.
Mala: Hair, sweda, purisha.
In case of poisoning, its decoction should be used after a proper stomach wash.

In general, mildly scented materials (Sugandhi dravyas) suppress pitta. Whereas intensely odourous materials (Gandha dravyas) suppress vata and kapha.

(180) MANAKANDA
Alocasia indica Scholt.

Kula : Suran kula.
Family : Araceae (cuckoo plant).
Latin name : Alocasia; indica = India.
English name : Great leaved callidium.
Sanskrit names : Manak, Mahapatra, Deerghadal, Mahacchada, Mahatpatra, Pankancha.
Botanical Description : A shrub resembles yam. Stalk - 7 to 18 cms. long and hard. Leaves - 0.75 to 1 mt. long, oval but heart shaped towords the stalk and straight towards the tip. Tuber - oblong, 13 to 20 cms. long. It blossoms in rainy season followed by fruiting.
Varieties : There are two varieties, 1) Punget and 2) sweet (medicinal use).
Habitat : All over India, specially Bihar and Bengal.
Chemical composition : Postassium oxalate, calcium carbonate and starch.
Properties :
Guru : guru, snigdha; **Rasa :** madhur; **Veerya :** sheeta; **Dosha :** vatapittashamak.
External uses : Hot leaves and turber are tied on inflammed area. Juice of roasted stalk is used as eardrops in earache and otorrhoea. Tuber ash mixed in oil is applied on numbness of the tongue.
Internal uses : Useful in vata disorders, ascites, constipation and piles.
Leaves and stalk have hemostatic property, hence used in bleeding disorders.Mixture of tuber 3 oz. + rice flour 16 tola + milk 24 tola + water 24 tola is cooked till water gets evaporated. This preparation is called Manamanda, which is given in anasarca.It is also used in splenomegaly, dysuria and as a general tonic.
Dose : Tuber powder - 2 to 4 gms; stalk and leafjuice - 12 to 24 ml.
Formulations : Manakadi gutika, Manamanda.
Srotogamitva :
Dosha : Vatapittaghna.
Dhatu : Rakta (leaves and stalk - hemostatic), splenomegaly.
Mala : Mutra (diuretic).
References -
'मानकंः स्यान्महापत्रः कथ्यन्ते तद्गुणआ अथ । मानकः शोथहृच्छीतो रक्तपित्तहरोऽलघुः ।। (भा. प्र.)
'मानकं स्वादु शीतं च गुरुचापि प्रकीर्त्तितम् ।' (सु. सू. ४६)
'पुराणं मानकं पिष्ट्वा द्विगुकृततण्डुलम् । साधितं क्षीरतोयाभ्यामभ्यसेत् पायसन्तु तत् ।
हन्ति वातोदरं शोथं ग्रहणीं पाण्डुतामपि । सिद्धो भिषग्भिराख्यातः प्रयोगोऽयं निरत्ययः ।। (भा. प्र.)

(181) MUCHKUNDA

Pterospermum suberifolium Lam.

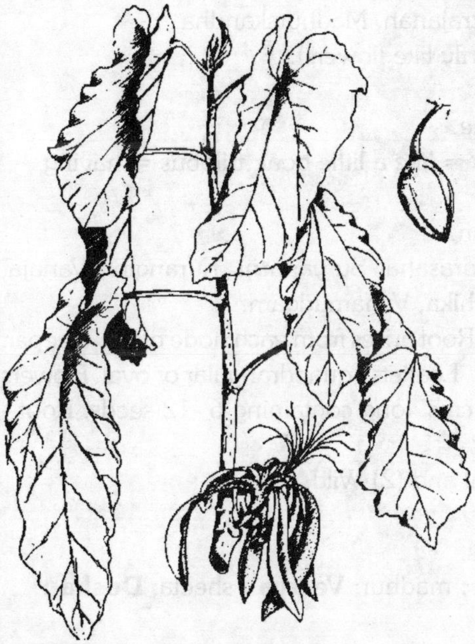

Kula: Pishachkarpas kula.

Family: Sterculiaceae.

Latin name: Pterospermum = Pteron = wing, spermum = seed ; suberifolium = cock like leaves.

Sanskrit names: Kshatravruksha, Chitrak, Prativishnuk, Bahupatra, Supushpa, Adhyarhi, Lakshmanav, Raktaprasav, Vasu.

Botanical Description: A tree with scented, brown flowers. Leaves - large, shield-like, (thus called kshatravruksha) upper surface green, lower is white. Shows vertical cracks on the bark. Trunk is brownish in colour. Branches - closely packed. Seeds are winged. Flowering occurs in summer.

Habitat: Orissa, Karnataka, Burma.

Properties:

Guna: ruksha; **Rasa:** kashaya, katu, tikta; **Vipak:** katu; **Veerya**: ushna; **Dosha:** tridoshahar, specially useful in vatakapha disorders.

External uses: Its local application is soothing and alleviates burning sensation in headache, bleeding piles and chicken pox.

Internal uses: Analgesic in vata diseases. Muchkunda is useful as an astringent in blood and bile related disorders. It controls bleeding in piles when given as a powder of flowers along with honey and sugar. It is also useful in bronchitis, asthma and skin diseases.

Srotogamitva:

Dosha: Kaphapittaghna.

Dhatu: Rakta (pittashamak), rasa (skin diseases).

Mala: Sweda.

Organ: Respiratory system.

Prabhav: Antitoxic.

References -

मुचकुन्द: शिरपीडापित्तास्रविषनाषन: ।।

मुचकुन्द: कटुतिक्त कफकासविनाशनश्च कण्ठकर: ।

त्वग्दोषशोफशमनो व्रणपामाविनाशनश्चैव ।।' (रा. नि.)

Not withstanding heavy and cotinuous rain, some plants wait for the autumn season to sprout.

(182) MUDGAPARNI
Phaseolous trilobus

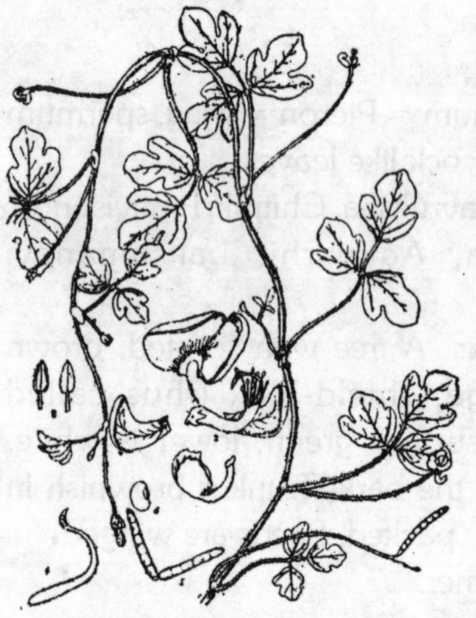

Gana : Jeevaneeya, Shukrajanan, Madhurskandha.
Kula : Shimbi kula (butterfly like flowers).
Family : Leguminoseae.
Subfamily : Papilionoseae.
Latin name : Phaseolous = like a little boat; trilobus = having three lobes.
English name : Wild bean.
Sanskrit names : Kshudrasaha, Suryaparni, Kurangini, Vanaja, Shimbi, Sinhi, Marjargandhika, Vanamudgam.
Botanical Description : Root arises from each node of the creeper. Leaves - trifoliate and hairy. Leaflets - quandrangular or oval. Flowers - yellow. Legume - 3 to 6 cms. long containing 6 -12 seeds. Root - very thick.
Varieties : Two - (1) Rural and (2) Wild.
Habitat : All over India.
Properties :
Guna : laghu, ruksha; **Rasa :** madhur, tikta; **Vipak :** madhur; **Veerya :** sheeta; **Dosha :** tridoshanashak, mainly vatapittashamak.
Uses : It is used locally in inflammation, ulcers and eye diseases. Tampoon made of it is kept in vagina in menorrhagia. Internally it is used in diarrhoea, dysentery, piles and spermatorrhoea. Vatashamak and raktagami are the specific actions of it.
Srotogamitva :
Dosha : Tridoshashamak.
Dhatu : Rakta (menorrhagia) (raktagami, vatashamak), shukra (spermatorrhoea).
Mala : Purisha (diarrhoea, dysentery).
Organs : Eyes and uterus.
References -
'अरण्यमुद्रजा वल्ली सशिम्बा पीतपुष्पका । मुद्गवल्ल्याभपर्णा या मुदूगपर्णिति सा स्मृता ।'
'मुदूगपर्णी हिमा रूक्षा तिक्ता स्वाद्वी च शुक्रला । चक्षुष्या क्षतशोथघ्नी ग्रहणीज्वरदाहनुत् ।।
दोषत्रयहरी लघ्वी ग्रहण्यर्शोतिसारहत् ।' (भा. प्र.)

(183) MUNDI
Sphaeranthus indicus Linn.

Gana: Medhya - Rasayan.
Kula: Bhrungaraj kula.
Family: Compositeae.
Latin name: Sphaeranthus = sphira = globelike, anthus = cranial; indicus = Indian or mollis =

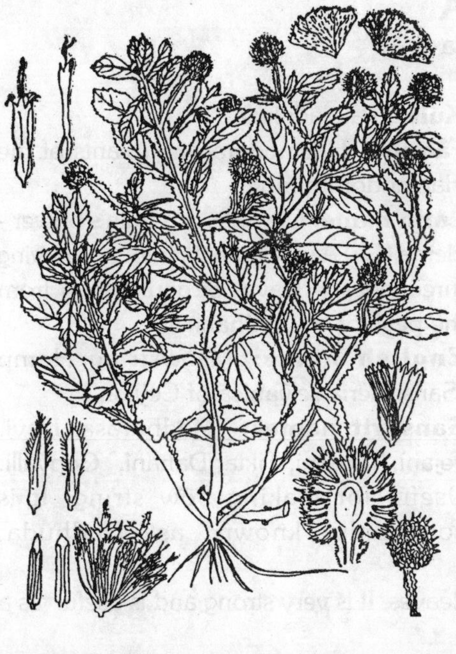

soft, usually meaning pubescent hairy like velvet.

Sanskrit names: Shravani, Tapodhana, Mundi, Bhikshu, Pawani, Shrimati, Tikta, Mahamundi.

Botanical Description: Mundi is a brain tonic, locally known as mudmudiya, karaguee, bad, tarapu. Mundi grows in rice fields after the crop is harvested. The shrub grows 15-30 cm. high and is scented. Leaves - round and composite without stalk and hairy like velvet, 3-6 cm. long, oblong shaped. Flower - stalk 12-18 cm. long, bears round inflorescence of violet colour. Flowering occurs in winter followed by fruiting. One of the varieties called mahashravani or mahamundi (Sphaeranthus africans) grows as a tree.

Chemical composition: Contains salt and brownish yellow volatile oil.

Properties:

Guna: laghu, ruksha; **Rasa:** tikta, katu, madhur; **Vipak:** madhur; **Veerya:** ushna;
Dosha: tridoshahar.

External use: Anti-inflammatory and analgesic.

Internal use: Being a nervine tonic and analgesic, it is useful in lethargy, epilepsy, other vata disorders. Paste of black pepper and mundi is given in headache and migraine.

It is an appetizer, digestive, laxative, hepatic stimulant and anthelmintic. Conditions like loss of appetite, hapatosplenic enlargement, jaundice, internal piles, and intestinal worms are treated with mundi. It is also used in cardiac debility, gout, erysepelas, oedema, lymphadenitis, chronic bronchitis and asthma. The oil of the roots is used as an aphrodisiac. Mundi is an excellent remedy in vata disorders. It is used in dysuria, pyuria, diabetes, skin disorders and fever.

Dose: Juice of the whole plant - 6 to 24 ml.; decoction - 50 to 100 ml.; powder - 0.5 to 1 gm.

References -

विष्वमुण्डी सुगन्धि च कदम्बाभफला स्थिरा । तृणकांगुलिवत्पत्रा -' (शि.)
'मुण्डी तिक्ता कटुः पाके वीर्योष्णा मधुरा लघुः । मेध्या गंडापचीकुष्ठकृमियोन्यर्तिपाण्डुनुत् ।।
श्लीपदारुच्यपस्मारप्लीहमेदोगुदार्त्तिहत् । महामुण्डी च तत्तुल्या गुणैक्ता महर्षिभिः .' (भा. प्र.)
मुण्डिका कटुतिक्तास्यादनिलास्त्रविनाशिनी । अपचीग्नी ह्यपस्मारगण्डश्लीपदनाशिनी । (ध. नि.)
'पीत्त्वा मुण्डितिकोत्थं स्वरसं मरिचावचूर्णितं चोष्णम् ।
भक्तादौ सप्ताहात् सूर्यावर्त्तार्धभेदको हन्यात् ।।' (शो.)

One wonders, who is more delicate, whether a flower or a human being? In the hot a flower does not wilt for at least six hours. Can an undraped man stand this heat for even six minutes?

(184) MURVA
Clematis triloba

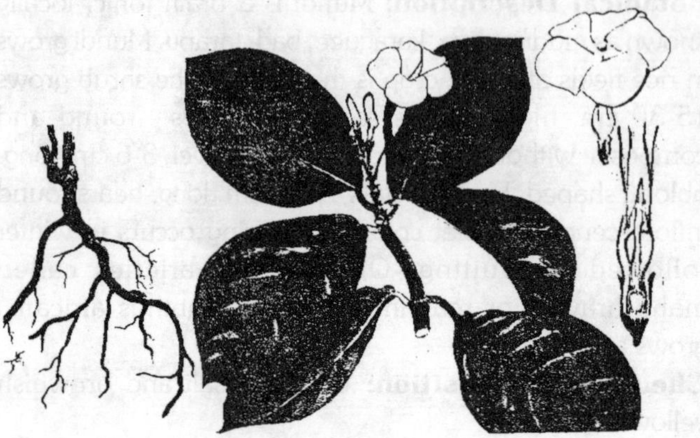

Kula: Patoladi kula.
Family: Haemodoraceae (plants of the Haemodorum tribe).
Latin name: Clematis = Virgin's bower - klema (Gk) A vine branch; triloba = having three lobes = leaves or gouriana = from the peak of Gauri Shankar.
English name: Bowstring Hemp (Sansevieria zelyanica of Ceylon.)
Sanskrit names: Madhurasa, Devi, Tejani, Triparni, Tikta, Dahani, Gopvalli. Useful for making bow string. It is commonly known as Dudhuda, Churanhar, Churnahar, Murhar, etc.
Botanical Description: It is a creeper and has trilobed leaves. It is very strong and is useful as a bow string.
Habitat: Grows everywhere.
Properties:
Guna: sara, guru; **Rasa:** madhur, tikta, kashay; **Veerya:** ushna; **Dosha:** kaphavatanashak.
Parts used: root.
Internal uses: It is used in bleeding disorders, diabetes, thirst, heart disease, itching, skin diseases, fever, vomiting and typhoid fever.
Srotogamitva:
Dosha: Tridoshanashak (kaphavatanashak).
Dhatu: Rasa (purifies breast milk), rakta (bleeding disorders), meda (antidiabetic).
Mala: Mutra.
References -
मूर्वासरागुरु :स्वादुस्तिक्ता पित्तास्त्रमेहनुत् । त्रिदोषतृष्णाहृद्रोगकण्डुकुष्ठज्वरापहा । (भा. प्र.)
मूर्वातिक्ताकषायोष्णाहृद्रोगकफवातहृत् वमिप्रमेह कुष्ठारिर्विषमज्वरनाशनी ।। (रा. नि.)

(185) MUSHALI
Asparagus adscendens Roxb.

Kula: Rasona kula.
Family: Liliaceae.
Gana: Shukrajanan.
Latin name: Asparagus-asper = rough,sharp to the touch ; adscendens = ascending.
Sanskrit names: Shveta, Musali, Mushali, Dholi.

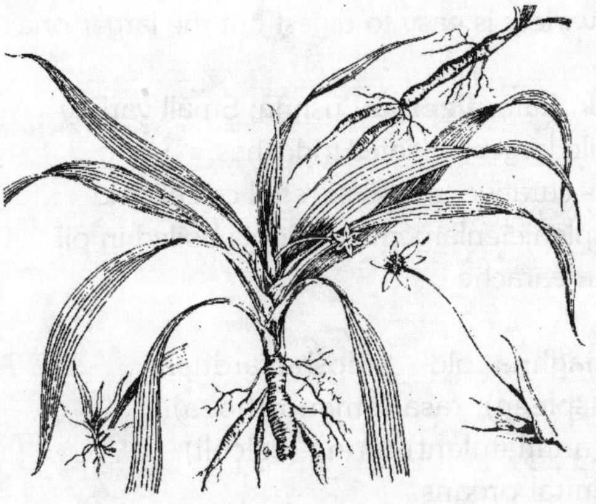

Botanical Description: A thorny shrub like Asparagus racemosus. Stem - long, tall, round and oily. Branches - greyish, hollow and ascending. It is full of thick and straight thorns and measuring 1 to 1.5 cm. Leaves - Stalk is long, hairy, round, measuring 1.5 - 4 cms and bearing 6-20 foliates in racemose form. Roots - oblong.

Varieties: 1) White - known as musali is described above and 2) Black - from Talmuli kula known as Curculigo orchioides.

Botanical description: Small shrub with 3-4 leaves, measuring 15 to 30 cm. long and linear. Flowers - yellow with petals in two rows. Seed - black and shining.

Properties:

Guna: guru, snigdha; **Rasa :** madhur, tikta; **Vipak :** madhur; **Veerya :** ushna; **Dosha:** tridoshahar (vatapittashamak).

Internal uses: It mainly acts on shukradhatu - spermatogenesis and aphrodisiac.

Black musali contains 43.5% starch and therefore is contraindicated in diabetes, but white variety can be used, as it is devoid of starch. It nourishes all the dhatus.

Dose: Root - 3 to 6 gms.

Formulations: Musalipak, Mushalyadiyog.

Srotogamitva:

Dosha: Tridoshahar but mainly vatapittashamak.

Dhatu: Shukra (spermatogenesis and aphrodisiac), all dhatus (rasayana, tonic); meda (white musali).

Mala: Purisha and mutra.

(186) MULAKAM

Raphanus sativus Linn.

Kula: Rajika kula.

Family: Cruciferaeae (petals make a cross.)

Latin name : Raphanus - radish-like, ra = quickly, phainomai = appear; sativus = cultivated.

English name : Garden radish, Turnip.

Sanskrit names: Mulak, Mulahva, Kandamula, Hastidanta, Haritparna, Ruchir, Teekshna, Mishra,Vyaktirasa.

Botanical Description : It is a shrub. Leaves - Long with serrated margins. Tuber - resembles elephant's tooth.

Varieties : 1) Chanakya mulak and 2) Nepal mulak.

Habitat : All over India, also grows at a height of 5000 mtrs. in Himalaya. Smaller variety is found towards Mahabaleshwar.

Chemical composition: Fresh radish contains 91% of water.

According to the science of colour, blue and yellow together make green. Fruits and leaves when matured and ripen become yellow. What happens to blue colour? Does it vanish?

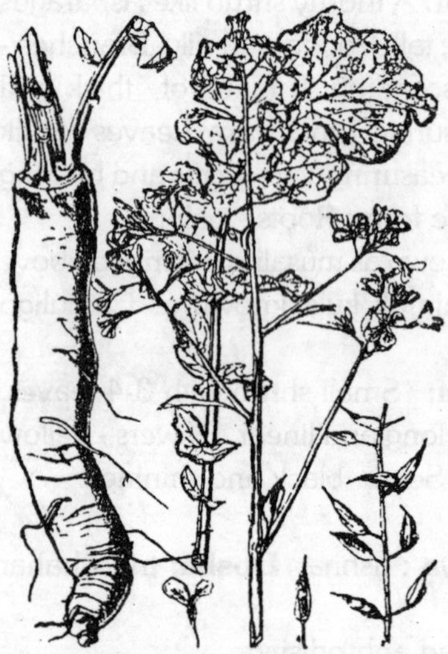

Properties : Smaller variety is easy to digest but the larger one is heavy to digest.

Rasa : katu ; **Vipak** :katu; **Veerya:** ushna; Small variety - alleviates tridoshas while larger - vitiates tridoshas.

Internal uses: Seed - curative, useful in renal calculi and amenorrhoea, hepatosplenic enlargement. Roots boiled in oil are used as ear drops in earache.

Srotogamitva :

Dosha : Dry - tridoshaghna, old - tridoshavardhak.

Dhatu : Rakta (liver, spleen); rasa (amenorrhoea).

Mala : Purishagami (antiflatulent), urine (calculi).

Organ : Liver and genital organs.

	Flower	Fruit
Dosha :	Kaphapittaghna	Kaphavataghna.
Dhatu :	Rakta.	
Organs :	Nose, larynx, eyes.	

References -

स्नेहसिद्धं तदेव स्यात् दोषत्रयविनाशनम् ।' (भा. प्र.)
'बालं दोषहरं वृद्धं त्रिदोषं, मारुतापहम् । स्नहसिद्धं, विशुष्कं तु मूलकं कफवातजित् ।।' (च. सू. २७)
'शुष्कं त्रिदोषशमनं शोथघ्नं गरजिल्लघु । तत्पुष्पं कफपित्तघ्नं तत्फलं कफवातजित् ।।' (रा. व.)
'मूलकं द्विविधं प्रोक्तं तत्रैकं लघुमूलकम् । शालामर्कटकं विस्त्रं शालेयं मरुसम्भवम् ।।
चाणक्यमूलकं तीक्ष्णं तथा मूलकपोतिका । नेपालमूलकं चान्यत्तद्भवेत् गजदन्तवत् ।।
लघुमूलं कटुष्णं स्याद्रुच्यं च लघु पाचनम् । दोषत्रयहरं स्वर्य ज्वरश्वासविनाशनम् ।।
नासिकाकण्ठरोगघ्नं नयनामयनाशनम् । महत्तदेव रुक्षोष्णं गुरु दोषत्रयप्रदम् ।।

(187) METHIKA

Trigonella foenum-graecum

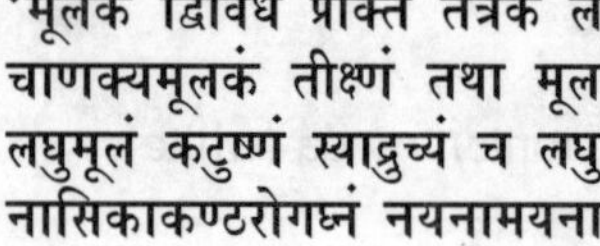

Kula : Methi kula.

Family : Papilionaceae.

Latin name : Trigonella - treis = three, gona = angle, little triangle; foenum = hay or grossum = large.

Sanskrit names : Methika, Methini, Deepani, Gandhaphala, Vallari, Manthya, Mishrapushpa, Kairavi, Peetbeeja.

Botanical Description: A shrub - 30 cms. high. Leaves-compound, trigonal. Flowers - small, pale yellow. Fruit - 5-6 cms. long, legume contains 10-20 seeds.

Properties:

Rasa : katu; **Vipak** : katu; **Veerya** : ushna; **Dosha** : vatakaphaghna.

Uses: Since it is an appetizer and carminative, it is useful in anorexia, loss of appetite and fever.

Women are advised to consume methi seeds in the post natal period to improve excretory and menstrual functions. It is used in dyspepsia, indigestion, rheumatoid arthritis and also as an aphrodisiac. Roasted seeds in the form of infusion are indicated in diarrhoea and small pox. Its porridge is used as galactogogue. Being astringent, roasted seeds along with dry grapes and common salt are given in diarrhoea. It is as potent as cod-liver oil because it contains phosphates, lecithin, nucleoalbumin. Seed powder or leaves pulp is used locally to reduce inflammation and hair fall. It is also used as lipolytic agent.

Parts used : Seed and whole plant.

Dose : Powder - 2 to 6 gms.

Srotogamitva:

Dosha : Vataghna, kaphaghna

Dhatu: Meda, asthi (hair fall), rasa (galactogogue).

Mala : Purisha (astringent).

Organ: Uterus.

References -

'मेथिका वातशमनी श्लेष्मघ्नी ज्वरनाशिनी ।।' (भा. प्र.)

(188) MESHASHRINGI

Gymnema sylvestree R. Br.

Kula: Arka kula.

Family: Asclepiadaceae.

Latin name: Gymnema = gymnos = naked; sylvestree = sylva wood land.

Sanskrit names: Meshashrungi, Vishani, Meshavalli, Ajashrungika, Madhunashini, Sarpadanshtra, Vartika, Chakshushya, Putrashreni.

Botanical Description: A herb bearing multiple branches and growing widely. Leaves - 3 to 7 cms. long, oval. Flowers - yellowish, in clusters. Fruits - 4 to 6 cm. long, hard, arrow shaped. One out of two legumes does not grow. Seeds - long, oval, flat, winged. Flowering occurs in autumn followed by fruiting in winter. The tongue becomes insensitive to sweet and bitter tastes for 1 to 2 hours after chewing the leaves of meshashringi.

Habitat: Konkan, Goa, Kerala, Madhya Pradesh.

Properties: Guna : laghu, ruksha; **Rasa:** kashaya; **Veerya:** ushna; **Dosha :** kaphavatashamak.

Chemical composition: Leaves contain resin, gymnemic acid, tartaric acid, enzymes etc.

External use: Application of leaves mixed with castor oil is useful in glandular swelling, hepatitis and splenic enlargement. Roots are used for application in snake bite.

Internal uses:

Its main action is seen on the digestive system.Being an appetizer, astringent and a hepatic stimulant, it helps to maintain the blood sugar to 0.12% by acting on pancreas, adrenal glands and the digestive glands. Hepatic stimulation leads indirectly to secretion of insulin from pancreas. This reduces the blood sugar and also the urinary sugar. These actions are obtained by using the leaves only and not by using extracts. Root has emetic properties similar to ipecac. It is useful in cardiac failure. Oral administration of seeds or roots in the form of smoking are used to relieve common cold and breathlessness. It is very useful in diabetes and calculi. A dose of 1-2 gms. of leaf powder with honey or cow's milk is given twice a day. It is useful in amenorrhoea, typhoid fever, general debility. Decoction of root is used in snake bite.

Dose: Leaf powder - 1 to 2 gms.; decoction of root - 40 to 80 ml.; powder - 1 to 3 gm.

Srotogamitva :

Dosha: Kaphaghna, vataghna.

Dhatu: Rakta (lowering blood sugar, liver stimulant), rasa (useful in amenorrhoea).

Mala: Mutra (lowers sugar, diabetes, calculus).

(189) MEDASAK

Litsea chinensis Lam.

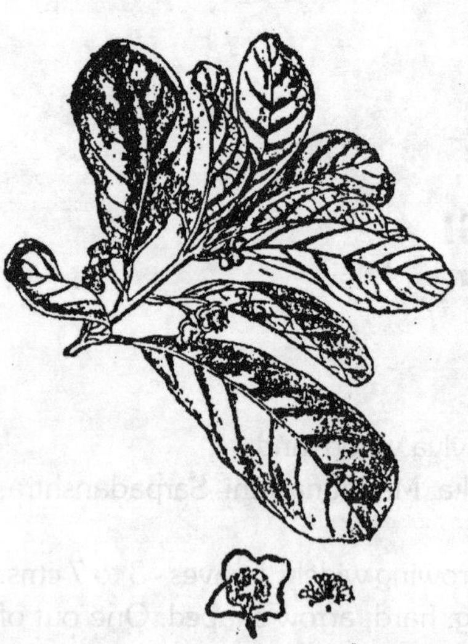

Kula: Karpur kula.

Family: Lauraceae.

Latin name: Litsea = Japanese name of the plant; chinesis = from China.

Sanskrit names: Karkameda, Medalakadi, Medalakavi, Meda.

Botanical Description: This evergreen tree grows 7 to 8 mt. high. Bark - 3 cm. thick, externally ash-grey but red inside, water turns slimy on immersing the bark in it. Leaves - 13 to16 cm. long and scented, 10 to 12 paired. Flowers - tiny, compound, spadix inflorescence, whitish yellow in colour. Fruits - are pea-like. The tree flowers in summer and fruits in rainy season.

Habitat: Forests of North India, Bengal, Dehradun, Mirzapur etc.

Chemical composition: Fruit contains oil. Tree contains laurototanin. By its property of snigdha, pichchil, katu, tikta, kashaya and ushna it is kaphavatashamak. Snigdha and pichchil gunas are superseded by its prabhav to act as kaphanashak.

External uses: Antiinflammatory property of bark and oil is useful in arthritis, fractures, contusions and joint stiffness.

Internal uses: It is vatashamak, analgesic, anticonvulsant and increases vascular tone. Therefore it is useful in sciatica, gout, backache and rheumatoid arthritis. It is used in loss of appetite, diarrhoea and ascites as it is katu, tikta, ushna, appetizer and astringent. Also useful in inflammation, oedema, bleeding, chronic cough, impotency and skin diseases.

Dose: Bark powder - 1 to 2 gms.

Srotogamitva:

Dosha: Kaphaghna, vataghna.

Dhatu: Majja (sciatica, backache), rakta (bleeding disorders), shukra (impotency).

Mala: Purisha (astringent).

References -

'मेदासक: सदापर्ण: गन्धपर्णश्च स स्मृत: । मध्यमाकृतिवृत्तश्च वन्यदेशोद्भवोऽपि च ।।
मेदासको लघु: स्निग्ध: कटुस्तिक्त: कषायक: । उष्णो वातकफौ हन्ति शोथशूलविनाशन: ।।
दीपन: स्तम्भनश्चैव सर्ववातविकारनुत् । अग्निमांद्याऽतिसारे च रक्तस्रावे च युज्यते ।।

(190) YUTHICA

Jasmin auriculata

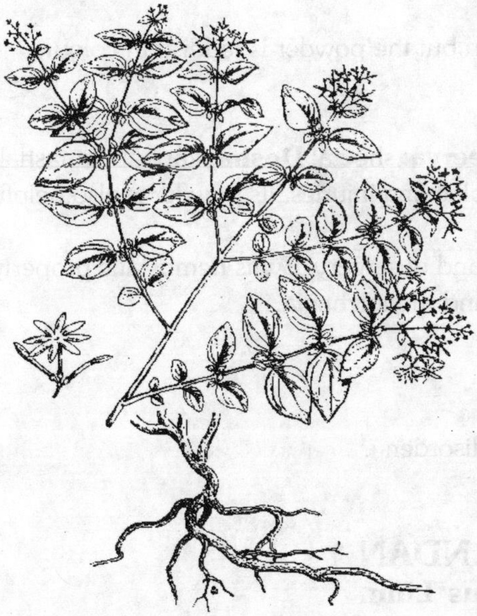

Kula: Prijatak kula.

Family: Oleaceae (Olive tree tribe).

Latin name: Jasmin = from Yasmine - Arabic name; auriculata = small eared.

English name: Jasmine.

Sanskrit names: Yuthica, Balpushpa, Pushpagandha, Ganojjwala, Ganika, Charumoda, Shikhandi, Swarnapushpika.

Varieties: Bhavamishra has described two varieties viz. white and yellow whereas Sushruta has described cream and snow white. A few other texts describe 3 varieties.

Botanical Description: Its creeper resembles the creeper of chameli. Leaves - compound, pentafoliated. Flowers - white or yellow in colour and have a very pleasant odour.

Habitat: All over India, predominantly in Bengal and Madras, Karnataka; Tamil women use yellow variety for cosmetic purposes.

Properties :

Guna:laghu; **Rasa:** tikta, kashaya, madhur; **Veerya:** sheeta; **Prabhav:** cardiotonic.

Uses: It is used in heart diseases, bleeding disorders, poisoning, skin diseases, stomatitis, gingivitis, eye disorders and ear, nose, throat conditions.

Dose: Juice of flowers - 10 to 20 ml.; decoction of leaves - 40 to 80 ml.

Srotogamitva:

Dosha: Pittaghna, kaphakarak, vatakarak.

Dhatu: Rakta (bleeding disorders, skin diseases).

Mala: Cleanses infected wounds.

Organ: Heart, respiratory organs.

References -

'यूथिका गणिकाऽम्बष्टा सा पीता हेमपुष्पिका । यूथीयुगं हिमं तिक्तं कटुपाकरसं लघु ।।
मधुरं तुवरं हृद्यं पित्तघ्नं कफवातलम् । व्रणास्रमुखदन्ताक्षिशिरोरोगविषापहम् ।।' (भा. प्र.)

Human beings love as pets the moving beings-animals. Would they also love the immobile beings-plants?

(191) RAKTANIRYAS
Daemenorops draco Blume.

Kula: Narikel kula.
Family: Palmae (Palm tribe).
Latin name: Daemenorops = evil spirit,very thorny climber; draco = dragon.
English name: Dragon's blood.
Sanskrit name: Raktaniryas.
Hindi: Khoonkharaba, Hiradokhae.
Botanical Description: Latex of the tree is bluish brown but the powder is reddish in colour.
Habitat: Arabia and Africa.
Properties:
Guna: laghu, ruksha; **Rasa:** kashaya; **Vipak:** katu; **Veerya:** sheeta; **Dosha:** kaphapittanashak.
External uses: Since it is a hemostat, it is used in fresh bleeding injuries. Its powder is also helpful for healing of chronic wounds.
Internal uses: Being astringent, it is useful in diarrhoea and dysentery. By its hemostatic property, it is useful in haemoptysis, haemetemesis, bleeding piles and menorrhagia.
Dose: Latex 1 to 1.5 gms.
Srotogamitva:
Dosha: Kaphaghna, pittaghna.
Dhatu: Rakta (hemostat), mansa (healing), (in bleeding disorders).
Mala: Purisha (astringent).

(192) RAKTACHANDAN
Pterocarpus santalinus Linn.

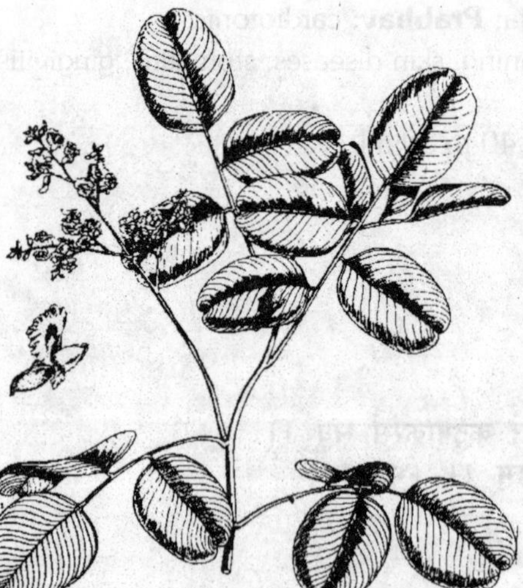

Kula: Shimbi kula.
Family: Leguminoseae.
Gana: Patoladi, Sarivadi, Priyangvadi, Pittaghna.
Latin name: Pterocarpus = ptero = winged, carpus = fruit; santalinus = sandal wood.
English name: Red sandal wood.
Sanskrit names: Kuchandan, Lohit, Harichandan, Raktasar, Tamrasar, Kshudrachandan, Arkachandan, Ranjan, Pravalphala, Surakta.
Botanical Description: A tree growing to a height of 5-10 mtrs. Bark is blackish grey. Trunk - externally white but red inside. Stalk bears flowers in all the directions. Legumes - 6 to 9 containing red seeds. Flowering and fruiting occurs in summer.
Habitat: South India, Karnataka.

Properties:
Guna: guru,ruksha; **Rasa:** madhur, tikta; **Vipak:** katu; **Veerya:** sheeta; **Dosha:** kaphapittashamak.
Uses: External application relieves oedema caused by kaphapitta. It is a refrigerant and hemostatic. It is useful in skin diseases, conjunctivitis and contusions, thirst, bleeding disorders, vomiting, fever, burning sensation, diarrhoea and poisoning.
Dose: Powder - 3 to 6 gms. Dolls made from its wood are sold in the market.
Srotogamitva:
Dosha: Kaphaghna, pittaghna.
Dhatu: Rakta, rasa, shukra (aphrodisiac).
Mala: Purisha (antidiarrhoeal).
Organ: Alimentary, lymphatic and circulatory systems.
References -
'रक्तं शीतं गुरु स्वादु च्छर्दितृष्णास्रपित्तहत् । तिक्तं नेत्रहितं वृष्यं ज्वरव्रणविषापहम् ।।' (भा. प्र.)
'रक्तचन्दनमतीव शीतलं तिक्तमीक्षगणगदास्रदोषनुत् ।
भूतपित्तकफकासज्वरभ्रान्तिजन्तुवमिजित्तृषापहम् ।।' (रा. नि.)

(193) RAJIKA
Brassica juncea Coss.

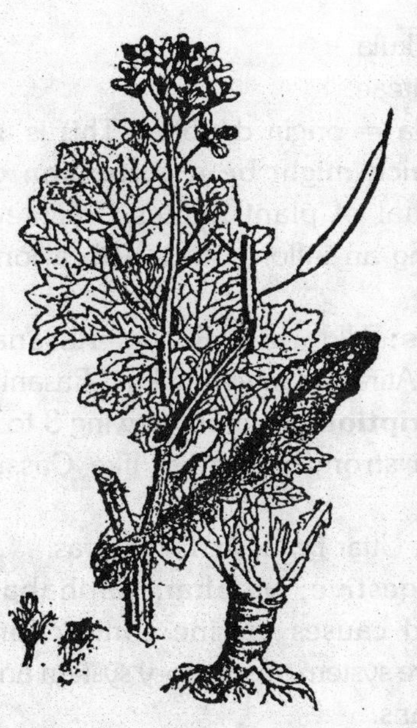

Kula: Rajika kula.
Family: Cruciferae.
Latin name: Brassica = Plautus = Latin name which includes 22 species; juncea = rushy - resembling rush, juncus).
Sanskrit names: Aasuri, Raktika, Rajkshavak, Krishnavarnak, Siddharthak.
Botanical Description: Perennial shrub, grows 6 to 9 cm. high, bears long leaves and yellow flowers which blossom in summer.
Habitat: All over India.
Chemical composition: It contains 20-25% stable oil. It yields a volatile oil on coming in contact with water.
Properties:
Guna: tikshna; **Rasa:** tikta; **Vipak:** katu; **Veerya:** ushna; **Dosha:** kaphavatashamak.
Uses: Paste of the seeds made in water and applied on the skin causes irritation. Rajika, when used in the form of oil, paste and decoction, is useful in many disorders of kapha and vata. Paste is made in a mortar in cold water, spread on a cloth and kept for 10 minutes over the affected part. Orally, it is useful in loss of appetite and anorexia. It is used as an emetic in treating internal poisoning. In acute and chronic dysentery, when the seeds are swallowed with water, they break inside the lumen of the intestine thereby clearing the luminal mucous and relieving griping pain. Its excessive use causes vitiation of pitta and therefore it should be used cautiously.

By carefully observing the types and location of plants and trees, one can identify the hidden mineral-wealth and the subterranean water-streams.

Srotogamitva:
Dosha: Kaphaghna, vataghna, pittakar.
Dhatu: Raktagami (spleen).
Mala: Purisha (worms).
Organ: Intestine.
Taila (Oil)
Dosha: Reduces vatadi doshas.
Dhatu: Raktagami.
Mala: Keshya.
References -
'राजी तु राजिकातीक्ष्णगन्धा क्षुज्जनिकासुरी । राजिका कफवातघ्नी तीक्ष्णोष्णारक्तपित्तकृत् किंचिद्रूक्षाग्निदा कण्डूकुष्टकोष्ठक्रिमीन् हरेत् ।।' (भा. प्र.)
'तीक्ष्णं तु राजिकातैलं ज्ञेयं वातादिदोषनुत् । शिशिर कटुक स्त्वच्चं केश्यं त्वग्दोषनाशनम् ।।' (रा. नि.)
आसुरी कटुतिक्तोष्णा वातप्लीहार्त्तिशूलनुत् । दाहपित्तप्रदा हन्तिकफगुल्मकृमिव्रणान् ।। (रा. नि.)

(194) RASANA
Inula racemosa Hook.

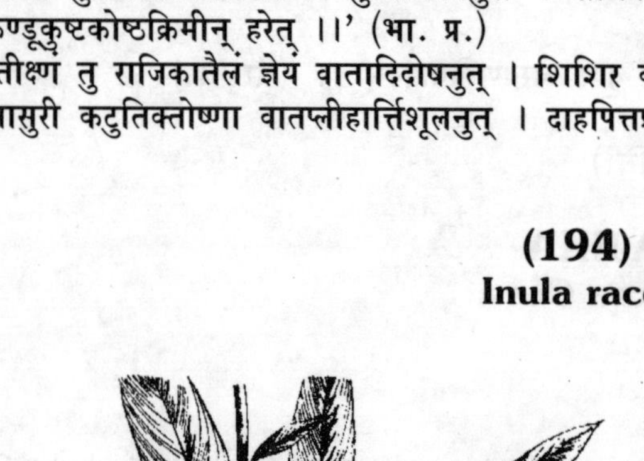

Kula: Bhrungaraj kula.
Family: Compositeae.
Latin name: Inula = origin doubtful. This is an ancient name which might be a corruption of Belenium - Manual of plant names Chichley; recemosa = having an inflorescence with a long undivided axis.
Sanskrit names: Uktarasa, Rasya, Rasana, Elaparni, Surasa, Atirasa, Gandhanakuli, Rasani.
Botanical Description: A shrub growing 3 to 6 cms. high. It is a strong purgative like Cassia angustifolia.
Habitat: Kashmir, Uttar Pradesh, Himalayas.
Properties: Digestive, vatahar, kaphahar, antiasthmatic and causes uterine contraction. Effective in digestive system, respiratory system and female genital organs.
Uses:
Digestive system : Flatulence, abdominal colic, indigestion.
Respiratory system: Asthma, bronchitis, pleuritis, chest pain.
Musculoskeletal system: Rheumatoid arthritis, vata disorders, tuberculosis.

Genital system: Amenorrhoea, dysmenorrhoea.
It is an antipyretic and is useful in skin diseases like itching, ring worm and eczema. In skin diseases, a paste of its roots prepared in cow's urine is applied. Its decoction is also used to wash the affected area. Rasana has a specific action in rheumatoid arthritis.

References -

रास्नामपाचनी तिक्त गुरुष्णा कफवातजित् ।
शोथ श्वास समीरास्त्र वातशूलोदरापहा ।
कास ज्वर विषाशीतिवातकामयहिध्महत् ।।' (भा. प्र.)

(195) RUMAMASTAKI
Pistacia lentiscus Linn.

Kula: Amra kula.
Family: Anacardiaceae.
Latin name: Pistacia = based on the Arabic name Foustag; lentiscus = mastich tree - gum or resin exuding from bark
English name : Mastich.
Synonyms: Rumimastagi, Mastagi, Alakrumi, Kundarrumi.
Botanical Description: A shrub which remains green perennially. Multiple incisions on the bark exude resin called and marketed as rumamastaki. Resin is white or yellow in colour, scented, in the form of round granules and slightly sweet to taste. Because of its stickiness, it is collected in a cloth, kept in water for some time, dried and then powdered.
Habitat: It is found along the Mediterrian coast i.e. Southern part of Europe and Northern Africa. It is transported to India through Iran and Afghanisthan.
Chemical composition: Masticic acid - 90% and masticin - 10%.
Properties:
Guna: laghu, ruksha; **Rasa:** madhur, kashaya; **Vipak:** madhur; **Veerya:** ushna; **Dosha:** vatapittashamak, kaphanissarak.
External use: It is used in oedema, for enhancing complexion and in bad breath. Keeping the powder of rumamastaki in mouth strengthens the gums and relieves bad breath.It is applied on the chest in pleuritis. It is used in loss of appetite, liver disorders, duodenitits, bronchitis, asthma, dysuria and dysmenorrhoea.
Dose: Resin - 1 to 3 gms.
Srotogamitva:
Dosha: Vataghna, pittaghna, kaphanissarak.
Dhatu: Rakta (liver,skin).
Mala: Mutra (dysuria), intestine.
Organ: Digestive and respiratory systems and uterus.

The ventral surface of the leaf and its dorsal can be used for two different purposes (e.g. the leaf of Samudrashopha- Argyria speciosa).

(196) ROHITAK

Tecomella undulata

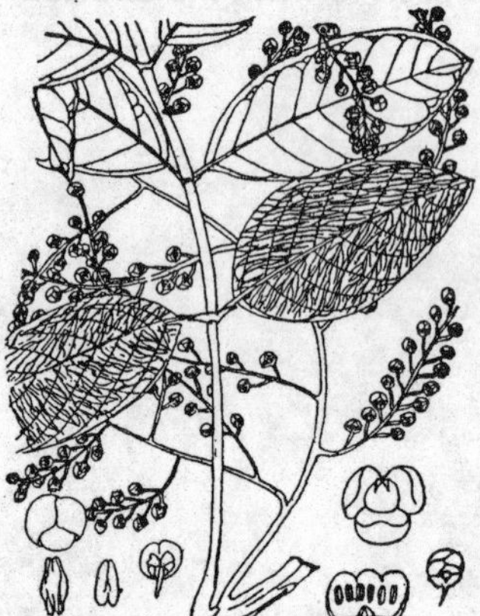

Kula: Shyonak kula.
Family: Bignoniaceae.
Latin name: Tecomella = from 'Tecoma' - Mexican name which is no longer a botanical name; undulata = wave-formed.
Sanskrit names: Rohitak, Rohit, Kushalmali, Sadaprasoon, Kutashalmali, Virochan, Shalmalik, Dadimpushpak.
White rohitak: Shwetarohit, Sita, Sitanga, Shuklarohit, Laxmivan, Janavallabha. (Specific action on spleen and lever).
Botanical Description: The tree grows 3 to 5 mtrs. high. Leaves - 15 to 18 cm. long, oval and flat tipped. This tree resembles pomegranate tree but bears legumes which are slightly bent and 24 cm. long. Seeds - winged, 3 cm. long. Flowering occurs in winter.
Habitat: Rajputana, Kathiawad, Kutch and Punjab.

Properties:
Guna: laghu, snigdha, katu; **Rasa:** tikta, kashaya; **Vipak:** katu; **Veerya:** sheeta; **Prabhav:** purgative; **Dosha:** kaphapittanasak.
Uses: Paste is applied on contusions. Juice is useful in conjunctivitis. When given internally, it acts on blood, spleen and liver and therefore is useful in loss of appetite, ascites, piles, and intestinal worms.
Dose: Bark decoction - 50 to 100 ml.; powder - 1 to 3 gms.
Preparations: Rohit kashtha, Rohitakadya choorna, Rohit ghrit, Rohitak loha.
Srotogamitva:
Dosha: Kaphaghna, pittaghna.
Dhatu: Rakta (liver, spleen); meda (diabetes, leucorrhoea).
Mala: Purisha.
Organs: Liver, spleen.
References -
'रोहीतको रोहितको रोही दाडिमपुष्पकः । रोहीतकः प्लीहघाती रुच्यो रक्तप्रसादनः ।।' (भा. प्र.)
'रोहीतको यकृत्प्लीहगुल्मोदरहरः सरः ।' (ध. नि.)
रोहीतकौ कटुस्निग्धौ कषायौ च सुशीतलौ । कृमिदोषव्रणप्लीहरक्तनेत्रामयापहौ ।।' (रा. नि.)

(197) ROHISHAM

Cymbopogon schoenanthus Linn.

Gana: Stanyajanan.
Kula: Yava kula.
Family: Gramineae.
Latin name: Cymbopogon = cymba = boot, andropogon = citratus; schoenanthus = aromatic - used in wines.

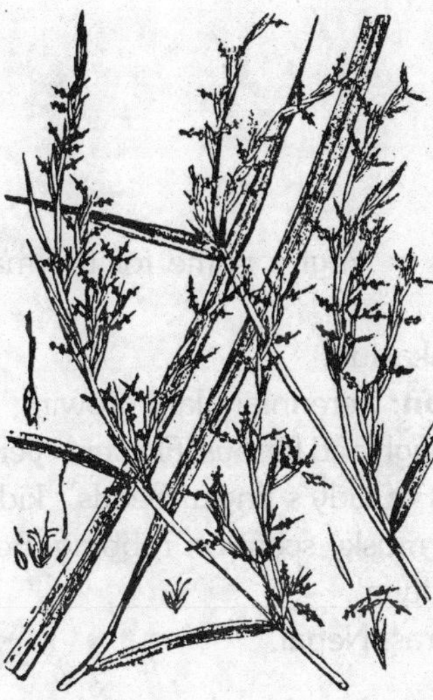

English names: Lemon grass, ginger grass, sweet rush.

Sanskrit names: Laghu rohisham - Kattruna, Saugandhik, Bhutee, Rohishtruna, Shyamak, Devajagdhak. **Deergha rohisham -** Rohishak, Drudhakand, Drudhacchada, Kutsit, Agiyadhas.

Botanical Description: A shrub, 1.5 to 2 mt. high with a slimy trunk. Leaves - brownish, tapering towards the end and have a rosy aroma. Inflorescence is enveloped in sepals. The plant blossoms in rainy season and fruits in winter. It looks like the shrub of rice from a distance.

Habitat: Punjab, Rajasthan, Uttar Pradesh, Bihar, Bengal, Southern India, Sri Lanka, Burma. It is found in northern parts of Nasik district of Maharashtra. The state auctions it for oil extraction.

Chemical composition: The leaves contain an aromatic oil (ganiol) which is brownish-blue, has a rose-like aroma and tastes like ginger.

Properties:

Guna: ruksha, laghu, tikshna; **Rasa:** katu, tikta; **Vipak:** katu; **Veerya:** ushna; **Dosha:** kaphavatashamak.

External uses: Analgesic and antiinflammatory action helps in rheumatoid arthritis, synovitis, dermatitis and alopecia.

Internal uses: Since rohisham is an appetizer, digestive, carminative and anthelmintic, it is useful in many disorders of the gastrointestinal tract. It is useful in cough, cold and asthma as it reduces the congestion of the respiratory tract. It acts as a galactogogue due to its rasa and raktagamitva. Rohisham is also used in dysuria. Since it is a diaphoretic, it is used in fever caused by kaphavata.

Parts used: Root, leaves and oil.

Dose: Decoction - 50 to 100 gm.; oil - 1 to 3 drops.

Srotogamitva:

Dosha: Kaphaghna, vataghna.

Dhatu: Rakta, rasa.

Mala: Mutra (urinary tract), sweda (diaphoretic).

Organ : Respiratory system, cough, bronchitis.

References -

'रोहिषं तुवरं तिक्तं कटुपाकं व्यपोहति । हत्कण्डुव्याधिरातास्त्रशूलकासकफज्वरान् ।।' (भा. प्र.)

'कत्तुणं श्वासकासघ्नं हद्रोगशमनं परम् । विसूच्यजीर्णशूलघ्नं कफवातास्त्रनाशम् ।।' (ध. नि.)

'कत्तुणं कटुकं तिक्तमुष्णं कटु विपाकतः । बलासवातरुधिरकण्डूहद्रोगनाशनम् ।।
कृमिकासज्वरश्वासशूलाजीर्णरुचिप्रणुत् । (कै. नि.)

The conch shell has to be put on a support for remaining stable; that the conch shell is important. Likewise gunas do take support of dravyas, but the gunas are important.

(198) LATAKASTURI
Hibiscus abelmoschus Linn.

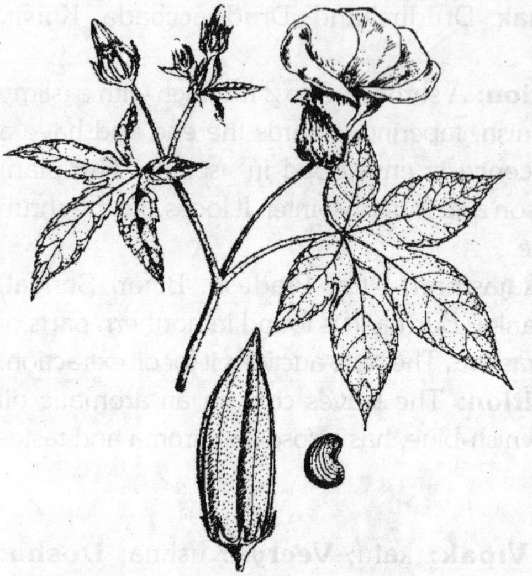

Kula: Karpas kula.
Family: Malvaceae.
Latin name: Hibiscus = Virgil's name for the marsh mallow; abelmoschus.
Sanskrit name: Latakasturi.
Botanical Description: Perennial plant growing 1 to 1.5 mtrs. high. Stalk is tough and fibrous. Flowers - yellow. Leaves - like the leaves of lady's finger. Seeds - kidney shaped and give out a musky scent on rubbing. Seeds are known as 'mushkadana'.
Habitat: Bengal, Madras, Nepal.
Properties:
Guna: laghu, ruksha; **Rasa:** ruksha, tikta, madhur, katu; **Vipak:** katu; **Veerya:** sheeta; **Dosha:** kaphapittashamak.
Uses: Being an appetizer, astringent and deodorant, it is useful in bad breath, anorexia, loss of appetite, diarrhoea, asthma, brochitis, dysuria and gonorrhoea. A fine powder of seeds is used in opthalmic conditions.
Srotogamitva:
Dosha: Kaphaghna, pittaghna.
Dhatu: Shukra (aphrodisiac), rasa.
Mala: Mutra.
Organ: Eye, stomach, urinary bladder.
References -
'लताकस्तूरिका तिक्ता स्वाद्वी वृष्या हिमा लघुः ।
चक्षुष्या दीपनी श्लेष्मतृष्णाबस्त्यास्यरोगहृत् ।।' (भा. प्र.)
'धार्यण्यास्येन वैशद्यरुचिसौगध्यमिच्छता । जातीकटुकपूगानां लवंगस्य फलानि च ।।' (च. सू. ५)
'जातीकटुकयोः फलम् ।... तिक्तं कटु कफापहम् । लघु तृष्णापहं वक्त्रक्लेददौर्गन्ध्य-
'नाशनम् । लताकस्तूरिका तद्वच्छीता वस्तिविशोधनी ।।' (सु. सू. ४६)

(199) LAJJALU
Mimosa pudica

Gana : Sandhaniya, Purishasangrahneeya, Priyangvadi, Ambasthadi.
Kula : Shimbi kula.
Family : Leguminoseae.
Latin name : Mimosa - mimos = mimic, sensitivity of the leaves.
English name : Sensitive plant, Humble plant.

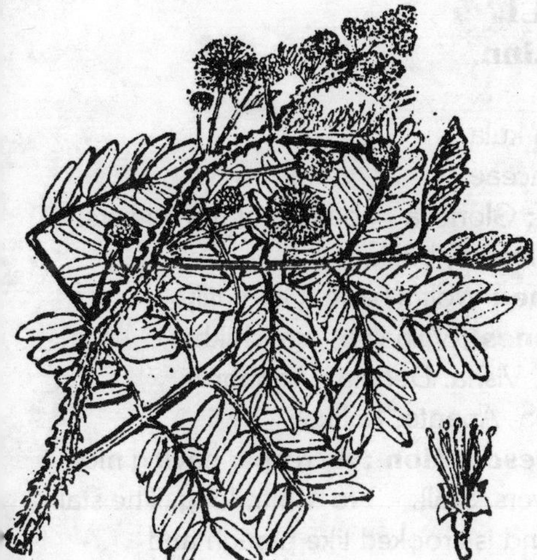

Sanskrit names : Lajjalu, Shamipatra, Samanga, Anjalikarika, Namaskari, Sparsharodanika.

Botanical Description : This thorny shrub grows 30 to 100 cms. in height. The stalk of the leaf is long and 4 leaves in the form of paw arise from it. Leaves - resemble that of khadir leaves and close up on touching, hence the name lajjalu, namaskari. Flowers - delicate and pink arise from the tip of flower stalk. They contain four big androceiums. Legumes - 1.5 to 2 cms. long and bear thorns. Each legume contains 3 to 4 seeds. The plant flowers in winter followed by fruiting.

It has one more small variety which grows 10-12 cms. high.

Habitat : It is said that this plant was originally found in Brazil and now it is seen all over India.

Properties :

Guna : laghu, ruksha; **Rasa** : kashaya, tikta; **Veerya** : sheeta; **Dosha** : kaphapittashamak. It is used internally as well as externally.

External uses : It has uniting, wound healing and hemostatic properties, hence is used in wounds, ulcers and fistulae.

Internal uses : It is a good astringent. It acts as a vasoconstrictor, thus providing relief in haemoptysis, menorrhagia and bleeding piles. Lajjalu is also a blood purifier and antiinflammatory. Because of its astringnt property, it is used in diarrhoea and dysentery. Seeds are particularly useful in prameha and diseases of the semen. It is also useful in fractures and poisons.

Parts used : Leaves and seeds.

Dose : Leafjuice - 10 to 20 ml.

Srotogsmitva :

Dosha : Kaphaghna, pittaghna.

Dhatu : Rakta (hemostatic - haemoptysis, haemorrhoids and menorrhagia); shukra (seeds - diseases of semen), asthi (uniting property).

Mala : Mutra (diabetes), purisha (diarrhoea, dysentery and colitis).

Organs : Uterus (menorrhagia).

References -

रक्तपादी शमीपत्रा स्पृक्का खदिरपत्रिका । स्पर्शात संकोचतां याति पुनश्च प्रसृता भवेत् ।।'

'लज्जालुः शीतलातिक्ताकषायाकफपित्तजित् । रक्तपित्तमतिसारंयोनिरोगान् विनाशयेत् ।।' (भा. प्र.)

'रक्तपादी कटुःशीता पित्तातिसारनाशिनी । शोफदाहश्रमश्वासव्रणकुष्ठकफास्रनुत् ।।' (रा. नि.)

Never forget the vibrations as these form the essence of life. Without vibrations what else is there from birth to death?

(200) LANGALI

Gloriosa superba Linn.

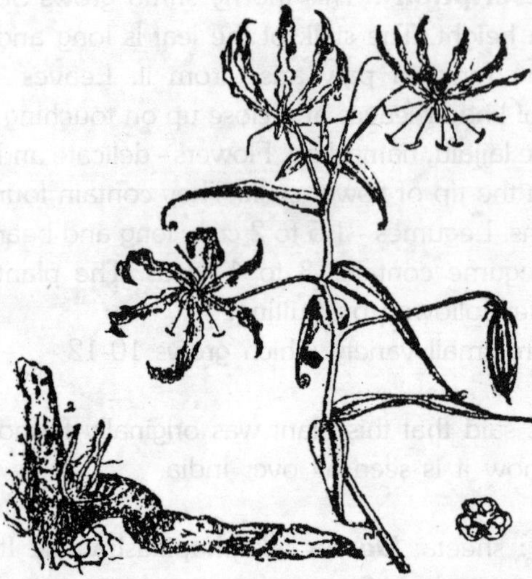

Kula : Rason kula.

Family : Liliaceae.

Latin name : Gloriosa = beauty of the flowers; superba = splendid, brilliant.

English name : Wolf's bane, Glory lilly.

Sanskrit names : Vishalya, Agnishikha, Garbhapatini, Visha, Deepta, Vranahrut, Swarnapushpa, Ananta, Kalikali.

Botanical Description : A creeper having nice attractive flowers. Stalk - 3 to 4 mtr. long. The stalk near the ground is crooked like plough and contracted distantly. Leaves - stalkless, 18 to 24 cms. long with hook like tip and climbs taking its support. Flowers - 9 to12 cms. in size, yellow and red towards periphery. Fruits - 9 to 12 inches in size. Tuber - round, flat and 3 cms long. It grows during monsoon and dries up as soon as rain stops.

Varieties : 1) Female - round tuber and 2) Male - flat and long tuber.

Habitat : Bengal , south India, Brahmadesh and Sri lanka.

Chemical composition : Tuber contains resin, superbine, gloriojine and starch.

Properties :

Guna : laghu, tikshna; **Rasa :** katu, tikta; **Veerya :** ushna; **Prabhav :** garbhapatan (abortefacient); **Dosha :** kaphavatashamak.

External uses : Locally abortefacient and vitiates blood. Its paste is applied on wounds, inflammations, lymphadenopathy, piles and scorpion sting. Its application on palms, soles, umbilicus and lumbar region eases the process of delivery and expulsion of placenta. Tuber kept in vagina acts as an abortefacient.

Internal uses : In low dose, it is useful in loss of appetite, pitta disorders, worms, dermatoses, typhoid and general debility.

Dose : For easy delivery and abortion - 3 to 6 ratti, otherwise in a low dose of 1 to 2 gms.

Srotogamitva :

Dosha : Kaphaghna, pittaghna and vataghna.

Dhatu : Rakta (dermatoses, piles).

Mala : Purisha (anthelmintic).

Organ : Uterus (abortifacient - local application on umbilicus, pelvis or palms and soles).

References -

'कलिहारी सरा कुष्ठशोफार्शोव्रणशूलजित् । सक्षारा श्लेष्मजित्तिका कटुका तुवरापि च ।।
तीक्षोष्णाकृमिहल्लध्वी पित्तला गर्भपातिनी ।' (भा. प्र.)
'लांगली कटुरुष्णा च कफवातविनाशिनी । तिक्ता सरा च श्वयथुगर्भशल्यव्रणापहा ।।'

'पाठालांगलिसिंहास्यमयूरकजटाः पृथक् । नाभिबस्तिभगालेपात् सुखं नारी प्रसूयते ।।'
'लांगलीमूलकल्केन वाऽस्याः पाणिपादतलमालिम्पेत् ।' (सु. शा. १०)

(201) LODHRA

Symplocos racemosa Roxb.

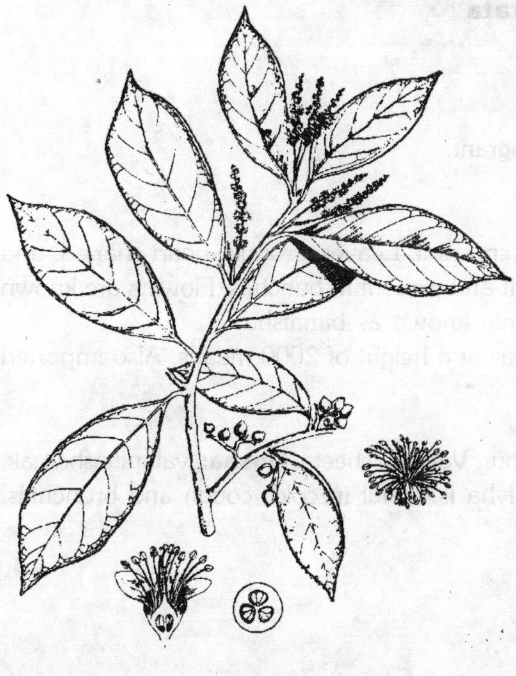

Gana : Artavashaman, Shonitasthapan, Sandhaneeya, Purishasangrahaneeya, Kashayaskandha, Lodhradi, Nyagrodhadi.
Kula : Rodhra Kula.
Family : Symplocaceae.
Latin name : Symplocos - symploca = connection, stems united at the base, sym = together; racemosa = racemed.
Sanskrit names : Lodhra, Rodhra, Shabarak, Tilwak, Tilakataru, Tiritak, Bhilli, Shambarpadap.
Botanical Description : Evergreen medium high tree. Leaves - round with a diameter of 9 to 15 cms. Flower stalk - 6 to 12 cms. long with yellow white flowers. Fruits - 1.5 cms. long and hard. Bark - red.
Another variety of lodhra is found in the Himalayas at the height of 1 - 3 thousand mtrs. which has bigger leaves, fruits and flowers compared to that of lodhra.
Habitat : North India, Malabar and Malaya.
Chemical Composition : It doesnot contain tanin.
Uses : Local application of the paste is useful in oedema, skin disorders, bleeding disorders, wounds, coujunctivitis and otorrhoea. It is used in tooth powder. It also enhances the complexion. Its astringent property helps in diarrhoea and dysentery. Being a vasoconstrictor, it is used in bleeding disorders and inflammations. Its decoction is used as vaginal douche in menorrhagia, leucorrhoea and endometritis. It is also useful in eye and skin disorders, fever, dysentery and vaginal disorders.
Lodhra mainly acts on rasa, rakta, meda dhatus and kapha dosha.
Dose : Decoction of bark - 50 to 100 ml; powder - 1 to 3 gms.
Formulations : Lodhrasar, Lodhradi Kadha.
Srotogamitva :
Dosha : Kaphaghna, pittaghna.
Dhatu : Meda (reduces meda), rakta (hemostat - bleeding disorders).
Mala : Purisha (astringent).
Organs : Intestines, eyes, vagina and uterus. (Lodhra is mainly effective in eye disorders).

If the plants are pest-laden and not healthy then how can one expect to desire health by using such plants?

References -
लोध्रो ग्राही लघुः शीतः चक्षु,यः कफपित्तनुत् ।
कषायो रक्तपितासृक् ज्वरातिसारशोथहृत् ।। (भा. प्र.)

(202) VANAPSIKA
Viola odorata

Kula: Banafsha kula.
Family: Violaceae (plants of the violet, Viola tribe).
Latin name: Viola = a Latin name; odorata = fragrant.
Indian name: Banafsha.
English name: Wild or sweet violet.
Botanical Description: The plant is hardly 8 to 9 cms. tall. Leaves - round, heart shaped, and with hairy undersurface. Flowers - blue, violet, fragrant and present in bunches. Flowers are known as gulbanafsha. Root - green in colour and commonly known as banafsha.
Habitat: From Kashmir to Western parts of Himalayas at a height of 2000 metres. Also imported from Iran.
Properties:
Guna: laghu,ruksha; **Rasa:** madhur, tikta; **Vipak:** madhur; **Veerya:** sheeta; **Dosha:** vatapittashamak.
Uses: Decoction of banafsha, yashtimadhu and gojivha is useful in cold, cough and bronchitis. Inhalation with its steam relieves throat pain.
Srotogamitva:
Dosha: Reduces pitta (shodhan), kapha (vamak).
Dhatu: Rakta (astringent).
Mala: Panchang (diaphoretic).

(203) VATA
Ficus bengalensis Linn.

Kula: Vata kula.
Family: Urticaceae.
Latin name: Ficus = the distorted form of the original Arabic word Fag; bengalensis = of Bengal - there is a huge Banyan tree in the botanical garden at Calcutta.
English name: Banyan tree (Banias used to have bazaar under this tree).
Sanskrit names: Raktapahla, Shungi, Kshiri, Vanaspati, Avarohi, Padrohan, Pakshyavas, Skandharuh, Mahacchaya.
Botanical Description : Banyan trees are huge and outspreading. Trunk is whitish grey in colour. Leaves - big, oval, 12 to 14 cms long, thick, turgid and darkgreen having 3 to 5 veins. Fruits - are red and round; they are not real fruits but contain innumerable minute flowers in them just like udumber (Ficus glomerata). Flowers bloom in spring and fruiting occurs in monsoon. The tree survives for many years.
Habitat: All over India.

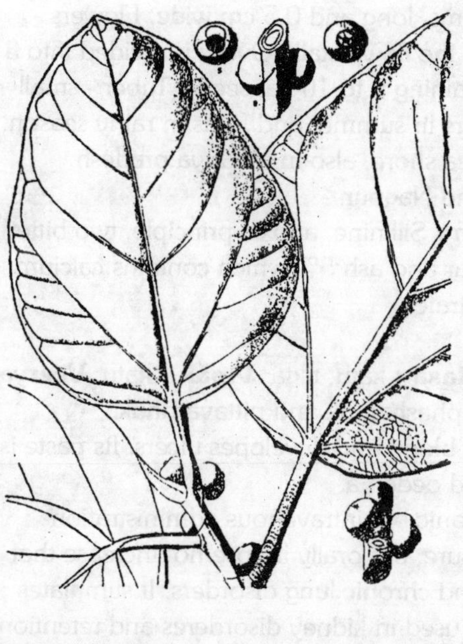

Chemical compostion: Skin and fruits (raw) contain 10% tannin.

Properties:

Guna: guru, ruksha; **Rasa:** kashaya; **Veerya:** sheeta; **Vipak:** katu; **Dosha :** kaphapittashamak.

External uses: The latex of vata is applied on wounds, cracked soles, synovitis, arthritis, lymphadenitis, otorrhoea, toothache, conjunctivitis and piles. Areal roots of vatavruksha in the form of paste is used to treat sagging breasts, skin diseases and skin ulcers. In synovitis and other inflammatory conditions, leaves are tied locally over the inflammed part.

Internal uses: The latex of vata is given orally to treat diarrhoea, amoebic dysentery and bacillary dysentery. In leucorrhoea and menorrhagia, the decoction of the bark is given as a douche. The latex of the tree is given with sugar as a remedy for premature ejaculation. Tender leaves of vata are used for grabhasthapan (anti abortifacient). Latex, bark, skin and fruits act as antidiabetic.

Dose: Decoction of bark - 50 to 100 ml.; powder - 3 to 6 gms.; latex - 10 to 20 drops.

Special Formulations: Nyagrodhadi choorna, Nyagrodhadya ghrit.

Srotogamativa:

Dosha: Kaphaghna, pittaghna.

Dhatu: Rakta (menorrhagia, complexion enhancer, bleeding disorders), shukra (delays ejaculation, tender leaves - garbhasthapan and punsavan), mansa-meda (wound healing).

Mala: Purish, mutra (astringent).

Organ: Uterus (menorrhagia, leucorrhoea, garbhasthapan).

References -

'वट:शीतो गुरुर्ग्राही कफपित्तव्रणापहः वर्ण्यो विसर्पदाहघ्नः कषायो योनिदोषहृत् ।।' (भा. प्र.)
वट:शीत:कषायश्च स्तम्भनो रूक्षणात्मकः । तथा तृष्णाच्छर्दिमूर्च्छारक्तपित्तविनाशनः ।।'
'गर्भदं वटशुंगं तु पिबेद् वन्ध्या रजस्वला । वारिणा शुक्लपक्षेहि पुष्येण च समाहतम् ।।' (शो.)
'वटांकुरा मसूराश्च प्रलेपात् व्यंगनाशनम् ।' (भा. प्र.)

(204) VANAPALANDU
Urginea indica

Kula : Rason kula.

Family : Liliaceae.

Latin name : Urginea, indica = Indian.

Sanskrit name : Kolakand.

English name : Indian squill.

Botanical Description : A herb resembling onion herb, bears flowers first followed by the

If the juice of a plant is used to give bhavana to the powder of same plant, then the gunas will definitely get enhanced.

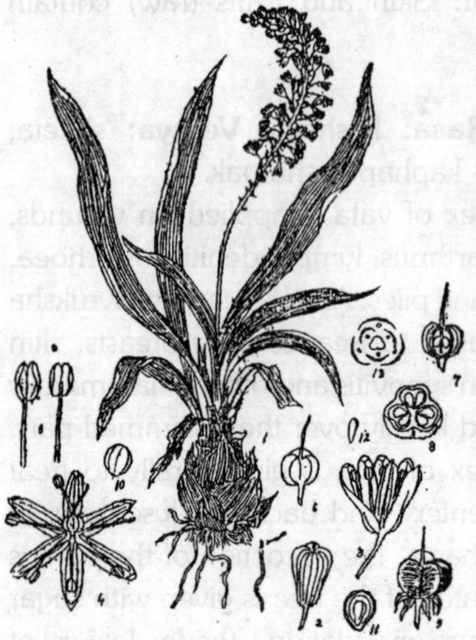

leaves. Leaves - 18 -50 cms. long and 0.5 cm wide. Flowers - white, bell like arise from the flowerstalk. Ovary is divided into 3 compartments each containing 5 to 10 flat seeds. Tuber - small like lemon. It bears flowers in summer and fruits in rainy season.

Habitat : Mainly near sea shore, also in Madhya pradesh, Simla, Punjab, Bengal and Nagpur.

Chemical composition : Sillinine, a toxic principle, two bitter principles, mucilage, sugar and ash 5% which contains calcium oxalate and crystals of citrate.

Properties :

Guna : tikshna, laghu; **Rasa :** katu, tikta; **Vipak :** katu; **Veerya :** ushna; **Dosha :** vatakaphashamak and pittavardhak.

External uses : Vitiates blood and developes ulcers. Its paste is used in skin disorders and oedema.

Internal uses : Cardiotonic but intravenous administration increases the blood pressure, but orally it dose not increase that much pressure. It is useful in chronic cold, chronic cough and chronic lung disorders. It stimulates renal tubules and thus increases urine formation, herce it is used in kidney disorderes and retention of urine. Being an emmenagogue it is used in dysmenorrhoea and ammenorrhoea. Also useful in pruritus and skin diseases.

Excretion : Through skin, lungs and kidneys.

Dose : Powder of tubers - 1 to 1.5 ratti, syrup - 30 to 60 drops, alcoholic extract - 5 to 30 drops. It is contrindicated in reflux oesophagitis, acute renal inflammation and acute cough, as it is irritant in nature.

New onion should be used. Its covering is removed, inner part is dried and used.

Srotogamitva :

Dosha : Vataghna, kaphaghna, pittakar.

Dhatu : Rakta (cardiotonic, expectorant, useful in pruritus and skin disorders), meda (useful in renal disorders), rasa (emmenagogue).

Mala : Mutra (useful in retention of urine) and excreted through skin, breath and urine.

(205) VANSHA
Bambusa bambos

Kula : Yava kula.

Family : Gramineae = plants of the Graminis, grass tribe.

Latin name : Bambusa = Indian name; bambos = derived from the name 'bamboo'.

English name : Common prickly bamboo.

Sanskrit names : Yavaphal, Trunaketu, Kantalu, Kantaki, Vanshi, Suparva, Trunadhwaj, Tejan, Keechak. It has two varieties, 1) hollow and 2) non - hollow.

Botanical Description : In female variety of bamboo, white juice gets accumulated in its hollow

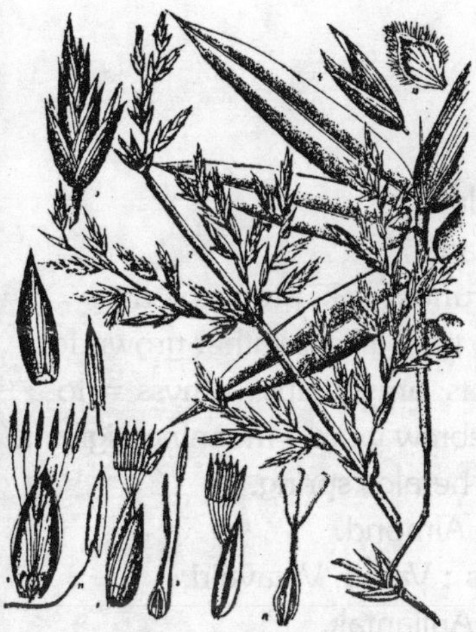

cavity, which is called as 'Vanshalochan'(bamboo manna). This tree grows 15-20 mtrs. high usually on islands. Stem - circumference is 30-40 cms. with distant nodes and the cavity between two nodes is hollow. Leaves - long with tapering ends. Flowers and Fruits - occur after 30 yrs. Flower stalk - long and branched. Flowers - homosexual. Fruit - resembles yava fruit and known as Vanshayav. It bears flowers and fruits in summer.

Varieties : It has many varieties.

Habitat : All over India, but mainly in Assam, Brahmadesh, Java and Sumatra.

Chemical composition : Vanshalochan contains 90% silica, potash, calciun carbonate, aluminium and yeast. (Artificial vanshalochan is available in the market which is not useful.)

Properties :

Guna : ruksha, laghu, tikshna; **Rasa :** madhur, kashaya; **Veerya :** sheeta but tender leaves and fruits - ushna.

Vanshalochan - kashaya, madhur, sheeta.

Root - kaphapittashamak, tender leaves and fruits - pittavardhak, vanshalochan - vatapittashamak.

Uses : Paste or ash of the roots is used locally in skin disorders, ringworn infection and dermatoses. Vanshalochan is used in vomiting, diarrhoea, heart diseaes, bleeding disorders, cough, asthma, chronic fever, pthisis and general debility. Decoction of leaves is useful is dysmenorrhoea and ammenorrhoea.

Fruit acts on meda dhatu and is useful in fat metabolism and obesity. Decoction of roots is given in rabies.

Parts used : Roots, leaves, tender leaves, fruit and vanshalochan.

Dose : Decoction - 15 to 100 ml; vanshalochan - 1to 3 gms.

Formulations : Sitopaladi churna, Talisadi churna.

Srotogamitva :

Dosha : Roots - kaphaghna, pittaghna; vanshalochan - vatapittaghna; tender leaves and fruits - pittakar.

Dhatu : Rasa (fever, dysmenorrhoea, thirst), rakta - (bleeding disorders), cough, dermatoses, aphrodisiac (vanshalochan), meda (brimhan - vanshalochan), meda (fat metabolism, antiobesity).

Mala : Purisha (astringent), mutra (diuretic).

References -

'वंशः सरो हिमः स्वादुः कषायो बस्तिशोधनः । छेदनः कफपित्तघ्नः कुष्टास्त्रवणशोथजित् ।।
तत्करीरः कटु पाकेरसे रूक्षो गुरुः सरः । कषायः कफहृत् स्वादुर्विदाही रातपित्तलः ।।
तदयवास्तु सरा रूक्षा कषायाः कटुपाकिनः । वातपित्तकरा उष्णा बद्धमूत्रा कफापहाः ।। (भा. प्र.)
'रूक्षः कषायानुरसो मधुरः कफपित्तहा । मेदःक्रिमिविषघ्नश्च वल्यो वेणुयवो मतः ।।' (च. सू. २७)
'वंशजा बृंहणी वृष्या बल्या स्वाद्वी च शीतला । तृष्णाकासज्वरश्वासक्षयपित्तास्त्रकामलाः ।।
हरेत् कुष्ठं व्रणं पाण्डुं कषाया वातकृच्छजित् ।' (भा. प्र.)

Even from the physical perspective, due to comparable basis of properties and activity, the mind may be able to differentiate between the minute constituents of the body.

(206) VATAM

Prunus amygdalus

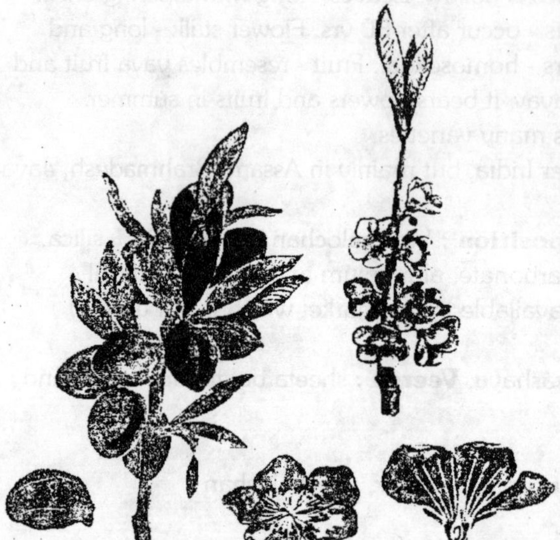

Kula : Taruni kula.

Family : Rosaceae.

Latin name : Prunus - Gk. proune, Lat. prunus = a palm tree, all spp either grown for fruits or ornaments; amygdalus - amyss = to lacerate, from Hebrew word - meaning vigilant. Its early blossom heralds spring.

English name : Almond.

Sanskrit names : Vatad, Vatavairi, Netropamaphal, Anilantak, Yugmashuktiputopam, Suphal. (Almond is contraindicted in bleeding disorders.)

Botanical Description : A medium high tree. Its unripe fruits are sweet and sour and are used as a vegetable. Seed - almond, its pulp is consumed.

Varieties : 1) Sweet and 2) Bitter (poisonous).

Habitat : Asia, Europe, Punjab and Kashmir.

Chemical Composition : It contains 56% stable oil and 25% proteins.

Properties :

Guna : guru, snigdha; **Rasa :** madhur; **Veerya :** ushna; **Dosha :** vatashamak, kaphapittavardhak.

Uses : Locally it cures skin disorders, pruritus and bacterial infections. It is also applied in vaginal pruritus. Oil of sweet almond is also used externally in skin disorders. Ashed rinds are used in toothpowder. Oil of sweet almond is massaged on the scalp to increase the stamina. Almond oil is used in various vata disorders, chronic constipation, dry cough, semen disorders, leucorrhoea and dysmenorrhoea. It is a good aphrodisiac, galactogogue and a health tonic. Also useful in dysuria and ikshumeha (as it does not contain starch). A preparation made from almond called badam pak is consumed during winter for weight gain and to increase the strength.

Parts used : Seed pulp and its oil.

Dose : Almonds - 7 to 11; oil - 2.5 to 10 tola.

Srotogamitva :

Dosha : Vataghna, kaphakar (contraindicated in pitta disorders).

Dhatu : Shukra (aphrodisiac), rasa (galactogogue, useful in dysmenorrhoea), rasayan (for weight gain) contrindicated in blood disorders.

Mala : Mutra (ikshumeha, dysuria), sweda (paste - antipruritic).

Local application of almond oil is effective in vaginal pruritus.

References -
'वातादो वातवैरी स्यान्नेत्रोपमफलस्तथा । वाताद उष्णः सुस्निग्धो वातघ्नः शुक्रकृद् गुरुः ।।
'वातादमज्जा मधुरो वृष्यः पित्तानिलापहः । स्निग्धोष्णः कफकृन्नेष्टो रक्तपित्तविकारिणाम् ।।' (भा. प्र.)
वातामा.... गुरुष्णास्निग्धमधुरा.... बलप्रदाः । (च. सू. २७)
वाताम... प्रभृतीनि । पित्तश्लेष्मकराण्याहुः स्निग्धोष्णानि गुरूणि च । बृंहणान्यनिलघ्नानि बल्यानि मधुराणि च ।।' (सु. सू. ४६)

(207) VARAHI
Dioscorides bulbifera

Kula : Varahkanda kula.
Family : Dioscoreaceae.
Latin name : Doiscorides = A Gk. physician; bulbifera = yielding bulbs or sativa = cultivated.
Sanskrit names : Vrushti, Varahi, Grushtika, Madhavi, Kanti, Vanamalini, Grushti, Saukari.
Botanical Description : It is a creeper with a slimy stalk having small nodes of about 3 cm. diameter in the angle of the leaf stalk. Leaves - compound, 6-18 cms. long and 5-12 cms. wide with pointed tips and 9 veins on them. The inflorescence of male flowers is 6 to 12 cms. long and that of female flowers is 12 to 30 cms. long. Fruits - triwinged. Seeds - also winged. Its tuber is used for medicinal purpose. It is grey with thick and long hair like pig's hair, but looks yellowish white when cut. Bhavaprakash has described another variety named charmakaraluk.
Habitat : Himalayas (at the height of 1650 mtrs.), Madhya pradesh and Konkan region.
Chemical composition : It cointains lot of starch.
Properties :
Guna : laghu, snigdha; **Rasa :** katu, tikta, madhur; **Vipak :** katu; **Veerya :** ushna; **Dosha :** tridoshahara.
External use : Oil heated with tubers is used in sinuses.
Internal uses : Being an appetizer, carminative and anthelmintic, it is used in loss of appetite, colic and worm infestations. It is also used in blood disorders, lymphadenitis, infertility, dermatoses, syphillis and general debility as it acts on rakta, meda and shukra dhatus.
Dose : Powdered tubers - 3 to 6 gms. with milk as an anupan.
Srotogamitva :
Dosha : Kaphavataghna, pittakarak.
Dhatu : Shukra (spermatogenic), rakta (dermatoses), all dhatus (rejuvenator and nutritive).
Mala : Mutra, purisha (anthelmintic).
References -
श्यामकर्कशवाराहवृषणाकारकंदका । ताम्बूलवल्लीछदना वाराही गुष्टिरुच्यते ।।' (कै. नि.)
'वाराहमूर्धवत् कंदो वाराहिकन्दसंज्ञितः । भिषजां तदलाभेन चर्मकारालुको मतः ।।' (वृन्द)
'शौकरो मधुरस्तिक्तः कटुको रसपाकयोः । शुक्रायुः स्वरवर्णआग्निबलपित्तविवर्धनः ।।
कफकुष्ठमरुन्मेहकृमीन् हन्ति रसायनम् ।' (कै. नि.)
वाराहकन्दः श्लेष्मघ्नः कटुको रसपाकतः । मेहकुष्टकृमिहरो बल्यो वृष्यो रसायनः ।।' (सु. सू. ४६)'
'वाराहीमूलचूर्णस्य शतं मधुपुतं क्रमात् । युवा स्यात् पयसा पीत्वा क्षीरान्नाज्यभुगादृतः ।। (शो.)

The modalities of pranayam, dharana, dhyana and namasmarana treat the corresponding body parts through the mind's attention being brought to these.

(208) VYAGHRANAKHI

Capparis zeylanica

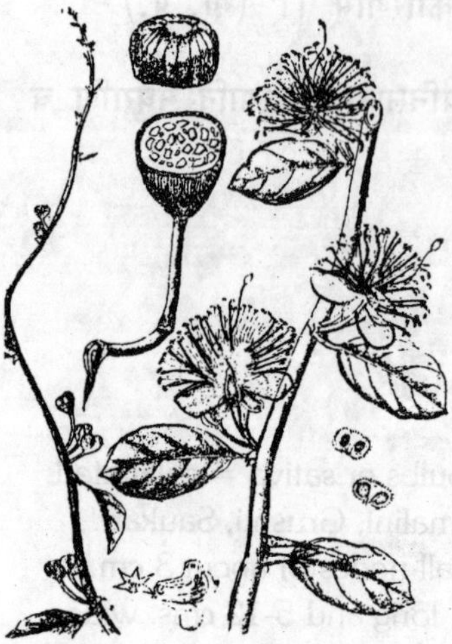

Kula : Varun kula.

Family : Capparis = from kabar - Arabic name; zeylanica = from ceylon.

Sanskrit names : Vyaghranakhi, Govindaphala.

Botanical Description : A bush with sharp thorns like the nails of tiger, hence the name vyaghranakhi (vyaghra = tiger, nakha = nail). Thorns arise along with the leaves. Fruits contain circular seeds.

Properties :

Guna : ruksha, laghu; **Rasa :** katu, tikta; **Vipak :** katu; **Veerya :** ushna; **Dosha :** vatakaphanashak.

Uses : Warm paste of roots is applied on inflammed and painful areas. Useful in abscesses.

Srotogamitva :

Dosha : Kaphaghna, vataghna.

Dhatu : Rakta (abscess, antiinflammatory).

Organ : Digestive system.

References -

गान्धारी कटुतिक्तोष्णा कफवातनिकृन्तनी ।
शोफघ्नी दीपनी रुच्या रक्तग्रन्थिरुजापहा ।।' (रा. नि.)

(209) VIKANKAT

Flacourtia ramoutchi Fam.

Kula : Vikankat kula.

Family : Flacourtiaceae.

Latin name : Flacourtia = after Mr. Etienne de Flacourt, Director of French East India company; ramoutchi = having many branches.

English name : Mauritius plum.

Sanskrit names : Sruvavruksha, Granthil, Swadukantak, Yagnyavruksha, Kantaki, Vyaghrapad, Vrukshakantakari.

Botanical Description : A small thorny tree resembling the tree of karamarda. Leaves - shiny, 9 cms. long, oval with serrated margins. Flowers - small, yellow or green in colour. Fruits - round, 2 cms. in diameter, slimy with pulp inside. Ripe fruits are purple or red in colour with small, numerous seeds.

Habitat : Himalayas, Bihar, Madhya Pradesh and Konkan region.

Properties : Fruit - appetizer and digestive, useful in jaundice and splenomegaly. **Bark -** astringent but diuretic.

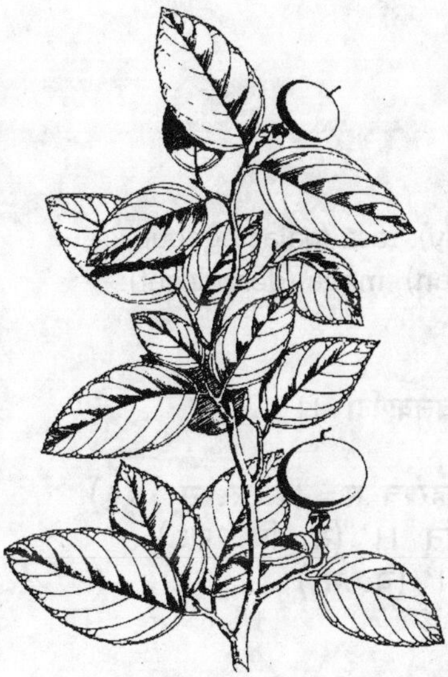

Srotogamitva :
Dosha : Tridoshaghna, pittasarak.
Dhatu : Rakta.
Mala : Purisha (purgative), bark - diuretic.
Organs : Stomach and intestines.
References -
विकंकतफलं पक्वं मधुरं सर्वदोषजित् ।। (भा. प्र. फलवर्ग)

(210) VIDARI

Pueraria tuberosa

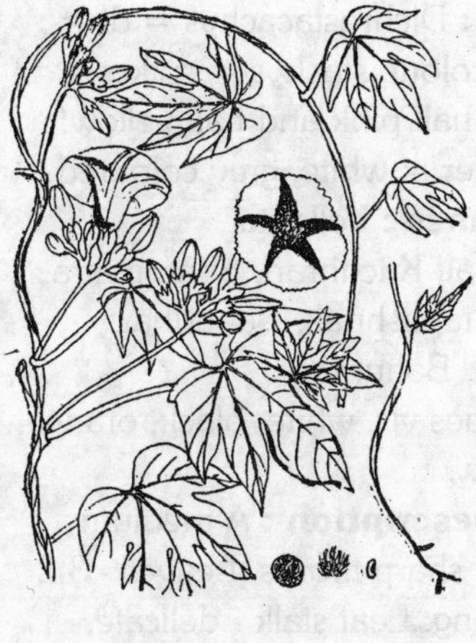

Kula : Shimbi kula.
Family : Leguminoseae.
Gana : Balya, Bruhan, Varnya, Kanthya, Snehopag, Madhurvarga, Vidarigandhadi, Vallipanchamoola, Pittashaman.
Latin name : Pueraria = after Mr. M.M.N. Puerari - scientist; tuberosa = tuberous rooted or Ipomoia digitata, I. paniculata.
Sanakrit names : Swadukanda, Sita, Ikshugandha, Payaswini, Vrushyakanda, Bhukushmandi, Shukla,Varada,Varahavadana.
Botanical Description : A wide spreading creeper. Its stalk has pores. Leaves - trifoliate, resembling the leaves of B. frondosa with 10-15 cms. long leaflets, pointed with dense hair on the lower surface. Inflorescence - purple. Fruits - 6 to 9 cms. long. Tubers - circular with a diameter of 30 to 40 cms. There is another variety called ksheervidari the tuber of which oozes out a thick latex on cutting it.
Habitat : Himalayas, Nepal, Bengal, Assam, Punjab and Konkan region.
Chemical composition : Resin, sugar and starch (in large quantity).
Properties:
Guna : guru, snigdha; **Rasa:** madhur; **Veerya :** sheeta; **Dosha :** vatapittashamak.
Uses : It is unctuous, anabolic, nutritive, cholagogue, carminative, cardiotonic, hemostatic, demulcent, aphrodisiac, galactogogue, diuretic, complexion enhancer and rejuvenator. Hence it is used to reduce intestinal dryness, in hepato-splenomegaly, cardiac debililty, bleeding disorders,

Just like the ultramicroscopic constituents of the body, mind too may have extremely minute components.

hoarseness of voice, cough, dysuria and pthisis.

Part used : Tuber.

Dose : Dried powder of tuber - 2 to 6 gms. with milk.

Srotogamitva :

Dosha : Vataghna, pittaghna (cholagogue).

Dhatu : Rakta (hemostatic, bleeding disorders, hepatosplenomegaly), rasa (galactogogue, complexion enhancer), shukra (aphrodisiac), mansa - meda (brimhan), meda (demulcent).

Mala : Mutra (diuretic).

References -

'विदारी मधुरा स्निग्धा बृंहणी स्तन्यशुक्रदा । शीता स्वर्या मूत्रला च जीवनी बलवर्णदा ।।
गुरुः पित्तास्त्रपवनदाहान् हन्ति रसायनम् ।' (भा. प्र.)
'मधुरो बृंहणओ वृष्यः शीतः स्वर्योऽतिमूत्रलः । विदारीकन्दो बल्यस्तु वातपित्तहरश्च सः ।। (स. सू. ४६)
चूर्ण विदार्याः सुकृतं स्वरसेनैव भावितम् । सर्पिर्मधुयुतं लीढवा दशस्त्रीरधिगच्छति ।।' (सु. चिं. २६)
पयस्तैलं घृतं चैव विदारीक्षुरसं मधु । संमूर्छ्च्य पाययेदैतत् विषमज्वरनाशनम् ।।' (च. स.)

(211) VEERATARU

Dichrostacachys cinerea

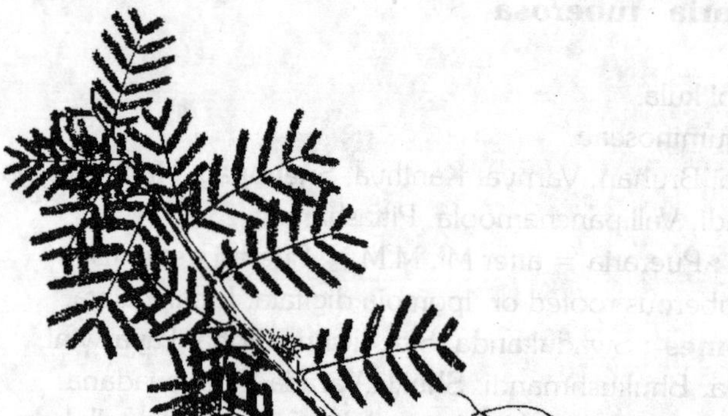

Kula : Shimbi kula.

Family : Leguminoseae.

Latin name : Dichrostacachys = di = two, chro = colour, stachys = spikes, inflorescence half pink and half yellow; cinerea - cinder = white, grey coloured.

Sanskrit names : Vellantar, Kshudhakushal, Krichhrari, Shamipatra, Kantaki, Lohitapushpak, Bahudhar, Granthiparna, Bahumool.

It has 5 varieties viz. white, black, orange, red and yellow.

Botanical Description : A medium high tree with sharp thorns. Leaves - 3.2 to 6.3 cms. long. Leaf stalk - delicate, hairy. Leaflets - nodes between 2 leaflets, 8-14 pairs. Flowers - resemble jasmine flowers, white, black, orange, red or yellow. Legumes - flat, grey and contain 6 to 10 seeds.

Habitat : Every where in dry regions.

Properties : Astringent, bitter.

Uses : Root is used in rheumatoid arthritis, disorders of spleen and kidney. Paste of tender leaves is used topically in eye disorders.

Srotogamitva :
Dosha : Kaphaghna, vataghna.
Dhatu : Rakta (acts on spleen).
Mala : Mutra (retention of urine, calculi), purisha (astringent).
References -
वेल्लन्तरो रसे पाके तिक्तस्तृष्णार्कफापहः ।
मूत्राघाताश्मजिद् ग्राही योनिमूत्रानिलार्तिजित् ।। (भा. प्र.)

(212) VRUKSHAMLA
Garcinia indica

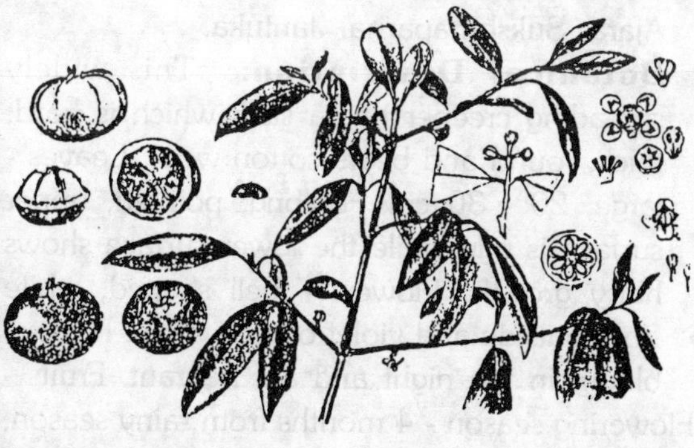

Kula: Nagkeshar kula.
Family: Guttifereae.
Latin name: Garcinia = after the name of Dr. Garcia; indica = Indian or G. Purpurea.
English name: Mate Mangosteen, Kokam butter tree, Red Mango.
Sanskrit names: Shakamla, Raktapurak, Amlashakh, Amlamahiruha, Puramla, Chudamla, Beejamla, Kaphamlak, Rasamla.
Botanical Description: This tree belonging to the nagkesar family is thin with the branches facing downwards. Leaves - tender, red, turn to dark green on maturity. This tree is bisexual. Fruits - of the size of orange, round and reddish. Pulp from the fruit is sour. Fruits devoid of seeds are marketed as kokam.
Habitat: This tree is prominantly found in Konkan, Kerala and Goa. It is also found in Malaysia, China and Singapore.
Chemical composition : Seeds contain 30% oil which is viscous and is sold as kokam oil.
Properties:
Guna: laghu, ruksha, amla; **Vipak:** amla; **Veerya:** ushna; **Dosha:** vatashamak and kaphapitta-vardhak.
Uses: Oil is used for healing ulcers especially in cracked soles. Syrup of fruits is used as a thirst quencher. It is a very good appetizer, cholagogue and improves peristalsis.
Srotogamitva:
Dosha: Raw fruit is vataghna, kaphapittavardhak. Ripe fruit - vataghna, kaphaghna.
Dhatu: Raktagami (hepatostimulant).
Mala: Purisha (astringent), anthelmintic.
Organs: Heart, intestine, digestive system.
References -
वृक्षाम्लाममम्लोष्णं वातघ्नं कफपित्तलम् । पक्वं तु गुरु संग्राहि मधुराम्लरसं तथा ।।
अल्पोष्णं रोचनं रूक्षं दीपनं वातनाशनम् । तृष्णार्शोग्रहणीगुल्मशूलहृद्रोगजन्तुजित् ।। (भा. प्र)
'वृक्षाम्लं ग्राहि रूक्षोष्णं वातश्लेष्मणि शस्यते ।' (च. सू. २७)

As Vaidyas often condition the plants for enhancing the treatment, it would be worthwhile to experiment with grafting as a type of conditioning and study the enhanced properties and therapeutic activity.

(213) VRUDDHADARU

Argyria speciosa

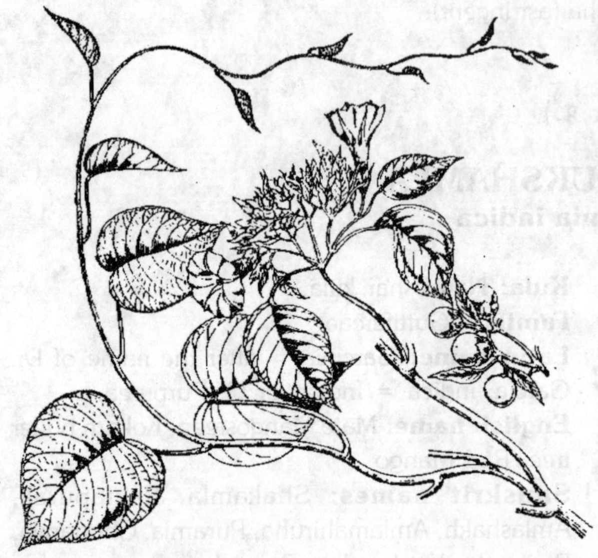

Gana: Adhobhagahara.
Kula: Trivrut kula.
Family: Convolvulaceae.
Latin name: Argyria = lower surface of the leaf is silvery white in colour; speciosa = showy, splendid, handsome.
Sanskrit names: Avegi,Vruddhapushphi, Ambika, Jeernadaru, Jeernafangi, Supushpi, Ajara, Sukshmaparna, Jantuka.
Botanical Description: This widely spreading creeper has a stalk which is hard, thick, round and bears cotton wool. Leaves - large, 20 - 30 cms. oblong, pointed, upper surface is oily while the lower surface shows hairy growth. Flowers - bell shaped, white from outside and violet or red within. Flowers bloom in the night and are fragrant. Fruits - oval, 3 cm. long, green, self breaking on ripening. Flowering season - 4 months from rainy season, followed by fruiting This creeper is usually planted in gardens.

Properties:
Guna: snighdha; **Rasa:** katu, tikta, kashaya; **Vipak** : madhur; **Veerya:** ushna; **Dosha:** kaphavatashamak; (Madhur vipaki inspite of katu, tikta, kashaya rasas.)
External uses: Application of the leaves is done as an antiinflammatory and wound healing. An interesting point to note is that when the lower hairy surface of the leaf is applied on the inflammed part, it accelerates suppuration while the upper smooth surface helps in wound healing.
Internal uses: It is used in vata diseases, heart diseases, cough (bronchitis), hoarseness of voice, diabetes mellitus, sexual weakness, tuberculosis and emaciaton.
Dose: Root and bark powder - 3 gms.; seed powder - 1/2 to 3/4 gms.
Srotogamitva:
Dosha: Kaphaghna, vataghna.
Dhatu: Majja, meda (diabetes), shukra, rasayan. It is a good brain tonic.
References -
'त्रिकोमकाण्डा सुबहुप्रताना फलेषु पीता कुसुमेषु रक्ता ।
'पत्रः सदुग्धैर्मुदुरोमवभ्दिस्ताग्बूलजष्वे: र्धनमूलकन्दे: ।।' (अ. स. टीका)
वृद्धदारु: कषायोण्ण: कटुस्तिक्तो रसायन: । वृष्यो वातामवातार्श:शोथमेहकफप्रत्: ।।
शुक्रायुर्बलमेधाग्निस्वरकान्तिकर: सर: ।' (भा. प्र.)
माषद्वयं तु तच्चूर्णं सर्पिषा सह योजयेत् । मासमात्रोपयोगेन मतिमान् जायते नर: ।।
मेधावी स्मृतिमांश्चैव वलीपलितवर्जित: ।' (भै. र.)

(अश्वगंधा दशपला तन्मात्रो वृद्धदारुक: । चूर्णीकृत्योभयं विद्वान् घृतभाण्डे निधापयेत् ।।
कर्षैकं पयसा पीत्वा नारीभिर्नैव तृप्यति । अगत्वा प्रमदां भूयाद्वलीपलितवर्जित: ।।' (शा.)

(214) SHANAPUSHPI
Crotalaria verrucosa

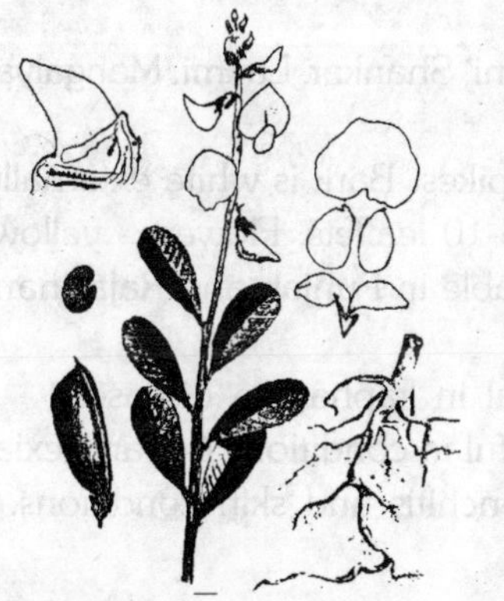

Kula: Shimbi kula.
Family: Leguminosae.
Upakula: Papilionaceae.
Latin name: Crotalaria = Krotalon = rattle, seeds rattling in the hollow of inflated pods, when mature; vernucosa = warted, covered with wart-like excrescences or C. angulosa.
English: Flax Hemp.
Sanskrit names: Shanapushpi, Bruhatpushpi, Shanghantika, Mahashana, Malyapushpi, Vamani, Katutiktaka, Ghanta.
Botanical Description: The herb is 1 to 1.5 mt. high. Leaves - thin, tender, ovoid, 12 - 13 cm.long . Flowers - 15 to 20 yellow flowers on a long stalk. Seeds - 10 to 20 in each legume. Dry legume maks a rattling sound.
Habitat: Southern India.
Properties:
Guna: laghu, ruksha, tikshna; **Rasa:** tikta, kashaya; **Vipak:** katu; **Veerya:** ushna; **Prabhav:** emetic.
Uses: Useful in kapahapitta diseases. Leaves are applied locally in oedema and skin diseases.It is an expectorant. Gargling of the decoction of the leaves is done in pharyngitis and stomatitis. Flowers are used in heart diseases and in bleeding disorders.
Dose: Root powder - 3 to 6gms; decoction of leaves - 6 to 12 ml.
Srotogamitva:
Dosha: Kaphaghna, pittaghna.
Dhatu: Rakta (skin diseases, bleeding disorders).
Mala: Emetic, (mala of kapha dosha).
Organs: Heart, liver, spleen.
References -
'शणपुष्पी स्मृता घण्टारवा शणसमाकृति: । शणपुष्पी कटुस्तिक्ता वामनी कफपित्तजित्, (भा. प्र)
शणपुष्पी रसे तिक्ता वामनी कफपित्तजित्। कषाया कण्ठहृद्रोगमुखरोगविनाशिनी ।।
'शणपुष्पी च बिम्बी च छर्दने ।' (च. सू. १)

The main spin off behind the ritual of gathering the leaves and flowers, during various Hindu festivals (Gauri, Ganapati and Mangalagauri) is to cultivate the plant-identifying skills of persons.

(215) SHAMI
Prosopis specigera

Kula: Shimbi kula.
Family: Leguminoseae.
Latin name: Prosopis = butter burr.; specigera = bearing spikes.
English name: Sponge tree.
Sanskrit names: Shami, Shankuphala, Keshahantri, Shivaphala, Ishani, Shankar, Laxmi, Mangalya, Papnashini.
Botanical Description: The tree is of medium height and bears spikes. Bark is white externally but yellow inside. Branches slanting downwards. Leaves - bearing 8-10 leaflets. Flowers - yellow. Legume 10-15 cm. long bearing seeds. Raw legume is used as vegetable in Punjab and Rajasthan.
Habitat: Gujarat and Rajasthan in India.
Properties: Shami is guru, ruksha, madhur and sheeta. It is useful in kaphapitta diseases.
Uses: Bark is used for local application in scorpion bite. It is also useful in conditions like anorexia, diarrhoea, dysentery, piles, haemetemesis, rheumatoid arthritis, bronchitis and skin conditions.
Srotogamitva:
Dosha: Kaphaghna, pittaghna.
Dhatu: Rakta (haemetemesis, vertigo, dermatitis).
Mala: Stool (astringent), keshaghna (fruit).
Organ: Respiratory tract (bronchitis), rheumatoid arthritis.
Specific use: Bark is used for application on scorpion bite.
References -
शमी तिक्ता कटुः शीता कषाया रोचनी लघुः ।
कफकासभ्रमश्वासकुष्ठार्शक्रिमिजित् स्मृता ।।' (भा. प्र.)
'गुरूष्णं मधुरं रूक्षंकेशघ्नं च शमीफलम् ।' (च. सू. २७)
'शमी रूक्षा कषाया च रक्तपित्तातिसारजित् ।।' (रा. नि.)

(216) SHATI
Hedychium spicatum

Gana: Shwashara, Hikkanigrahana.
Latin name: Hedychium = Hedys = sweet, chion = snow, sweet scented snow, white flowers of this plant are fragrant; spicatum = spiked (or Curcuma zedoaria or zemburet).
English name: Long Zedoary, R. Zedoary.
Sanskrit names: Kachur, Gandhamul, Dravida, Karsha, Gandhasar, Jatil, Sthoolkanda, Sati, Gandha.
Botanical Description: This is a perennial shurb. Tubers are thick, oblong and potato-like. The tubers are scented. Dried pieces of the tubers are available in the market. Leaves - 30 cm. long and slightly broader. Flower stalk has branches and bears white flowers which have soft cilia on them. Ovary - round. The plant bears flowers and fruits in rainy season.

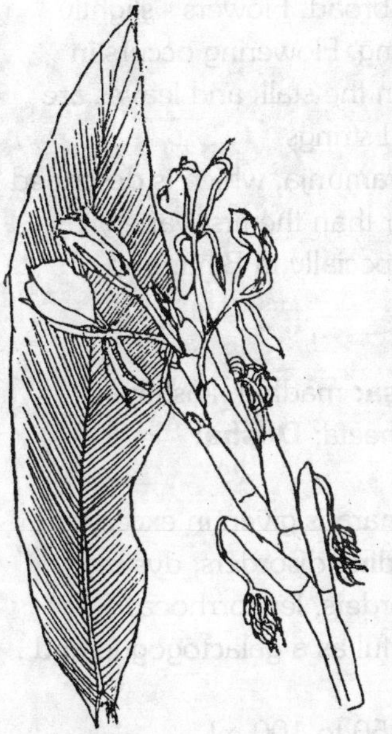

Habitat: Himalaya, Kumaon, Nepal, Bhutan.

Properties:

Guna: laghu, tikshna; **Rasa:** katu, tikta, kashay; **Vipak:** katu; **Veerya:** ushna; **Dosha:** kaphavatanashak.

External use: It is used for application in arthritis and wounds. In dental diseases, it is used for application on the teeth as a tooth powder. Shati mixed with oil is used for fumigation to remove bad odour. Its application is done on alopecia and its nasal administration is done in diseases of the head.

Internal use: Since it is an appetizer, digestive, analgesic and astringent, it is useful in anorexia, vomiting, indigestion, colicy pain and diarrhoea. It is also used in cough, cold, asthma, hiccups, skin diseases, diseases of the blood and in pyrexia. Its fumigation is done in hiccups.

Dose: Powder of the tuber - 1 to 3 gms.

Formulations: Shatyadi churna, Shatyadi kwath.

Srogamitva:

Dosha: Kaphaghna, vataghna.

Dhatu: Rakta (purifier), rasa (febrifuge), meda (ligaments, fumigation in hiccups).

Mala: Purisha (ama digestive, astringent), hair (alopecia).

Organs: Very useful in cleansing the mouth.

References -

'शटी पलाशी पड्ग्रन्था सुव्रता गन्धमूलिका । गन्धारिका गन्धवपूर्वधूः पृथुपलाशिका ।।
भवेद्गन्धपलाशी तु कषाया ग्राहिणी लघुः । तिक्ता तीक्ष्णाच कटुकानुष्णास्यमलनाशिनी ।।
शोथकासवणश्वासशूलहिध्मग्रहापहा ।' (भा. प्र.)
'शटी स्यात् कटुतीक्ष्णोष्णा सन्निपातज्वरापहा । कफास्त्रव्रणकासघ्नी वक्त्रशुद्धिविधायिनी ।। (ध. नि.)
'शटी तिक्ता कटुस्तीच्या कषाक्ष्णा ग्राहिणी लघुः । अनुष्णा मुखवैरस्यमलदौर्गन्ध्यनाशनी ।।
दोषकासव्रणश्वासशूलहिध्मज्वरापहा ।' (कै. नि.)

(217) SHAR

Sacchrum munja Roxb.

Kula : Yava kula.

Family : Gramineae (grass-like).

Gana : Trunapanchamoola.

Latin name : Sacchrum = sugar producing; munja = Indian name.

Sanskrit names : Bann, Ikshu, Sayak, Kshur. **Another variety -** Ikshur, Munja, Kanda, Tirkansa.

Botaniocal Description: This is a shrub which usually grows near the banks of rivers and survives for many years. It appears like sugarcane. Stalk - is 3 to 4 mtrs. long and is divided into many segments by small tubers. Each segment is long and slender. Leaves - thin, flat, 1 to 1.5

Could the cause of one disease be the treatment of another disease and the treatment of one disease be the cause of another disease (?)

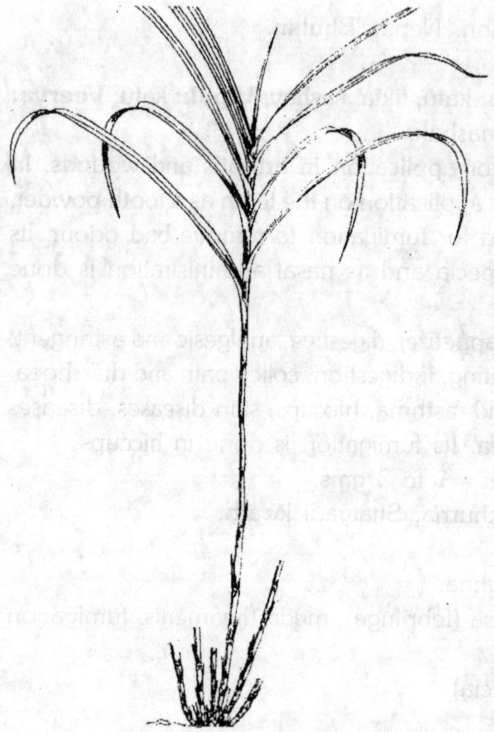

mtrs. long and 6 to 9 cms. broad. Flowers - slightly brownish but white on drying. Flowering occurs in spring. Fibres obtained from the stalk and leaves are uesd in making threads and strings.

Varieties : Two - 1) Bhadramunja, which is described here and 2) Munja, smaller than the first variety.

Habitat : All over India especially in Bihar and Bengal.

Properties:

Guna: laghu, snigdha, **Rasa:** madhur, kashaya; **Vipak :** madur; **Veerya:** sheeta; **Dosha:** tridoshashamak.

Uses : Water boiled with shara is given in excessive thirst. It is also used in bleeding disorders, dysuria, burning sensation, eye disorders, leucorrhoea, erysepelas etc. It is also useful as a galactogogue and aphrodisiac.

Dose : Decoction of root - 50 to 100 ml.

Formulation : Trunapanchamoola.

Srotogamitva :

Dosha: Tridoshashamak.

Dhatu : Rakta (bleeding disorders, burning sensation, menorrhagia, erysepelas), rasa (galactogogue), shukra.

Mala : Mutra (dysuria).

References -

'मुंजयं तु मधुरं तुवरं शिशिरं तथा । दाहतृष्णाविसर्पास्त्रमूत्रकृच्छ्राक्षिरोगहृत् ।।
दोषत्रयहरं वृष्यं मेखलासूपयुज्यते ।' (भा. प्र.)

(218) SHINSHAPA

Dalbergia sissoo

Gana: Kashaya skandha.

Kula: Shimbi kula.

Family: Leguminoseae.

Latin name: Dalbergia = Mr. Nicholas Dalberg; sissoo = from the Indian name shisav, or D. latifolia.

English name: Black wood, Rose wood.

Sanskrit names: Mahashyama, Krishnasara, Tikshnasara, Kapila, Krishnashinshapa, Varan, Guru, Picchila, Angarsara, Mandalpatrika, Ugmapatrika.

Varieties: 1) Black, 2) Yellow and 2) White (abortifacient).

Botanical Description: The tree grows to 15 - 20 mtrs. in height. Its synonyms like krishnasara

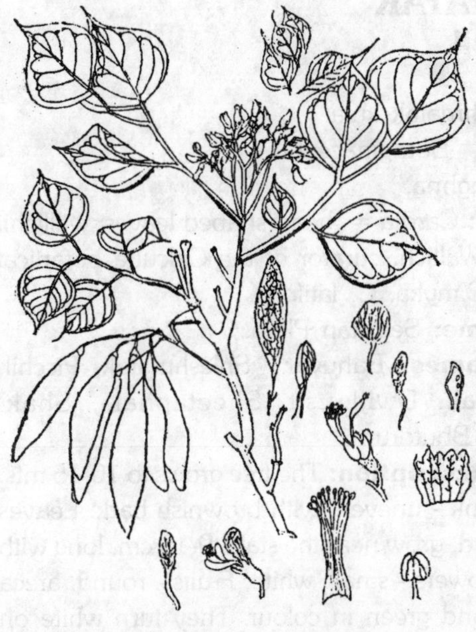

and shyamla are suggestive of its appearance. It is also known as shisham, shishu, sisam, rosewood etc. Trunk - sturdy and round. Bark is fissured. Core is thick, hard and blackish in colour (good for making furniture). Branches - tender, pointing downwards. Stalk of leaf - long, wavy with 3-5 leaflets. Flowers - small, yellowish or whitish. Legume - thin with a single seed. On chewing a thin branch, the colour changes from white to yellow and finally it becomes red.

Varieties: 1) Krishnasara and 2) Kapilsara ?

Properties:

Guna: laghu, ruksha; **Rasa:** kashaya, katu, tikta; **Vipak:** katu, **Veerya:** ushna.

Uses: Since it pacifies all the three doshas, it is used in dermatoses, as an anthelmintic and a wound cleanser. Root - constipative. Leaves - appetizer, antimenorrhagic. Trunk - blood purifier, anti-inflammatory and is useful in dysmenorrhoea and menstrual disorders. Decoction of the leaves is used in burning sensation, while in fever, decoction of the trunk is used.

Parts used: Leaves, trunk, bark, root.

Doses: Decoction of leaves - 12 to 24 ml.; powder - 3 to 6 gms.

Srotogamitva:

Dosha: Tridoshashamak.

Dhatu: Rakta (leaves - hemostat, trunk - shodhak), meda (diabetes), rasa (dysmenorrhoea).

Mala: Mutra.

Organ: Uterus (abortifacient), bastigami.

References -

शिंशपा कृष्णसारा स्यात् वृत्तपत्राऽणुपुष्पका । शिंबिफला गुच्छपुष्पा तद्वत् कपिलशिंशपा ।।' (शि.)
'शिंशपा पिच्छिला श्यामा कृष्णसारा च सा गुरुः । कपिला सैव मुनिभिर्भस्मगर्भेति कीर्त्तिता ।।'
शिंशपा कटुका तिक्ता कषाया शोथहारिणी । उष्णवीर्या हरेन्मेदःकुष्ठश्वित्रवमिक्रिमीन् ।।
बस्तिरुग्णदाहास्रबलासान् गर्भपातिनी ।'' (भा. प्र.)
'कटुष्णं कण्डुदोषघ्नं बस्तिरोगविनाशनम् । शिंशापायुगलं वर्ण्य हिक्काशोथविसर्पजित् ।।' (ध. नि.)
शिंशापासारस्नेहास्तिक्तकटुकषाया दुष्टव्रणशोधनाः कृमिकफकुष्ठानिलहराश्च ।' (सु. सू. ५४)
'उदकाद्द्विगुणं क्षीरं शिंशपासारसंयुतम् । तत् क्षीरशेषं क्वथितं पेयं सर्वज्वरापहम् ।।'
वसामेहिनं शिंशपाकषायम् ।')

A detailed consideration of dosha-dushya in the patient is important not only for the diagnosis of the disease but also for the treatment.

(219) SHLESHMATAK
Cardia wallichii

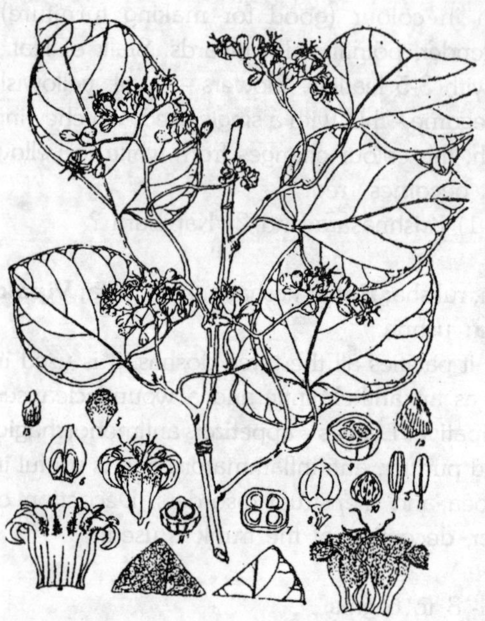

Kula: Shleshmatak kula.
Family: Boraginaceae.
Gana: Vishaghna.
Latin name: Cardia = heart shaped leaves; wallichii = after Dr. Wallich, curator of the Calcutta botanical gardens or C.myka, C. latifolia.
English name: Sepistan Plum.
Sanskrit names: Bahuvar, Shleshmatak, Picchil, Bhutvrukshak, Dwijkutsit, Sheetaphal, Shak, Karbudarak, Bhutdrum.
Botanical Description: The tree grows to 10-15 mts. in height.Trunk - uneven, with brownish bark. Leaves - heart-shaped, grow near the stalk, 9-15 cm. long with 3-5 veins. Flowers - small, white. Fruits - round, areca nut-shaped and green in colour. They turn white on ripening. Fruit pulp - slimy with single seed. Flowering occurs in summer followed by fruiting. Gujarati community uses its fruits for making pickles. Cardia dicotoma, a smaller variety, is found in Punjab.
Habitat: All over India. Does not grow above 1650 mt. sea level.
Properties:
Guna: snigdha, guru, pichchil; **Rasa:** madhur; **Vipak:** madhur; **Veerya:** sheeta. **Fruit:** tikta, **Vipak:** katu. **Bark:** kaphapittashamak; **Fruits:** vatapittashamak but kaphavardhak.
External uses: Decoction of skin is used in poisoning, ulcers and otorrhoea in the form of drops or paste or wash.
Internal uses: The astringent and anthelmintic property of bark helps in dysentery and intestinal worms. Intestinal dryness is reduced by ripe fruits, also useful to reduce or dilute the toxic or drastic effect of purgatives. Fruits - syrup is used in haemetemesis, dry cough, rhinorrhoea, nephritis, azoospermia and fever.
Dose: Bark decoction - 12 to 24 ml. (useful in skin disorders); for fruit sherbat, 6 to 10 gms. of fruits are used.
Formulations: Shleshmatak panak.
Srotogamitva:
Dosha: Vataghna, pittaghna, kaphavardhak.
Dhatu: Rakta, shukra.
Mala: Urine (dysuria), hair.
Internally: Shamak.

References -

बहुवारस्तु शीतः स्वादुद्दालो बहुवारकः । शेलः श्लेष्मातकश्चापि पिच्छिलो भूतवृक्षकः ।।'
बहुवारो विषस्फोटव्रणवीसर्पकुष्ठनुत् । मधुरस्तुवरस्तिवतः केश्यश्च कफपित्तकृत् ।।
फलमामं तु विष्टम्भि रूक्षं पित्तकफास्रजित् । तत्पक्वं मधुरं स्निग्धं श्लेष्मलं शीतलं गुरु ।।' (भा. प्र.)
श्लेष्मातकः कटुहिमो मधुरः कषायः स्वादुश्च पाचनकरः कृमिशूलहारी ।
आमास्रदोषमलरोधबहुव्रणार्ति विस्फोटशान्तिकरणः कफकारकश्च ।।' (रा. नि.)

(220) SHAILEYA
Parmelia perlata

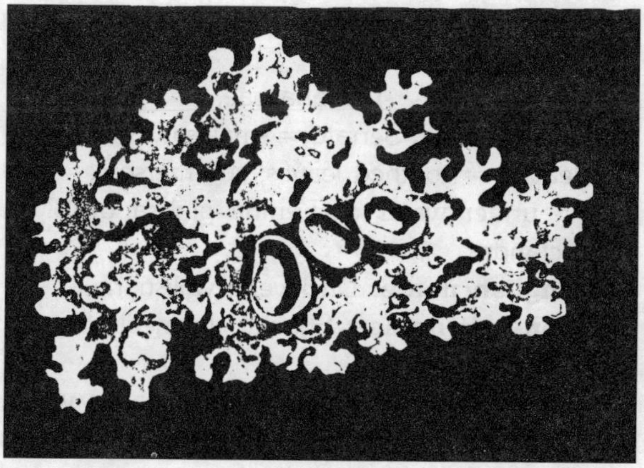

Kula: Shaileya kula.
Family: Lichenes, Parmaliaceae.
Latin name: Parmelia = shield; perlata = very broad.
Sanskrit names: Vruddhapalit, Jeernapalit, Vruddha, Kalanusaryak, Sthavir, Shiladadru, Shilapushpa, Shilodbhav.
Habitat: Himalaya, Punjab, Iran etc. Also grows on old wooden walls and stones. It should be used after purification.
Botanical Description: A small shrub growing on old trees, house walls and stone mines. Outer trunk is greenish black but internally it is white. On uprooting the whole plant, it appears like a fruit which emits a typical smell. Only fresh and fragrant flowers are used in medicine.
Chemical compostion: It contains a yellow pigment, gum, starch, lichenine and kryosophenic acid.
Properties:
Guna: laghu, snigdha; **Rasa:** tikta, kashaya; **Vipak:** katu; **Veerya:** sheeta; **Prabhav:** cardiostimulant and pittashamak.
External use: Anti-inflammatory, relieves itching and pain. It is usd in wounds, headache, itching and skin disorders in the form of paste. Warm paste is applied on the back, hip and lower abdomen region in renal failure to act as a diuretic.
Internal use: Its action as an appetizer and astringent makes it useful in the conditions like thirst, loss of appetite, diarrhoea and dysentery. Its valatile property acts as an antiflatulent. It is also useful in cardiac debility, blood disorders and bronchitis.
Dose: In calculi and renal failure, a decoction of 6 gms of the plant is given along with sugar and cumin seed powder. It might be acting on the binding material of the calculi. Panchang is used. Powder is given in a dose of 6 - 12 gms. and decoction 24 - 40 ml.
Srotogamitva:
Dosha: Kaphaghna, pittaghna.

The indriyas that perceive gunas also perceive the opposite gunas.

Dhatu: Meda, rakta (bleeding disorders).
Mala: Mutra (lithotripsic action).
References -
'शैलेयं तु शिलापुष्पं वृद्धं कालानुसार्यकम् । शैलेयं शीतलं हृद्यं कफपित्तहरं लघु ।
कण्डू कुष्ठाश्मरीदाहविषहृल्लासरक्तजित्' (भा. प्र.)
'शैलेयं शिशिरं तिक्तं सुगन्धि कफपित्तजित् । दाहतृष्णावमिश्वासव्रणदोषविनाशनम् । ।' (रा. नि.)

(221) SHAIVAL
Serratophyllum submersom

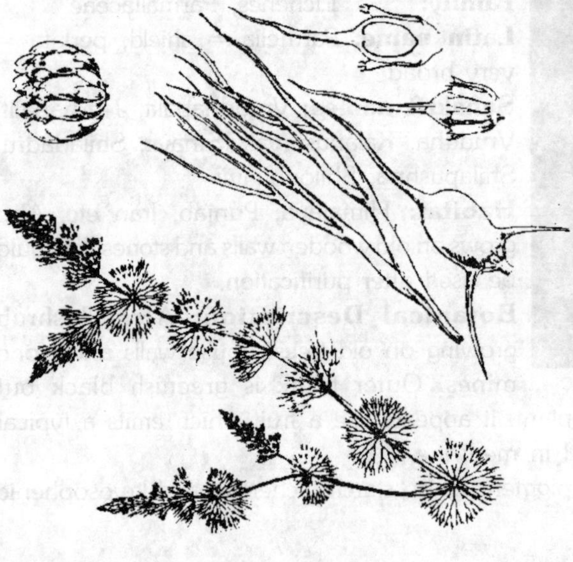

Kula: Shaival kula.
Family: Lemanaceae.
Latin name: Serrato = small saw, phyllum = leaved = toothed leaves; sub-mersom = sub = under water or Lemna globsa or Blyxa octandra.
English name: Duckweed vallisnaria.
Sanskrit names: Shaival, Jalaneeli, Sheval, Jalaj, Shevalum.
Habitat: Grows in plenty under shallow water. Does not grow below 1 ft. depth as sun rays do not reach to that depth.
Botanical Description: It is formed and found in different ponds and lakes, grows over stones in shallow water, leaves form a thick over the water surface which appears greenish blue and hence the name jalaneeli.

Habitat: Everywhere in India.
Properties:
Guna: laghu, snigdha; **Rasa:** kashaya, tikta, madhur; **Vipak:** katu; **Veerya:** sheeta, tridoshashamak, specially acts on pitta (since it grows in contact with water).
External uses: Its paste is used in burning sensation on the skin and in bleeding piles, as it has hemostatic and refrigerant effects.
Internal uses: It is used in thirst, dysentery, bleeding disorders, fever and burning sensation.
Dose: Decoction - 12 to 24 ml.
Parts used: Panchang.
Srotogamitva:
Dosha: Tridoshashamak, pittaghna.
Dhatu: Rakta.
Mala: Purisha (dysentery).

References -
शैवालं तुवरं तिक्तं मधुरं शीतलं लघु । स्निग्धं दाहतृषापित्तरक्तज्वरहरं परम् ।।' (भा. प्र.)
'शैवालं शीतलं स्निग्धं सन्तापव्रणनाशनम् ।' (रा. नि.')

(222) SHRUNGATAK

Trapa bispinosa

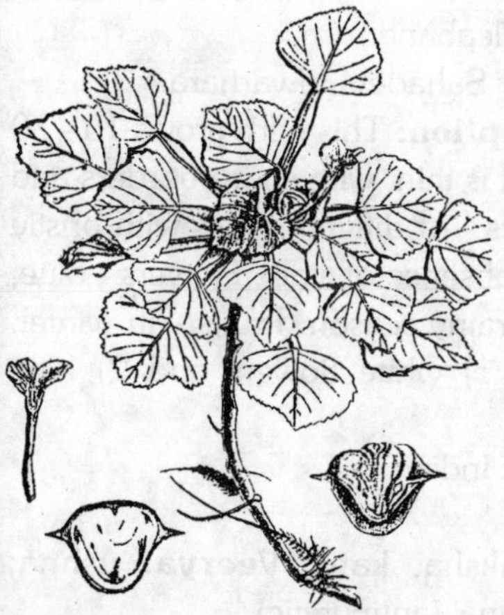

Kula: Shrungatak kula.
Family: Onagraceae.
Latin name: Trapa = an ancient weapon - Kalkitrapa - with four spikes; bispinosa = having two spines.
English name: Indian waterchestnut, water caltrap.
Sanskrit names: Shrungatak, Jalaphal, Trikonphali, Shrungruha, Jalavalli, Vishani, Shrungahva, Kaseruka, Ambukanda.
Botanical Description: This creeper grows in water. Leaves - round with red veins, serrated border, 6 - 9 cms. broad. Stalk of leaves - 12 -18 cms. long and brownish. Fruit - triangular, with spines at two ends, greenish from outside with white pulp. Flowering occurs in rainy season and fruiting in autumn.
Another variety with four spines (Trapa incisa) is also found.

Habitat: It is found in different lakes all over India. Fruit contains starch and manganese in large amounts.

Properties:
Guna: guru, ruksha; **Rasa:** madhur, kashaya; **Veerya:** sheeta; **Dosha:** tridoshashamak - especially pittashamak.

Uses: External application has a soothing effect. It improves taste and acts as an astringent, aphrodisiac, diuretic and a rejuvenating agent. It is used in thirst, anroexia, diarrhoea, dysentery, haemetemesis, loss of libido, abortion and dysuria.

Dose: 3 to 6 gms.

Srotogamitva:
Dosha: Tridoshashamak, pittashamak, kaphaghna.
Dhatu: Rakta, shukra (aphrodisiac).
Mala: Mutra (diuretic), purisha (astringent).
Organ: Uterus.

References -
'श्रृंगाटकं जलफलं त्रिकोणफलमित्यपि । श्रृंगाटकं हिमं स्वादु गुरु वृष्यं कषायकम् ।।
ग्राहि शुक्रानिलश्लेष्मप्रदंदाहास्रपित्तनुत् ।' (भा. प्र.)
'श्रृंगाटकः शोणितपित्तहारी गुरुः सरो वृष्यतमो विशेषात् ।
त्रिदोषतापश्रमदोषहारी रुचिप्रदो मेहनदार्ढ्यहेतुः ।।' (रा. नि.)
'श्रृंङ्गाटकं बिसं द्राक्षा कशेरु मधुकं सिता ।
यथासंख्यं प्रयोक्तव्याः गर्भस्त्रावे पयोयुताः ।।' (सु. शा. १०)

I have experienced that in Europe and Australia, the common Indian plants are not seen. The flora is entirely different on these continents.

(223) SAHADEVI
Vernonia cineria Len.

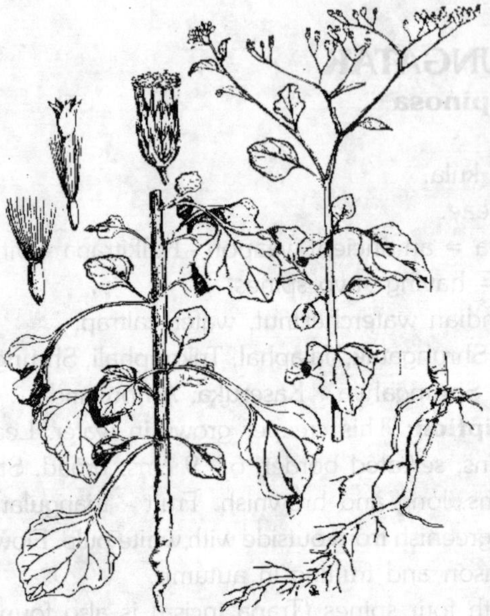

Kula: Bhrungaraj kula.
Family: Compositeae.
Latin name: Vernonia = of the spring; cineria = cinder coloured.
English name: Fleabane.
Sanskrit names: Sahadevi, Jwarhara.
Botanical Description: This herb grows 15 - 30 cms. in high. Stalk is thin, with sharp borders and bristly hairs. Leaves - of different sizes with bristly hair on them and absence of stalk. Flowers - blue, purple, appear in rainy season. Fruits - in winter.
Varieties: Two - 1) white flowers and 2) blue flowers.
Habitat: All over India.
Properties:
Guna: laghu, ruksha, katu; **Veerya:** ushna;
Prabhav: jwaraghna (antipyretic).

Uses: It is used externally as well as internally. Externally, it is used in quaternary fever by tying its root with scalp hair and rubbing its juice on the skin. Paste of the leaves is applied on conjunctivitis and guinea worm. Its laxative, anthelmintic, blood purifying and diaphoretic properties make it useful in piles, intestinal worms, blood disorders, skin diseases, fever and renal calculi. Insects do not stay around this plant.
Dose: Panchang and roots are used; syrup - 12 to 24 ml.; decoction - 50 to 100 ml.
Srotogamitva:
Dosha: Vataghna.
Dhatu: Saptadhatu, majja, rakta, mansa.
Mala: Sweda, mutra (diuretic, lithotripsic).
Prabhav: Quaternary fever (antipyretic).
References -
'दण्डोत्पला सहदेवी विषमज्वरनाशिनी । सहदेवी द्विधा प्रोक्ता श्वेता नीला च पुष्पतः ।।
द्वयंचैकान्तरं हन्ति भक्षणात् धारणादपि । निद्राकरा धृता शीर्षे नीला सिध्म विनाशिनी ।।'
'सहदेवीकृता पिण्डी सर्वविस्फोटनाशिनी ।' (शो.)
'स्वरसैः सहदेव्या वा सिद्धं तैलं ज्वरं जयेत् ।' (वै. म.)
'सहदेवीशिफा बद्धा श्वेतसूत्रेण कन्यया । निहन्ति दक्षिणे पाणौ ज्वरभूतग्रहादिकान् ।।'
'ज्वरं हन्ति शिरोबद्धा सहदेवीजटा यथा ।' (च. सू. २६)

(224) SARAL

Pinus-cedrus deodar Roxb. Sargent.

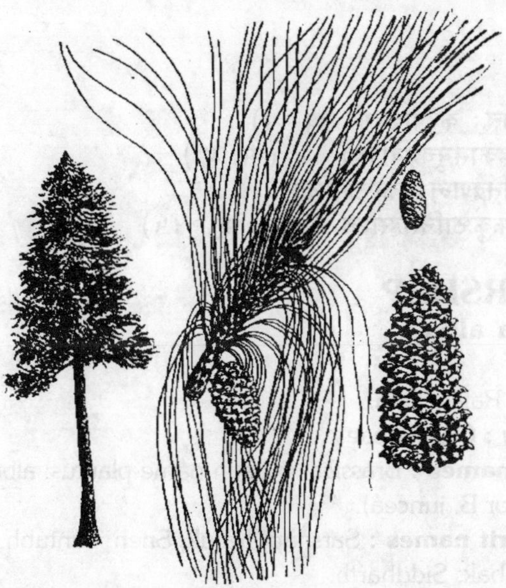

Kula: Deodar kula.
Family: Conifereae.
Gana: Purishavirajaneeya, Shleshmaputihar, Eladi (S.)
Latin name: Pinus = from latin pinus = pine, cedrus = Arabic, kedron = power; deodar = Sanskrit name or P. Longifolia.
English name: Long lived pine, cheer pine.
Sanskrit names: Putikashtha, Pittadrum, Deepvruksha, Snigdhadaru, Marichapatrak, Surabhidaruk, Bhadradaru, Amardaru.
Botanical Description: This tree attains a height of 70 - 90 mtrs. Diameter of the trunk is around 12 mtrs. Bark is 3 to 6 cms. thick with brownish red colour. Core is whitish yellow externally and reddish from inside. Leaves - pointed, 15 - 36 cm. long, bent towards the ground and grow in bunches. Flowers - 1.5 cm. long. Fruits - hard, round. Seeds - 1.5 to 3 cm. oblong. Flowering occurs in summer and fruiting in rainy season. Leaves fall off in winter followed by growth of new leaves later.
Habitat: Himalaya at the height of 1-2 thousand mtrs.
Chemical composition: It has a latex called gandhabijora (also called shriveshthak, shrivas, saralniryas), turpentine oil (20%).
Properties:
Guna: laghu, tikshna, snigdha; **Rasa:** katu, tikta, madhur; **Vipak:** katu; **Veerya:** ushna; **Dosha:** kaphavatashamak.
External uses: It is antibacterial and anticoagulant. Local application of oil removes maggots from wounds. Turpentine oil mixed with camphor is useful in arthritis, pulmonary oedema, chest pain and flatulence. Gandhabijora mixed with castor oil is applied on abscess.
Internal uses: It stimulates the nerves and also acts as a hepatostimulant. Its appetizer and laxative properties are useful in digestive disorders, gall stones, helminthiasis, especially tape worms, peptic ulcer, typhoid fever and intestinal obstruction (as enema).
Respiratory system: Acute and chronic bronchitis, tuberculosis.
Reproductive and Urinary system: In gonorrhoea and cystitis (gandhabijora), leucorrhoea.
Skin: Useful in skin diseases as it is excreted through skin.
Dose: Powder - 1 to 3 gm.; biroja - 1 to 2 gm.; oil - 3 to 10 drops. Overdose causes diarrhoea, vomiting, paralysis and sensory loss.

In any branch of knowledge, first a larger group is studied and then the constituent individuals are studied. This is the sequence of obtaining knowledge and Nyaya darshan follows the same.

Srotogamitva:
Dosha: Kaphaghna, vataghna.
Dhatu: Majja (stimulant), rakta.
Mala: Purisha (anthelmintic), sweda, mutra.
Organ: Antitussive in respiratory tract.
References -
'सरल: पीतवृक्ष: स्यात्तथा सुरभिदारुक: । सरलो मधुरस्तिक्त: कटुपाकरसो लघु: ।।
स्निग्धोष्ण: कर्णकण्ठाक्षिरोगक्षोरहर:स्मृत । कफानिलस्वेददाहकासमूर्च्छविापह: ।।' (भा. प्र.)
सरल: कटुतिक्तोष्ण: कफवातविनाशन: । त्वग्दोषथोकड्वर्तिव्रणघ्न: कोष्ठशुद्धिद: ।।'
'सरल सारस्नेहास्तिक्तकटुकषाया: दुष्टव्रणशोधना:' कृमिकफकुष्ठानिलहराश्च ।' (सु. सू. ४५)

(225) SARSHAP
Brassica alba

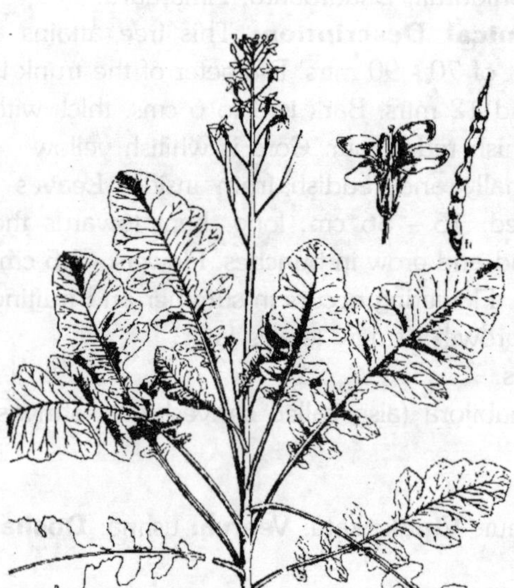

Kula : Rajika kula.
Family : Crucifereae.
Latin names : Brassica = Latin name plautus; alba = white (or B. juncea).
Sanskrit names : Sarshap, Katuk, Sneh, Tantubh, Kadambak, Siddharth.
Botanical Description : Annual herb 30-90 cms. high. Leaves - 30 to 45 cms. long. Flowers - yellow. Fruit - small containing yellow or red seeds.
Varieties : 1) White (Siddharth) - superior and 2) Red.
Habitat : All over India.
Chemical composition : Seeds contain 23-25% stable oil.
Properties :
Guna : tikshna (seed and oil), snigdha (vegetable), ruksha; **Rasa :** katu, tikta; **Vipak :** katu; **Veerya :** ushna; **Dosha :** vatakaphashamak and pittavardhak.
External uses : Seeds - lekhan, enhances complexion and cures dermatoses. Oil - antibaterial and analgesic.
Internal uses : Appetizer. It is one of the best medicines for splenomegaly. It is also an aphrodisiac and emmenagogue. In pyorrhoea, gargles of its oil mixed with salt are useful. Vegetable prepared from the leaves is considered to be harmful (vitiates all the three doshas).
Srotogamitva :
Dosha : Kaphaghna, vataghna, pittavardhak (vegetable - tridoshakar).
Dhatu : Raktagami (vitiates blood, causes bleeding disorders).
Mala : Purisha (constipative), mutra.

Organ : Spleen.

Sarshap oil

Dosha : Pittavardhak, kaphaghna, vataghna.

Dhatu : Rakta (vitiation), shukraghna, rakta (useful in splenomegaly).

Mala : Purisha (anthelmintic).

Organ : Harmful to eyes.

(There is no medicine other than sarshap oil which is effective in splenomegaly.)

References -

'सर्षपः कटुकस्नेहस्तुन्तुभश्च कदम्बकः । गौरस्तु सर्षपः प्राज्ञैः सिद्धार्थ इति कथ्यते ।।
सर्षस्तु रसे पाके कटुः स्निग्धः सतिक्तकः । तीक्ष्णोष्णः कफवातघ्नो रक्तपित्ताभिवर्धनः ।।
रक्षोहरो जयेत् कण्डूकुष्ठकोष्ठक्रिमिग्रहान् । यथा रक्तस्तथा गौरः किन्तु गौरो बरो मतः ।।'
'विदाहि बद्धविण्मूत्रं रूक्षं तीक्ष्णोष्णमेव च । त्रिदोषं शाकम् ।। (सु. सू. ४६)
'सर्षपशाकं शाकानाम् (अहिततमम)' (च. सू. २५)
कटुष्णं सार्षपं तैल रक्तपित्तप्रदूषणम् । कफशुक्रानिलहरं कण्डूकोठविनाशनम् ।।' (च. सू. २७)
कटुपाकमचक्षुष्यं स्निग्धोष्णं बहुपित्तलम् । कृमिघ्नं सार्षपं तैलंकण्डूकुष्ठापहं लघु ।।' (सु. सू.)
कटुतैलोपदेशं तु वक्ष्यामि प्लीहनाशनम् । नातः परतरं किञ्चिदौषध प्लीहशान्तये ।।'

(226) SWARNAKSHIRI

Argemone mexicana

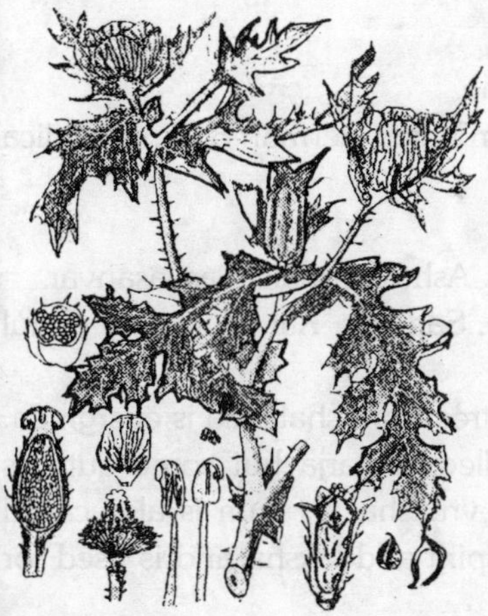

Gana : Bhedaneeya (C.); Adhobhagahar, Shyamadi, Vranashodhan (S.).

Kula : Ahifen kula.

Latin name : Argemone - Gk word Argema = cataract of the eye. This was a reputed cure; mexicana = of Mexico.

English name : Yellow thistle, Prickly or Mexican poppy.

Sanskrit names : Kanchanakshiri, Peetadhattur, Swarnadugdha, Rukmini, Kanchani, Hemanga, Kshiragarbna, Dugdhika, Tiktadugdhika.

Botanical Description : A thorny shrub 6-9 cms. high and oozes yellow latex if cut anywhere. Leaves - long, thorny with irregular margins and white striations. Flowers - yellow with five tender petals. Fruit - round, 3-5cms. in size. Seed - like mustard seeds, black and numerous. They make noise like alcotol when put in the fire.

Habitat : All over India, but mainly on islands.

Chemical composition : Leaf and fruit contain berberine , while seeds contain 22% stable oil and 49% albumin.

External uses : Latex, juice and seed oil has wound cleaning and healing properties and cure dermatoses. Root ground into paste is applied on inflammation and scorpion sting. Local application of an oil or paste of seeds is useful in osteoarthritis.

Mixture of 1 drop of latex and ghee is used as an eyedrops in nightbindness and ulcers in the eye -

There is no organic disease which does not have its origin in one of the rasas like madhur etc.

Gana Nighantu.

Internal uses : Being a laxative, extract of the whole plant or seed oil is used in constipation, flatulence and abdominal pain. 3 to 4 gms of powdered roots is given in taperworm infestation. (It dose not develope laxation always but causes nausea and sometimes vomiting.)

Latex - is useful in blood disorders, syphillis, oedema, dysuria, pyuria, caculi, dermatoses and typhoid. Powdered seeds - useful in cold, cough and asthma.

Dose : Powdered roots - 1 to 2 gms; powdered seeds - 2 to 3 gms; latex - 10 to 12 drops; oil - 25 to 40 drops and juice - 5 to 10 ml.

Srotogamitva :

Dosha : Kaphaghna, pittaghna.

Dhatu : Rakta (blood disorders and dermatoses - latex), rasa (cough).

Mala : Mutra (dysuria, pyuria, calculi), purisha (laxative, useful in taperworms).

Organ : Intestines.

References -

'हेमाहा रेचनी तिक्ता भेदन्युत्क्लेशकारिणी । कृमिकण्डू विषानाहकफपित्तास्रकुष्ठनुत् ।।' (भा. प्र.)

'स्वर्णक्षीरी हिमा तिक्ता कृमिपित्तकफापहा । मूत्रकृच्छ्राश्मरीशोफदाहज्वरहरा परा ।।' (रा. न.)

(227) SARJA

Vateria indica

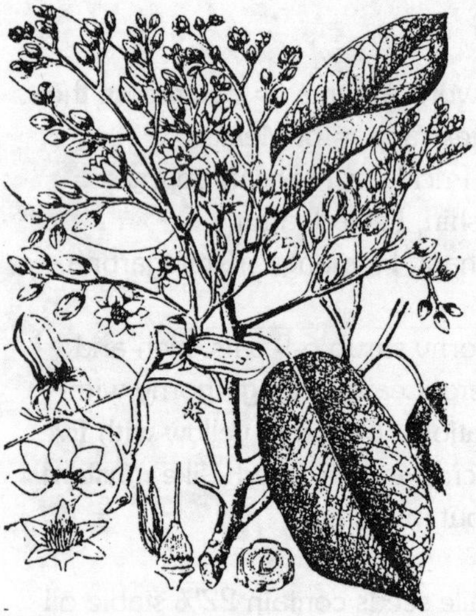

Kula: Shal kula.

Family: Dipterocarpaceae.

Latin name: Vateria = Abraham Vater, German Botanist; indica = of India or Shorea robusta.

English name: Sal tree.

Sanskrit names: Shal, Sarja, Ashwakarnak, Sasyasanvar.

Gum: Devdhoop,Yakshadhoop, Sarjaras, Ral (extremely useful in ulcers and burns).

Botanical Description: This tree from shal kula is evergreen. The tree which gives ral is called as sarja but some authors consider it as a variety of shal vruksha. Its gum is also called chandras which is mixed with spirit and laksha and is used for polishing wooden furniture.

Chemical composition: Its seeds contain 49.2% oil.

Uses: By its oleation, stimulant and analgesic properties, it is useful in chronic rheumatic arthritis. Gum is used for fumigation.

Srotogamitva:

Dosha: Pittaghna, vataghna, kaphaghna.

Dhatu: Rakta (dermatoses, bleeding disorders).

Mala: Stool (constipative, antidiarrhoeal).

Organs: Intestine.

References -
सर्जस्तु तुवरस्तिक्तः हिमः स्निग्धोऽतिसारजित् ।
पित्तास्यदोषकुष्ठघ्नः कण्डूविस्फोटवातजित् ।। (रा. नि.)

(228) SALLAKI
Boswellia serrata

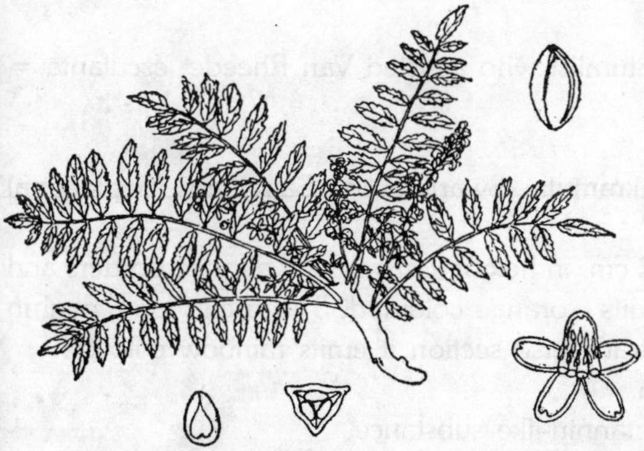

Kula: Guggul kula.
Family: Burseraceae.
Latin name: Boswellia = after Dr. Boswel, Edinburgh; serrata = saw toothed or B. thurifera yielding Frankincense or B. glabra (hairless).
English name: Benzoin, Indian olibanum.
Sanskrit names: Shallaki, Gajabhakshya, Suvaha, Surabhi, Rasa, Maharuna, Kunduraki, Vallaki, Bahustrava. (Its gum is called gandhabiroja or kundaruka).
Botanical Desription: The tree of sallaki is 8 to 10 mtrs. high. Bark is thin and it peels off easily from its stem. Leaves resemble neem leaves. Flowers - are small, scented and white in colour. Ovary is tripartate. Fruit - contains single seed. Gum oozes on peeling the skin. It turns milky on rubbing with water. Five different types of gum is used in Unani system of medicine.
Habitat: Maharashtra (Eastern part), Madhya Pradesh, Rajasthan, South India, Nepal, Marathwada and Himalaya.
Properties:
Guna: laghu, ruksha; **Rasa:** tikta, madhur, kashaya; **Vipak:** katu; **Veerya:** sheeta.
Gum: tikshna, katu, anushna.
Uses: Useful in disorders caused by kaphapitta. Paste is applied in rheumatoid arthritis and cervical adenitis; ointment is used in chronic ulcers. In eye diseases, it is used by mixing with honey. It is an appetizer and digestive, therefore useful in bad breath, loss of appetite, diarrhoea, dysentery, It is used in chronic cough in the form of smoking. Colour of the stool is restored to normal due to its action on pitta. Also useful in gonorrhoea and sexual weakness.
Srotogamitva:
Dosha: Kaphaghna, pittaghna.
Dhatu: Meda, shukra, mansa.
Mala: Purish (diarrhoea, dysentery), astringent, urine (dysuria), sweda (stimulates sweating).
Organs: Joints, respiratory tract.
References -
'शल्लकी गजभक्षा च सुवहा सुरभी रसा । महेरुणा कुन्दुरुकी वल्लकी च बहुस्रवा ।।
शल्लकी तुवरा शीता पित्तश्लेष्मातिसारजित् । रक्तपित्तव्रणहरी पुष्टिकृत् समुदीरिता ।। (भा. प्र.)

Charaka has insisted that the knowledge of drayva should not be done in a lopsilid manner. It should be done with name, form and properties as well as with all the three together.

'कुन्दरुर्मधुरस्तिक्तस्तीक्ष्णः त्वच्यः कटुहरेत् । ज्वरस्वेदग्रहालक्ष्मीमुखरोगकफनिलान् ।।' (भा. प्र.)
'शल्लकी तिक्तमधुरा ग्राहिणी परा । कुष्ठास्रकफवातार्शोव्रणदोषार्त्तिनाशिनी ।।'
'कुन्दुरुः कटुकस्तिक्तो वातश्लेष्मामयापहः । पाने लेपे च शिशिरः प्रदरामयशान्तिकृत् ।' (ध. नि.)

(229) SAPTACHAKRA
Casearia esculanta

Kula: Saptachakra kula.
Family: Samydaceae.
Latin name: Casearia = after Mr. Caserius - Naturalist who assisted Van Rheede; esculanta = tasty or Salacia prinoides.
English name: Wild coryfruit (winterberry like).
Sanskrit names: Saptachakra, Saptaranga, Vakramula, Swarnamula, Saptakapi (Septagonal shape on transverse section).
Botanical Description: A shrub growing 6 to 12 cm. in height. Leaves with dentate borders and are asymmetrical. Flowers - greenish in colour. Fruits - orange coloured, 3 to 6 cm. long, oval in shape. Root - externally golden coloured but in transverse section it emits rainbow colours.
Habitat: Kerala, Maharashtra, Coorg, Shi Lanka.
Chemical properties: Astringent bark contains tannin-like substance.
Properties:
Guna: laghu, ruksha, tikshna; **Rasa:** tikta, kashya; **Vipak:** katu; **Veerya:** ushna.
Uses: Saptachakra is useful in kaphavata disorders. It also purifies pitta. Local application of root paste reduces the inflammation of piles. Being appetizer, digestive, laxative, hepatostimulant and cholagogue, it is useful in loss of appetite, liver enlargement, jaundice and piles. It reduces the blood disorders. It acts as rasayana in restoring the normalcy in diabetes and polyuria. It helps in reducing excessive sweating by emulsifying fatty tissue.
Dose: Root powder - 1 to 2gms.; rasayana 0.5 to 1gm; decoction - 3 to 6 gms.
Srotogamitva:
Dosha: Kaphaghna, vataghna, pitta purification.
Dhatu: Rakta (antidiabetic - hepatic stimulant), meda (metabolism), rasayana.
Mala: Mutra (diabetes, polyuria).
Organs: Rakta, meda, urinary system.

(230) SILHAK
Altingia excelsa

Kula: Silhak kula.
Family: Hamamelidaceae (American witch havel).
Latin name: Altingia = of the lofty places; excelsa = distinguished, lofty or liquid amber orientalis (Noronda).
English names: Liquid storax, Rose malloes, liquid amber.

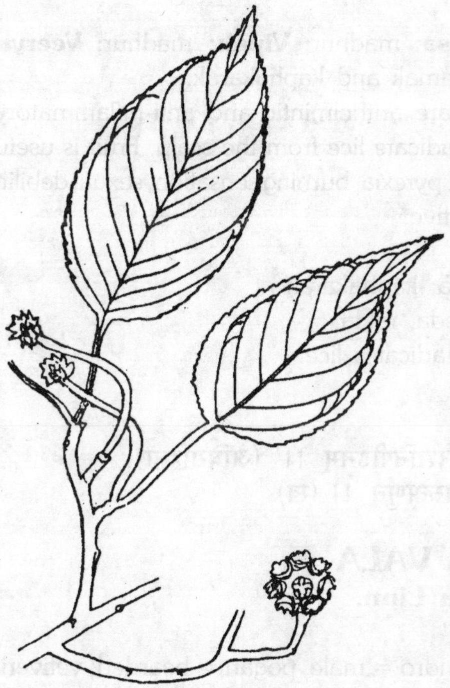

Sanskrit names: Turushka, Kapitail, Silhak, Yavandeshaj, Kapi. Available commercially as shila rasa.

Botanical Description: When cuts are made on the trunk, it oozes out a white sticky substance which immediately becomes viscous like honey. Greyish black in colour, on preserving for a long time, it becomes scented like a rose. It is soft, oily and submerges in water.

Habitat: Arabia, Asia minor, Burma, Bhutan, Malaysia, China, Assam.

Properties:

Guna: snigdha, laghu, tikta; **Rasa:** katu, madhur; **Vipak:** katu; **Veerya:** ushna; **Dosha:** vatakaphashamak.

Uses: The oil is used for bath to relieve itching, vata disorders and ulcers. It acts as an expectorant and pulmonary tonic in chronic bronchitis, asthma and tuberculosis when given with honey. It is a rasayana and aphrodisiac, useful in pyuria and dysuria.

Srotogamitva:

Dosha: Kaphaghna, vataghna.

Dhatu: Shukra (aphrodisiac), rasa (dysmenorrhoea), rasayana, rakta (pulmonary tonic, dermatoses), meda (reduces excessive sweating).

Mala: Mutra (dysuria, pyuria), reduces excessive sweating.

Organs: Respiratory system (cough, dyspnoea, tuberculosis).

References -

'सिल्हकस्तु तुरुष्कः स्याद्यतो यवनदेशजः । कपितैलं स चारुयातं तथा च कपिनामकः ।।
सिल्हकः कटुकः स्वादु स्निग्धोष्णः शुक्रकान्तिकृत् । वृष्यः कण्ठ्यः स्वेदकुष्ठज्वरदाहग्रहापहः ।। (भा. प्र.)
'तुरुष्कः सुरभिस्तिक्तः स्निग्धश्च कुष्ठजित् । कफवातश्मरीमूत्राघातश्वासज्वरार्त्तिजित् (रा. नि.)

(231) SITAPHALAM
Anona squamosa

Kula: Sitaphala kula.

Family: Anonaceae.

Latin name: Anona = word from native name; squamosa = scaly.

Sanskrit names: Sitaphalam, Krishnabeejam, Parushphalam, Gandagatra.

Botanical Description: This tree grows 3 to 5 mts. high and is well known to all Indians. (Its origin is in South America). Leaves - 6-9 cms. long and resemble guauva leaves. Flowers - 3 cms. long and always with three petals. Fruit - fleshy and contains multiple oblong seeds. Surface of the fruit shows round blebs. Anona reticulata (Ramphala) belongs to the same family but is smooth externally.

Water is usually Avyakta, whichever plant it enters, it imbibes the rasa of that plant.

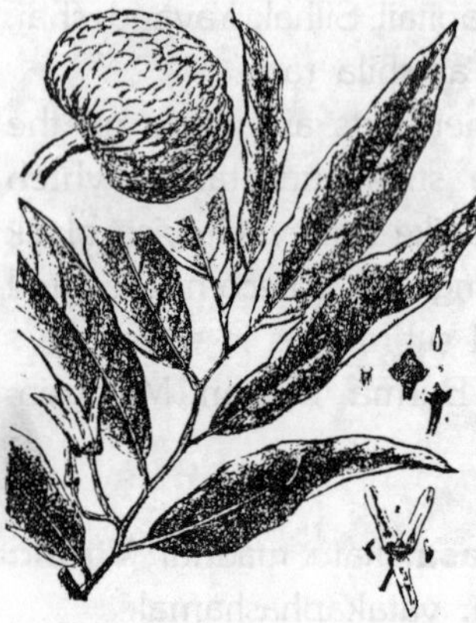

Properties:

Guna: laghu, snigdha; **Rasa:** madhur; **Vipak:** madhur; **Veerya:** sheeta; **Dosha:** vatapittashamak and kaphakarak.

Uses : Leaves and seeds are anthelmintic and anti-inflammatory. Paste of leaves is used to eradicate lice from the scalp. Fruit is useful in bleeding disorders, dysuria, pyrexia, burning sensation, sexual debility and thirst. Ripe fruit is laxative.

Srotogamitva:

Dosha: Vataghna, pittaghna, kaphakarak.

Dhatu: Shukra, mansa, meda, rakta.

Mala: Purisha (laxative), eradicates lice.

Organ: Heart.

References -

गण्डगात्रं हिमं वृष्यं वातपित्तनिषूदनम् । श्लेष्मलं तर्षशमनं वान्त्युक्लेशनिपीडनम् ।।' (अत्रिसंहिता)
सीताफलं सु मधुरं शीतं हृद्यं बलप्रदम् । बृंहणं शुक्रलं दाहरक्तपित्तमरुत्व्रणुत् ।। (स्व)

(232) SUGANDHA VALA

Andropogan vetiveria Linn.

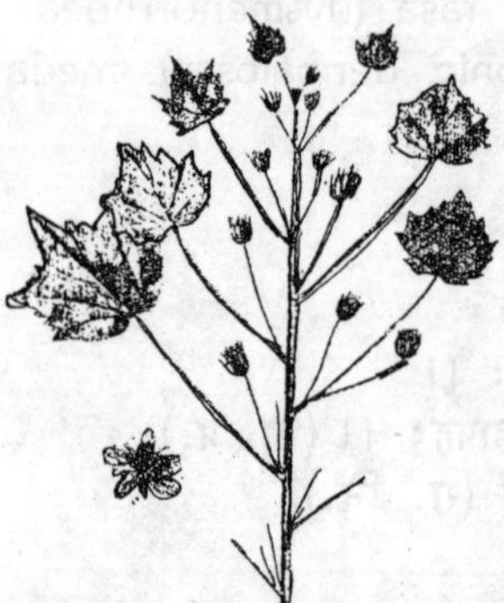

Latin name: Andropogan = Andro = male, pogan = bearded; vetiveria or muricatus = full of rough, short, sharp points or zizanioidus.

Sanskrit names: Hviber, Barhishta, Udichya, Kesha, Ambu, Keshya, Lalanapriya, Kuntaloshir.

Properties:

Guna: laghu, sheeta, stimulates appetite, digestive.

Habitat: Uttar Pradesh, Sindh, Burma.

Botanical Description: It is a shrub; rhizome is black externally but yellow white inside. Very useful in kapha pitta disorders.

Part used : Root.

Dose: 1 to 3 gms.

Srotogamitva:

Dosha: Kaphapittaghna.

Dhatu: Rakta, rasa (fever).

Mala: Mutra, sweda.

(233) SUDARSHAN

Refer to plant No. 130 (Nagdamani).

(234) SURANJAN
Colchicum luteum Baker.

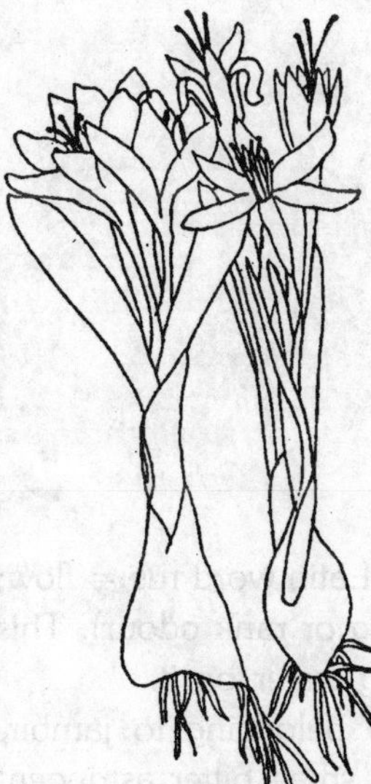

Kula: Rason kula.
Family: Liliaceae (Plants of the lily tribe).
Latin name: Colchicum = Autumn Corcus - from the name of a country called Colchis in Asia minor; luteum = yellow.
Sanskrit name: Suranjan.
It has three varieties -
1) White - Sweet, used orally, found in Iran and called surinjan-e-shiri.
2) Yellow - Small, bitter, called surajan-e-talkh. Orally used. Found in Kashmir, Punjab, Afghanisthan. Contains colchicine.
3) Black - Poisonous, used only externally.
Properties:
Guna: laghu, ruksha; **Rasa:** tikta; **Vipak:** katu; **Veerya:** ushna; **Dosha:** kaphavatashamak.
External use: The black variety is used externally. It is useful in inflammation as an analgesic. An application of saffron + egg + suranjan is done in arthritis. Its powder is applied on wounds for quick healing.
Internal use: It is used in sciatica as it reduces vata. Being pittashamak, it is useful in ascites. White variety is used in debility and impotency. Suranjan is useful in urinary and skin conditions.
Dose: Tikta suranjan - 120 to 360 mgm.; sweet - 1 to 3 gms.; satva (harantutia) - 60 mgm. Overdose - intoxicant.
Formulation: Majune Surinjan.
Srotogamitva:
Dosha: Kaphaghna, vataghna.
Dhatu: Mansa; majja, rakta, shukra.
Mala : Emetic, purgative, mutra (dysuria).

(235) SURPUNNAG
Ochrocarpus longifolia

Kula: Nagkesar kula.
Family: Guttifereae.
Latin name: Ochro-carpus = yellowish white fruit; longi-folius = long leaved.
Sanskrit names: Nameru, Surpunnag, Sureshta, Surparnica, Surtunga.
Botanical Description: Bark is brownish grey in colour. Flowers - resemble Mimusops elingi with a single seed. Raw tender flowers are marketed as Mesua ferrea.
Habitat: South Konkan, Kerala, Karnataka; grows near sea-shore.
Properties: Properties are similar to those of Mesua ferrea. **Guna:** laghu, ruksha; **Rasa:** amla,

In Amarkosha, the gardens are called Vana and Upavana. However, the garden in front of the homes of either minister or prostitute is called only a "Vruksha vatika".

kashaya, tikta; **Vipak:** katu; **Veerya:** ushna. It is kaphapitta shamak, deodorant and nervine tonic.

Srotogamitva:

Dosha: Pittaghna, kaphaghna.

Dhatu: Majja, meda.

Mala: Sweda, purisha.

Organ: Brain.

References -

पुन्नागः सूरपर्णिका सुगंधिपुष्पयुक्ता दक्षिणापंथ 'सूरपित' नाम्ना प्रसिद्धा । (डल्हण)

(236) SUDDAB

Ruta graveolens

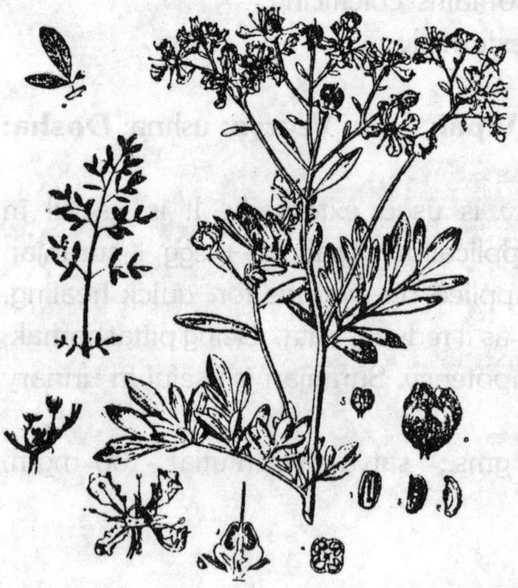

Kula: Jambir kula.

Family: Rutaceae (Rue-like).

Latin name: Ruta = rue - from the Latin word rus = flow; graveolens = herb of grace (of strong or rank odour). This plant emits odour even on sprinkling water on it.

Botanical Description: This shrub belonging to jambir-kula grows 3-6 cms high. Leaves - thin, small, bitter, astringent and foul smelling. Flowers - small, yellowish in colour. Fruits tripartite with three seeds differentiated.

Habitat: India, Iran, Afghanistan.

Chemical composition: It has a volatile oil containing sulphur.

Properties:

Guna: laghu, ruksha, tikshna; **Rasa:** kashaya; **Vipak:** katu; **Veerya:** ushna, useful in kaphavata diseases.

External use: Local application is antibacterial and rubifacient. It is effective in earache, otorrhoea and vata diseases, also useful in snake and scorpion bite.

Internal use: It is useful in tetanus and epilepsy (especially useful in women and children in the form of decoction).

Respiratory system: In children it is used for chronic cold and cough.

Digestive system: Useful in flatulence, abdominal colic, and intestinal worms.

Urogenital system: In women, it is useful in conditions like obstructed labour, amenorrhoea, renal failure, skin conditions etc.

Temperature: In fever, it stimulates sweating and urination. Leaves are used.

Srotogamitva:

Dosha: Kaphaghna, vataghna, pittakar.

Dhatu: Rasa (amenorrhoea), majja (tetanus - vata diseases).

Mala: Mutra, sweda, purisha (helminthiasis).

Organs: Repiratory system, alimentary system (flatulence).

Prabhav: Antitoxic - snake and scropion bites.

(237) SNUHI

Euphorbia nerifolia Linn.

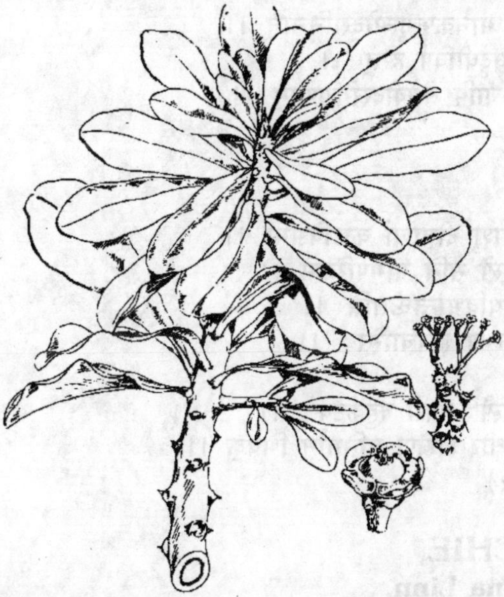

Gana: Virechan (C.), Adhobhaghara (S.)
Kula: Erand kula.
Family: Euphorbiaceae (name of the scientist).
Latin name: Euphorbia = after Euphorbus = physician; nerifolia = neri = oleander like, folia = leaves or E. nivulia or E. antiquorum.
English name: Common milk hage.
Sanskrit names: Snuk, Snuhi, Mahavruksha, Guda, Nistrinshapatrak, Samantdugdha, Gandir, Vajrakantak, Sudha.
Botanical Description: Shrub is small with trunk and branches bearing thorns. Leaves - 30-60 cms. thick and fleshy. Flowers - yellowish. Seeds - flat, leaves shred during winter. Flowering and fruiting occurs in summer. It has six hundred varieties like tridhari, chaudhari, sabarkande etc. Charakacharya has divided it into (a) alpakantak and (b) bahukantak. The latter variety is considered to be superior. Latex is usually collected at the end of winter from a plant which is 2 to 3 years old.
Habitat: All over India, Sikkim, Bhutan.
Chemical composition: Euphorban, resin, gum, rubber, calcium maleate etc.
Properties:
Guna: laghu, snigdha, tikshna; **Rasa:** katu; **Vipak:** katu; **Veerya:** ushna; **Dosha:** kaphavatahara.
External use: Leaves are useful in inflammatory conditions. **Decoction -** drops are used in earache. **Latex -** useful in skin diseases, toothache, impotency, piles and in preparation of ksharsutra.
Internal uses: Digestive system - in the process of shodhan, it is used as a purgative, if the patient can tolerate strong purgatives. Also useful in ascites, hepatosplenic enlargement, anaemia, leucoderma, diabetes mellitus, schizophrenia, syphilis, rheumatoid arthritis and gout. Juice of snuhi mixed with honey, salt and borax is used in bronchitis and asthma.
Root is useful as an antidote to poisons of plant origin.
Dose: Root powder - 250 to 500 mgm.; juice of the stem - 12 to 24 ml.; leaf juice - 2 to 5 drops; latex - 20 to 125 mgm. (It causes diarrhoea).
Formulations: Vajrakshar, Snuhyadi taila.
Srotogamitva:
Dosha: Kaphaghna, vataghna, pittashodhan.
Dhatu: Shodhan of rasa, rakta, mansa, meda, mejja. Therefore useful in hepatosplenic enlargement, anaemia, leucoderma, diabetes, schizohprenia. Rakta (syphilis).
Mala: Purisha (diarrhoea), mutra (calculus).

Aquatic plants are rich in their constituents at night. These should be collected during night only.

Organs: Intestine.

Latex is a drastic purgative and therefore it should be used cautiously.

References -

'सेहुण्डो रेचनस्तीक्ष्णो दीपनः कटुको गुडः । शूलामाष्ठीलिकाध्मानकफगुल्मोदरानिलान् ।।
उन्मादमेहकुष्ठार्शः शोथमेदोश्मपाण्डुताः । व्रणशोथज्वरप्लीहविषदूषीविपं हरेत् ।।
उष्णवीर्यं स्नुहीक्षीरं स्निग्धं च कटुकं लघु । गुल्मिनां कुष्ठिनां चापि तथैवोदररोगिणाम् ।।
हितमेतद्विरेकार्थे ये चान्ये दीर्घरोगिणः (भा. प्र.)
'स्नुक्पयस्तीव्रविरेचनानाम् श्रेष्ठम् ।' (च. सू. २५)
(स्नुहीक्षीरं विरेचने ।' (च. सू. १))
'विरेचनानां सर्वेषां सुधा तीक्ष्णतमा मता । संघातं हि भिनत्त्याशु दोषाणां कष्टविभ्रमा ।।
तस्मान्नैषा मृदौ कोष्ठे प्रयोक्तव्या कदाचन । न दोषनिचये चाल्पे सति मार्गपरिक्रमे ।।
पाण्डुरोगोदरे गुल्मे कुष्ठे दूषीविषार्दिते । श्वयथौ मधुमेहे च दोषविभ्रान्तच्छेतसि ।।
रोगैरेवंविधैर्ग्रस्तं ज्ञात्वा सप्राणमातुरम् । प्रयोजयेन्महावृक्षं सम्यक् स ह्यवचारितः ।।
सद्यो हरति दोषाणां महान्तमपि संचयम् ।' (च. क. १०)
'द्विविधः स मतो यश्च बहुभिश्चैव कंटकैः । सुतीक्ष्णैः कंटकैरल्पैः प्रवरो बहुकंटकः ।।
सनाम्ना स्नुग्गुडानन्दा सुधा निस्त्रिंशपत्रकः । तं विपाट्याहरेत् क्षीर शस्त्रेण मतिमान् भिषक् ।।
द्विवर्षं वा त्रिवर्षं वा शिशिरान्ते विशेषतः ।' (वा. क. अ. २)

(238) SUCHIE
Atropa belladona Linn.

Kula: Kantakari kula.

Family: Solanaceae (plants of the night shade - Solanum tribe).

Latin name: Atropa = atro = dark blackish; bella - donna = bellus = beautiful, donna = donum = gift, present.

Sanskrit names: Sag-angur, Angurshapha, Suchi, Girbuti, Zalakphala.

Botanical Description: Shrub grows 12-15 cm. high, stem is broad but soft. Leaves are particularly thick in the middle and thin peripherally. Fresh leaves are ciliated while the older ones are not. Fruit - blackish, shining. Root - 30 cm. long, 3 to 6 cm. thick and fleshy.

Habitat: In the Himalayas at the height of over 4000 mtrs.

Chemical composition: It contains atropin and hyosciamine.

Properties:

Guna: laghu, ruksha; **Rasa:** tikta and katu; **Vipak:** katu; **Veerya:** ushna; **Prabhav:** madak; **Dosha:** kaphavataghna and pittavardhak. It is poisonous, therefore can cause adverse effects.

External uses: When mixed with alcohol and applied on the skin, it causes analgesic effects because of absorption from the skin. Blood vessels of the skin are dilated after initial vasoconstriction. It causes dilatation of the pupil when used as eye drops. It is therefore contraindicated in increased intraoccular pressure. It is used externally in inflammatory ulcers, glandular swelling and joint pains. It is also useful in conjunctivitis.

Internal uses: It has a sedative effect, causes analgesia and produces delirium. It reduces the salivary secretion and therefore used in loss of appetite and excessive salivation. Though it is a sedative, it has beneficial effects on the heart. Therefore it is used in cardiac debility, heart pain and irregular pulse.

Respiratory system: Useful in bronchitis, asthma and hiccups.

Urinary system: Without increasing the output, it improves the process of urine formation and therefore useful in bed wetting and renal colic due to calculus.

Reproductive system: It is a spermicidal and reduces sweating and breast milk secretion. It cause tissue destruction. It is used as an antidote in morphine and aconite poisoning.

When misused, it causes dryness of mouth, dilatation of pupil, loss of eye sight, dehydration, dysuria, difficulty in deglutition and skin rashes. This condition should be treated by emesis, purgation, stomach wash, morphine and aconite preparations, stimulants and artificial respiration for revival of the patient. Children can tolerate it but is contraindicated in old age, pittaprakruti and excessive pitta dosha.

Srotogamitva:

Dosha: Kaphaghna, vataghna, pittakar.

Dhatu: Rakta, majja, dhatu - destruction, rasa (suppression of breast milk.)

Mala: Saliva (suppression), sweda (suppression), analgesic in renal calculus.

Organ: Heart.

Prabhav: Somnelence.

(239) SURAN

Amorphophallus campanulatus Roxb.

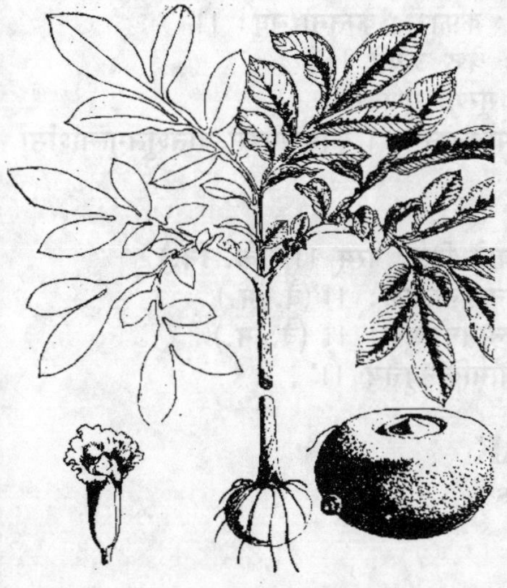

Kula: Suran kula.

Family: Araceae (Plants of the Cackoo tribe).

Latin name: Amorphophallus = A= not, morphus = shape, phallus = sword guard; campanulatus = bell shaped or Arum campanulatum.

English names: Telugu Potato, Telinga potato Tacca.

Sanskrit names: Arshoghna, Kanda, Kandarha, Suvritta, Vatari, Kandasuran, Sthulkandak, Tivrakandak, Ruchyakandak.

Botanical Description: This is a shrub with a life span of one year but the tuber remains under the soil for a longer period. It grows to a height of 30-60 cms. It bears many white raised germinating spots.Tuber - centrally depressed, having a diameter of 18 - 30 cms., hemispherical, bearing umbrella-type leaves, tripartate in the begining with tips showing faint greenish colour. Flowers - homosexual, stamen is of brown colour. Fruit - red coloured containing 2-3 seeds. Flowering occurs in rainy season followed by fruiting.

Varieties: There are two varieties viz. 1) cultivated and 2) wild (A. sylvalicus) or madanmasta The latter variety grows in the forests on its own. White and brownish are the other two varieties. Amongst

Prana-vayu induces spitting and apan vayu induces the force required for defecation. Both these vayus act on two different ends of the body.

these two, brownish is used in medicine, the other variety is used as a vegetable for consumption. It is considered to be the best amongst the vegetables of the kanda variety.
Habitat: All over India.
Chemical composition: It contains calcium oxalate. It causes itching which is seen more with the use of the wild variety.
Properties:
Guna: laghu, ruksha, tikshna; **Vipak:** katu; **Veerya:** ushna; **Prabhav:** arshoghna; **Dosha:** vatakaphashamak.
External uses : In inflammed joints and elephantiasis, it is applied locally by mixing with honey.
Internal use : Since it is apprtizer, digestive, hepatostimulant, laxative, analgesic, anti haemorrhoidal and anthelmintic, it is helpful in anorexia, loss of appetite and hepatosplenomegaly. It is used specially in piles caused by vitiation of vatakapha. Besides, it is also useful in bronchitis, asthma, sterility and ammenorrhoea.
Dose: Tuber - 1 to 3 gms. Suran is contraindicated in bleeding disorders and skin disorders because of its ushna property. To overcome its adverse effects, butter milk, lemon juice and tamarind should be used.
Srotogamitva:
Dosha: Vataghna, kaphaghna, pittavardhak.
Dhatu: Rakta (hepatosplenomegaly), shukra (aphrodisiac), meda.
Mala: Purisha (constipative but useful in piles).
Organs: The entire digestive system.
References -
'सूरणो दीपनो रूक्षः कषायः कण्डुकृत् कटुः । विष्टंभ्भी विशदो रुच्यः कफोर्शः कृन्तनो लघुः ।।
विशेषादर्शसे पथ्यः प्लीहगुल्मविनाशनः । सर्वेषां कन्दशाकानां सूरणः श्रेष्ठ उच्यते ।।
'दद्रूणां कुष्ठिनां रक्तपित्तिनां न हितो हि सः । सन्धानयोगे सप्राप्तः सूरणो गुणवत्तरः ।।
सूरणो गुदकीलहा ।' (सु. सू. ४६) 'सूरणः कटुको रुच्यो दीपनः पाचनस्तथा । कृमिदोषहरो वातशूलगुल्मार्शसां हितः ।।
'श्वासः कासः च प्लीहानं निवारयति सेवितः ।' (ध. नि.)
वनसूरणकन्दस्तु विशेषादर्शसां हितः । गुल्मे स्थौल्ये तथा वाते श्लेष्मवाते हितः परम् ।।' (कै. नि.)
'मासमेकमनन्नाशी सूरणं भक्षयेत् सुखम् । तक्रानुपानमाश्वर्शोनिर्मलोन्मूलनोत्सुकः ।।'(बै. म.)
'मासमेकमनन्नाशी सूरणं भक्षयेत् सुखम् । तक्रानुपानमाश्वर्शोनिर्मलोन्मूलनोत्सुकः ।। (बै. म.)
'मृल्लिप्तं सौरणं कम्दं क्त्वाग्नौ पुटपाकवत् । अद्यात् सतैललवर्णं दुर्नामविनिवृत्तये ।।'

(240) SAIREYAK
Barleria prionitis

Kula: Vasa kula.
Family: Acantheceae. Plants of the bears foot. (Acanthium = thorn).
Latin name: 1) Whitish yellow - Barleria = named after Rev. J. Barrelier of Paris; prionitis = sawlike. 2) Whitish red - Barleria cristita (= crested.) 3) Blue - Barleria strigosa (= bristled).
Sanskrit names: Dashi, Sairiyak, Koranda, Saireya, Kurantak (yellow kuranta), Artagal (blue koranta), Mrudukantak, Zintica.

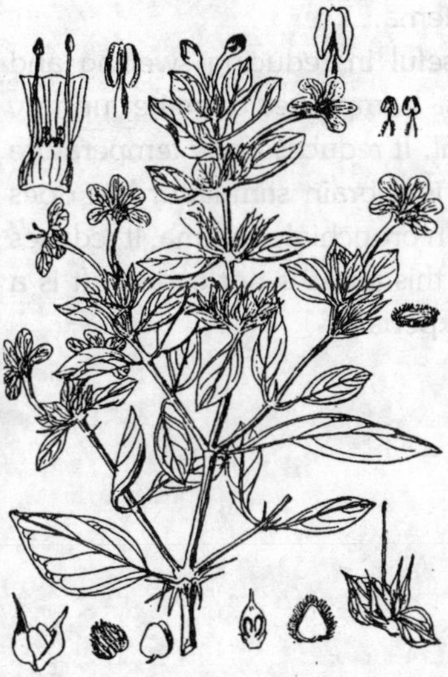

Botanical Description: This shrub grows 0.5 to 2 mtrs. high and bears multiple thorny branches. Leaves - resemble the leaves of Adhatoda vasica measuirng 12 cm x 2 cm. Flowers - whitish, yellowish, brown and blue. Each ovary contains 2 flat oval seeds.
Habitat: Tropical hilly area, Maharashtra, Tamilnadu, Assam, Punjab, Sri lanka. The yellow variety is seen everywhere.
Properties:
Guna: laghu, tikta, **Rasa:** madhur, slightly amla; **Vipak:** katu; **Veerya:** ushna; **Dosha:** kaphavatashamak.
External uses: Reduces inflammation. Leaves are applied for healing of ulcers, urticaria, boils and lymphadenitis. A preparation of oil made from this plant is used in greying of hair and ulcers. Juice of leaves is applied for toothache.
Internal uses: It increases vascular tone and is therefore useful in blood disorders, gout, syphilis, anasarca, rhinorrhoea and bronchitis with expectoration especially in children. Juice of the leaves of white sahachar mixed with Viola odorata is useful in spermatorrhoea. Root powder is used for brushing the teeth in tooth ache. Decoction of the leaves is used as antipyretic.
Dose: Leaf juice - 10 to 20ml.; decoction - 50 to 100 ml.
Srotogamitva:
Dosha: Kaphaghna, vataghna.
Dhatu: Rakta (leucoderma, gout), spermatorrhoea, rasa (antipyretic).
Mala: Hair (dying).
Organs: Respiratory tract (bronchitis).
References -
'सैरेयकः श्वेतपुष्पः सैरेयः कटसारिका । सहचरः आर्तगलः स च झिष्ट्यपि कथ्यते ।।
'कुरण्टकोऽत्र पीते स्याद्रक्ते कुरबकः स्मृतः । नीले बाणा द्वयोरुक्तो दासी चार्तगलश्च सः ।।
सैरेयः कुष्ठवातास्त्रकफकण्डुविषापहः । तिक्तोण्णो मधुरोऽनम्लः सुस्निग्धः केशरंजनः ।।'

(241) SOMA
Ephedra gerardiana Rich.

Family: Ephedraceae.
Latin name: Ephedra = sea grapes, horse tail; gerardiana = after John Girard.
English name: Ephedra.
Habitat: Himalayas at the height of 2000 - 5000 mtrs.
Parts used: Trunk, panchang.
Collection period: Spring.
Botanical Description: Shrub.
Dose: Decoction - 20 to 50 ml.
Properties: Digestive, laxative, diuretic, hepatic stimulant, antipyretic, neurostimulator, vatahara,

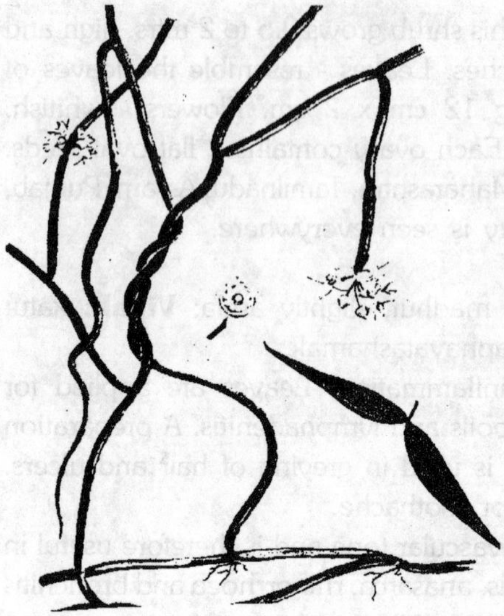

ama digestive, reduces oedema.

Uses: 1) Decoction is useful in reducing swelling and pain of rheumatoid arthritis. It improves appetite, urinary output and bowel movement. It reduces body temperature in fever. 2) Like alcohol, it is a brain stimulator but does not produce intoxication. 3) In bronchial ashthma, it reduces dyspnoea. (The identity of this plant is not certain. It is a subject of debate among experts).

(242) HARAMAL

Paganum harmal Linn.

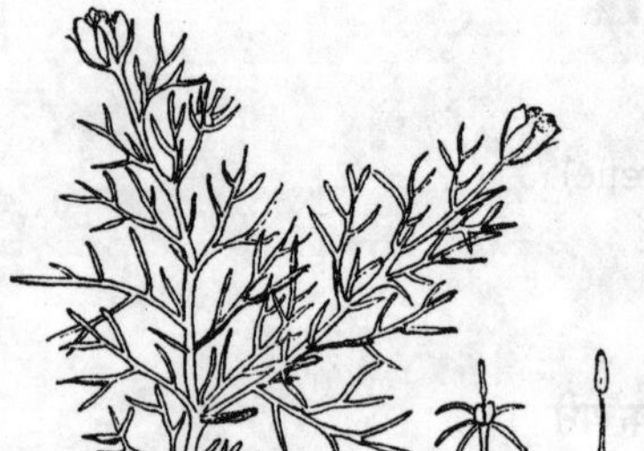

Kula: Jambir kula.

Family: Rutaceae.

Latin name: Paganum = rustic - belonging to the country; harmal = from the name Harmal.

English name: Syrian Rue.

Botanical Description: This shrub, 0.5 to 1 mt. in height, has a life span of many years. Leaves - 6-9 cm. long, equidistant. Flowers - white, arising from the angle of the leaves. 12 to 15 stamens are distributes in two circles. Fruits - round, trilobulated, easily breakable, contain three black seeds with a strong fragrance. It is said that seeds are used for extinguishing fire. Out of the two varieties, brownish variety is very useful.

Habitat: Arabasthan, Iran, Sindh, Kashmir, Punjab, North India, West India.

Properties:

Guna: laghu, ruksha; **Rasa:** tikta; **Vipak:** katu; **Veerya:** ushna; **Dosha:** kaphavatashamak, pittavardhak.

Uses: It is used as an analgesic, antibacterial, antiflatulent, anthelmintic, blood purifier, expectorant, oxytropic, galactogogue, emmenagogue and anticonvulsant. Medicated oil is used in earache.

Dose: 1 to 3 gms. Excess dose causes burning, euphoria, addiction and nausea. Drugs of madhur and amla properties are used for relieving the symptoms.

Srotogamitva:
Dosha: Kaphaghna, vataghna, pittavardhak.
Dhatu: Majja, rakta, rasa.
Mala: Purisha (anthelmintic).
Organ: Uterus (contraction). Treatment should be done cautiously.

(243) HARIDRU
Adina cordifolia Roxb.

Kula: Manjistha kula.
Family: Rubiaceae (plants of the rubia, madder).
Latin name: Adina = adinos = crowded, flowers being disposed in heads; cordifolio = cordi = heart, folia = leaves.
Sanskrit names: Peetadaru, Kadambak, Dhulikadamb, Haridru, Peetkashtha, Peetaksupushpa, Suravha, Peetakadrum, Shriman.
Botanical Description: This tree grows 8-10 mt. high. It is commonly known as haldu or haldarva. Leaf stalk is 2 - 6 cm. long. Leaves - 12 - 28 cm. in diameter, round, heart shaped and with pointed ends. Flowers - yellow, bloom in autumn. Fruit - resembles betel nut and contains five seeds. Fruiting occurs in summer. Bark of the trunk is greyish white externally. Internally, it is yellow but it turns brownish black with proceeding age.
Habitat: Western parts of India, foot hills of Himalayas; bark contains a bitter principle.
Properties:
Guna: laghu, ruksha **Rasa:** tikta; **Vipak:** katu **Veerya:** sheeta; **Dosha** : kaphapitta shamak, therefore useful in diseases caused by kaphapitta.
External uses: Due to its cleansing and healing property of ulcers, it is used in skin diseases, ulcers, discolouration and dermatoses.
Internal uses: Like many other dravyas of bitter rasa, it is a powerful appetizer. It helps in digestion of ama and secretion of bile but causes constipation and acts as an anthelmintic. Therefore, it is useful in conditions like loss of appetite, indigestion, thirst, liver disorders, dysentery and intestinal worms. Since it is a haematinic, it is used in blood disorders.
Parts used: Bark and leaves are used for medicinal purposes.
Dose: Decoction: 50 to 100 ml.; juice: 10 to 20 ml.; powder: 2 to 3 gms.
Srotogamitva:
Dosha: Kaphaghna, pittaghna.
Dhatu: Rakta.
Mala: Cholagogue, constipative and anthelmintic.
Organs: Liver, spleen, stomach.
References -
'हरिद्रुको महावृक्षोकदम्बाभफलो गिरौ । भवेत् वृत्तदल: पीतकाष्ठ: श्रीमान् सुदारक: ।।' (शि.)
'हरिद्रु: पीतलस्तिक्तो मंगल्य: पित्तवान्तिजित् ।
अंगकान्तिकरो बल्यो नानात्वग्दोषनाशन: ।।' (रा. नि.)

The Ayurvedic treatises of Charaka, Sushruta and Vagbhatta cover not only the subject matter but also have an aesthetic dimension.

(244) HAPUSHA

Juniperus communis Linn.

Kula: Hapusha kula.

Family: Cupressaceae or Coniferae.

Latin name: Juniperus = rough, Latin name of Junipes (Celtic word Junperus = rough); communis = commonly growing in society or Thivetia nerifolia (leaves like Oleander nerium).

Sanskrit names : Hapusha, Vapusha, Vistra, Para, Ashvatthaphala, Matsyagandha, Plihahantri, Vishaghni, Dhwankshanashini.

Botanical Description: It is a shrub. Leaves resemble the leaves of Cannabis sativa. Fruits - blackish, round, small, containing three seeds. Bhavprakash has classified it into two as ashwatthaphala and bruhatphala.

Habitat: Western and northen parts of Himalayas, Nepal, Bhutan and Iran. It grows over the height of 4000 mtrs.

Chemical composition: Fruits contain 50% volatile oil, fructose, oxalic acid etc.

Properties:

Guna: guru, ruksha,tikshna; **Rasa:** katu, tikta; **Vipak:** katu; **Veerya:** ushna; **Dosha:** kapahavatashamak.

External uses: It has antiinflammatory and ulcer healing properties because of which it is used in skin disorders and ulcers. It is applied externally on the penis in loss of libido while the juice is used in deafness.

Internal uses: As it stimulates the nerves, it is used in paralysis and nervous disorders. Since it is an appetizer, carminative, mildly astringent and anthelmintic, it is used in loss of appetite, abdominal pain, piles, dysentery, intestinal worms and ascites. It is useful in bronchitis, asthma, dysmenorrhoea, leucorrhoea and gonorrhoea.

Part used: Fruit.

Dose: Fruit-powder - 3 to 5gms.; oil - 1 to 2 drops for improving appetite and 4 to 6 drops as a diuretic.

Srotogamitva:

Dosha: Kaphaghna, vataghna.

Dhatu: Rakta, rasa, mansa, majja, rasa (dysmenorrhoea and amenorrhoea).

Mala: Purisha (laxative, anthelmintic), mutra.

Organ: Respiratory tract (bronchitis and asthma).

References -

'हपुषा दीपनी तिक्ता कटूष्णा तुवरा गुरुः । पित्तोदरसमीरार्शोग्रहणीगुल्मशूलहृत् ।।' (भा. प्र.)

हपुषा कटुतिक्तोष्णा गुरुर्वातबलासजित् । प्रदरोदरविड्बन्धशूलगुल्मार्शसां हिता ।।' (रा. नि.)

(245) HANSRAJ
Adiantum lunulatum

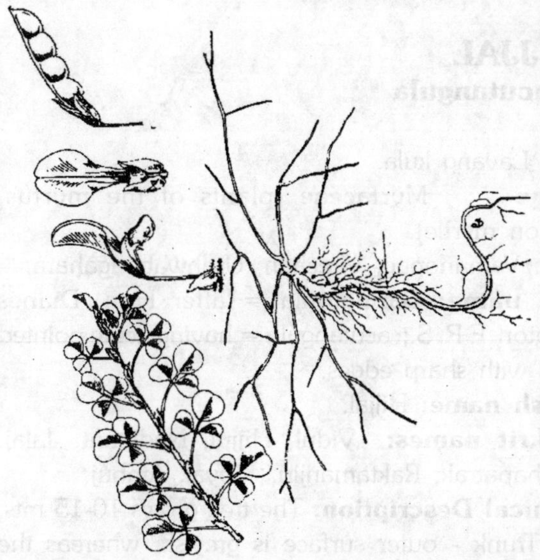

Kula: Hansraj kula.
Family: Polypodiaceae.
Gana: Kanthya, Madhurskandha (C.); Vidarigandhadi (S.)
Latin name: Adiantum = adiantos = dry, lunulatum = crescent, half moon shaped.
English name: Maiden hair.
Sanskrit names: Vishwagandhi, Tripadi, Hansapadi, Dhrutmandalika, Hansapadakarpatra, Raktalajjalu.
Botanical Description: This is a shrub growing 3 to 6 cms. in height. Root - tender, brownish. Branches - thin. Leaves - small, soft with round dentate borders; under surface of the leaves bears a reproductive organ through which the new plant grows. It dose not bear flowers.
Habitat: Marshy lands, cold hilly areas.

Properties:
Guna: guru, snigdha; **Rasa:** madhur, tikta, kashaya; **Vipak:** madhur; **Veerya:** sheeta;
Dosha: Vatapittashamak and kaphanissarak.
External uses: Since it is a refrigerant, antidote and has wound healing properties, it is used in urticaria, plague and spider poisoning to reduce swelling, pain and burning sensation.
Internal uses: Due to its astringent property, it is used in diarrhoea and intestinal worms. It is useful in bleeding disorders and other blood disorders since it is pittashamak. It is useful in pneumonitis, rhinitis, bronchitis and asthma since it is an expectorant. As it is vatapittashamak, it helps in dysuria by increasing urine flow.
Dose: Panchang juice - 5 to 10 ml.; panchang powder - 1 to 3 gms.
Srotogamitva:
Dosha: Vataghna, pittaghna, kaphanissarak.
Dhatu: Rakta (bleeding disorders).
Mala: Mutra (diuretic).
Prabhav: Antidote for poisons.
Srotas: Respiratory system - bronchitis.
References -
'हंसपादी गुरुः शीता हन्ति रक्तविषव्रणान् । विसर्पदाहातीसारलूताभूताग्निरोहिणी ॥' (भा. प्र.)
'हंसपादी हिमा गुर्वो रोपणी हन्ति शोणितम् । दाहातीसारवीसर्पलूताशोथविषव्रणान् ॥' (के. नि.)

Many formulations using guggulu as the base have made it possible not only to preserve their gunas but also to maintain their potency for twenty years (!)

(246) HINSTRA (JATAMANSI)

This plant is described in Part 1 / Sr. No. 63

(247)HIJJAL

Baringtonia acutangula

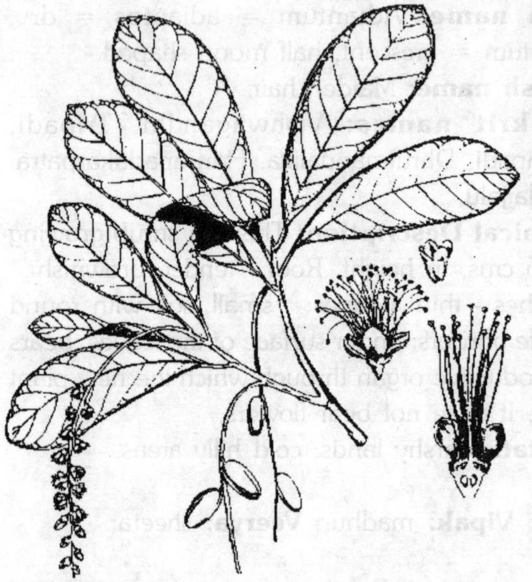

Kula: Lavang kula.

Family: Myrtaceae (plants of the myrtus, common myrtle).

Gana: Vamanopag, Virechan, Urdhwabhagahara.

Latin name: Baringtonia = after Hon. Dianes Barington F. R. S.; acutangula = having acute pointed angles with sharp edges.

English name: Hijjal.

Sanskrit names: Vidul, Hijjul, Nadikant, Jalaj, Deerghapatrak, Raktamanjiri, Toyaj, Ambuj.

Botanical Description: The tree grows 10-15 mts. high. Trunk - outer surface is greyish, whereas the inner one is white in colour. Leaves - 15 x 6 cm, oblong. Flowers - brownish, with 30 cm. long stalk. Fruits 6 - 12 cm. x 3 - 5 cm, centrally thick.

Habitat: Himalayas, bank of the Yamuna, Ayodhya, Bengal, Central and Southern India and Burma. Water turns foamy due to its saponin content.

Properties:

Guna: laghu,ruksha,tikshna; **Rasa:** tikta, katu, madhur; **Vipak:** katu; **Veerya:** ushna.

Prabhav: emetic; **Dosha:** kaphapittashodhan, vatashaman.

Seeds are analgesic, lekhan and are especially used for nasya. Paste prepared from the seeds is locally applied to relieve pain. In eye diseases and jaundice, it is used as an eye ointment. Hijjal is useful as an emetic in diseases caused by kapha and as a purgative in pitta diseases. It is therefore used in ascites, intestinal worms and diarrhoea. Since it is a blood purifier, it is used in blood disorders. Also useful in bronchitis and asthma. Mixture of hijjal powder + Vitex nigundo + sugar is useful in typhoid, splenic enlargement and chronic fever.

Dose: Fruit powder - 3 to 6 gms. (emetic); 0.5 to 1 gm. for other indications; leaf juice 10 to 20 ml.

Srotogamitva:

Dosha: Kapha (shodhan), pitta (shodhan), vata (shaman).

Dhatu: Rakta (cough, dyspnoea, enlargement of the spleen); rasa (dysmenorrhoea).

Mala: Mutra (pyuria, dysuria); purisha (anthelmintic).

Organ: Uterine contraction (obstructed labour and dysmenorrhoea).

References -

'फलं समुद्रस्य कटूष्णकारि वातापहं भूतनिरोधकारि ।
त्रिदोषदावानलदोषहारि कफामयभ्रांतिविरोधकारि ।।'
'हिज्जल: कटुरुष्णश्च पवित्रो भूतनाशन: । वातामयहरो नानाग्रहसंचारदोषजित् ।।' (रा. नि.)
'जलवेतसवद्वेद्यो हिज्जलोऽयं विषापह: ।' (भा. प्र.)
जलेन घृष्ट्वा पीं चेत् कृमिनाशकरं परम् । तदेव चांजितं नेत्रे कामलां नाशयेत् ध्रुवम् ।। (रा. नि.)
'दलोत्थ: स्वरस: पेयो हिज्जलस्य समाक्षिक: । जयत्याममतीसारम् ।।' (च. द.)
'हिज्जलस्य फलं घ्रष्ट्वा पानीये नित्यमञ्जनम् ।
चक्षु:स्त्रावे प्रशान्त्यर्थं कार्यमेतन्महौषधम् ।।' (बंगसेन)

(248) HRUTPATRI
Digitalis purpurea

Kula: Katuka kula.
Family: Scrophulariaceae (plants of the scrophularia, fig wort).
Latin name: Digitalis = finger shape of flowers; purpurea = purple.
English name: Digitalis.
Sanskrit names: Hrutpatri, Tilpushpi.
Botanical Description: This shurb grows 1 to 1.25 mtrs. in height. Leaves - 12 to 30 cm. long and 6 to 18 cm. broad. The upper surface of the leaves is green while the under surface is white with cilia. Lamina of the leaf is dentate. Flower stalk - 40 cm. long, bearing 60 to 70 flowers of yellowish violet colour. Fruits - small with plenty of seeds. Flowering and fruiting occurs in the month of June.
Habitat: India, Europe, America, grows at a height of 1000 - 3000 mtrs.
Properties:
Guna: laghu, ruksha; **Rasa:** tikta; **Vipak:** katu; **Veerya:** ushna; **Dosha:** kaphavatashamak and pittavardhak.
External use: It creates intense irritation when applied on the skin.
Internal use: On prolonged use, it causes nauses. Alcohol extract acts faster. It acts faster when administered rectally. It has specific activity on the heart. It slows down the heart rate, increases the contraction of the cardiac muscles, increases the refractory period, increases the blood pressure and therefore it is useful in cardiac debility and oedema.
Its kaphaghna action is seen in bronchitis, asthma and pulmonary oedema. By improving the renal blood flow, it improves the renal filtration and urine formation in 48 hrs.
It is also useful in sterility and dysmenorrhoea, high fever and cardiac debility.
Excessive dose causes vomiting, diarrhoea, anaemia, headache and bradycardia. This condition is treated by stomach wash, coffee, alcoholic stimulants, fomentation and bed rest.
Srotogamitva:
Dosha: Kaphaghna, vataghna, pittavardhak.
Dhatu: Rakta, meda, shukra.
Mala: Mutra (diuretic).
Organ: Heart, uterine contraction.

In a mango fruit, rasas get transformed first it is astringent, later it is sour and finally sweet. The steady presence of Prithvi-dravya is responsible for inducing all these rasas.

PART IV

DRAVYAS OF ANIMAL ORIGIN AND OTHERS

INTRODUCTION

The following chapters deal with the properties of a few dravyas of animal origin. Generally, these dravyas act on the body by showing gamitva on the corresponding parts of the human body. These dravyas then bring about an increase in those body constituents which have similar properties. This concept has been explained in the Sharir sthana of Charaka samhita.

Following this principle, various remedies can be prescribed. For example, blood or meat soup and especially liver soup should be used in diseases related to blood loss. Similarly, cow's urine and goat's urine in mutrakshaya and praval (corals) and oyster shells etc. are used in asthikshaya. Here also, the concept of dosha-dhatu-mala is important. For example, udid has properties similar to kapha dosha,mansa and shukra dhatus and purisha. Therefore udid causes an increase in all these. Every dravya should be considered in this way, in relation to human beings.

Various types of agni present within the body perform the function of converting all these dravyas into various body constituents.

1. JALAVARGA

Taiteryopnishad has described the genesis of jala mahabhoota after the genesis of agni (teja) mahabhoota in the process of cosmogenesis. Jala (water) is absolutely essential for maintaining life of all living systems.

Sanskrit names : Paneeya, salil, neer, keelal, jala, ambu, aap, vaar, vaari, uda, daka, ka, toy, paya, paath, jeevan, vana, aṃbha, arna, amrut, ghanrasa, saril, kamal, bhuvan, kabandh, kamandh, jeevaneeya, naar, ksheer, shambar, meghapushpa. (There are 32 synonyms for jala).

There are numerous types of water and they can be differentiated into natural and unnatural types. (Kaup, saras, tadag, chaundya, prasravan, audbhid, vapi and nadey are the further eight subtypes of water).

The water which falls on the earth from the sky is only of one type. But while falling from the sky and even after falling, certain conditionings do occur on the water which bring about a change in its properties depending on the desha (type of land) and kala (season). Water imbibes the properties of the land with which it comes in contact. Even different seasons bring about a change in the properties and actions of water. Water is usually pure in the month of Ashwin while in the rainy season it is generally impure.

If the colour of the land is white then it gives astringent taste to water.

If it is yellowish then it gives a bitter taste to water.

If the land has kapil varna, then the water becomes alkaline.

If the land has more of salts then the water becomes salty.

In mountain regions the water becomes pungent.

If the land is black in colour then it gives sweet taste to water.

Even though water has been described as an exceptionally useful substance and evethough it is called jeevan, tarpan, hridya and buddhiprabodhan, yet its efficacy depends on individual constitution of the consumer and the amount consumed.

Therefore, it is wrong to say that water can be consumed in any quantity, at any time and in whatever manner one thinks is correct. It has been said that even a healthy person should drink water judiciously (पिबेत् स्वस्थोऽपिच अल्पश:) then in conditions of diseases, it becomes even more important to think about the comsumption of water.

Simple boiled water can be used as a remedy for diarrhoea, fever and cough. In fever, when there is excessive thirst, water, in which heated iron rod has been dipped several times, is used as a remedy. This reduces fever and excessive thirst.

Diseases caused due to indiscriminate use of water can be cured simply by controlling the amount of water ingested.

Those people who suffer from diseases of kapha and especially those who have chest congestion can have relief by not drinking water in the evening after 6 p.m. till afternoon, the next day.

The sanskrit word for water is 'aap' and it is always used in the plural. (Even in Hindi, the same usage is seen).

The conditioning done on water by repeatedly dipping heated metals like gold in it creates special properties in it without causing any change in the dravya-guna-karma of the metal. The tongue has been called 'aapya' because throughout the 24 hours of the day, it is constantly moistened with water. Thus, if this perfusion stops even for a moment then the person starts showing symptoms of 'ojakshaya' and this 'oja' can be reinstated simply by giving a spoonful of water. Such is the position of water in human life and therefore water is called jeevan. (जीवनं तर्पणं हृद्यं … वा. सू. अ ५-१)

Properties of water might change depending on the container. For example, water kept in a copper vessel. Water shares a producer-product relationship with the rasa dhatu of the body. Even then, for water to get imbibed in the body as rasa dhatu, it is absolutely essential that it is first acted upon by the rasa dhatvagni. Without that it will not get incorporated in the rasa dhatu. If water is drunk in large qunatities then it causes diarrhoea. Water does not have any rasa of its own.

There can be innumerable grades in the rasa-anurasa of water depending on the action of land, seasons, moon, sun, soil, wind etc. If water is not taken appropriately then it can act as a poison.

There is a belief that underground reservoirs of water are generally found in the vicinity of certain trees. Can these trees be considered jaleeya? For example - umbar, jambul. If water is heated then it loses its taste but if it is poured repeatedly from one container into another container from a height, then its taste returns. This water does not increase kapha. Water flowing in a river splashes against stones, water descending from a water fall gets purified. It is observed that water obtained from other sources gets putrid but Ganga's water never becomes putrid. Water stored in cool places devoid of sunlight is more likely to cause filariasis.

A major portion of this earth and living systems is made up of water. Therefore, the well being of this world and of human beings is not possible without water.

Water falling from the sky during rainy season, if stored properly, can be very useful. Water therefore has an exceptionally important place in the life of all living beings.

2. DUGDHAVARGA

Milk, which is a dravya included in the jeevaneeya varga, is of eight types as described by Charakacharya.

The eight types of milk are those obtained from sheep, goat, cow, buffalo, camel, elephant, horse and human. Even though the properties and actions of all these are generally same, yet, each one has its own specific properties.

Generally - Milk is sweet,unctuous, cold, prenana (increases rasa dhatu), bruhan (increases mansa dhatu), vrushya (increases shukra dhatu), medhya (improves memory), balya (increases strength), manaskar,jeevaneeya (raktagami, raktavahasrotogami and a potent pacifier of pitta), sandhanak (catalyses healing of fractures), sarvasatmya (useful for all age groups), shaman as well as shodhan (depending on the amount, prakriti and condition), trishnaghna (cures excessive thirst), deepan, useful for emaciated and debilitated patients as also in anaemia (which causes laxity of all dhatus along with ojakshaya), amlapitta (hyperacidity), shotha (oedema),gulma, udar, shodhan and yet useful in diarrhoea.

Milk is contraindicated in acute fever but is extremely important in chronic fever. Useful in burning sensation, especially in inflammatory conditions. Useful as a purgative in constipation. Similarly useful in reproductive system and in seminal disorders. Milk acts as a diuretic on the urinary system. From the point of view of doshas, it is vata-pitta shamak.

It can be used as nasya(nasal administration),for topical application, for avgaah (full body or locally), as an emetic, for asthapanbasti, as a purgative and for various procedures like snehan etc.

Milk has an exceptional importance in health and also in treating diseases, yet there are contraindications also .Though milk is good for health, there are certain conditions and certain diseases in which it is contraindicated.

Properties and actions of each type of milk

1) Sheep's milk : It is not good to taste, yet it is ushna and pacifies vata diseases. It increases hiccups, dyspnoea, kapha and pitta. Sheep's milk is the least indicated milk among all the types of milk. Sheep's nose has a continuous discharge. From the point of view of the sheep , this may be natural but it may be the reason why its milk is not very good for human consumption.

2) Goat's milk : Goats drink lesser amount of water. They undergo a lot of physical exertion and eat various plants having pungent and bitter tastes. Because of this, their milk is easy to digest and is useful in kshaya, fever, dyspnoea, bleeding disorders and diarrhoea.

3) Cow's milk : It is jeevaneeya (performs the function of rakta dhatu), rasayana (nourishes all the dhatus), useful for emaciated and debilitated people, increases intellect, strength, acts as a galactogogue and laxative. Apart from this, it is useful in exhaustion, giddiness, intoxication, asthma, cough, excessive thirst and excessive hunger, chronic fever, dysuria and bleeding disorders. Cow's milk is naturally slightly yellow in colour. It increases oja dhatu.

4) Buffalo's milk : It is sheeta veerya and heavy to digest. It is very useful for those who experience excessive hunger and also have insomnia.

5) Camel's milk : It is slightly ushna, ununctuous, salty, light and is deepan. Because of these properties, it is useful in vata, kapha, abdominal distention, helminthiasis,oedema, ascitis and haemorrhoids.

6) Elephant's milk : It is the best dravya for building the body as strong as an elephant's body.

7) Horse's milk : Milk of animals like horse and donkey is very ushna and therefore, it is light, mildly salty and slightly sour.

8) Human milk : It is vata-pitta shamak and is very useful in raktapitta, inflammation due to injury and various eye disorders. It can be used as a nasya and also for tarpan.

If milk is consumed without heating then it is heavy and causes excessive viscosity in the body. But if it is heated at lower temperature for a longer period then its properties are altered and does not cause viscosity. But again, if it is heated strongly, it becomes heavy to digest. Fresh milk is extremely good for health. In fact, proper care about the cleanliness has to be taken.

No substance is absolutely useful or absolutely harmful. This point of view is supported by the universally accepted principle that `No two individuals are identical'. The beneficial or harmful effects of all dravyas differ from person to person. Milk may not suit a particular person but if it is necessary for him, then not only milk but any other dravya can be given after proper conditioning.

Ayurveda has not accepted biased or absolute opinions about milk or any other dravya including poisonous dravyas.

Those people who experience excessive chest congestion with expectoration during night time should be given hot milk with turmeric or jaggery before bed time. This stops production of kapha in the body. These conditionings of milk are very useful.

In the west as well as in the far eastern countries, only cold milk is used. Pregnant women are rightly advised large quantity of milk for their nutrition as well as well-being of the foetus. Milk is called 'lac', 'mulgere' in Latin. The sanskrit names are ksheer, dugdha, paya, stanya, stantyodbhava, amrut, piyush, jeeva, atma, jeevaneeya.

Eventhough milk is similar to all the dhatus of the body, it produces shukra immediately. As a result, it increases oja.

1) Milk drunk in the morning is vrushya, bruhan and agnivardhak.
2) Milk taken in the afternoon produces kapha, increases strength and relieves dysuria.
3) Milk taken at night cures many ailments.

1) In childhood, milk - increases agni.
2) In youth, milk - increases strength.
3) In old age, milk - increases veerya.

Cow's milk should be consumed in the morning whereas buffalo's milk in the evening. Even though milk is extremely beneficial, it is not compatible with salt, food items made from flour, black gram, moong, rhizomes etc.

Milk boiled with various medicines has been used as a remedy in various ailments.

Depending on the disease, prakriti and condition of the patient, parpati kalpa can be given to a patient and then milk can be taken in any amount to produce the effect of rasayana. In ascites, a diet consisting of only milk is advised for six months. (The author has obtained similar results with vardhamaan pippali). In jvara, when the doshas are pakva and are aggravated,virechan (purgation)is indicated. But other dravyas cannot be given in fever.In such a situation, milk should be used as a purgative.

In diarrhoea, when there is aam along with abdominal spasm, milk boiled with mustard is indicated.

There is a difference between the milk obtained from wild and domesticated animals. The latter yield milk which is heavy to digest whereas wild animals have light milk.

If milk is heated to a very high temperature and then immediately cooled (pasteurisation), it does not sour for a long time. Such milk can be stored in paper cartons under refrigeration, for about a week.

References -

'क्षीरं जीवनीयानाम् ।' 'क्षीरघृताभ्यासो रसायनानाम् ।' (च. सू. २५)
'अजाक्षीरं शोषघ्नस्तन्यसात्म्यसांग्राहिकरक्तपित्तप्रशमनानाम् । 'महिषीक्षीरं स्वप्नजननानाम् ।' अविक्षीरं श्लेष्मपित्तजननानाम् ।' (च. सू. २५)
'गोक्षीरं क्षीराणाम् (हिततमम्), अविक्षीरं क्षीराणाम् (अहिततमम्)' (च. सू. २५)
'प्रायशो मधुरं स्निग्धं शीतं स्तन्यं पयो मतम् । प्रीणनं बृंहणं वृष्यं मेध्यं बल्यं मनस्करम् ।।
जीवनीयं श्रमहरं श्वासकासनिबर्हणम् । हन्ति शोणितपित्तं च सन्धानं विहतस्य च ।।
सर्वप्राणभृतां सात्म्यं शमनं शोधनं तथा । तृष्णाघ्नं दीपनीयं च श्रेष्ठं क्षीणक्षतेषुच ।।

पाण्डुरोगेऽम्लपित्ते च शोषे गुल्मे तथोदरे । अतिसारे ज्वरे दाहे श्वयथौ च विशेषतः ।।
योनिशुक्रप्रदोषेषु मूत्रेषु प्रदरेषु च । पुरीषे ग्रथिते पथ्यं वातपित्तविकारिणामृ ।।
नस्यलेपावगाहेषु वमनास्थापनेषु च । विरेचने स्नेहने च पयः सर्वत्र युज्यते ।।' (च. सू. १)
तत्र सर्वमेव क्षीरं सर्वप्राणभृतामप्रतिषिद्धं जातिसात्म्यत्वात्, वातपित्तशोणितमानसेष्वपि विकारेष्वविरुद्धं, जीर्णज्वरकासश्वासशोषक्षयगुल्मोन्मादोदरमूर्च्छाभ्रम मददाहपिपासाहृद्बस्ति दोषपाण्डुरोगग्रहणीदोषार्शः शूलोदावर्त्तातिसारप्रवाहिकायोनिरोगगर्भास्त्रावरक्त पित्तश्रमक्लमहरं पाप्मापहं बल्यं वृष्यं वाजीकरणं रसायनं मेध्यं वयःस्थापनमायुष्यं जीवनं बृंहणं संधानंवमनविरेचनास्थापनं तुल्यगुणत्त्वाच्चौजसो वर्धनं बालवृद्धक्षतक्षीणानां क्षुद् व्यवायव्यायामकर्शितानां च पथ्यतमम् ।' (सु. सू. ४५)
'स्वादु शीतं मृदु स्निग्धं बहलं श्लक्ष्णपिच्छिलमृ । गुरु मन्दं प्रसन्नंच गव्यं दशगुणं पयः ।।
तदेवं गुणमेवौजः सामान्यदभिवर्धयेत् । प्रवरं जीवनीयानां क्षीरमुक्तंरसायनम् ।। (च. सू. २७)
'उपवासाध्वभाष्यस्त्रीमारुतातपकर्मभिः । क्लान्तानामनुपानार्थं पयः पथ्यं यथामृतम् ।।' (च.सू.२७)
'केवलं तु पयस्तस्याः शृतं वाऽशृतमेव वा । शर्करांक्षौद्रसर्पिभिर्युक्तं तद् वृष्यमुत्तमम् ।।' (च. चि. २)
जीर्णज्वराणां सर्वेषां पयः प्रशमनं परम् । पेयं तदुष्णं शीतं वा यथास्वं भेषजैः शृतम् ।। (च. चि. ३)
'पयसः प्रयोगो विषमज्वरे ।' (च. चि. ३)

3. GHRITVARGA

Ghrit is not only included in the annavarga but it is also used as the best remedy for pitta disorders and vata-pitta disorders. Ghrit is best among all snehanas used internally. Since ghrit has a natural tendency to accept and imbibe various conditionings, its properties and actions become more evident when combined with other dravyas. Therefore the preparation of medicated ghrit is extensively used in Ayurveda not only in vata-pitta disorders but also in almost all diseases. Though ghrit has properties contrary to those of pitta, yet it is agnideepan, increases intellect, memory, strength, eyesight and increases shukra dhatu also.

It is extremely useful for people of all age groups, increases fertility, improves complexion of the skin, produces tenderness, improves voice and is bruhan. It increases oja. Ghrit is very useful for such patients who have undergone trauma, surgery, burns and emaciation. Ghrit is also useful for increasing the strength of all the senses.

Medicated ghrit can be used in erysepelas, poisoning, psychosis, oedema, displeasure, fever etc. Ghrit is the best dravya among all dravyas useful for sustaining life.

Ghrit has different actions when licked and when swallowed. For example, when licked, it is pitta shamak whereas when swallowed, it pacifies vata. It is the best antidote for all poisons. The clear upper layer of ghrit is easy to digest as it is ununctuous. The word 'ajya' means melted ghrit.

Ghrit is very useful for persons of vata prakriti and pitta prakriti. It doesnot increase kapha as well. Puranghrit (10 year old ghrit) is very useful in psychosis, epilepsy, fainting, diseases of the head, ears and eyes and is very useful in healing wounds.

It can be used for nasal administration, massage, oral administration, enema etc.

Ghrit is madhur, has madhur vipak and is sheeta veerya.

The melting point of ghrit is 33 to 37°C. It contains more oxgen than other oils. Cow's ghrit is considered the best whereas sheep's ghrit is considered harmful.

Ghrit is again subdivided into various types depending on the conditioning and time of storage.

Ksheerghrit : Ghrit prepared by heating cream which is extracted directly from milk is called ksheerghrit.

Haiyangveen : Cream extracted directly from milk is called haiyangveen.

Sadyoghrit : Ghrit which is immediately obtained by heating butter is called sadyoghrit.

Ghrit : The same sadyoghrit, when solidifies, is called ghrit.

Ajya : Ghrit, when melted by mild heating, is called ajya.

Ghritmanda : The upper layer of ghrit which remains in a melted state for years is called ghritmanda.

Jeerna-Puran-Ghrit : 10 years old ghrit is called puran ghrit.

Kumbha Ghrit : 100 years old ghrit is called kumbha ghrit.

Maha Ghrit : 111 years old ghrit is called maha ghrit.

Stored ghrit becomes progressively solidified because its water content goes on decreasing progressively. Maha ghrit becomes hard like a stone. It has to be boiled in water and then used. It increases strength and intellect. It is considered austere and relieves bhootabadha.

Properties and actions of ghrit :

1) Cow : sweet, madhur vipaki, sheeta, pacifies vata-pitta, anti-toxin, very useful to the eyes, and increases strength. (People staying in Konkan and tribal people call cow's ghrit as cow's oil).

2) Goat : increases agni, is light to digest, useful to the eyes, increases strength, useful in pthysis, cough and asthma.

3) Buffalo : sweet, heavy to digest, cures raktapitta, increases kapha, pacifies vata-pitta and is extremely sheeta.

4) Camel : katu vipaki, useful in oedema, poisoning and as antihelminthic. It is deepan, pacifies kapha-vata, dermatosis, useful in tumour and ascites.

5) Sheep : light to digest, does not vitiate pitta, useful in kapha, vata, vaginal diseases, pthysis and tremors.

6) Horse's and Donkey's Ghrit : is easy to digest, ushna veerya, astringent, relieves kapha, deepan and causes retention of urine.

7) Human milk Ghrit : is extremely beneficial and is useful in increasing the growth of the body, increases the agni and acts as an antitoxin. It is light to digest.

(How is ghrit prepared from human milk is not known, but it is not available currently).

8) Elephant's Ghrit : is astringent, bitter and causes retention of urine and faeces. It is deepan and easy to digest. Useful in kapha, dermatoses, toxins and parasites.

Ghrit obtained by churning milk acts as an astringent and is useful in raktapitta, vertigo, fainting and eye diseases.

Supernatent ghrit is sweet to taste and relieves pain in the pelvis, ears, eyes and head. It is used in enema, nasal administration and for akshipuran. The upper layer of ghrit is light and is useful for giving anuvasan and matrabasti in fever.

Oil is not to be consumed on the day of fasting. But ghrit can be taken. But it is not easily available and is costly also. Therefore human ingenuity has given the superior name of ghrit to hydrogenated oils. But the properties do not change by simply changing the name. Yet, such artificial ghrit is being used.

The proportion of ghrit in the milk of kapila (brick-red coloured) cow is high. Compared to this, the proportion is lower in black cow's milk. If butter is boiled, filtered and then kept undisturbed, it gets solidified. If betel leaves are added to it then it imparts a particular colour to the ghrit. Cow's ghrit is yellowish in colour. Ghrit is not used in Europe and Australia.

Such is the importance of milk-ghrit. In facial paralysis, butter is more useful than ghrit. Ayurveda has indicated the use of medicated ghrit in almost all diseases.

References -

'घृतं पित्तानिलहरं रसशुक्रौजसां हितम् । निर्वापणं मृदुकरं स्वरवर्णप्रसादनम् ।। (च. सू. १३)
वातपित्तप्रकृतयो वातपित्तविकारिणः । चक्षुःकामाःक्षतःक्षीणाःवृद्धाःबालास्तथाऽबलाः ।।
आयुःप्रकर्षकामाश्च बलवर्णस्वरार्थिनः । पुष्टिकामाः प्रजाकामाः सौकुमार्यार्थिनश्च ये ।।
दीप्त्यौजःस्मृतिमेधाग्निबुद्धीन्द्रियबलार्थिनः । पिबेयुः सर्पिरार्ताश्च दाहशस्त्रविषाग्निभिः ।।' (च. सू. १३)
'सर्पिर्वातपित्तप्रशमनानाम् ।' समघृतसक्तुप्राशाभ्यासो वृष्योदावर्त्तहराणाम् ।' (च. सू. २५०
'गव्यं सर्पि; सर्पिषाम् (हिततमम्), आविकं सर्पिः सर्पिषाम् (अहिततमम्)' (च. सू. २६)
'स्मृतिबुद्ध्यग्निशुक्रौजःकफमेदोविवर्धनम् । सर्वस्नेहोत्तमं सर्पिमधुर रसपाकयोः ।।' (च. सू. २७)
'शस्तं धीस्मृतिमेधाग्निबलायुः शुक्रचक्षुषाम् । बालवृद्धप्रजाकान्तिसौकुमार्यस्वरार्थिनाम् ।।
क्षतक्षीणपरीसर्पशस्त्राग्निग्लपितात्मनाम् । वातपित्तविषोन्मादशोषालक्ष्मीज्वरापहम् ।।
स्नेहानामुत्तमं शीतं वयसः स्थापनं परम् ।' (अ. हृ. सू. ५)
'यथा प्रज्वलितं वेश्म परिषिञ्चन्ति वारिणा । नराः शान्तिमभिप्रेत्य तथा जीर्णज्वरे घृतम् ।।
स्नेहाद् वातं शमयति शैत्यात् पित्त नियच्छति । घृतं तुल्यगुणं दोषं संस्कारात्तु जयेत् कफम् ।।
नान्यः स्नेहस्तथा कश्चित् संस्कारमनुवर्त्तते । यथा सर्पिरतः सर्पिः सर्वस्नेहोत्तमं मतम् ।।' (च. नि. १)
'सर्पिः खल्वेवमेव पित्त जयति, माधुर्याच्छैत्यान्मन्दवीर्यत्वाच्च, पित्तं ह्यमधुरमुष्णं तीक्ष्णं च । (च. वि. १)

4. MADHUVARGA

The etymology of the word `madhu' is as follows - मन्यते एतम् इति मधु ।
Ayurveda has described honey as the best medicine for kapha.

Properties : Sweet, astringent aftertaste, ununctuous, cold, light, viscous, yogavahi, mild, subtle, vishada.

Actions : Increases the agni, improves complexion and voice, increases softness of the skin, cardiac tonic, aphrodisiac, facilitates reunion of bones in fractures, removes vitiated doshas, improves wound healing, promotes mental health, cleanses all the srotas, acts as an astringent, improves vision, produces a sense of well-being, pervades the minute srotas of the body, increases appetite and facilitates formation of asavas and arishtas.

Action on doshas : Pacifies all the three doshas, acts on kapha through its lightness, and pacifies vata-pitta by its viscocity, sweet and astringent properties (Vagbhatta-honey increases vata).

Action on diseases : Diabetes, hiccups, asthma, cough, diarrhoea, vomiting-excessive thirst, helminthiasis, toxin, dermatosis, jaundice, haemorrhoids, pruritus, abdominal distention, diseases of the throat, uneasiness, intoxication, burning sensation, constipation.

Dhatugamitva : Meda, shukra, majja (beneficial to the eyes, improves intellect.)

Honey is included among those dravyas which can be consumed regularly. In India, it has been considered only as a medicine. Sushrutacharya has described eight types of honey. (During

Charakacharya's era, four were known namely makshik, bhramar, kshaudra and pautik). By the time Sushruta samhita was written, four new types came to be known viz. chatra, aardhya, daal and auddalak.

The English name is honey while the Latin name is mel.

1) Makshik : Honey collected by big, brickred, wild bees is called makshik. This honey is lighter than kshaudra honey and is considered to be the best. Useful in diseases like asthma.

2) Bhramar : Honey which is collected by a blue-black garden bee is called bhramar. It is viscous, sweet and heavy.

3) Kshaudra : Honey collected by small honey bees is called kshaudra. This honey is sheeta, light and lekhana.

4) Pautik : Honey collected by yellowish bees which sit on sweets is called pautik. It is ununctuous, ushna, toxic and therefore, it causes vatarakta, raktapitta, intoxication and causes burning.

5) Chatra : The shape of the bee-hive is like an umbrella. This honey bee lives in cold regions and it likes the nectar of mahuva tree. This honey has sweet vipak, is heavy, cold and is useful in raktapitta, leucoderma, diabetes and worms.

6) Aardhya : This type of honey is collected by bees which are reddish yellow in colour and are found in the wild. It relieves kapha and pitta.

7) Daal : This honey bee is very small in size and it builds its bee hive in the leaves of trees. The word 'dal' means leaves. Honey collected on leaves is called daal. It is astringent, ushna veerya, sour, increases pitta, ununctuous, pungent vipaki, and is useful in vomiting and diabetes.

8) Auddalak : Honey collected by small, brickred insects in a hive. It is astringent, increases strength, bitter to taste, but pungent vipaki, does not vitiate vata, increases appetite and improves voice, and is useful in dermatosis and toxins.

Ama : Freshly collected honey by honey bees is apakva and should not be used.

Pakva : Honey collected by honey bees in a closed bee hive is pakva and is called madhyam (better type of honey).

New : Pakva honey as collected by the above method is madhyam (of better quality).

Old : One year old honey is pakva and is considered the best.

Chemical composition of honey : Glucose 84.9%, formic acid; sucrose 2.69%, alkaloids 0.12%, water 10.03%, nitrogen 1.29%. Specific gravity - 1.36.

Characteristics of best quality honey :

1) Sinks in water 2) flies do not sit on it 3) a dog does not lick good honey 4) if honey is poured on a vertically held cloth, then it does not wet the cloth but instead flows along its surface 5) burns like oil 6) if applied in the eyes, causes irritation.

Appearance : Sometimes, air bubbles are trapped inside honey and therefore it appears frothy.

Testing of honey by the five senses :

1) Appearance : Honey should have a yellowish tint similar to that of cow's ghrit. As the honey becomes older, its colour changes. It changes with seasons also. The appearance of honey doesnot aid much in testing its purity.

2) Rasa : The taste of honey depends on the taste of the nectar collected from various flowers. Honey is sweet to taste and has an astringent aftertaste. We can obtain honey which is collected from the flowers of the same tree.

Honey may initially contain various rasas apart from sweet taste and astringent aftertaste but they are not refined. They remain unmanifested, only sweet and astringent tastes being manifest.

3) Odour : On burning, honey should not give out a bad odour. (Sugar gives such bad odour). Honey has its own characteristic strong odour. Dogs, who have a strong sense of smell, stay away from honey. Honey is useful in masking the odour of castor oil and cod liver oil.

4) Consistency : Viscous honey becomes thin on heating. If a drop of honey is held between two fingers and pressed then pure honey will become thinner whereas honey contaminated with sugar or jaggery becomes more viscous.

5) Sound on heating : The proportion of water in honey is 10.03% but is totally a part of honey. Therefore, when unadulterated honey is put in a flame, it doesnot produce any crackling sound. A wick of cotton dipped in honey, like the one dipped in oil or ghee, burns without producing any sound.

Honey : Many plants have nectar in their flowers. Honey bees are always attracted towards this nectar. They suck this nectar and store it in their bee hive. After a few days, they stop collecting nectar. Pure honey can be obtained from this bee hive by centrifugation. Such honey will not contain eggs of the bees and other unwanted constituents of the hive. Wax is obtained in this method of extracting honey. Wax is used internally in a disease called bhasmak (characterized by excessive hunger) and also externally for application as an ointment.

If such honey is stored, then after a few days, crystals of sugar get precipitated. The properties of this sugar are similar to those of honey.

'Ajeerna' caused by honey is very severe. Honey is the best remedy for ulcers caused due to vitiation of meda dhatu.

References -

'मधु संदधाति' मधुश्लेष्मपित्तप्रशमनानाम् ।' (च. सू. २७)
'तल्लघुत्वात् कफघ्नं पैच्छिल्यान्माधुर्यात् कषायभावाच्च वातपित्तघ्नम् ।
बृंहणीयं मधु नवं नातिश्लेष्महरं सरम् । मेद:स्थौल्यापहं ग्राहि पुराणमतिलेखनम् ।।
दोषलयापहं पक्वमामम्लं त्रिदोषकृत् । तद्युक्तं विविधैर्योगैर्निहन्यादामयान् बहून् ।।
नानाद्रव्यात्मकत्वाच्च योगवाहि परं मधु ।' (सु. सू. ४५)

5. IKSHUVARGA

Sugarcane : is sweet, madhur vipaki, heavy, sheeta veerya, unctuous, nutritive, aphrodisiac, diuretic, produces parasites and kapha and pacifies raktapitta.

Types : Paundrak, bheeruk, vanshak, shwetaporak, kantar, tapas, kashthekshu, suchipatrak, nepal, deerghapatra, neelpor, koshakrit are the twelve types mentioned in Sushruta samhita. There might have been only two types in the Charaka era. These are paundrak and vanshak. Another type, named shataparvak has also been described by Vagbhatta.

Apart from these, manogupta, raktekshu, krushnekshu, sukumar, venuniswan, karkotak, shwetekshu, karankeshu, asipatra, madhutrun etc. are also its synonyms.

Jaggery, kakvi and sugar are used in preparing medicines. All these three are prepared from sugarcane.

Paundrak sugarcane is the best among all. Sushrutacharya has described the properties and actions of all the types of sugarcane.

Paundrak and Bheeruk : Sheeta, sweet, unctuous, nutritive, produces kapha, heavy and aphrodisiac.

Vanshak, Kantar and Tapas : have the same properties but they have some amount of salty taste in it.

Shwetporak : has similar properties as vanshak but is slightly ushna and produces vata.

Kasthekshu : similar to vanshak but it vitiates vata.

Soochipatra, Nepal, Neelpor, Deerghapatrak : These three types of sugarcane are vata vardhak, they pacify kapha pitta, are mildly astringent and cause burning sensation.

Koshakar : is guru, sheeta, pacifies raktapitta and is useful in pthysis.

Sugarcane : is extremely sweet in the roots, the sweetness continues in the stem as well, whereas the apex part is slightly salty.

If sugarcane juice is directly consumed without using the juice machine then it doesnot cause pitta, increases kapha, pacifies vata-pitta, cleanses the mouth and is aphrodisiac.

Juice extracted by machine is heavy to digest and produces constipation.

If sugarcane juice is heated and boiled then it becomes heavy, laxative, unctuous, slightly teekshna and alleviates kapha-vata.

Vishwamitra had discovered sugarcane ages ago and named it as sweet-grass.

It is said that if a patient of jaundice sucks pieces of sugarcane, then they become yellow in colour. Vagbhatta has included jaggery in madhurvarga but sugar has not been included!

The part of surgarcane towards the roots is very sweet, the central part is less sweet whereas the upper most part is salty. Sugarcane belongs to the family Graminae.

English name : Sugarcane,

Latin name : Saccharum officinarum.

Sanskrit names : Ikshu, deerghacchad, bhoomirasa, gudmoola, asipatra, madhutrun.

Types : Paundrak, kantar, bheeruk, vanshak, shwetporak, tapsekshu, kashthekshu, suchipatrak, naipal, deerghapatra, neelpor, borad, shatpatra, panduk, vetra, kodrav, kavni.

References -

'इक्षवो रक्तपित्तघ्ना बल्या वृष्या कफप्रदाः । स्वादुपाकरसाः स्निग्धाः गुरवो मूत्रलाः हिमाः । (भा. प्र.)
इक्षवो मधुरा मधुरविपाका गुरवः शीताः स्निग्धाः बल्याः वृष्याः मूत्रलाः रक्तपित्तप्रशमनाः कृमिकरोश्चेति ।' (सु. सू. ४५)

'मत्स्यण्डिका-खण्ड-शर्करा विमलजाता उत्तरोत्तरं शीताः स्निग्धाः गुरुतराः मधुरतराः वृष्याः रक्तपित्तप्रशमनास्तृष्णाप्रशमनाश्च ।' (सु. सू. ४५)

6. TAILAVARGA

The etymology of the word 'taila' is 'efleueesodYeJeb lewueced'. Even if it so, oil obtained from various grains, seeds and other parts are all included under 'taila'. Charakacharya has said that there are two sources of oil (1) plant source and (2) animal source. Among these, oils obtained from plant source fall within tailavarga. In Konkan, cow's ghrit is called cow's oil.

Oil can be extraced from the following parts of plants (1) roots (2) tubors (3) bark (4) leaves (5) flowers (6) fruits (7) pulp (8) skin of the fruit and (9) seeds.

Ayurveda in general, and Sushrutacharya in particular, has given a long list of plants from which oil can be extracted. Nearly 60 different plants yield oils.

English name : oil, **Latin name** : oleum.

These oils are of two types, non-volatile (fixed) and volatile. Those which are viscous, having a mild odour and which are extracted by crushing or boiling are called fixed oils (non-volatile). Contrary to this, those oils which evapourate on keeping them open are called volatile oils. Oils are extracted by various procedures :

1) Crushing (hot and cold)
2) Distillation
3) Boiling
4) Steam

Use of oil has rejuvenating properites. Those who undergo regular oil massage do not suffer premature aging and their excercise tolerance also increases.

Oil extracted from different dravyas have varying properties and actions. Oil is extracted from the following plants - erand, sarshap, uma, kusumbh, danty, moolak, rakshoghna, karanj, arishta, shigru, suryaphool, ingudi, peelu, shankhini, neep, saral, aguru, deodar, shinshapasar, tuvarak, bhallatak, jyotishmati, bibhitak, atimuktak, akrod, narikel, moha, kinkan, kakdi, ervaru, kohla, bhokar, charoli, kashmari, palas beeja, til.

Sesamum oil is the best remedy for all wounds. It keeps the wounds clean, non-infected and soft and therefore it becomes easier to take stitches.

Internal and external use of oil has been indicated in almost all diseases. But it has been particularly indicated in diseases caused by vata. Oil is the best remedy for diseases of vata. Basti (enema) is the most effective treatment for vata. Therefore oil enema is a very effective treatment for vata.

7. MADYAVARGA

Ayurveda has indicated the use of madyavarga in diseases as well as in health. Following are the general properties of liquor - all the three types of liqour (paushtik, mardvik and madhur) cause pitta, are acidic, improve appetite, deepan, bhedan, alleviate kapha and vata, cardiotonic, purify basti, light to digest, vidahi (produces burning sensation), ushna veerya, enhances the working of the senses, vikashi and enhances the excretion of urine and stools.

Following are the types of madya mardvik, kharjur, sura, shwetasura, prasanna, kudhanyasura, madhulika, akshiki, kohli, jagal, bakkas, gudsidhu, sharkarsidhu, pakvarasasidhu, apakvarasasidhu, akshik, jambav, surasav, madhvasav, mairey, ikshurasasav, madhuk and pushpayonisidhu. Apart from this, asavas are prepared from taproots/ tubers, roots and flowers. Each of these have varying properties.

Liquor, again is of new and old types and they have different properties. New liquor is not considered beneficial. Liquor becomes old after one year. This liquor should be used for treating diseases.

English name : Spiritous Liquor.

If liquor is consumed then meat has to be eaten and vice versa. In colloquial language it is called 'eating and drinking'.

Liquor should always be consumed in small quantity along with unctuous diet, meat etc. If consumed appropriately, it acts like elixir but if it is taken inappropriately then it acts like poison. If taken judiciously it is beneficial but then the person begins to calculate. People start thinking that if a small quantity of liquor makes them feel so good then a larger quantity would make them feel even better ! It is universally known that liquor has ill-effects on the liver. Once cirrhosis-like changes appear in the liver, the person loses self-control. This is so because apart from its innumerable functions, the liver also aids in maintaining self restraint. The etymology of the word यकृत (liver) denotes this function. यं - संयमं करोति इति यकृत् ।

Once this self restraint is lost, all the ill-effects follow. Man is also to be blamed because when he indulges in excessive drinking, it produces a sense of well-being along with psychological elevation and a 'kick'. He thinks that if he feels good with one peg then more pegs would be even better. This is where he commits a big mistake. No doubt that liquor has some beneficial properties just as poisons also have some beneficial effects.

But just as poisons are to be taken in exact doses only, liquor also should be taken in proportion only. But poisons also are tolerated well after prolonged use and the same amount may be inadequate.

Liquor is also used as a treatment for disorders caused by excessive liquor. Of course, the liquuor is prepared from different source. But the diseases caused by liquor can be counteracted only by liquor as it possesses gamitva on the affected srotas. The concept of gamitva is widely used in Ayurveda.

8. SHOOKADHANYAVARGA (GRAMINAE)

Dhanyavarga has been subdivided into shookadhanyavarga (having husks) and shamidhanyavarga (having legumes).

In the shookadhanya varga, various types of rice like rakta, mahan, kalam, shakunahrit, saramukh, deerghashooka, rodhrashook, sugandhak, patang, tapaneeya, yavak, hayan, paansu, bashpa, naishadhak are included. Similarly, various types of wheat like shashtik, mahavrihi, krishnavrihi, jatumukh, kukkutand, kapal, paravatak, shookar, varak, uddalak, ujjval, cheen, sharad, dardur, gandhan, kuruvind, patal are also included. Also rale, hareek, ransali, save, yava, vanshajyava, gahu are also included.

Shookadhanya is important in diet whereas shamidhanya is useful as an appetizer.

Raktashali is the most important among shookadhanyavarga.

'Shooka' means the husk on that particular grain. When the husk is not peeled off, it is called 'beeja' and when the husk is peeled off, it is called 'tandul'. For example, this is the difference between apamarga beeja and apamarga tandul. Beeja has the capacity to reproduce whereas a tandul loses this capacity.

Shookadhanyas are lighter to digest compared to shimbidhanyas.

9. SHAMIDHANYAVARGA (SHIMBIDHANYA) (LEGUMINOSAE) (BEANS)

This type of dhanyavarga grows in legumes. It includes moonga, toor, masoor, vatana, chawli, kilith, pavta, udid, teel, alasi, kardai etc. The legumes contain one or more seeds. The legumes of these plants peel off by themselves except those of two plants (bahava and bhuimoonga). Shimbivarga is mostly used in diet as an appetizer. There are methods of peeling off the legumes. The legumes of vatana, moonga etc. break from both the sides and the seeds are thrown out. Mohri, shiras break from both the sides from bottom towards the top, but the seeds remain attached to one of the coverings. The legumes of lady's finger break from many sides. There are many pores on the fruits of opium. Shimbivarga is then subdivided into three types depending on the morphology of the flowers :-

1) Aparajita varga (gokarna)
2) Pootikaranjadi (sagargota)
3) Babbuladi (babul)

Aushadhi shimbi phala include gokarna, palas, jyesthamadhu, gunja, agasti, neel, taag, khulkhula, salvan, pithvan, khajkuhili, pangara, sharpunkha ,bavchi, mudgaparni, mashparni, shisav, sagargota, chinch, kanchan etc.

Sanskrit names : Shameej, shimbij, shimbibhava, soopya, vaidal.

Properties and actions : :These are usually sweet to taste but ununctuous, astringent, katu vipaki, increase vata, reduce kapha-pitta, produce retention of urine and faeces and are sheeta by nature. All shamidhanya except moonga and masoor cause abdominal distention. Among them, vatana is extremely vatal. This shimbi varga is ruksha, vatal, sweet to taste and sheeta. It reduces agni, pureesh, veerya and kapha.

Shookadhanya as well as shimbidhanya become lighter to digest when they are one year old.

10. MANSAVARGA

Eight types of meat are included in mansavarga.

Mrigya, vaishkarik, pratud : These three come under the classification of jangal mansa.

Bileshay, prasah : These come under the category of sadharan mansa.

Mahamrigya, apchar, maatsya : These three are included in the category of anoop mansa.

1) Mrigya varga : This varga includes the meat of deer, antelope, kurar, ruksha, gokarna, mrigmatruk, rabbit, elk, charushka, sharabh etc. The meat of kalvit is considered to be the best among this group.

2) Vaishkarik varga : (Animals which find their prey after digging the ground) - Quail, wild sparrow, vartir, wild cock, cock, pingla, upchakra, chakor, kurubahu, vartak, vartika, partridge, krakar, peacock, cock, bakar, gonarda, girivartika, sarpad, indrabh, varat etc. are the animals included in this group. The meat of lava and tittir is the best in this group.

3) Pratud varga : (Animals which use their beaks to gather food) - Jeevanjeevak, datsyooh (crow), kalvat, parrot, sarika, lattha, cuckoo, pigeon, sparrow etc.

4) Bileshay varga : (Animals residing in burrows) - Frog, iguana, snake, porcupine etc. are included in this group.

5) Prasah varga : Cow, donkey, mule, camel, cheetah, horse, lion, bear, monkey, cat, rat, tiger, wolf, mangoose, hyena, fox, jackal, falcon, blue jay, dog, crow, hawk, vulture, owl, black sparrow, dhoomika, madhuha etc. are the animals included in this varga. This varga includes animals as well as birds.

5) Mahamrig varga : Wild boar, buffalo, nagun, rohit, elephant, wild horses, wild cow, rhinoceros, wild ox etc. are the animals of this group.

7) Apchar varga : Swan, heron, duck, crane, karduva, cock, balaka, kurti, chakravak, madgu, karkocha etc. are included in this varga.

8) Maatsya varga : Rohit, pathin, tortoise, kumbhir, crab, oyster, conch, udra, snail, shafari, bamb, chandrika, chulooki, alligator, crocodile, shiras, timingil, raji, chilichim etc. are included in this group.

Since goat and sheep have mixed characteristics, they fall in more than one group.

In Ayurvedic scriptures, the word 'rasa' implies 'mansa rasa' (meat soup) at many places.

Edible meat : Fresh, pure and meat of young animals is the best.

Non-edible meat : The meat of animals which died due to diseases, toxins or which die a natural death should not be consumed. Similarly, meat of extremely emaciated or extremely obese animals should not be consumed.

Heavy (to digest) meat : Meat on the anterior side of male animals and that of pregnant animals is heavy to digest.

Light (to digest) meat : In four legged animals, meat of female animals is lighter to digest whereas in birds, meat of male birds is lighter.

Progressively heavier meat :

1) Stomach - waist - back - thighs - shoulders - head (thus the meat of the head region is the heaviest.)

2) Amashaya is heavier than pakvashaya.

3) Rakta - mansa - meda - asthi - majja - shukra (shukra dhatu is the heaviest to digest).

4) Flesh - testis penis bladder liver anus (anus is the heaviest to digest).

Some of the animals included in these eight groups are useful in certain specific disease conditions. For example, in conditions involving mansa kshaya, the meat of carnivorous animals is very useful. This is so because this meat optimises the agni of mansa dhatu and facilitates its acceptance by the body. In no other disease has non-vegetarian diet been so strongly recommended by Ayurveda.

References -

'मांसं बृंहणीयानाम् ।' रसस्तर्पणीयानाम् । क्रव्यादरसाभ्यासो ग्रहणीदोषशोषाशोध्नानाम् ।.' (च. सू. २५)
शरीरबृंहणे नान्यदाद्यं मांसाद् विशिष्यते ।' (च. सू. २७)
क्षये मांसरसः परम् ।' (च. सू. २७)
तस्मान्मांसमाप्यायते मांसेन भूयस्तरमन्येभ्यः शरीरधातुभ्यः ।' (च. शा. ६)
गत्वा स्नात्वा पयः पीत्वा रसं चानुशयीत ना । तथाऽस्याप्यायते भूयः शुक्रं च बलमेव च ।।' (च. चि. २)
'शुष्वते ज्ञीणमांसाय कल्पितानि विधानवित् । दद्यान्मांसादमांसानि बृंहणानि विशेषत्ः ।।
मांसेनोपचितांगानां मांसं मांसकरं परम् । तीक्ष्णोष्णलाघवाच्स्तं विशेषान्मृगपक्षिणाम् ।।'

'मांसमेवाश्नतः शोषो माध्वीकं पिबतोऽनुच । नियतानल्पचित्तस्य चिरं काये न तिष्ठति ।।' (च. चि. ८)
'बर्हितित्तिदक्षाणां हंसानां शूकरोष्ट्रयोः । खरगोमहिषाणां च मांसं मांसकरं परम् ।।' (च. चि. ८)
'मांसाशिनां च मांसानि भक्षयेद् विधिविन्नरः । विशुद्धमनसस्तस्य मांसं मांसेन वर्धते ।।' (सु. चि. १)

11. LAVANAVARGA

Following lavanas (salts) fall in the lavana varga (1) saindhav (2) padelon (3) bidlavana (4) samudra (5) audbhid (6) kale and (7) sambar.

These salts are generally sookshmagami (can pervade all the minute channels of the body), reduce the viscosity of kapha-pitta, laxative, pacify vata, digestive, ushna, appetizers and increase kapha-pitta. Lavana must be used in the preferential order as given above. When panchalavana are indicated, the first five salts given in the list must be used. When tripatu are indicated, the first three in the list must be used.

Saindhav

Properties : Slightly sweet to taste, light and not ushna (multani namak, now-a-days even this salt is produced artificially).

Actions : Aphrodisiac, cardiotonic, pacifies all the three doshas, useful to the eyes, not so ushna, does not produce burning sensation and increases the agni. This is the best in lavana varga.

Latin name : Sodium chloride, impure rock salt. In all preparations, when the specific type of salt to be used is not mentioned, saindhav should be used.

Padelon

Properties : Light, having a pleasant odour, has pungent vipak.

Actions : Cardiotonic, carminative, laxative, increases the agni and improves appetite.

Latin name : Sodium chloride, black salt.

Bidlavan

Properties : Light, sanchal lavana.

Actions : Carminative, increases agni, laxative, relieves flatulance, abdominal colic and reduces heaviness of stomach.

It is artificial. 28 kgs of sambar salt + 20 ounces of amla churna, when burnt together give 24 kgs. of bidlon.

Samudra

Properties : Madhur vipaki, heavy.

Actions : Produces kleda in the body.

English name : Tablesalt, common salt.

Latin name : Sodia Muras (The famous salt satyagraha of Mahatma Gandhi was carried out for this salt).

Audbhid

Properties : Bitter, pungent, corrosive, salty.

Actions : Increases kapha.

English name : Fossil salt.

Latin name: Pot. Nitre.

Kale

Properties : Light, increases pitta and pacifies kapha - vata (Bangadkhar).

Actions : Hridya, carminative, laxative, increases agni and appetite.

English name : Black salt.

Sambar (Romak)

Properties : Light, very corrossive, increases pitta greatly.

Actions : Produces kshar-like actions.

(Salt from the salt lake of Ruma near Sambar in Ajmer).

Charakacharya has given exceptional importance to lavana rasa probably due to the following two reasons -

1) If the amount of salt is too much then it supersedes all other tastes.

2) If any of the remaining five rasas are in excess in a particular food item, then this can be corrected by adding some salt.

References -

लवणमन्नद्रव्यरुचिकाराणाम् श्रेष्ठम् ।’ (च. सू. २५)
‘रोचनं लवणं सर्व पाकि स्त्रंस्यनिलापहम् ।’ (च. सू. २७)
‘लवणो रसः पाचनो क्लेदनो दीपनः च्यावनः छेदनो भेदनः तीक्ष्णः सरो विकासी अधःस्त्रंसी अवकाशकरो स्तंभबंधसंघातविधमनः वातहरः सर्वरसप्रत्यनीकभूतः आस्यमास्त्रवयति कफं विष्यंदयति मार्गान् विशोधयति सर्वशरीरावयवान् मृदूकरोति रोचयति आहारमाहारयोगी ।’ (च. सु. २६)
‘लवणं पुनरौष्ण्यतैक्ष्ण्योपपन्नमनतिगुर्वनतिस्निग्धमुपक्लेदिविस्त्रं सनसमर्थमन्नद्रव्यरुचिकरम् । आपातभद्रं प्रयोगसमसाद्गुण्यात् दोषसंचयानुबन्धम् । तद्रोचनपाचनोपक्लेदनविस्त्रंसनार्थमुपयुज्यते ।’ (च. वि. १)
स एवंगुणोऽप्येक एवात्यर्थमुपयुज्यमानः पित्तं कपयति, रक्तं वर्धयति, तर्षयति, मूर्च्छयति, तापयति, दारयति, कृष्णाति मांसानि, प्रगालयति कुष्ठानि, विषं वर्धयति, शोफान् स्फोटयति, दन्तांश्च्यावयति, पुंस्त्वमुपहन्ति, इन्द्रियाण्युपरुणद्धि, वलीपलितखालित्यमापादयति, अपि च
लोहितपित्ताम्लपित्तवीसर्पवातरक्तविचर्चिकेन्द्रलुप्तप्रभृतीन् विकारान् उपजनयत् ।’ (च. सू. २६)
‘तदत्यर्थमुपयुज्यमानं ग्लानिशैथिल्यदौर्बल्याभिनिवृत्तिकरं शरीरस्य भवति । ... ये ह्यतिलवणसात्म्याः पुरुषास्तेषामपि खालित्येन्द्रलुप्तपालित्यानि वलयश्चाकाले भवन्ति ।’
‘प्रायो लवणं पित्तलमचक्षुव्यंमन्यत्र सैन्धवात्’ (अ. स. सू. १८)
‘रोचनं दीपनं वृष्यं चक्षुष्यमविदाहि च ।
त्रिदोषघ्नं समधुरं सैन्धवं लवणोत्तमम् ।।’ (च. सू. २७)
‘चक्षुष्यं सैन्धवं हृद्यं रुच्यं लघ्वग्निदीपनम् ।
स्निग्धं सुमधुरं वृष्यं शीतं दोषघ्नमुत्तमम् ।।’ (सु. सू. ४६)
‘सैन्धवं लवणं स्वादु दीपनं पाचनं लघु ।
स्निग्धं रुच्यं हिमं वृष्यं सूक्ष्मं नेत्र्यं त्रिदोषहृत् ।।’ (भा. प्र.)
रुचकं रोचनं भेदि दीपनं पाचनं परम् । सस्नेहं वातुनुन्नातिपित्तलं विशदं लघु ।। (भा. प्र.)
लघु सौवर्चलं पाके वीर्योष्णं विशदं कटु । गुल्मशूलविबन्धघ्नं हृद्यं सुरभि रोचनम् ।।’ (सु. सू. ४६)
सौक्ष्म्यादौष्ण्याल्लघुत्वाच सौगन्धाच्च रुचिप्रदम् । सौवर्चलं विवन्धघ्नं हृद्यमुद्गारशोधिच । (च. सू. २७)
विडं सक्षारमूर्ध्वाधः कफवातानुलोमनम् । दीपनं लघु तीक्ष्णोष्णं रुक्षं रूच्यं व्यवायि च ।
विवन्धानाहविष्टम्भोदर्दगौरवशूलनुत् ।’ (भा. प्र.)
‘सक्षारं दीपनं सूक्ष्मं शूलहृद्रोगनाशनम् ।
रोचनं तीक्ष्णमुष्णं च बिडं वातानुलोमनम् ।। (सु. सू. ४६)
‘तैक्ष्ण्यादौष्ण्याद् व्यवायित्वाद् दीपनं शूलनाशनम् ।

ऊर्ध्वं चाधश्च वातानामानुलोम्यकरं विडम् ।।' (च. सू. २७)
सामुद्रं मधुरं पाके नात्युष्णमविदाहि तत् ।
भेदनं स्निग्धमीषच्च शूलघ्नं नातिपित्तलम् ।। (सु. सू. ४६)
सामुद्रं मधुरं पाके सतिक्तं मधुरं गुरु । नात्युष्ण दीपनं भेदि सक्षारमविदाहि च ।।
श्लेष्मलं वातनुत्तिक्तमरूक्षं नातिशीतलम् ।' (मा. ध.)
'गडाख्यं लघु वातघ्नमत्युष्णं भेदि पित्तलम् ।
तीक्ष्णोष्णं चापि सूक्ष्मं चाभीष्यन्दि कटुपाकि च ।।' (भा. प्र.)
'रोमकं तीक्ष्णमत्युष्णं व्यवायि कटुपाकि च ।
वातघ्नं लघु विष्यन्दि सूक्ष्मं विड्भेदि मूत्रलम् ।।' (सु. सू. ४६)
'सतिक्तं कटु सक्षारं विद्याल्लवणमौदभिदम् ।' (सु. सू. ४६)
'सतिक्तकटु सक्षारं तीक्ष्णमुत्क्लेदि चौद्भिदम् ।' (च. सू. २७)

PART V

DRAVYAS OF ANIMAL ORIGIN ETC. (CONTD.)

1. KASTURI

Sanskrit names : Darpa, Kasturika, Nabhi, Kasturi, Gandhavallik, Mrigandaj, Vedhamukhya, Mrignabhi, Mrigmad, Sahasrabhit. **Hindi :** Kasturi, **Arabic :** Misk, **Persian :** Mushk.

English name : Musk.

Appearance : In the male deer of kasturi mrig (Fam. Ruminentia; Mosehu moschiferus) there is a small ovoid cyst near the umbilicus. White hair grow on this cyst and there is a punctum in the centre. The inside of this cyst contains a black coloured, granular and extremely fragrant substance. This substance is called kasturi. It is white in colour and slightly fluid for 1 to 2 years but later it becomes black and solidified. (One has to be cautious about artificial musk available in the market.)

Types : Depending on the habitat of the musk deer, Bhavprakash has described three types of kasturi.

1) Kamroopiya : It is black in colour and is considered to be the best.

2) Nepali : It is bluish in colour and is of intermediate quality.

3) Kashmiri : It is slightly reddish in colour and is of inferior quality.

Habitat : The musk deer is seen in the Himalayan forests of Russia, China, Central Asia, Tibet, Nepal, Bhutan, Assam and Kashmir at a height of 2 to 3 thousand metres. Musk is obtained by killing the deer and removing the cyst found near the umbilicus. During mating season, the musk of the deer becomes extremely fragrant.

Chemical composition : Musk contains ammonia, olein, cholesterol, fats, wax, gelatin etc. It also contains a viscous, colourless oil called muskon.

Pure, unadulterated musk is blackish in colour, fragrant, does not dissolve in water, does not burn completely in a flame and gives an odour similar to that of burning leather.

Properties : Laghu, ruksha, bitter, pungent, katu vipaki and ushna veerya. It pacifies kapha - vata.

External use : Removes bad odour, cold, stiffness and acts as an anti-depressant.

Internal use : Alleviates mental weakness and is extremely useful in psychosis, epilepsy, convulsions, paresis, coma etc.

Digestive system : It is deepan and pachan and therefore it is useful in ama, colic and agnimandya.

Circulatory system : Acts as a cardiotonic, provides strength to heart and other vital organs during fever.

Respiratory system : Useful in cough, asthma, whooping cough and other coughs caused by vata.

Reproductive system : It is a potent aphrodisiac. Due to its anti-toxin action, it reduces the effects of toxins on vital organs.

Dose : 60 to 120 mg.

Formulatons : Kasturibhairav, Kasturibhushan, Mrigmadasav etc.

Srotogamitva :

Dosha : Kapha - vata.

Dhatu : Shrukra (aphrodisiac); rasa, rakta (pachan).

Mala : Reduces the foul odour of stools and sweat.

References -

कामरूपोद्भवा कृष्णा नैपाली नीलवर्णयुक् । काश्मीरे कपिलच्छाया कस्तूरी त्रिविधा स्मृता ।।
कामरूपोद्भवा श्रेष्ठा नैपाली मध्यमा भवेत् । काश्मीरदेशसंभूता कस्तूरी अधमा स्मृता ।।
कस्तरिका कटुस्तिक्ता क्षारोष्णा शुक्रला गुरुः । कफवातविषच्छर्दिशीतदौर्गंध्य शोषहृत् ।। (भा. प्र.)
या गन्धं केतकीनां वहति भृशतरं वर्णतः पिंगलाभा ।
स्वादे तिक्ता कटूष्णा लघु परितुलिता मर्दिता चिक्कणा स्यात् ।।
दग्धा नो याति भस्म चिमचिमीकुरुते चर्मगन्धा हुताशे,
सा शुद्धा शोभनीया वरमृगतनुजा राजयोग्या प्रदिष्टा ।।'
करतलजलमध्ये स्थापनीया महभ्दिः पुनरपि तदवश्यं चिन्तनीयं मुहुर्तम् ।।
यदि भवथि च रक्तं तज्जलं पीतवर्ण न भवति मृगनाभिः कृत्रिमोऽयं विकारः ।। (कै. नि.)

2. GOROCHANA

Sanskrit names : Rochana, Gorochan, Hajrulbakar, Sangagaab, Gavrohan.

English name- Gall stone (of a cow or bull).

Appearance : This is a biliary calculus formed in the gall bladder of cow or a bull. It is yellowish in colour and has a mild fragrance.

Properties : Laghu, ruksha, bitter, katu vipaki, ushna veerya. Gorochana pacifies kapha-vata and acts as a cholagogue.

External use : When applied externally, it acts as an anti-inflammatory agent and therefore it is applied on leucoderma, haemorrhoids etc. It is also used as a topical application in the eyes.

Internal use : Very effective in epilepsy. Approximately 2 grams of gorochana given daily with rose water for a few days cures epilepsy. The seizures do not recur after that.

Digestive system : Since it is deepan, anuloman and cholegogue, it is useful as a digestive and is used in constipation, sluggishness of the liver, anaemia and jaundice.

Circulatory system : It is used in oedema, enlarged cervical lymph nodes and also in measles.

Reproductive system : It is rasa - raktagami and therefore used in dysmenorrhoea and amenorrhoea.

Urinary system : Useful in dysuria and in urinary calculus.

Satmikaran : Useful in debility, especially of children.

Dose : 250 to 750 mgs.

Formulations : Balarka rasa.

Srotogamitva :

Dosha : Kapha , vata, pitta (cholagogue).

Dhatu : Rakta-meda (leucoderma, sluggishness of the liver, anaemia, jaundice, oedema, cervical lymphnodes); rasa (dysmenorrhoea, amenorrhoea) prevents miscarriages.

Mala : Mutra (dysuria-litholytic).

Prabhav : Anti-toxin.
Manovahasrotas : Epilepsy, psychosis.

3. POOTI (KHATIKA)

It is white in colour and is tasteless and odourless. It is of two types (1) khati and (2) gaur khati. Its chemical formula is $CaCO_3$ .Khatika is sweet, astringent, bitter, sheeta veerya and alleviates kapha-pitta.

Uses : When used externally, it acts as an astringent and absorptive.
Internally, it reduces acidity and acts as an astringent in diarrhoea. Khatika (chalk) is used in ointments. Similarly, it is also used in tooth powders. Its astringent action strengthens the teeth and reduces bleeding from the gums. It is especially useful in diarrhoea accompanied by green-coloured stools. It is generally used in diarrhoea, hyperacidity and corrosive toxins. It can be given in a dose of 1 to 3 grams. Ama pitta causes green-coloured stools and khatika is useful in it.

Srotogamitva
Dosha : Alleviates kapha pitta.
Dhatu : Rakta.
Mala : Causes retention of stools and reduces sweat.
References -
'खटिका दाहास्रजिच्छीता मधुरा विषशोथजित् ।' (भा. प्र.)
'खटिका शिशिरा तिक्ता मधुरा शोथनाशिनी । पित्तप्रशमनी कामं विविधव्रणरोपणी'
'कफदाहास्रदोषघ्नी नेत्रामयनिषूदनी । हरिद्वर्णातिसारघ्नी स्वेदातिस्रावहारिणी ।।' (र. त.)

4. MRIGSHRING

The horns of various animals have properties and actions similar to bones. These can be used internally as well as externally. Externally, powdered horn is used for local application and for dhoopana (fumigaton). For internal use, bhasmas have to be prepared so that it is absorbed by the body. The most commonly used horns are mrig (deer) shring and sambar shring.

External uses : The fumes of mrigshring are given for inhalation to patients of hiccups and asthma. This clears the respiratory system and reduces congestion. Sambarshring, when boiled with milk and applied on the inflammed part, reduces the pain and swelling. It is also used as a topical application in the eyes.

Internal uses : Mrigshring bhasma - when given with honey and ghee, is useful in cough, asthma and hiccups. Mrigshring bhasma is well-known as a remedy for weakness of the heart and rajayakshma.

Srotogamitva
Dosha : Tridoshaghna.
Dhatu : Rasa (pranavaha srotas, lungs); rakta (reduces inflammation).
Organ : Heart.

References -
'एकद्विशफशृंगाणि.... । सर्वाण्येकैकशो वापि दग्ध्वा क्षौद्रघृतान्वितम् ।।
चूर्ण लिहन् जयेत् कासं हिक्कां श्वासं च दारूणम् ।' (च. चि. १७)
'युञ्ज्याद् धूं शालनिर्यासजातं नैपालं वा गोविषाणोद्भवं वा ।' (सु. उ. ५०)

5. AGNIJAR (AMBER)

English name : Ambergris.
Sanskrit names : Agnijar, Tundamaya, Amber, Shahab.
Amber is a pathological growth (cyst) found in the intestine of a marine animal called sperm whale. This animal eats a special type of plant and as a result it dies after becoming weak. Its body is carried to the shore. The cyst is then removed from the stomach and it is made available as amber. Sometimes, amber is obtained after hunting the animal. Freshly removed amber has a natural faecal odour. On drying it in the sun, the bad odour disappears and it develops a peculiar fragrance. It is black on the surface but whitish from within. Its melting point is 145°F and boiling point is 212°F. Amber is insoluble in water but soluble in alcohol and oil. When mixed with hot spirit, a white granular compound called amberin (85%) is obtained.
Properties and actions : Laghu, ruksha, katu vipaki and ushna veerya. Amber is tridoshaghna and pacifies kapha-vata in particular.
Internal uses : Since it is a brain tonic, it is helpful in mental weakness, paresis, Bell's palsy, fainting, psychosis, epilepsy and other vata disorders.
Digestive system : Due to its deepan, pachan, anuloman and astringent action, it is used in abdominal colic and grahani roga.
Other systems : Cardiotonic, aphrodisiac, general tonic and alleviates cold. Therefore, it is used in weakness of the heart, impotency, chronic cold and rigors and also in debility.
Dose : 120 to 360 mg.
Srotogamitva
Dosha : Tridoshaghna but particulaly kapha - vata.
Dhatu : Majja (weakness of majja); shukra (aphrodisiac); especially useful in vata disorders of majja dhatu.
Mala : Purisha (grahi).
Manovaha srotas : Psychosis, epilepsy, fainting.
References -
'अग्निजारस्त्रिदोषघ्नो धनुर्वातादिवातनुत् । वर्धनो रसवीर्यस्य दीपनो जारणस्तथा ।।' (र.च)
'स्यादग्निजारः कटुरुष्णवीर्यस्तुन्दामयो वातकफापहश्च ।
'पित्तप्रदः सोऽधिकसन्निपातशूलार्तिशीतामयनाशनश्च ।।' (रा. नि.)

6. MUKTA (MOTI)

Latin name : Avicula, Mytilus margaritiferus.
Bhavprakash has included this under the group of navaratna.
Sanskrit names : Mauktik, Shuktisambhavam, Bhooshanarhatam, Shreshtha, Luloo, Marvareed.
English name : Pearl.
Pearl should be white, shiny, heavy, without any pores and symmetrical. It is an animal product which is formed in oyster shells in the seas off Persia, Sri Lanka and in the sea of Saurashtra near Jamnagar. It contains huge amount of calcium.
Properties and actions : Laghu, ruksha, sweet, madhur vipaki, aphrodisiac and sheeta veerya. Mauktik pacifies all the three doshas - through its light and ununctuous properties, it pacifies kapha, by madhur vipak it pacifies vata and by its sheeta veerya, pacifies pitta.
External use : In diseases of the eyes, mukta pishti is used along with honey for topical application.
Internal use : It increases memory as it is a brain tonic. It is also useful in psychosis, epilepsy and headache caused by pitta. Mauktik is extremely useful in insomnia caused by vata-pitta. It is one of the medicines which are constantly required in practice of Ayurveda.
Digestive system : It is sheeta, yet deepan to liver and is astringent, it is useful in agnimandya, liver diseases, raktatisara, bleeding piles and grahani.
Circulatory system : Very useful in diseases of respiratory system like cough, asthma, urahkshat, parshwashool and tuberculosis. Agnimandya and night sweats seen in tuberculosis are reduced by it and the patient gains weight.
Reproductive system : Acts as an aphrodisiac. Useful in shukrameha, menorrhagia and leucorrhoea.
Skin : Useful in conditions of excessive sweating, bad odour due to sweat and acts as an antidepressant. Mauktik acts as a rasayana in pyrexia, debility, tuberculosis, fractures and also in menorrhagia, anaemia, wounds and diarrhoea. Muktapishti is best used for any type of burning sensation, internally or externally. It is also useful in weakness of eyesight. It is majjagami and nourishes majja dhatu.
Antitoxic property : Should be used in lead poisoning.
Dose : 60 to 120 gm (Mauktik should be directly used in the form of fine powder (pishti) instead of using mauktik bhasma which is prepared in a furnace. Mauktik bhasma is not different from fine powder of oyster shells. Formulations like Muktapanchamrit, Kamdoodha, Vasantkusumar etc. contain mauktik.)
References -
'मौक्तिकं शीतलं वृष्यं चक्षुष्यं बलपुष्टिदम् ।' (भा. प्र.)
मौक्तिकं सुमधुरं सुशीतलं दृष्टिरोगशमनं विषापहरम्
राजयक्ष्मपरिकोपनाशनं क्षीणवीर्यबलपुष्टिवर्धनम् ।।' (रा. नि.)
'कफपित्तक्षयध्वंसि कासश्वासाग्निमांद्यनुत् ।
पुष्टिदं वृष्यमायुष्यं दाहघ्नं मौक्तिकं मतम् ।।' (र. चू.)

7. PRAVAL

English name : Coral.

Latin name : Corallium rubrum (rubrum = red)

Bhavprakash has included it under the group of maharatna. Praval is the fossil of a marine animal. It becomes harder and increasingly red as time passes. The lower portion of praval is called 'praval mool' and the upper portion is called 'praval shakha'. Praval is found in abundance in the seas of Eastern Australia.

Sanskrit names : Vidrum, laga, pala, pakhala, marja, busud, kama, marga, corallium rubrum, coral, angarak, mani, ambodhipallav, bhaumratna, raktang, raktankur etc. Praval having a bright colour, round in shape, without uneven curves, without any cracks, heavy in weight and which does not change its colour even after rubbing it against a stone is considered to be the best. Praval having opposite characteristics should not be used.

Chemical composition : Calcium carbonate 83%, magnesium carbonate 3.5%, iron -4.5%, organic compounds 8%.

Properties and actions : Laghu, ruksha, sweet, slightly sour, madhur vipaki, sheeta veerya, praval is tridoshahara.

External use : Useful in eye diseases and in wounds by its lekhana and avasadana properties.

Internal uses : Useful in those conditions in which brain tonic activity is required.

Digestive system : Reduces hyperacidity and is deepan, pachan, astringent. Through these actions, it is useful in acid-peptic disorders, diarrhoea accompanied with bleeding, bleeding piles and ulcerations in the intestine.

Respiratory system : Useful in various ailments of the respiratory system like chronic rhinitis, cough, asthma and tuberculosis.

Circulatory system : Useful in weakness of the heart, diseases of raktadhatu and raktapitta.

Reproductive system : Aphrodisiac, useful in shukra meha.

Urinary system : Due to its diuretic property, it is used in dysuria caused by kapha.

Skin : Since it modifies sweat secretion, it is helpful in excessive sweating and night sweats associated with tuberculosis. Useful in pyrexia, exhaustion, tuberculosis and toxins.

Dose : Praval pishti, Praval bhasma - 120 to 360 mg. (Praval panchamrut is especially useful in acid-peptic disorders). (The seas near the East coast of Australia are abundant in Praval).

Srotogamitva :

Dosha : Tridosha-vata, kapha.

Dhatu : Majja (brain tonic), rakta (raktapitta, bleeding piles, acid-peptic diseases); shukra (aphrodisiac, shukrameha).

Mala : Purisha (astringent); mutra (diuretic, useful in dysuria caused by kapha); sweda (useful in excessive sweating, night sweats in tuberculosis).

References -

'पक्वबिम्बीफलच्छायं वृत्तायतमवक्रकम् । स्निग्धमव्रणकं स्थूलं प्रवालं सप्तधा शुभम् ।
पाण्डुरं धूसरं रूक्षं सव्रणं कोरकान्वितम् । निर्भारं च तथा सूक्ष्मं प्रवालं नेष्यतेऽष्टधा ।।' (र. चू.)
'बालार्ककिरणा रक्ता सागरसलिलोद्भवा लता यास्ति ।

न त्यजति निजरूचिं निकपे घृष्टापि सा स्मृता जात्या ।।' (भा. प्र.)
'प्रवालं सुमृतं क्षारं मधुरं मधु शीतलम् । दीपनं पाचनं चैव दृष्टिरोगनिषूदनम् ।।
त्रिदोषशमनं बल्यं विशेषात् कफवातनुत् । क्षयकासहरं चैव रक्तपित्तप्रणाशनम् ।।
स्वेदातिनिर्गमहरं रात्रिस्वेदहरं परम् । विषघ्नं भूतशमनं वीर्यवर्णविवर्धनम् ।।' (र..) त

8. SHANKHA

English name : Conch.
Latin name : Tritonium (a special marine insect). It is included in the category of upratna. Shankha is the shell of a particular marine insect.
Sanskrit names : Kambu, Varibhava, Jalaj, Deerghaniswan, Suswara, Deerghanad, Dhaval, Shrivibhushan. Shankha which is big, heavy, white and without any pores is considered to be the best. Shankha which has a shine like moon should be used.
Chemical composition : It contains calcium and other salts.
Properties and actions : Laghu, ruksha, teekshna, pungent, katu vipaki, cold to touch but ushna veerya. It pacifies kapha-vata.
External uses: Used in eye diseases for topical application. If powdered shankha and hartal are applied topically then this mixture acts as a hair remover.
Internal uses : Reduces hyperacidity, deepan, pachan, anuloman. Due to these properties, it is used in agnimandya, ajeerna, abdominal colic, hyperacidity, gulma, grahani and enlargement of liver and spleen.
Respiratory system : Useful in cough and dyspnoea caused by kapha.
Dose : 250 to 500 mg.
Formulations : Shankha vati, Chandrodaya varti.
Srotogamitva :
Dosha : Vataghna, kaphaghna.
Dhatu : Rasa, rakta, mansa, meda (pachan, liver- spleen enlargement).
Mala : Pureesh (astringent, grahani).
Organ : Stomach (nutritive, pacifies kapha, reduces dyspnoea).
References -
शंखक्षारो हिमोग्राही ग्रहणीरोगनाशनः ।
नेत्रपुष्पहरो वर्ण्यस्तारुण्यपिटिकाप्रणुत् ।। (भा. प्र.)

9. SHUKTI

English name : Pearl oyster.
Latin name : Avicula.
Sanskrit names : Muktasfota, abdhimandooki.
This substance, which is included in the category of upratna, is produced in rivers and seas. The shukti (oyster) of the sea in which mukta (pearl) is formed is called mukta shukti. Shukti found in the river is called jala shukti. Shukti should be large and should have a shiny reddish colour.
Chemical composition : It contains some amount of calcium.

Properties and actions : Laghu, ruksha, sweet, madhur vipaki, sheeta veerya, shukti is tridoshaghna. Its properties are similar to mauktik but it is less effective. If mauktik is unavailable then shukti is used as a subtitute but it is not as effective in treating various types of burning sensations. Useful in asthma, heart diseases and abdominal pain. Its bhasma is used as a very good deepan.
Srotogamitva :
Dosha : Tridoshaghna.
Dhatu : Rasa, rakta, majja, (raktapitta, burning sensation).
Mala : It reduces the foul smell of various malas.

10. SHAMBOOK

It is the shell of a particular marine insect.
English name : Snail.
Latin name : Gastropoda (that which moves on its stomach).
Sanskrit names : Kshullak, Kshudrashankha, Shambook, Nakhashankhak.
Shambook also is a shell of a particular insect. This insect lives in deep pot-holes. Shambook which is hard, dark brown in colour, has striations on it and is whitish on its inner side should be used for medicinal purposes.
Source : Though it is found every where in India, it is abundant in marshy lands.
Chemical composition : It contains calcium carbonate 85 to 95% and also calcium phosphate, magnesium phosphate, magnesium sulphate, iron and silica.
Properties and actions : Bitter, pungent, ushna, deepan, pachan, anuloman. Because of these properties, it is useful in ajeerna (indigestion), parinam shoola (ulcers), gulma etc. The insect is very useful in debilitating diseases of children.
Dose : 250 to 500 mg.
Formulation : Shambookadi gutika.
Srotogamitva :
Dhatu : Rakta.
Mala : Purisha (grahi).

11. VARATIKA

Varatika is the shell of a marine animal.
Sanskrit names : Kapardika, Kaudi, Badua, Kajak, Kharmohra.
Latin name : Cypria moneta.
Appearance : Yellow coloured varatika having a cyst on the dorsal side, 3 to 4 gms. in weight and which is pointed is considered to be the best.
Chemical composition : It contains calcium phosphate, calcium carbonate, flouride, magnesium phosphate, manganese, sodium chloride etc.
Properties and actions : Laghu, ruksha, teekshna, pungent, bitter, katu vipaki and ushna veerya. It pacifies kapha-vata.
External use : Used as a topical application in eye diseases and skin diseases. Kapardika bhasma

is also used topically in wounds and otalgia.

Internal uses :

Digestive system : Deepan, pachan, bhedan and grahi. Due to these properties, it is used in agnimandya, ajeerna, parinam shoola, grahani and gulma.

Respiratory system : Used in cough caused by kapha-vata.

Dose : 250 to 500 mg.

Formulation : Brihat Loknath Rasa.

Srotogamitva :

Dosha : Kaphaghna, vataghna.

Dhatu : Rasa, raktagami, vrushya.

Mala : Purisha.

Organ : Eyes (internally and externally).

References -

'कपर्दः कटुतिक्तोष्णः कर्णशूलव्रणापहः । गुल्मशूलामयघ्नश्च नेत्रदोषनिकृन्तनः ।।' (धा. नि.)

'परिणामादिशूलघ्नी ग्रहणीक्षयनाशिनी । कटूष्णा दीपनी वृष्या नेत्र्या वातकफापहा ।।' (र. चू.)

APPENDICES

GLOSSARY

A

Aap : water (one of the five mahabhootas).
Aapya : made up of or constituted by aap mahabhoota.
Abhav : non - existence, nullity, absence.
Abhishyandi : that which causes obstruction of the channels because of sliminess and heaviness.
Abhyang : rubbing with unctuous substances, inunction, massage.
Abhyas : repeated reading, study or use; inculcation of a truth conveyed in sacred writing by repetition.
Acharya : teacher, scholar.
Achchapan sneha : administration of pure oil or ghee without adding any medicines to it.
Achetan : without life force, inanimate.
Achetan dravyas : inanimate substances (inorganic).
Adan kala : procurement period; the period of the year in which the energy of the living beings and other non-living material on the earth gets absorbed.
Adhikaran : support.
Adhyavata : a disorder of the nervous system characterised by altered muscle tone.
Adi : 1. beginning, commencement; a firstling. 2. used in the sense of etc. like vatadi doshas meaning all the doshas including vata, pitta and kapha.
Adibhautik : those miseries and diseases which arise out of external objects.
Agneya : made up of or constituted by agni.
Agni : 1. fire (one of the panchamahabhootas). 2. the term generally used in Ayurveda to indicate the power of digestion. In a broad sense, it implies all the digestive and metabolic functions of the body.
Agni bala : the strength (intensity) of agni.
Agni deepak : that which stimulates the agni (appetite).
Agnidagdha : burns.
Agnimandya : weakness of agni, loss of appetite.
Agnivardhak : that which increases agni (digestion).
Ahankar : the third of the eight producers or sources of creation, viz. the conceit or conception of individuality, individualization.
Ahar : food, nourishment, diet.
Ahar dravya : a substance used as food.
Akash : a free or open space, vacuity, the ether, sky or atmosphere (one of the panchamahabhootas).
Akasheeya : made up of or constituted by akash.
Akshepakaghna : anti-convulsant.
Akshepjanak : convulsant.
Akshipuran : putting eyedrops.
Alpa : little, less, scanty.
Ama : literally, this term means " uncooked material." In the context of Ayurveda, it means the product of improper digestion and metabolism.

Amapachan : that which digests ama.
Amashaya : stomach.
Amavata : disease caused by ama, rheumatic disease.
Ambu : water.
Amla : sour (one of the six rasas).
Amlapitta : acid peptic disease.
Andaj : born of an egg, oviparous.
Angamardaprashaman : alleviating body ache, malaise.
Anna : food.
Anoop desha : wet, marshy land.
Ansaruja : a condition characterised by pain in the scapula.
Antardah : deep burning sensation.
Antarmarga : literally means "the inner path". In Ayurveda, it means one of the three paths through which the disease affects the body namely the digestive tract.
Antarvidradhi : deep abscess.
Antaschetan : living beings in whom the life force is not evident (inner animation, life force within).
Antra : intestine.
Anuman : logically arrived at conclusion or inference.
Anupan : vehicle of medication, which has to be taken along with the medicine.
Anuvasan : a medicated enema prepared by adding oil to it. Sometimes ghee, muscle fat and bone marrow are added to it.
Anuvasanopag : that which supports the action of anuvasan.
Apachi : enlargement of soft / suppurated and discharging glands of the neck.
Apadesha : the second step in a syllogism (i.e. statement of the reason).
Apan vayu : one of the five sub-types of vayu in the body. It is situated in the lower abdomen and controls excretion.
Apara : distant, inferior, lower.
Apasmar : epilepsy.
Apathya : unsuitable, inconsistent or unwholesome diet and activities in particular diseases.
Apta : An enanlightened authority free from the effect of rajas and tamas who guides perfectly.
Apta vakya : words (of advice) from an apta.
Aptopadesha : advice given by an apta.
Arbud : a tumour.
Ardit : facial palsy.
Arohini : climbing creeper.
Arsha : haemorrhoids, piles.
Arshoghna : that which cures piles.
Artava : literally,this term means a seasonal or periodical phenomena. In women, it implies the menstrual flow. This term is often used to mean the ovum (stri beeja) which is responsible for conception.
Artavjanan : emmenagogue.
Artavshaman : that which regulates menstruation and pacifies abnormalities of menstruation.

Artha : the objects of the senses.
Ashmaribhedan : lithotrypsic.
Ashtanghridaya : compilation by Vagbhatta (junior), one of the vriddhatrayis.
Ashtangsangraha : compilation by Vagbhatta (senior).
Ashukari : a substance which acts speedily by spreading instantly in the body.
Ashukaritva : the property of ashukari.
Ashwinikumar : the mythological twin brothers who were the physicians of the gods.
Asravisruti : blood letting.
Asthapan : one of the two types of medicated enema in which usually decoctions are used.
Asthi : bones (one of the seven dhatus).
Asthisandhanak : that which facilitates union of fractured bones.
Asthapanopag : that which supports the action of asthapan.
Atharva veda : one of the four vedas.
Atisar : diarrhoea.
Atma : soul.
Atma gunas : those gunas which are characteristics of the soul.
Audbhid : dravyas which penetrate the earth and come out as plants.
Aushadhi : medicinal plant, medicine.
Aushadhi dravya : medicinal substance.
Aushnya : heat.
Avabhasini : the first among the seven layers of skin.
Avidahi : that which does not imbalance pachak pitta.
Avrushya : that which reduces potency.
Avrutta : covering.
Avyakta : the unevolved, primary germ of nature, primordial element or productive principle whence all the phenomena of the material world are developed. Also called moola prakriti.
Ayurveda : the science of health or medicine. It is classed among sacred sciences and is considered as a supplement of the Atharva veda.

B

Bahirantaschetan : living beings in whom the life force is very evident; animation seen externally.
Bahirmarg : literally meaning "the external path", one of the three paths through which the disease affects the body namely the skin and the seven dhatus.
Bahuruja : pain in the shoulders.
Bahuvarshayu : plants which survive for many years.
Bala : strength, functional capacity.
Balya : strengthening; that which raises the functional capacity.
Basti : the word basti means urinary bladder. Medicated enema which was administered in old days with the help of the bladder of animals is also called basti.
Beeja : seed.
Bhaga : portion, area.

Bhagandar : anorectal fistula.
Bhasmak : a disease of the digestive system characterised by unsatiable hunger in spite of repeated food intake.
Bhaum : made up of or constituted by prithvi mahabhoota, pertaining to bhumi (earth).
Bhava padarth : existential phenomena.
Bhavana : a process in which a medicinal substance is impregnated with the juice of another medicinal substance.
Bhedaneeya : purgative.
Bodhak kapha : one of the five sub-types of kapha which is situated in the mouth and helps in perception of taste.
Brahma : universal spirit, creator.
Bruhan : anabolism.
Bruhaneeya : a substance which has anabolic effect.
Buddhi : intellect.

C

Chaitanya : animation, life force.
Chakrapani : a commentator on Charaka samhita.
Chakshurendriya : the sense of sight.
Chakshushya : beneficial to the eyes.
Chala : moving, trembling or shaking.
Charaka samhita : compilation by Charaka. This volume is reverred as the most authentic text on Ayurveda.
Charaka/Charakacharya : an ancient Ayurvedic scholar who compiled Charaka samhita which is one of the vriddhatrayis.
Chardi : vomiting.
Chardi nigrahan : medicines which control vomiting, anti-emetic.
Charma : skin.
Charmadal : a skin disease characterised by itching, eruptions.
Chedaneeya : that which cuts and splits off.
Chetan : life force.
Chetan dravya : organic substance.
Chikitsa : treatment, cure.
Churna : powder.

D

Daha : burning sensation.
Dahaprashaman : that which alleviates burning sensation.
Dakshinavartini : a creeper turning towards the right.
Dakshinayana : southern solstice.
Dant : teeth.

Dantya : beneficial to the teeth.
Darshanshastra : the science of views, doctrines or philosophical systems.
Daurbalya : weakness.
Deepan : stimulation of digestive functions.
Deepeneeya : stimulant of digestive functions.
Desha : a word denoting a country, region or place.
Dharan : providing support.
Dharana : collection or concentration of the mind (joined with the retention of breath).
Dharma : this term is generally used for religion. In Ayurveda, it means innate tendency or property.
Dhatu : a constituent, element or essential ingredient of the body; tissue.
Dhatubala : strength of the dhatus.
Dhatupradushan : vitiation of dhatus.
Dhatushaithilya : weakness or laxity of the dhatus.
Dhruti : firmness, constancy, resolution, will.
Dhyana : meditation, thought, reflection.
Disha : direction (cardinal points).
Dolayantra : an apparatus used in purification procedures of drugs.
Dooshya : that which gets vitiated by the doshas namely the dhatus.
Dosha : literally means vice or fault. In Ayurveda, it means the three humours of the body namely vata, pitta and kapha which vitiate the dhatus.
Doshabala : strength of the dosha.
Doshaghna : that which ameliorates doshas.
Doshanashak : that which alleviates doshas.
Doshaprashaman : amelioration of doshas.
Doshavardhak : that which increases the doshas.
Dravya : substance.
Dravyagunakarmavignyan : science of the properties and actions of substances.
Drushtighna : that which harms the eyesight.
Dukha : sorrow, pain, discomfort.
Dukhasahatva : stress tolerance.
Durgandha : foul smell.
Dwesha : jealousy.
Dwivarshayu : plant living for two years.

F

Firang : syphilis.

G

Galaganda : tumour on the side of the neck or goitre.
Gamitva : the property of going or moving towards a particular part in the body, tropism.

Gandamala : cervical lymphadenitis.
Gandha : smell.
Garbha : foetus.
Garbhapatan : abortive.
Garbhashaysankochak : oxytocic.
Garbhotpadak : that which promotes conception.
Ghranendriya : the sense of smell.
Ghrita : ghee (clarified butter).
Gnyan : knowledge, enlightenment.
Grahani : 1. the small intestine or that part of the alimentary canal which is the site of pachak agni. 2. a disease which affects the small intestine and is charaterised by tinismus, foul smelling stools and mucous in the stools.
Grahi : drugs which stimulate digestion and absorption of fluids in the body. Generally this means a drug which causes constipation.
Greeshma : summer.
Grudhrasi : sciatica.
Guda : anus.
Gudabhransha : rectal prolapse.
Guhyapushpa : hidden flowers.
Gulma : 1. a shrub. 2. a glandular enlargement or a lump in the abdomen constituted by doshas.
Gulmini : creeper.
Guna : property.
Gunakarmashastra : science of properties and actions.
Gunavad : a doctrine which considers guna as the most important attribute of a substance.
Gunavadi : one who is a believer in gunavad.
Guru : heavy, that which is digested slowly.
Gurvadi : gunas like guru etc.

H

Hemant : winter.
Hetu : cause of disease.
Hikka : hiccups.
Hikkanigrahan : control of hiccups, drugs that control hiccups.
Hima : 1. cold (one of the twenty gurvadi gunas). 2. cold infusion.
Hridayottejak : cardiac stimulant.
Hridbalya : cardiotonic.
Hridruja : cardiac pain.
Hridya : cardiotonic, that which pleases the mind and senses.

I

Ichcha : wish, desire.

Ikshu : sugarcane.
Ikshumeha : a type of prameha (diabetes).
Indriya : faculty of sense, organ of sense.
Indriyartha : object of sense.

J

Jala : water (one of the panchamahabhootas).
Jalaj : produced or born or living or growing in water.
Jangal : arid land, sparingly grown with trees and plants (though not infertile).
Jangam : of or pertaining to animate living beings.
Jara : senility.
Jarayuj : viviparous.
Jeevaneeya : that which promotes longevity and optimises all the vital constituents and functions of the body.
Jeevaneeya gana : group of jeevaneeya substances.
Jeevaneeya karma : jeevaneeya action.
Jeevatma : soul.
Jivha : tongue.
Jvara : fever.
Jvarahara : that which alleviates fever, febrifuge.

K

Kala : time or season.
Kalka : pulp made from fresh plants.
Kalpana : forming, imagining or composing preparations of medications.
Kamala : jaundice.
Kandara : tendons.
Kandughna : antipruritic.
Kanthya : demulcent, beneficial to voice, larynx, throat.
Kapha : one of the three doshas.
Kaphadurgandhihar : that which alleviates foul smell of kapha.
Kaphaghna : that which alleviates kapha.
Karan dravya : causative substance.
Karma : drug action, biodynamic effect of drug.
Karnya : beneficial to the ears.
Karshya : emaciation.
Karya dravya : resultant substance.
Kasahara : drugs that alleviate cough.
Kashaya : 1) astringent taste (one of the six rasas); 2) decoction.
Kashtasadhya : diseases which are cured with relative difficulty.
Kathina : hard (one of the twenty gurvadi gunas).

Katu : pungent (one of the six rasas).
Kesha : hair.
Keshanashan : that which removes hair.
Keshavardhak : stimulant of hair growth.
Keshya : beneficial to hair growth.
Khara : rough (guna).
Kleda : slimy.
Kopan : vitiation of doshas.
Koshtha : 1. torso with its viscera. 2. applied to sensitivity of gastrointestinal digestion and motility.
Krumi : parasite, worms.
Krumighna : anthelmintic, antiparasitic.
Krura koshtha : costive bowels unaffected by strong purgatives.
Krushata : leanness, thinness.
Kshar : alkaline extract of plant.
Kshar karma : a procedure involving the use of kshar.
Kshaya : pthisis.
Ksheer : milk, latex.
Kshup : shrub
Kushtha : dermatoses.
Kushthaghna : anti-dermatoses.
Kwath : decoction.

L

Laghav : property of lightness.
Laghu : light (guna); easy to digest.
Laghutar : lighter.
Lahi : a light prepartion made from rice which is used in diarrhoea.
Lakshana : symptoms, signs.
Langhan : fasting.
Lasika : lymph.
Lata : creeper.
Lavana : salt; salty in taste (one of the six rasas).
Lehya : lickable, to be licked up or eaten by licking.
Lekhan : scratching, scraping, scarifying.
Leknaneeya : substances that bring about lekhan.
Lepa : anything smeared on, ointment, medicinal paste for topical use.
Lepan : that which smears or anoints.
Ling : signs and symptoms of diseases.
Loha : iron.
Loma : hairs on the body other than scalp, face and pubis.

M

Madakari : intoxicating.
Madan : maddening, intoxicating.
Madhur : sweet (one of the six rasas.)
Madhurakshaman : that which alleviates glycosuria.
Madhurya : the quality of sweetness.
Madhyam marg : literally means "the middle path". In Ayurveda, it means one of the three athways through which diseases affect the body namely the vital organs and joints.
Madya : alcoholic beverage.
Mahabharat : a great epic poem written by sage Vyasa narrating the contests of descendants of Bharat.
Mahabhoota : element of which the universe is composed.
Mahat-tatva : literally means "the great principle". According to the Sankhya philosophy, it is the second of the 23 principles produced from prakriti and so called as the great source of Ahankara (self consciousness).
Mahavruksha : a large tree.
Majja : marrow (sixth among the seven dhatus of the body).
Mala : any bodily excretion.
Malapachan : that which digests the malas (unmetabolised products).
Malayana : the paths of excretions.
Mana : mind (in its widest sense as applied to all the mental powers).
Mansa : flesh, muscle tissue (third among the seven dhatus of the body).
Mansagami : acting on the mansa dhatu, having tropism for mansa dhatu.
Mansavardhak : that which increases mansa dhatu.
Mardav : the quality of softness.
Mardavkar : that which produces softness.
Marma : a mortal spot or a vulnerable point (Ayurveda has described 107 such mortal spots).
Meda : fatty tissue.
Medakshaya : reduction of fatty tissue.
Medhya : causing or generating intelligence, mental vigour or power.
Medodosha : diseases caused by dyslipidemia.
Medopachak : digesting fatty tissue.
Moola prakriti : see avyakta.
Moolarohini : creeper climbing by rootlets.
Mrudu : soft (one of the twenty gunas).
Mukhadurgandhinashak : that which stops bad breath.
Mukharoga : diseases of the oral cavity.
Mukhavaishadyakar : that which cleanses the mouth.
Murchha : fainting.
Murdhavikar : diseases of the supraclavicular region.
Mutra : urine.
Mutraghat : anuria.

Mutrakruchchra : painful discharge of urine, a class of urinary affections of which eight kinds are enumerated.
Mutrasangrahaneeya : that which reduces urine excretion.
Mutravirajaneeya : that which restores the normal colour of urine.
Mutrayana : the path of urine excretion.

N

Nabhas : made up of or constituted by akash mahabhoota.
Nabhi : umbilicus.
Nadi : pulse.
Nakha : nail.
Nakshatra : an asterism or constellation through which the moon passes, a lunar mansion.
Namasmarana : the glorification or incessant repetition of the name of a god.
Nashak : destroying, annihilating, removing.
Nasya : nasal insufflation.
Nidrajanak : that which induces sleep.
Nighantu : compilation of synonyms.
Nitya : eternal.
Nityatva : eternity.
Niyama : the fixed order of things.
Niyatkalikjvarpratibandhak : anti-malarial, anti-periodic.
Nyaya darshan : a system of philosophy delivered by Gautama (it is one of the six darshanas).

O

Oja : the ultimate essence of dhatus, specifically shukra.
Ojabala : the strength or power of oja.
Oshadhi : an annual plant or herb which dies after becoming ripe.

P

Pachan : digestion (this word is also used for substances which are digestive).
Padarth : substance.
Padarthvignyan : science of substances.
Padarthvignyanshastra : that branch of knowledge which deals with the science of substances.
Padmakantak : a type of skin disease.
Pak : digestion, assimilation of food.
Pakva : digested or assimilated food.
Pakvashaya : the large intestine.
Pakvatisar : diarrhoea without mucous secretion.
Panchabhautik : made up of or constituted by the panchamhabhootas.
Panchamahabhootas : the five elements that make up the universe viz. vayu, akash, teja, aap

and prithvi.
Panchamahabhootatmak : made up of or constituted by the panchamahabhootas.
Panchakarma : the five types of therapeutic procedures used in Ayurveda for removal of doshas from the body.
Panchang : the five parts (usually used in the context of plants where it means the five parts of plants viz. roots, stem, leaves, flowers and fruits).
Panchashodhan : another word for panchakarma.
Panchatanmatra : the five subtle rudiments of the panchamahabhootas.
Panchavidh : of five types.
Panchendriya : the five senses.
Panduroga : anaemia.
Para : distant.
Paradi : the gunas including para etc.
Pariman : measure.
Parmanu : an infinitesimal particle or atom (30 are said to form a mote in a sun beam).
Parshwashoolaghna : that which alleviates lateral chest pain.
Parthiv : 1. made up of or constituted by prithvi mahabhoota. 2. earthly, belonging to the earth, minerals.
Pathya : regimen of diet in a particular disease.
Patrarohini : creeper climbing by leaves.
Peenas : purulent sinusitis.
Peshi : tissue.
Phalavarga : class of fruits.
Phant : hot infusion.
Phuphus : lungs.
Pichchila : viscous, sticky.
Pitta : one of the three doshas.
Pittasarak : producing excessive pitta, inducing sara guna of pitta, cholagogue.
Pittashamak : pacifying pitta.
Pleeha : spleen.
Prabhav : a specific action distinct to that particular substance.
Pradhan : important, prominent or dominant.
Prajasthapan : promoting fertility.
Prakopa : vitiation.
Prakopak : that which causes vitiation.
Prakriti : 1. the original nature, character, constitution or temper of a person. 2. the original producer of (or rather passive power of creating) the material world.
Praman : a means of acquiring sound knowledge, any proof or testimony or evidence.
Prameha : this term is generally used for diabetes (In Ayurveda, this term is applied to a group of 20 urinary diseases including diabetes).
Prana : 1. life force. 2. one of the five sub-types of vayu.
Pranavahasrotas : the respiratory system.
Pranayam : a technique in yoga which uses deep breathing exercises for achieving control of the

mind.
Prasad : the clear, pure or refined state of any dhatu.
Prasarini : spreading creeper.
Praspand : vibrations.
Pratishyay : rhinitis.
Pratyaksha : directly demonstrable evidence.
Pravahika : dysentery.
Preenan : pleasing, delighting or satisfying.
Prithvi : earth, one of the five mahabhootas.
Punarvasu Atreya : a sage who learnt Ayurveda from other sages and taught it to his disciples. The Charaka samhita which is available today is derived from his teachings.
Puran : filling.
Purish : stools, faeces.
Purishajanan : that which increases the bulk of stools.
Purishakshapanak : that which reduces the bulk of stools.
Purishasangrahaneeya : that which increases solid consistency of the stools.
Purishavirajaneeya : that which restores the normal colour of stools.
Pushti : nourishment.

R

Raja : an attribute of mental constitution - the other two being satva and tama.
Rajayakshma : tuberculosis.
Rakta : blood, one of the seven dhatus of the body.
Raktapitta : bleeding disorders.
Raktaprasadak : that which purifies blood.
Raktavruddhi : Functional and quantitative improvement of blood.
Rasa : 1. a dhatu circulating continuously throughout the body and the first among the seven dhatus of the body. 2. juice of any medicine. 3. taste - perceived by the tongue. 4. mercury.
Rasadi dhatus : the dhatus including rasa etc.
Rasapradhan : a substance in which its taste is dominant.
Rasayana : a substance which alleviates old age and diseases and promotes vitality; adaptogen.
Rasendriya : the sense of taste.
Raukshya : the quality of dryness.
Ritu : season.
Rochan : appetiser.
Roga : disease.
Roga nidan : diagnosis.
Roga samprapti : pathogenesis.
Rogotpatti : genesis of diseases.
Roopa : shape, appearance.
Rudhir : blood, a synonym of rakta.
Rugna : patient, the diseased.
Ruksha : dry.

Ruksha lahi : a preparation made from rice which is used to control diarrhoea.
Rukshan : producing dryness.

S

Sadharan : a type of land intermediate between marshy and arid lands.
Saindhav : rock salt.
Samadosha : diseases which involve ama in their pathogenesis.
Saman : 1. one of the five sub-types of vata dosha which aids in digestion. 2. commonality.
Samanvaya : conjunction or union.
Samanya : the attribute of commonality.
Samanya gunas : a class of gunas.
Samhita : writings, ideas, concepts or sutras put together (volume).
Sammoorchana : the act of congealing or thickening, increasing, spreading or accumulating.
Samprapti : pathogenesis.
Samyoga : joining together or placing together; combination.
Sandhaneeya : 1. that which facilitates reunion of fractures. 2. substances that aid in fermentation.
Sandra : thick, dense, viscid.
Sangnyasthapan : that which restores consciousness.
Sankhya : accurate measure, limiting factor for many entities - number, weight etc.
Sankhya darshan : an ancient school of philosophy which considers the universe to be made up of 24 elements.
Sannipat : concommitant vitiation of all the three doshas.
Sanshodhan : purification of body elements by appropriate removal of vitiated doshas.
Sanshodhan dravyas : substances which remove the vitiated doshas from the body.
Sanskar : proper conditioning.
Sanskrit : an ancient Indian language in which Ayurveda is written.
Sant : saintly.
Santapnivarak : that which alleviates fever or burning sensation.
Sara : 1. fluid, liquid (one of the twenty gunas). 2. cathartic, purgative, laxative.
Satkaryavad : a principle of Sankhya darshan which believes in the necessary existence of an effect (as inherent in a cause).
Satmikaran : an agent which induces satmya.
Satmya : body-compatible not leading to a disturbance.
Satva : a quality of mental constitution others being raja and tama.
Saukshmya : minuteness, subtlety.
Shabda : sound.
Shaitya : quality and feeling of coldness.
Shakti : power, strength, force.
Shaman : that which pacifies the doshas without removing them from the body.
Sharad : autumn.
Sharir : body (physical).

Sharirshastra : anatomy.
Sharirvignyan : the science of the body.
Shastra : science - often used for traditional knowledge.
Sheeta : cold.
Sheeta dharma : coldness.
Sheeta lahi : a formulation made from rice which is used for controlling diarrhoea.
Sheeta prashaman : substances that alleviate cold.
Sheeta shakti : the power of cold.
Shilajit : a mineral medicinal substance (asphaltum).
Shimbi dhanya : substances that grow in legumes (mainly pulses).
Shirahshool : headache.
Shirovirechan : removal of doshas from the head by nasal administration of medicines.
Shirovirechanopag : substances that help in shirovirechan.
Shishir : winter.
Shivambu : one's own urine.
Shlakshna : smooth (one of the twenty gunas).
Shlipad : filariasis.
Shodhan : purification.
Shodhan dravyas : substances that are used for shodhan.
Shok : grief.
Shonitprashaman : substances that pacify the doshas of the blood.
Shonitsthapan : hemostatic.
Shoolaprashaman : analgesic substances.
Shosh : 1. dryness of mouth. 2. pthisis.
Shoth : oedema, inflammation.
Shothahara : that which reduces swelling.
Shramahara : removing fatigue.
Shreekhand : a sweet prepartion made from curds.
Shrut : decoction.
Shruti : knowledge obtained by hearing.
Shukra : semen (the last of the seven dhatus of the body).
Shukra nashan : that which destroys semen.
Shukra shodhan : that which purifies semen.
Shukraghna : that which destroys shukra.
Shwasa : breathlessness.
Shwasahara : substances which relieve breathlessness.
Shwitra : leucoderma.
Siddhant : a principle.
Sidhma : a type of skin disease.
Sira : blood vessels.
Sira shaithilya : laxity of blood vessels.
Skandharuja : pain in the shoulders.
Smashru : moustache, beard, axillary and pubic hair.

Smruti : retentive memory.
Snayu : muscle / ligament.
Sneha : oleogenous substance.
Snehan : oleation; a procedure in panchakarma which involves oleation.
Snehopag : substances that aid in snehan.
Snigdha : oily (one of the twenty gunas).
Somal : arsenic.
Sootrarohini : thread - like climbing creeper.
Sransan : laxative.
Stabdhagatrata : stiffness of the body.
Stambhak : that which causes stambhan.
Stambhan : withholding body fluids.
Stanya : breast milk.
Stanyajanan : substances that stimulate production of breast milk.
Stanyakshapan : galactofuge.
Stanyashodhan : substances that purify breast milk.
Sthairya : quality of stillness; stability, firmness.
Sthavar : substances obtained from immobile sources (plants, minerals etc.).
Sthira : steady, stable.
Sthitapragnyata : balanced, non-attached; an attribute of personality.
Sthoola : coarse, thick, heavy.
Sthoulya : obesity.
Sthoulyanashan : anti-obesity.
Sugandh : fragrance.
Sugandhi : fragrant.
Sukha : happiness, pleasure.
Sukhasadhya : diseases which can be cured with relative ease.
Sukshma : minute, subtle (one of the twenty gunas).
Sutra : aphorism, lines in a samhita depicting ideas and concepts.
Sutra sthana : that section of a samhita (usually the first) which explains the basic ideas and concepts of its subject in aphorisms.
Swasthavritta : a healthy life style suggested by Ayurveda.
Swasthya : the state of health.
Sweda : perspiration, sweat.
Sweda dushti : vitiation of sweat.
Swedaj : caused or produced by perspiration.
Swedajanan : diaphoretic.
Swedal : that which causes perspiration.
Swedan : causing perspiration (fomentation).
Swedavahasrotas : sweat glands and ducts.
Swedayan : the path of excretion of sweat.
Swedopag : substances that aid in swedan (i.e. causing perspiration).

T

Taijas : made up of or constituted by teja mahabhoota.
Tamas : darkness; a quality of mental constitution others being raja and satva.
Tanmatra : rudimentary or subtle elements from which the five mahabhootas or grosser elements are formed.
Tarpan : satiety.
Teevra : sharp, fast acting, very potent.
Teja : light, fire (one of the five mahabhootas).
Teja samyoga : combination of a dravya with teja mahabhoota causing change.
Tikshna : hot, fast acting.
Tikta : bitter.
Tridosha : the three doshas - vata, pitta and kapha.
Tridoshaj : produced by all the three doshas.
Triguna : three gunas - satva, raja and tamas.
Trishna : thirst, craving.
Trishnanigrahan : removing (assuaging) thirst.
Trupti : satiation.
Truptighna : that which removes satiation.
Tvacha : skin.
Tvagindriya : the sense of touch.
Tvak : skin.

U

Udar : 1. abdomen 2. diseases of the abdomen, especially ascites.
Udard : urticaria.
Udardaprashaman : that which alleviates urticaria.
Udavarta : a group of symptoms caused by witholding natural urges.
Udbhid : plants sprouting from the earth.
Unduk : caecum.
Unmad : mania.
Upadhatu : a by-product during the formation of dhatu from which nothing new is formed.
Upashamaneeya : substances that pacify doshas.
Urahkshat : disease characterized by cavities / lesions in the lungs.
Ushna : hot, heat.
Ushna dharma : the property of hotness.
Uttar tantra : section of a samhita (usually the last) in which usually miscellaneous subjects are discussed.
Uttarayana : northern solstice.

V

Vahan : flow; production, maintenance and destruction of dhatus.
Vaidya : a physician who practises Ayurveda.
Vaidyak : the practice of Ayurveda.
Vaikarik : one of the three ahankars in the Sankhya darshan.
Vaisheshik gunas : special (specific) gunas of the senses, namely shabda, sparsha, roopa, rasa and aandha.
Vajikaran : aphrodisiac, increasing male reproductive functions.
Valkal : bark of tree.
Vaman : emesis.
Valli : creeper.
Vamanopag : substances that aid in emesis.
Vamavartini : creeper growing with tropism to the left.
Vanaspati : plants with minute flowers which cannot be seen - apushpa.
Vanaspatya : plants with visible flowers and fruits - sapushpa.
Vardhak : causing increase.
Varga : class.
Varnya : that which improves complexion.
Varsha : monsoon, rainy season.
Vasant : spring season.
Vata : one of the three doshas, also called vayu.
Vata vruddhi : increase in vata.
Vatanashak : alleviating vata .
Vatanulomak : substances that facilitate normal downward passage of vata in the body.
Vatarakta : gout.
Vayahsthapan : anti-aging.
Vayaveeya : made up of or constituted by vayu.
Vayu : 1. air, wind - one of the five mahabhootas. 2. one of the three doshas of the body, also called vata.
Vedana : pain, discomfort.
Vedanasthapan : analgesic.
Veerya : 1. potency 2. semen.
Veerudh : plants growing as creepers.
Veeryapradhan : substances in which veerya is the primary phenomenon.
Vibandhanashak : alleviating constipation.
Vibhaga : section, part.
Vichar : thought, mental attitude, consideration.
Vidagdha : burnt, inflammed, turned sour.
Vidahi : substances that cause burning and inflammation.
Vidradhi : abscess.
Vignyan : science.
Vihar : life style.

Vikashi : substances that cause laxity of joints of the body and depletion of oja.
Vikrant : strong, victorious.
Vikriti : vitiation, pathology.
Vimal : clear, pure, without any impurities.
Vipak : post digestion metabolic state.
Virechak : purgative.
Virechan : purgation.
Virechanopag : substances that aid in purgation.
Visarga kala : bestowal period; that part of the year in which the strength of all living forms increases.
Visarpa : erysepalas.
Visha : poison.
Vishad : clear, pure.
Vishaghna : antidote.
Vishaushadhi : medicines prepared from poisons.
Viman sthana : a section in a samhita in which clinical examination is discussed in detail.
Vishaya : sense object.
Vishesha : specificity, peculiarity.
Vranaropan : that which facilitates healing of wounds.
Vranashodhan : that which cleanses wounds.
Vruddhatva : senility.
Vruksha : tree.
Vrushya : aphrodisiac.
Vrushyatva : potency.

Y

Yakrut : liver.
Yakrutottejak : liver stimulant.
Yapya : diseases which cannot be cured but can be controlled by continuous medication.
Yogavahi : a substance which when combined with another substance imbibes in itself the properties and actions of the other substance.
Yonidosha : gynaecological disorders.
Yuka : lice.
Yukti : skilfully deviced stratagem, application or practice.
Yukti praman : a mode of authenticating knowledge which uses yukti.

MEDICINAL PLANTS AND INDICATIONS

Agnidagdha : Ral ointment, Tugakshiryadi ointment.
Amlapitta : Pravalpanchamrut, Asparagus racemosus, Cynodon dactylon.
Antardah : Anjan, Callicarpa macrophylla, Nordostachys jatamansi, kamaladi gana.
Arshoghna : Semecarpus anacardium (dry piles), Holerrhena antidysentrica, buttermilk, Amorphophallus campanulatus, Plumbago zeylanica, dry ginger, Aconitum heterophyllum, Terminalia chebula.
Antarvidradhi : Moringa oleifera (bark), varunadi gana.
Ashmaribhedan : Berginia ligulata, Crataeva nurvala, Dolichos biflorus, varunadi, vellantaradi gana.
Anuvasanopag : Inula racemosa, Cedrus deodar, Randia dumetorum, Tribulus terrestris, Premna integrifolia, madankutajadi gana.
Angamardaprashaman : Vidaryadi gana.
Apasmar : Brahmikalpa.
Ansaruja : Mocha rasa nasya.
Ardit : Fresh butter.
Atisar : Holerrhena antidysenterica (bark), priyangvadi gana, ambashthadi gana, Aconitum heterophyllum.
Asthisandhanak : Vicisus quadrangularis (juice), formulations of coral etc.
Agnivardhak : Ginger, ginger + salt, Aconitum heterophyllum, Plumbago zeylanica, Piper nigrum, Cuminum cyminum, Trachispermum amami, varunadi.
Amapachan : Mustadi varga, Carica papaya, Raphanus sativus, Plumbago zeylanica, Curcuma longa, Aconitum heterophyllum, Swertia chirata.
Asthapanopag : Operculina terpethum, Aegle marmelos, Piper longum, Acorus calamus, Randia dumetorum.
Artavajanan : Hemp plant, Sesamum indicum, Abroma augusta, Clerodendron serratum, Bambusa bambos.
Artavashaman : Symplocos racemosa, Saraca indica, Eupatorium triplinerve, Hibiscus rosa-sinensis.
Akshepjanak : Strychnos nux-vomica.
Akshepakaghna : Betula utilis.
Adhyavata : Vachadi gana.
Udard : Diospyros tomentosa, Buchanania latifolia, Acasia catechu, Alstonia scholaris, Terminalia arjuna, Piper nigrum + ghee, juice of Garcinia indica.
Udar : Milk and urine of camel.
Unmad : Preserved or old ghee of ten years.
Kaphaghna : Vaman, honey, asanadi, varunadi, aragwadhadi, arkadi, mushkakadi, surasadi, mustadi and vatsakadi gana.
Kanthya : Hemidesmus indicus, root of sugarcane, Glycerrhiza glabra, piper longum, raisins, Pueraria tuberosa, Solanum xanthocarpum, Solanum indicum, leaves of Abrus precatorius, Adiantum lunulatum, Alpinia galanga.
Kushthaghna : Acasia catechu, blood letting, Embelia ribes, krumighna yoga, Semecarpus

anacardium, Cassia fistula, Vitex negundo, Psoralea corylifolia, Cassia tora, asanadi gana.

Kandughna : Santalum alba, Cassia fistula, Pongamia glabra, Azadirachta indica, Capsicum annuum, mustard seeds, Cuminum cyminum.

Krumighna : Embelia ribes (krumiprakriti vighat), Mallotus philippinensis, Mucuna pruriens, Vitex negundo, Ipomoea reniformis, Balanites aegyptica, asanadi, surasadi gana.

Kaphavata : Terminalia chebula.

Kaphameda : Varunadi, ushakadi, rodhradi, arkadi gana.

Kaphapittaghna : Guduchyadi gana.

Kaphadurgandhihar : Cedrus deodar, Eucalyptus citriodora.

Karnya : Crinum asiaticum, Erithrina variegata.

Kasahar : Solanum xanthocarpum, Terminalia belerica, raisins, Terminalia chebula, Piper longum, Rhus succedania, Phyllanthus urinaria, vidaryadi gana.

Keshya : Eclipta alba, Cocos nucifera, Sesamum indicum, Indigofera tinctoria.

Keshanashan : Balanites aegyptica (fruit), paste of calcium carbonate + yellow arsenic.

Karshya : Flesh, santarpan, sleep.

Kamala : Patoladi gana.

Gandamala : Bauhinia variegata.

Garbhashaysankochak : Aristolochia indica, Abroma augusta, Carum carvi, Gloriosa superba, Ruta graveolens, Paganum harmal.

Garbhotpadak : Shukra.

Grahi : Myristica fragrans, Coleus amboinicus, nyagrodhadi gana.

Gulma : Varanadi, ushakadi gana.

Gar : Gold formulations.

Grahani : Buttermilk, Holerrhena antidysenterica, Semecarpus anacardium, parpatikalpa.

Garbhapatan : Gloriosa superba.

Gudabhransha : Mustak taila, ash of flowers of Canabis sativa, T - bandage.

Grudhrasi : Castor oil.

Chakshushya : Triphala with ghee and honey, Symplocos racemosa, rasanjan (preparation made from Berberis aristata), Cassia absus, nasya, anjan, tarpan, Coptis teeta, Strychnos potatorum.

Chhardinigrahan : Rice puffs, licking Santalam alba + Emblica officinalis, Eugenia jambolana, Mangifera indica, Citrus medica, Crocus sativus, Punica granatum, vidaryadi gana.

Chhedan : Terminalia belerica, Adhatoda vasica, Piper nigrum, Abies webbiana, Syzygium aromaticum, Cinnamomum zeylonica, Glycerrhiza glabra, Viola odorata.

Jeevaneeya : Jeevak, Rushabhak, Listea chinensis, kakoli, ksheerkakoli, Ureria picta, Desmodium gangeticum, Leptadenia reticulata, haematinics, padmakadi gana.

Jwarahar : Cyperus rotundus+Fumeria parviflora, dashamoola, Hemidesmus indicus, Rubia cordifolia, Grewia asiatica, triphala.

Truptighna : Dry ginger, Piper officinarum, Emblia ribes, Acorus calamus, Cyperus rotundus, Piper longum.

Trushanigrahan : Dry ginger, Alhaji maurorum, shadangodak.

Dukhasahatva : Exercise.

Deepan : Panchakola, Garcinia pedunculata, Piper nigrum, Carum roxburghianum, Semecarpus anacardium, Ferula foetida.

Dahaprashaman : Santalum alba, Gmelina arboria (fruit), Glycerrhiza glabra, sugar, Nelumbo nucifera, Hemidesmus indicus, Serrato submersom, Andropogan muricatus.
Dantya : Mimusops elingi, Zanthoxylon alatum, Saraca indica (bark), triphala, dry ginger, Acasia catechu, black sesame.
Drushtighna : Fried recipes of wheat.
Dharan : Bones.
Nasya : Achyranthes aspera (seeds), Celastrus paniculata, Piper nigrum, Piper longum, Emblia ribes, Moringa oleifera (seeds), mustard seeds, velladi gana.
Nidrajanan : Buffalo's milk, Withania somnifera, Lawsonia inermis, pearl, Rauwolfia serpentina, Herpestis monniera.
Niyatkalik jvarpratibandhak : Alstonia scholaris, Caesalpinia crista, Calotropis procera, Ocimum sanctum, quinine.
Pachan : Mustadi gana.
Pakvatisar : Priyangvadi, ambashtadi gana.
Peenas : Vatsakadi gana.
Puran : Majjadhatu enhancing drugs.
Preenan : Milk, drugs increasing rasa dhatu, padmakadi gana.
Pratishyay : Shrikhand (Amarkosha), snehan, nasya, surasadi gana.
Prameha : Shilajit (rasayan), Emblica officinalis + Curcuma longa, asanadi gana.
Pleehagami : Tecomella undulata, Piper longum, Aloe vera.
Purishasangrahaneeya : Mango seed, Oroxylum indicum, Symplocos racemosa, mocharasa, Mimosa pudica, Woodfordia floribunda (flower).
Purishavirajaneeya : Eugenia jambolana, Cinnamomum Zeylonica, Madhuka indica, Sesamum indicum, Ficus religosa, Boswellia serrata.
Purishakshapanak : Milk, fruit juice, butter milk.
Purishajanan : Pulses, leafy vegetables, horse gram, yava.
Prajasthapan : Herpestis monniera, Asparagus racemosus, Sapindus trifoliatus, Cynodon dactylon, Nelumbo nucifera, masanumasik kashay (decoction of certain dravyas which are specifically indicated for each month of pregnancy).
Pittashamak : Ghee, durvadi gana, nyagrodadhi, padmakadi, sarivadi gana.
Pittasarak : Virechan, Picrorrhiza kurroa, cow's urine, Berberidae podophyllum, Aloe vera.
Pittakaphaghna : Patoladi gana.
Parshwashoolaghna : Inula racemosa.
Firang : Black powder of triphala (wounds).
Balya : Pueraria tuberosa, Withania somnifera, Sida cordifolia, Desmodium gangeticum.
Bruhaniya : Gmelina arboria, vidaryadi, padmakadi gana.
Bahuruja : Mocharasa nasya.
Bhedaneeya : Operculina turpethum, Ipomoea hederacea, Citrulus colocynthis, Picrorrhiza kurroa, Mallotus phillippinensis.
Medavrut vata : Commiphora mukul.
Mutraghat : Tribulus terretris, Dendropthoe falcata, Bergenia ligulata, trunapanchamool, parushakadi, varunadi, vellantaradi gana.
Mutravirajaneeya : Nelumbo nucifera, Glycerrhiza glabra, Callicarpa macrophylla, Woodfordia

floribunda (flowers).
Mutrasangrahaneeya : Panchapallav, Aegle marmelos, Bauhinia racemosa.
Murdhavikar : Nasya.
Murchha : Cold water, cool air, shade.
Medodosha : Arkadi gana, asanadi gana, varunadi gana.
Medhya : Convolvulus pluricaulis, Centella asiatica, Celastrus paniculata, Benincasa hispida.
Madakari : Morphine, Canabis sativa, Hyocymus reticulata, Datura seeds.
Mukhadurgandhinashak : Hibiscus abelmoschus, Syzygium aromaticum, Myristica fragrans.
Mukhavaishadyakar : Betel leaf, dry ginger.
Malapachan : Mustadi gana.
Madhurakshaman : Gymnema sylvestree, Coccinia indica, Eugenia jambolana (seed), Aegle marmelos.
Mukha roga : Nasya, Kaval, blood letting.
Yakrutgami : Jeevaneeya.
Yuka : Oil of Cedrus deodar.
Yoni dosha : Rodhradi gana, mustadi gana, nyagrodhadi gana.
Rasayana : Terminalia chebula, Emblica officinalis, Tinospora cordifolia, Semecarpus anacardium, Embelia ribes, Piper longum, Allium sativum, Argyria speciosa.
Raktavardhan : Jeevaneeya gana.
Rochan : Mango, Carissa congesta, Zizyphus jujuba, Garcinia indica, Garcinia pedunculata, Punica granatum, Citrus medica.
Raktapitta : Adhatoda vasica (panchang), Mimosa pudica, sarivadi gana, nyagrodhadi gana.
Raktaprasadak : Padmakadi gana.
Lekhaneeya : Cyperus rotundus, Saussurea luppa, Curcuma longa, Acorus calamus, Aconitum heterophyllum, Picrorrhiza kurroa, Plumbago zeylanica, Pongamia glabra.
Lalaprasekjanan : Capsicum annum, Anacyclus pyrethrom.
Lepan : Flesh.
Vayahsthapan : Emblica officinalis, Tinospora cordifolia, Terminalia chebula, Leptadenia reticulata, Centella asiatica, Desmodium gangeticum.
Vranashodhan : Triphala + Commiphora mukul, honey, Azadirachta indica, Curcuma longa, old ghee, arkadi gana, surasadi.
Vranaropan : Honey, Sesamum indicum.
Vamanopag : Honey, Glycerrhiza glabra, Randia dumetorum, Bauhinia variegata, Piper longum, salt, Acorus calamus, mustard seeds, Luffa echinata, madanadi gana.
Varnya : Santalum alba, Andropogon muricatus, Rubia cordifolia, Hemidesmus indicus, Glycerrhiza glabra, saffron, rodhradi gana, Pandanus tectorius.
Vishaghna : Albizzia lebbek, Curcuma longa, Rubia cordifolia, Vitex negundo, Strychnos potatorum, Cinnamomum zeylonica, gold, patoladi, rodhradi, aragwadhadi gana.
Virechanopag : Raisins, Gmelina arboria, Grewia asiatica, triphala, Salvadora persica, nikumbhadi gana.
Vedanasthapana : Shorea robusta, Myrica nagi, Anthocephalus indicus, Saraca indica, Hyocymus reticulata, Ricinus communis, Commiphora mukul.
Vrushya : Withania somnifera, Abrus precatorius (leaves), Amorphophallus sylvalicus, padmakad

gana.
Vatanashan : Allium sativum, basti, oil, bhadradarvadi gana, veertaradi gana, vidaryadi gana.
Vatarakta : Commiphora mukul.
Vidradhi : Blood letting (acute), Moringa oleifera (decoction of bark).
Vishthambhi : Artocarpus heterophyllus.
Vidahi : Withania somnifera, mustard seeds.
Vatanuloman : Peppermint, bidlavana, Mentha spicate, Ricinus communis, Anethum sowa, Gardenia gummifera.
Vikasi : Areca catachu.
Vatapittaghna : Vidaryadi gana, padmakadi gana.
Vruddhatva : Milk + ghee, Emblica officinalis, Terminalia chebula.
Shukrashodhan : Saussurea luppa, Anthocephalus indicus, Myrica nagi, Asterocantha longifolia Andropogon muricatus.
Shukraghna : Acasia catechu, mushkakadi gana.
Shukrajanan : Mucuna pruriens, Withania somnifera, jeevaneeya varga, Asparagus racemosus, Astercantha longifolia, Asparagus adscendens.
Shwitra : Asanadi gana.
Shirahshool : Varunadi gana.
Shoth : Boerhavia diffusa, Swertia chirata + dry ginger.
Shok : Liquor.
Shosh : Liquor (made from grains), meat, milk.
Shwasahar : Inula racemosa, Cinnamomum zeylonica, Ferula foetida, Ocimum sanctum, Phyllanthus niruri, vidaryadi, surasadi gana.
Shramahar : Liquor, bath, raisins, Phoenix sylvestris, Punica granatum, Grewia asiatica, sugarcane, rice.
Sheetaprashaman : Aquilaria agallocha, Valerian wallichi, dry ginger, Acorus calamus, cumin seeds, Solanum xanthocarpum, Premna integrifolia, Piper longum, Oroxylum indicum, coconut.
Shirovirechanopag : Velladi gana.
Shothahar : Dashamoola, Boervhia diffusa, dry ginger, Swertia chirata, cow's urine.
Shoolaprashaman : Panchakola, Carum roxburghianum, Cuminum cyminum, cumin seeds, Lepidium sativum, subja.
Shonitastapan : Honey, Gycerrhiza glabra, mocharasa, Symplocos racemosa, sugar, red ochre, rice puffs.
Stanyajanan : Crataeva nurvala, rice, trunapanchamool, Arundo donax, Cymbopogon schoenanthus.
Stanyashodhan : Cocculus hirsutus, shashthyadi yog (V. Uttartantra).
Sthoulyanashan : Berberis aristata, exercise, shilajit, Commiphora mukul, varunadi, ushakadi gana, butter milk.
Sandhaneeya : Lac, madhukadi ten plants (Ch. Sutrasthan), nyagrodhadi gana.
Sransan : Cassia fistula, Cassia angustifolia.
Stanyakshapanak : Mallika.
Snehopag : Raisins, Glycerrhiza glabra, Pueraria tuberosa, Listea chinensis, Cordia wallichii, kakoli, ksheerkakoli.

Swedopag : Moringa oleifera, Ricinus communis, Calotropis procera, Boerhavia diffusa, Sesamum indicum, Dolichos biflorus.
Sangnyasthapan : Ferula foetida, Acorus calamus, Nordostachys jatamansi, Anjelica glouca, Anthocephalus indicus.
Sara : Figs, Linon usitaitisimum, jaggery.
Stambhan : Woodfordia floribunda (flowers), Acacia arabica, Helicteres isora.
Santapnivarak : Santalum alba, Vernonia cineria, pearl.
Skandharuja : Mocharasa nasya.
Stabdhagatrata : Swedan.
Sthairya : Exercise.
Hikkanigrahan : Hedychium spicatum, Inula racemosa, Zizyphus jujuba (fruitpulp), Solanum xanthocarpum, Piper longum, Solanum indicum, Dendropthoe falcata.
Hridya : Mango, Zizyphus jujuba, Carissa congesta, Garcinia indica, Garcinia pedunculata, Citrus medica.
Hridbalya : Terminalia arjuna, Cinamomum camphora, Digitalis purpurea, Urginea indica, Parmelia perlata, coffee, vidaryadi gana.
Hridruja : Shyamadi gana.
Sarvaroga (all diseases) : Shilajit, vasant kalpa.

INDEX OF SANSKRIT NAMES OF PLANTS

Part IV & V

INDEX OF BOTANICAL NAMES OF PLANTS

LIST OF REGIONAL NAMES OF PLANTS

Sr. No.	Sanskrit Name	Botanical Name	Hindi	Marathi	Gujarati
1.	Agnimantha	Premna integrifolia Linn.	Arni, Agethu, Ganiyar	Airan	Arani
2.	Aguru	Aquilaria agallocha Roxb.	Agar	Agar	Agar
3.	Ajmoda	Carum roxburghianum D.C. Sprague	Ajamoda	-	Deepyak Ajamod
4.	Ativisha	Aconitum heterophyllum Wall.	Atees	Ativish	Ativish
5.	Aparajita	Clitoria terneata Linn.	Aprajit	Gokarna	Kaligarani, Kalikoyal
6.	Apamarga	Achyranthes aspera Linn.	Chidchidi	Aghada	Aghedo
7.	Arka	Calotropis procera Ait. R. Br.	Akvan, Aak, Madar	Rui	Aakado
8.	Arjuna	Terminalia arjuna W.& A.	Arjun, Kahu, Kahua	Sardhol	Arjun
9.	Ashwagandha	Withania somnifera Dunal.	Asagandh	Dhorgunja, Aaskandh	Aasangh, Ghoda-ahan
10.	Ashoka	Saraca indica Linn.	Ashok	Ashok	Ashok
11.	Ahifen	Papaver somnifera Linn.	Afim	Afoo	Afin
12.	Amalaki	Emblica officinalis Gaertn.	Anvala	Avala	Anvala
13.	Aragvadha	Cassia fistula Linn.	Amaltas	Bahava	Garmalo
14.	Ardrak	Zinziber officinale Rose.	Sonth	Ale	Sunth, Adu
15.	Indravaruni	Cirtulus colocynthis Schrad.	Indrayan	Kaduvr-undavan	Indravana
16.	Udumbar	Ficus racemosa Linn.	Gular	Umbar	Umbarado
17.	Usheeram	Andropogon muricatus Retz.	Khas	Kala vala	Valo
18.	Erand	Ricinus communis Linn.	Andi, Rendi	Erandi	Erandiyo
19.	Ela	Elettaria cardmomum Maton.	Ilaichi	Velachi	Elcha
20.	Katuka	Picrorrhiza kurroa Royle ex Benth.	Kutaki	Kutaki	Kadu
21.	Kantakari	Solanum xanthocarpum Schrad.	Bhatakataiya, Chhoti kateri	Ringni	Bhonyringani
22.	Kapikachhu	Mucuna pruriens Hook	Koncha, Kevanch	Khajkuhili	Kaucha, Kavach
23.	Karkatshringi	Rhus succedania Linn.	Kakadsingi	Kakadshingi	-
24.	Karpoor	Cinamomum camphora Nees & eherm	Karpoor	Kapoor	Kapoor
25.	Karanja	Pongamia glabra Linn-Mess.	Dithouri	Karanj	Karanj
26.	Karaveer	Narium indicum Mill.	Kaner, Kanail	Kanher	Kanher
27.	Kanchanar	Bauhinia variegata Linn.	Kachanar	Kanchan	Champakati

Bengali	Tamil	Telugu	Punjabi	Arabic	Persian
Ganibhari	Thalanji	Nelichett	-		-
Agaru	Agalichand	Aguee	-	-	-
Mayur,	Brahmakusha	Amati, Oman		Karafs-e-hindi	Karafs-e-hindi
Randhuni				Basmoda	Basmoda
Aataeech	Atibidyam	Atibasa	Patees, Batees	-	Bajjituraki
Aparajita	Kakkanam	Diten	-	-	-
-	Najurivi	Apamargam	-	-	Kharevajgun
Aakand	Erakham	Mandaramu	Aka	Ushar	Kharak
-	Marutai	Tellamaddi	Jamura	-	-
Ashwagandha	Amakulong	Piniru	-		-
Ashok	Ashodham	Ashokamu		-	-
Afim	-	-	-	Afyoon	-
Amalaki, Amla	Nellikai	Ushiriki	-		Amlaj, Amla
Sondal	Kondre	Aragwadhamu	Girdanali	Khiyarshambar	
Sonth, Ada	Shukku, Inji	Allam	-	Janjbeel	Shangveer, Adharakh
Rakhalshasa	Petikari	Paparbudam	Kaudtumbha	Hanjal	Kharbuj-e-valkh
Yagnyadumbar	Kharasa	Raeega	-	Jamaij	Anjeer-e-adam, Anjeer-e-ahamak
Khaskhas, Benaghas	Vettiver	Veltivellu	-		
Gherenda	Amannakku	Eramuduku	-	Virva	Bedanjeer
Elach	Elam	Elakulu		Kakul-e-kunver	Ilaichi surkha
Katki	Kadugu, Rohini	Katuki	Kaud	Kharbak-e-hindi	Kharabk-e-hindi
Kantikari	Kandankantiri	Kooda	Kandiyari	Badanjan barri	Vadangan barri
Alakushi	Punaikakali	Nadook	-		-
Kankadashrungi	Kankadashrugi	Kankadashrungi	-		-
Karpoor	Karpooram	Karpooram	-	Kafoor	Kapoor
Dahar karanj	Puggum	Kanagu	-	-	-
Karavi	Alari	Jannerat	-	Sammulhimar	
Kanchan	Mandarai	Devkanchanamu	-		

Sr. No.	Sanskrit Name	Botanical Name	Hindi	Marathi	Gujarati
28.	Kiratatikta	Swertia chirata Buch-Aam.	Chirayata	Kadechirait	Kariyatu
29.	Kutaja	Holerrhena antidysenterica Wall.	Kud, Kudaiya	Kuda	Kudo
30.	Kupeelu	Strychnos nux-vomica Linn.	Kuchala	Kuchla	Zerkuchla
31.	Kumari	Aloe vera Linn.	Elua, Musabbar	Korphad	Elio
32.	Kushtham	Saussurea lappa Clarke.	Kuth	Kushtha, Upalet	Kath, Upalet
33.	Kushmand	Benincasa hispida Thum.	Petha, Bhaua	Bhuikohla	Bhuru kohlu
34.	Krishnajeerak	Carum carvi Linn.	Shahajira	Kale jeere	Shahajeeru
35.	Khadir	Acacia catechu Willd.	Khair	Khair	Kher
36.	Guggulu	Commiphora mukul Hook ex stocks	Gugal	Guggul	Gugal
37.	Guduchi	Tinospora cordifolia Willd-Mierss	Giloy, Gurach	Gulvel	Galo
38.	Gokshur	Tribulus terrestris Linn.	Hathchikar	Gokharu	Nanha Gokharu
39.	Gandhaprasarani	Paederia foetida Linn.	Pasaran, Gandhaprasarani	Hiranvel	Gandhan
40.	Gambhari	Gmelina ardoria Linn.	Gambhar	Shivan	Shivan,Savan
41.	Chandana	Santalum alba Linn.	Saphet chandan	Chandan	Sukhad
42.	Changeri	Oxalis corniculata Linn.	Teen patiyan	Ambuti	
43.	Chitrak	Plumbago zeylanica Linn.	Chita	Chitrak	Chitro
44.	Jatamansi	Nordostachys jatamansi DC.	Balchhad, Jatamansi	Jatamansi	Jatamansi
45.	Jatiphalam	Myristica fragrans Houtt.	Jaiphal	Jaiphal	-
46.	Jeerak	Cuminum cyminum Linn.	Jeera	Pandhare Jeere	Jeeru
47.	Jyotishmati	Celastrus paniculata Willd.	Malkangani	Malkangoni	Malkangani
48.	Jambu	Eugenia jambolana Lam.	Jamun	Jambhul	Jambu
49.	Talispatram	Abies webbiana Lindle.	Talishpatra	Talispatra	
50.	Trivrutta	Operculina terpethum Linn.	Nishoth, Pitohari	Nishottar	Nasottar
51.	Tulsi	Ocimum sanctum Linn.	Tulsi	Tulas	Tulsi
52.	Tuvaraka	Hydnocarpus wightiana Blume.	Chaulmogra, Papeeta	Kadu kavath	-
53.	Tejovha	Zantho-xylon alatum Roxb.	Tejbal	Tejbal	-
54.	Twak	Cinnamomum zeylonica Blume	Dalchini, Vaj	Dalchni	Taj
55.	Dadim	Punica granatum Linn.	Anar	Dalimba	Dadam
56.	Daruharidra	Berberis aristata DC.	Daruhaldi, Kashmal	Daruhalad	Daruhaldar
57.	Devadaru	Cedrus deodar Roxb-Loud	Deodaru	Deodar	
58.	Dronapushpi	Leucas cephalotus Spreng	Guma	Tumba,	Kubo

Bengali	Tamil	Telugu	Punjabi	Arabic	Persian
Chireta	Neelvembu	Neelvem	Charaita	Kasabujajreera	Nainihabandi
Kurachi	Vennalai	Kakkodies		Shajralisanul asafirul murr	Darakhtajavan kunjshka talkh
Kunchila	Yettikotai	Mushtivittalu		Ajaraki, Habbul,	Kuchula
-		-	-	Sibra	Shabayar
Kud	Koshtham, Gostan	Kushtham	-	Kust-e-hindi	Kust-e-talkh
Kumda	-	Gummadi	-	Vaduv	Mahadab
Shajeera	Shimai shiragam	Sheema, Jilakar	-	Kammanasvad	Jeer-e-syah
Khayer	Kachukahi	Podalmanu	Kher	-	-
-	Gukkal, Gukkul	Maishakshi Gubulu	-	Mukkul	-
Gulanch	Shinilkodi	Tippatigo	-	Gulanch	-
Gokhari	Nerunaji	-	Bhakada	Hasak	-
Gandhabhaduliya	Pinari Sangai	Savirel	-		-
Gamar	Gumadi	Padmagomaru	Gambhari		-
-	Sandanmarabh	Gadhapuchekka		Sandal-e-abyaj	Sandal-e-Saphet
Amrul	Puliyarai	Pulchit	Khattibuti		
Chitta	Chittir	Telchitra	-	Sheetraj	Sheetar
-			-	Subulutibba	Narad hindi
				Subul-e-hindi	
Jaiphal	Jaikei	Jajikey	-	Joujbuva	Joujbuya
Jeere	Cheerakam	Jeelkari	-	Cummum, Abyaj	Jeer-e-saphet
-	Valulavai	-	-	Tailan	-
Kaljam	Shambu, Naval	Neredu	Jamlu		
Talispatra	Talispatri	Talispatri	-		-
Teundi	Shivaai, Chivatai	Tegad	-	Turbud	-
Kaltulsi	Tulsi	Gapparachetta	-	-	-
Choulmogra	Bharvattai, Advibadamu		-		Biranj mogra
Nepali dhane			-	Fagira khababa khandan	Kababa dahan Kushada
Daruchini	Caruya	Sanlifu		Darsini	Darchini
Dadimba	Madalai chetti	Danimma	-	Rumman	Anar
-	Marpanjal	Kasturi pappu	Jounsar	-	Darchoba
Deodaru		Deodari	Diyar		
Alakasa	-	Puyappatosi	-	-	-

Sr. No.	Sanskrit Name	Botanical Name	Hindi	Marathi	Gujarati
				Kumbha	
59.	Danti	Balio spermum montanum Arg.	Danti	Danti	
60.	Dhattura	Dhattura stramonium Linn.	Dhatura	Dhotra	Dhatturo
61.	Dhataki	Woodfordia floribunda Salisb	Dhay	Dhaiti	Dhavni
62.	Dhanyakam	Coriandrum sativum Linn.	Dhaniyan	Dhane	Dhana
63.	Nagakesar	Mesua ferrea Benth + Hook	Peela Nagakesar	Nagachafa	Peelu Nagakesar
64.	Nagbala	Grewia hirsuta Vahl	Gudsharkara	Nagabala	Gangeti
65.	Nimba	Azadirachta indica Linn.	Neem	Kadunimba	Limdo
66.	Nimbuka	Citrus acida	Kagji nimbu	Kagdi limbu	Kagdi limbu
67.	Nirgundi	Vitex negundo Linn.	Samhalu, Meudi	Nirgud	Nagod, Nagad
68.	Patol	Trichosanthes dioica Roxb	Parval	Kadu padval	Parval
69.	Palasha	Butea frondosa Lam-kutze.	Tak,Tes	Palas	Khakhro
70.	Patala	Stereospermum suaveolens Dc.	Padal, Adhakapari	Padal	Padal
71.	Patha	Cissempelus pareira Linn.	Padh	Pahadvel, Vasanvel	Venavel, Kalipatha
72.	Parsik yawani	Hyocymus reticulata Linn.	Khurasani ajwayan	Khurasani owa	Khurasani ajmo
73.	Pippali	Piper longum Linn.	Pipal	Lendi pimpli	Pipar
74.	Punarnava	Boer lhavia diffusa Linn.	Gadhpurana, Gandahibindo	Ghetuli	Rati Satodi, Basedo
75.	Pushkarmoola	Inula racemosa Hook-F	Poharmool	Pokharmool	-
76.	Prushniparni	Ureria picta Desv.	Pithavan	Pithavan, Dav Ranbhal	Peethavan
77.	Baladway	Sida cordifolia Linn.	Bariyar, Khirainti	Chikna	Bal, Baladana
78.	Bakuchi	Psoralea corylifolia Linn.	Bakuchi, Bavachi	Bavachi	-
79.	Brahmi	Herpestis monniera H.B.K.	Jalabrahmi, Jalaneem, Brahmi	Brahmi	-
80.	Bibheetaka	Terminalia belerica Roxb.	Baheda, Bhaira	Beheda	Baheda, Bhaira
81.	Bilva	Aegle marmelos Corr.	Bel	Bel	Bili
82.	Bruhati	Solanum indicum Linn.	Badi Kateri, Banbhanta	Dorli	Ubhi Ringni
83.	Bhallataka	Semecarpus anacardium Linn.	Bhilava	Bibba	Bhilamo
84.	Bhanga	Canabis sativa Linn.	Bhang	Bhang	Bhang
85.	Bharngi	Clerodendron serratum Linn.	Bharangi, Babhanaiti	Bharang	Bharangi
86.	Bhrungraj	Eclipta alba Hask.	Bhangra, Bhagaraiya	Maka	Bhangro

Bengali	Tamil	Telugu	Punjabi	Arabic	Persian
Hafoon	-	Amadam	-	-	-
Dhautura	-	Unmetta	Dhattur	-	-
-	Dhairi jargi	Sirinji	Dhavi	-	Dhava
Dhane	Katamalli	Danyalu	-	Kujvar	Kashnij
Nageshwar	Villuttu champakam	Nagachampakam	-	Miskurumman	Nar-e-mushk
Gorakshachakule	-	-	-	-	-
Banmethi					
Neem	Bembu, Vempu	-	Nimba	Ajad darakbt-ul-hind	Ajad dorakht-e-hindi
Patilebu	Elumicche	Nimma	-	-	Leemu
Nishinda	Nouchi	Tellavavili	-	Aslak	Panjagusta
Patol	Kambuyudalai	Kambapatala	-	-	-
Palash	Murukku	Madug	-	-	-
Parul	Padri	Kaligottu	-	-	-
Ekleja	Appatta	Pada	-	-	-
-	Kurasani momam	Kurasani yamani	Khurasani-ajwain	Bajulbajja	Tukhmabang
Pipul	Tipli	Pipul	Madhan	Darphilaphil	Philphijdaraj
Punarnava, Gadapunya	Sukuetti	Afatasamidi	-	Handakuki	-
-	-	-	-	-	-
Chakule, Shankarjata	Kolaponna	Kolku ponna	-	-	-
Bedela	Paniyar	Tela antis	Kharyati	-	-
Havuch	Karpokarishi	Bhavanchi	Bavachi	-	-
Brahmishak, Udhabini	Neerabrahmi	Shambranichettu	-	-	-
Bayda	Akkam	Tai	-	Balilaj	Balil
Vel	Aluvidyam	Bilwamu	Bil	Safarjal-e-hindi	Behahindi
Vyakud	Papparamalli	Tellamoolak	-	-	Katai kalaun
Bhela	Senkottui	Fidivittalu	Bhalanva	Habbul kalba kinnab	Baladur kinnab
Bhang, Siddhi	-	-	-	Kinnab	Kinnab
Bamunhati	-	-	-		-
Bhimraj	Kaikeshi	Galgara	Bhangra	Kadimulambit	-

Sr. No.	Sanskrit Name	Botanical Name	Hindi	Marathi	Gujarati
87.	Madanphala	Randia dumetorum Lamk.	Mainphal	Gelphal	Mindhal
88.	Madhuyashti	Glycerrhiza glabra Linn.	Mulethi, Jethimadh	Jyeshthamadh	Jethimadh
89.	Maricha	Piper nigrum Linn.	Kalimircha, Golmircha, Mirich	Kali Miri	Mari
90.	Mishreya	Anethum sowa Kurz.	Soya	Balanshep	Suwa
91.	Mustak	Cyperus rotundus Linn.	Motha, Nagarmotha	Nagarmotha	Nagarmoth, Muth
92.	Manjishtha	Rubia cordifolia Linn.	Manjith	Manjishta	Majith
93.	Mandookparni	Centella asiatica Urbn.	-	Karivana	Khadbrahmi
94.	Yavani	Trachispermum amami Linn-Sprague.	Ajwayan	Owa	Ajmo
95.	Yawasa	Alhaji maurorum Desv.	Jawasa	Dhamasa	Jawaso
96.	Rasona	Allium sativum Linn.	Lahasun	Lasun	Lasan
97.	Latakaranj	Caesalpinia bondue Roxb.	Kantakarej, Karanjuva	Sagargota	Kankach
98.	Lavang	Syzygium aromaticum Merr.	Lavang, Loung	Lavang	Laving
99.	Lodhra	Symplocos racemosa Roxb.	Lodh	Lodhra	Lodhar
100.	Vacha	Acorus calamus Linn.	Vach	Vekhand	Vaj, Ghadavaj
101.	Vatsanabh	Aconitum ferox Wall.	Vishnag, Bachnag	Vachnag	Bachnag
102.	Varun	Crataeva nurvala Roxb.	Baruna, Varna	Varun	Vayvarno,Varano
103.	Vasa	Adhatoda vasica Nees.	Adusa, Bakas	Adulsa	Arduso
104.	Vidang	Emblia ribes Burm. F.	Vayvidang, Bhabirang	Vavding, Ilingi,Apatbar	Vavding
105.	Shatapushpa	Foeniculum vulgare Gaertn.	Sounf	Badishep	Variyali
106.	Shatavari	Asparagus racemosus Willd.	Satavar	Shatavari	Shatavari
107.	Sharapunkha	Tephrosia purpurea Linn.	Sarfonkha	Unhali	Sharapankho
108.	Shal	Shorea robusta Gaertn.	Sal, Sakhu	Ralecha vruksha	Ralnu jhad
109.	Shaliparni	Desmodium gangeticum DC.	Sarivan	Salvan, Dav, Ranbhai	Salvan
110.	Shalmali	Salmelia malabarica Scott & Endl.	Semal, Semar	Katesvar, Savar	Shemlo, Simulo
111.	Shigru	Moringa oleifera Lam.	Sahijan	Shevga	Saragvo, Sekto
112.	Shireesh	Albizzia lebbek Benth.	Siris	Shirish	Sarasdo
113.	Shyonak	Oroxylum indicum Vent.	Sonapatha	Tentu	Ardusho
114.	Shankhapushpi	Convolvulus pluricaulis Chois.	Shankhahuli	Shankhapushpi	Shankhavali
115.	Saptaparna	Alstonia scholaris R.Br.	Chhitvan,	Satvan	Satvan

Bengali	Tamil	Telugu	Punjabi	Arabic	Persian
Mayanaphal	Marukkalam	Mang	-	Joujul	-
Yashtimadhu	Atimadhuram	Yashtimadhukam	-	Aslussas	Bekhamruk
Gol marich	Milagu	Miriyalu	-	Filfil aswad	Filfil syah
Shaluka	Shatakuppi, Virai	Shatakuppivittalu	-	Shibbin	-
Muta	Muthakach	Tungugandalavim	-	Soad Kufi	Mushk-e-jamm
Manjishtha	Mandittu	Tamravalli	-	Fuvva	Runas, Rodak
Thulkadi	Vanjar kiri	Manukbrahmi	-	-	-
Joman	Aman	Oman	-	Cunulmuluki	Nankhvah
Jawasa	-	-	-	Haaj	Kharshutur
Rashun	-	-	Thum	Soom, Foom	Seer
Batakaranj	Gach chakakai	Gach chakakaya	-	-	-
Lavang	Kirambu	Karavallu	-	-	-
Lodh	Velli	Lodhug-chettu	Pathani lodh	-	-
-	-	-	Charch	Vajjauddulvaj	Karunak, Agar-e-turki
Kathavish	-	-	-	-	-
Varun, Varungachha	Mavilingam	Magalingam		-	-
Bakas	Edhatod	Adasara	-	-	-
Bidag	Vayu vilamagam	Vayu vilamagam	Bavding	-	-
Mouri	Shoumbu	Sopu	Sonf	Rajiyanaj	Rajiyan, Badiyan
Shatamali	Sadavari	Challa	-	-	-
Banneel	Kamukkivelai	Vempali	Sarpankh	-	-
Shal	Talur, Kungilium	Jalarichetta	-	-	-
Shalpani	-	Kolkuponna	-	-	-
Shimul	Shalvadhu	Burug	-	-	-
-	Murangai	Munaga	-	-	-
Shirish	Dirasanvedhi	Dirsan	-	Sultan-ul-ashjar	-
Shona	Vangamaram	Dundillam	-	-	-
Dankuni	-	-	-	-	-
Chhatim	Elillaippalai	Edakulriti	Satouna	-	-

Sr. No.	Sanskrit Name	Botanical Name	Hindi	Marathi	Gujarati
116.	Sarpagandha	Rauwolfia serpentina Benth Ez Kurzaa.	Chatium, Satouna Chhota chand, Pagalki buti, Chandmarva	Hadaki, Adakai	Amelpadi
117.	Sariva	Hemidesmus indicus R.Br.	Anatamool, Kapoori	Upalsari	Upalsari, Kapoormadhuri
118.	Haridra	Curcuma longa Linn.	Haldi	Halad	Haldar
119.	Haritaki	Terminalia chebula Retz.	Harad,Harre	Hirda	Harad, Himej
120.	Hingu	Ferula foetida Linn.	Hing	Hing	Hing, Badharani

Bengali	Tamil	Telugu	Punjabi	Arabic	Persian
Chandar, Chhota Chond	Chivanmel podi	Patalagandhi	-	-	-
Anantmool, Kapoori	Nannari	Muktapulgm	-	-	-
Halud	Majjal	Pasupu	-	Urukussafar	Jarad, Chob
Haritaki	Kandakai	Kandukar	-	Halilaj	Halil
-	Prungayam	Idu	-	Hiltit	Angajad

INDEX OF COMMON FORMULATIONS

RECOMMENDED READING

(Compiled by Dr. Ashok D. B. Vaidya)

1 Aiyer KN and M Koammal, Pharmacognosy of Ayurveda Drugs, Univ. Kerala, Trivandrum, 1963.

2 Atal CK and BM Kapur, Cultivation and Utilisation of Medicinal Plants RRL, Jammu, 1982.

3 Avery G S (Ed), Drug Treatment, ADIS Press, Sydney 1997.

4 Balick M J, Elisabetsky E, Laird S (Eds), Medicinal Resources of the Tropical Forest – Biodiversity and its importance to Human Health, Columbia University Press, New York 1975.

5 Bazaz YPS (Ed), Biotechnology in Agriculture and Forestry, Vol. 15, Medicinal and Aromatic Plants, Springer-Verlag, Berlin 1991.

6 Bep – Oliver Bever, Medicinal Plants of Tropical West Africa, Cambridge University Press, Cambridge, 1986.

7 Bhaishajya Ratnavali (Ed), RD Shastri, Chowkhamba Sanskrit Sansthan, Varanasi, 1985.

8 Bhattacharya S, Chiranjiva Aushadhi, Anand Publishers, Calcutta.

9 Bhavan's S.P.A.R.C., Selected Medicinal Plants of India. - A Monograph of identity, safety and clinical usage. CHEMEXCIL, Mumbai 1992.

10 Bhavaprakash Nighantu, Sastu Sahitya, Ahmedabad.

11 Bianchini F and F Corbetta, Health Plants of the World : Atlas of Medicinal Plants, Newsweek Books , New York 1975.

12 Bisset NG (Ed), Herbal Drugs and Phytopharmacenticals, Medpharm Scientific Pub lishers, Stuttgart, 1993.

13 Bole PV and Vaghani Y, Field Guide to the Common Trees of India, WWF, Oxford University Press, New Delhi, 1986.

14 Bose KG, Pharmacopoeia Indica , Bose Laboratories, Calcutta, 1928.

15 Bradley PR (Ed), British Herbal Compendium, British Herbal Medicine Association,

16 Bruenton J, Pharmacognosy, Phytochemistry of Medicinal Plants, Lavosier, Paris, 1995. Dorset, 1992.

17 Caius JF and KS Mhaskar, The Medicinal and Poisonous Plants of India, Scientific Publishers, Jodhpur, 1986.

18 Chadwick D J and J. Marsh, Bioactive Compounds from Plants, Wiley, Chichester, 1990.

19 Chang HM and PPH But (Eds), Pharmacology and Application of Chinese Materia Medica, World Scientific, Singapore, 1986.

20 Charaka- Samhita, (Ed), GS Pandeya, Chowkhambha Sanskrit Sansthan, Varanasi, 1983.

21 Chopra RN, Indigeneous Drugs of India, Academic Publishers, Calcutta 1982.

22 Chopra RN, Nayar SL, Chopra IC, Glossary of Indian Medicinal plants, CSIR, New Delhi, 1956.

23 Cowen JC, Flowering Trees and Shrubs of India, Thacker, Mumbai, 1965.
24 Cutler DF, Recent Trends in Plant Anatomy, Tata McGraw-Hill, New Delhi, 1972.
25 Dahanukar SA and UM Thatte, Ayurveda Revisited, Popular Prakashan, Mumbai.
26 Dandiya PC and S B Vohra, Research and Development of Indigenous Drugs, IHMMR, New Delhi, 1988.
27 Dash B, Basic Principles of Ayurveda, Concept, New Delhi 1980.
28 Datta SC and B Mukherji, Pharmacognosy of Indian Root and Rhizomes Drugs, Govt. of India Press, Calcutta, 1950.
29 Datta SC and B Mukherji, Pharmacognosy of Leaf Drugs, Govt. of India Press, Calcutta, 1958.
30 Desai VG, Aushadhi-Sangraha, JT Acharya, Mumbai, 1927.
31 Dhanwantari Nighantu (Eds), PV Sharma and GR Sharma, Chowkhambha Orientalia, Varanasi, 1982.
32 Duke JA, Handbook of Medicinal Herbs, CRC Press, Algonac, 1985.
33 Dutt U C and King G, Materia Medica of Hindus, Calcutta, 1900.
34 Dwivedi VN, Aushadhi Vigyan Shastra, Vaidyanath Ayurveda Bhavan, Nagpur, 1970.
35 Dymock W et al, Pharmacographia Indica Regan Paul, London, 1890.
36 European Pharmacopoiea, Maisonneeuva, Saint – Ruffine, 1997.
37 Frawley D and V Lad, The Yoga of Herbs: An Ayurvedic Guide to Herbal Medicine, Lotus, 1998.
38 Gerson S, Health Essentials: Ayurveda: The Ancient Indian Healing Art, Element, Shaftsbury, 1993.
39 Goodman and Gilman's The Pharmacological Basis of Therapeutics (Ed), A.G.Goodman Gilman, Ninth Edn., McGraw–Hill, New York, 1996.
40 Graves G, Medicinal Plants, Bracken Books, London, 1990.
41 Handa SS and MK Kaul (Eds), Supplement to Cultivation & Utilization of Medicinal Plants RRL, Jammu, 1996.
42 Handa SS and V K Kapoor, Pharmacognosy, Vallabh Prakashan, New Delhi, 1988.
43 Handbook of Domestic Medicines and Common Ayurvedic Remedies, CCRIMH, New Delhi, 1979.
44 Holmstedt B and Liljestrand G, Readings in Pharmacology, Pergamon Press, London, 1963.
45 Hooker JD, Flora of British India, Reeve & Co. London, 1879.
46 Indian Herbal Pharmacopoeia, Vol. 1, Vol. 2, IDMA & RRL, Mumbai, 1998, 1999.
47 Indraji J, Vanaspati-Shastra, Pravin Prakashan, Rajkot, 1998.
48 Jain SK, Medicinal plants, National Book Trust, New Delhi, 1968.
49 Jain SK, Vanaspati Kosha, Rajakamal Prakashan, Delhi, 1965.
50 Kapoor LD, Handbook of Ayurveda Medicinal Plants, CRC Press, Miami, 1990.
51 Kashyap–Samhita (Ed), S Vidyalankar, Chowkhambha Sanskrit Sansthan, Varanasi, 1988.
52 Keville K, The Illustrated Herb Encyclopedia, Mallard Press, New York, 1991.
53 Keys JD, Chinese Herbs, Their Botany, Chemistry and Pharmacodynomics, CE Tuttle and Co. Rutland, Vermont, Tokyo, 1976.

54 Khory RN and NN Katrak, MateriaMedica of India and Their Therapeutics, Neeraj Publishers, New Delhi, 1980.
55 Kirtikar KR and BD Basu, Indian Medicinal Plants, Mahendrapal Singh, Dehradun, 1985.
56 Kloppenberg J, First the Seed: The Political Economy of Plant Biotechnology, Cam bridge University Press, New York, 1987.
57 Krantz JC, Historical Medical Classics Involving New Drugs, Williams and Williams, Philadelphia, 1974.
58 Krishnamurthy KH, A Source Book of Indian Medicine – An Anthology, B. R. Publish ing Co., Delhi.
59 Kulkarni R D, Principles of Pharmacology in Ayurveda, Kulkarni, Mumbai, 1977.
60 Kurup PNV, Handbook of Medicinal Plants, CCRIMH, New Delhi, 1977.
61 Lele RD, Ayurveda and Modern Medicine, Bharatiya Vidya Bhavan, Mumbai, 1986.
62 Lewis WH and MPE Elwin-Lewis Medical Botany, Wiley, New York, 1977.
63 Madhava Nidana, Chowkhambha Orientalia, Varanasi, 1987.
64 Maheshwari P and U Singh, Dictionary of Economic Plants of India, I.C.A.R, New Delhi, 1965.
65 Manske RHF (Ed), The Alkaloids, Academic press, New York, 1955.
66 Maurice M Iwu, Handbook of African Medicinal Plants, CRC Press, Tokyo, 1993.
67 Metcalfe CR and L Chalk, Anatomy of Dicotyledons, Clarendon, Oxford, 1950.
68 Mitra R, Bibliography on Pharmacognosy of Medicinal Plants, NBRI, CSIR, Lucknow, 1983.
69 Mukherji B, The Indian Pharmaceuticals Codex – Indigenous Drugs, CSIR, New Delhi, 1953.
70 Nadkarni KM, Indian Materia Medica , Popular Prakashan 3rd Edn., Mumbai, 1976.
71 Newall CA, Anderson LA and Phillipson J D Herbal Medicines: A Guide For Healthcare Professionals, The Pharmaceutical Press, London, 1996.
72 Nodine JM and P E Siegler (Eds), Animal and Clinical Pharmacologic Techniques in Drug Evaluation, Vol. 1, Yearsbook Medical Publishers Inc., Chicago, 1964.
73 Pade SP, Aryabhisak, Sastu-Sahitya, Ahmedabad, 1932.
74 Paranjpe AS, A History of Pharmacology, MMJ, Pune, 1961- 62.
75 Perry LM, Medicinal Plants of East and Southeast Asia, The MIT Press, Boston, 1980.
76 Pharmacopoeia of India, Govt. of India, New Delhi, 2nd Edn., 1966.
77 Pharmacopoeia of the People's Republic of China (English Edition), Guandong Sci ence and Technology Press, Guangzhon, 1989.
78 Quality Control Methods for Medicinal Plant Materials, WHO, Geneva, 1992.
79 Raghunathan K and R. Mitra, Phramacognosy of Indigenous drugs, CCRAS, New Delhi, 1982.
80 Randhwa NS and Parmar BS (Eds), Neem Research and Development, Society of Pesticide Science, 1993.
81 Rastogi RP and Mehrotra BN, Compendium of Indian Medicinal Plants, Vol. 1 (1960-1969), Vol 2 (1970-1979), CDRI, CSIR, New Delhi, 1991.
82 Riley M, Maori Healing and Herbal, Viking Seven Seas, Paraparaumu, NZ, 1994.

83 Sathaye B, Practical Exemplified Elaboration of Padartha Vidnyana (Ayurveda), Suhasini Sathaye, Goa.

84 Satoskar RS, Bhandarkar SD and Ainapure SS, Pharmacology and Pharmacothera peutics, Popular Prakashan, Mumbai, 16th Edn., 1999.

85 Satyavati GV et al, Medicinal Plans of India, Indian Council of Medical Research, New Delhi, 1976.

86 Schmutterer H and KRS Ascher (Eds), Proceedings of 3rd International Neem Confer ence, Nairobi, 1987.

87 Shah CS and JS Qadry, A Text Book of Pharmacognosy, BS Shah Prakashan, Ahmedabad, 1976.

88 Sharma PV, Dravyagunavignyan, Chaukhambha Sanskrit Sansthan, Varanasi, 4th Edn., 1978.

89 Shiv Sharma, Realms of Ayurveda, Arnold, Heinemann, New York, 1979.

90 Sivarajan VV and I. Balchandran, Ayurvedic Drugs and Their Plant Source, Oxford & IBH, New Delhi, 1991.

91 Standardisation of Single Drugs of Unani Medicine, CCRUM, New Delhi, 1987.

92 Sudarshan SR, Yellapa Reddy AN, Gowda B, Oshadhi Kosha, (Cylopedia of Indian Medicinal Plants), Kalpataru Research Academy, Bangalore, 1993.

93 Sushruta Samhita (Ed), JT Acharya, Chawkhambha Orientalia, Varanasi, 1980.

94 Sutaria RN, A Text Book of Systematic Botany, Khadayata, Ahmedabad, 1969.

95 Svoboda R E, Prakriti, Your Ayurvedic Constitution, Motilal Banarasidas, New Delhi, 1993.

96 The Ayurvedic Pharmacopoeia of India, Ministry of Health and Family Planning, New Delhi, 1989.

97 The Useful Plants of India, CSIR, New Delhi, 1986.

98 The Wealth of India, C.S.I.R, New Delhi.

99 Trease GE and W.C. Evans, Pharmacognosy, Balliere Tindal, Eastbourne, 1983.

100 Udupa KN, Advances in Research in Indian Medicine, B.H.U., Varanasi, 1970.

101 Vagbhatta - Ashtangahridaya, Sastu Sahitya, Ahmedabad, 1966.

102 Wagner H, Bladt S and Zgainski EM, Plant Drug Analysis, Springer-Verlag, Berlin, 1984.

103 Wagner H, Hikino H, and N R Farsworth (Eds), Economic and Medicinal Plants, Re search Academic Press, London, 1965.

104 Wallis T H, Text Book of Pharmacognosy, Churchill, 5th Edn, London, 1967.

105 Warrier G and D Gunawant, The Complete Illustrated Guide to Ayurveda, Element, Shaftsbury, 1997.

106 Warrier PK (Ed), Indian Medicinal Plants, Orient Longman, Madras, 1994.

107 Weiss S and G Weiss, Growing and Using The Healing Herbs, Wings Book, New York, 1992.

108 Wijesekara ROB, The Medicinal Plant Industry, CRC Press, Boca Raton, 1991.

109 Zeichmeister L, Progress in Chemistry of Natural Products, Springer-Verlag, Berlin, 1989.

110 Zenk MH, El- Shagi H, Stockight J et al, Plant Tissue Culture and its Biotechnological Applications, Springer-Verlag, Berlin, 1977.

WEBSITES OF INTEREST

(Compiled by Dr. Ashok D. B. Vaidya)

Major Search Engines :

http://www.altavista.com
http://www.cyberall.com
http://www.khoj.com
http://www.ask.com
http://www.google.com
http://www.excite.com
http://www.metacrawler.com

Other Websites :

http://www.stneasy.cas.org	(Napralert) Data Base
http://www.medplant.in.com	
http://www.biosis.org.home.html	
http://www.chiron-h.com/global herb/	Global/Herb software
http://www.cas.org	Chemical Abstract
http://www.metalab.unc.edu/herbmed/	Herbal News
http://www.nlm.nih.gov	US National Library of Medicine
http://www.ncbi.nlm.nih.gov	PubMed/Medline
http://www.bl.uk	British Library
http://www.search.harvard.edu	Harvard University
http://www.amedio.com	Selected Medical Topics
http://www.ayurvedaindia.org	Basics in Ayurveda
http://www.ayurveda.com	US Ayurveda Institute
http://www.arthritis.org/search	Arthritis Queries
http://www.cancertrials.nci.nih.gov	Cancer Trials
http://www.DiabetesWebsite.com	Diabetes Data
http://www.sierracheb.org	Environment, Biotech
http://www.britannica.com	Encyclopedia Britanica
http://www.fda.gov	US Food & Drug Administration
http://www.faseb.org/genetics/	Genetics Data
http://www.healthlibrary.com	India Medical
http://www.herbalgram.org	Excellent Links
http://www.herbsociety.org	Membership Advantages
http://www.herbs.org	Herbal Research
http://www.mayohealth.org	Mayo Clinic Education
http://www.intelihealth.com	USP, Doctor Queries
http://www.reutershealth.com	Health News
http://www.medmatrix.org	Good Links

http://www.idma_assn.org	Indian Drug Manufacturers Association
http://www.medivisionindia.com	
http://www.MDSPEAK.com	A Major India Site
http://www.nimh.nlm.nih.gov	Mental Health (US)
http://www.neuroguide.com	Neurosciences
http://www.who.int	World Health Organisation
http://www.eatright.org	Nutrition and Diet
http://www.pain-education.com.au	
http://www.pharmachemguide.com	
http://www.researchgrant.com	How to write grant application
http://www.researchpaper.com	Guide to paper writing
http://www.telehealth.net	
http://www.who.ch/dmp/ed1-10.htm	Essential Drugs
http://www.yale.edu	Yale University
http://www.chemistry.gsu.edu/post-docs	Nupronet
http://www.bmj.com	British Medical Journal
http://www.botany.net/IDB	
http://www.cellbio.com	Cell Biology
http://www.ChemWeb.com	
http://www.audoboninstitute.org	
http://www.internets.com/mednets	
http://www.uselessknowledge.com	

CAUTION

Medications from the medicinal plants, based merely on data in this textbook, are not to be formulated and tried by unqualified persons. This textbook is meant for the students, teachers, scientists, vaidyas and clinicians in Ayurveda, Complementary Medicine or Phytopharmacology. Standard formulations and dosage-forms based on these plants are manufactured by the licensed manufacturers in India, as approved by the Drug Control Administration. These can be used by Ayurvedic Physicians for their patients. The publishers and the Academic Committee of Bhavan's SPARC cannot assume responsibility for the effects of any unauthorized use of medicinal plants mentioned in the textbook.

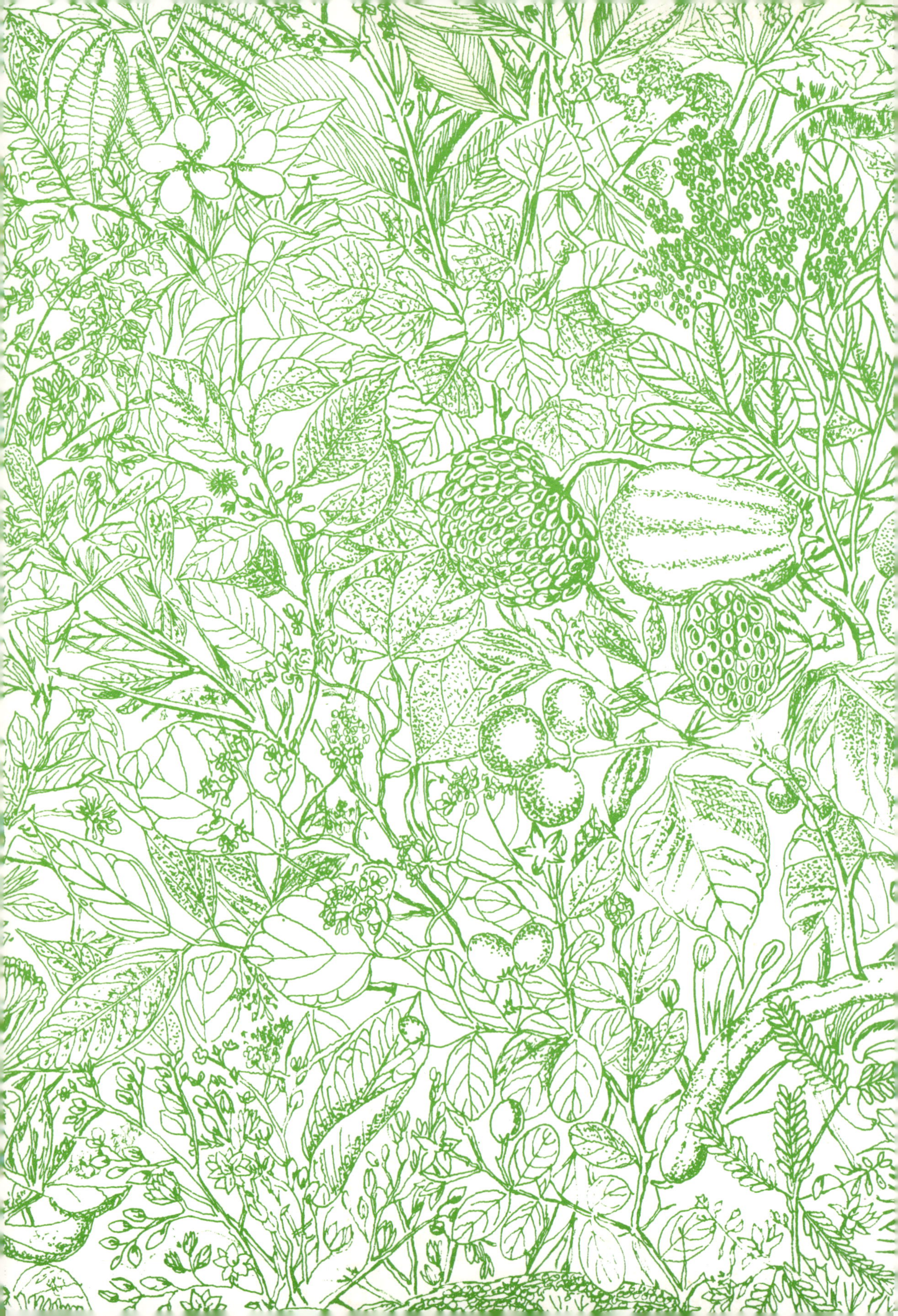